The chart on the inside back cover shows compatibility guidelines for administering drugs intravenously. Guidelines assume drugs are in 5% dextrose, 0.9% sodium chloride, or mixtures of dextrose and sodium chloride. Check that each of the drugs you are combining is compatible with the solution used.

Compatibility depends on many factors, including:

- Order of mixing
- Relative concentrations
- Speed of mixing
- Degree of agitation of the solution.

If any physical change is noted, do not administer the solution. Changes include precipitation, discoloration, foaming, or hazing.

You can reduce the uncertainty by using separate piggybacks for each drug rather than mixing the drugs in one solution. This allows for individual dose adjustment and avoids possible concentration-dependent incompatibilities.

Drugs reported to be visually compatible are included here as compatible. There is no reliable data for the mixing of three or more drugs. In combinations for which conflicting or inconclusive data are available, ask your pharmacist before mixing.

This chart was modified with permission from data provided by the University of Michigan Hospital Drug Information Service.

- *The chart does not include all potential admixture incompatibilities—always check with your pharmacist first.*

Calculations:
IV administration

Two common formulas are used to calculate IV rate in drops per minute. The drop factor is found on the tubing package.

$$\text{drops/min} = \frac{\text{cc/hr}}{60} \times \text{drop factor}$$

$$\text{drops/min} = \frac{\text{vol to be infused}}{\text{hours allotted} \times 60} \times \text{drop factor}$$

Common rates can be found in this table:

Hrs to infuse 1000 cc	cc/hr	Drop factors		
		10	*15*	*20*
		resulting in drops/min:		
6	166	27	40	55
8	125	20	30	42
10	100	16	25	33
12	80	13	20	27

- IV compatibility tables may also be found on pages 33–35, following a general discussion on intravenous administration of medications.
- A compatibility chart for IM injections is found on page 30, along with diagrams of injection sites on pages 12–13 and a general discussion on intramuscular injections as a method for administering medications.

Rosalinda Alfaro-LeFevre, MSN, RN
President, NDNP Consultants
Malvern, Pennsylvania

Marcia E. Blicharz, EdD, MSN, RNC
Curriculum Coordinator
School of Nursing, Trenton State College
Trenton, New Jersey

Nancy M. Flynn, MSN, RNC
Clinical Educator, Bryn Mawr Hospital
Bryn Mawr, Pennsylvania

Mary Jo Boyer, MSN, RN
Assistant Director of Nursing and Allied Health,
Delaware County Community College
Media, Pennsylvania

Drug Handbook

A Nursing Process Approach

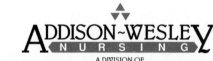

ADDISON~WESLEY
NURSING
A DIVISION OF
THE BENJAMIN/CUMMINGS PUBLISHING COMPANY, INC.

Redwood City, California ◆ Menlo Park, California ◆ Reading, Massachusetts ◆ New York
Don Mills, Ontario ◆ Wokingham, U.K. ◆ Amsterdam ◆ Bonn ◆ Sydney ◆ Singapore
Tokyo ◆ Madrid ◆ San Juan

For my husband. - R.A.L.

For my family. - M.E.B.

For my supportive family. - N.F.

For my family. - M.J.B.

Sponsoring editor: Pat Coryell
Executive editor: Debra Hunter
Assistant editor: Devra Lerman
Outside production service: Johnstone Associates
Text designer: Paul Quin
Cover designer: John Martucci
Cover photograph: Adam Hart-Davis, SPL/Photo Researchers
Compositor: Auto-Graphics, Inc.

The authors and publishers have exerted every effort to ensure that drug selections and dosages set forth in this text are in accord with current recommendations and practice at the time of publication. However, in view of ongoing research, changes in government regulations, and the constant flow of information relating to drug therapy and drug reactions, the reader is urged to check the package insert for each drug for any change in indications of dosage and for added warnings and precautions. This is particularly important where the recommended agent is a new and/or infrequently used drug. Mention of a particular generic or brand name drug is not an endorsement or an implication that it is preferable to other named or unnamed agents.

Library of Congress Cataloging-in-Publication Data

Drug handbook: a nursing process approach / R. Alfaro-LeFevre . . . [et al.]
  p. cm.
  Includes bibliographical references and index.
  ISBN 0-201-09278-6
  1. Drugs—Handbooks, manuals, etc. 2. Nursing—Handbooks, manuals, etc. I. Alfaro-LeFevre, R.
  [DNLM: 1. Drug Therapy—handbooks. 2. Drug Therapy—nurses, instruction. 3. Drugs— handbooks. 4. Drugs—nurses' instruction. 5. Nursing Process—handbooks. QV 39 D79365]
RM301.12.D78   1992
615.5´8—dc20
DNLM/DLC   91-31703
for Library of Congress   CIP

ISBN 0-201-09278-6

  2 3 4 5 6 7 8 9 10 — DO — 95 94 93 92

Addison-Wesley Nursing
A Division of The Benjamin/Cummings Publishing Company, Inc.
390 Bridge Parkway, Redwood City, California 94065

Contents

vii
How to Use This Book

How to Use This Book

Your time is precious

Nurses have to learn and apply a tremendous amount of information in a very short period of time. Later, when they are working in the clinical setting, they need to be able to recall and use much of that information immediately.

You need simple clinical tools

For these reasons, we have designed and written this book with two goals:

1 To clearly and simply present the most important information on the safe and effective administration of common drugs.

2 To show how you can ensure goal-oriented, quality management of individual medication regimens through specific applications of the nursing process.

You need reminders of special concerns

Children, pregnant or nursing women, and the elderly often have needs different from those generally required for adults. Such special concerns are clearly distinguished, beginning with a cautions grid in each drug listing that highlights concerns. A ✋ device under contraindications identifies relevant information.

Three useful sections

To achieve these goals, the book is divided into three color-coded sections. Each section is described in more detail on the following pages as well as in the brief introduction at the front of the section.

I Nursing Process and Medication Administration

Including injection site diagrams, dosage calculation charts, IV rate charts, and both IV and IM compatibility tables, this handy compendium of checklists, examples, and procedures helps you apply nursing process to the effective administration of medications.

II Classification Overviews

Key concepts help you understand the workings and use of basic functional and chemical classifications of drugs. Use overviews with prototype drug descriptions and individual drug listings to get a firm understanding of basic drug types.

If you can't find a class you want, check the front of Section II; there you will find a cross-reference list of classes and subclasses, along with references to prototype drugs where applicable.

III Drugs

Alphabetical organiztion provides quick retrieval of specific clinically important information on the most commonly used drugs. Clearly presented and consistently organized for easy use on the nursing floor.

If you don't know the generic name of a brand, check the index; it will give you the generic name, which you can then look up alphabetically in Section III.

Abbreviations

Lists of FDA pregnancy classes, schedule of controlled substances, categories of side effects, abbreviations, and NANDA nursing diagnoses begin on page xv.

Nursing Process and Medication Administration

Practical and concise

Packed with checklists, specific guidelines, and sample care plans, these few pages are your on-site review for all the steps in the nursing process, from assessment through evaluation.

Nursing process at your fingertips

Specific information on application of nursing process in the clinical setting is as valuable for focusing student learning as it is for giving experienced nurses all the important nursing process information at their fingertips.

Framework for using drug-specific information

This process-based approach to clinical nursing gives you a reliable context for using specific medication information. Teamed up with the drug information in Section III, guidelines and checklists help you apply pharmacological information and meet individual needs.

Administration procedures

In addition, a summary section provides important data on all the routes of drug administration:

♦ Guidelines for all major medication routes.

♦ Common sites for IM injections, including those specific to children, with formulas for computing dosages and drip rates.

♦ Compatibility charts for both IM and IV drugs (also shown on the endpapers).

Assessment

♦ Prepares you to interview the individual and significant others, with tips for how to meet the needs of children and the elderly.

♦ Gives guidelines for conducting an appropriate physical examination.

♦ Helps you evaluate the drug information at hand and find the resources needed to complete the information you need.

Diagnosis

♦ Discusses nursing diagnoses as they relate to medication regimens and the importance of identifying and dealing with collaborative problems.

♦ Gives concrete examples for clustering data to identify nursing diagnoses and collaborative problems.

Planning

♦ Discusses the need to identify goals and outcome criteria.

♦ Shows you how to individualize and prioritize the plan of care.

♦ Presents guidelines for scheduling and documenting the medication regimen.

♦ Introduces the clinical concept of nursing judgment and drug-specific interventions.

Implementation

♦ Reviews safety procedures for administering all medications.

♦ Includes important charting criteria for both medication records and nursing notes.

♦ Stresses the need for ongoing assessment of responses to medications.

Evaluation

♦ Offers questions to help you focus on determning goal achievement and modifying the care plan.

♦ Provides sample nursing care plans and discusses how they can help you maintain an effective medication regimen.

♦ Includes checklists for evaluating medication knowledge and helping prevent drug accidents.

Applying the nursing process Because nursing care is not given in isolation but in the busy clinical setting, information must be readily accessible and easy to follow. This book provides summaries of nursing tools and procedures in concise, straightforward, immediately useable forms.

Checklists These summarize key points and help you give comprehensive care. Topics include questions a nursing drug manual should answer, consulting about medication information, evaluating knowledge of the medication regimen, preventing drug-related accidents in the home, and what to do if a child accidentally ingests a medication.

Guidelines Helpful pointers guide you through complex clinical activities. Topics include interviews (with special guidelines for children and the elderly), coordinating and scheduling the medication regimen, preventing common medication errors, special administration considerations for children and the elderly, and charting.

Examples Theory is reinforced with concrete examples. Clinical situations show you how to set priorities. Sample care plans are included for the most common diagnoses associated with medications—Knowledge deficit: medication regimen, and Impaired home maintenance management. (Resolving these diagnoses reduces the likelihood of the diagnosis, Potential for injury.)

Injection site diagrams A complete and succinct procedures section summarizes important concerns for each route of medication administration. For injections, clear identification of injection sites for charting purposes is teamed with straightforward injection site diagrams, including special sites for children.

Safety Check:
Before giving medications

Ask yourself the following questions:

1 **Has the physician clearly written:**
   ☐ The name of the medication.
   ☐ The dose and route of administration.
   ☐ The frequency or conditions of administration.
   ☐ The length of time the medication is to be

2 **Interview parents and child together, then ask additional questions separately.** This can provide information about how the parents and child interact, and can allow expression of different points of view.

3 **Use terminology that the child can understand.**

4 **Consider use of play therapy or role play** to encourage the child to relate his or her feelings about taking medications.

4   Assessment

☐ Check the label when you tak dose from storage.
☐ Check the label immediate it.
   ☐ Check the label again as unit dose wrapper.

6 **Is the drug properly lab**

the physical examination and review of diagnostic studies and to gather the data that is pertinent to medication administration.

Guidelines:
Gathering data about physical status

1 **Begin by recording accurate age, he and weight.** These are important in de ing safe drug dosage.

2 **Document vital signs:** temperature respirations, and blood pressure.

intended. While the nurse alone is not accountable for achieving the therapeutic goal, you must answer the questions "What specific ben eficial effects are anticipated by giving the medication to this specific individual?" and "How do I know if the medication is worki The drug information in this book will he you determine these answers, because it therapeutic goals and outcome criteria drug (check any drug for an example).

Scheduling the Medication Regimen
Proper scheduling of the medication plays a major role in the success of tion treatment plan. All medicatio patient will be taking should be s and timing of doses should be s that optimum beneficial effect achieved. The following guide

Example:
Setting priorities for monitoring for potential complications

You have someone who has just begun receiving intravenous nitroglycerin. Because of the rapid response to IV administration and the potency of nitroglycerin and its effect on the cardiovascular system, you know you must assign a high priority to monitoring and documenting blood pressure and pain level every 5 minutes.

Example:
Setting priorities for timing of medications

You have someone scheduled to receive an antibiotic four times a day for a severe infection. The routine qid times for medications are 10-2-6-10. Because of the importance of maintaining adequate antibiotic blood levels, you

10   Planning

Dorsogluteal site

Ventrogluteal site

Iliac crest

Anterior superior iliac spine

Ventrogluteal injection site

Posterior superior iliac spine

Dorsogluteal injection site

Greater trochanter

Sciatic nerve

Key concepts

Here are summarized the central ideas that can unlock your understanding of broad classes of drugs: how the class works, when the drugs are most frequently used, and how they are administered. Use these overviews when learning or reviewing general uses and effects of a class.

Clear presentation

The simple narrative style of this section makes even complicated matters easy to understand. And the brevity of the text means that you get the most important information quickly.

Theoretical grounding

Once you master key concepts for each class, you will be able to apply this information when learning about individual or new drugs in the class.

Classifications are organized alphabetically so they're easy to find. At the beginning of Section II, a cross-reference list helps you find classes and subclasses covered in the section and refers you to prototype drugs for classes where there are no overviews.

Prototypes Identifies the most commonly used drugs at the beginning of each overview. Prototypes are especially useful when learning about drug classifications for the first time.

Drugs listed by subclass Lists the drugs within the classification that can be found in the drug section (Section III). Complete lists of brand names are found in Section III. The index provides a cross-reference from brand names to the relevant generic drug name.

◆ For specifics, refer to the individual drug in Section III.

OVERVIE

dose may be repeated every 10–15 minutes 3 doses. If angina is unrelieved the param should be called.

• Encourage keeping a record of pattern angina attacks; stress that an increase quency or severity should be reported.

• Point out the need to pace activitie stress (emotional and physical), and rest periods.

• Advise changing positions slowly dizziness.

• Stress that discontinuing antia abruptly could precipitate coron

Contraindications/Precautions

Contraindicated in history of hypersensitivity to the drug or to a closely related drug; possibly also in congestive heart failure (CHF), bradycardia, heart block, hypotension, severe anemia, head trauma, cerebral hemorrhage, glaucoma, and asthma.

Side effects/Adverse reactions

Hypersensitivity: rash, pruritus, hypotension. **Skin:** **CNS:** headache, dizziness, weakness. **GI:** flushing. **CV:** orthostatic hypotension. gastrointestinal disorders.

ing venous return and left ventricula Nitroglycerin is the drug of choice fo ment of acute attacks.

2 Calcium channel blockers act di indirectly on the heart by inhibit of calcium ions across the cell m cardiac and smooth muscle celle influx of calcium causes these more slowly, thereby decreasi and increasing vasodilation.

3 Beta-adrenergic blockers heart by blocking the hear pathetic (adrenergic) stim ing the rate and force of

Use/Therapeutic goal:
Prevention or resolutio the heart (angina).
Therapeutic goal: In oxygenation and ac blood pressure. O pain relief, and, f absence of or sig and intensity of improvement i

Dose range/A
The choice o patient's cli route of ad effects, an patient.
Depend given s nitroc main

Wh usu bl s

OVERVIEW

explain that taking iron with ascorbic acid increases absorption.

• Stress the importance of adequate intake of iron-rich foods (red meats, fish, spinach).

• Warn that iron overdose can be lethal; stress the need to call poison center or emergency room immediately if overdose is suspected.

• Encourage drinking plenty of fluids (unless contraindicated by disease), eating plenty of fruit and fiber, and exercising daily to prevent constipation. Advise checking with physician about taking stool softeners or laxatives.

• Before administering, or for more information, see individual drug.

Antianginals

Prototypes: nitroglycerin, verapamil, propranolol hydrochloride

Nitrates
erythrityl tetranitrate (Cardilate)
isosorbide dinitrate (Isordil)
nitroglycerin (Nitrostat)
pentaerythritol tetranitrate (Peritrate)

Calcium channel blockers (see separate overview)
diltiazem hydrochloride (Cardizem)
nicardipine hydrochloride (Cardene)
nifedipine (Procardia, ◆Adalat P.A.)
verapamil (Calan, ◆Cordilox Oral)

Beta-adrenergic blockers (see separate overview)
atenolol (Tenormin, ◆Noten)
metoprolol tartrate (Lopressor, ◆◆Betaloc)
nadolol (Corgard)
propranolol hydrochloride (Inderal, ◆Apo-propranolol, ◆Deralin)

Action Antianginals prevent and treat coronary ischemia and chest pain that occurs when oxygen supply does not meet myocardial demand:

• They increase the supply of oxygen to the heart by dilating coronary arteries and increasing coronary blood flow and tissue perfusion.

• They decrease the demand for oxygen by decreasing the workload of the heart (either by reducing left ventricular end diastolic pressure and systemic vascular resistance or by slowing heart rate and force of contraction).

Other notable hemodynamic effects include a decrease in venous return and blood pressure.

Antianginals may be categorized into three groups, depending on action.

tes act indirectly on the heart by dilating teries (improving coronary perfu peripheral veins (decrea

- ◆ Classification Overviews are organized using the same categories as the individual drugs in Section III.

  Here you find the core information common to drugs in the class.

Action Explains how these drugs produce therapeutic effects and describes differences in the action of various subclasses.

Use Supplies common indications, therapeutic goals, and outcome criteria.

Dose Provides general guidelines for how the medications are usually administered.

Contraindications/Precautions Lets you know when a drug should be withheld or given with caution.

Side effects Lists additional common effects of drugs in this class.

Nursing implications Suggests possible *Nursing diagnoses* (see complete list of NANDA diagnoses on page xvii), then gives key nursing interventions and charting reminders.

Patient & family teaching/Home care Suggests possible *Nursing diagnoses,* then presents keys to safe and effective home administration and discusses supporting holistic measures.

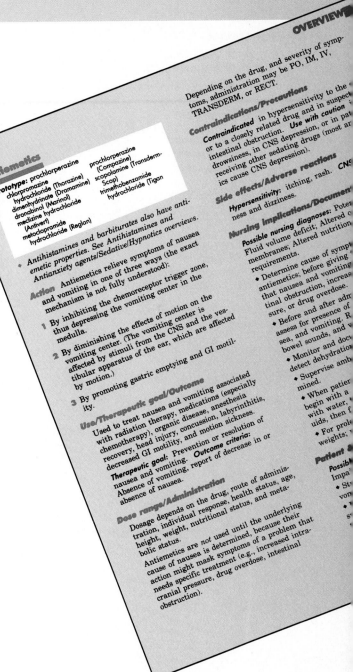

OVERVIEW

Antiemetics

Prototype: prochlorperazine
chlorpromazine hydrochloride (Thorazine)
dimenhydrinate (Dramamine)
dronabinol (Marinol)
meclizine hydrochloride (Antivert)
metoclopramide hydrochloride (Reglan)
prochlorperazine (Compazine)
scopolamine (Transderm-Scop)
trimethobenzamide hydrochloride (Tigan)

- ◆ Antihistamines and barbiturates also have antiemetic properties. See Antihistamines and Antianxiety agents/Sedative/Hypnotics overviews.

Action Antiemetics relieve symptoms of nausea and vomiting in one of three ways (the exact mechanism is not fully understood):

1 By inhibiting the chemoreceptor trigger zone, thus depressing the vomiting center in the medulla.

2 By diminishing the effects of motion on the vomiting center. (The vomiting center is affected by stimuli from the CNS and the vestibular apparatus of the ear, which are affected by motion.)

3 By promoting gastric emptying and GI motility.

Use/Therapeutic goal/Outcome
Used to treat nausea and vomiting associated with radiation therapy, medications (especially chemotherapy), organic disease, anesthesia recovery, head injury, concussion, labyrinthitis, decreased GI motility, and motion sickness. *Therapeutic goal:* Prevention or resolution of nausea and vomiting. *Outcome criteria:* Absence of vomiting, report of decrease in or absence of nausea.

Dose range/Administration
Dosage depends on the drug, route of administration, individual response, health status, age, height, weight, nutritional status, and metabolic status.
Antiemetics are *not* used until the underlying cause of nausea is determined, because their action might mask symptoms of a problem that needs specific treatment (e.g., increased intracranial pressure, drug overdose, intestinal obstruction).

Depending on the drug, and severity of symptoms, administration may be PO, IM, IV, TRANSDERM, or RECT.

Contraindications/Precautions
Contraindicated in hypersensitivity to the drug or to a closely related drug and in suspected intestinal obstruction. *Use with caution* in drowsiness, in CNS depression, or in patients receiving other sedating drugs (most antiemetics cause CNS depression).

Side effects/Adverse reactions
Hypersensitivity: itching, rash. CNS: ... ness and dizziness.

Nursing implications/Documentation
Possible nursing diagnoses: Potential for ... Fluid volume deficit; Altered oral ... membranes; Altered nutrition ... requirements.

- ◆ Determine cause of symptoms ... antiemetics; before giving ... that nausea and vomiting ... tinal obstruction, increased ... sure, or drug overdose.
- ◆ Before and after administration ... assess for presence of ... sea, and vomiting. Record ... bowel sounds, and watch ...
- ◆ Monitor and document ... detect dehydration ...
- ◆ Supervise ambu... mined.
- ◆ When patient ... begin with a ... with water, then ... uids, then f...
- ◆ For prolo... weights; ...

Patient &
Possib...
Impa...
- ◆ St...
vom...
- ◆ ...
sw...

A quick reference for clinical use

For easy use in the clinical setting, the information for each drug is organized to answer the following questions:

1 *What does this drug do?*

2 *Why is this drug indicated?*
   What is the therapeutic goal?
   How will I know if it is working?

3 *Is the prescribed dose within normal range?*
   How is this drug given?

4 *Is there any reason why I should not give this drug to this person?*
   Are there some people who require close monitoring when getting this drug?

5 *What adverse reactions and side effects should I watch for?*

6 *What should I monitor?*
   How should I intervene?
   What should I record?

7 *What do I need to teach?*

Generic name These are followed by phonetic pronunciations.

Brand names These follow the **full generic name,** including U.S., Canadian, and Australian brands. ♦ indicates drugs available in Canada only, and ♣ indicates Australia only.

Class Refers to the common chemical or functional classes to which the drug belongs. Overviews for many of the important classifications are given in Section II.

If this drug is a **prototype** in its class or subclass, a star ★ indicates that it is one of the most frequently used drugs of its type.

Antidote Lists the generic name of the antidote, if any. Check the guidelines on overdose management following Section III (pages have a red edge).

Cautions Presented in a standard grid, showing special concerns for children, pregnant or nursing mothers, and the elderly.

PEDS ♨ See the precautions for children in the contraindications section. **OK** No documented problems for children.

PREG Lists the FDA categories of drug safety (list on page xv). ♨ indicates that the drug has more than one pregnancy category, which can be found in the contraindications section.

GERI ♨ See the precautions for the elderly in the contraindications section. **OK** No documented problems for the elderly.

CONTROLLED SUBSTANCE class, if any, appears to the right of the cautions grid (list on page xv).

bup-ren-or′ feen

buprenorphine

buprenorphine hydrochloride: Buprenex, ♣Temgesic
Injection
Class: Narcotic analgesic
Antidote: Naloxone hydrochloride (Narcan)   CONTROLLED SUBSTANCE V

PEDS   PREG   GERI
♨   C   ♨

Action Alters both perception of and response to pain by binding to opiate receptors at various sites in the CNS. This drug is approximately 30 times more potent than morphine sulfate (0.3 mg is equal to 10 mg of morphine) and 250 times more potent than meperidine (0.3 mg is equal to 75 mg of morphine).

Use/Therapeutic goal/Outcome Moderate to severe pain: Relief of pain. **Outcome criteria:** Report of comfort; absence of signs of pain (grimacing, frowning, restlessness, reluctance to move or cough) with increase in signs of comfort (relaxed facial expression, decreased restlessness, improved ability to move or cough); blood pressure and pulse within normal limits when compared to baseline.

Dose range/Administration
Interaction alert: Other CNS depressants, alcohol, sedatives, hypnotics, antipsychotics and skeletal muscle relaxants increase effects. May antagonize action of other narcotics.
♨ IM, IV: 0.3 mg to 0.6 mg q6h prn or [...]clock. [...] doses slowly. SC route is [...]reased dosage for the [...]irations and

alcoholism; a[...]
toxic psycho[...]
♨ Use with ca[...]
the elderly [...]
pregnant w[...]
years has n[...]

Side effects/[...]
Hypersensitiv[...]
depression, d[...]
sedation, diz[...]
euphoria. C[...]
hypotension, [...]
hypoventilat[...]

Nursing impl[...]
Possible nurs[...]
Potential for[...]
• Have patie[...]
before and a[...]
and record i[...]
• Monitor cl[...]
keep side ra[...]
allowed out [...]
• Give pain [...]
• Be aware [...]
dence may a[...]
appear up to[...]
ued.
• For narcot[...]
for abstinen[...]
narcotic ant[...]

Patient & fa[...]
Possible nurs[...]
alterations; [...]
• Stress the [...]
before it is s[...]
• Advise tho[...]
from activiti[...]
[...]k assistan[...]

Action

What does this drug do?

Provides a concise explanation of how the drug produces therapeutic effects. Where pertinent, details additional important information about action (e.g., pharmacokinetics).

Use/Therapeutic goal/Outcome

Why is this drug indicated?
What is the therapeutic goal?
How will I know if it is working?

Includes the use and corresponding therapeutic goal, followed by *Outcome criteria,* stating the signs that indicate goal achievement.

Dose range/Administration

Is the prescribed dose within normal range?
How is this drug given?

Interaction alert Highlights drug interactions or incompatibilities that may enhance or retard the drug's effects or increase the risk of side effects, toxicity, or overdose.

♦ 🌢 indicates the drug should be taken with or after food. 🗗 indicates the drug should be taken on an empty stomach. Be sure to read statements following symbols for clarification.

♦ Comprehensive information on dosage and administration, including dosages for children and the elderly, where available.

Clinical alert Helps you prepare and administer the drug, including information on the forms in which it is available. This section also lists critical precautions for possibly severe adverse reactions.

more ▶

Dose range/Administration

Interaction alert: CNS effects may be additive to those of alcohol, barbiturates, and other CNS depressants. Use cautiously with anticholinergics and MAO inhibitors, or within 14 days after discontinuation of MAO inhibitors.

Adult: PO: 10–20 mg tid. Not to exceed 60 mg/day or 2–3

PREG **B**

Clinical alert: weeks of therapy.

Contraindications/Precautions

Contraindicated in hypersensitivity to cyclobenzaprine, and in acute recovery-phase myocardial infarction, dysrhythmias, heart block, conduction disturbances, congestive heart failure, or hyperthyroidism. *Use with caution* in history of urinary retention, angle

♦ Advise against operating machinery or combining with CNS depressants especially if drowsiness is present.

♦ Warn that dry mouth may occur; using ice chips, sugarless gum, or for relief.

♦ Explain the importance of con cian before taking OTC medica effects develop.

♦ Point out the importance o and high-fiber foods to prev

♦ Stress the importance of treatment plan, including of therapy (e.g., relaxatio

♦ See *Skeletal-muscle rela information.*

Side effects/Adverse reactions

Hypersensitivity: rash. CV: facial flus tachycardia. CNS: tingling of the e dizziness. GI: nausea, heartburn. doses may prolong bleeding time. ing.

Nursing implications/Documen

Possible nursing diagnoses: Acti Pain.

♦ Document baseline circulat ence and quality of periphe color, and temperature) and monitor periodically there

♦ Monitor for dizziness, tion until response is de

Patient & family tea

Possible nursing diagn Impaired home mai

♦ Advise taking cy to reduce GI symp

♦ Stress that im ally gradual wi apy is necessa

♦ Explain the to reduce diz usually sub

♦ See *Antian*

C

do not abate, or *any* new signs and symptoms of discomfort that might indicate superinfection (medication regimen may have to be changed).

♦ Advise drinking 2–3 L of fluids daily to maintain adequate hydration (especially important if fever exists).

♦ Stress the importance of taking antibiotics for the entire time prescribed, even if signs and symptoms abate.

♦ See *Anti-infectives overview for more information.*

sye-klan'de-late

cyclandelate

Cyclan, Cyclospasmol, Cydel
Class: Vasodilator, peripheral

PEDS 🤚 PREG **C** GERI 🤚

Action Dilates blood vessels by producing a direct papaverine-like relaxation of smooth muscle. There is no significant effect upon blood pressure and heart rate.

Use/Therapeutic goal/Outcome
Occlusive vascular disease and vasospastic conditions (arteriosclerosis obliterans, intermittent claudication, nocturnal leg cramps, and Raynaud's disease): Promotion of circulation and increased activity tolerance. *Outcome criteria:* Improvement of pulse volume, skin color and temperature; report of decreased pain; evidence of increased activity tolerance.

Dose range/Administration
🌢 Give with food or milk to reduce GI distress.

Adult: PO: Initially, 200–400 mg qid. After clinical response, reduce by 200 mg increments to 400–800 mg/day in 2–4 divided doses.

PREG **C**

Contraindications/Precautions
Contraindicated in hypersensitivity to cyclandelate. *Use with caution* in obliterative coronary artery or cerebrovascular disease, bleeding disorders, hypertension, or glaucoma. 🤚 Use with caution for the elderly. Safe use for children and pregnant or nursing mothers has not been established.

---

cyclobe

cyclober
Class: Antis

PEI

Ac

Contraindications/Precautions

Is there any reason why I should not give this drug to this person?
Are there some people who require close monitoring when getting this drug?

The FDA pregnancy category is repeated here. **Contraindicated** Lists instances in which the drug should be withheld and the physician notified. **Use with caution** Lists conditions under which you should pay special attention to dosages and watch especially carefully for side effects, overdose, or toxicity.

🖐 Highlights considerations for children, pregnant or nursing mothers, and the elderly.

Side effects/Adverse reactions

What adverse reactions and side effects should I watch for?

Begins with **Hypersensitivity** reactions, to assist in early recognition of these responses. Other reactions are then listed by body system in order of common occurrence (see the list of systems on the next page).

◆ If serious adverse reactions or hypersensitivity occur, see the guidelines for overdose management and anaphylaxis management at the end of Section III (pp. 733 and 734, marked with a red stripe).

Nursing implications/Documentation

What should I monitor?
How should I intervene?
What should I record?

Suggests possible **Nursing diagnoses** that might be present in individuals requiring this drug (a complete list of NANDA diagnoses is on page xvii).

◆ Lists key nursing interventions that help promote the desired therapeutic effect and minimize adverse reactions.

◆ Identifies holistic interventions that promote therapeutic effects.

◆ Gives key data that should be recorded.

Patient & family teaching/Home care

What do I need to teach?

Suggests possible **Nursing diagnoses** for home care.

◆ Bulleted points describe nursing interventions that help individuals and their families learn to safely use medications and effectively manage the medication regimen.

◆ Holistic measures are included to support therapeutic goals, enhance the effectiveness of the medication, and help avoid adverse reactions.

◆ Cross-references at the end of the listing direct you to overviews or other drugs for important additional information.

Contraindications/Precautions

Contraindicated in hypersensitivity to hydromorphone, and in increased intracranial pressure or status asthmaticus. **Use with caution** in respiratory depression, increased cerebrospinal fluid pressure, hepatic or renal disease, hypothyroidism, shock, Addison's disease, alcoholism, seizures, head injury, severe CNS depression, brain tumor, bronchial asthma, and COPD.

🖐 Safe dose for children must be individualized by physician. Use with caution for the elderly or debilitated. Safe use for pregnant or nursing mothers has not been established (preg D for high dosage at term; otherwise, preg C).

Side effects/Adverse reactions

Hypersensitivity: (rare) rashes, hives, itching, facial swelling. **CNS:** euphoria, mood changes, convulsions with large doses, extreme somnolence, coma, physical dependence. **Resp:** respiratory depression. **CV:** hypotension, bradycardia. **GI:** nausea, vomiting, constipation, ileus. **GU:** urinary retention. **Skin:** induration from repeated subcutaneous injections. **MS:** skeletal-muscle flaccidity.

Nursing implications/Documentation

Possible nursing diagnoses: Pain; Anxiety; Potential for injury; Constipation.
◆ Have patient rate pain on a scale of 1–10 before and after medication is given; report and record inadequate pain control.
◆ Ascertain that there is not an acute abdominal problem before giving hydromorphone (may mask or worsen pain of cholecystitis, obstruction, or appendicitis).
◆ Document pulse, respirations, and blood pressure immediately before and 1 hr after administration.
◆ Monitor closely for risk factors for injury; keep side rails up and supervise ambulation if allowed out of bed.
◆ Give before pain is severe for best effects.
◆ Document and monitor bowel function to prevent constipation; provide adequate fluid and ... atives before problem is severe.
... al for psychic and physi-... d use (withdrawal ... orphine, bu...

Patient & family teaching/Home c...

Possible nursing diagnoses: Sensory/pe... alterations; Knowledge deficit.
◆ Explain the rationale for reporti... discomfort before it is severe.
◆ Advise ambulatory patients to ... activities that require alertness... assistance if there is any quest... to get out of bed (e.g., if there ... light headedness).
◆ Explain procedures briefly ... terms.
◆ Warn not to exceed pres... of overdose, dependence, ... (instead of increasing do... tory pain relief should ...
◆ Stress that alcohol a... sants may cause exce...
◆ See Narcotic and no... overview for more i...

hydroxocobala...

Alpha-Ruvite, Cod...
Class: Vitamin B ...
min

PEDS	PREG
OK	A

Action Prom... olism and ... coenzym... duction... nucleo... meth...

Use/T... Vi... ni... r...

Schedules and abbreviations

FDA categories of drug safety for pregnant women

A *Generally considered safe.*
Studies have failed to show risk to fetus in the first trimester of pregnancy. There is no evidence of harm in later trimesters.

B *No demonstrated risk.*
If risk has been demonstrated in animal studies, there are no adequate studies to predict risk to pregnant women or their fetuses. If no risk has been demonstrated in animals, neither has any risk been demonstrated in human studies.

C *Some risk possible, weigh advantages.*
Animal studies have shown adverse effects to the fetus, but there is insufficient data to predict risk to pregnant women or their fetuses. In some situations, the need for use during pregnancy may outweigh the possible risk to the fetus.

D *Risk shown, weigh advantages.*
Risk to the human fetus has been shown in clinical investigations or post-marketing surveillance. In some situations, the need for use during pregnancy may still outweigh risk to the fetus.

X *Generally contraindicated.*
Risk to the human fetus has been clearly documented in human studies, clinical investigation, or post-marketing surveillance. Risks to the fetus outweigh any need for use during pregnancy.

NR No category has been assigned (not rated).

🖑 The drug has more than one category, usually depending upon trimester. Refer to the contraindications section.

Schedule of controlled substances

I *Containers marked C-I* 🍁 *Schedule H*
High potential for abuse; no accepted medical use.

II *Containers marked C-II* 🍁 *Schedule F*
High potential for abuse, but has accepted medical uses. Possibly strong physical and psychological dependence.

III *Containers marked C-III* 🍁 *Schedule F*
Less potential for abuse; accepted medical uses. Some risk of physical/psychological dependence.

IV *Containers marked CIV* 🍁 *Schedule F*
Low potential for abuse; accepted medical uses. Mild physical/psychological dependence possible.

V Little potential for abuse; accepted medical uses. Some mild physical/psychological dependence possible.

Categories of side effects

In each drug listing, hypersensitivity reactions are listed first, and then the affected systems in the order in which effects are most frequently observed.

Hypersensitivity Side effects that indicate allergy or hypersensitivity.
CNS Side effects on the central nervous system.
CV Cardiovascular side effects.
Ear Adverse reactions affecting the ear and hearing.
Eye Side effects on the eye and vision.
GI Gastrointestinal side effects.
GU Genitourinary side effects.
Hem Side effects noted upon examination of a blood specimen.
MS Side effects on the musculoskeletal system.
Resp Side effects on breathing and the respiratory system.
Skin Side effects noted upon examination of the skin.
Misc Side effects that do not fit in another category.

Abbreviations

ABG arterial blood gas

AIDS acquired immune deficiency syndrome

ADL activities of daily living

APTT activated partial thromboplastin time

ALT alanine aminotransferase

AST aspartate aminotransferase

bid twice a day *(bis in die)*

BUN blood urea and nitrogen

CAI carbonic anhydrase inhibitor

CBC complete blood count

CHF congestive heart failure

CNS central nervous system

CO cardiac output

COPD chronic obstructive pulmonary disease

CPK creatinine phosphokinase

CPR cardiopulmonary resuscitation

CV cardiovascular

CVA cerebrovascular accident

CVP central venous pressure

D5W dextrose 5% in water

EEG electroencephalogram

EKG electrocardiogram

FBS fasting blood sugar

FDA U.S. Food and Drug Administration

FEV forced end expiratory volume; FEV1, after 1 min

g gram(s)

GI gastrointestinal

gr grain(s)

gt(t) drop(s) *(gutta)*

GU genitourinary

h hour(s)

Hct hematocrit

HDL high-density lipoprotein, a type of cholesterol

Hem hemotology; used to indicate side effects noted on examination of a blood specimen

Hgb hemoglobin

GERI geriatric

HIV human immunodeficiency virus

hr hour(s)

hs at bedtime *(hora somni)*

IM intramuscular injections, medication administration

Inhal inhalation

IU international unit(s)

IPPB intermittent positive pressure breathing

IV intravenous, medication administration

kg kilogram(s)

KVO keep vein open

L liter(s)

LDH lactate dehydrogenase

LDL low-density lipoprotein, a type of cholesterol

m² square meter(s)

MAO monoamine oxidase

MAOI MAO inhibitor

mcg microgram(s)

mEq milli-equivalent(s)

mg milligram(s)

MI myocardial infarction

min minute(s)

Misc miscellaneous, for side effects not included in other systems

ml milliliter(s)

mon month(s)

MS musculoskeletal

NaCl sodium chloride

NPO nothing by mouth *(nulla per os)*

NS normal saline solution, 0.9% sodium chloride in water

NSAID nonsteroidal anti-inflammatory drug

OTC over-the-counter or non-prescription medication

PAP pulmonary artery pressure

pc after meals *(post cibum)*

PCWP pulmonary capillary wedge pressure

PED pediatric

PREG FDA pregnancy category

prn as needed *(pro re nata)*

PT prothrombin time

PTT partial thromboplastin time

PVC premature ventricular contraction

PVR peripheral vascular resistance

PWP pulmonary wedge pressure

PO oral, medication administration by mouth *(per os)*

q every, as q4h, every 4 hours *(quaque)*

qd daily *(quaque die)*

qid 4 times a day *(quater in die)*

qod every other day

RBC red blood cell count

Rect rectal, medication administration

REM rapid eye movement, a sleep indicator

Resp respiratory

SC subcutaneous injections

SGOT serum glutamic-oxaloacetic transaminase

SGPT serum glutamic-pyruvic tansaminase

SL sublingual, oral medication administration

ss one-half *(semis)*

STAT immediately *(statim)*

TCA tricyclic antidepressant

tid 3 times a day *(ter in die)*

T₃ triiodothyronine

T₄ thyroxine

U unit(s)

WBC white blood cell count

wk week(s)

yr year(s)

> greater than, over

< less than, under

NANDA-approved nursing diagnoses

Approved nursing diagnoses from the North American Nursing Diagnosis Association. In 1992, the label *high risk for* replaced the label *potential for;* text references may still refer to *potential.* Other phrasing also changed slightly.

Activity intolerance
—, high risk for
Adjustment, impaired
Airway clearance, ineffective
Anxiety
Aspiration, high risk for
Body image disturbance
Body temperature, high risk for altered
Breastfeeding, effective
—, ineffective
Breathing pattern, ineffective
Communication, impaired verbal
Constipation
—, colonic
—, perceived
Decisional conflict (specify)
Decreased cardiac output
Defensive coping
Denial, ineffective
Diarrhea
Disuse syndrome, high risk for
Diversional activity deficit
Dysreflexia
Family coping, compromised, ineffective
—, disabling, ineffective
—, potential for growth
Family processes, altered
Fatigue

Fear
Fluid volume deficit
—, high risk for
Fluid volume excess
Gas exchange, impaired
Grieving, anticipatory
—, dysfunctional
Growth and development, altered
Health maintenance, altered
Health-seeking behaviors (specify)
Home maintenance management, impaired
Hopelessness
Hyperthermia
Hypothermia
Incontinence, bowel
—, functional
—, reflex
—, stress
—, total
—, urge
Individual coping, ineffective
Infection, high risk for
Injury, high risk for
Knowledge deficit (specify)
Noncompliance (specify)
Nutrition, altered: less than body requirements
—: more than body requirements
—: high risk for more than body requirements
Oral mucous membrane, altered
Pain
—, chronic
Parental role conflict
Parenting, altered
—: high risk for
Personal identity disturbance
Physical mobility, impaired
Poisoning, high risk for
Post-trauma response

Powerlessness
Protection, altered
Rape-trauma syndrome
—: compound reaction
—: silent reaction
Role performance, altered
Self-care deficit: bathing/hygiene
—: dressing/grooming
—: feeding
—: toileting
Self-esteem, disturbance
—, low: chronic
—, low: situational
Sensory/perceptual alterations (specify: visual, auditory, kinesthetic, gustatory, tactile, olfactory)
Sexual dysfunction
Sexuality, altered patterns
Skin integrity, impaired
—: high risk for
Sleep pattern disturbance
Social interaction, impaired
Social isolation
Spiritual distress (distress of the human spirit)
Suffocation, high risk for
Swallowing, impaired
Thermoregulation, ineffective
Thought processes, altered
Tissue integrity, impaired
Tissue perfusion, altered (specify type: renal, cerebral, cardio-pulmonary, gastrointestinal, peripheral)
Trauma, high risk for
Unilateral neglect
Urinary elimination, altered
Urinary retention
Violence, high risk for: self-directed or directed at others

Acknowledgments

Review Board

Ledjie Ballard, MSN, RN, CRNA, Chief Nurse Anesthetist, Group Health Cooperative, Eastside Hospital, Seattle, WA

Anne Curtis, RN, MSN, ONC, Oncology Clinical Specialist, Bryn Mawr Hospital, Bryn Mawr, PA

Patricia A. Fenn, MD, Chief, Section of Rheumatology, Bryn Mawr Hospital, Bryn Mawr, PA

Bruce Fox, RPh, President, Fox Pharm Consultants, Chadds Ford, PA

Arthur L. Hupka, PhD, Chairman, Department of Pharmacology and Toxicology, Ponce School of Medicine, Ponce, Puerto Rico

Stephen A. Walker, PharmD, Assistant Director of Pharmacy, Drug Information, and Clinical Services, Lankenau Hospital, Philadelphia, PA

Contributors

Ruth A. Benfield, MSN, RNCS, Associate Professor of Nursing, Montgomery County Community College, Blue Bell, PA

Carol Fetterman Blauth, MSN, RNC, Staff Development Educator, Mercer Medical Center, Trenton, NJ

Kathleen Lovell Bratby, MSN, RN, Supervisor, Brunswick Hospital Center, Amityville, NY and Adjunct Faculty, School of Nursing, State University of New York at Stony Brook

Margaret Ann Daingerfield, MA, RN, Former Staff Nurse, Critical Care Burn Unit, St. Barnabas Medical Center, Livingston, NJ

Ann Delengowski, MSN, RN, Oncology Clinical Nurse Specialist, Thomas Jefferson University Hospital, Philadelphia, PA

Patricia B. Evans, MSN, MEd, RNC, Curriculum Coordinator, Chester County Hospital School of Nursing, West Chester, PA

Marlene Joy Goodwin-Scappa, MSN, RN, Cardiovascular Clinical Specialist, Adjunct Faculty, School of Nursing, Trenton State College, Trenton, NJ

Mary Ellen Heintzelman, MS, RN, Former Assistant Professor of Nursing, East Stroudsburg University, East Stroudsburg, PA, and Consultant, Occupational Health

Marlene Kahn, MSN, RNC, Medical-Surgical Instructor, Chester County Hospital School of Nursing, West Chester, PA

Janice E. Malloy, MSN, RN, Clinical Nurse Specialist, Thomas Jefferson University Hospital, Philadelphia, PA

Renee Martin, MSN, RNC, Student, Villanova Law School, Chester Springs, PA

Cheryl Meyer, MSN, RN, Assistant Professor of Nursing, Delaware County Community College, Media, PA

Bruce P. Mericle, MSN, RN, Assistant Professor, School of Nursing, Trenton State College, Trenton, NJ

Deborah A. Pezzella, MSN, CCRN, Clinical Specialist, Critical Care, Germantown Hospital and Medical Center, Philadelphia, PA

Eileen M. Roche, DNSc, RNC, Assistant Professor of Nursing, Widener University, Chester, PA

Susan Rokita, OCN, MSN, RN, Oncology Clinical Nurse, Milton S. Hershey Medical Center, Hershey, PA

Patricia L. Ryan, MSN, RNC, Assistant Professor of Nursing, Gwynedd-Mercy College, Gwynedd Valley, PA

Donna Steele, MA, RN, Assistant Professor, University of Medicine and Dentistry of New Jersey, Newark, NJ

Virginia Stemhagen, MA, RN, Director, School of Nursing, Mercer Medical Center, Trenton, NJ

Cindy Stern, OCN, MSN, RN, Oncology Clinical Nurse Specialist, Thomas Jefferson University Hospital, Philadelphia, PA

Wanda May Webb, MSN, RN, Level I Coordinator, Brandywine Hospital School of Nursing, Coatesville, PA

Carol Zack, MS, RN, Associate Professor, Wilkes University, Wilkes-Barre, PA

Margaret E. Zazo, MSN, MS, RN, Nursing Instructor, Brandywine School of Nursing, Coatesville, PA

Reviewers

Claude Agostini, RPh, Donald Armstrong, MD, Matthew Astroff, MD, Steven G. Atcheson, MD, Julie Barton, MD, Mary Kay Beasley, RN, Terry Bellevou, BSN, RN, Nancy Bensen, MSN, RN, Barbara Bogdan,

MSN, Patricia E. Brien, MSN, MEd, BSN, Sharon Brim, BSN, RN, Douglas K. Brown, MD, Jannet M. Carmichael, PharmD, Scott Charland, PharmD, Nancy Conrad, EdD, MSN, RN, P. Howard Cummings, EdD, RN, Anne Curtis, MSN, RN, Carleen M. Derenthal, Susan deWit, MSN, RN, Laurel Eisenhauer, PhD, RN, Joann M. Eland, PhD, RN, James M. Ellison, MD, Elizabeth Ferrigno, RPh, Sherry W. Fox, CNRN, MS, BSN, Glen Fine, MS-ACP, MBA, Stephen Fox, MD, Timothy Fox, MD, Polly Gardner, CCRN, MN, RN, Krissy Gorman, RPh, Jerry Gould, PharmD, Susan K. Grant, CCRN, MS, RN, Charles Huberty, RPh, Renee S. Hyde, MSN, BSN, Steven LaPorte, MD, Robert Julien, PhD, MD, Charlotte D. Kain, EdD, RNC, Karri Kitchens, OCN, RN, Beth Larren, Janet Lederer, MN, RN, Hilde Leigh, RN, Linda L. Lilley, MSN, BSN, Barbara MacDermott, MS, BS, Bruce MacNeill, RRT, Kathleen R. Mahoney, MSN, Mildred Marion, Esther Matassarin-Jacobs, OCN, PhD, RN, Joan G. Mattioli, RN, Geoffry McEnany, MSN, BSN, Marylou Medlin, RN, Luana Nedich, RPh, Judy Nelson, RN, Michael J. Norvell, PharmD, John O'Hara, MD, Barbara O'Reilly, RN, Phelps Potter, MD, Vicki G. Pritchard, CIC, MSN, Carol Proctor, RRT, RPFT, David Reinke, PhD, Linda Robinson, MSN, RN, CS, Mary W. Rode, MSN, RN, Michael Saruk, MD, Constance Sechrist, RN, Anjana N. Shah, MD, Hardy Sorkin, MD, Charles Staddon, MD, Katherine Stefos, PhD, Shirley Stokes, CNAA, MSN, MAEd, RN, Christine Szychlinski, Suzanne M. Thornley, PharmD, Karen Tietze, PharmD, Richard Tolin, MD, David Treveno, MD, Barbara Vassallo, EdD, MSN, BSN, Daniel Wallace, MD, Janet R. Weber, MSN, RN, Fred Weinblatt, MD, John R. White, Jr., PharmD, John Willens, MD, Gregory Williams, MD, and Ann Woodworth, RCVT, RN.

Special thanks

We have dedicated this book to our families, in appreciation for their support and their acceptance of the limitations on family life that were necessary to write this book.

Our special thanks go to the following people who, because of their knowledge, expertise, and unfailing support during various stages of this book, helped us to move forward to completion: Thomas Flynn, Ann Peterman, Nat and Louise Rochester, Heidi Laird, Ledjie Ballard, Diane Verity, Leslie Culp, Constance Sechrist, Becky Resh, Elizabeth Ferrigno, Stephen Walker, Bruce Fox, Debra Hunter, Pat Coryell, Devra Lerman, and Grace Wong.

We want especially to commend Paul Quin and Judy Johnstone for pulling together the final stages of production. Their attention to detail, commitment to quality, and willingness to take the necessary time was over and above what any authors could ask.

1

Assessment:
Focusing data collection on the medication regimen

Focus Assessment

Performing a nursing assessment that focuses on gathering specific data about an individual's medication regimen includes gathering two types of information:

1 Information about the **person** to receive the medications

2 Information about the **medications**

Information about the person to receive the medications must be obtained from a complete nursing assessment. This includes gathering **subjective data** (what the patient **states**) by interviewing the patient and significant others, and gathering **objective data** (what you **observe**) by performing a physical examination and reviewing results of diagnostic studies. Additional information may be obtained by reviewing previous medical records, especially medication records.

Information about drugs is usually gathered from the literature (pharmacology references, package inserts) and from consultations with experts (nurses, pharmacists, physicians). Let's take a look at how to gain accurate, pertinent data about both medications and the people who will be taking them.

The Interview:
Asking the right questions

A focused, in-depth nursing interview is essential to determining how to safely and effectively administer medications. Each individual is unique and is likely to have a personal viewpoint concerning taking medications. Some people view medications as "fix-it pills"—they believe medicines can fix anything, and "the more you take the better." Others view them as poisons that should be avoided as long as "you're not feeling bad."

Taking the time to have an open and honest discussion about how your patients **take** medications and how they **feel** about taking them can make the difference between success and failure. It will help you to get to know your patients as individuals, which will be valuable later when you are determining how they are responding to their medications. Early warning signs of complications due to the prescribed medications may come in the form of very subtle changes: changes that may be so subtle that only someone who knows the person will notice. It is also not unusual for patients to be the first to sense that something is not "quite right." Establishing a good rapport makes it easier for them to communicate uneasy feelings. You, as the nurse, will then be alerted to look for signs and symptoms that indicate there may be a problem.

Keeping in mind the importance of performing a focused, in-depth interview, the following offers guidelines for asking questions that focus on gathering data about the individual's medication regimen.

Guidelines:
Focusing the interview on taking medications

1 **Take the time to get to know the person.** People are more open when they feel more at ease. Include a family member or significant other in discussions about the medication regimen. In emergency situations, obtain a minimum history of allergies and current medications.

2 **Explain that the purpose of the interview is to discuss how the person feels he or she reacts to medications** (what works, what doesn't work) so best therapeutic effects can be attained.

3 **Explore the person's lifestyle and how it might be affected by taking medications.** Examine diet, occupation, daily activities, religion, recreation, responsibilities, family, friends, sense of well-being, and financial and spiritual resources.

4 **Determine history of present and past illnesses.**

5 **Examine present and past medication history:**

◆ **Ask about allergies or adverse reactions to medications.** If these are reported, ask for a description of what happened.

◆ **Assess knowledge of current medications:** what is taken and why, what dose is taken, who prescribed the medication(s), how doses are taken, whether the medications are working, and whether there are any side effects. Be sure to include questions about over-the-counter (OTC) medicines, as well as holistic or folk remedies. If there is a written record of the medications, ask to see this. If there is *any* doubt about the patient's reliability, have a family member bring in medications from home.

◆ *Be aware that if there is more than one prescribing physician, there is a greater risk of drug interactions and incompatibilities. One physician may be unaware that another physician is also prescribing for the patient.*

◆ **Determine past medications.** Ask the same questions about past medications as you did about current medications.

◆ **Ask how the individual feels about taking medicines** and whether taking them will interfere with daily lifestyle.

6 **For women of child-bearing age, determine whether there is a possibility of pregnancy or if the woman is currently lactating.** Many drugs taken by mothers affect fetal development or nursing infants because they cross the placenta or are present in the breast milk.

7 **Terminate the interview by summarizing** what has been discussed **and by encouraging the person** to voice opinions, ask questions, and let you know how he or she is feeling.

◆ Interviewing children

1 **Establish a rapport with parents and child.** Children often need more time to establish trust.

2 **Interview parents and child together, then ask additional questions separately.** This can provide information about how the parents and child interact, and can allow expression of different points of view.

3 **Use terminology that the child can understand.**

4 **Consider use of play therapy or role play** to encourage the child to relate his or her feelings about taking medications.

5 **Determine techniques or aids** that can be used at home to facilitate taking medications.

◆ Interviewing the elderly

1 **Ascertain that the person can hear what you are saying.** Many elderly people suffer some degree of hearing loss.

2 **Ensure that necessary visual and hearing aids are being worn.**

3 **Provide plenty of light and minimize noise.**

4 **If the person seems confused, talk slowly** and use simple terms.

5 **Determine the most frequent caregivers.** Try to interview both the person and the caregivers together, then separately. Allow for varying points of view and for assessment of patient-caregiver interaction.

6 **Determine the names of all attending physicians.** The elderly often have multiple system problems and may have several prescribing physicians.

7 **Identify strategies or products** that can be used at home to guard against forgetting to take medications.

The Physical Exam:
Assessing physical status

Since drugs are chemicals that will alter how the body functions, it is vital that you complete a physical examination and review diagnostic studies before starting any medication regimen. This **baseline physical examination** is necessary to be sure that the medication is indeed indicated and that there are **no contraindications** to its administration; it also helps identify potential problems and clearly assess changes after administering the medication. When patients are unable to communicate, their physical status is a key factor in determining beneficial or adverse medication effects. The following guidelines will help you to focus the physical examination and review of diagnostic studies and to gather the data that is pertinent to medication administration.

Guidelines:
Gathering data about physical status

1 **Begin by recording accurate age, height, and weight.** These are important in determining safe drug dosage.

2 **Document vital signs:** temperature, pulse, respirations, and blood pressure.

3 Perform a complete physical examination. Include a review of systems: neurological, respiratory, cardiovascular, circulatory, gastrointestinal, genitourinary, musculoskeletal, and integumentary (skin).

◆ *For IM or IV administration (or if drug abuse is suspected), special attention should be given to assessment of the muscles, skin, and veins.*

4 Check results of diagnostic studies that indicate liver and kidney function. These are the organs of metabolism and excretion of most drugs. Examine the values of SGOT, LDH, bilirubin, alkaline phosphatase, BUN, and creatinine.

5 Check drug-specific diagnostic studies. For example, if a patient is going to be taking an anticoagulant, check the prothrombin time. (For drug-specific diagnostic studies, see the *Nursing implications/Documentation* section under the drug listing).

6 If the patient is already taking medications, determine how he or she is responding. The letters in the mnemonic *TACT* help you remember to check the following:

T Therapeutic effect

A Adverse reactions and side effects

C Contraindications

T Toxicity and overdose

This gives a new dimension to the statement "Assess with *tact* when you give medications."

◆ Assessing children

1 Ascertain actual age (for children under 3 years, convert age to months), height, and weight. (Most medications are ordered on basis of body weight and age.)

2 Try to take vital signs when the child is calm because respiration and heart rate increase with stress or exercise. If possible, sit with the child and assess pulse and respirations without his or her knowledge.

3 Allow children to handle examination equipment (e.g., stethoscope) and to try the techniques themselves. For the very young, you might want to make a game of the examination; for older children, make it an opportunity for learning.

◆ Assessing the elderly

1 Determine accurate height and weight instead of asking the patient to supply information that might not be current. If the person is frail, a chair scale or bedscale may be necessary.

2 Assess mental status, memory, motor skills, and ability to follow simple instructions.

3 Monitor diagnostic studies closely. The elderly are more likely to be susceptible to adverse effects of medications.

The Drug Regimen:
Gathering information

Gathering information about the medications that the patient is taking is as important as gathering information about the patient. You must ascertain exactly what drugs are currently on the medication regimen. (This may have been determined during the nursing interview, but must be validated by checking physician's orders.) The physician's written orders (or prescriptions) should specify the following information about each drug:

❑ The patient's name and address

❑ The date of the order or prescription

❑ The drug name (generic or brand name)

❑ The dosage and route of administration

❑ The frequency of administration (when the medication should be given)

❑ The length of time the patient is to continue taking the medication (this may be determined by hospital policies)

If this information is not clear, you should contact the physician and ask him to clarify the order. Failure to clarify an unclear order is considered negligence and could result in harm to the patient.

Information about Specific Drugs

Once you have determined the medications that your patient is to receive, you must determine exactly how each medication works, how each is likely to alter body functioning, and what factors may influence its action. Drug information can be obtained in two ways:

1 By studying the available literature (pharmacology texts, drug manuals, journal articles, package inserts)

2 By consulting other qualified health care professionals (pharmacists, physicians, nurses)

Choosing Appropriate
Pharmacological References

Today's nurse is faced with the problem of choosing among many pharmacology texts and references. Should you use the ones the doctors use? How about the ones the pharmacists use? Surely these books contain everything! Unfortunately, this is not so. Although many of these books provide helpful information, they were not written to meet the needs of nurses.

You should choose references that provide drug information that *nurses* need to know: patient education, nursing diagnoses, documentation, home care, as well as the information available in the *Physician's Desk Reference* (*PDR*). We have designed this book to provide the information that you, as a nurse, need to meet the ever-growing demands of nursing practice. However, to help you evaluate other literature for nursing use, the following checklist outlines common questions a nursing drug manual should answer about medications.

Checklist:
Questions a nursing drug manual should answer

❑ What are the generic and brand names of the drug?

❑ Why is this drug usually given?

❑ How does this drug work and how is it likely to change my patient's current state of functioning?

❑ When is this drug contraindicated?

❑ What is the safe dose range and method of administration?

❑ Does this drug interact with food or with other drugs?

❑ What side effects, adverse reactions, and potential complications might be experienced when taking this drug?

❑ Are there special considerations for giving this drug to children, pregnant or nursing mothers, or the elderly?

❑ What potential nursing diagnoses might be seen in individuals taking this drug?

❑ How can I monitor for therapeutic effects, side effects, adverse reactions, and toxicity?

❑ What nursing interventions help promote therapeutic effects and reduce side effects and adverse reactions?

❑ How can I prevent complications and help people cope with side effects?

❑ What data is important to document when using this drug?

❑ What should I teach about this drug, and how can I prepare people to take it at home?

Consulting Qualified
Health Care Professionals

Because of the incredible rate of change of available drug preparations, and because of the complexity of some patient situations, you will at times need to consult a qualified health care professional (physician, pharmacist, nurse) to supplement the information that is available in the literature. In addition, you may need information about a new drug that is not yet covered in the literature. Information from consultations can be as valuable as information from published sources. Whenever the usual references do not answer your specific questions about a medication, you should seek consultation.

Checklist:
Consulting about medication information

❑ **Don't ask just anyone.** Find a reliable resource person. Ask the nursing supervisor to help you to locate an expert. *Rationale:* Be sure that you are asking the most qualified professional.

❑ **Do ask the person's name and document who gave you the information.** You may want to keep a personal log. *Rationale:* You need to be sure who gave you the information in case there are questions later.

❑ **Don't just accept someone's word when he or she gives you information.** Ask "Can you tell me what reference you are using?" or "Can you send me the information?" *Rationale:* This will help validate the information and you can learn more by reading the reference.

❑ **Do check with more than one professional if you are not sure.** *Rationale:* This will help you ensure that the information is correct.

❑ **Don't give the medication if you don't have all the information necessary to do so safely.** Notify the supervisor or head nurse that you lack sufficient information to give this drug safely. *Rationale:* You are the one who is accountable for giving the medication, and you should not give it if you are unsure about its safety.

2

Diagnosis:
Identifying nursing diagnoses and collaborative problems

Nursing Diagnoses and Collaborative Problems

Once you have gathered data about your patient and the medications, you are ready to identify nursing diagnoses and collaborative problems.

The nursing diagnoses deal with the *human response* of your patient and are treatable through independent nursing interventions. Often these problems are associated with learning about medications, preventing injury or discomfort, and managing the medications at home.

On the other hand, collaborative problems cannot be treated by independent nursing interventions alone. They require the nurse to collaborate with the physician (or other qualified health care professional) to initiate appropriate definitive treatment (Carpenito, 1991). For example, if you perform a nursing assessment and note that a patient who is receiving an antibiotic might be developing a rash, you would need to report this immediately to the physician. Together you would decide what actions must be taken, depending on the severity of the reaction and the need for antibiotics.

The following section discusses how to identify nursing diagnoses (human responses) and collaborative problems (potential complications) associated with medication administration.

Identifying Nursing Diagnoses

Nursing diagnoses focus on the human responses of individuals, families, and groups, and their use encourages nurses to meet those human needs once considered as "nice to do if there's time." Today's standards mandate that nurses make nursing diagnoses and identify nursing interventions that promote, maintain, and restore health. For example, it is no longer considered "nice" to teach patients about their medications, it is standard procedure. If your patient doesn't know about medications, and you fail to identify the problem or teach the necessary information, then you are providing substandard nursing care. Nurses must become skilled in recognizing and treating actual and potential nursing diagnoses frequently associated with drug therapy.

The North American Nursing Diagnosis Association (NANDA) has compiled a list of nursing diagnoses accepted for study and clinical testing (listed in the Preface). Analysis of patient and medication data may suggest the presence of one of these nursing diagnoses. Grouping nursing assessments with drug information will make you aware of patterns that suggest a specific nursing diagnosis. Note the following example:

Example:
Clustering patient and drug data to formulate a nursing diagnosis

Data

◆ States "no bowel movement in 3 days."

◆ States "full feeling in stomach."

◆ Medication record documents that the patient has been taking codeine 30 mg q4h around the clock for 2 days.

◆ Drug manual lists constipation as a common side effect of codeine.

Nursing Diagnosis: *Constipation related to codeine* as manifested by statements of "no bowel movement in 3 days" and "full feeling in stomach," and documented course of codeine for 2 days.

Common Nursing Diagnoses Associated wtih Medications

People who are taking medications are at risk for several nursing diagnoses. Some nursing diagnoses are related to a side effect or action of the medication (e.g., *Potential for injury* related to postural hypotension side effect of propranolol, or *Constipation* related to side effect of codeine); others arise because the patient has just begun drug therapy (e.g., *Knowledge deficit*), or because the medication regimen is somewhat complicated for home management (e.g., *Impaired home maintenance management*). There are three nursing diagnoses that seem especially linked with medication administration in general:

1 *Potential for injury*

2 *Knowledge deficit*

3 *Impaired home maintenance management*

Potential for injury is a frequent diagnosis, and often occurs because of specific actions or side effects of medication. It may more often be related to problems associated with *Knowledge deficit* and *Impaired home maintenance management*, for which detailed care plans are given at the end of Chapter 5. As you read the care plans, note that resolving problems associated with *Knowledge deficit* and *Impaired home maintenance management* often reduces the risk of *Potential for injury*.

Identifying Collaborative Problems and Potential Complications

Collaborative problems are actual or potential pathophysiologic complications that may result from diagnostic, monitoring, or treatment-related situations. The nurse's role in dealing with these potential complications is that of monitoring to detect their onset and status, of implementing protocols and physician-prescribed interventions, and of collaborating with the appropriate health care professionals for definitive treatment. For example, for a patient receiving medication, the nurse's role is to:

1 **Monitor** to detect early signs and symptoms of potential medical complications that may result from taking medications, including allergic reactions (e.g., a rash on a patient receiving an antibiotic), untoward side effects (e.g., respiratory depression in a person receiving a sedative), and overdose or toxicity (e.g., nausea and vomiting in a person taking digoxin).

2 **Withhold the medication** if there is any question that it should be given, contact the physician, and provide supportive measures as needed (these may be as simple as asking the patient to remain in bed with the side rails up, or as complicated as sounding the cardiac arrest alarm).

3 **Implement nursing interventions** to reduce the incidence of potential complications (e.g., if you were giving a patient anticoagulants, you would take extra care when giving injections).

The nurse's role in monitoring for early detection of drug-related complications cannot be overemphasized. In fact, the sole reason for many hospitalizations is to ensure early detection and treatment of drug-related complications by having expert nursing observation and documentation.

Identifying drug-related complications involves analyzing patient and medication information. For example, take a look at how the following information about a 71-year-old woman who is taking heparin has been grouped to identify the potential complication of *hemorrhage*. Then study the checklist, provided to assist you in identifying common potential drug-related complications.

Example:
Clustering patient and drug data to identify collaborative problems/potential complications

Data

♦ The patient is a female, age 71.

♦ She is receiving heparin 5,000 units q6h SC.

♦ Drug information includes a warning that women over 65 are more likely to experience hemorrhage as an adverse reaction.

Collaborative Problem: *Potential complication: hemorrhage* as evidenced by documented regimen of heparin 5,000 units q6h for this female who is over 65.

Checklist:
Identifying potential complications

1 **Potential complication: allergic response**

❑ Check for allergies to the drug, closely related drugs, or substances used to prepare the drug. Also determine if the patient has a history of being an "allergic person." People who have multiple allergies are more likely than people without allergies to have allergic reactions to medications.

2 **Potential complication: adverse reaction**

❑ Ascertain that the individual does not have any of the signs, symptoms, or illnesses listed under the *Contraindications/precautions* section for the drug(s) you are about to administer. Be sure that you consider age, weight, and special precautions for pregnant or nursing mothers.

❑ Examine data for history of preexisting conditions that may precipitate adverse reactions or influence drug dosage. (For example, a person with a history of ulcers may react adversely to aspirin by bleeding.)

❑ Study the *Side effects/Adverse reactions* section for the drug to be sure that you are aware of the reactions that have happened to other people taking the same drug. (Any patient is at risk for these, especially when they are beginning therapy).

**3 Potential complication:
drug incompatibility/interaction**

❏ Consider all the medications that are being taken and check drug information for incompatibilities or interactions.

4 Potential complication: toxicity/overdosage

❏ Monitor diagnostic studies for abnormal liver and kidney function (SGOT, LDH, alkaline phosphatase, BUN, creatinine), because the body's ability to metabolize and excrete medications depends greatly on liver and kidney function.

❏ Monitor serum drug levels, if applicable. (See individual drugs for other signs and symptoms of toxicity or overdosage.)

❏ Check other medications that have been given to determine whether one may potentiate another. (For example, a person who has received a narcotic may be oversedated when given a routine medication for sleep.)

3

Planning:

Setting priorities, determining goals, documenting the medication schedule, identifying nursing interventions, and documenting the care plan

Once you have identified nursing diagnoses and collaborative problems, you are ready to plan nursing care. Planning involves setting priorities, determining goals, scheduling and documenting the medication regimen, and identifying nursing interventions to promote therapeutic effects and minimize side effects and adverse reactions.

Setting Priorities

Since you can't do everything at once, set priorities by determining what **must** be done first, and what can wait until later. You need to set priorities for nursing diagnoses, for monitoring for potential complications, and for timing of medications.

Example:
Setting priorities for nursing diagnoses

You have a patient with two nursing diagnoses, *Knowledge deficit: insulin injection technique* and *Disturbance in self-concept* related to newly diagnosed diabetes. You would probably do well to work on the problem of *Disturbance in self-concept* before you work on teaching how to give an injection.

Example:
Setting priorities for monitoring for potential complications

You have someone who has just begun receiving intravenous nitroglycerin. Because of the rapid response to IV administration and the potency of nitroglycerin and its effect on the cardiovascular system, you know you must assign a high priority to monitoring and documenting blood pressure and pain level every 5 minutes.

Example:
Setting priorities for timing of medications

You have someone scheduled to receive an antibiotic four times a day for a severe infection. The routine qid times for medications are 10-2-6-10. Because of the importance of maintaining adequate antibiotic blood levels, you

should clarify with the physician and assign around-the-clock times, such as a 6-12-6-12 schedule, even if it means waking the patient. In this situation, the need for maintaining a good blood level of the antibiotic has to take a priority over the person's need for undisturbed sleep.

Determining Goals and Outcome Criteria

For every nursing diagnosis you identify, you should determine a client-centered goal to direct nursing care and to serve as an evaluation criterion later when evaluating the success of the plan of care. For example, for the nursing diagnosis of *Knowledge deficit: insulin injection technique*, you may set a goal of "Will demonstrate sterile self-injection of insulin by 9/18." This goal will direct you to teach insulin injection technique by 9/18, and will also help you evaluate the plan of care (on 9/18 determine whether the individual can self-inject insulin).

It is also important to determine the therapeutic goal of medications and the outcome criteria that indicate the drug is working as intended. While the nurse alone is not accountable for achieving the therapeutic goal, you must answer the questions "What specific beneficial effects are anticipated by giving the medication to this specific individual?" and "How do I know if the medication is working?" The drug information in this book will help you determine these answers, because it lists therapeutic goals and outcome criteria for each drug (check any drug for an example).

Scheduling the Medication Regimen

Proper scheduling of the medication regimen plays a major role in the success of the medication treatment plan. All medications the patient will be taking should be considered, and timing of doses should be scheduled so that optimum beneficial effects can be achieved. The following guidelines are suggested to help you in coordinating and scheduling the medication regimen.

Guidelines:
Coordinating and scheduling medications

1 **Consider all medications to be taken, as well as the patient's daily schedule.**

2 **Avoid drug interactions by separating the administration times of drugs that are likely to interact or potentiate one another.** For example, avoid giving a tranquilizer and a sedative at the same time, unless this has been determined to be necessary.

3 **Schedule doses to avoid food-drug interactions, to promote beneficial effects, and to minimize side effects.** Give medications with or without food as suggested by the drug information, and set administration times to maintain desired serum drug levels.

4 **Whenever possible, schedule doses for the convenience of the patient.** For example, routine doses of diuretics should not be given late at night when the patient is trying to sleep.

Documenting

Once you have determined how to coordinate and schedule drug administration, it must be documented clearly on the medication record to provide easy access to information about the medication regimen. This medication record is a very important piece of nursing documentation; all of the vital information about the patient's medications can be found in one place. Keeping the information in one place reduces the likelihood that a consulting physician or another nurse will overlook important data.

Because the format of medication records varies from institution to institution, you will have to become familiar with your facility's policies and procedures for documenting medications. Despite the variability in format and design, all medication records should provide the information necessary to answer the following important questions.

Checklist:
Questions that the medication record should answer

❏ What is the age, height, weight, and diet of this patient?

❏ What is this patient allergic to?

❏ What medications has this person received?

❏ What medications is the person yet to receive?

❏ What drugs may be given prn, and for what reasons?

❏ What medications are "one time only" or "stat" drugs?

❏ What is the dose, route of administration, and time of each dose?

❏ When was each medication ordered (start date), and when will each be discontinued (stop date)?

❏ What doses have been withheld?

❏ Who transcribed or checked the medication order?

❏ Who administered each dose?

❏ What was the site of each injection?

This may be noted by writing a number which corresponds to an injection site. See example: codes for injection sites on page 12.

Adjunctive (Drug-specific) Nursing Interventions

Adjunctive nursing interventions are those independent nursing interventions performed specifically because the patient is receiving a certain medication. These interventions are performed to promote therapeutic effects of a medication, to provide for safety, to reduce the incidence of side effects and adverse reactions, and to monitor for detection of potential medication-related complications.

There are three types of adjunctive nursing interventions:

1 **Assessment interventions** are those activities nurses perform to monitor for problems related to the medication regimen.

2 **Teaching interventions** are those activities nurses perform to promote knowledge of the medication regimen.

3 **Action interventions** are those activities that nurses perform or assist the patient in performing to enhance the action of the drug or to minimize expected side effects. Putting up siderails for safety, or helping a patient get out of bed when the patient has received a sedative, are examples of action interventions.

Turn to page 14 for more examples of adjunctive interventions.

Guidelines:
Codes for injection sites

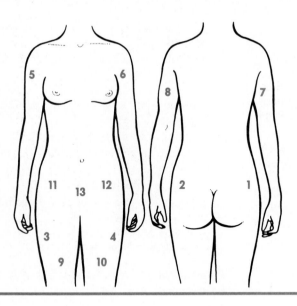

1 Right gluteal IM
2 Left gluteal IM
3 Right lateral thigh IM
4 Left lateral thigh IM
5 Right deltoid IM
6 Left deltoid IM
7 Right arm SC
8 Left arm SC
9 Right anterior thigh IM
10 Left anterior thigh IM
11 Right lower abdomen SC
12 Left lower abdomen SC
13 Mid lower abdomen SC

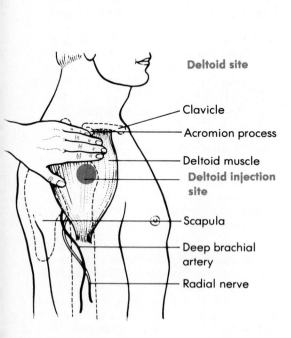

Deltoid site

Clavicle
Acromion process
Deltoid muscle
Deltoid injection site
Scapula
Deep brachial artery
Radial nerve

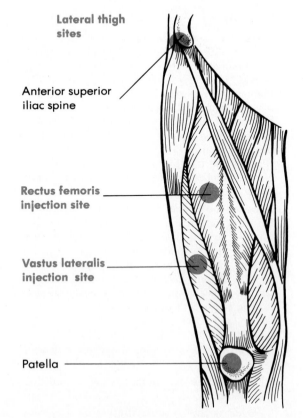

Lateral thigh sites

Anterior superior iliac spine

Rectus femoris injection site

Vastus lateralis injection site

Patella

Ventrogluteal site

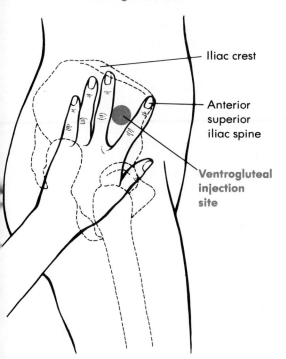

Iliac crest

Anterior superior iliac spine

Ventrogluteal injection site

Dorsogluteal site

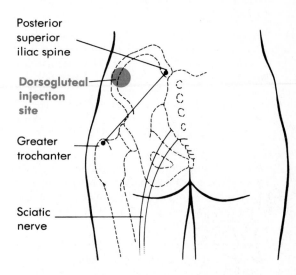

Posterior superior iliac spine

Dorsogluteal injection site

Greater trochanter

Sciatic nerve

Pediatric injection sites

Deltoid injection site

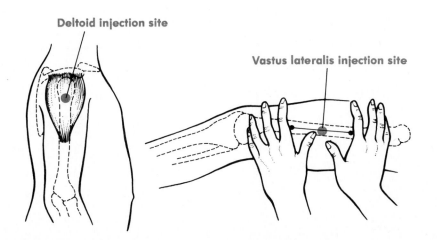

Vastus lateralis injection site

Dorsogluteal injection site

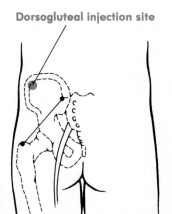

Examples:
Adjunctive (drug-specific) nursing interventions

♦ **Putting up side rails after administering a sedative.** *Rationale:* Provides for safety; the patient may become disoriented from the medication.

♦ **Exploring with a patient why he or she feels anxious and helping him or her identify things to allay the anxiety before giving a tranquilizer.** *Rationale:* Enhances expected therapeutic effects of the medication by helping the person use inner strength to reduce anxiety. Often, this may even *eliminate* the need for a tranquilizer.

♦ **Explaining the reason that a pain medication will be given,** e.g., to enable him or her to perform coughing and deep breathing exercises better. *Rationale:* Promotes clinical goal of therapy because the patient is aware of the reason for medication.

♦ **Planning for increased exercise, fluids, and dietary intake of roughage when a patient is taking a drug that may cause constipation.** *Rationale:* Minimizes the side effect of constipation.

♦ **Explaining that it is important for the patient to let you know if the medication makes him or her feel dizzy, and to call for assistance if this occurs.** *Rationale:* Promotes early detection of side effects and provides for safety.

♦ **Teaching a woman in labor relaxation techniques, in addition to giving her medication for pain.** *Rationale:* Enhances expected therapeutic effects by reducing nervous and muscular tension.

♦ **Recording frequent blood pressures of a patient who has just begun taking an antihypertensive medication.** *Rationale:* Monitors the potential complication of hypotension.

Identifying Adjunctive Interventions

The importance of these types of independent nursing interventions cannot be underestimated: they can even reduce the need for some medications. For example, someone who requests a sleeping pill may receive a similar effect if the nurse takes the time to discuss the reasons for the inability to fall asleep, or even to give a relaxing back rub. Nurses must view the whole picture and employ holistic, nonchemical interventions to enhance the intended effect of the medicine—and perhaps even eliminate the need for a particular medication.

The *Nursing interventions/Documentation* and *Patient & family teaching/Home care* sections will help you identify drug-specific adjunctive nursing interventions. The care plans for *Knowledge deficit: medications* and *Impaired home maintenance management* will also help you determine independent nursing interventions that promote a therapeutic medication regimen.

4

Implementation:
Administering medications safely and effectively

Performing Ongoing Assessments

Your ability to perform ongoing assessments **before** giving any medication is essential to administering medications safely and effectively. These assessments are necessary to be sure that there are no contraindications to giving the drug, to help predict possible untoward reactions, and (in some cases) to determine whether the drug is still indicated. If you give a drug without assessing the patient, and the patient's assessment data indicates that the drug obviously should be withheld, it may harm the patient, and you would be as accountable as the physician.

◆ *In fact, if the order was appropriate when the physician saw the patient, but inappropriate when you* **gave** *the medication because of a change in clinical status, you may be the only one who is accountable.*

The physician prescribes medications, but legally, the nurse is responsible for assessing the patient before drug administration to be sure that there are no signs and symptoms that indicate that the drug should be withheld. Although nurses (with the exception of some *nurse practitioners*) are restricted by law from prescribing drugs, nurses are accountable for:

1 clarifying orders that are unclear,

2 questioning doses that are excessive, and

3 withholding doses and **notifying the physician** whenever there is a question whether the drug should be given.

Assessing current status helps you anticipate how a patient may react to a medication. For example, you may read in a drug manual that the onset of action of an intramuscular narcotic occurs within 30 minutes, and the duration of action is 2 to 3 hours. While this may be true as an average, individuals may react differently depending on their other medications and their age, height, weight, and health status. Use drug information as a guide to predicting effects; use **your assessment skills** before giving medications to individualize the medication regimen to special needs.

Finally, because of the unpredictability of individual reactions, make it a rule:

◆ *Give all first doses with caution, and with close attention to patient status after drug administration.*

Perform a safety check like that shown on the next page before giving any medication.

Monitoring Responses and Detecting Complications

Performing ongoing assessments **after** medication administration is the key to determining how the patient is responding to a medication, and to detecting potential complications early. These assessments will help you determine whether someone is experiencing the **desired therapeutic effect**, whether there are any **side effects** or **adverse reactions** that may need to be managed, and even whether the drug should be continued.

◆ **It is useless to give a medication that is not working.**

◆ **It is even worse to continue giving a medication that causes more problems than it relieves.**

Within each drug listing, the *Use/Therapeutic goal/Outcome* section tells you how to determine if your patient is experiencing the desired therapeutic effects. The *Nursing implications/Documentation* and *Patient & family teaching/Home care* sections help you determine what you should monitor to assure early detection of side effects or adverse reactions.

Preventing Medication Errors

Because of the ever-present possibility of human error, preventing medication errors is a major concern of nurses. Many mistakes can be prevented by checking for human error that could occur at crucial points in the process of the physician prescribing, the pharmacist dispensing, and the nurse administering medications.

Safety Check:
Before giving medications

Ask yourself the following questions:

1 Has the physician clearly written:

❏ The name of the medication.

❏ The dose and route of administration.

❏ The frequency or conditions of administration.

❏ The length of time the medication is to be taken. (*This may be determined by standard hospital policy.*)

❏ **Has a nurse initialed** that the physician's order was properly transcribed?

2 Is this medication order still valid?

❏ Check expiration dates.

❏ Also ensure that the order has been rewritten if the patient has just returned from the operating room.

◆ *All medication orders are usually canceled when a patient goes to the operating room, and new orders must be written when the patient returns.*

3 Why is this drug indicated for this specific patient?

4 Is this the correct time to give this medication?

❏ Have I checked the time that the last dose was given?

5 Have I checked the medication label three times to be sure that I have the right medication?

❏ Check the label when taking the medication from storage.

❏ Check the label before preparing the medication.

❏ Check the label again when replacing the medication in storage.

For unit doses:

❏ Check the label when you take the unit dose from storage.

❏ Check the label immediately before opening it.

❏ Check the label again as you discard the unit dose wrapper.

6 Is the drug properly labeled, and does it appear as it should?

❏ Unit doses and new bottles should be intact and free from evidence of tampering (seals should be intact).

❏ Most parenteral medications should be clear, rather than look cloudy or contain crystals.

❏ Pills, tablets, and capsules should be free from evidence of dirt or moisture.

7 Do I have the right patient?

❏ Is the name on the identification bracelet the same as the name on the physician's order sheet?

❏ Does the name on the medication bottle match the identification bracelet?

8 Is the dose and route of administration appropriate for this patient?

❏ Is dose within the recommended limits?

❏ Is patient allowed or able to tolerate this route?

9 Does this individual exhibit any signs and symptoms that indicate that this drug should not be given?

❏ Has the patient received any **other** medications that may affect how this drug will act?

❏ Are there procedures planned that may influence whether this medication should be given (e.g., when insulin is ordered and the individual is not allowed to eat because of lab studies)?

Crucial Points:
Key times to check for human error

1 When the physician prescribes the order.
☐ Is the order clear, appropriate, and within usual dose range?

2 When the nurse or unit clerk transcribes.
☐ Does the transcription match the order?

3 When the pharmacist dispenses the drug.
☐ Does the label match the order?

4 When you take the medicine out of the medicine drawer or cabinet.
☐ Did you check the label when you picked up the medication?
☐ Did you check the label when you withdrew the medication?
☐ Did you check the label when you returned the medication or discarded the packaging?

5 When you administer the medication.
☐ Do you have the right patient for this medication?
☐ Have you assessed the patient?
☐ Are you following correct procedures?

When nurses administer medications, they are the *last chance* that a previous error of the physician, the pharmacist, the clerk, or another nurse may be detected.

The Safety Check: Before giving medications offers detailed questions that should be asked before giving a medication to reduce the incidence of error. The following guidelines will also help prevent medication errors.

Guidelines:
Preventing common medication errors

1 **Be careful with decimal points.** For example:
♦ Write *0.2* instead of *.2* (*.2* could lose its decimal point and be read as *2*).
♦ Never write *2.0* for *2* (*2.0* could lose its decimal point and become *20*).

2 **Never assume familiarity with the packaging or appearance of a drug. Read labels!**
♦ Different drugs can look the same, and packaging can change.

3 **If a patient questions his medications, double-check the order** directly with the physician's order.

♦ Encourage individuals to learn their medication regimen; they can provide additional safety checks.

4 **Keep unit doses in their original containers** until you and the medications are at the patient's bedside.

5 **Don't leave medications at the bedside** unless specifically ordered by the physician.

6 **When giving injections to children or restless individuals, obtain assistance** to position the patient.

7 **Be aware of high-risk situations.**
♦ People over 60 years old are disproportionately involved in errors.
♦ Errors in parenteral medications can cause more serious consequences because of the rapid onset of drug action.

8 **Use a reliable formula for calculating dosage**, and keep it handy.
♦ To calculate the number of cc or tablets that make up a prescribed dose, use the following formula (make sure the doses are all in the same unit of measure):

$$\frac{\text{Prescribed dose}}{\text{Dose per cc or tablet}} = \frac{\text{How many cc or}}{\text{tablets to give}}$$

Administering medications to children

1 Ascertain safe pediatric dose range based on recommendations for pediatric dosage in the literature. Depending on the drug, use an appropriate method of calculation. Dosage may be based on any of the following:
♦ Body surface area, see *Nomogram: Estimating body surface area* on p. 19
♦ Body weight
♦ Age
♦ Clark's Rule:
Child dose = Adult dose × Child wt (lb)/150
or   Adult dose × Child wt (kg)/70

2 Consider age and developmental differences that may influence drug distribution, rate of absorption, and rate of elimination.
♦ Infants and young children have immature kidney and liver function, and therefore are more susceptible to nephrotoxicity and hepatotoxicity, as well as drug toxicity itself.
♦ The gastrointestinal tracts of infants have higher pH (are more alkaline) than those of adults. This may hasten or prolong drug absorption, depending on the medication.

- Infants and young children absorb topical medications more quickly than adults because the epidermis is thinner.
- Drugs usually have greater bioavailability in children because they bind less extensively with plasma proteins.
- Infants and young children should receive lateral thigh IM injections, because the gluteal and deltoid muscles are underdeveloped.
- When giving ear drops to children under three, pull the outer ear backward before insertion; for older children, pull the outer ear upward and backward.

3 Individualize nursing interventions depending on the child's developmental age and ability to understand and communicate.
- Take the time to earn the child's trust, and include significant others in planning and administering nursing care; tell child of intent to administer medication just before actual administration (children have a poor sense of time, and anticipation can upset them).
- Allow the child to express negative feelings and acknowledge that you understand what he or she is saying; allow parents to offer support.
- Reinforce the fact that the medication is necessary "to make you better." Although it may feel like punishment, or it may taste bad, it is to help, not harm the child.
- Explain to the child that you realize how difficult it is to be brave—even if the child cries or fights during medication administration. Ask the child if there is someone or something that would help him or her be brave.
- Praise positive behaviors, and use appropriate rewards, such as hugs and stickers.
- If the child cannot or will not cooperate with IM or IV drug administration, acquire the assistance necessary to restrain the child adequately for safe administration. Do not scold the child for resisting painful administration; simply restrain the child appropriately.
- Avoid mixing PO meds with essential foods; use jelly or pudding.
- Acquire devices to make measuring and administering more acceptable to children (e.g., favorite cup for liquid medication).

Administering medications to the elderly

1 Check the drug literature to determine whether there are special precautions for the elderly. Physiological changes due to aging and chronic disease states can increase or decrease response to a drug.

2 Be aware that in the elderly, certain medications can have effects opposite from those intended. For example, a sleeping pill may cause excitement.

3 Monitor closely for hepatic or renal toxicity and for drug toxicity itself. Many elderly people have decreased liver and kidney function.

4 Assess ability to swallow; crush medications and administer with strained food if appropriate.

5 Observe carefully for changes in mental status (confusion), since these are often early warnings of toxicity and adverse reactions.

6 Expect lower doses or frequency of administration of some drugs. Decreased renal function of elderly patients prolongs the drug half-life.

7 Do not administer injections in immobile limbs.

Using Correct Procedures

A major factor in the safe administration of medications is that of following correct administration procedures. Your ability to use good technique and follow safe procedures when giving medications by the various routes of administration is as important as your ability to decide whether a medication order is acceptable (see Chapter 6, *Guidelines for Procedures*).

Making Nursing Judgments

The nurse's responsibility to monitor clinical status while administering medications implies that the nurse is also responsible for making judgments about the data collected during the ongoing nursing assessments. This means that the nurse must

1 Analyze the data

2 Take appropriate action

3 Report and document significant data and actions taken.

For example, if while giving a drug known to lower blood pressure, you note that a person's blood pressure has become unusually low, your responsibility is to withhold the next dose, document the withheld dose and the reason, and report to the physician that the dose was withheld.

Nomogram:
Estimating body surface area and computing child dose

Place the edge of a card (or other straight edge) with one end on child's height, the other on the child's weight. Where the edge of the card crosses the center column, you can read the body surface area (m²).

For children of normal height and weight, use these quick reference columns to find body surface area (m²) by weight in pounds (left chart) or kilograms (right chart).

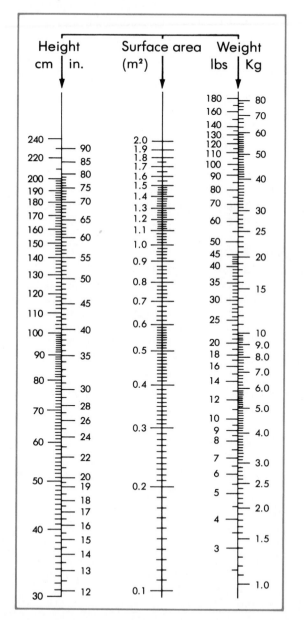

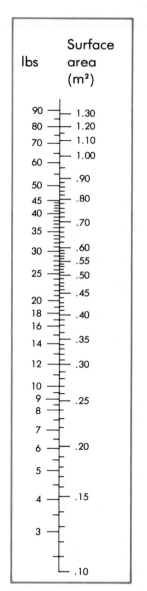

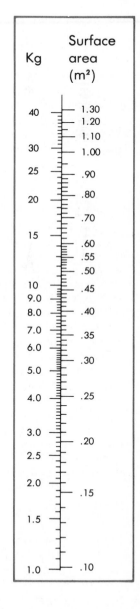

When you have found body surface area (m²) using one of the above charts, substitute it in this formula to convert adult dose to the specific child dose:

$$\text{Child dose} = \text{Adult dose} \times \frac{\text{Body surface area (m}^2\text{)}}{1.7}$$

Nurses are frequently responsible for choosing the appropriate drug, dose, and route of administration for "prn" pain medications and sedatives. Physicians may order as many as three or four different drugs to be given depending on the severity of the situation. The nurse must choose the most appropriate drug, based on the individual's status. For example, on a surgical unit you might have to choose between a strong intramuscular and a weak oral analgesic for pain. It is your responsibility to administer the most appropriate medication. You make a judgment and give the drug that best achieves the desired response with the least chance of adverse reaction or side effects.

The ability to make this type of judgment depends on your nursing knowledge and clinical expertise. If you are unsure about making these judgments, you should consult a more qualified nurse, the physician who prescribed the drug, or a pharmacist.

Performing Adjunctive (Drug-specific) Nursing Interventions

Safe and effective administration of medications depends not only upon your ability to monitor reactions to medications and to make nursing judgments, but also upon your ability to implement interventions: to teach about medications, to reduce side effects and adverse reactions, to provide for safety, and to promote therapeutic effects. Examples of interventions can be found in Chapter 3 on p. 14.

You will be expected to implement adjunctive interventions. They are considered standard nursing interventions performed for any patient receiving a specific medication.

Adjunctive interventions may not be documented on the care plan; instead they may be found in the nursing standards and policy and procedure manual of the agency where you are working and in drug manuals. For example, most institutions require (and nursing drug manuals state) that bedside rails must be placed in the upright position after a patient receives a sedative. It is your responsibility to be familiar with the nursing interventions in the standards, policies, and procedures of your institution and the interventions listed in drug manuals.

These interventions should be performed consistently whenever a medication is given. The *Nursing implications/Documentation* and *Patient & family teaching/Home care* sections

for each drug help you identify drug-specific adjunctive nursing interventions.

Charting

Charting of medications, responses to medications, and nursing interventions has become increasingly important over the past decade. Charting serves three purposes:

1 **Communicating and monitoring health status and response to medications.**

2 **Providing a legal document** that might be reviewed in a court of law. Your documentation of the medications you gave, responses to the medication, and the nursing assessments and interventions performed may answer the question, "Has this individual received acceptable quality care?"

3 **Assuring quality.** Written records are essential for evaluating the quality and efficiency of the care given.

When you chart about medications, you use two kinds of records: the medication record, and nursing notes.

Guidelines:
Charting on the medication record

The exact manner in which you chart on the medication record is determined by the policies and procedures of the institution where you are working. However, these guidelines apply to all charting on medication records.

1 Chart the medication as soon **after** you give it as possible.

2 Write letters and numbers clearly, or you may contribute to errors.

3 If you chart your initials, be sure that your full signature is on file.

4 Chart injection sites for each parenteral medication that you give. This is usually done with a code number as given in *Guidelines: Codes for injection sites* on page 12.

5 Don't chart a medication that another nurse gave.

6 Follow hospital policy for omitted doses or doses given at unscheduled times (usually the dose is circled, with additional comments on the nurses' notes).

Guidelines:
Charting in nurses' notes

Nurses' notes provide a place to chart additional explanatory information about medications; they clarify and complement what you have charted on the medication record. Although double documentation (charting the same thing in two places) should be avoided, additional significant documentation about an individual's response to medication and interventions employed should be described in the nurses' notes (for example, charting "Reports nausea after administration of iron").

If the response to the medication is as expected, some institutions do not require charting about medication in the nurses' notes; initialing the doses given is all that is required.

These guidelines will help you identify what to chart about medications on the nursing notes to clarify and complement what has been charted on the medication record.

1 If a drug dose has been withheld or vomited, it should be circled on the medication record, and you should chart **what happened** on the nursing notes.

For example, "Laxative withheld because patient has been having loose stools," or "Vomited 5 minutes after digoxin was given. Dr. LeFevre notified."

2 If someone is receiving medications that significantly affect blood pressure, pulse rate, respiration, or temperature, document vital signs **before and after** medication administration, and as frequently thereafter as necessary.

3 Chart ongoing assessment findings that describe responses to new or potent medications. Chart **what you observed**, including side effects and adverse reactions, **what you did**, and **how the patient responded**.

For example, "Lidocaine running at 2 mg per min. Patient complains of slight dizziness. Blood pressure stable. Notified Dr. O'Hara. Lidocaine decreased to 1 mg per min per Dr.'s order. Patient now denies dizziness. No increase in PVCs noted."

4 Document significant adjunctive nursing interventions that you have performed to provide for safety, promote therapeutic effects, or minimize side effects of medications. Also chart the **response** to your interventions.

For example, "Explored reasons for anxiety, but he seems unable to pinpoint cause of anxiety. Serax given, but still restless. Bedside rails up."

5

Evaluation:
Examining the effectiveness of the medication regimen and providing quality assurance

When nurses talk about the evaluation phase of the nursing process, they usually are referring to evaluation of the nursing care plan (i.e., evaluation of goal achievement for nursing diagnoses). However, this section focuses on evaluating the **effectiveness of the medication regimen.** (For information on evaluating the nursing care plan, the reader is directed to nursing process and fundamentals texts.)

Examining the Effectiveness of the Medication Regimen

Examining the effectiveness of the medication regimen begins with determining whether the individual is achieving therapeutic goals. For example, with insulin doses, you would examine the recorded blood sugars, ask about episodes of signs of hypoglycemia, and determine whether there has been a consistent control of blood sugars. The outcome criteria for each drug indicate which data will tell you whether the therapeutic goal for that medication is being achieved.

If assessment data demonstrate therapeutic goal achievement, and the individual does not demonstrate adverse effects, then the medication regimen is working and should be continued without change. If the therapeutic goal is not achieved, or if new problems arise, then it is time to examine the factors that are affecting the medication regimen and make some changes. The following checklist will assist you in determining variables that may affect the success of the medication regimen. Once you have identified these variables, you will be able to make the necessary changes.

Checklist:
Evaluating the medication regimen

❑ Is your original clinical assessment correct and complete? Have you missed something?

❑ How does the individual feel the medicines are working?

❑ What factors does the person feel are helping or hindering achievement of therapeutic effects?

❑ Are unresolved nursing diagnoses impeding the response (e.g., *Ineffective coping* related to excessive independence and problems with asking for help).

❑ Did you set appropriate priorities?

❑ Were the medications, doses, routes, and times appropriate for this specific situation and patient?

❑ Were adjunctive nursing interventions that promote therapeutic effects, minimize side effects and adverse reactions, and provide for safety identified and implemented?

Providing Quality Assurance

Performing quality assurance studies that examine the quality and efficiency of nursing care during medication administration involves the study of medical and nursing records and medication error forms. Most nurses understand the importance of clear, accurate medication records and nurses' notes. However, many feel threatened by medication error forms or *incident reports* (also called *risk management forms*).

◆ *Remember that medication error forms do not become a part of the patient's medical record. They are hospital records that are usually kept by the quality assurance department or risk management nurse.*

Making a medication error—for whatever reason—is extremely upsetting. Documenting the error often elicits intense negative feelings and, perhaps, even shame, despite the cause of the error. However, when these feelings are overcome and nurses objectively state the facts, medication error forms can become valuable tools in examining factors that contributed to errors. Once these factors are identified, nursing policies and procedures can be revised to reduce errors and promote safe, effective medication regimens.

The next page begins the sample care plans for knowledge deficit: the medication regimen and Impaired home maintenance management.

♦ Some nurses may prefer to use this diagnosis as an etiologic factor (e.g., Impaired home maintenance management related to lack of knowledge).

Assessment

❑ **Determine who will be responsible for administering medications.** Include appropriate significant others. *Rationale:* All individuals involved in implementing the medication regimen should be included because their knowledge will contribute to the success of the plan. If the patient is a child, or is incapable of learning, the teaching plan should focus on the caregiver.

❑ **Examine physical, emotional, and psychological status.** *Rationale:* If the person is too ill or too upset, formal teaching should be deferred. However, the person is never too ill for you to briefly explain procedures as they occur. For example, say "I'm giving you medication to help you rest" when administering a medication to a semiconscious, restless individual.

❑ **Identify factors that may impede learning** (e.g., fatigue, pain, denial, anger, fear, problems with cognition, poor reading skills). *Rationale:* This will help you set priorities. For example, a frightened person's fear must be dealt with before you can begin teaching that person. Identifying other factors (such as poor reading skills) will help you determine alternative teaching strategies (such as using pictures rather than written text for a person who cannot read).

❑ **Explore whether taking the medications is viewed as important.** *Rationale:* Whether the patient (and family) values the importance of taking the medications is likely to be a major factor in their desire to learn.

❑ **Determine factors that may impede the willingness to follow the medication regimen:**
   ♦ Ascertain whether there are personal feelings or spiritual beliefs that oppose taking medications.
   ♦ Identify concerns about adverse side effects of the medications.
   ♦ Examine individual coping mechanisms if the medication requires lifestyle changes.

♦ Determine whether there are financial or social pressures or other priorities that interfere with taking the medications.
Rationale: Problems interfering with the willingness to take medications should be resolved or reduced before the plan is implemented.

❑ **Assess for physical and mental handicaps:**
   ♦ Observe the person's ability to follow simple instructions.
   ♦ Assess for problems with short-term and long-term memory, and for evidence of confusion.
   ♦ Assess for vision, hearing, or motor impairment.
Rationale: Physical and mental handicaps are major factors that reduce one's ability to follow a medication regimen.

❑ **Examine previous knowledge.** Ask what is known about the medications. Determine if written and verbal instructions for the medication regimen have been given. (See *Checklist: Evaluation of knowledge of medication regimen* at the end of this care plan.) *Rationale:* Once you have identified what the person already knows, then you can determine the content of the teaching plan. It is frustrating and useless to waste time "learning" things that are already known. Written instructions reinforce learning.

❑ **If the person is already taking medications,** ask how the medication regimen is followed. *Rationale:* People often have their own methods of taking medications. The nurse should not interfere with techniques that are not detrimental to the person's health.

❑ **Examine readiness to learn.** Ask what things about medications are important to learn and whether there are any specific questions. *Rationale:* Some people may be frightened by hearing every detail about drug therapy—every possible side effect—and want to know only what is absolutely necessary.

❑ **If the person is concerned about side effects or adverse reactions, explain that he or she will be closely monitored,** and the drug discontinued if the adverse reactions are worse than the disease. Teach ways of minimizing the incidence of side effects and adverse reactions. *Rationale:* Learning ways to avoid reactions and side effects helps people minimize their occurrence and gives people a feeling of control over their lives.

Client goal/Outcome criteria

♦ *These ideal goals must be individualized depending on the nursing assessment. The person should be allowed to refer to written material when relating the information.*

The person (or caregiver) will relate (or demonstrate) how to follow the prescribed medication regimen. This includes the ability to

❑ List the name and dose of each medication.

❑ Relate why each medication is necessary.

❑ Relate when to take each medication.

❑ Demonstrate or describe how to take each medication.

❑ Explain how each medication should be stored.

❑ Relate how to determine if each medication is working.

❑ List foods and/or drugs to be avoided.

❑ State the length of time it will be necessary to take each medication.

❑ Relate how to observe for side effects, adverse reactions, and allergic reactions.

❑ Identify ways of preventing side effects and adverse reactions.

❑ Explain what to do if side effects or adverse reactions occur.

❑ Relate whether a dose may be skipped and when.

❑ Describe activities that should be avoided while on each medication.

❑ Relate where written information about each medication can be found.

Planning/Implementation

❑ **Individualize goals and interventions depending on problems and strengths identified during assessment** (see goals above). *Rationale:* Goals and interventions must be client-specific. Including strengths will increase the efficiency of the plan of care.

❑ **Provide written and verbal summaries of important information, especially things that should be reported (e.g., side effects, pregnancy, new symptoms).** *Rationale:* For those who can read, written information is vital for referral and review during learning, and for later reference.

❑ **If the medication regimen requires lifelong changes,** encourage the person to view the short term; that is, to deal with problems as they come, one day at a time. *Rationale:* Addressing problems as they come helps to reduce feelings of being overwhelmed.

❑ **If the person has financial pressures, social pressures, or other priorities that interfere with taking medications, stress the fact that in the long run, taking medications will improve health, prevent additional cost of illness, and help the individual meet other priorities.** Secure financial support and help at home if possible. Consult with physician to see if less expensive generic drugs can replace brand name drugs. *Rationale:* Putting things in perspective and viewing the long-term benefits help point out the importance of following the medication regimen. Using available human and financial resources helps reduce social and financial pressures.

❑ **For people with visual or motor problems, acquire visual or physical aids for convenience.** For example, for the elderly, use large print instructions, and don't use child-proof lids. (See also care plan for *Impaired home maintenance management.*) *Rationale:* These types of aids are valuable tools that help people become self-reliant.

❑ **If the person has trouble remembering to take medications, simplify the medication regimen as much as possible.** For example, schedule doses to coincide with daily activities, such as meals, or consider the availability of sustained-release preparations or injected medications that last longer. *Rationale:* Finding ways to remember to take medications and keeping the medication regimen as simple as possible are the keys to compliance.

❑ **Have the person demonstrate or relate what is known at the beginning and end of teaching sessions.** *Rationale:* Comparisons of knowledge before and after sessions will help you determine what has been learned and whether the person is ready for new information.

• *The person should be allowed to refer to written information if necessary. Circle "yes" or "no" as indicated. List comments following each item.*

Yes No Lists names and doses of each medication

Comments:

Yes No Relates when to take each medication

Comments:

Yes No Demonstrates or relates how to take each medication

Comments:

Yes No Relates why each medication is necessary

Comments:

Yes No Explains how each medication should be stored

Comments:

Yes No Relates how to determine if the medication(s) are working

Comments:

Yes No Lists food and drugs to be avoided

Comments:

Yes No States the length of time he or she will need to take each medication

Comments:

Yes No Verbalizes how to observe for side effects and adverse reactions

Comments:

Yes No Verbalizes how to prevent side effects and adverse reactions

Comments:

Yes No Explains what to do if side effects or adverse reactions occur

Comments:

Yes No Relates if and when doses can be skipped

Comments:

Yes No Describes activities that should be avoided when on the medication

Comments:

Yes No Relates where written information about the medications can be found

Comments:

Evaluation

❑ **Compare individual behavior with the outcome criteria identified during the planning phase.** (See *Checklist: Evaluation of knowledge of medication regimen*, above.) **Rationale:** Comparisons between stated goals and individual behavior indicate the progress of goal achievement.

❑ **If goals are not achieved, reassess the entire plan of care.** Determine factors that are impeding progress and revise the plan. **Rationale:** An unsuccessful plan should not be allowed to continue without careful analysis.

❑ **If goals are achieved**, terminate the plan of care, and stress your availability as a resource person who can answer questions that might arise. **Rationale:** It is the goal of nursing to promote independence and encourage self-care. Some people, however, need to be given permission to contact the nurse again, even though the plan has officially been terminated.

Nursing Care Plan
Impaired home maintenance management: medication regimen

Assessment

☐ **Explain that the purpose of examining how the medications are administered at home is to make the medication regimen safer and easier to follow.** Also encourage the person to offer suggestions or ideas as the plan is developed. *Rationale:* This may help to motivate the person to identify ways to make following the medication regimen safer and more convenient. Asking for suggestions helps the person to take an active part in determining the plan of care.

☐ **Assess for knowledge deficit** (see previous care plan). *Rationale:* The person must be knowledgeable about the medication regimen before he or she can assist in determining how to manage the medication regimen at home.

☐ **Consider household members and frequent visitors when determining safe medication storage areas.** (see *Checklist: Preventing drug-related accidents in the home* following this care plan.) *Rationale:* Special consideration for safety must be employed if there are children or impaired individuals at the home.

☐ **Assess whether the medications are stored at the recommended temperature and are protected from light** (if applicable). *Rationale:* Medications should be stored as directed to maintain potency.

☐ **Assess environment for factors that make medication administration safer and more convenient.** For example, a pitcher of water and medications on a nightstand is helpful for a bedridden patient who must be alone for a time. *Rationale:* A little ingenuity can go a long way to provide convenience and safety.

☐ **Examine how hazardous wastes such as needles and syringes are disposed.** *Rationale:* Proper disposal is important for safety.

☐ **Determine if the person or family can relate what to do if an emergency occurs.** (See *Checklist: What to do if a child ingests a medication*, following this care plan.) *Rationale:* In spite of all precautions, accidents may happen, and the person and family should be prepared.

Client goal/Outcome criteria

♦ *These criteria should be individualized based on the nursing assessment.*

The person (or caregiver) will relate (or demonstrate) the safe management of the medication regimen at home, including how to:

☐ Store medications properly to maintain potency and provide for safety and convenience.

☐ Adapt the environment for safety and convenience.

☐ Use assistive devices that make medication administration easier (if appropriate).

☐ Use cues at home that remind the patient to take medications.

☐ Dispose of hazardous trash safely.

☐ Prevent drug-related accidents.

☐ Call for help in an emergency.

Planning/Implementation

☐ **If the person lacks knowledge about the medication regimen, see care plan for Knowledge deficit: medication regimen.** *Rationale:* Knowledge of the medication regimen is essential to home maintenance management.

☐ **Individualize goals and nursing interventions depending on the problems and strengths identified during the nursing assessment.** For example,

♦ Give significant others responsibilities as indicated.

♦ Teach how to childproof the home, and how to store medications safely.

♦ Help identify ways to remember when to take medications. For example, encourage using a written schedule, or timing doses with common activities such as eating meals.

♦ Adapt environment for safer and easier drug administration.

♦ If the person is physically impaired, acquire assistive devices to help administer medications.

♦ Help the person provide for safe disposal of hazardous waste.

Checklist:
Preventing drug-related accidents in the home

Yes No Are all medications out of children's reach?

Yes No Are there childproof caps on all medications? (May not be required for the elderly or debilitated.)

Yes No Is each medication in the original container, and labeled with the name of person, name of drug, dose, expiration date, and instructions for use?

Yes No Have any medications, including OTC medications, expired?

Yes No Are needles and syringes safely out of the reach of children?

Yes No Are hazardous wastes, needles, and syringes being safely disposed?

Yes No Have children been warned of the danger of playing with medications, needles, and syringes?

Yes No Are the poison control and emergency aid phone numbers readily available by the phone, and does everyone know how to use them?

Yes No Is syrup of ipecac on hand?

Checklist:
If a child accidentally ingests a medication

❏ Remain calm and examine the child's mouth for residual pills. Remove them if possible.

❏ If the child is in distress or is unconscious, call for emergency aid (ambulance), stay with the child, and have someone else (if possible) call the poison control center.

❏ If the skin or eyes are irritated, rinse with cool water immediately.

❏ If the child is in satisfactory condition, take the container or label to the phone and call the poison control number immediately. **Do not wait for symptoms to appear!**

❏ Proceed as directed by the poison control center.

♦ Advise keeping written instructions by the telephone with emergency instructions.

Rationale: Instructions should be readily available.

Evaluation

❏ **Compare behaviors with the goals and outcome criteria that you have identified.** *Rationale:* Comparing stated goals with what the patient is able to relate or demonstrate indicates the progress of goal achievement.

❏ **Modify or terminate the plan of care as indicated.** *Rationale:* Unsuccessful plans should be modified to minimize factors that inhibit progress. If identified outcome criteria are met, then the person should be encouraged to be self-reliant and self-directive in seeking health care assistance.

6

Guidelines for Procedures:
Administering medications

Oral Route:
General guidelines for all oral medications

♦ Determine whether the medication should be given with food or on an empty stomach.

♦ Hold oral medications if the patient is vomiting or has become unresponsive, and notify physician.

♦ Ascertain whether the drug has specific storage requirements.

Tablets and capsules

♦ Do not break tablets unless they are scored. (May cause incorrect dose.)

♦ Do not break capsules or mix their contents with foods or fluids unless drug information indicates this is acceptable. (May affect drug potency, affect drug action, or cause GI irritation.)

♦ Never open or crush sustained-release preparations; stress the need to swallow them whole, rather than to chew them. (May affect drug potency and action.)

♦ Instruct the patient to put sublingual medications under the tongue until they are absorbed, and to avoid drinking anything for 30 min. (May affect drug potency and action.)

♦ Instruct the patient to keep buccal tablets between the upper gum and the cheek until they are completely absorbed.

Liquids

♦ Shake all suspensions well until all the particles are completely dispersed.

♦ Dilute emulsions, if necessary.

♦ Do not dilute elixirs—give full strength. Keep in mind that elixirs usually contain alcohol to dissolve water insoluble drugs; do not give to recovering alcoholics.

♦ Mix strong-tasting solutions (e.g., potassium chloride) with water or juice, unless contraindicated by diet. Give chilled to make solution more palatable.

Nasogastric or gastrostomy tube

♦ Determine whether the drug is affected by tube feedings. Plan doses accordingly (tube feeding may have to be interrupted).

♦ If possible, place the patient in a sitting position.

♦ Assess for proper position of the tube. Introduce air into tube and listen over the stomach for sounds of the air entering. Hold the dose if you are not certain that the tube is positioned in the stomach.

♦ Stop the feeding and administer medication in the following manner:

1. Pour 5–10 cc of water into a syringe. Insert syringe into tube and allow the water to flow into the tube by gravity (clears the tube).

2. Pinch tube before all the water has entered it and add the medication to the syringe.

3. Unpinch the tube and allow the medication to enter. Repinch the tubing before all the medication has entered.

4. Add 5–10 cc of water to flush the medication into the stomach; allow all of this to enter the tube.

5. Clamp or continue tube feeding as indicated.

Parenteral route:
Subcutaneous and intramuscular injections

♦ Be aware that SC and IM routes usually increase drug effect and hasten onset of action when compared to the oral route.

♦ Select needle length and gauge according to the amount of fat and muscle at the injection site, and the viscosity of the medication.

♦ Use sterile technique for withdrawing and injecting medication.

♦ Allow an air bubble (0.2 to 0.3 cc) in the syringe to be injected with the medication. This helps prevent the drug from leaking into the surrounding tissues.

♦ Check medication records for previous injection sites and rotate injection sites as much as possible.

* Choose an injection site that is free of bruises, tenderness, or injury; cleanse injection sites with alcohol sponges before and after drug administration.

* Aspirate into the syringe after needle is inserted to ensure that the needle has not entered a vessel. If blood does enter the syringe, withdraw the needle, discard the needle and syringe, and administer a new dose.

* **Insert needles quickly** to minimize pain, and **inject fluid slowly** to maximize drug absorption.

* Gently massage injection site to promote absorption. (May be contraindicated with some solutions. Check individual drugs.)

* Chart injection sites on the medication record or nursing notes according to agency policy.

* More on subcutaneous injections

* Bunch the tissue and hold it (to maximize the amount of adipose tissue at the injection site) as you insert the needle at a *45-degree angle*. Aspirate, then keep tissue bunched as you inject the fluid and withdraw the needle.

* If you are giving the injection to a grossly obese patient, or if the injection is of heparin or insulin, insert the needle at a *90-degree angle*.

* More on intramuscular injections

* Spread the skin (to minimize the amount of adipose tissue at the injection site and to make the muscle more accessible), and insert the needle at a *90-degree angle*. Aspirate, then keep the skin spread until the fluid has been injected.

* For Z-track injections, displace skin, subcutaneous tissue, and fat laterally. Insert needle, inject fluid, and release tissue while withdrawing needle.

* For those with liver disease, receiving heparin, or with bleeding tendencies, avoid IM injections.

* *See Compatibility: Drugs for IM injection (p. 30) and Guidelines: Codes for injection sites (p. 12).*

Intravenous administration

* Be aware that IV administration will produce immediate potent effects. When giving a medication by either continuous drip or bolus, administer *slowly* until patient response is ascertained (see individual drugs for recommended rates of infusion).

* Maintain sterile technique for withdrawing medications, adding medications, changing bottles, bags, or tubing, and changing IV dressings.

* Use the smallest bore needle that will successfully infuse the solution. (The size will depend on the viscosity of the solution).

* Start IVs in the most distal vein (farthest from the heart) that will accept the needle chosen for infusion. Avoid compromised limbs and lower extremity sites, unless specifically authorized by physician.

* Be aware that hypertonic IV solutions (e.g., highly concentrated hyperalimentation solutions) must *never* be infused into peripheral veins (a central venous line is required).

* Expel air from syringes and tubing before IV administration (some tubings have air filters).

* When adding a medication to a solution, affix a label that states the name of the drug, the date and time it was added, and the name of the nurse who added the medication (as soon as the medication has been added, not before; advance notation has been known to contribute to errors).

* Record intake and output for patients receiving continuous IVs; report imbalances.

* Listen to lung sounds; report changes.

* Follow hospital policies for tubing changes, dressing changes, and documentation of IV site assessments.

* Discontinue sites that are red, inflamed, or edematous, or sites that lack good blood return. Report signs of phlebitis to physician.

* Use an IV pump or controller for children and for solutions that need precisely calculated administration. (If the solution is irritating to tissues, a *controller* rather than a *pump* will minimize the risk of extravasation. Controllers use gravity to infuse the fluid, and therefore, an alarm is more likely to sound if the catheter slips out of the vein. Pumps deliver fluid by positive pressure.)

* Be aware that flushing blocked IV lines may cause emboli.

* *See Compatibility: Drugs for IV administration and Calculations: IV administration (pp. 33– 35).*

* Heparin locks

* After ascertaining that the catheter is in the vein, maintain patency by flushing gently with

Compatibility: Drugs for IM injection

★ Physically compatible
☆ Compatible in syringe for 15 minutes only
● Incompatible
Blank means no data is available

	atropine	chlorpromazine	cimetidine	codeine	dexamethasone	diphenhydramine	droperidol	fentanyl	glycopyrrolate	hydrocortisone	hydromorphone	hydroxyzine	meperidine	methylprednisolone	metoclopramide	morphine	pentazocine	prednisolone	prochlorperazine	promethazine	scopolamine
amobarbital	●	●	●	●	●	●	●	●	●	●	●	●	●	●	●	●	●	●	●	●	●
atropine		☆	★			☆	☆	☆	★		☆	☆	☆		☆	☆	☆		☆	☆	☆
benztropine	●	●	●	●	●	●	●	●	●	●	●	●	●	●	●	●	●	●	●	●	●
chlordiazepoxide	●	●	●	●	●	●	●	●	●	●	●	●	●	●	●	●	●	●	●	●	●
chlorpromazine	☆			★		☆	☆	☆	★		☆	☆	☆	●	☆	☆	☆		☆	☆	☆
cimetidine	★																				
codeine		★							★			★	☆						★		
dexamethasone						●			★	●	★							★	●	●	
diazepam	●	●	●	●	●	●	●	●	●	●	●	●	●	●	●	●	●	●	●	●	●
diphenhydramine	☆	☆			●		☆	☆	★		☆	☆	☆	●	☆	☆	☆	★	☆	☆	☆
droperidol	☆	☆			☆			☆	★		☆	☆			☆	☆	☆		☆	☆	☆
fentanyl	☆	☆				☆	☆		★		☆	☆	☆		☆	☆	☆		☆	☆	☆
glycopyrrolate	★	★		★	★	★	★	★			★	★	★	●		★	●		★	★	★
haloperidol	●	●	●	●	●	●	●	●	●	●	●	●	●	●	●	●	●	●	●	●	●
hydrocortisone					●	●		●										★	●	●	
hydromorphone	☆	☆			☆		☆	☆	★				☆	●			☆			☆	☆
hydroxyzine	☆	☆		★		☆	☆	☆	★		☆				☆	☆	☆	★	☆	☆	☆
meperidine	☆	☆		☆		☆	☆	☆	★		●	☆			☆	●	☆		☆	☆	☆
methylprednisolone		●				●		●							★	●					
metoclopramide	☆	☆			★	☆	☆	☆			☆	☆	☆	★		☆	☆		☆	☆	☆
morphine	☆	☆				☆	☆	☆	★			☆	●		☆		☆		☆	☆	☆
pentazocine	☆	☆				☆	☆	☆	●		☆	☆	☆		☆	☆			☆	★	☆
pentobarbital	●	●	●	●	●	●	●	●	●	●	●	●	●	●	●	●	●	●	●	●	●
phenobarbital	●	●	●	●	●	●	●	●	●	●	●	●	●	●	●	●	●	●	●	●	●
phenytoin	●	●	●	●	●	●	●	●	●	●	●	●	●	●	●	●	●	●	●	●	●
prednisolone					★	★				★		★							●	●	
prochlorperazine	☆	☆		★	●	☆	☆	☆	★	●	●	☆	☆			☆	☆	●		☆	☆
prometazine	☆	☆		●	●	☆	☆	☆	★	●	☆	☆	☆		☆	☆	★		☆		☆
ritodrine	●	●	●	●	●	●	●	●	●	●	●	●	●	●	●	●	●	●	●	●	●
scopolamine	☆	☆				☆	☆	☆	★		☆	☆	☆		☆	☆	☆		☆	☆	
secobarbital	●	●	●	●	●	●	●	●	●	●	●	●	●	●	●	●	●	●	●	●	●

Adapted from Schlafer, p. 1370. Source: University of Michigan Hospitals.

a low-dose heparin or normal saline solution at least every 12 hours (follow hospital policy).

♦ When you give a medication through the heparin lock, use the SASH method (saline flush, antibiotic or medication, saline flush, heparin flush).

♦ **Central venous lines**

♦ Always check for X-ray confirmation of proper catheter position before using central venous line. (Hemothorax and pneumothorax are common complications of insertion of central venous catheters.)

♦ Check for good blood return and monitor for infiltration (check for swelling around the neck, axillary region, and shoulder, and for pain or difficulty with breathing).

♦ Prevent thrombus formation by using an infusion device that sounds an alarm if the fluid runs out or stops infusing; flush unused ports of multilumen catheters with heparin (follow agency policies).

♦ Monitor for and report signs of infection (drainage at site, fever, chills); expect that a culture will be ordered, and that the central line may have to be removed.

♦ Follow hospital policies for changing containers and tubings and redressing insertion site.

♦ Use slide clamp on central catheter to prevent air embolism when changing IV tubing. Tape all connections.

Nasal Route:
General guidelines for nasal administration

♦ Use equipment for only one patient and keep it clean to prevent infection.

♦ Provide tissues and ask the person to blow the nose gently before nasal application.

♦ Rinse dropper or tip of spray container after use and dry with paper towel.

Nasal sprays

♦ Have the person hold his or her head upright, and sniff up forcefully while the spray container is squeezed.

♦ Spray once or twice as directed in each nostril.

♦ Allow 3–5 min for spray to work, then repeat if indicated. (Person may blow nose after 3–5 min.)

Nose drops

♦ If possible, have the person sit with head tilted backwards. (If patient is lying down and this is not contraindicated, hyperextend the neck by placing a pillow under the shoulders.)

♦ Insert dropper slightly less than 1/2 inch into the nostril and instill drop(s).

♦ Ask the person to maintain a head-back position for 1–2 min so that the medication can be absorbed.

Oral inhalation

♦ Shake inhaler well before administering.

♦ Place inhaler in mouth (or 2 finger-breadths from mouth, depending on policy), and have the person exhale completely. A spacer device is available for those who cannot coordinate inhalation with dose delivery.

♦ Dispense dose by pushing on inhaler as the patient inhales a long slow breath.

♦ Have the person hold breath for 10–15 sec before exhaling.

♦ Wait 2 min before using inhaler again.

Other Routes:
Eye drops

♦ Give the person a separate tissue for each eye.

♦ Use eye droppers and squeeze containers for only one patient.

♦ Have the person lie down or sit with head tilted back.

♦ Draw down the skin below the eye to expose the lower conjunctival sac and instill drop(s) as ordered; avoid touching the cornea (may cause corneal damage and discomfort).

♦ Ask the person to keep eye(s) closed for 1–2 min after medication is applied to promote absorption.

Eye ointments

♦ Follow eye drop guidelines, but insert approximately 1/2 inch of ointment (or ordered amount) along the conjunctival sac.

♦ Explain that vision may be blurred for a few minutes after application.

Ear drops

♦ Warm the medication to body temperature before administration. (Either hold the bottle in your hands for a few minutes, or run warm water over the bottle.)

♦ Use droppers on only one patient.

♦ Have the person lie with ear up, ready for drops.

• For adults, pull the external part of the ear upward and backward, point the dropper in the direction of the eardrum, and instill drops as ordered. (For children under 3 years simply pull the external ear backward.)

• Ask the person to stay on his or her side for a few minutes after instillation to promote absorption. Apply a cotton ball if ordered.

Skin medications

• If the skin is broken, use sterile technique.

• Check with the physician whether to cleanse the area before applying the medication, and what to use to cleanse.

• Use gloved fingers or tongue depressor to remove ointments from jars (never bare hands).

• Using gloves, apply medication as indicated (rub with firm strokes, pat, spray, paint). Use thin layers unless otherwise ordered.

• *For application of nitroglycerin, see drug.*

Rectal medications

• Use rectal medications with extreme caution on cardiac patients, because of the risk of vagal stimulation.

• Have the individual lie on the left side and encourage deep breaths and relaxation.

• For suppositories, use a lubricant, such as petrolatum, and with a glove, gently insert suppository beyond the internal sphincter (approximately 2 inches). The patient should lie on the side for 20 min after insertion to prevent inadvertent expulsion; for infants, hold buttocks together.

• For retention enemas, encourage the person to try to move bowels before administering the enema to promote absorption. Administer slowly at body temperature, using low pressure to avoid stimulating evacuation response. After you give the enema, instruct the person to lie flat on back and hold it for at least 30 min.

Vaginal medications

• For vaginal suppository or cream, have the patient in the lithotomy position (flat on back with knees drawn up and legs spread apart) and, using gloves, insert into the vagina.

• Administer at bedtime, or have the woman lie with hips elevated for 5 min and remain in bed for 30 min after insertion to promote absorption and prevent loss of medication.

Urethral medications

• Maintain aseptic technique at all times.

• For continuous bladder irrigation, affix labels to bottles stating the drug name, dose, time drug was added, and name of the nurse who added it; monitor intake and output carefully.

• Monitor closely for infection and septic shock, especially in the elderly, who are more susceptible.

• For chemotherapeutic or special medication instillation, refer to policies.

Compatibility:
Drugs for IV administration

The next two pages show compatibility guidelines for administering drugs intravenously. Guidelines assume drugs are in 5% dextrose, 0.9% sodium chloride, or mixtures of dextrose and sodium chloride. Check that each of the drugs you are combining is compatible with the solution used.

Compatibility depends on many factors, including:

* Order of mixing
* Relative concentrations
* Speed of mixing
* Degree of agitation of the solution.

If any physical change is noted, do not administer the solution. Changes include precipitation, discoloration, foaming, or hazing.

You can reduce the uncertainty by using separate piggybacks for each drug rather than mixing the drugs in one solution. This allows for individual dose adjustment and avoids possible concentration-dependent incompatibilities.

Drugs reported to be visually compatible are included here as compatible. There is no reliable data for the mixing of three or more drugs. In combinations for which conflicting or inconclusive data are available, ask your pharmacist before mixing.

This chart was modified with permission from data provided by the University of Michigan Hospital Drug Information Service.

* *The chart does not include all potential admixture incompatibilities—always check with your pharmacist first.*

Calculations:
IV administration

Two common formulas are used to calculate IV rate in drops per minute. The drop factor is found on the tubing package.

$$\text{drops/min} = \frac{\text{cc/hr}}{60} \times \text{drop factor}$$

$$\text{drops/min} = \frac{\text{vol to be infused}}{\text{hours allotted} \times 60} \times \text{drop factor}$$

Common rates can be found in this table:

Hrs to infuse 1000 cc	cc/hr	Drop factors		
		10	15	20
		resulting in drops/min:		
6	166	27	40	55
8	125	20	30	42
10	100	16	25	33
12	80	13	20	27

Compatibility of drugs for IV administration

★ Compatible at Y-site
24 Number of hours compatible
☆ Compatible in syringe for 15 minutes only
○ Conflicting information
● Incompatible
Blank means no data is available

	amikacin	aminophyll.	ampicillin	calcium chl.	calcium glu.	cefamandole	cefazolin	cefoperazone	cefotaxime	cefoxitin	cephalothin	cephapirin	chloramphen.	cimetidine	clindamycin	dexameth.	diazepam	digoxin	dobutamine	dopamine	furosemide	gentamicin	heparin
amikacin		★	●	24	24		8	●	●	●	●	●	24	24	★	24	●				●		●
aminophylline	★		★	24	★		○		●			●	★	24	●	24	●	24	★	○	8	24	○
ampicillin	●	★		●	●	24						●		24			●				★	●	★
calcium chloride	24		●			●						24	24				●			★	24		
calcium gluconate	24	24	●									24	24		●	●	●			●			24
cefamandole		★		●	●		●		●					24	★		●					●	★
cefazolin	8	○	24		●							24		○	24	24	●			●			24
cefoperazone																	●						
cefotaxime	●	●												24	★		●					●	
cefoxitin	●													★	24		●					●	8
cephalothin	●	●			●									24	○	24	●				24		24
cephapirin	●	★		24	24									24	★		●						24
chloramphenicol	24	24	●	24	24	24					24	24				24	●	24		24	24		24
cimetidine	24	●	24			●	○			★	○	★			★	★	●	★	24		★	★	24
clindamycin	★	●			●	24	24		24	24	24			★			●					24	24
dexamethasone	24	24			●	★	24							24	★		●						★
diazepam	●	●	●	●	●	●	●	●	●	●	●	●	●	●	●	●		●	●	●	●	●	●
digoxin		24												24	★		●		24				★
dobutamine		★		★			●		●		●			24			●	24			★		
dopamine		○	★	24					24			24		★			●		★			★	24
furosemide	●	8												★			●					●	●
gentamicin		24	●			●	●		●		●	●		★	24		●				★		●
heparin	●	○	★		24	24	★	24		8	24	24	24	24	24	★	●	●	★	●	24	★	
hydrocortisone sodium phosphate	24	24			●						○	★	●				●					●	○
lidocaine	24		24	24	○	●			24			24		24	★		24	●	24	★	24	●	24
magnesium sulfate	★		★	○	○	○	★	★	★	★	★	★		★		★				★		★	★
mannitol	24				24				24		8	24							24	20			
morphine sulfate	★	●	★				★	★	★	★		★	★	★	☆	★	●		★			★	●
multivitamins/12		●	★	24	24	★	★	★		★				★			●					●	★
nafcillin		●											24			24	●			●			24
nitroglycerin		★															●		★	24			
nitroprusside	●	●	●	●	●	●	●	●	●	●	●	●	●	○	●	●	●	●	●	●	●	●	
norepinephrine	24	●	●	24	24							●		★			●			★	★		24
oxytocin	★	24	★			★	24	★	★	★	★	24			★		●					★	★
penicillin gk+	8	★		24	24		24				24	●		★	24	24	●			●	6		○
phenobarbital	24	24	●	24	24		24				24			●	●	●	●						24
phentolamine																	●		★				
phenytoin	●	●	●	●		●	●					●		●	●		●		●	●		●	●
potassium chloride	24	24	24	24	24	24	24						24	24	24	24	★		★	24	24	★	24
procainamide		24		24										24			●		★				★
ranitidine	★		★			★	★				★			★	★	★	●	★			★	★	
sodium bicarbonate	24	24	●						●	24	24	24	24	24			●						★
tobramycin					★	●								24		24	●			24		●	
trimethoprim/sulfamethoxazole																	●						
vancomycin	★	●			24									●	★		●		●				●
verapamil	★	○	★	★	★	★	★	★		★	★	★	★	★	★	★	★	●	★	★	★	★	★

♦ See page 33 for notes and cautions.

Drug	hydrocort. s.p.	lidocaine	magnes. sulf.	mannitol	metoclopramide	metronidazole	morphine sulf.	multivit./12	nafcillin	nitroglycerin	nitroprusside	norepinephrine	oxytocin	penicillin gk⁺	phenobarbital	phentolamine	phenytoin	potassium chl.	procainamide	ranitidine	sodium bicarb.	tobramycin	trimeth./sulf.	vancomycin	verapamil
amikacin	24	24	★	24		24	★				●	24	★	8	24			●	24	★	24	●		★	★
aminophylline	24	24			24	24	●		●	★	●	●		24	★	24		●	24	24		24		●	○
ampicillin			★		●	○	★	★			●	●	★		●			●	24	★	●				★
calcium chloride		24	○				24				●	24			24	24		●	24		●				★
calcium gluconate	●	24	○		★		24				●	24			24	24		●	24	24	●			24	★
cefamandole		○	○	24			●	★	★		●			★				●	24	★					★
cefazolin		●	★				●	★	★		●			24	24	24		●	24	★					★
cefoperazone			★					★	★		●			★				●							★
cefotaxime			★					★			●			★				●							★
cefoxitin		24	★	24				★	★		●			★				●			★	24			★
cephalothin	○	○	★				●	★	★		●		○	★	○			●	24	★					★
cephapirin	★		★	8				★			●		●	★	24	24		●	24			24			★
chloramphenicol	●	24	★	24	●	24	★		24		●		24	●				●	24	24			●		★
cimetidine		★			○	24	☆	★	24		○	★		★	●			●	24			24		★	★
clindamycin		★		24	24	★					●			★	24	●		●	24		★	24			★
dexamethasone		24			24				24		●				24			●	★			★			★
diazepam	●	●	●	●	●	●	●	●	●	●	●	●	●	●	●	●	●	●	●	●	●	●	●	●	●
digoxin		24									●							●	★	★					★
dobutamine		★	★				★			●		★		●		★		●	24	★		●			★
dopamine		24		24								24	★	6				●	24						★
furosemide			●	20			●			★	●							●	★						★
gentamicin		●			24	★	★	●			●			★				●		★		●			★
heparin	○	24	★		24	24	●			24	●	24	★	○	24			●	24	★		★		●	★
hydrocortisone sodium phosphate				24							●				24	●								●	★
lidocaine				24					★		●	●			24	24		●	24	24	★	○			★
magnesium sulfate				24	★		24	★			●	24	24	★				●	24		●	★	★	★	★
mannitol					24						●				10			●	●						★
morphine sulfate					24	★			★		●				★	●		●	24		●	★	★	★	★
multivitamins/12			24		24						●				★			●	24		●	★			★
nafcillin			★				★				●	★	★					●	24		○				○
nitroglycerin		★									●							●							★
nitroprusside	●	●	●	●	●	●	●	●	●		●	●		●	●	●	●	●	●	○	●	●	●	●	○
norepinephrine		●	24						★		●			24	●			●	24	★					★
oxytocin			24				★				●				●			●	24			★	★	★	★
penicillin gk⁺	24	24	★	10		24	★	★			●				●			●	24	24	★	6		●	★
phenobarbital	●	24					●				●	●		●				●		24	●			●	★
phentolamine											●	24						●							★
phenytoin	●	●	●	●	●	●	●	●	●	●	●	●	●	●	●	●	●	●	●	●	●	●	●	●	○
potassium chloride		24	24		●	24		24	24	24	●	24	24	24					24	★	24	24		24	○
procainamide		24									●				●	24		●						24	★
ranitidine		★							★		○		★		★			●	★			24		★	
sodium bicarbonate		○	●		●		●	●	○		●			6				●	24					●	○
tobramycin		24		★	24				★		●		★					●	24				●		★
trimethoprim/sulfamethoxazole		★							★		●					★		●							●
vancomycin	●		★					★			●				★	●		●	24	24	★		●		★
verapamil	★	★	★	★	★		★		○	★		★	★	★	★	★	○		○	○	★	○	★	●	

For specific information, refer to individual drug in Section III.

Classification overviews are useful in learning or reviewing general uses and effects of major drug groups, including how the class works, when the drugs are most frequently used, and how they are usually administered. Classifications are alphabetically ordered for easy accessibility.

Prototypes Most commonly used drugs of this class and its subclasses are listed at the top.

Drugs A listing by subclass of drugs that can be found in Section III; includes a common brand name.

Action Explains how the class produces therapeutic effects and describes differences in actions of subclasses.

Use Lists common indications.

Dose administration Provides general guidelines for drug administration.

Contraindication/Precautions Lets you know when doses should be withheld or given with caution.

Side effects Additional common effects of drugs in the class.

Nursing implications Suggests possible **Nursing diagnoses,** then gives key nursing interventions and charting reminders.

Patient & family teaching/Home care Suggests possible **Nursing diagnoses,** then presents keys to safe and effective home administration and discusses supporting holistic measures

♦ **Before administering any medication, check the individual drug listing in Section III.**

Contraindications/Precautions
Contraindicated in history of hypersensitivity to the drug or to a closely related drug; possibly also in congestive heart failure (CHF), bradycardia, heart block, hypotension, severe anemia, head trauma, cerebral hemorrhage, glaucoma, and asthma.

Side effects/Adverse reactions
Hypersensitivity: rash, pruritus, hypotension. **CNS:** headache, dizziness, weakness. **Skin:** flushing. **CV:** orthostatic hypotension. **GI:** gastrointestinal disorders.

Nursing implications/Documentation
Possible nursing diagnoses: Potential for injury; Activity intolerance, Anxiety.
• Give sublingual doses of nitroglycerin at the

dose may be repeated every 10–15 minutes for 3 doses. If angina is unrelieved the paramedics should be called.
• Encourage keeping a record of pattern of angina attacks; stress that an increase in frequency or severity should be reported.
• Point out the need to pace activities, avoid stress (emotional and physical), and plan for rest periods.
• Advise changing positions slowly to avoid dizziness.
• Stress that discontinuing antianginal abruptly could precipitate coronary vasospasm.
• Warn that drinking alcohol may cause flushing and hypotension.
• Emphasize that nitrates can be inactivated if exposed to moisture, heat, or air.

---

explain that taking iron with ascorbic acid increases absorption.
• Stress the importance of adequate intake of iron-rich foods (red meats, fish, spinach).
• Warn that iron overdose can be lethal; stress the need to call poison center or emergency room immediately if overdose is suspected.
• Encourage drinking plenty of fluids (unless contraindicated by disease), eating plenty of fruit and fiber, and exercising daily to prevent constipation. Advise checking with physician about taking stool softeners or laxatives.
• Before administering, or for more information, see individual drug.

Antianginals

Prototypes: nitroglycerin, verapamil, propranolol hydrochloride

Nitrates
erythrityl tetranitrate (Cardilate)
isosorbide dinitrate (Isordil)

nitroglycerin (Nitrostat)
pentaerythritol tetranitrate (Peritrate)

Calcium channel blockers (see separate overview)
diltiazem hydrochloride (Cardizem)
nicardipine hydrochloride (Cardene)

nifedipine (Procardia, ♦Adalat P.A.)
verapamil (Calan, ♦Cordilox Oral)

Beta-adrenergic blockers (see separate overview)
atenolol (Tenormin, ♦Noten)
metoprolol tartrate (Lopressor, ♦♦Betaloc)
nadolol (Corgard)

propranolol hydrochloride (Inderal, ♦Apo-propranolol, ♦Deralin)

Action Antianginals prevent and treat coronary ischemia and chest pain that occurs when oxygen supply does not meet myocardial demand:
• They increase the supply of oxygen to the heart by dilating coronary arteries and increasing coronary blood flow and tissue perfusion.
• They decrease the demand for oxygen by decreasing the workload of the heart (either by reducing left ventricular end diastolic pressure and systemic vascular resistance or by slowing heart rate and force of contraction).
Other notable hemodynamic effects include a decrease in venous return and blood pressure.
Antianginals may be categorized into three groups, depending on action:
1 **Nitrates** act indirectly on the heart by dilating coronary arteries (improving coronary perfusion) and by dilating peripheral veins (decreas-

ing venous return and left ventricular volume). Nitroglycerin is the drug of choice for treatment of acute attacks.
2 **Calcium channel blockers** act directly and indirectly on the heart by inhibiting the influx of calcium ions across the cell membrane of cardiac and smooth muscle cells. The slow influx of calcium causes these cells to contract more slowly, thereby decreasing contractility and increasing vasodilation.
3 **Beta-adrenergic blockers** act directly on the heart by blocking the heart's response to sympathetic (adrenergic) stimulation, thus reducing the rate and force of contraction.

Use/Therapeutic goal/Outcome
Prevention or resolution ischemic attacks the heart (angina).
Therapeutic goal: Improvement in myocardial oxygenation and activity tolerance; reduced blood pressure. **Outcome criteria:** Relief of pain relief, and, for long-term treatment, absence of or significantly decreased frequency and intensity of anginal attacks, with improvement in activity tolerance.

Dose range/Administration
The choice of agent and dosage depend on patient's clinical status, individual drug, route of administration, incidence of side effects, and the age, height, and weight of the patient.
Depending on the drug, antianginals may be given SL, PO, and IV; e.g., sublingual nitroglycerin may be administered for long-term maintenance.
When these drugs are given IV, they are usually placed on monitors, and their blood pressure checked frequently until stable.
⚠ The elderly usually require lower doses. Only verapamil and nifedipine have been approved for children.
Clinical alert: Overdose of any of these drugs requires emergency equipment. Doses are titrated to age, height, and weight), and heart rate to titrate dosage, depend

List of classification overviews

♦ *Classifications listed in bold print are found in alphabetical order in the following pages. Alternative names for classifications are listed to help you find information more quickly.*

Adrenergics (sympathomimetics)

Adrenocorticosteroids

Analgesics, *see* **Narcotic and non-narcotic analgesics**

Androgens and anabolic steroids, *see drugs:* danazol, ethylestrenol, fluoxymesterone, methyltesterone, nandrolone, oxandrolone, oxymetholone, testosterone

Anesthetics, *see* **Local anesthetics**

Antacids, *see drugs:* aluminum hydroxide, aluminum and magnesium, calcium carbonate, magaldrate, simethicone

Antianemics

Antianginals

Antianxiety agents, sedatives, and hypnotics

Antiarrhythmics

Antibiotics, *see* **Anti-infectives**

Anticholinergics (parasympatholytics)

Anticoagulants and thrombolytic enzymes

Anticonvulsants

Antidepressants

Antidiabetics (hypoglycemics)

Antidiarrheals, *see drugs:* diphenoxylate with atropine, kaolin with pectin, loperamide, octreotide acetate

Antiemetics

Antifungals, *see* **Anti-infectives**

Antihistamines

Antihypertensives

Anti-infectives

Antilipemics

Antimanic agents, *see drug:* lithium

Antineoplastics

Antiparasitics, *see* **Anti-infectives**

Antiparkinsons

Antipsychotics

Antipyretics, *see* **Narcotic and non-narcotic analgesics**

Antithyroid agents, *see* **Thyroid hormone antagonists**

Antituberculars, *see* **Anti-infectives**

Antitussives, expectorants, and mucolytics

Antiulcer agents, *see* **Histamine₂ antagonists**

Antivirals, *see* **Anti-infectives**

Beta-adrenergic blockers

Bronchodilators

Calcium channel blockers

Cardiac glycosides, *see drug:* digoxin

Cerebral stimulants

Chemotherapeutic agents, *see* **Antineoplastics**

Cholinergics

CNS stimulants, *see* **Cerebral stimulants**

Diuretics

Expectorants, *see* **Antitussives, expectorants, and mucolytics**

Glucocorticoids, *see* **Adrenocorticosteroids**

Histamine₂ antagonists

Hormones, *see* **Thyroid hormones** and drugs: danazol, testosterone, estrogens, insulin, oxytocin

Hypnotics, *see* **Antianxiety agents, sedatives, and hypnotics**

Hypoglycemics, *see* **Antidiabetics**

Immunosuppressants

Inotropic agents, *see drugs:* amrinone, digoxin, dobutamine, dopamine, isoproterenol

Iron products, *see* **Antianemics**

Laxatives

Lipid-lowering agents, *see* **Antilipemics**

Local anesthetics

Mucolytics, *see* **Antitussives, expectorants, and mucolytics**

Narcotic and non-narcotic analgesics

Neuromuscular blockers *see drugs:* atracurium, gallamine, metocurine, pancuronium, succinylcholine, tubocurarine, vecuronium

Nonsteroidal anti-inflammatory drugs (NSAIDs)

Parasympatholytics, *see* **Anticholinergics**

Salicylates, *see* **Narcotic and non-narcotic analgesics**

Sedatives and hypnotics, *see* **Antianxiety agents, sedatives, and hypnotics**

Skeletal-muscle relaxants

Steroids, *see* **Adrenocorticosteroids**

Stool softeners, *see* **Laxatives**

Sympathomimetics, *see* **Adrenergics**

Thyroid hormone antagonists

Thyroid hormones

Thrombolytic enzymes, *see* **Anticoagulants and thrombolytic enzymes**

Vasopressors, *see drugs:* dopamine, ephedrine, isoproterenol, metaraminol, norepinephrine, phenylephrine

Adrenergics (sympathomimetics)

Prototypes: epinephrine, isoproterenol, norepinephrine, phenylephrine

albuterol (Proventil)
albuterol sulfate (★Respolin Inhaler)
bitolterol mesylate (Tornalate)
dobutamine hydrochloride (Dobutrex)
dopamine hydrochloride (Intropin)
ephedrine hcl (♥Fedrine)
ephedrine sulfate (Ephed II)
epinephrine (Bronkaid)
epinephrine bitartrate (AsthmaHaler)
epinephrine hydrochloride (Sus—Phrine)
ethylnorepinephrine (Bronkephrine)
isoetharine (Bronkosol)
isoproterenol (Aerolone)

isoproterenol hydrochloride (Isuprel)
isoproterenol sulfate (Medihaler-ISO)
metaproterenol sulfate (Alupent)
metaraminol bitartrate (Aramine)
norepinephrine bitartrate injection (LevoPhed)
phenylephrine hydrochloride (Neo-Synephrine)
pseudoephedrine hydrochloride (Sudafed)
pseudoephedrine sulfate (Afrinol Repetabs)
ritodrine hydrochloride (Yutopar)
terbutaline sulfate (Brethine)

♦ *See also Cerebral Stimulants and Broncho-dilators overviews.*

Action Adrenergics (sympathomimetics) mimic the fight-or-flight response of the sympathetic nervous system by either stimulating the receptors or causing the release of epinephrine and norepinephrine. Epinephrine and norepinephrine are neurotransmitters that mediate sympathetic nervous system activity.

Adrenergics act in one of two ways:

1 **Direct-acting adrenergics** (e.g., epinephrine) stimulate alpha- or beta-adrenergic receptors, or both.

2 **Mixed-acting adrenergics** (e.g., ephedrine) do three things: they directly (but weakly) stimulate alpha- and beta-adrenergic receptors, they cause the release of norepinephrine from sympathetic nerve endings, and (to a lesser extent) they stimulate the release of epinephrine from the adrenal medulla.

These drugs differ in their selectivity for stimulating adrenergic sites. Some produce a generalized sympathetic response; other, more selective drugs, produce only a partial response. Nonselective adrenergics stimulate *all* alpha- and beta-adrenergic receptors. Selective adrenergics stimulate *all* alpha- and *some* beta-adrenergic receptors, or *only* beta receptors. The more selective the drug, the higher the likelihood of desired response with few side effects. Stimulation of alpha-adrenergic receptors produces vasoconstriction, reduction in

blood flow, increased systemic blood pressure, and pupillary dilation. Stimulation of beta-1 receptors increases rate and force of heart contraction, speed of impulse conduction, and generation of impulses. Stimulation of beta-2 receptors relaxes bronchial and genitourinary smooth muscle, dilates skeletal muscle in blood vessels, and increases blood glucose levels.

Use/Therapeutic goal/Outcome

These drugs have many, varied uses, including the following: heart failure (dobutamine, dopamine, epinephrine, isoproterenol), hypotension (dopamine, metaraminol bitartrate, phenylephrine), poor renal perfusion (dopamine), paroxysmal supraventricular tachycardia (phenylephrine), nasal stuffiness (phenylephrine, ephedrine, pseudoephedrine), allergic responses (epinephrine), eye examinations and open-angle glaucoma (epinephrine); prolongation of spinal or local anesthesia (phenylephrine, epinephrine); premature labor (ritodrine hydrochloride, terbutaline sulfate), and bronchodilation (albuterol, isoproterenol).

♦ *For therapeutic goals and outcome criteria, see individual drugs.*

Dose range/Administration

Dose and route of administration depend on the drug, the indication, and the individual's response, age, height, weight, and health state. Potency and specific effects vary significantly from drug to drug, making it difficult to generalize about dose range and administration. However, the following key points are important to remember when administering any adrenergic.

When giving SC doses, aspirate carefully before injecting to avoid directly introducing drug into a blood vessel.

Only qualified critical-care nurses give these drugs IV, because of the potential for severe cardiovascular effects. Continuous infusion rates are carefully titrated by using an IV rate controller, the patient is attached to a heart monitor, and blood pressure is closely monitored (every 2–5 min until stable, then every 15–60 min, depending on clinical status). Some hospitals have standing policies and procedures for IV adrenergic administration; check these before starting the medication.

🖐 **Children and the elderly are often exceptionally sensitive to sympathomimetics; they require lower doses and their responses must be carefully monitored.**

Epinephrine is frequently given to children for bronchospasms or allergic reactions.

Contraindications/Precautions

Contraindicated in hypersensitivity to the drug or to a closely related drug, in a narrow-angle glaucoma, and in monoamine oxidase inhibitor (MAOI) therapy. *Systemic adrenergics are contraindicated* in hypertension, history of stroke, peripheral vascular disease, tachycardia, frequent ectopy, severe bradycardia, heart block, ischemic heart disease, and hypovolemia. *Use with caution* in diabetes or prostatic hypertrophy.

✋ **Use with caution in children and the elderly. For safe use for pregnant or nursing mothers, see individual drugs.**

Side effects/Adverse reactions

Hypersensitivity: exaggeration of side effects. *CV:* palpitations, tachycardia, frequent ectopy, hypertension, chest pain. *CNS:* stimulation, headache, nervousness, restlessness, apprehension, tremors. *GI:* nausea, vomiting. *GU:* urinary retention.

Nursing implications/Documentation

Possible nursing diagnoses: Potential for injury; Urinary retention; Anxiety.

♦ Record lung sounds, respirations, pulse, and blood pressure, before and after administration, until response is determined; then as frequently as indicated by condition.

♦ Monitor for CNS side effects (e.g., tremors, restlessness) that may increase risk of injury; during IV administration, keep the person in bed with side rails up and call bell in reach.

♦ Monitor for urinary retention, especially in men > 40 yrs.

♦ For diabetics, monitor blood sugar closely (insulin requirements may increase).

Patient & family teaching/Home care

Possible nursing diagnoses: Anxiety; Fear; Knowledge deficit; Impaired home maintenance management.

♦ Explain that, because they mimic the body's response to stress, these drugs may cause feelings of anxiety or fear.

♦ Reassure that the patient will be closely monitored to fine-tune dose for optimum response.

♦ Stress the importance of reporting palpitations, rapid or irregular pulse, or chest pain immediately.

♦ Caution against using OTC drugs without physician's approval because of potential adverse interactions.

♦ *Before administering, or for more information, see individual drugs.*

Adrenocorticosteroids

Prototypes: cortisone, prednisone

Naturally occurring steroids

cortisone acetate (Cortone)	hydrocortisone sodium phosphate (Hydrocortone Phosphate)
hydrocortisone (Hydrocortone)	
hydrocortisone acetate (Cortifoam)	hydrocortisone sodium succinate (Solu-Cortef)
hydrocortisone cypionate (Cortef)	

Synthetic steroids

beclomethasone dipropionate (Vanceril)	prednisolone sodium phosphate (Pediapred)
dexamethasone (Decadron)	prednisolone steaglate (Sintisone)
dexamethasone acetate (Decadron L.A.)	prednisolone tebutate (Predalone TBA)
dexamethasone sodium phosphate (Dexasone)	prednisone (Deltasone)
methylprednisolone (Medrol)	triamcinolone (Aristocort)
methylprednisolone acetate (Depo-Medrol)	triamcinolone acetonide (Kenaject)
methylprednisolone sodium succinate (Solu-Medrol)	triamcinolone diacetate (Articulose-L.A.)
prednisolone (Delta-Cortef)	triamcinolone hexacetonide (Aristospan Intra-articular)
prednisolone acetate (Predicort)	

Action Medicinal (exogenous) adrenocorticosteroids increase blood levels of adrenocorticosteroid hormones that are normally secreted by the cortex of the adrenal gland. These natural and synthetic agents are also called *corticosteroids* or *steroids*. They influence almost all body systems by affecting fluid and electrolyte balance and metabolic activities of the musculoskeletal, cardiovascular, central nervous, gastrointestinal, endocrine, and hematologic system.

Steroids are divided into two different groups, depending on chemical structure and chief physiologic action:

1 Mineralocorticoids influence fluid and electrolyte balance by promoting reabsorption of sodium and excretion of potassium in the renal tubules.

2 Glucocorticoids promote metabolism of carbohydrates, proteins, and fats by regulating metabolic pathways.

However, most therapeutic agents have both glucocorticoid and mineralocorticoid properties.

Naturally occurring steroids (cortisone and hydrocortisone), given in physiologic doses for adrenocortical insufficiency restore normal hormone levels, promoting fluid and electrolyte balance and normal metabolism.

Synthetic glucocorticoid hormones, given in pharmacologic (supraphysiologic) doses provide anti-inflammatory, anti-allergic, and anti-immune actions. These drugs suppress inflammation by inhibiting accumulation of inflammatory cells, reducing dilation and permeability of capillaries, and inhibiting the release of chemical mediators of inflammation. They suppress the allergic and immune responses by inhibiting cell-mediated immune reactions.

Use/Therapeutic goal/Outcome

Naturally occurring steroids (cortisone and hydrocortisone) are used systemically for replacement therapy of primary or secondary adrenal insufficiency. Hydrocortisone is used systemically in the treatment of shock to increase cardiac output, blood pressure, and blood flow to the kidneys.

Synthetic steroids are used in the treatment of a variety of problems and diseases: inflammatory diseases, such as rheumatic and collagen disorders; diseases of the respiratory tract, intestinal tract, nervous system, eyes, and skin; allergies; hematologic diseases and malignancies (see Antineoplastics overview). Dexamethasone is frequently given to suppress inflammation after trauma or surgery of the head, nose, mouth, neck, and spinal cord, with the therapeutic goal of suppression of swelling and minimization of pathology (secondary to pressure from the swelling).

◆ This criterion is not always measurable; because of their well-known effectiveness, steroids are often used prophylactically; research has demonstrated that these drugs reduce swelling and improve recovery.

◆ *For therapeutic goals and outcome criteria, see individual drugs.*

Dose range/Administration

The choice of agent and dosage depends on severity, prognosis, probable duration of the disease and the response and tolerance of the person being treated. *Physiologic doses* are used to replace deficient adrenal cortex secretions. *Pharmacologic doses* may be massive,

high, or moderate, depending on the acuity of the disease.

Depending on the drug and indication, steroids are given by the following routes: PO, IM, IV, SC, intradermal, INHAL (oral or nasal), RECT (suppository, enema, or instillation), OPTH, otic, topical, or (by physician) intralesional or into the joint (intrabursal or intra-articular). If systemic effects are not desired, nonsystemic routes are preferable (although systemic absorption is *possible* with these routes).

PO doses are given with food or milk to reduce gastric irritation.

IM injections are not given in the deltoid muscle, but rather deep into the gluteal muscles to lessen the possibility of muscle atrophy.

Short-term, high-dose therapy is usually discontinued rapidly, using "step-down" dosage. When discontinuing long-term steroid therapy, dose is *tapered* slowly. The presence of exogenous corticosteroids in the blood suppresses the adrenal cortex, which then decreases its production of *endogenous* corticosteroids (negative feedback effect). Recovery from adrenal suppression may take as long as 1 yr after treatment is discontinued.

Interaction alert: Steroids may alter the dose requirement of many medications. Oral anticoagulants and antidiabetics may need to be increased. Steroids may diminish antibody response to vaccines and toxoids and promote neurologic complications. Potassium-depleting diuretics may cause severe hypokalemia. Steroid doses may also need adjustment if they are given with drugs that alter *steroid* metabolism or absorption (e.g., antacids, phenytoin, phenobarbital, ephedrine, rifampin, cholestyramine, and colestipol).

Contraindications/Precautions

Contraindicated in hypersensitivity to the drug or to preservatives or propellants present in some preparations; and in active peptic ulcer disease, tuberculosis, and fungal or herpetic infections. *Use with caution* in AIDS, hypertension, congestive heart failure (CHF), diabetes mellitus, glaucoma, hypothyroidism, osteoporosis, myasthenia gravis, thrombophlebitis, and history of bleeding ulcers or mental illness.

Use with caution for pregnant or nursing mothers, and for children (steroids may alter growth and development), and for the

elderly (who are more susceptible to side effects and adverse reactions).

Side effects/Adverse reactions

Hypersensitivity: rash, hives, hypotension, respiratory distress or anaphylaxis. *CNS:* euphoria, restlessness, insomnia, hallucinations, depression, psychosis. *Eye:* glaucoma, cataracts. *MS:* impaired growth in children. *CV:* thrombophlebitis, embolism, irregular heartbeat. *GI:* increased appetite, gastric ulcer, oral candidiasis. *Misc:* hyperglycemia, withdrawal syndrome. *With prolonged use: Skin:* acne, increased hair growth, thin and shiny skin, ecchymoses or petechiae, delayed wound healing. *GI:* nausea or vomiting, bleeding, pancreatitis. *MS:* osteoporosis; pain in hip, back, ribs, arms or legs; muscle wasting. *CV:* hypertension, edema, hypokalemia. *GU:* menstrual irregularity. *Misc:* increased susceptibility to infection; cushingoid appearance (moon-face and buffalo hump); withdrawal syndrome or acute adrenal insufficiency.

Nursing implications/Documentation

Possible nursing diagnoses: Pain; Altered thought processes; Potential for infection; Impaired skin integrity; Impaired tissue integrity; Body image disturbance; Impaired physical mobility; Fluid volume excess; Altered oral mucous membrane.

◆ Record baseline weight, blood pressure, CBC, and electrolyte levels; check periodically if therapy is prolonged.

◆ Give PO doses with food or milk to minimize gastric distress.

◆ Assess for edema, weight gain, or hypertension; keep a flowsheet of weight and vital signs.

◆ Monitor for and report signs of hypokalemia (e.g., muscle cramping or weakness, paresthesias, palpitations, fatigue, nausea, polyuria).

◆ Observe for and report mental changes, especially in patients with history of mental or emotional problems.

◆ Monitor for signs and symptoms of hyperglycemia, especially diabetics (these drugs often cause problems with glycemic control).

◆ After surgery, examine closely for wound dehiscence (splitting at suture line) resulting from delayed healing; give adequate support with coughing and ambulation.

◆ During withdrawal from long-term therapy, assess for symptoms of adrenal insufficiency (e.g., nausea, dyspnea, fever, hypotension, myalgia,and hypoglycemia).

◆ For topical use, enhance absorption by applying medication to clean, moist surfaces and by covering wound with occlusive dressing.

◆ Be aware that systemic side effects may occur with topical use.

◆ With long-term therapy in children, assess effect on growth and development.

Patient & family teaching/Home care

Possible nursing diagnoses: Knowledge deficit; Impaired home maintenance management.

◆ Point out the importance of taking PO doses with food and of reporting abdominal pain.

◆ Explain the need to restrict sodium intake and to notify physician of edema or excessive weight gain.

◆ Advise avoiding exposure to infections; warn that corticosteroids may mask usual signs of infection.

◆ Emphasize the need to notify physician of infection, trauma, or other stressful situations (may alter dose requirements).

◆ With long-term therapy, suggest wearing a medical alert tag that warns of the need for extra steroids during acute stress or illness.

◆ Caution against having immunizations, vaccinations, and skin tests because of decreased antibody response.

◆ Stress the importance of remaining under close medical supervision and of having blood tests as frequently as recommended.

◆ Warn against using alcohol and medications that may cause gastric bleeding (e.g., aspirin, ibuprofen).

◆ Advise eating potassium-rich foods regularly, especially if diuretics are being taken.

◆ Warn those taking digitalis that nausea, slow pulse, and weakness must be reported immediately (steroids may affect digitalis requirements).

◆ Advise against using OTC or prescription medications without consulting primary physician.

◆ Caution not to discontinue steroids against medical advice, and to adhere to prescribed dose schedule.

◆ Warn that the body may require as much as 1 yr to readjust after long-term corticosteroid therapy is discontinued.

◆ With rectal use, advise reporting rectal bleeding, pain, burning, itching, or other signs of irritation.

◆ With injection into joints, explain the need to avoid stress or strain on joint, even though pain and swelling are relieved.

◆ Caution females that menstrual irregularities may occur; advise discussing birth control method with gynecologist.

◆ To prevent osteoporosis, suggest a diet with adequate protein, calcium, and vitamin D to minimize bone loss.

◆ *Before administering, or for more information, see individual drugs.*

Antianemics

Prototype: ferrous sulfate

Iron products
ferrous gluconate (Fergon)   iron dextran (Hydextran)
ferrous sulfate (Feosol)

Biological response modifier/hormone
erythropoietin (Epogen)

Action Antianemics act in two very different ways:

1 **Iron products** increase the amount of circulating hemoglobin by replacing deficient supplies of iron, an essential component of hemoglobin.

2 **Erythropoietin** increase the amount of circulating red blood cells by replacing deficient supplies of erythropoietin, a hormone produced in the kidneys that stimulates production of red blood cells in the bone marrow. Erythropoietin is not effective unless iron stores are adequate.

Use/Therapeutic goal/Outcome

Iron products: Used in the treatment of anemia caused by iron deficiency. **Therapeutic goal:** Increase in circulating hemoglobin. **Outcome criteria:** Hemoglobin levels within normal range (females, 12–16 g/100 ml; males, 14–18 g/100 ml).

Erythropoietin: Used in the treatment of anemia associated with deficient erythropoietin levels in end-stage renal disease. **Outcome criteria:** Hematocrit of 28–36%.

Dose range/Administration

Factors that influence dosage and administration include the underlying cause of the anemia, individual responses, route of administration, and the individual's health state, age, height, weight, and nutritional status.

Iron products (except iron dextran): Given PO.

🖐 **Give with or after meals, if GI distress is noted, although food reduces absorption by one-half to one-third.**

Iron dextran: IM via Z-track injection; rarely given IV because of the severity of associated side affects.

Clinical alert: Be careful to prevent overdosage of iron, which can be lethal.

🖐 **Iron is frequently taken during pregnancy and lactation and may be given with caution (because of risk of overdose) to children and the elderly.**

Erythropoietin: SC or IV, under strict medical supervision.

Contraindications/Precautions

Iron products contraindicated in hypersensitivity to the drug or to a closely related drug.

Erythropoietin contraindicated for any use other than erythropoietin deficiency.

Side effects/Adverse reactions

Iron products: Hypersensitivity: skin rash, hives, trouble breathing. **GI:** (When taken PO): nausea, abdominal discomfort, constipation, black-green coloration of stools.

Erythropoietin: See erythropoietin drug monograph.

Nursing implications/Documentation

Possible nursing diagnoses: Activity intolerance; Constipation.

◆ Monitor hemoglobin and hematocrit closely (frequency determined by severity of illness).

◆ Provide for a balance between rest and activity.

◆ Monitor and record bowel elimination; ensure adequate fluid and fiber intake.

Patient & family teaching/Home care

Possible nursing diagnoses: Knowledge deficit; Impaired home maintenance management.

◆ Point out the need to take iron products after meals or at bedtime if GI distress is noted;

explain that taking iron with ascorbic acid increases absorption.

◆ Stress the importance of adequate intake of iron–rich foods (red meats, fish, spinach).

◆ Warn that iron overdose can be lethal; stress the need to call poison center or emergency room immediately if overdose is suspected.

◆ Encourage drinking plenty of fluids (unless contraindicated by disease), eating plenty of fruit and fiber, and exercising daily to prevent constipation. Advise checking with physician about taking stool softeners or laxatives.

◆ *Before administering, or for more information, see individual drug.*

Antianginals

Prototypes: nitroglycerin, verapamil, propranolol hydrochloride

Nitrates
erythrityl tetranitrate (Cardilate)
isosorbide dinitrate (Isordil)
nitroglycerin (Nitrostat)
pentaerythritol tetranitrate (Peritrate)

Calcium channel blockers (see separate overview)
diltiazem hydrochloride (Cardizem)
nicardipine hydrochloride (Cardene)
nifedipine (Procardia, ♣Adalat P.A.)
verapamil (Calan, ♣Cordilox Oral)

Beta-adrenergic blockers (see separate overview)
atenolol (Tenormin, ♣Noten)
metoprolol tartrate (Lopressor, ♣♣Betaloc)
nadolol (Corgard)
propranolol hydrochloride (Inderal, ♣Apo-propranolol, ♣Deralin)

Action Antianginals prevent and treat coronary ischemia and chest pain that occurs when oxygen supply does not meet myocardial demand:

◆ **They increase the supply of oxygen to the heart by dilating coronary arteries and increasing coronary blood flow and tissue perfusion.**

◆ **They decrease the demand for oxygen by decreasing the workload of the heart (either by reducing left ventricular end diastolic pressure and systemic vascular resistance or by slowing heart rate and force of contraction).**

Other notable hemodynamic effects include a decrease in venous return and blood pressure.

Antianginals may be categorized into three groups, depending on action:

1 **Nitrates** act indirectly on the heart by dilating coronary arteries (improving coronary perfusion) and by dilating peripheral veins (decreasing venous return and left ventricular volume). Nitroglycerin is the drug of choice for treatment of acute attacks.

2 **Calcium channel blockers** act directly and indirectly on the heart by inhibiting the influx of calcium ions across the cell membrane of cardiac and smooth muscle cells. The slow influx of calcium causes these cells to contract more slowly, thereby decreasing contractility and increasing vasodilation.

3 **Beta-adrenergic blockers** act directly on the heart by blocking the heart's response to sympathetic (adrenergic) stimulation, thus reducing the rate and force of contraction.

Use/Therapeutic goal/Outcome

Prevention or resolution of ischemic attacks of the heart (angina).

Therapeutic goal: Improvement in myocardial oxygenation and activity tolerance; reduction of blood pressure. *Outcome criteria:* Report of pain relief, and, for long-term treatment, absence of or significantly decreased frequency and intensity of anginal attacks, with an improvement in activity tolerance.

Dose range/Administration

The choice of agent and dosage depends on the patient's clinical status, individual response, route of administration, incidence of side effects, and the age, height, and weight of the patient.

Depending on the drug, antianginals can be given SL, PO, and IV; continuous low-dose nitroglycerin may be applied to the skin for maintenance.

When these drugs are given IV, the patient is usually placed on the cardiac monitor, and blood pressure checked every 5 min until it is stable.

🖑 **The elderly usually require lower doses. Only verapamil and nitroglycerin are approved for use in children.**

Clinical alert: Only qualified nurses are to give these drugs intravenously. Keep resuscitative equipment nearby. Give careful consideration to age, height, weight, (IV dosage is based on weight), and health state. Blood pressure, heart rate, and intensity of chest pain are used to titrate doses. Lower doses may be necessary, depending on individual responses.

Contraindications/Precautions

Contraindicated in history of hypersensitivity to the drug or to a closely related drug; possibly also in congestive heart failure (CHF), bradycardia, heart block, hypotension, severe anemia, head trauma, cerebral hemorrhage, glaucoma, and asthma.

Side effects/Adverse reactions

Hypersensitivity: rash, pruritus, hypotension. **CNS:** headache, dizziness, weakness. **Skin:** flushing. **CV:** orthostatic hypotension. **GI:** gastrointestinal disorders.

Nursing implications/Documentation

Possible nursing diagnoses: Potential for injury; Activity intolerance; Anxiety.

♦ Give sublingual doses of nitroglycerin at the first sign of angina; have the patient rate pain on a 1-to-10 scale immediately before and 5 minutes after administration.

♦ Record pulse and blood pressure before and after administering drug.

♦ Monitor for and report headache (a side effect usually relieved by mild analgesics; tolerance of headache usually develops with long-term use).

♦ Observe for postural hypotension; take blood pressure in both arms; (sitting and standing if possible).

♦ Supervise ambulation until response is determined.

♦ Coordinate care to provide frequent rest periods.

♦ Be aware that nitrates are inactivated when exposed to heat, moisture, and air (should be discarded 6 months after opening).

Patient & family teaching/Home care

Possible nursing diagnoses: Fear; Knowledge deficit; Impaired home maintenance management.

♦ Explain that antianginals help reduce the workload of the heart and improve coronary blood supply.

♦ Stress the need to follow dose regimen closely (the drug should be taken at the same time each day).

♦ Emphasize the importance of ongoing medical follow-up.

♦ Explain than an extra sublingual dose of nitroglycerin may be necessary during stress or at night (if angina is nocturnal); teach that

dose may be repeated every 5 minutes for 3 doses. If angina is unrelieved the paramedics should be called.

♦ Encourage keeping a record of pattern of angina attacks; stress that an increase in frequency or severity should be reported.

♦ Point out the need to pace activities, avoid stress (emotional and physical), and plan for rest periods.

♦ Advise changing positions slowly to avoid dizziness.

♦ Stress that discontinuing antianginals abruptly could precipitate coronary vasospasm.

♦ Warn that drinking alcohol may cause fainting and hypotension.

♦ Emphasize that nitrates can be ineffective if exposed to moisture, heat, or air (keep in a cool, dark place).

♦ Encourage significant others to learn CPR; explain that survival rate of cardiac arrest is greatly increased when CPR is initiated immediately.

♦ *Before administering, or for more information, see individual drug.*

Antianxiety agents/ sedatives/hypnotics

Prototypes: diazepam, diphenhydramine, phenobarbital

✔ Drugs checked below are likely to produce profound sleep.

Antihistamines

diphenhydramine hydrochloride (Benadryl)
doxylamine succinate (Unisom)

hydroxyzine hydrochloride (Atarax)
promethazine hydrochloride (Phenergan)

Benzodiazepines

alprazolam (Xanax)
✔chlordiazepoxide (Libritabs)
chlordiazepoxide hydrochloride (Librium)
clorazepate dipotassium (Tranxene)
diazepam (Valium)
✔flurazepam hydrochloride (Dalmane)

halazepam (Paxipam)
lorazepam (Ativan)
✔midazolam hydrochloride (Versed)
oxazepam (Serax)
prazepam (Centrax)
✔temazepam (Restoril)
✔triazolam (Halcion)

Barbiturates

✔pentobarbital (Nembutal)
✔pentobarbital sodium (Nembutal Sodium)
phenobarbital (Barbita)

phenobarbital sodium (Luminal Sodium)
✔secobarbital sodium (Seconal)

Miscellaneous agents

buspirone hydrochloride (BuSpar)

✔chloral hydrate (Noctec)
✔paraldehyde (Paral)

Action Antianxiety agents (tranquilizers), sedatives, and hypotics produce CNS depression, and induce relaxation or sleep, depending on dosage, route of administration, and individual response. Lower doses (sedative doses) usually promote relaxation and *allow* sleep, whereas higher doses (hypnotic doses) *produce* sleep. Although it is unclear exactly how these drugs work, it is believed that they interfere with nerve impulse transmission in the reticular activating system (responsible for sleep and arousal mechanisms). Benzodiazepines also have some additional anticholinergic action, especially when injected or taken in high doses.

These drugs vary in onset and duration of action. For example, pentobarbital has a rapid onset of action (10–15 min) but a short duration of action (peak effect in 2–4 hr). Phenobarbital has a slow onset of action (60 min) and a long duration of action (peak effect in 10–12 hr).

Some of these drugs have additional significant actions. Clorazepate dipotassium, diazepam, and phenobarbital reduce skeletal muscle tension (see Skeletal muscle relaxants overview). Phenobarbital, diazepam, lorazepam, and secobarbital have anticonvulsant actions (see Anticonvulsants overview). For the major actions of antihistamines, see that overview.

Use/Therapeutic goal/Outcome

While some of these drugs have uses that are addressed in other overviews, this overview will address two main uses:

1 Treatment of anxiety or insomnia on a short-term basis.

2 Sedation before and during uncomfortable procedures.

Therapeutic goal: Promotion of relaxation, sleep, and effective coping. **Outcome criteria:** Report of feeling more calm, resting well, and coping more effectively; decrease in pulse rate, blood pressure, and motor movement (e.g., restlessness, pacing); observable signs of drowsiness and sleep.

Dose range/Administration

Dosage varies greatly, depending on the drug, indication, route of administration, response, age, height, weight, and health state. Some of these drugs are much more potent than others;

for example, the dose of triazolam is only a small fraction of a milligram (0.25–0.5 mg), but the dose of secobarbital is 100 mg. Some of these drugs can be given only PO; others can be given IM, IV, or RECT (suppository).

Clinical alert: Because of the risk of *respiratory depression*, only qualified personnel administer these drugs IV. A professional (physician, nurse anesthetist, respiratory therapist) who is qualified to perform endotracheal intubation should be nearby, and resuscitation equipment and emergency drugs should be readily available.

Benzodiazepines have nearly replaced barbiturates because they are believed to be safer (they produce less ataxia and have less overall depressant and cumulative effect).

Antihistamines frequently are purchased without a prescription and used for insomnia without consulting a physician. Some OTC medications are marketed as sleep aids (e.g., doxylamine), whereas others are marketed as allergy and cold medications (diphenhydramine). All may be taken to aid sleep.

Children and the elderly usually require lower doses because the effects are more profound, usually take longer to wear off, and sometimes cause paradoxical excitement. Recent studies indicate that the lingering and cumulative effects of tranquilizers, sedatives, and hypnotics can cause falls in the elderly. This suggests that short-acting drugs (e.g., lorazepam) may be safer for the elderly than the long-acting drugs (e.g., diazepam).

All of these drugs (except the antihistamines) have a potential for psychologic and physical dependence. They should be taken only on a short-term basis, under medical supervision, and their use should be minimized by teaching and using holistic measures to promote relaxation and sleep (later in this overview).

These drugs are never withdrawn abruptly after long-term treatment because of the risk of severe adverse effects.

Contraindications/Precautions

Contraindicated in hypersensitivity to the specific agent or a closely related agent and in impaired consciousness, respiratory depression, severe respiratory disease (unless the patient is intubated), shock, undiagnosed neurologic disorders, porphyria, and history of drug abuse.

Use with caution and with close monitoring in suicidal tendencies.

Benzodiazepines, because they have additional anticholinergic actions, are also *contraindicated* in glaucoma, paralytic ileus, and prostatic hypertrophy.

👉 **All of these drugs are contraindicated for pregnant or nursing mothers (unless taken for seizures). Use with caution for children and the elderly.**

Side effects/Adverse reactions

Hypersensitivity: pruritus, rash, hypotension. *CNS:* impaired judgment, lingering or excessive drowsiness, dizziness, hangover, confusion, paradoxical excitement. *CV:* decreased heart rate and blood pressure. *Misc:* side effects of abrupt withdrawal include disturbed sleep, insomnia, anxiety, delirium, muscle twitching, tremors, seizures, fever.

Nursing implications/Documentation

Possible nursing diagnoses: Potential for injury; Sensory/perceptual alterations (visual and auditory); Sleep pattern disturbance.

♦ Document mental status before administration, monitor patient activity closely *after* administration, and employ appropriate measures to ensure safety (e.g., side rails up, call bell within reach, no unsupervised smoking).

♦ Provide an environment conducive to rest (decrease noises, and lower lights; offer reading materials).

♦ Be sure that PO doses are swallowed (not hoarded).

♦ Recognize that these drugs do not provide pain relief (patient may need an analgesic as well).

♦ Monitor for and report signs of overdosage (slurred speech, continued somnolence, respiratory depression, confusion) and tolerance (increased anxiety or wakefulness).

♦ Use holistic measures to promote relaxation and sleep (see following).

Patient & family teaching/Home care

Possible nursing diagnoses: Knowledge deficit; Ineffective coping (family and individual); Impaired home maintenance management.

♦ Stress that drug tolerance and dependence can occur and that the drug is used only when holistic measures (e.g., quiet music, relaxation techniques) are ineffective.

♦ Emphasize that the effects of alcohol and other CNS depressants may be potentiated; these must be avoided.

♦ Reinforce the need to consult with physician before using OTC drugs, and the importance of returning for medical follow-up; caution against abruptly discontinuing any of these agents after long-term use.

♦ Advise avoidance of driving and other potentially hazardous activities while under the effects of the medication.

♦ Warn that these drugs have potential for abuse, and should only be taken under medical supervision.

♦ Teach holistic measures that promote relaxation and sleep (see following).

♦ *Before administering, or for more information, see individual drugs.*

Holistic Measures
that promote relaxation and sleep

1 Help the individual recognize factors that are contributing to insomnia. Some common factors are: inability to unwind after physical or mental activity, lack of knowledge of relaxation techniques, ineffective problem-solving skills, pain, use of caffeine or alcohol late in the day.

2 Teach interventions that help promote sleep:

♦ Allow time for unwinding and relaxing before sleep (avoid physically or mentally stimulating activities just before bedtime).

♦ Use relaxation techniques (mental imagery, soft music, reading, back rub, warm bath, warm milk).

♦ Avoid catnapping, and stick to a schedule for retiring and rising (even when you don't feel tired or don't feel like getting up).

♦ Avoid alcohol and caffeine after 4 PM (sometimes complete abstinence is recommended).

♦ Plan for optimal pain relief at night (may require analgesic).

3 Point out the importance of daily exercise in promoting rest, and encourage establishing a program for getting enough exercise (e.g., daily walks).

4 Assist the person to cope with periodic insomnia:

♦ Stress that alcohol must not be used as a sedative.

◆ Explain that the body can go for periods of time with minimal sleep (many people sleep less than 6 hrs a night).

◆ Encourage doing something relaxing or productive when unable to sleep (getting up and doing something for an hour can be more relaxing than tossing and turning).

Antiarrhythmics

Prototypes: quinidine, lidocaine hydrochloride, propranolol hydrochloride, verapamil, digoxin

Class IA
disopyramide phosphate (Norpace, ♣Rythmodan LA)
procainamide hydrochloride (Procan SR)
quinidine gluconate (Quinaglute, ♣Quinate), quinidine polygalacturonate (Cardioquin)
quinidine sulfate (Quinidex)

Class IB
lidocaine hydrochloride (Xylocaine, ♣▲Xylocard)
mexiletine hydrochloride (Mexitil)
phenytoin sodium (Dilantin, see Anticonvulsants overview)
tocainide hydrochloride (Tonocard)

Class IC
encainide hydrochloride (Enkaid)
flecainide acetate (Tambocor)
propafenone hydrochloride (Rythmol)

Class II (Beta-blockers see overview)
acebutolol hydrochloride (Sectral, ♣Monitan)
atenolol (Tenormin, ▲Noten)
esmolol hydrochloride (Brevibloc)
metoprolol tartrate (Lopressor, ♣▲Betaloc)
propranolol hydrochloride (Inderal, ♣Apo-Propranolol, ▲Deralin)
timolol maleate (Blocadren, ♣Apo-Timol)

Class III
amiodarone hydrochloride (Cordarone)
bretylium tosylate (Bretylol, ♣▲Bretylate)

Class IV (Calcium channel blockers, see overview)
verapamil hydrochloride (Calan, ▲Veradil)

Miscellaneous agents
amrinone lactate (Inocor)
atropine sulfate (see Anticholinergics overview)
digitoxin (Crystodigin)
digoxin (Lanoxin)
edrophonium chloride (Tensilon, see cholinergics overview)

Action Most antiarrhythmics prevent or correct heart rhythms that deviate from normal sinus rhythm by altering the movement of one or more ions (Na^+, K^+, Ca^{2+}) across myocardial cell membranes. These drugs correct the abnormal electrophysiology of the dysrhythmic heart by reducing automaticity, slowing conduction, increasing the duration of the refractory period, or producing a combination of these responses.

Antiarrhythmics are grouped into six classes, depending on their action and effect on cardiac electrical properties:

IA **Class IA sodium channel blockers** suppress automaticity by prolonging action potential duration and effective refractory periods. (This action decreases the likelihood that premature stimulation will induce muscle contraction.) These drugs inhibit spontaneous depolarization by raising the threshold. (Many drugs in class IA have an anticholinergic effect on the vagus nerve, which may interfere with their primary antiarrhythmic action on the atria. Pretreatment with digitalis is common before these drugs are used for atrial fibrillation or flutter.)

IB **Class IB sodium channel blockers** decrease action potential duration and prolong effective refractory period, especially in the Purkinje fibers; they increase threshold and decrease automaticity.

IC **Class IC sodium channel blockers** significantly depress automaticity by slowing spontaneous depolarization.

II **Class II beta-blockers** suppress automaticity and slow impulse conduction by an antagonistic effect on cardiac response to catecholamines.

III **Class III drugs** prolong action potential duration and effective refractory period in the ventricles and Purkinje fibers, resulting in an "antifibrillation" action.

IV **Class IV calcium channel blockers** slow impulse conduction and prolong effective refractory periods, especially in the AV node.

◆ *Important drugs that do not conform to these categories are listed as miscellaneous agents (atropine, amrinone, digitoxin, digoxin, and edrophonium). Each of these agents is unique and has important actions and uses in addition to antiarrhythmic properties; detailed information is given under the individual drug.*

Antiarrhythmics may be used whenever arrhythmias or risk factors for arrhythmias are present. Arrhythmias jeopardize the heart's ability to pump enough blood for adequate tissue perfusion. The word *arrhythmia* (without rhythm) is often used interchangeably with *dysrhythmia* (disturbed rhythm). The risk of arrhythmias is increased in myocardial infarction, anesthesia, electrolyte imbalance, acid-base imbalances, hypotension, and oxygenation problems.

Most arrhythmias involve one of the following abnormalities:

1 Altered automaticity/impulse generation. The normal rate of the sinoatrial (SA) node may be altered, or impulses may be generated by *ectopic* (abnormal) sites, such as the AV node or in the myocardium of the ventricles, rather than by the SA node.

2 Altered impulse conduction. Impulses may be conducted too slowly, too quickly, or in the wrong direction through the heart.

3 Altered automaticity/impulse generation and altered impulse conduction.

Use/Therapeutic goal/Outcome

Used to treat or prevent arrhythmias. ***Therapeutic goal:*** Promotion of normal sinus rhythm with regular ventricular response. ***Outcome criteria:*** Normal sinus rhythm with regular ventricular response on EKG; acceptable arrhythmia control within limits determined by physician; (in presence of a pacemaker) 1:1 pacing and regular ventricular rhythm demonstrated on EKG.

Dose range/Administration

Although antiarrhythmics within the same classes have similar actions, these drugs are quite different from one another; therefore, doses and routes of administration vary. Most antiarrhythmics are taken PO, except in acute situations, when they are given IV. When used for arrhythmias, atropine, bretylium, and lidocaine are given only IV. During IV administration of any antiarrhythmic, the patient *must* be placed on a cardiac monitor, and resuscitation drugs and equipment must be readily available.

Clinical alert: Arrhythmias are aggravated by oxygen deprivation, acid-base imbalances, and electrolyte imbalances; therefore, actions to correct these problems *must* be taken before (optimally) or during antiarrhythmic administration. Often, improving oxygenation and correcting acid-base or electrolyte imbalances reduce or eliminate the need for antiarrhythmics.

The choice of antiarrhythmic depends on the severity of the arrhythmia, on the drug's ability to control the specific type of arrhythmia (for example, quinidine is effective in atrial

fibrillation), and the presence of contraindications (for example, propranolol is not be given in congestive heart failure [CHF]).

Choosing the best antiarrhythmic and optimal dose is often quite difficult. What works for one individual may not work for another. All antiarrhythmics can potentially induce other arrhythmias, make the current arrhythmia worse, or cause problems with blood pressure. Because individual responses are often unpredictable, patients starting antiarrhythmics or undergoing dose adjustment must be closely monitored for any changes in cardiovascular status. Sometimes outpatient monitoring is possible; however, many patients are admitted to the hospital solely for monitoring of cardiovascular status during periods of dose adjustment.

Contraindications/Precautions

Contraindicated in hypersensitivity to the drug or a closely related drug, possibly in cardiac, renal, or hepatic failure or in heart block (unless a mechanical pacemaker is present), and (for IV) when there is no immediate IV site, cardiac monitor, or resuscitative drugs and equipment nearby. ***Use with caution*** in diabetes and hypertension.

Use with caution for children (the safety of drugs has not been established) and the elderly. Children and the elderly usually require lower doses. Safety of use for nursing or pregnant mothers should be checked with each drug.

Side effects/Adverse reactions

Hypersensitivity: rash, difficulty in breathing, exaggerated side effects. ***CV:*** worsening of arrhythmia, new arrhythmias, hypotension, EKG changes. ***CNS:*** dizziness, lightheadedness, apprehension. ***GI:*** nausea.

Nursing implications/Documentation

Possible nursing diagnoses: Potential for injury; Activity intolerance.

◆ Report immediately if there are problems with oxygenation, acid-base balance, or electrolyte imbalance (especially hypokalemia); monitor all patients closely for hypokalemia (a common, but serious, problem).

◆ Withhold dose and report if, after administration of an antiarrhythmic, any of the following occurs: a significant drop in blood pressure, bradycardia, worsening of the arrhythmia, or evidence of new arrhythmias.

♦ Monitor closely for dizziness or lightheadedness; keep patient in bed or supervise ambulation until response is determined.

♦ Allow for a balance of rest and activity.

♦ Ensure comprehensive monitoring of cardiovascular status by assessing blood pressure, heart rate, respiratory rate, lung sounds, peripheral pulses, intake and output, and activity tolerance frequently; record assessments at least every 4 hours during periods of dose adjustment.

Patient & family teaching/Home care

Possible nursing diagnoses: Anxiety; Fear; Knowledge deficit; Altered patterns of sexuality; Impaired home maintenance management.

♦ Stress that antiarrhythmics improve the heart's pumping efficiency by controlling irregular heartbeat; reinforce the need to return for ongoing medical follow-up.

♦ Point out the need to take these drugs exactly on time and to avoid "doubling up" on doses without physician's approval (doubling up on doses of some of these drugs can cause severe adverse effects).

♦ Explain that close monitoring of cardiovascular status is necessary to fine-tune dosage, to detect adverse effects early, and to ensure optimal response with minimal dosage.

♦ Encourage voicing of fears or concerns so that these issues can be addressed.

♦ Teach how to take pulse and blood pressure; stress that accurate self-assessment of pulse and blood pressure can ensure early detection of potential complications and promote peace of mind that the heart is working well.

♦ Explore sexual concerns; encourage seeking counseling as needed.

♦ Offer family members the opportunity to learn CPR; point out that early initiation of CPR by laymen has saved many lives.

♦ *Before administering, or for more information, see individual drugs.*

Anticholinergics (parasympatholytics)

Prototype: atropine sulfate
atropine sulfate (see   benztropine mesylate
  Antiarrhythmics overview)   (Cogentin)

biperiden (Akineton)
glycopyrrolate (Robinul)
ipratropium bromide
  (Atrovent)
procyclidine hydrochloride
  (Kemadrin)

propantheline bromide (Pro-
  Pantheline, ♣ Pantheline,
  ✦Propanthel)
scopolamine (see antiemetics
  overview)
trihexyphenidyl
  hydrochloride (Artane)

Action Anticholinergics (parasympatholytics) block parasympathetic influences by inhibiting the actions of the neurotransmitter acetylcholine at many peripheral (and central) receptor sites. Anticholinergics affect smooth muscles, cardiac muscles, and secretory glands, producing the following effects on organs and systems:

1 **Eye:** pupillary dilation (mydriasis) and loss of near vision (cycloplegia) due to relaxation of the iris, radial muscle, and ciliary muscle; decreased tearing due to suppression of the lacrimal glands.

2 **CNS:** In adults, some anticholinergics (e.g., atropine) have little CNS effect; others (e.g., scopolamine) have a sedative effect. Some individuals, especially the elderly and very young, experience a paradoxical excitation when given anticholinergics.

3 **Resp:** Decreased bronchial secretions; relaxation of airway passages.

4 **CV:** Increased speed of impulse conduction and heart rate, due to vagus nerve inhibition.

5 **GI:** Decreased salivary and gastric acid secretions and intestinal motility; some (e.g., scopolamine) reduce nausea.

6 **GU:** Impaired urination due to inhibition of muscles responsible for urination (causes relaxation of the detrusor muscle of the bladder and contraction of the trigone muscle and sphinctor). There is also impaired erection.

7 **Skin:** Decreased ability to sweat (inhibiting the individual's ability to reduce body temperature during fever, exercise, or periods of increased environmental temperature).

Many drugs that are not used primarily as anticholinergics have anticholinergic actions (some bensodiazepines, antiarrhythmics, antihistamines, sedatives, hypnotics; most tricylic antidepressants and antiparkinsonian agents; and almost all antipsychotics).

Use/Therapeutic goal/Outcome

Although anticholinergics have had many applications, many of their uses are declining. For example, their function in preoperative medication is to reduce secretions; the need for this has decreased with the availability of better anesthetics that are not as irritating to the bronchi. Anticholinergic therapy for peptic ulcer disease has almost been replaced by histamine blockers. See Histamine$_2$ antagonists overview. Today's most common uses, therapeutic goals, and outcome criteria are listed below. For additional uses check individual drugs.

Diarrhea, irritable or spastic bowel disorders (diverticulitis, colitis): Therapeutic goal: Decrease in GI motility, promotion of normal bowel elimination. ***Outcome criteria:*** Reported absence of diarrhea, reduction of abdominal pain, normal bowel movements.

Bradycardia: Therapeutic goal: Counteraction of vagal response, promotion of normal sinus rhythm. ***Outcome criteria:*** Return of normal sinus rhythm, pulse > 60, absence of symptoms of shock (no feeling of fainting, systolic blood pressure > 100 mm Hg).

Ophthalmic examination: Therapeutic goal: Dilation of pupils, prevention of changes in lens shape, facilitation of visualization of eye structures, facilitation of refraction measurement. ***Outcome criteria:*** Enlargement of pupils, absence of pupillary reaction to light.

Preoperative medication: Therapeutic goal: reduction in salivary and bronchial secretions, prevention of bradycardia. ***Outcome criteria:*** report of feeling "dry" or thirsty, dry mouth, heart rate > 60.

Motion sickness: Therapeutic goal: prevention of nausea. ***Outcome criteria:*** reported absence of nausea.

Bronchospasm: Therapeutic goal: Bronchodilation, improvement in air movement. ***Outcome criteria:*** Increased forced expiratory volume (FEV), decreased wheezing, report of breathing easier.

Dose range/Administration

Dosage and route of administration depend on the drug, indication, response, age, height, weight, and health state. Children and the elderly and debilitated usually require lower doses.

Depending on the drug and the indication, anticholinergics are given PO, IM, IV, OPTH, or transdermally. Although many anticholinergics are prescription drugs, many OTC medications used for motion sickness, hay fever, and colds contain anticholinergics or drugs that have anticholinergic properties.

Give oral anticholinergics 30–60 min before meals, because food interferes with their absorption.

Because these drugs can influence absorption of other medications by decreasing GI motility, separate doses of anticholinergic drugs from doses of other medications by 1–2 hours.

Contraindications/Precautions

Contraindicated in hypersensitivity to the drug and in narrow-angle glaucoma; tachycardia; ischemic heart disease; hyperthyroidism; urinary obstruction; surgery or inflammation of the urinary tract; recent bowel surgery; bowel inflammation, obstruction, or hypomotility. ***Use with caution*** in myasthemia gravis.

Use with caution in the elderly and children (some anticholinergics are contraindicated for children). Anticholinergics are used for pregnant or nursing mothers only if benefits outweigh risks.

Side effects/Adverse reactions

Hypersensitivity: rash, wheezing, difficulty in breathing. ***Eye:*** enlargement of pupils, decreased pupillary reaction to light, blurred vision, photophobia, decreased tearing (may cause eye irritation). ***Resp:*** thickening and plugging of mucus. ***CV:*** tachycardia, tachyarrhythmias, paradoxical bradycardia (after parenteral administration), hypotension. ***GI:*** decreased bowel motility, paralytic ileus, dry mouth, constipation. ***GU:*** urinary hesitance and retention. ***Misc:*** muscle weakness.

Nursing implications/Documentation

Possible nursing diagnoses: Constipation; Urinary retention; Potential for injury; Altered oral mucous membranes.

♦ Advise taking oral doses 30–60 minutes before meals.

♦ Before giving any anticholinergic, ascertain that there is no history of glaucoma; withhold dose and report immediately if eye pain is noted after administration.

♦ Monitor elimination patterns until response is determined; document bowel movements and urinary output. Increase fluid and fiber intake to avoid constipation.

♦ Observe for vision problems and for paradoxical CNS excitement (may increase risk of injury); employ safety precautions as needed.

♦ Provide ice chips, fluids, and special mouth care to relieve dry mouth.

Patient & family teaching/Home care

Possible nursing diagnoses: Knowledge deficit; Impaired home maintenance management.

◆ Point out that these drugs may cause sensitivity to light and difficultly in judging distances; caution individual to avoid driving until vision is stable. Stress the importance of reporting persistent eye problems or pain.

◆ Explain that ice chips and sips of water help relieve dry mouth; encourage use of lip emollient or petrolatum to prevent cracked lips.

◆ Stress the need to avoid OTC medications unless they are approved by physician, because many have anticholinergic actions.

◆ Warn that because sweating is inhibited, the individual is at risk for heat exhaustion in hot environments.

◆ *Before administering, or for more information, see individual drugs.*

Anticoagulants and thrombolytic enzymes

Prototypes: heparin sodium, warfarin, streptokinase

Anticoagulants

heparin calcium (Calciparine, ♣Calcilean, ♠Caprin)
heparin sodium (Heparin Lock Flush Solution, ♣Hepalean, ♠Uniparin)

warfarin sodium (Coumadin, ♣Warfilone Sodium)

Thrombolytic enzymes

alteplase-tPA (Activase, ♠Actilyse)
anistreplase (Eminase)

streptokinase (Streptase)
urokinase (Abbokinase, ♠Ukidan)

Action Although both anticoagulants and thrombolytic enzymes put the patient at risk for bleeding, they have very different actions:

1 **Anticoagulants** delay coagulation and prevent formation and extension of thrombi (but do not dissolve existing clots) by inhibiting thrombin formation (either directly in the blood or indirectly through inhibition of prothrombin synthesis in the liver).

Heparin, a direct-acting anticoagulant, delays coagulation rapidly by combining in the blood with an alpha globulin (heparin cofactor) to form a potent antithrombin.

Warfarin, by contrast, acts indirectly by inhibiting vitamin K-dependent clotting factors (II, VII, IX, and X); only after 16–48 hours is clotting ability significantly affected.

Heparin causes an increase in partial thromboplastin time (PTT); warfarin causes an increase in prothrombin time (PT). An increase in the PTT or PT decreases the risk of thrombi formation but increases the risk of bleeding. For this reason, the PT and PTT must be monitored closely to minimize the risk of thrombus formation *and* bleeding (see Dose range/Administration).

2 **Thrombolytic enzymes** directly dissolve thrombi by binding to the fibrin in the clot and converting plasminogen to plasmin, the enzyme that degrades fibrin.

Although dissolving thrombi in large vessels that supply vital tissues is beneficial, these enzymes can also dissolve clots that are necessary to prevent bleeding. Because of the risk of hemorrhage, thrombolytic enzymes are used only for very specific situations and patients.

Use/Therapeutic goal/Outcome

Anticoagulants: Used in the treatment of disorders or situations where there may be a high risk for thrombus and embolus formation: phlebitis, pulmonary embolus, myocardial infarction, atrial fibrillation, peripheral vascular disease, cardiac and vascular surgery, cerebral thrombosis, kidney dialysis, and prolonged immobility. Heparin is usually used during the acute phase of illness, whereas warfarin is used for long-term prevention of thrombus formation.

Therapeutic goal: Prevention of thrombus or embolus formation. **Outcome criteria:** PTT (heparin) of 1.5–2 times the normal value; PT (warfarin) of 1.5–2 times the normal value (physician determines therapeutic range, which varies according to clinical status); signs of adequate tissue perfusion (palpable peripheral pulses, absence of pain, absence of additional neurologic deficits, warm extremities with good capillary refill).

Low-dose heparin flush: Maintenance of patency of IV heparin locks and arterial lines. **Outcome criteria:** Good blood return in the line (for heparin locks).

Thrombolytic enzymes: Used in specific emergency situations; e.g., to dissolve thrombi occluding the coronary arteries and to prevent extension of myocardial infarction (alteplase and streptokinase) to dissolve pulmonary and venous emboli (streptokinase and urokinase). **Therapeutic goal:** Dissolution of existing thrombi or emboli and reestablishment of perfusion of ischemic tissues. **Outcome criteria:** Signs and symptoms of reperfusion of the affected vessels and tissues (absence of pain, return of pulses and color).

Dose range/Administration

Anticoagulants may be given PO (warfarin) or parenterally (heparin). Heparin is *never* given IM; it is given IV or SC. Because heparin is extremely irritating to the tissues, the guidelines for SC injection are very specific (see Nursing implications/Documentation for heparin). The dose range of anticoagulants depends on the indication (prophylaxis or treatment), drug, route of administration, and the patient response. Dosage is determined by monitoring the PTT (for heparin) and PT (for warfarin). PTs or PTTs are drawn at the same time every day, with special consideration to the time of the last dose of anticoagulant.

Thrombolytic enzymes may be given IV or into the coronary artery (by physician). The specific dose range and method of administration depends on the onset of symptoms, indications, and the patient's clinical status. Most agencies have clearly defined protocols and policies for method of administration. Often, while thrombolytic enzymes are being given to dissolve existing clots, heparin is also being given intravenously to prevent formation of new clots.

The use of anticoagulants is routine for many nurse generalists. However, thrombolytic enzymes are given *only* by physicians and nurses who are well educated in the necessary monitoring and treatment techniques.

Contraindications/Precautions

Anticoagulants: **Contraindicated** in hypersensitivity to the drug; active bleeding or conditions that cause bleeding tendency (e.g., hemophilia, fragile blood vessels); blood dyscrasias, anticipated surgery; recent surgery of the eye, brain, or spinal cord; threatened abortions; GI ulcers; open wounds, subacute bacterial endocarditis; pericarditis; severe hypertension; advanced renal or hepatic disease.

🖐 **Use with caution in the elderly or debilitated because they may be more sensitive to the drug's effects, placing them at higher risk for hemorrhage. Use heparin with caution for children, and give only IV (not SC). Use with caution for pregnant or nursing mothers; in some situations, they are contraindicated.**

Thrombolytic enzymes: Specific contraindications and precautions are numerous; see individual drug.

🖐 **Contraindicated for the elderly (>75) because of the high incidence of cerebral hemorrhage. Safe use for children and pregnant or nursing mothers has not been established.**

Side effects/Adverse reactions

Anticoagulants: **Hypersensitivity:** fever, runny nose, headache, nausea, vomiting, shortness of breath, rash, itching, tearing, anaphylaxis. **Hem:** bleeding (can range from slight bruising to hemorrhage).

Thrombolytic enzymes: **Hypersensitivity:** flushing, headache, muscle pain, nausea, rash, itching, difficulty in breathing, anaphylaxis. Reactions can be severe; when streptokinase and urokinase are given, some protocols routinely include giving diphenhydramine first. **Hem:** hemorrhage (either internal or external).

Nursing implications/Documentation

Possible nursing diagnoses: Potential for injury; Pain.

◆ **For anticoagulants**

◆ Assess for history of bleeding conditions before giving first dose.

◆ Check for baseline PTT and PT lab results before giving first dose, and monitor to ascertain therapeutic range daily until maintenance dose is established.

◆ Schedule PTTs or PTs at appropriate times, depending on when anticoagulant doses are given.

◆ Before giving next dose, report PTT and PT that are not within therapeutic range because of the potential for thrombus formation (if *below* therapeutic range) or bleeding (if *above* therapeutic range).

◆ Record anticoagulant therapy where all medications are charted to avoid an oversight that the patient is being anticoagulated. Use a flow sheet for monitoring PTT and PT levels to ascertain that dosage is safe.

◆ Monitor closely for occult or overt bleeding: check gums for bleeding, assess skin for bruising, and observe for tarry stools, GI bleeding, or hematuria (may signify onset of hemorrhage).

◆ Report signs of fever or skin rash immediately (may signify severe complications).

◆ Ensure that anticoagulant therapy is discontinued or reversed before surgical or invasive procedures.

♦ **For thrombolytic enzymes**

♦ Keep in mind that these drugs are given only by nurses and physicians who are well educated in every aspect of the necessary monitoring and treatment techniques.

♦ Be aware that allergic responses to streptokinase and urokinase are common and sometimes severe.

♦ Keep patients in bed with side rails up.

♦ Monitor closely for neurological complications (secondary to cerebral hemorrhage) and for signs of bleeding at other site (assess abdomen, urine, puncture sites).

♦ *See individual drugs; implications are numerous, and documentation requirements are very specific.*

Patient & family teaching/Home care

Possible nursing diagnoses: Anxiety; Fear; Knowledge deficit.

♦ **For anticoagulants**

♦ Explain that aspirin, other salicylates and ibuprofen also have anticoagulant effects and therefore must be avoided.

♦ Warn against using OTC drugs unless they are specifically approved by physician.

♦ Stress the importance of taking doses at the same time every day without missing doses and of recording each dose as soon as it is taken. (If a dose is forgotten, it should be taken as soon as possible.)

♦ Emphasize that abdominal or flank pain, heavy menstrual flow, or signs and symptoms of bleeding (e.g., bruising, blood in urine or stools) must be reported immediately.

♦ Teach the importance of notifying the dentist and other physicians that anticoagulants are being taken.

♦ Recommend use of a soft tooth brush and an electric razor to prevent injury.

♦ Warn against performing activities that may result in falls, cuts, bumps, or bruises.

♦ **For thrombolytic enzymes**

♦ Explain that close monitoring of vital signs and (for use in emergency treatment of coronary occlusion) EKG is necessary to monitor response to medication.

♦ Point out that close monitoring also helps to detect early signs of side effects which can then be treated.

♦ Stress the need to keep nurses informed of new symptoms or "strange sensations" in case they are medication-related.

♦ *Before administering, or for more information, see individual drug.*

Anticonvulsants

Prototypes: diazepam, ethosuximide, phenobarbital, phenytoin

Barbiturates
mephobarbital (Mebaral)	primidone (Mysoline,
phenobarbital (Luminal)	♥Sertan)

Benzodiazepines
clonazepam (Klonopin)	lorazepam (Ativan)
diazepam (Valium)	

Hydantoins
ethotoin (Peganone)	phenytoin (Dilantin)
mephenytoin (Mesantoin)	

Succinimides
ethosuximide (Zarontin)	phensuximide (Milontin)
methsuximide (Celontin)	

Miscellaneous agents
acetazolamide sodium (Diamox)	phenacemide (Phenurone)
carbamazepine (Tegretol, ♥Mazepine, ♣Teril)	valproic acid (Depakene)
magnesium sulfate	valproate sodium (♣Epilim)
paraldehyde (Paral)	divalproex sodium (Depakote, ♥Epival, ♣Valcote)

Action Anticonvulsants suppress the initial stage of the seizure (raise the seizure threshold) and/or *reduce the spread* of seizures by depressing abnormal neuronal discharges in the CNS. Although anticonvulsants do not *cure* the underlying cause of seizures, they are believed to limit seizures in one of several ways: by depressing the motor cortex, by altering the levels of neurotransmitters, or by stabilizing neuronal membranes (they control the movement of sodium ions across the cell membrane during conduction of a nerve impulse).

The barbiturates and benzodiazepines have significant CNS depressant effects (see Antianxiety Agents, Sedatives, and Hypnotics classification overview). Phenytoin has antiarrhythmic actions (see Antiarrhythmics classification overview). Carbamazepine is often effective in affective disorders and chronic pain.

Use/Therapeutic goal/Outcome

Treatment of various types of seizures, as shown in the table on the opposite page.

Therapeutic goal: In long-term therapy: Prevention or limitation of seizures with minimal side effects. *In acute situations*: Cessation of seizure episode. *Outcome criteria:* Serum drug levels within therapeutic range; absence of (or significant decrease in) seizure episodes; absent or minimal side effects.

Seizure type

Anticonvulsant ● used, ★ preferred, R used in refractory cases (when seizures are not controlled by other drugs)

Hydantoins: ethotoin	●		●		
mephenytoin	R		R	R	
phenytoin	★		●	●	★
Barbiturates: mephobarbital	●	●			
phenobarbital	★		●	●	●
primidone	●		●	●	
Succinimides: ethosuximide			★		
methosuximide			R		
phensuximide			R		
Benzodiazepines: clonazepam			●		
diazepam					★
Others: acetazolamide	●	●			
carbamazepine	★			★	
phenacemide				R	
valproic acid	●	●		●	

magnesium sulfate: used for magnesium deficiency-related seizures.

paraldehyde: used for alcohol withdrawal-related seizures.

Dose range/Administration

● The dose range and route of administration is highly individualized, depending on the severity of the seizures, the drug, individual responses, and age, height, and weight.

● The choice of agent depends on the type of seizure, rather than the cause. Determining the appropriate therapy often involves trials of several different drugs or combinations of drugs.

● Seizures that are not controlled by a specific drug are considered refractory to that drug, and other, sometimes less desirable, drugs must be used.

● The incidence of side effects may also influence the choice and dose of anticonvulsant. To reduce the incidence of side effects, anticonvulsant therapy is usually initiated at the lowest effective dose while serum drug levels are carefully monitored. Usually, the initial dose is one-quarter to one-third the required maintenance dose. When anticonvulsants are discontinued, dosage is reduced gradually (sudden withdrawal is likely to cause an increase in the frequency and severity of seizures).

◆ Most anticonvulsants are given PO. Acetazolamide, clonazepam, magnesium sulfate, paraldehyde, phenobarbital, and phenytoin may be given parenterally (either IM or IV; check individual drugs).

◆ Many other drugs alter the seizure threshold and may decrease the effectiveness of anticonvulsants. For this reason, whenever any medication is added or deleted from the medication regimen, patients should be carefully monitored for increased risk of seizures.

Contraindications/Precautions

Contraindicated in hypersensitivity to the drug and in bone marrow depression and blood dyscrasias. Other contraindications differ from drug to drug. *Use with caution* in severe liver or kidney disease (dose may require adjustment) and coagulation problems.

Give with caution during pregnancy. Anticonvulsants, especially the hydantoins, are a risk to the fetus. The risk of harm from withdrawing the medication should be weighed against the risk of continuing the medication. In any case, the mother should be informed of the risks for herself and the fetus. Safety of use of these drugs for children and the elderly should be checked with each drug. Children and the elderly are at higher risk for hepatotoxicity and other untoward effects.

Side effects/Adverse reactions

Hypersensitivity: excessive side effects, mild to severe rashes. *CNS:* sluggishness, drowsiness, ataxia, sedation, slurred speech. *GI:* gingival hyperplasia (hydantoins), lip enlargement (children taking hydantoins), nausea, constipation. *Hem:* leukopenia, agranulocytosis. *Skin:* hirsutism, acne.

Nursing implications/Documentation

Possible nursing diagnoses: Potential for injury; Altered oral mucous membranes.

• Obtain and record a detailed **history of seizures** (type, frequency, duration, usual time they occur, precipitating factors, presence of an aura); initiate seizure precautions as indicated.

• Schedule doses at regular intervals to maintain a steady serum drug level.

• Keep a flow sheet of anticonvulsant **serum drug levels**; report levels that are not within therapeutic range.

• Assess oral mucous membrances for inflammation; provide special mouth care as indicated.

• Observe for over sedation, ataxia, and problems with coordination; report these side effects, and initiate appropriate safety precautions.

• For prolonged therapy, monitor CBC and liver function tests periodically; report signs of hematological side effects (persistent fatigue, sore throat, fever, infections).

• Monitor pregnant women for increased risk of seizures (may require dose increase); after delivery, observe neonates for anticonvulsant side effects (e.g., increased risk of bleeding).

• For parenteral route, record **vital signs** before and after medication is given until response is determined.

Patient & family teaching/Home care

Possible nursing diagnoses: Knowledge deficit; Impaired home maintenance management; Ineffective coping (individual and family).

• Stress the need to take anticonvulsants on time and (if necessary) around the clock to maintain steady drug levels; advise following instructions to take with or without food.

• Warn that stopping anticonvulsants suddenly may increase the frequency and severity of seizures; emphasize the need for ongoing medical follow-up.

• Teach significant others how to protect the individual during a seizure; in severe cases, help develop a plan for getting help and treatment immediately (e.g., teach how to maintain respirations and to call emergency medical services).

• Caution that alcohol may reduce drug effectiveness.

• Caution against driving or participating in other activities that require alertness until response is determined (many anticonvulsants initially cause drowsiness).

• Advise wearing a medical alert bracelet that states the type of seizures and medications.

• Encourage individuals and families to verbalize feelings and concerns; assist in identifying ways to cope with the uncertainty of seizure disorders (e.g., refer to support groups, such as the Epilepsy Foundation of America and the National Head Injury Foundation).

• *Before administering, or for more information, see individual drugs.*

Antidepressants

Prototype: imipramine hydrochloride

Tricyclic antidepressants

amitriptyline hydrochloride (Elavil, ♣Levate)
amoxapine (Asendin)
desipramine hydrochloride (Norpramin)
doxepin hydrochloride (Sinequan, ♣Triadopin)
imipramine hydrochloride (Tofranil, ♣Impril)

imipramine pamoate (Tofranil-PM)
maprotiline hydrochloride (Ludiomil)
nortriptyline hydrochloride (Aventyl)
protriptyline hydrochloride (Vivactil, ♣Triptil)
trimipramine maleate (Surmontil, ♣Apo-Trimip)

Monoamine oxidase inhibitors

isocarboxazid (Marplan)
phenelzine sulfate (Nardil)

tranylcypromine sulfate (Parnate)

Atypical antidepressants

bupropion hydrochloride (Wellbutrin)
clomipramine hydrochloride (Anafranil)—antiobsessional drug (see individual drug monograph).

fluoxetine hydrochloride (Prozac)
lithium—most common use is for bipolar disorder (see individual drug monograph).
trazodone hydrochloride (Desyrel)

Action Antidepressants appear to relieve depression by affecting the brain levels of the neurotransmitters norepinephrine, serotonin, and dopamine. The precise mechanism is unclear; theoretically, an imbalance of these neurotransmitters results in depression.

Antidepressants are grouped into three major categories:

1 **Tricyclic antidepressants (TCAs)** named for their 3-ring chemical structures, are the most commonly prescribed. They decrease neurotransmitters uptake, thus increasing neurotransmitter level (and effect) at the synapse.

2 **Monoamine oxidase inhibitors (MAOIs)** inhibit neurotransmitter breakdown which also increases neurotransmitter concentration.

3 **Atypical antidepressants** are more closely related to the TCAs than the MAOIs, but their

chemical structures, indications, and side effects are dissimilar.

Use/Therapeutic goal/Outcome

Symptoms associated with depression (sleep, mood, appetite, and psychomotor activity disturbances; feelings of hopelessness, helplessness, and worthlessness). **Therapeutic goal:** Promotion of well-being, alleviation of symptoms of depression. **Outcome criteria:** Report of sleeping better, coping better, and improved sense of well-being; demonstration of more normal appetite, sleep patterns, mood, social interaction, and activity level.

Phobias: Therapeutic goal: Prevention of episodes of extreme fear, promotion of coping with daily living. **Outcome criteria:** Report of less fear and better ability to cope with daily activities.

Obsessive-compulsive disorders: Therapeutic goal: Elimination of excessive compulsive behaviors. **Outcome criteria:** Demonstration of absence of compulsive behaviors, report of decreased anxiety.

Dose range/Administration

Dosage and administration depend on the drug, indication, individual response, age, height, weight, and nutritional status. Previous response to a particular drug and undesirable side effects of each drug must be considered (a drug that was successful in the past is likely to be successful now). The dosage of all antidepressants is titrated carefully, with close monitoring of response (full response may not occur for 2–4 weeks).

Most antidepressants are available in tablets or capsules. Some are available as liquid to be given PO; amitriptyline and imipramine are available for IM injection.

Interaction alert: MAOIs have potentially fatal drug-drug and food-drug interactions and, therefore, are used when other antidepressants (and ECT) have failed. Check with the pharmacist for potential interactions before giving these drugs with any other medication. If a new drug that interacts with MAOIs is to be started, the MAOI is discontinued at least 2 weeks before the first dose of the new drug is given (it takes 2 weeks for the effect of the MAOI to wear off). Tyramine-rich foods and beverages must be avoided (in general, as foods age, ferment, or degrade, their tyramine content increases). **Tyramine-rich foods: Dairy:** cheese; aged and strong varieties, sour cream,

yogurt. **Fruits/vegetables:** avocados, bananas, fava beans, canned figs, raisins. **Alcohol:** beer, chianti, and sherry wine. **Meats:** liver, pickled herring, salami, sausage, tenderized meat. **Misc:** caffeine (coffees, colas, teas), chocolate, licorice, soy sauce, yeast.

Contraindications/Precautions

Contraindicated in hypersensitivity to the drug. **Use with caution** in patients with suicidal tendencies (all antidepressants are toxic in high doses, and fatal intentional doses are common).

TCAs: Contraindicated in the acute recovery phase of myocardial infarction, prostatic hypertrophy, and convulsive disorders. **Use with caution** in increased ocular pressure, narrow-angle glaucoma, urinary retention, hyperthyroidism, and hepatic disease.

MAOIs: Contraindicated in severe renal or hepatic disease, cerebrovascular or cardiovascular disease, congestive heart failure (CHF), hypertension, severe headaches, pheochromocytoma, agitation, schizophrenia, within 1–2 weeks of anesthesia, and with many drugs and foods: sympathomimetics, TCAs, and tyramine-rich foods can precipitate hypertensive crisis, a rapid, potentially fatal increase in blood pressure. **Use with caution** in impaired renal function, diabetes, epilepsy, parkinsonism, and hyperthyroidism.

🤚 **Use antidepressants with caution for pregnant and nursing mothers and the elderly. MAOIs are contraindicated for children under 16 years and the elderly.**

Side effects/Adverse reactions

Hypersensitivity: rash, petechiae, urticaria. **CV:** orthostatic hypotension, hypertension, tachycardia, and (for MAOIs) cardiac arrhythmias. **CNS:** anxiety, ataxia, sedation, confusion, insomnia, overstimulation, headache, dizziness, extrapyramidal symptoms (including tardive dyskinesia), and (for MAOIs) fatigue, memory problems, tremors and twitching. **Eye:** blurred vision. **GI:** dry mouth, diarrhea, constipation, paralytic ileus, anorexia, increased appetite, weight gain, abdominal cramps, and (for MAOIs) nausea, hepatotoxicity. **Skin:** decreased or increased sweating, photosensitivity. **Hem:** agranulocytosis. **GU:** urinary retention, prostatic hypertrophy, acute renal failure, and (for MAOIs) difficulty in urination, impotence.

Nursing implications/Documentation

Possible nursing diagnoses: Potential for injury; Constipation; Altered oral mucous membrane.

♦ Be sure that PO doses are swallowed (not hoarded).

♦ Monitor for orthostatic hypotension, dizziness, and drowsiness; supervise ambulation until response is established.

♦ Record intake and output; observe for dehydration or urinary retention; provide special mouth care.

♦ Monitor for and report suicidal tendencies, increased depression, or excessive drowsiness (may require change in medication).

♦ Prevent constipation by monitoring bowel movements and providing adequate fiber and fluid intake; offer laxatives or stool softeners before problems becomes severe.

Patient & family teaching/Home care

Possible nursing diagnoses: Ineffective coping (family and individual); Sleep pattern disturbance; Impaired home maintenance management.

♦ Stress that these drugs reduce the depression that is interfering with effective decision making and coping. Reassure patient that when depression lessens, healthy changes will be easier to make.

♦ Explain that side effects may occur immediately, but usually diminish after a few weeks; however, beneficial (antidepressant) effects may not be felt for 2–4 weeks.

♦ Explain that changing position slowly will help prevent dizziness.

♦ Point out the role of adequate nutrition, exercise, and sleep in combating depression.

♦ Emphasize that the effects of alcohol, sedatives, and tranquilizers may be potentiated.

♦ Advise consulting with physician before using OTC drugs; stress the need for ongoing for medical follow-up.

♦ Recommend that continued depression be reported and that physician be consulted before increasing dose (may increase side effects) or stopping drug (depression may recur).

♦ Advise avoidance of driving and other potentially hazardous activities until response is established.

♦ Suggest using ice chips, hard candy, or gum to relieve dry mouth; stress the need for good mouth care.

♦ Warn women to report immediately if pregnancy is planned or suspected.

♦ *Before administering, or for more information, see individual drugs.*

Antidiabetics (hypoglycemics)

Prototypes: tolbutamide, insulin

Oral hypoglycemics (sulfonylureas)

acetohexamide (Dymelor)	glyburide (Micronase)
chlorpropamide (Diabinese)	tolazamide (Tolinase)
glipizide (Glucotrol)	tolbutamide (Orinase)

Insulins

Rapid-Acting

regular insulin (Novolin R) prompt zinc suspension insulin (Semilente)

Intermediate-Acting

isophane insulin suspension/ NPH (NPH iletin I) insulin zinc suspension (Humulin L)

Long-Acting

protamine zinc suspension/ PZI (Protamine Zinc and PZI)

extended zinc suspension (Ultralente)

Insulin Mixture

isophane insulin suspension and regular insulin (Novolin 70/30)

♦ *Beef, pork, and human insulins are available.*

Action Antidiabetic agents (hypoglycemics) reduce blood sugar and regulate the metabolism of carbohydrates, proteins, and fats in two very different ways.

1 Oral hypoglycemics (sulfonylureas) stimulate the beta cells of the pancreas to release insulin. Oral hypoglycemics are effective only when the pancreas still has some functioning beta cells.

Oral hypoglycemics are used as an adjunct to diet and weight control in the treatment of type II, or non–insulin-dependent diabetes mellitus (NIDDM).

2 Parenteral antidiabetics (insulin) are medicinal (exogenous) sources of insulin, used when the pancreas cannot produce enough insulin to metabolize glucose intake.

Insulin is used to treat type I, or insulin-dependent diabetes mellitus (IDDM), and for type II diabetes when oral hypoglycemics, diet, and weight control are ineffective; during periods of stress (e.g., illness, surgery, or emotional stress) that temporarily increases insulin requirements; or during pregnancy, when oral hypoglycemics pose a risk to the fetus and insulin requirements may be greater.

Also nondiabetics may require additional insulin during parenteral nutrition (hyperalimentation) because the infusion of high caloric IV fluids significantly increases insulin requirements. These requirements are sometimes too great for even a normal pancreas.

Insulin is a hormone that is necessary for life. Although the exact mechanism of action is not fully understood, it is known that insulin has 3 major actions:

- **It converts carbohydrates to energy** by allowing glucose to pass from the bloodstream into muscle cells, increasing glucose oxidation *and* conversion to glycogen for storage.

- **It promotes protein synthesis** by moving amino acids into cells.

- **It prevents the breakdown of fats** as a source of energy by promoting carbohydrate metabolism and increasing the conversion of glucose to fat for storage.

Because insulin plays a vital role in metabolism, it is often thought of as the key to the fuels that supply cells with the energy to survive. Without insulin, cells die of starvation.

Oral hypoglycemics and insulins vary significantly in onset, peak, and duration of action (pharmacokinetics). Knowing the onset, peak, and duration of the specific antidiabetic agent is essential to promoting desirable effects (blood sugar control) and preventing undesirable effects (*hypo*glycemia and *hyper*glycemia). The adjacent table lists the action times of oral hypoglycemics and insulins.

Use/Therapeutic goal/Outcome

Used to treat diabetes and hyperglycemia. **Therapeutic goal:** Promotion of glycemic control. **Outcome criteria:** Absence of clinical symptoms of hypoglycemia (confusion, shakiness, weakness, diaphoresis, apprehension), blood glucose studies that demonstrate normal glucose levels (a fasting blood sugar (FBS) of 100–140 mg/dl is considered good control; FBS of 140–200 mg/dl is considered fair control; during pregnancy, FBS of 60–80 mg/dl is preferred).

Dose range/Administration

Dose is highly individualized depending on the type of hypoglycemic agent; route of administration; age, height, and weight; degree of pancreatic function; response (e.g., some individuals are sensitive to insulin; the elderly may be resistant to insulin); nutrient intake (increased caloric intake increases insulin requirements);

activity level (exercise decreases insulin requirements); and additional stressors (illness, surgery, emotional stress, pregnancy) that may increase insulin requirements. The source (beef, pork, human), purity, and concentration of insulin are very important, as is the condition of the injection site (insulin injected into lipoatrophied or lipohypertrophied tissue is not absorbed as well as that injected into healthier tissues; some diabetics may be tempted to use these unhealthy injection sites because the injection is less painful).

Pharmacokinetics

Oral hypoglycemic	Half-life	Duration
Acetohexamide	4–6 hr	6–12 hr
Chlorpropamide	36 hr	> 60 hr
Glipizide	3–4 hr	12–24 hr
Glyburide	10 hr	24 hr
Tolazamide	7 hr	36 hr
Tolbutamide	4–6 hr	6–12 hr

Insulin	Onset	Peak	Duration
Regular insulin	½–1 hr	2–5 hr	5–8 hr
Prompt insulin zinc suspension	1–2 hr	5–10 hr	12–16 hr
Isophane insulin suspension/NPH	1–2 hr	4–12 hr	24–28 hr
Insulin zinc suspension	1–3 hr	6–15 hr	24–28 hr
Protamine zinc insulin/PZI	4–8 hr	14–24 hr	> 36 hr
Extended insulin zinc suspension	4–8 hr	10–30 hr	> 36 hr
Isophane insulin suspension and Regular insulin (human)	¼–1 hr	2–8 hr	24 hr

Adapted from Marshal Schlafer and Elaine Marieb: *The Nurse, Pharmacology, and Drug Therapy* (Redwood City, CA: Addison-Wesley, 1989). pp.911, 922.

Insulin must be given parenterally (SC or IV) because it is degraded by the digestive system. Only regular insulin can be given intravenously, (dose adjustment may be necessary for continuous infusion initially; insulin binds to bags and tubing). Because insulin irritates tissues and frequent injections are required, SC insulin is given at specific sites with special technique (see guidelines in this overview).

Concentrations are U-40, U-100, and U-500 (U-400 is being researched). Fewer than 2 per-

Guidelines:
Injection sites for insulins

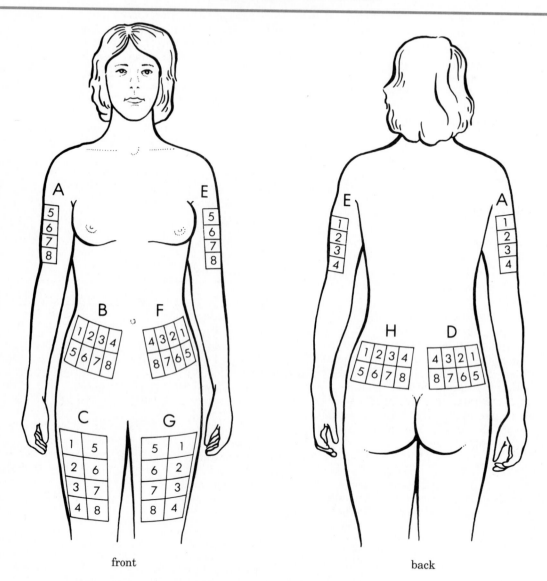

front   back

- ◆ Injection sites should be about 1 inch apart.
- ◆ Mark sites on plastic overlay as you use them.
- ◆ Rotate sites in a regular pattern, either in order within each area, or using all 1 sites first, then all 2 sites, etc.
- ◆ Avoid using the same site more often than every 4–6 weeks.
- ◆ When hospitalized, request nurses to inject sites you normally cannot reach.

Adapted from Marshal Schlafer and Elaine Marieb, *The Nurse, Pharmacology, and Drug Therapy* (Redwood City, CA: Addison-Wesley, 1989), p.916.

cent of diabetics use U-40. Most use U-100; insulin-resistant diabetics use U-500 because they require large doses. Insulin syringes used must match concentration (U-40/ml, U-100/ml, and U-500/ml).

Species sources (types): **Beef or pork insulin** is derived from the pancreas of cows or pigs, respectively. **Semisynthetic human insulin** is produced by converting pork insulin enzymatically. **Biosynthetic human insulin** is made by recombinant DNA technology from *Escherichia coli* bacteria. "Human" insulins are structurally identical to natural human insulin.

Human insulins induce less antigen formation, act more predictably, and provide better glucose control. For this reason, human insulin is indicated in those who are allergic to beef or pork, newly diagnosed Type I diabetics, pregnant Type II diabetics (gestational diabetes), individuals who only need insulin for a temporary period (e.g., after surgery), insulin-resistant diabetics, individuals with lipoatrophy or lipohypertrophy, or diabetics who refuse pork or beef products for religious or ethical reasons.

Often, different types of insulins must be mixed to give optimal glycemic control. Regular insulin can be mixed with most other kinds of insulin, but insulins of different species sources cannot be mixed together. Compatibility for any mixture must be confirmed with the pharmacist or package insert.

Achieving glycemic control: Managing insulin doses to achieve glycemic control depends on timely administration of doses (usually before meals), close monitoring of blood sugar, and the patient's ability to follow the prescribed diet. Because changes in blood sugar are not always symptomatic, the importance of close monitoring of blood sugar (by laboratory studies or blood glucose meter readings) cannot be overstated. Depending on the health state and severity of diabetes, blood sugar is checked from 2–4 times a day (when healthy) to every hour (in severe illness).

Stable diabetics usually receive insulin at the same times every day (e.g., before breakfast, or before breakfast and dinner); however, during illness or periods of dose adjustment, the physician may order *sliding-scale* insulin doses: blood sugars are read at the set times, and regular insulin is given according to the glucose levels and the physicians orders.

Even in healthy diabetics, insulin dosage may change from day to day without obvious reason; daily dose adjustments based on blood sugar readings may be necessary. By adjusting doses to meet varying daily requirements under the guidance of physicians and clinical nurse specialists, many diabetics have learned to regulate their own insulin doses by checking blood sugar with a blood glucose meter at set times during the day, and then adjusting the dose accordingly. Those who have not learned to do this need knowledgeable and professional support; sometimes, they require frequent visits by a nurse. Nurses who help diabetics in the home should remember that insulin is available without prescription in most states, allowing for easy replacement of lost or defective vials.

Interaction alert: Alcohol, nonsteroidal anti-inflammatory drugs (NSAIDs), salicylates, steroids, beta-blockers, tetracyclines, antipsychotics, thyroid hormones and antagonists, diuretics, and many other medications alter insulin requirements. For this reason, blood sugars are monitored even more closely whenever a medication is added or deleted from the medication regimen.

Contraindications/Precautions

Contraindicated in severe hypersensitivity to the drug or its components (pork or beef) and in hypoglycemia.

Use with caution for children and the elderly because of unpredictable responses. The elderly's insulin requirements are also more likely to be altered by other medications. Oral antidiabetics are contraindicated for pregnant women (human insulin is usually required).

Side effects/Adverse reactions

Incidence of side effects for oral hypoglycemics is usually low and dose-related; with some, alcohol may induce a disulfiram-like reaction. The most common side effect of both oral hypoglycemics and insulin is hyper-insulinism, causing hypokalemia and hypoglycemia (tachycardia, arrhythmias, headache, visual disturbances, sweating, shakiness, apprehension, confusion, drowsiness, unconsciousness). Insulin hypersensitivity may cause local inflammation, and a mild generalized rash; with beef and pork insulin, lipoatrophy and lipohypertrophy.

Nursing implications/Documentation

Possible nursing diagnoses: Potential for injury; Impaired skin integrity; Impaired tissue integrity; Altered nutrition: more than body requirements; Altered nutrition: less than body requirements.

♦ Ascertain baseline blood sugar before giving first dose and monitor closely thereafter; check blood sugar 30 min before each meal and at bedtime before hs snack; keep a flow sheet of blood sugars; report trends or isolated episodes of hyperglycemia or hypoglycemia.

♦ Monitor food intake; notify physician when the person is not eating.

♦ Recognize that diabetics are at risk for electrolyte imbalances, kidney failure, cardiac disease, vascular disease, GI symptoms (nausea, vomiting, constipation, diarrhea), and neuropathy; monitor electrolytes (especially potassium), BUN, and creatinine *carefully*, and report abnormalities.

♦ Monitor and record daily weight and intake and output, especially during periods of illness; notify physician of significant weight change or significant discrepancies in intake and output.

♦ If signs of *hypo*glycemia (shakiness, sweating, sudden weakness, pale skin, anxiety, confusion, nervousness) are noted, confirm by blood glucose meter reading, and then give 15 g of a fast-acting carbohydrate: 4 oz of fruit juice, 4–6 pieces of hard candy, 1 Tbsp of sugar or honey. If blood glucose meter is not immediately available, give carbohydrate, and check glucose level later; if the patient is unconscious, report immediately, provide support, and have D50W for injection ready for administration.

♦ If signs of *hyper*glycemia (extreme thirst, frequent urination, fruity breath, lethargy, coma) are noted, confirm by blood glucose meter reading, and report immediately to physician; expect IV administration of regular insulin and NS (for rehydration). Before beginning an insulin infusion, prime the tubing with 50–100 ml of solution to bind insulin to tubing.

♦ Stress that those with type I diabetes, particularly children, are more prone to ketoacidosis than those with type II diabetes; during stress or illness, they should have urine checked for ketones when blood sugar is greater than 240 mg/dl.

♦ For nursing interventions that apply to insulin or oral antidiabetics only, see individual drugs.

Patient & family teaching/Home care

Possible nursing diagnoses: Knowledge deficit; Impaired home maintenance management.

♦ Explain that antidiabetic agents control blood sugar but do not cure diabetes; stress that careful regulation of diet and antidiabetic agents, based on monitoring of blood sugars and ongoing medical follow-up, can help promote health and prevent the long-term complications of diabetes (heart and kidney disease, blindness).

♦ Point out that diet, activity, illness, and emotional stress may greatly affect insulin requirements (especially in children); advise that hypoglycemia may be caused by excessive exercise, profuse sweating, skipped or delayed meals, or decreased carbohydrate intake.

♦ Stress the need to eat everything on meal plan, especially carbohydrates, but to avoid concentrated sweets.

♦ When injections are needed, provide chart with plastic cover on which the patient can mark injection sites (see sample in this overview); stress need to rotate injection sites to avoid hardening of tissue.

♦ Point out that increased insulin dosage may be needed during illness, despite inability to tolerate food; advise notifying physician if illness occurs.

♦ Teach the signs and symptoms of hypoglycemia and hyperglycemia and what to do if these occur.

♦ Advise reporting persistent symptoms of nausea, vomiting, fatigue, thirst, and frequent urination.

♦ Suggest carrying some form of fast-acting carbohydrate (e.g., small box of raisins) for treatment of hypoglycemia.

♦ Warn against drinking alcohol and using OTC drugs without physician's approval.

♦ For patient and family teaching that applies only to insulin or only to oral antidiabetics, see individual drugs.

♦ Before administering, or for more information, see individual drugs.

Antiemetics

Prototype: prochlorperazine

chlorpromazine
  hydrochloride (Thorazine)
dimenhydrinate (Dramamine)
dronabinol (Marinol)
meclizine hydrochloride
  (Antivert)
metoclopramide
  hydrochloride (Reglan)

prochlorperazine
  (Compazine)
scopolamine (Transderm-
  Scop)
trimethobenzamide
  hydrochloride (Tigan

♦ *Antihistamines and barbiturates also have anti-emetic properties. See Antihistamines and Antianxiety agents/Sedative/Hypnotics overviews.*

Action Antiemetics relieve symptoms of nausea and vomiting in one of three ways (the exact mechanism is not fully understood):

1 By inhibiting the chemoreceptor trigger zone, thus depressing the vomiting center in the medulla.

2 By diminishing the effects of motion on the vomiting center. (The vomiting center is affected by stimuli from the CNS and the vestibular apparatus of the ear, which are affected by motion.)

3 By promoting gastric emptying and GI motility.

Use/Therapeutic goal/Outcome

Used to treat nausea and vomiting associated with radiation therapy, medications (especially chemotherapy), organic disease, anesthesia recovery, head injury, concussion, labyrinthitis, decreased GI motility, and motion sickness.

Therapeutic goal: Prevention or resolution of nausea and vomiting. **Outcome criteria:** Absence of vomiting, report of decrease in or absence of nausea.

Dose range/Administration

Dosage depends on the drug, route of administration, individual response, health status, age, height, weight, nutritional status, and metabolic status.

Antiemetics are *not* used until the underlying cause of nausea is determined, because their action might mask symptoms of a problem that needs specific treatment (e.g., increased intracranial pressure, drug overdose, intestinal obstruction).

Depending on the drug, and severity of symptoms, administration may be PO, IM, IV, TRANSDERM, or RECT.

Contraindications/Precautions

Contraindicated in hypersensitivity to the drug or to a closely related drug and in suspected intestinal obstruction. **Use with caution** in drowsiness, in CNS depression, or in patients receiving other sedating drugs (most antiemetics cause CNS depression).

Side effects/Adverse reactions

Hypersensitivity: itching, rash. **CNS:** drowsiness and dizziness.

Nursing implications/Documentation

Possible nursing diagnoses: Potential for injury; Fluid volume deficit; Altered oral mucous membranes; Altered nutrition: less than body requirements.

♦ Determine cause of symptoms before giving antiemetics; before giving first dose, ascertain that nausea and vomiting are not due to intestinal obstruction, increased intracranial pressure, or drug overdose.

♦ Before and after administering antiemetics, assess for presence of bowel sounds, pain, nausea, and vomiting. Report onset of absence of bowel sounds, and withhold dose.

♦ Monitor and document intake and output to detect dehydration. Offer frequent mouth care.

♦ Supervise ambulation until response is determined.

♦ When patient is able to tolerate liquids, begin with a small amount of ice chips; follow with water, then clear liquids, then full liquids, then food.

♦ For prolonged antiemetic use, record daily weights; report weight loss.

Patient & family teaching/Home care

Possible nursing diagnoses: Knowledge deficit; Impaired home maintenance management.

♦ Stress the need to report persistent nausea, vomiting, or abdominal discomfort.

♦ Explain that avoiding fatty foods and eating smaller, more frequent meals may reduce nausea.

♦ Point out the need to drink clear liquids when nausea abates; caution to advance diet slowly to full liquids and then to food.

▶

Antiemetics 63

• Advise against use of alcohol or other CNS depressants.

• Warn against driving or other activities that require mental alertness until response is established.

• Emphasize the need to maintain good mouth care, especially when not taking liquids by mouth.

◆ *Before administering, or for more information, see individual drug.*

Antihistamines

Prototype: diphenhydramine hydrochloride

H_1-receptor antagonists

Ethylenediamine derivatives
  tripelennamine citrate (PBZ)   tripelennamine
                                     hydrochloride (PBZ-SR)

Ethanolamine derivatives (aminoacyl ethers)
  carbinoxamine maleate   diphenhydramine
    (Clistin)   hydrochloride (Benadryl)
  clemastine fumarate (Tavist) doxylamine succinate
                                 (Unisom)

Propylamine derivatives (alkylamines)
  brompheniramine maleate   dexchlorpheniramine
    (Dimetane)   maleate (Polaramine)
  chlorpheniramine maleate   triprolidine hydrochloride
    (Chlor-Trimeton)   (Actidil)

Phenothiazine derivatives
  methdilazine hydrochloride   trimeprazine tartrate
    (✦Dilosyn, Tacaryl)   (✦Penectyl, Temaril)
  promethazine hydrochloride
    (✦Histanil, Phenergan)

Miscellaneous H_1-receptor Antagonists
  astemizole (Hismanal)   cyproheptadine
  azatadine maleate   hydrochloride (Periactin)
    (Optimine, ✦Zadine)   terfenadine (Seldane,
                                 ✦Teldane)

Inhibitor of Histamine Release
  cromolyn sodium (Intal,
    ✦IntalSpincaps, Opticrom)

Action Antihistamines prevent but do not reverse histamine-mediated responses. Most act by competing for H_1-receptor sites of effector cells (only cromolyn sodium inhibits histamine release). The most common histamine-mediated responses are antigen-antibody reactions, commonly known as hypersensitivity or allergic reactions. Histamine is a naturally occurring protein that is produced and stored mainly in mast cells and released in hypersensitivity, anaphylactic, and inflammatory reactions.

Because of their chemical structure and their CNS depressant effects, some antihistamines also have antiemetic, sedative, and anticholin-

ergic actions. These actions and uses are addressed in the respective overviews. Terfenadine and astemizole are newer antihistamines that apparently do not cross the blood-brain barrier and thus cause little or no sedation. Some antihistamines (e.g., diphenhydramine) have antipruritic and local anesthetic effects.

Use/Therapeutic goal/Outcome

Most common use is in treatment of chronic and acute hypersensitivity reactions. Hypersensitivity symptoms may be mild (runny nose, sneezing, pruritus, rash, tearing) to severe (difficulty in breathing, generalized swelling, hypotension, anaphylaxis).

Therapeutic goal: Prevention or reduction of annoying or harmful hypersensitivity symptoms. **Outcome criteria:** Report and demonstration of relief of hypersensitivity symptoms, clearing of air passages, vital signs within normal limits.

Dose range/Administration

Dosage depends on the severity of the reaction, drug, route of administration, individual response, age, height, and weight.

Children and the elderly usually require lower doses.

Some antihistamines are administered only PO in the form of tablets, suspensions, or syrups. Others may be given topically, IM, or IV (parenteral administration is used most often for acute reactions). Cromolyn is the only antihistamine that is inhaled. Administration of topical antihistamines is limited to 7 days or less. Some antihistamines are given with milk or food to decrease GI symptoms; others are given on an empty stomach with a full glass of water (for individual drugs).

The choice of agent for treatment of chronic allergies varies with individual responses. One individual may respond well to a medication and experience minimal side effects, whereas another may experience profound side effects that require discontinuation of the medication. A trial of several drugs may be necessary to achieve relief of symptoms with few side effects. Terfenadine and astemizole have been very useful in the treatment of chronic or seasonal allergic symptoms because they produce little or no sedation.

In severe acute reactions, antihistamines alone do not control symptoms; usually, diphenhydramine is given with epinephrine and dexamethasone.

Because antihistamines do not reverse allergic reactions, they are most effective if given before anticipated contact with allergens or at the earliest onset of symptoms (antihistamines taken at earliest onset of symptoms minimize the reaction by preventing effects of additional histamine release).

Many individuals cope with allergies by taking OTC preparations at times of anticipated risk (e.g., when pollen counts are high, when in contact with animals) and by using a combination of medical and holistic approaches (see Patient and Family Teaching/Home Care).

In the hospital setting, many physicians prescribe diphenhydramine to be given before medications that might stimulate histamine-mediated responses or before administration of blood to patients at risk for blood reactions (e.g., patients who have a rare blood type that is difficult to match or who have received multiple transfusions).

Contraindications/Precautions

Contraindicated in hypersensitivity to the drug; in glaucoma, lower respiratory obstruction, and emphysema; and in those taking monoamine oxidate inhibitors (MAOIs). **Use with caution** in CNS depression, seizure disorders, cardiovascular disease, prostatic hypertrophy, or obstructive bowel or bladder disease.

Bronchial asthma: There is conflicting information about antihistamine use in bronchial asthma. Traditional guidelines advise against using antihistamines to treat lower respiratory tract symptoms, including asthma; according to the American Academy of Allergy and Immunology, however, antihistamines may be given with caution provided that no previous adverse response has occurred.

Contraindicated for pregnant or nursing mothers unless benefits clearly outweigh risks. Use with caution for children and the elderly, who are more susceptible to CNS effects of sedation, ataxia, and paradoxical excitement.

Side effects/Adverse reactions

Hypersensitivity: excessive side effects and (for topical use) rash. **CNS:** drowsiness, sedation, ataxia, paradoxical stimulation, abnormal involuntary movement of muscles or limbs (extrapyramidal effects). **CV:** tachycardia, hypotension. **GI:** dry mouth, anorexia, constipation, diarrhea. **GU:** urinary hesitance or retention.

Nursing implications/Documentation

Possible nursing diagnoses: Potential for injury; Ineffective airway clearance; Urinary retention; Fluid volume deficit; Potential for infection.

◆ Determine and record known allergens; provide an environment free from allergens (especially sleeping areas).

◆ Monitor lung sounds; report increased wheezing or shortness of breath immediately.

◆ Monitor sputum production closely; report purulent or foul-smelling sputum or increased sputum production.

◆ Ensure adequate hydration by providing at least 2000 ml fluids per day; record daily intake.

◆ If drug is given parenterally, monitor for dizziness and hypotension; supervise ambulation until response is determined.

◆ Report excessive sedation, ataxia, confusion, or paradoxical excitement (may indicate toxicity or adverse reaction).

◆ If urinary hesitance or retention is noted, have the individual void before dose is given.

Patient & family teaching/Home care

Possible nursing diagnoses: Knowledge deficit; Impaired home maintenance management.

◆ Stress that antihistamines prevent but do not reverse hypersensitivity reactions and that antihistamines work best if taken before or at onset of symptoms; emphasize that if symptoms have already appeared, improvement will take time.

◆ For chronic allergies, point out the importance of a comprehensive medical and holistic approach to reducing reactions (keeping the environment free from allergens, using air conditioning, learning biofeedback interventions during asthma attacks, maintaining ongoing medical follow-up with an allergy specialist).

◆ For acute hypersensitivity reactions (e.g., bee stings), stress the need to seek immediate medical attention; advise consulting with a physician to determine whether desensitization is needed and to develop a plan about what to do if stings occur (e.g., self-administer epinephrine and call paramedics).

• Stress the need to report increasing shortness of breath or tachypnea; advise calling the paramedics if the reaction is acute.

• Advise reporting persistent symptoms of inflammation; explain that these may indicate early signs of infection.

• Emphasize that doses must not be increased without physician's approval; point out that concomitant alcohol use may cause excessive sedation and coordination problems.

• Stress that unless the patient is taking a "nondrowsiness formula" antihistamine, such as terfenadine or astemizole, the patient must not drive until response is determined.

• Warn nursing mothers that antihistamines may reduce milk flow and be passed on to the infant in breast milk.

• Caution those with hypertension against using OTC antihistamines without physician's approval (may cause increase in blood pressure).

◆ *Before administering, or for more information, see individual drugs.*

Antihypertensives

Prototypes: clonidine, trimethaphan camsylate, reserpine, prazosin hydrochloride, verapamil hydrochloride, labetalol, propranolol hydrochloride, hydralazine, captopril

Central adrenergic agonists
clonidine (Catapres, ♣Dixarit)
guanabenz acetate (Wytensin)
guanfacine hydrochloride (Tenex)
Methyldopa (Aldomet, ♣Dopamet)

Ganglionic blockers
trimethaphan camsylate (Arfonad)

Peripherally acting catecholamine depleters
guandrel sulfate (Hylorel)
guanethidine monosulfate (Ismelin)
reserpine (Serpasil)

Alpha-adrenergic blockers
prazosin hydrochloride (Minipress)
terazosin hydrochloride (Hytrin)

Calcium channel blockers (see separate overview)
Diltiazem hydrochloride (Cardizem)
Nicardipine hydrochloride (Cardene)
Nifedipine (Procardia)
Verapamil hydrochloride (Calan)

Beta-blockers (see separate overview)
acebutolol hydrochloride (Sectral, ♣Monitan)
atenolol (Tenormin, ♠Noten)
carteolol hydrochloride (Cartrol)
labetalol (a combined alpha- and beta-adrenergic blocker) (Trandate, ♠Presolol)
metoprolol tartrate (Lopressor, ♣♠Betaloc)

nadolol (Corgard)
penbutolol sulfate (Levatol)
pindolol (Visken)
propranolol hydrochloride (Inderal)
timolol maleate (Blocadren, ♣Apo-Timol)

Vascular smooth muscle relaxants
diazoxide (Hyperstat)
hydralazine (Apresoline, ♣Novo-Hylazin, ♠Supres)
minoxidil (Loniten)
sodium nitroprusside (Nipride)

Angiotensin-converting enzyme (ACE) inhibitors
captopril (Capoten)
enalapril maleate (Vasotec, ♣♠Amprace)
lisinopril (Prinivil)

Diuretics (see separate overview)

Action Antihypertensives lower blood pressure in one or more ways:

◆ **Reduce heart rate, myocardial contractility and cardiac output (reducing the force of circulating blood exerted upon the vessel wall).**

◆ **Reduce the tone of arterial smooth muscle, causing dilation of blood vessels (decreasing the pressure of the blood vessel walls on the circulating volume).**

◆ **Reduce circulating blood volume (blocking reabsorption of water and electrolytes by the kidney).**

Antihypertensives may be classified into nine groups, depending on their main site of action.

1 **Central adrenergic agonists** inhibit vasoconstriction by stimulating the cardiovascular centers of the brain, causing decreased outflow of sympathetic vasoconstrictor impulses (the arterial walls will then exert less pressure on the blood) and decreased outflow of cardioaccelerator impulses (the heart rate will be reduced).

2 **Ganglionic blockers** reduce sympathetic stimulation of the heart and blood vessels. However, they produce such profound reductions in blood pressure that they are employed **only in emergencies**.

3 **Peripherally acting catecholamine depleters** reduce vascular wall tone by reducing sympathetic nervous system stimulation of blood vessels. They decrease peripheral resistance and blood pressure by blocking the release or re-uptake of norepinephrine. Because reserpine depletes norepinephrine in the CNS (as well as peripherally), it reduces blood flow in the brain and is more likely to be associated with adverse CNS effects.

4 **Alpha-adrenergic blockers** decrease vascular resistance and reduce blood pressure by block-

ing vascular alpha-1 adrenergic receptors, promoting vasodilation.

5 Calcium channel blockers decrease peripheral resistance by reducing smooth muscle contractility and by decreasing heart rate and contractility (see separate overview).

6 Beta-blockers block the transmission of nerve impulse at the beta-adrenergic receptors of the sympathetic nervous system and depress excessive renin secretion in the kidney (see separate overview).

7 Vascular smooth muscle relaxants dilate blood vessels by relaxing the muscles of the vessel wall. They have a direct action on the peripheral arterioles.

8 Angiotensin converting enzyme (ACE) inhibitors are different from all other antihypertensive drugs. They inhibit angiotensin converting enzyme, blocking the conversion of angiotensin I to the very potent vasoconstrictor angiotensin II; they also reduce secretion of aldosterone (the hormone that causes kidneys to reabsorb sodium and water), preventing sodium and water retention and reducing peripheral vascular resistance (PVR), central venous pressure (CVP), and pulmonary capillary wedge pressure (PCWP).

9 Diuretics act on the renal tubules to promote sodium and water excretion. As a result, intravascular fluid volume decreases, and blood pressure is reduced.

◆ Monoamine oxidase inhibitors (MAOIs) have an antihypertensive effect but are rarely given for this use because of potentially fatal food and drug interactions. They are not covered in this overview.

Use/Therapeutic goal/Outcome

Used to treat hypertension. *Therapeutic goal:* stable blood pressure within normal range and tolerated by the patient (some patients need a slightly elevated blood pressure for satisfactory perfusion of vital organs). *Outcome criteria:* diastolic blood pressure < 90 mm Hg, with no clinical signs or symptoms of shock (urine output > 25 ml/hr, satisfactory peripheral pulses, absence of restlessness/confusion).

Dose range/Administration

Dosage depends on the drug, route of administration, individual response, degree of hypertension, incidence of side effects, age, height,

weight, and health status. Concomitant use of other drugs that affect blood pressure may also influence dose range.

Often, finding the best drug (or combination of drugs) and optimal dose involves a trial-and-error period in which certain antihypertensives are tried alone or together. As a rule, dosage is usually started at the lowest level and then gradually increased as the patient is monitored for blood pressure control and incidence of side effects. If one drug is unsatisfactory because of poor control or excessive side effects, another drug may be substituted or added until the desired effect is achieved.

Antihypertensives are usually given PO. Hypertensive crisis requires IV route treatment to immediately reduce blood pressure.

Contraindications/Precautions

Contraindicated in hypersensitivity to the drug or to a related drug and in hypotension.

Side effects/Adverse reactions

Hypersensitivity: itching, rashes, and urticaria. **CV:** hypotension, bradycardia, congestive heart failure (CHF), fever. **CNS:** dizziness, syncope, libido changes. **GI:** dry mouth. **Skin:** edema. **GU:** impotence.

Nursing implications/Documentation

Possible nursing diagnoses: Activity intolerance; Fatigue; Potential for injury; Altered oral mucous membrane.

◆ Assess mental status, and document pulse and blood pressure (if possible, lying, sitting, and standing, in both arms) before administration, and frequently thereafter until response is determined.

◆ Consult with physician to determine desired therapeutic range for blood pressure (be aware that some patients may require a slightly elevated blood pressure to perfuse vital organs).

◆ Ascertain that baseline blood sugar, CBC, electrolytes, BUN, creatinine, uric acid, and liver function studies are obtained before giving first dose; report abnormalities and monitor closely thereafter.

◆ Monitor for hypersensitivity reactions and for confusion, dizziness, arrhythmias, and hypotension; if these occur, withhold drug, and report immediately.

◆ Supervise ambulation until response is determined; allow for rest periods with activity.

♦ Monitor and document daily weights, and intake and output; report significant negative or positive balance.

♦ Be aware that many of these drugs cause dry mouth; provide frequent mouth care.

Patient & family teaching/Home care

Possible nursing diagnoses: Knowledge deficit; Impaired home maintenance management; Altered sexuality patterns.

♦ Explain the importance of taking antihypertensives exactly as prescribed, even when feeling well; explore individual's feelings concerning ability to follow medication regimen.

♦ Emphasize the importance of good medical follow-up.

♦ Explain that these drugs reduce "wear and tear" on blood vessels and improve longevity and health.

♦ Teach how to monitor pulse and blood pressure; instruct patient to report syncope, hypertension or hypotension, and persistent dizziness.

♦ Advise changing positions slowly to avoid dizziness.

♦ Encourage monitoring weight daily and reporting sudden weight gain (likely to be fluid retention).

♦ Warn against drinking alcohol or taking **any** OTC drugs unless these are approved by the physician (some interactions can cause severe reactions).

♦ Advise avoiding driving and hazardous activities until response is determined (drug may cause drowsiness).

♦ Be aware that many of these drugs may alter sexual ability; explore concerns, and consult with a specialist if necessary.

♦ Discuss holistic measures of enhancing effect of antihypertensives (weight control, reduction of dietary salt intake, daily exercise, stress-reduction techniques).

♦ *Before administering, or for more information, see individual drug.*

Anti-infectives

Prototypes: penicillin G, cefazolin, sulfisoxazole, tetracycline, erythromycin, gentamicin, amphotericin B, acyclovir

Antibiotics

Penicillins

amdinocillin (Coactin)
amoxicillin (Polymox)
amoxicillin/clavulanate potassium (Augmentin)

ampicillin sodium/sulbactam sodium (Unasyn)
ampicillin trihydrate (Principen)
azlocillin sodium (Azlin)
bacampicillin hydrochloride (Spectrobid)
carbenicillin disodium (Geopen)
carbenicillin indanyl sodium (Geocillin)
cloxacillin sodium (Tegopen)
cyclacillin (Cyclapen-W)
dicloxacillin sodium (Dynapen)
methicillin sodium (Staphcillin)
mezlocillin sodium (Mezlin)

nafcillin sodium (Unipen)
oxacillin sodium (Prostaphlin)
penicillin G, benzathine (Bicillin L-A)
penicillin G, potassium (Pfizerpen)
penicillin G, procaine (Wycillin)
penicillin G, sodium (Cystapen)
penicillin V potassium (Pen-Vee K)
piperacillin sodium (Pipracil)
ticarcillin disodium (Ticar)
ticarcillin disodium/ clavulanate potassium (Timentin)

Cephalosporins

cefaclor (Ceclor)
cefadroxil monohydrate (Duricef)
cefamandole nafate (Mandol)
cefazolin sodium (Ancef)
cefonicid sodium (Monocid)
cefoperazone sodium (Cefobid)
ceforanide (Precef)
cefotaxime sodium (Claforan)
cefotetan disodium (Cefotan)

cefoxitin sodium (Mefoxin)
ceftazidime (Fortaz)
ceftizoxime sodium (Cefizox)
ceftriaxone sodium (Rocephin)
cefuroxime axetil (Ceftin)
cefuroxime sodium (Zinacef)
cephalexin monohydrate (Keflex)
cephalothin sodium (Keflin)
cephapirin sodium (Cefadyl)
cephradine (Anspor)
moxalactam (Moxam)

Sulfonamides

co-trimoxazole (sulfamethoxazole/ trimethoprim) (Bactrim)
sulfacetamide sodium 10% (Bleph-10 Liquifilm Ophthalmic)
sulfacetamide sodium 15% (Isopto Cetamide Ophthalmic)

sulfacetamide sodium 30% (Sodium Sulamyd 30% Ophthalmic)
sulfadiazine (Microsulfon)
sulfamethoxazole (Gantanol)
sulfasalazine (Azulfidine)
sulfisoxazole (Gantrisin)

Tetracyclines

demeclocycline hydro- chloride (Declomycin)
doxycycline hyclate, monohydrate (Vibramycin)

minocycline hydrochloride (Minocin)
oxytetracycline (Terramycin)
tetracycline hydrochloride (Achromycin)

Urinary tract drugs

cinoxacin (Cinobac)
methenamine hippurate (Urex)
methenamine mandelate (Mandelamine)

nalidixic acid (NegGram)
nitrofurantoin (Macrodantin)
norfloxacin (Noroxin)
ofloxacin (Floxin)

Aminoglycosides

amikacin sulfate (Amikin)
gentamicin sulfate (Garamycin)
kanamycin sulfate (Kantrex)

neomycin sulfate (Mycifradin)
streptomycin sulfate
tobramycin sulfate (Nebcin)

Antituberculars

capreomycin sulfate (Capastat)
cycloserine (Seromycin)
ethambutol hydrochloride (Myambutol)

isoniazid (Nydrazid)
pyrazinamide (Tebrazid)
rifampin (Rifadin)

Miscellaneous drugs
  aztreonam (Azactam)
  chloramphenicol
    (Chloromycetin)
  ciprofloxacin (Cipro)
  clindamycin hydrochloride,
    palmitate hydrochloride,
    phosphate (Cleocin)
  erythromycin (Erythrocin)
  imipenem/cilastatin sodium
    (Primaxin)

  mupirocin (Bactroban)
  pentamidine isethionate
    (Pentam 300)
  spectinomycin
    dihydrochloride (Trobicin)
  trimethoprim (Proloprim)
  vancomycin hydrochloride
    (Vancocin)

Antifungals

  amphotericin B (Fungizone)
  fluconazole (Diflucan)
  flucytosine (Ancobon)
  griseofulvin (Fulvicin-U/F)

  ketoconazole (Nizoral)
  miconazole (Monistat)
  nystatin (Nilstat)

Antivirals

  acyclovir sodium (Zovirax)
  amantadine hydrochloride
    (Symmetrel)

  gancyclovir (Cytovene)
  zidovudine (Retrovir)

Antiparasitics

Amebicides/Trichomonacides
  iodoquinol (Diquinol)
  metronidazole (Flagyl)

  metronidazole hydrochloride
    (Flagyl I.V.)

Anthelmintics
  mebendazole (Vermox)
  pyrantel pamoate
    (Antiminth)
  pyrantel embonate
    (Combantin)

  quinacrine hydrochloride
    (Atabrine)
  thiabendazole (Mintezol)

Action Anti-infectives kill bacteria (bactericidal action) or limit their growth (bacteriostatic action) either by interfering with the cell wall of microorganisms, or by interfering with the intracellular metabolism. **Broad-spectrum** anti-infectives are effective against many different microorganisms. **Narrow-spectrum** anti-infectives are effective against a few specific microorganisms.

Anti-infectives are classified into four major groups, depending on their effectiveness against pathogenic organisms:

1 **Antibiotics:** effective against bacteria

2 **Antifungals:** effective against fungi

3 **Antivirals:** effective against viruses

4 **Antiparasitics:** effective against parasites

Three factors influence an anti-infective's ability to fight a specific infection:

♦ **Sensitivity, or vulnerability, of the organism** to the anti-infective (some organisms are resistant to certain anti-infectives).

♦ **Concentration of the anti-infective** at the site of infection. This is determined by the characteristics of the drug itself and by the

dose and route of administration. For example, IV administration provides high blood concentrations of the anti-infective.

♦ **Immune defenses and health state of the individual** receiving the anti-infective. For example, a patient whose immune system is failing may not be able to eliminate infection completely, even if potent anti-infectives are given.

Use/Therapeutic goal/Outcome

Used to treat or prevent infections. Optimally, the drug used is known to act against the microorganism cultured from a patient specimen. While awaiting culture results, the physician may prescribe an anti-infective that is likely to be effective (empirical treatment). Once sensitivity results are obtained, a more specific anti-infective may be indicated. **Therapeutic goal:** Elimination of pathogenic bacteria; prevention or resolution of infection. **Outcome criteria:** Absence of pathogen growth on cultures; absence of signs and symptoms of infection (increased WBC, fever, pain, redness, swelling, drainage); improved X rays; and (if cultures are not taken) absence of signs and symptoms of infection when the recommended course of required anti-infective has been completed.

Dose range/Administration

Dosage and administration depend on the severity of infection, potency of the anti-infective, route of administration, age, height, weight, and health state. Patients with decreased renal function often require reduced dosages and close monitoring (BUN and creatinine and drug levels) during therapy. A few antibiotics exhibit a narrow therapeutic/toxicity range (e.g., vancomycin and the aminoglycosides). When these drugs are given, the physician usually orders peak and trough levels (see guidelines on the following page).

Contraindications/Precautions

Contraindicated in history of hypersensitivity to the drug or to a closely related drug and possibly in renal or hepatic failure.

Side effects/Adverse reactions

Hypersensitivity: hives, rash, pruritus, and difficulty in breathing (may signify the onset of anaphylaxis). **GI:** diarrhea, nausea, vomiting, abdominal pain, anorexia.

Guidelines:
Peak and trough levels for anti-infectives

Peak and trough levels are determined from blood samples drawn at specific times to ensure that the concentration of the anti-infective is within the therapeutic range. **Blood for peak levels** is drawn when the concentration of drug is expected to be highest (timing depends on drug, route of administration, and patient status). **Blood for trough levels** is drawn when the concentration of drug is expected to be lowest (immediately before a dose is given).

Monitoring:
When peak and trough levels are needed

Monitoring anti-infective blood levels may be necessary in two situations:

1 When the difference between the anti-infective's therapeutic and toxic concentration is small (the drug has a narrow margin of safety).

2 When the patient's ability to metabolize and excrete medications is unpredictable (e.g., because of kidney disease or dialysis).

Scheduling:
When to draw the blood

Although some situations vary, general practice is to draw blood for peak levels 30 min after the completion of an IV infusion, 1 hr after an IM dose, and 1–2 hrs after a PO dose. Trough levels are drawn immediately before a dose.

Response:
If peak and trough levels are abnormal

Report abnormal peak and trough levels to the physician, who can then make the necessary medication adjustment.

Nursing implications/Documentation

Possible nursing diagnoses: Potential for infection; Diarrhea; Fluid volume deficit.

• Obtain necessary cultures and baseline laboratory results (CBC, electrolytes, BUN, creatinine, liver function studies) before starting anti-infectives; monitor closely thereafter if therapy is prolonged.

• Determine if the person has ever had an unusual reaction to a medication. (Be aware that hypersensitivity reactions are likely in a person who has multiple allergies, who is allergic to a closely related drug, or who has a family member with an allergy to the drug.)

• Plan to give doses of anti-infectives at equal time intervals around the clock (if possible) to maintain steady blood levels; also consider whether best results are obtained when the drug is taken with or without food.

• Give IV doses intermittently, and monitor closely for signs of phlebitis (pain, redness, swelling, heat).

• Give IM doses deep into large muscle masses to minimize pain.

• If hypersensitivity reaction occurs, withhold next dose, report to physician; document signs and symptoms and actions taken; and clearly mark chart and medication record with "allergy" notation.

• Document status of clinical signs and symptoms of infection; monitor WBC count; report to physician if no improvement occurs within 24–72 hrs, depending on severity of infection.

• If therapy is prolonged, monitor for, document, and report signs of superinfection, a common side effect (signs and symptoms include vaginal discharge, fever, sore mouth and throat, diarrhea).

• Notify physician if liver or kidney function tests (LDH, AST/SGOT, alkaline phosphatase, BUN, creatinine) indicate deterioration in condition.

• Provide preferred fluids, and monitor and document intake and output to ensure adequate hydration; report persistent negative or positive balance.

• Keep oral suspensions refrigerated, and shake them well before using. (In addition, many IV anti-infectives must be refrigerated —check manufacturer's recommendations.)

• Monitor peak and trough serum anti-infective levels (if ordered) for therapeutic and toxic blood levels.

Patient & family teaching/Home care

Possible nursing diagnoses: Knowledge deficit; Impaired home maintenance management.

◆ Stress the importance of taking the anti-infective for the entire length of time prescribed, even if signs and symptoms abate; reinforce the importance of taking the medication as prescribed (on time, and with or without food).

◆ Teach the signs and symptoms of hypersensitivity reaction (rash, pruritus, wheezing, difficulty in breathing); caution to withhold dose and notify physician immediately if these appear.

◆ Advise reporting persistent or new symptoms (fever, sore throat, diarrhea), because they may indicate a need for a change in antibiotic.

◆ Point out the need to drink at least 2-4 quarts of liquid daily, unless doing so is contraindicated by heart or kidney disease.

◆ *Before administering, or for more information, see individual drug.*

Antilipemics

Prototypes: Cholestyramine, Clofibrate

Drugs that lower serum cholesterol

cholestyramine (Questran)	dextrothyroxine sodium
colestipol hydrochloride	(Choloxin)
(Colestid)	lovastatin (Mevacor)
	probucol (Lorelco)

Drugs that lower serum triglyceride

clofibrate (Atromid-S,	gemfibrozil (Lopid)
✦Claripex)	niacin (Nicobid)

Action Antilipemics reduce serum cholesterol and/or triglycerides by various mechanisms. Cholestyramine and colestipol bind with bile acids (precursors of cholesterol); the nonabsorbable compound is then excreted in feces. The other agents have very different actions, and vary in their effectiveness for lowering specific lipoproteins (low-density lipoproteins [LDL], very-low-density lipoproteins [VLDL], high-density lipoproteins [HDL]) and triglycerides.

Use/Therapeutic goal/Outcome

Used to reduce serum lipids when dietary modification alone has failed (dietary restrictions should be tried for 2–3 months before starting antilipemics). **Therapeutic goal:** Maintaining normal serum lipid levels (thereby reducing risk factors for atherosclerosis). **Outcome criteria:** Within 3 months, serum triglyceride and LDL-cholesterol levels are within normal range, with improved HDL-cholesterol ratios. If there is no improvement after 3 months, the drugs are discontinued.

Dose range/Administration

Antilipemics are given as part of a holistic program of diet and exercise to control cholesterol. All antilipemics are given PO. Dosage depends on the drug, the severity of hyperlipidemia, individual response, and occurrence of side effects. Some of these drugs are powders that must be mixed in a liquid (preferably in juice to mask taste) rather than taken dry. Taking the powder dry can cause esophageal irritation or obstruction.

Interaction alert: Cholestyramine and colestipol decrease absorption of almost all other oral drugs; therefore, give these drugs 1 hr before or 4 hrs after other medications.

🖐 **Safety of long-term antilipemic therapy in children is not established. Therefore, children's doses are small initially and increased only if necessary.**

Contraindications/Precautions

Contraindicated in hypersensitivity to the drug. Cholestyramine and colestipol are contraindicated also in severe constipation and fat-soluble vitamin deficiency. Other contraindications can be found in the individual drug monographs. **Use with caution** in history of GI disorders, peptic ulcer disease, arrhythmias, hypertension, bleeding disorders, or impaired liver or kidney function.

🖐 **Safe use for children and pregnant or nursing mothers has not been established.**

Side effects/Adverse reactions

Hypersensitivity: pruritus, rash. **GI:** nausea, vomiting, constipation, diarrhea, anorexia.

🖐 **Because these drugs vary in action, each has its own additional side effects. (See individual drug listings.)**

Nursing implications/Documentation

Possible nursing diagnoses: Constipation; Altered nutrition: more than body requirements.

◆ Assess dietary habits, and identify ways of reducing cholesterol intake (e.g., using margarine instead of butter).

◆ Check baseline serum cholesterol levels, triglyceride levels, and liver function studies; monitor periodically thereafter (drug may need to be discontinued if there is no change, a paradoxical increase in cholesterol levels, or alteration in liver function).

♦ Monitor and document bowel elimination to detect constipation or diarrhea; establish a plan to prevent constipation; report diarrhea to physician.

♦ Monitor for and report persistent GI symptoms.

♦ Report signs of tachycardia, jaundice, or bleeding tendencies immediately.

Patient & family teaching/Home care

Possible nursing diagnoses: Knowledge deficit; Ineffective individual coping; Impaired home maintenance management.

♦ Explain that this drug reduces blood cholesterol levels and decreases the risk of cardiovascular disease.

♦ Point out the need to reduce other cardiac risk factors (obesity, smoking, high-cholesterol diet, sedentary life-style), and help develop a plan to cope with changes in daily living.

♦ Advise reporting persistent diarrhea, other GI symptoms, palpitations, and bleeding or bruising tendencies.

♦ Discuss the role of adequate hydration, fiber intake, and exercise in preventing constipation.

♦ Stress that lowering cholesterol levels requires life-long commitment, medical follow-up, and life-style changes.

♦ *Before administering, or for more information, see individual drugs.*

Antineoplastics

Prototypes: cyclophosphamide, doxorubicin, methotrexate, vincristine

Alkylating agents
busulfan (Myleran)
carboplatin (Paraplatin)
carmustine (BiCNU)
chlorambucil (Leukeran)
cisplatin / *cis*-platinum (Platinol)
cyclophosphamide (Cytoxan)
dacarbazine / DTIC (DTIC-Dome)
ifosfamide (Ifex)

lomustine / CCNU (CeeNU)
mechlorethamine hydrochloride / nitrogen mustard (Mustargen)
melphalan (Alkeran)
streptozocin (Zanosar)
triethylenethiophosphoramide (Thiotepa)
uracil mustard (Uracil Mustard)

Antitumor antibiotics
bleomycin sulfate (Blenoxane)
dactinomycin / actinomycin D (Cosmegen)

daunorubicin hydrochloride (Cerubidine)
doxorubicin hydrochloride (Adriamycin)
mitomycin (Mutamycin)

mitoxantrone hydrochloride (Novantrone)
plicamycin / mithramycin (Mithracin)

procarbazine hydrochloride (Matulane)

Antimetabolites
cytarabine / ara-C / cytosine arabinoside (Cytosar-U)
fluorouracil / 5-fluorouracil / 5-FU (Adrucil)
floxuridine (FUDR)

hydroxyurea (Hydrea)
mercaptopurine (6-MP)
methotrexate (Folex)
thioguanine / 6-thioguanine / 6-TG (♦Lanvis)

Hormonal agents
aminoglutethimide (Cytadren)
cortisone acetate (Cortone Acetate)
dexamethasone (Decadron)
flutamide (Eulexin)
hydrocortisone sodium succinate (Solu-Cortef)
leuprolide acetate (Lupron)

megestrol acetate (Megace)
methylprednisolone sodium succinate (Solu-Medrol)
mitotane (Lysodren)
prednisone (Cortalone)
tamoxifen citrate (Nolvadex)
testolactone (Teslac)
trilostane (Modrastane)

Plant alkaloids
vinblastine sulfate (Velban)
vincristine sulfate (Oncovin)

vindesine sulfate (Eldisine)

Miscellaneous agents
amsacrine / m-AMSA (♦Amsidyl)
asparaginase / L-asparaginase (Elspar)
erwinia asparaginase / porton asparaginase
etoposide / VP-16 (VePesid)

interferon alfa-2a (Roferon-A)
interferon alfa-2b (Intron A)
levamisole (Ergamisol)
teniposide / VM-26 (♦Vumon)

♦ *See Adrenocorticosteroids overview for additional information about cortisone acetate, dexamethasone, hydrocortisone sodium succinate, and prednisone.*

Action All antineoplastic agents except hormonal agents affect the cell cycle. This series of orderly biochemical events encompasses the life span of a cell from formation until its division into two new cells. Some agents are especially effective in altering cell growth at a specific phase of the cell cycle and are called *cell cycle-specific* (CCS) antineoplastic agents. *Cell cycle-nonspecific* (CCNS) antineoplastic agents are effective at any point in the cell cycle and destroy both growing and resting (dormant) cells.

All antineoplastic agents except hormonal agents are *cytotoxic* (they poison the cell) and destroy both normal and abnormal cells. These agents are most effective against cells with a rapid growth rate (cancer, bone marrow, GI lining, hair follicles, ova, and sperm). These drugs are usually most effective against cancer in its earliest stages, because cancer cells often grow at their most rapid rate at the beginning of the disease.

The cell cycle:

M phase/most vulnerable
Mitosis (the cell divides)

G$_2$ phase
Pre-miotic interval

G$_0$/G$_1$ phase   S phase/vulnerable
Resting   DNA synthesis

8 hrs   10 hrs   2 hrs

Cancer cells and other fast-growing cells
can complete a cycle in less than a day.   1/2 hr

48 hrs   20 hrs   10 hrs

The slowest-growing cells take over 3 days   1 hr
to complete a cycle, and the vulnerable S
and M phases are proportionally shorter.

Antineoplastics may be classified into six
categories:

1 Alkylating agents, the first known anticancer
drugs, are effective in all phases of the cell
cycle (cell cycle-nonspecific), and prevent cell
growth primarily by damaging deoxyribonu-
cleic acid (DNA). They are called *alkylating
agents* because they damage the cell by insert-
ing alkyl groups into DNA, ribonucleic acid
(RNA), proteins, and other macromolecules.

2 Antitumor antibiotic agents destroy tumor
cells by interfering with the synthesis of DNA,
RNA, or both (some of these drugs are cell
cycle-specific, and some are cell cycle-
nonspecific). These drugs are not used for
infections because they are highly toxic.

3 Antimetabolites are primarily effective during
the S phase of the cell cycle, when DNA is
synthesized. These drugs are incorporated into
DNA or RNA molecules; they substitute
purines and pyrimidines in normal metabolic
pathways for nucleic acid synthesis and form
defective molecules that are unable to synthesize the necessary proteins for cellular function. Antimetabolites are classified into three
groups: purine antagonists, pyrimidine antagonists, and folate antagonists. They are most
effective for rapidly growing tumors.

4 Hormonal agents are effective against tumors
that need a favorable hormonal environment to
grow. These include **hormonal drugs** (estrogens, progestins, androgens), **antihormonal
drugs** (antiestrogens, antiadrenal,
gonadotropin-releasing agents), and **adreno-**

corticosteroids. All may be given to reduce
the rate of tumor growth, although hormonal
agents have no direct cytotoxic effect and cannot cure cancer. The choice of drug is determined by the type of hormonal environment
that is favorable for tumor growth; the intent
of drug therapy is to change the hormonal
environment to one that is unfavorable for
growth. If the cancer thrives on estrogen, for
example, an antiestrogen agent or an androgen
may be given.

♦ *Adrenocorticosteroids combat certain cancers
(leukemias, lymphomas, Hodgkin's disease, and
some breast cancers) by stopping DNA
synthesis, interfering with mitosis and cellular
protein synthesis, and enhancing the body's
response to other antineoplastic agents. See
Adrenocorticosteroids overview.*

5 Plant alkaloids (plant derivatives) are cell
cycle-specific drugs that work mainly during
the M phase (mitosis). Their activity in the G
and S phases is limited. Each of these drugs
has different uses and toxicities.

6 Miscellaneous agents include investigational
drugs and biologic response modifiers. Each
drug has unique properties.

Use/Therapeutic goal/Outcome

Used to treat various cancers, alone or in combination with other drugs, surgery, and/or radiation treatment. ***Therapeutic goal:*** Reduction
or elimination of the rapid, uncontrolled proliferation of abnormal cells (unlike normal cells,
cancer cells reproduce without maintaining an
equilibrium between cell death and the production of new cells). ***Outcome criteria:*** Tumor or
disease regression or stabilization on radiologic
and physical examination and (for leukemias)
an absence of blasts upon microscopic examination of peripheral blood specimens (if there is
an absence of blasts in the peripheral blood, an
examination of the bone marrow may be performed; absence of these immature cells in the
bone marrow specimen further demonstrates
goal achievement).

Dose range/Administration

Clinical alert: Except for the hormonal agents, all of these drugs are given only by nurses who are knowledgeable in the comprehensive management of the administration of chemotherapeutic agents. Before preparing and giving these drugs, the nurse must become familiar with the individual agency's relevant protocols and policies. Because many of these drugs are carcinogens, gloves or double gloves are worn during preparation and administration, and the agents are not prepared or administered by pregnant women.

Dosage is highly individualized depending on the drug, route of administration, age, height, weight, health status, and other important factors, including: type of cancer; stage of cancer (different doses and regimens may be prescribed at different stages of the disease and for maintenance); resistance of the cancer to therapy (some cancers have a natural resistance or develop a resistance to certain antineoplastics); concomitant use of other antineoplastics; prior treatment with radiation therapy; and presence of signs of toxicity.

Because all of these drugs (except hormonal agents) are cytotoxic to normal cells as well as cancer cells, there is a very small margin between the dose that is needed to destroy the cancer cells and the dose that destroys normal cells (most significantly, bone marrow). For this reason, dosage is determined after comprehensive physical examination, including hematologic studies, and a careful weighing of the risks against the benefits of giving the drug. The patient is carefully monitored, and doses are withheld until the patient has sufficiently recovered from toxicities of previous doses. Often these drugs are not given if the white blood count (WBC) is less than 4000/mm^3 or if the platelet count is less than 100,000/mm^3 (these results indicate severe bone marrow depression). However, these parameters vary, depending on health status and the drug. Other signs of toxicity, such as electrolyte imbalances, GI symptoms, or elevated creatinine, BUN, and liver function studies, may also require that the medication be withheld.

Many of these drugs are given in combination with other antineoplastic drugs or after radiation therapy or surgery. They are often given according to an established protocol or regimen that has been found effective for the particular type of cancer. For example, a combination of cyclophosphamide, doxorubicin, methotrexate,

and procarbazine has been successful in treating lung cancer.

Depending on the drug, the most common routes of administration for antineoplastics are PO, SC, IM, or IV. Careful attention must be given to giving IV doses exactly as prescribed: Some of these drugs are *vesicants*, i.e., they are so irritating that extravasation (seepage from the vein) can cause blistering and even necrosis of tissues surrounding infusion vessels. Although not all of these drugs are vesicants, most are irritating to tissues. All sites of chemotherapy administration are carefully assessed prior to administration to ascertain that the needle or catheter is in the vein (that there is good blood return) and during administration for early detection of extravasation. The rule is to **prevent** extravasation from happening in the first place. If it does occur, the drug must be stopped immediately, the physician notified, and protocols for treatment initiated. These protocols are very specific; they may include application of heat or cold and the administration of a medication that counteracts the damaging effect of the antineoplastic agent. The medication may be applied topically or injected into the area of extravasation.

Some antineoplastic agents may also be injected intrathecally or directly into the tumor by the physician. Some are instilled intracavitarily (for example, into the bladder).

Contraindications/Precautions

Contraindicated in hypersensitivity to the drug and in severe bone marrow depression or toxicity, also (for many drugs) if the patient has received radiation therapy within the previous 4 weeks. **Use with caution** for the debilitated, pre-existing bone marrow depression, malignant infiltration of the kidney or bone marrow, and in liver dysfunction.

🖐 **Contraindicated for nursing mothers and in the first trimester of pregnancy (safety for use during the second two trimesters has not been established). The safety of some of these drugs for children has not been established; those that are given to children are given with caution. Use with caution for the elderly and debilitated (often given in reduced dosage).**

Side effects/Adverse reactions

Hypersensitivity: pruritus, rash, chills, fever, breathing problems, anaphylaxis. **Hem:** leukopenia, thrombocytopenia, agranulocytosis, anemia (all a result of bone marrow depression), hyperuricemia, electrolyte imbalances. *GI:* anorexia, nausea, vomiting, diarrhea, mucositis, enteritis, abdominal pain, intestinal ulcers, paralytic ileus, hepatotoxicity. *CV:* congestive heart failure (CHF), arrhythmias. *GU:* renal failure, amenorrhea, azoospermia, sterility. *Skin:* alopecia, dermatitis, erythema; (in extravasation) pain, redness, swelling, sloughing of skin. *CNS:* confusion, weakness, dizziness, headache, malaise, depression. *Misc:* fever, immunosuppression (increased risk of viral, bacterial, and fungal infections, especially opportunistic viruses such as herpes and cytomegalovirus), carcinogenesis and mutagenesis (especially alkylating agents).

Nursing implications/Documentation

Possible nursing diagnoses: Potential for infection; Altered oral mucous membrane; Fluid volume deficit; Fear; Diarrhea; Potential for injury; Altered nutrition: less than body requirements; Fatigue.

- **Before giving an antineoplastic agent check protocols, policies, and physician's orders to be sure that all necessary laboratory results have been received before giving ordered dose. These studies are likely to include the following:**

☐ Studies that demonstrate level of bone marrow function: hemoglobin, hematocrit, RBC, WBC with differential, and platelet count.

☐ Studies that demonstrate level of kidney function: serum BUN, creatinine, and creatinine clearance studies (blood and urine study).

☐ Studies that demonstrate level of liver function: serum bilirubin, LDH, AST/SGOT, ALT/SGPT, alkaline phosphatase.

☐ Studies that demonstrate balance or imbalance of body chemistry/metabolic processes: serum sodium, potassium, chloride, total carbon dioxide, calcium, magnesium, glucose, phosphorous, albumin, total protein.

☐ Additional studies that are specifically necessary for certain drugs/patient problems (e.g., creatine phosphokinase [CPK] when there is a potential for cardiac problems).

- If there are abnormalities in the above studies, withhold drug, and report (the physician may cancel or modify the dose).

- Document vital signs and weight; report abnormalities or sudden weight loss or gain.

- Follow protocol, policies, and physicians' orders for prevention and treatment of nausea, vomiting, and hypersensitivity reactions. Recognize that often pre-administration and post-administration IV therapy will be given to ensure adequate hydration. Expect that an antiemetic (e.g., metoclopramide), an anti-inflammatory (e.g., dexamethasone), and an antihistamine (e.g., diphenhydramine) might be ordered to be given 30–60 min before antineoplastic agent administration.

- **During and following administration of an antineoplastic agent:**

- Monitor vital signs and physical status closely to detect early signs and symptoms of adverse reactions.

- Document temperature at least daily (more often with certain drugs); report temperature greater than 101°F that lasts more than 4 hrs.

- Minimize incidence of nausea and vomiting by giving prescribed antiemetics on time, providing a quiet environment, decreasing stimuli that may trigger the vomiting center, and modifying diet as needed; check whether the drug should be given in divided doses, with food, on an empty stomach, or at bedtime to reduce nausea.

- Consult with dietician to provide adequate nutrition (supplements may be required).

- Ascertain adequate hydration and nutrition by monitoring and documenting episodes of diarrhea, daily weight, and intake and output; report weight loss or fluid imbalance. Recognize that damage to the kidneys due to hyperuricemia resulting from rapid destruction of cells may be prevented by an intake of at least 2 L/day.

- Report persistent diarrhea, administer prn antidiarrheals, and consult with dietician to obtain a diet plan to reduce diarrhea.

- When WBCs are low, discourage visitors and hospital personnel with colds from coming in close contact with the patient (reverse isolation may be required); monitor closely for, and report, early signs of infection (e.g., elevated temperature); use aseptic technique when caring for any open skin areas.

- When platelets are low, prevent risk of bleeding by avoiding IM injections, using a cotton swab rather than a toothbrush for mouth care, and avoiding rectal temperatures; monitor for and report signs of bleeding (check urine and stools for occult blood).

• When hemoglobin is low, provide frequent rest periods.

• Monitor mouth and rectum for inflammation (mucositis); provide special mouth and perianal care as needed. If mouth pain is present, consult with physician to obtain an order for anesthetic viscous xylocaine (can be swished and swallowed).

• Observe skin for dry, red, or cracked areas; keep areas clean, apply lotion as necessary, and establish a schedule for massaging and repositioning.

• Monitor mental status; report confusion or extreme drowsiness or depression; institute measures to ensure safety (e.g., keep side rails up).

Patient & family teaching/Home care

Possible nursing diagnoses: Family coping (potential for growth); Ineffective family coping (disabling/compromised); Hopelessness; Body image disturbance; Self-esteem disturbance; Knowledge deficit; Impaired home maintenance management.

• Help maintain a positive attitude by keeping treatment goals in mind; acknowledge that undergoing chemotherapy is hard on the body, mind, and spirit, but emphasize that once the regimen is completed, the odds for recovery are much better.

• Explain that antineoplastics often cause significant side effects because they affect not only cancer cells but also bone marrow, hair follicles, GI tract cells, ova, and sperm. Reassure that with close monitoring, adverse affects can be limited by early detection and treatment.

• Provide a list of symptoms that should be reported immediately: fever (over 100°F); chills; sweating, especially at night; diarrhea; burning upon urination; severe cough or sore throat; hives or rashes; unusual bleeding or bruising (teach to check stools, urine, gums); persistent dizziness, fatigue, flu-like symptoms; (for IV therapy) pain, redness, swelling at the site of infusion.

• Teach the importance of special mouth care with a cotton swab (not toothbrush) and of avoiding injury when platelet count is low.

• If WBCs are low, advise to avoid crowded areas and friends, children, and family with colds or flu-like symptoms.

• Stress the need to avoid OTC drugs and alcohol unless these are specifically approved by the physician.

• Point out the need to monitor weight and report significant weight loss or gain (> 7 pounds) within 3 days.

• Emphasize that hair loss is transient, and explore feelings, concerns, and methods of coping (hats, wigs); consult with physician and patient to determine whether tourniquets or ice should be applied to the scalp before, during, or after drug administration (check for policy or protocol for management).

• Advise that fertility may be affected by chemotherapy (fertility may increase as cancer goes into remission or decrease from the chemotherapy); advise discussing birth control measures with physician.

• Caution that administration of vaccines should be avoided (because of decreased resistance) and that contact with children who have recently taken oral polio vaccine should also be avoided.

• Stress that changes in body image are *temporary* (once the chemotherapy regimen is completed, the individual will regain hair and be better able to control weight; some will need to gain, some will need to lose).

• Provide phone numbers of support groups (e.g., American Cancer Society) and written literature that can help people find ways to cope with the day-to-day problems of living with cancer and chemotherapy.

• *Before administering, or for more information, see individual drug.*

Antiparkinsons

Prototype: levodopa

Dopamine precursors
levodopa (Levopa)   carbidopa-levodopa (Sinemet)

Dopamine-releasing agents
amantadine hydrochloride (Symmetrel, ♣Amantadine HCl)

Dopamine receptor agonists
bromocriptine mesylate (Parlodel)   selegiline hydrochloride (Eldepryl)
pergolide mesylate (Permax)

Action   Antiparkinson (dopaminergic) agents control parkinsonian and extrapyramidal symptoms by promoting the natural balance of the neurotransmitters acetylcholine and dopamine in the CNS (dopamine deficiency results in excessive acetylcholine action). The symptoms of Parkinson's disease are probably caused by depleted supplies of dopamine.

The conversion of levodopa to dopamine in the extrapyramidal centers of the brain reverses the deficiency in dopamine. Carbidopa is added to the preparation to reduce the amount of levodopa required; it prevents peripheral metabolism of levodopa. Amantadine increases the release of dopamine from presynaptic nerve endings, delays dopamine uptake, and may have anticholinergic actions. Bromocriptine, pergolide, and selegiline directly stimulate dopamine receptors in the extrapyramidal centers and in the hypothalamus.

- *Anticholinergics also have antiparkinsonian actions. They inhibit acetylcholine, thus reducing the cholinergic-to-dopaminergic ratio toward normal. See Anticholinergics overview.*

Use/Therapeutic goal/Outcome

Used to treat Parkinson's disease and to control symptoms of drug-induced extrapyramidal disorders. *Therapeutic goal*: Promotion of normal motor function. *Outcome criteria:* Absence of (or significant decrease in) tremors, rigidity, akinesia, drooling; improvement in gait, balance, posture, speech, and handwriting.

Dose range/Administration

The dose range is variable and highly individualized, depending on the drug and the individual response, severity of symptoms, age, height, and weight.

These drugs are given after food, to reduce GI symptoms and promote absorption.

Interaction alert: Pyridoxine, monoamine oxidase inhibitors (MAOIs), benzodiazepines, phenytoin, phenothiazines, and haloperidol may antagonize the effects of levodopa.

Contraindications/Precautions

Contraindicated in hypersensitivity to the drug, ergot derivatives, or tartrazine (which may be present in some brands); and in narrow-angle glaucoma, psychosis, MAOI therapy. *Use with caution* in cardiac disease, pyloric obstruction, or prostatic enlargement.

Safe use for pregnant or nursing mothers and for children has not been established.

Side effects/Adverse reactions

Hypersensitivity: rash, flushing, dermatitis, ergotism. *CV:* orthostatic hypotension arrhythmias. *GI:* nausea, vomiting, dry mouth, constipation. *CNS:* confusion, abnormal involuntary movements. *GU:* urinary retention. *Eye:* blurred vision.

Nursing implications/Documentation

Possible nursing diagnoses: Impaired physical mobility; Constipation; Potential for injury.

- Establish baseline profile of abilities and disabilities to differentiate disease symptoms from drug-induced adverse reactions.
- Monitor vital signs, especially during dosage adjustment; report and document significant changes.
- Report side effects promptly, especially muscle twitching and spasmodic winking (early signs of overdosage).
- Supervise ambulation until response is determined.
- Monitor bowel function, and provide adequate fluids and fiber; give stool softeners and laxatives before problem becomes severe.
- Report signs of deteriorating mental status or psychosis (may require discontinuing the medication).

Patient & family teaching/Home care

Possible nursing diagnoses: Knowledge deficit; Impaired home maintenance management.

- Explain that it may take several months to achieve maximum effect.
- Teach that avoiding high-protein foods or concentrated proteins at one meal enhances effects (levodopa competes with amino acids for transport to the brain).
- Stress the need for ongoing medical follow-up; warn that suddenly stopping these drugs may cause parkinsonian crisis 1–3 days later.
- If patient experiences insomnia, suggest taking last dose earlier in the day.
- Caution to change position slowly to prevent orthostatic hypotension and dizziness.
- Point out that driving and other activities that require alertness should be avoided until response is determined (drug may initially cause drowsiness).
- Teach the need to prevent constipation through daily exercise and adequate fluid and fiber intake.

- *Before administering, or for more information, see individual drugs.*

Antipsychotics

Prototype: chlorpromazine hydrochloride

Phenothiazines

acetophenazine maleate (Tindal)

chlorpromazine hydrochloride (Thorazine, ♣Chlorpromanyl)

fluphenazine decanoate, enanthate, and hydrochoride (Prolixin)

mesoridazine besylate (Serentil)

perphenazine (Trilafon, ♣Phenazine)

thioridazine hydrochloride (Mellaril, ♣Apo-Thioridazine)

trifluoperazine hydrochloride (Stelazine, ♣Calmazine)

Thioxanthenes

chlorprothixene (Taractan, ♣Tarasan)

thiothixene hydrochloride (Navane)

Butyrophenones

haloperidol (Haldol, ♣Peridol)

Dibenzoxazepines

loxapine hydrochloride and succinate (Loxitane, ♣Loxapac)

Dibenzodiazapines

clozapine (Clozaril)

Dihydroindolones

molindone hydrochloride (Moban)

◆ *For information on lithium carbonate and reserpine, see individual drug.*

Action   Antipsychotics relieve symptoms of psychoses (in particular, aggressiveness and hostility, anxiety, hyperactivity, sleep disturbances, hallucinations, delusions, paranoia, and withdrawal), which are thought to be related to abnormal dopaminergic or alpha-adrenergic activity in the CNS. The causes of these symptoms have not been determined with certainty; therefore, an antipsychotic mechanism has not been precisely determined. It probably involves antagonism or interference with dopamine (or, for some drugs, alpha-adrenergic) transmission in the CNS. Their side effects are related to these actions and to anticholinergic and serotonergic actions in the CNS and peripheral nervous system.

Antipsychotics may be classified by chemical structure into six major categories:

1 **Phenothiazines**

2 **Thioxanthenes**

3 **Butyrophenones**

4 **Dibenzoxazepines**

5 **Dibenzodiazapines**

6 **Dihydroindolones**

These structural differences cause variations in potency, duration of action, and tendency to promote certain side effects. At usual dosages, low-potency antipsychotics (e.g., phenothiazines) are more likely to cause sedation but are less likely to cause extrapyramidal side effects. Potent antipsychotics (e.g., haloperidol, a butyrophenone) are less sedating but are more likely to produce extrapyramidal side effects early in treatment.

Use/Therapeutic goal/Outcome

Used to treat schizophrenia and other psychotic disorders. ***Therapeutic goal:*** Promotion of reality orientation, elimination of hyperactivity and agitation. ***Outcome criteria:*** Demonstration of better reality orientation, problem-solving ability, and improved interpersonal interactions; decreased hyperactivity and agitation.

◆ *The phenothiazines may also be used as antiemetics and as sedatives. See Antiemetics and Antianxiety agents, Sedatives, and Hypnotics overviews.*

Dose range/Administration

Dosage depends on the drug, severity of illness, concomitant use of other medications, individual response, age, height, and weight. Factors that influence the choice of agent and dosage include physician preferences, previous response, and the incidence of side effects. High doses may be required early in treatment, but for maintenance therapy they are titrated to the lowest effective dose.

Contraindications/Precautions

Contraindicated in hypersensitivity to the drug and in prostatic hypertrophy and urinary obstruction. ***Use with caution*** in suicidal tendencies, and in liver or kidney disease.

🖑 **Contraindicated for pregnant and nursing mothers. Use with caution for children and the elderly.**

Side effects/Adverse reactions

Hypersensitivity: rash, abdominal pain, jaundice (probably a hepatic hypersensitivity reaction; most commonly seen with chlorpromazine), blood dyscrasias. ***CV:*** orthostatic hypotension, hypertension, palpitations. ***CNS:*** drowsiness;

extrapyramidal reactions (including pseudopar-kinsonism, akathisia, acute dystonia), tardive dyskinesia, and neuroleptic malignant syn-drome. *Eye:* blurred vision, photophobia. *Resp:* nasal congestion, dyspnea. *Hem:* hyperglycemia. *GI:* dry mouth, constipation, diarrhea, weight gain. *Skin:* photosensitivity, gray-blue pigmentation. *GU:* prostatitis, uri-nary retention, urinary frequency, impaired ejaculation, impotence, priapism, amenorrhea. *Misc:* gynocomastia, galactorrhea, fever.

Nursing implications/Documentation

Possible nursing diagnoses: Altered thought pro-cesses; Potential for injury; Constipation; Altered oral mucous membrane; Urinary reten-tion.

✦ Ascertain that CBC, BUN, creatinine, and liver function studies have been performed before giving first dose, and check these peri-odically thereafter.

✦ Be sure that PO doses are swallowed (not hoarded).

✦ Monitor for orthostatic hypotension, dizzi-ness, and drowsiness; supervise activities until response has been determined.

✦ Record weight every 2 weeks; report signifi-cant weight gain or loss.

✦ Provide special mouth care; observe for and report oral ulcers.

✦ Prevent constipation by monitoring bowel movements and by ensuring adequate fiber and fluid intake; offer laxatives or stool soften-ers before problem becomes severe.

✦ Monitor for urinary retention; report persis-tent retention.

✦ Report persistent sore throat, fever, and mal-aise (these may be signs of agranulocytosis); report muscle rigidity, high fever, respiratory distress, tachycardia, or tremors (may indicate neuroleptic malignant syndrome).

Patient & family teaching/Home care

Possible nursing diagnoses: Sleep pattern dis-turbance; Knowledge deficit; Impaired home maintenance management.

✦ Emphasize the need to continue medication, even when feeling well.

✦ Explain that changing positions slowly will help prevent dizziness.

✦ Stress that the effects of alcohol, sedatives, and tranquilizers may be potentiated.

✦ Caution to consult with physician before using OTC drugs; stress the need for ongoing medical follow-up.

✦ Provide a list of side effects that should be reported: involuntary movements, muscular rigidity, tremor, fever, respiratory distress, tachycardia, persistent sore throat.

✦ Point out that doses should not be increased or stopped without checking with physician.

✦ Caution to wear sunscreen (Number 15), pro-tective clothing, and sunglasses when in the sun.

✦ Advise avoiding driving and other potentially hazardous activities until response has been established.

✦ Suggest using ice chips, hard candy, or gum to relieve dry mouth; stress the need for good mouth care.

✦ Warn women to report if pregnancy is planned or suspected.

✦ *Before administering, or for more information, see individual drugs.*

Antitussives/expectorants

Prototypes: acetylcysteine, guaifenesin

Antitussives

benzonatate (Tessalon)	diphenhydramine
codeine	hydrochloride (Benadryl)
dextromethorphan	
hydrobromide (Benylin	
DM)	

Expectorants and Mucolytics

acetylcysteine (Mucomyst, ❦ ♣ Parvolex)	iodinated glycerol (Organidin)
ammonium chloride	potassium iodide (SSKI)
guaifenesin (Robitussin)	terpin hydrate

Action *Antitussives* suppress coughing centrally by depressing the cough center in the medulla or peripherally by inhibiting pulmonary stretch, thus decreasing impulses to the cough center.

Expectorants and mucolytics facilitate expulsion of mucus by reducing its viscosity, adhesive-ness, and surface tension and by promoting secretion from mucous membranes.

✦ *Codeine and hydrocodone are narcotics (see Analgesics overview). Diphenhydramine is an antihistamine (see Antihistamines overview).*

Use/Therapeutic goal/Outcome

Antitussives: Used to suppress nonproductive or excessive coughing (excessive coughing jars bronchial tissues and predisposes individuals to bronchial inflammation). *Therapeutic goal:* Reduction of coughing, promotion of rest, and prevention of inflammation of the bronchial tree. *Outcome criteria:* Absence of (or decrease in) coughing.

Expectorants: Used to facilitate productive coughs. *Therapeutic goal:* Enhance removal of respiratory tract secretions. *Outcome criteria:* Improved ability to cough up mucus; clearing of lung fields after coughing.

Dose range/Administration

Dosage depends on the drug, individual responses, age, height, and weight.

Guaifenesin is the only FDA-approved expectorant. The efficacy of ammonium chloride, iodinated glycerol, potassium iodide, and terpin hydrate has not been established.

Give antitussives after meals. Give expectorants before meals, and encourage the patient to cough up excessive mucus before eating (coughing on a full stomach may induce vomiting).

Contraindications/Precautions

Contraindicated in hypersensitivity to the drugs.

Side effects/Adverse reactions

Hypersensitivity: pruritus, rash. Because each drug is unique, specific side effects are detailed under the individual drug.

Nursing implications/Documentation

Possible nursing diagnoses: Ineffective airway clearance; Fluid volume deficit; Potential for infection.

◆ Monitor lungs sounds and color, odor, and character of sputum production; report purulent, foul-smelling, or increased production of sputum.

◆ Report sudden onset of shortness of breath immediately.

◆ Record temperature, pulse, and respiration 4 times a day; report elevations to physician.

◆ Ensure adequate hydration by providing at least 2000 cc fluids daily; record daily intake.

◆ Consult with physician about using a humidifier.

◆ Provide mouth care after session of expectorating mucus.

Patient & family teaching/Home care

Possible nursing diagnoses: Knowledge deficit; Impaired home maintenance management.

◆ Stress the need to take antitussives after meals.

◆ Point out that taking expectorants and working to clear lungs *before meals* helps promote expectoration without causing nausea; teach to cough effectively.

◆ Teach the importance of maintaining adequate hydration; advise asking physician about using a humidifier.

◆ Caution to report if onset of (or increase in) shortness of breath occurs with activity.

◆ For smokers, reinforce that smoking should be avoided, at least until well again.

◆ *Before administering, or for more information, see individual drugs.*

Beta-adrenergic blockers

Prototype: propranolol

Selective beta-blockers

acebutolol (Sectral)	metoprolol tartrate
atenolol (Tenormin)	(Lopressor)
esmolol hydrochloride	
(Brevibloc)	

Nonselective beta-blockers

carteolol hydrochloride	penbutolol sulfate (Levatol)
(Cartrol)	pindolol (Visken)
labetalol hydrochloride	propranolol hydrochloride
(Normodyne)	(Inderal)
nadolol (Corgard)	timolol maleate (Blocadren)

Action Most beta-adrenergic blockers (betablockers) inhibit the fight-or-flight response of the sympathetic nervous system; that is, they decrease the rate and force of cardiac contraction and reduce blood pressure by blocking the action of norepinephrine and epinephrine (adrenergic neurotransmitters). Norepinephrine and epinephrine promote transmission of impulses that make the heart beat faster and with greater force and cause the blood vessels to constrict. When a beta-blocker competes with norepinephrine and epinephrine at the adrenergic receptor sites, it interrupts these impulses.

Beta-blockers delay atrioventricular conduction, decrease heart rate, and decrease force of contraction, thereby reducing myocardial oxygen demand (antianginal action). Propranolol, and to a lesser extent metoprolol, have a membrane-stabilizing, "quinidine-like" effect (which relates to their antiarrhythmic action). By decreasing plasma renin secretion in the kidney, beta-blockers prevent the formation of angiotensin II, a very potent vasoconstrictor, and the secretion of aldosterone. Through this action, beta-blockers prevent sodium and water retention and peripheral vasoconstriction (antihypertensive action).

♦ *See overviews of Antianginals, Antiarrhythmics, and Antihypertensives for additional information.*

Beta-blockers are classified according to the sites they block:

1 **Beta-1 (selective) beta-blockers** block only receptors in cardiac tissue.

2 **Beta-2 (nonselective) beta-blockers** block receptors located both in cardiac tissue and in other tissues (mainly in the bronchi, vascular smooth muscle, and uterus).

Beta-1 blocker cardioselectivity is dose-dependent. At low doses beta-1 blockers block mainly beta-1 (cardiac) sites. At high doses, beta-1 blockers also block beta-2 receptor sites, increasing airway resistance in the bronchioles (causing bronchoconstriction) and inhibiting vasodilation of peripheral blood vessels. Because beta-blockers inhibit the fight-or-flight response, people who take these agents may not have the usual physiologic response to stress (e.g., heart rate may not rise with fever, diabetic shock, or hypotension).

Use/Therapeutic goal/Outcome

Beta-blockers may be used to treat the following: hypertension, angina, arrhythmias, migraine conditions, idiopathic hypertrophic subaortic stenosis (IHSS), mitral valve prolapse (MVP), glaucoma, pheochromocytoma, hyperthyroidism. They are also used to reduce post-myocardial infarction mortality. The most common uses and corresponding therapeutic goals and outcome criteria are listed below.

Hypertension. **Therapeutic goal:** blood pressure stable, within normal range, and tolerated by the patient. **Outcome criteria:** diastolic blood pressure < 90 mm Hg; absence of headache and visual disturbances.

Angina. **Therapeutic goal:** decrease in oxygen demand of the myocardium. **Outcome criteria:** report of decrease in or absence of chest pain, increased exercise tolerance.

Arrhythmias. **Therapeutic goal:** control of tachyarrhythmias and ectopy. **Outcome criteria:**

absence of or reduction in tachyarrhythmias and ectopy.

Migraine headache. **Therapeutic goal:** prevention of cerebral vasodilation. **Outcome criteria:** report of decrease in or absence of headache.

Dose range/Administration

Dosage depends on the drug, severity of the problem, route of administration, individual response, health status, age, height, weight, and nutritional status. Impaired renal or hepatic function may alter dose requirements. Measurement of heart rate and blood pressure are generally used as a guide to titrating doses. Most beta-blockers are given twice daily; some are effective when given once a day.

Contraindications/Precautions

Contraindicated in hypersensitivity to the drug and in cardiogenic shock, sinus bradycardia, second- or third-degree heart block, PR interval > 0.24 seconds, overt congestive heart failure (CHF), and pulmonary disease. **Use with caution** in diabetes and severe liver disease. Beta blockers are not to be discontinued abruptly.

👋 **Use with caution for pregnant and nursing mothers.**

Side effects/Adverse reactions

Hypersensitivity: rash, pruritus. **CV:** bradycardia, hypotension, CHF, cold extremities, edema, peripheral vascular disease. **GI:** nausea, vomiting, diarrhea, constipation, dry mouth. **CNS:** fatigue, vivid dreams, depression, insomnia, nervousness, vertigo, paresthesias. **Resp:** dyspnea, asthma-like symptoms, increased airway resistance, bronchospasm. **Hem:** hyperglycemia, hypoglycemia. **MS:** joint and muscle pain.

Nursing implications/Documentation

Possible nursing diagnoses: Activity intolerance; Fatigue; Potential for injury.

♦ Assess mental status; document pulse and blood pressure (if possible, lying, sitting, and standing, in both arms) prior to administration and frequently thereafter until response is determined.

♦ Consult with physician to determine desired therapeutic range for blood pressure and heart rate (be aware that parameters for withholding the medication are written by physician).

OVERVIEW

• Ascertain that baseline CBC, electrolytes, BUN, creatinine, and liver function studies have been obtained before giving first dose; report abnormalities, and monitor closely thereafter.

• Monitor for hypersensitivity reactions and for symptoms of confusion, dizziness, bradycardia, CHF, and hypotension; if these occur, withhold drug, and report immediately.

• If drug is given IV, keep patient in bed with side rails up; once patient is allowed out of bed, supervise ambulation until response is determined.

• Allow for a balance between rest and activity.

• Monitor and document daily weight and intake and output; report significant negative or positive balance.

Patient & family teaching/Home care

Possible nursing diagnoses: Knowledge deficit; Impaired home maintenance management.

• Explain the importance of taking these drugs exactly as prescribed, even when feeling well; warn not to discontinue beta-blockers abruptly (may precipitate angina or arrhythmias).

• Emphasize the importance of good medical follow-up. Explain that the drug reduces "wear and tear" on blood vessels, reduces the workload of the heart, and improves longevity and health.

• Explore feelings concerning ability to follow medication regimen.

• Teach how to monitor pulse and blood pressure; stress the need to report syncope, hypertension or hypotension, or persistent dizziness; provide pulse and blood pressure parameters for withholding medication.

• Advise changing positions slowly to avoid dizziness.

• Encourage daily monitoring of weight and reporting sudden weight gain (likely to be fluid retention).

• Warn against drinking alcohol or taking OTC drugs without physician's approval (some interactions can cause severe reactions).

• Advise against excessive exposure to cold; stress that persistent coldness in feet or hands must be reported.

• Discuss holistic measures of enhancing effect of antihypertensives and antianginals includ-

ing weight control, salt reduction, daily exercise, and stress-reduction techniques.

• *Before administering, or for more information, see individual drug.*

Bronchodilators

Prototype: theophylline
albuterol (Proventil)
aminophylline (♦Corophyllin)
bitolterol mesylate (Tornalate)
ephedrine hydrochloride (Fedrine)
ephedrine sulfate (Ephed II)
epinephrine (Bronkaid)
epinephrine bitartrate (AsthmaHaler)
epinephrine hydrochloride (Sus-Phrine)
ipratropium bromide (Atrovent)
isoetharine hydrochloride (Bronkosol)
isoetharine mesylate (Bronkometer)
isoproterenol (Isuprel)
isoproterenol hydrochloride (Isuprel Hydrochloride)
isoproterenol sulfate (Medihaler-Iso)
metaproterenol sulfate (Alupent)
pirbuterol acetate (Maxair)
terbutaline sulfate (Brethine)
theophylline (Theo-Dur)

• **Many of these drugs are also adrenergics. Their specific use as bronchodilators is addressed here.**

Action Brochodilators prevent or reverse bronchospasm by relaxing the smooth muscles of the bronchial walls:

1 **Aminophylline and theophylline** increase tissue concentration of cyclic adenosine monophosphate (c-AMP).

2 The adrenergics mimic the sympathetic nervous system acting on beta-2 adrenergic receptors in the bronchioles.

Bronchodilators also stimulate the heart and CNS because of their sympathomimetic action.

Use/Therapeutic goal/Outcome

Used to treat bronchospasm associated with asthma, obstructive airway disease, and bronchitis. *Therapeutic goal:* Relief of bronchospasm, improvement in air movement. *Outcome criteria:* Clearing of lung fields upon auscultation, increase in FEV_1, report of breathing more easily, satisfactory arterial blood gases and oxygen saturation.

Dose range/Administration

Dosage depends on the drug, route of administration, health state, age, height, weight, nutritional status, metabolic status, severity of side effects (e.g., tachycardia, arrhythmias), and individual absorption rates. Depending on the drug and the severity of the problem, these drugs are administered PO, SC, IM, IV, RECT, and INHAL. Absorption of suppository form is highly erratic and unpredictable.

Contraindications/Precautions

Contraindicated in hypersensitivity to the drug or to a closely related drug and in preexisting dysrhythmias. **Use with caution** in cardiac problems.

Side effects/Adverse reactions

Hypersensitivity: dizziness, flushing, rash, hives, swelling of face, lips, or eyelids, difficulty breathing. **CNS:** headache, tremors, nervousness. **CV:** tachycardia, dysrhythmias.

Nursing implications/Documentation

Possible nursing diagnoses: Ineffective airway clearance; Potential for injury; Activity intolerance.

♦ Auscultate lungs before and after administration; document sputum production and response.

♦ Monitor closely for tachycardia and dysrhythmias; if these are significant, withhold drug, and report.

♦ Pace activity to allow for rest periods.

♦ Observe for dizziness; if this is present, keep patient in bed during treatment.

Patient & family teaching/Home care

Possible nursing diagnoses: Knowledge deficit; Impaired home maintenance management; Anxiety; Fear.

♦ Explore factors that cause asthma attacks (environmental, emotional), and teach holistic measures for reducing stress and how to cope with panic response.

♦ Instruct the patient to report palpitations or an increase in dyspnea; teach pursed lip and diaphragmatic breathing.

♦ Have the patient demonstrate method of administration (inhalation, injection, or suppository) before discharge.

♦ Warn against taking OTC drugs without checking with physician because of risk of interaction.

♦ Explain the importance of maintaining adequate hydration.

♦ Encourage verbalizing fears and concerns. Point out that having difficulty in breathing can add to feelings of anxiety and fear. If these feelings are not expressed, they can compound the problem; if they are expressed, the nurse can better help the patient.

♦ *Before administering, or for more information, see individual drug.*

Calcium channel blockers

Prototype: verapamil
diltiazem hydrochloride (Cardizem)
nicardipine (Cardene)
nifedipine (Procardia)
nimodipine (Nimotop)
verapamil hydrochloride (Calan)

Action Calcium channel blockers dilate vascular smooth muscle (including coronary arteries), decrease myocardial contractility, decrease heart rate, slow atrioventricular conduction, and reduce cardiac oxygen demand by preventing calcium ions from entering cells. Calcium channels are specialized pores located within the cell membrane that regulate the entry of calcium ions. In cardiac tissue and vascular smooth muscle, the influx of calcium ions is critical to cell function and muscle contraction. Blockage of calcium alters cell behavior. Calcium channel blockers differ from one another in their ability to block calcium channels at specific locations. Verapamil and diltiazem block calcium channels in vascular smooth muscle and in the heart. Nifedipine, nicardipine, and nimodipine act primarily on calcium channels of the vascular smooth muscle.

Use/Therapeutic goal/Outcome

Calcium channel blockers may be used to treat the following: hypertension, angina, arrhythmias, and subarachnoid hemorrhage (nimodipine only). They are new agents whose therapeutic potential is yet to be fully revealed. Other uses under investigation include prophylaxis for migraine headache and treatment of manic-depressive disorders, Raynaud's disease, asthma, cardiomyopathies, esophageal disorders and preterm labor.

Some common approved uses and corresponding therapeutic goals and outcome criteria are listed below.

Hypertension. Therapeutic goal: blood pressure stable, within normal range, and tolerated by patient. **Outcome criteria:** blood pressure within normal limits; absence of headache and visual disturbance.

Angina. Therapeutic goal: decreased oxygen demand of the myocardium. **Outcome criteria:**

reported decrease in or absence of chest pain, increased exercise tolerance.

Arrhythmias. Therapeutic goal: control of tachyarrhythmias. ***Outcome criteria:*** Absence of tachyarrhythmias.

Subarachnoid hemorrhage. Therapeutic goal: Improvement in neurologic deficits. ***Outcome criteria:*** increased level of consciousness, return of motor function.

Dose range/Administration

Dosage depends on the drug, indication, age, height, weight, and severity of condition and response tolerance. Heart rate, blood pressure, and intensity of chest pain are generally used as a guide to dosage titration. Other factors that influence dosage are route of administration (PO or IV) and use of other medications that enhance or decrease drug action. Impaired hepatic function may alter dosage requirements.

👋 **Children and the elderly usually require lower doses.**

Contraindications/Precautions

Contraindicated in hypersensitivity to the drug and in cardiogenic shock, sinus bradycardia, second- or third-degree heart block, advanced congestive heart failure (CHF), and symptomatic hypotension. ***Use with caution*** in hepatic or renal disease and in patients who are also receiving digitalis and beta-blockers.

Side effects/Adverse reactions

Hypersensitivity: rash, pruritus, extreme hypotension. ***CV:*** bradycardia, hypotension, CHF, edema. ***GI:*** nausea, constipation. ***CNS:*** fatigue, dizziness, headache. ***Misc:*** elevated liver enzymes.

Nursing implications/Documentation

Possible nursing diagnoses: Activity intolerance; Fatigue; Potential for injury.

◆ Assess mental status, and document pulse and blood pressure (if possible, lying, sitting, and standing, in both arms) before administration and frequently thereafter until response is determined.

◆ Consult with physician to determine desired therapeutic range for blood pressure and heart rate (be aware that parameters for withholding the medication are written by physician).

◆ Ascertain that baseline CBC, electrolytes, BUN, creatinine, and liver function studies are obtained before giving first dose; report abnormalities, and monitor closely thereafter.

◆ Monitor for hypersensitivity reactions and for symptoms of confusion, dizziness, bradycardia, CHF, or hypotension; if these occur, withhold drug, and report immediately.

◆ If drug is given IV, keep patient in bed with side rails up; once patient is allowed out of bed, supervise ambulation until response is determined.

◆ Monitor and document daily weight and intake and output; report significant negative or positive balance.

Patient & family teaching/Home care

Possible nursing diagnoses: Knowledge deficit; Impaired home maintenance management; Noncompliance.

◆ Explain the importance of taking these drugs exactly as prescribed, even when feeling well; warn not to discontinue calcium channel blockers abruptly (may exacerbate signs and symptoms).

◆ Emphasize the need for ongoing medical follow-up; explain that the drug reduces "wear and tear" on blood vessels, reduces the workload of the heart, and improves longevity and health.

◆ Teach how to monitor pulse and blood pressure; emphasize the need to report syncope, bradycardia, hypertension or hypotension, or persistent dizziness; provide pulse and blood pressure parameters for withholding medication.

◆ Advise changing positions slowly to avoid dizziness.

◆ Encourage daily monitoring of weight and reporting sudden weight gain (likely to be fluid retention).

◆ *Before administering, or for more information, see individual drugs.*

Cerebral stimulants

Prototype: dextroamphetamine sulfate
- amphetamine sulfate
- caffeine (Vivarin)
- dextroamphetamine sulfate (Dexedrine)
- methamphetamine hydrochloride (Desoxyn)
- methylphenidate hydrochloride (Ritalin)
- pemoline (Cylert)

Action Central nervous system (CNS) stimulants release stored norepinephrine from nerve terminals, resulting in respiratory stimulation, appetite suppression, increased energy, increased mental alertness, and improved spirits. In adults, there is a stimulant effect; in children with Attention Deficit Disorders with Hyperactivity (ADDH), there usually is a paradoxical calming effect. Peripherally, cerebral stimulants cause vasoconstriction, pupillary dilation, and constriction of the urinary sphincter. Caffeine is a phosphorodiesterase inhibitor (its mechanism differs), but it has central and respiratory stimulant actions also.

Use/Therapeutic goal/Outcome

Amphetamines and methylphenidate are used to treat narcolepsy. *Therapeutic goal:* prevention of sleep episodes. *Outcome criteria:* Absence of (or decrease in) episodes of narcolepsy.

For children > 6 yrs: Amphetamines, methylphenidate, and pemoline are used to treat ADDH. *Therapeutic goal:* improvement of attention span. *Outcome criteria:* Increased ability to sit still, concentrate, and pay attention.

Amphetamines may be prescribed for short-term appetite suppression. Caffeine is often used as a self-prescribed stimulant.

Dose range/Administration

The effects of doses of these drugs are highly individual. Dose range depends on the drug, the indication, and individual responses. Age, height, weight, and health status also affect dosage. Children, and many adults, are very sensitive to cerebral stimulants. To prevent insomnia, the last dose of these drugs is given in the early afternoon, no later than 6 hours before bedtime. Extended-release form should be taken early in the a.m., 10–14 hours before bedtime.

🖐 **Children receiving cerebral stimulants for treatment of ADDH usually undergo periodic "drug holidays" to determine whether the drug is still necessary. Dosage is decreased as children approach puberty and discontinued after puberty.**

Caffeine is commonly found in beverages and OTC medications. Caffeine in beverages (coffee, tea, or cola) is the most commonly used stimulant among adults. Excessive amounts are sometimes consumed to combat fatigue and promote alertness. Today, caffeine use is discouraged because of the potential long-term cardiovascular effects. **Amphetamines** and the other related cerebral stimulants are controlled substances that have a high potential for drug addiction and abuse. They are given only by prescription, under strict medical supervision.

Contraindications/Precautions

Contraindicated in hypersensitivity or intolerance to cerebral stimulants and in hypertension, angina, cardiovascular disease, hyperthyroidism, glaucoma, or history of drug abuse.

🖐 **Most are contraindicated for children under 6 years and pregnant or nursing mothers. Only used for narcolepsy in the elderly; use with caution.**

Side effects/Adverse reactions

Hypersensitivity: itching, rashes. **CNS:** insomnia, restlessness, hyperactivity, nervousness, headache, tremors, twitches. **CV:** palpitations, tachycardia. **GI:** nausea, vomiting, constipation. **Misc:** drug dependence, tolerance.

Nursing implications/Documentation

Possible nursing diagnoses: Altered thought processes; Sleep pattern disturbance; Constipation; Altered nutrition: less than body requirements.

◆ Question carefully regarding use of OTC drugs and beverages containing caffeine.

◆ Monitor attention span and ability to concentrate, and report and document changes in status (dosage may need adjustment).

◆ Document blood pressure at least daily when beginning therapy, and periodically once stabilized.

◆ Document daily weight, and record food intake to ensure adequate nutrition; provide decaffeinated beverages.

◆ Prevent side effect of constipation by monitoring bowel movements, ensuring adequate hydration, and providing fruits, juices, and vegetables (use laxatives only when necessary).

◆ Monitor for sleep pattern disturbance, and avoid giving doses within 6 hours of bedtime.

Patient & family teaching/Home care

Possible nursing diagnoses: Knowledge deficit; Impaired home maintenance management.

◆ Explain that amphetamines have a high potential for abuse and should be taken only as prescribed under continuous medical supervision.

◆ If the drug is used as an appetite suppressant, stress the importance of enrolling in behavior modification weight reduction program.

♦ Stress the importance of reading labels and avoiding caffeine (may increase stimulant effects).

♦ Emphasize that side effect of constipation can be avoided by drinking plenty of fluids, eating fruits and fiber, ensuring adequate exercise, and using mild laxatives when necessary.

♦ If caffeine is used as a stimulant, explore reasons for feeling the need for a stimulant, and discuss holistic measures of promoting health (getting proper rest and exercise).

♦ For children, teach the need to monitor physical and mental growth and the need to report failure to grow or extremes in behavior (dosage may require adjustment).

♦ Point out the need for gradual withdrawal with tapering of doses to avoid withdrawal symptoms (headache, fatigue, depression).

Before administering, or for more information, see individual drug.

♦

Cholinergics

> **Prototype:** neostigmine
> ambenonium chloride (Mytelase)
> bethanechol chloride (Urecholine)
> edrophonium chloride (Tensilon)
> methacholine chloride (Provocholine)
> neostigmine bromide
> neostigmine methylsulfate (Prostigmin)
> physostigmine salicylate (Antilirium)
> pilocarpine (Isopto Carpine)
> pyridostigmine bromide (Mestinon)

Action When given in required doses, cholinergics (parasympathomimetics) promote muscle tone and function by increasing the concentration of the neurotransmitter acetylcholine at postganglionic parasympathetic receptors or by stimulating the receptors directly. Acetylcholine transmits nerve impulses from nerve cells to muscle cells (neuromuscular junctions). Excessive or deficient acetylcholine may cause *neuromuscular blockade*: If doses are greater than required or less than required, muscle tone and function may be *reduced*, even paralyzed.

Cholinergics are either direct acting or indirect acting:

♦ **Direct-acting cholinergics** stimulate the cholinergic receptors.

♦ **Indirect-acting cholinergics** prevent the breakdown of acetylcholine by inhibiting the enzyme cholinesterase at skeletal neuromuscular junctions.

Cholinergics mimic the parasympathetic nervous system, conserving energy and producing the following effects on organs or systems (many of these effects are blocked by atropine):

Eye: pupillary constriction (miosis), increased tearing, decreased night vision, impaired distance vision (myopia).

Resp: Increased bronchial secretions, constriction of airway passages.

CV: Decreased speed of cardiac impulse conduction and heart rate, possible reflex tachycardia and decrease in blood pressure.

GI: Increased salivary secretions, gastric secretions, intestinal motility.

GU: Stimulation of urination (cholinergics constrict the detrusor muscle of the bladder and relax the trigone muscle and sphincter).

Skin: Increased sweating, flushing.

Use/Therapeutic goal/Outcome

Cholinergics have many, varied uses including those for urinary retention (bethanechol and neostigmine), glaucoma (pilocarpine), myasthenia gravis (ambenonium chloride, pyridostigmine bromide, neostigmine, edrophonium chloride —for diagnosis only), reversal of anesthesia (edrophonium chloride), abdominal distention and ileus (neostigmine and bethanechol), supraventricular tachycardia (edrophonium chloride), diagnosis of asthma (methacholine), CNS toxicity associated with overdose of anticholinergics and tricyclic antidepressants (physostigmine salicylate).

♦ *For therapeutic goals and outcome criteria, see individual drugs.*

Dose range/Administration

Dosage and route of administration depend on the drug, indication, and the individual's response, age, height, weight, and health state. Depending on the drug and the indication, cholinergics may be given PO, SC, IM, IV, INHAL, or OPTH. Not all of these drugs can be given by all of these routes; for example, bethanechol chloride is *never* given IM or IV.

Clinical alert: When used to treat myasthenia gravis, give cholinergics *exactly on time* to maintain therapeutic levels and avoid cholinergic crisis. Remember that in myasthenia gravis there is a very fine line between therapeutic range and toxic range. Always keep atropine nearby to reverse cholinergic crisis, especially during systemic administration. Give PO doses with food.

Contraindications/Precautions

Contraindicated in hypersensitivity to the drug and (for systemic use), in cerebrovascular disease, seizures, obstructive lung diseases, bradycardia, heart block, hyperthyroidism, intestinal or urinary obstruction, peptic ulcer disease, and Parkinson's disease.

☜ **Use with caution in the elderly because of the increased risk of tachycardia, hypotension, and angina.**

Side effects/Adverse reactions

Hypersensitivity: skin rash. **Eye:** tearing, photophobia, problems with distance vision (these reactions are associated with systemic administration; side effects of ophthalmic administration are rare). **CNS:** dizziness, lightheadedness, tremors. **CV:** bradycardia or tachycardia, dysrhythmias, hypotension. **GI:** nausea, vomiting, cramping. **GU:** urinary frequency, uterine cramping.

Nursing implications/Documentation

Possible nursing diagnoses: Altered patterns of urinary elimination; Potential for injury.

◆ Ascertain whether the patient is taking other cholinergics (may increase risk of cholinergic crisis) or anticholinergics (may inhibit desired action—check labels of OTC medications).

◆ Observe carefully for dizziness and lightheadedness, especially after parenteral administration; supervise ambulation until response is determined.

◆ Document pulse and blood pressure daily when beginning systemic therapy; report abnormalities.

◆ For bedridden patients, keep bedpan close at hand (they may experience urinary frequency).

◆ Report signs of excessive cholinergic activity (bradycardia, tachycardia, bronchoconstriction, flushing, sweating, dizziness, diarrhea, cramps).

Patient & family teaching/Home care

Possible nursing diagnoses: Knowledge deficit; Impaired home maintenance management.

◆ Advise taking these drugs with food to reduce GI symptoms.

◆ Stress the need to take these drugs on time, exactly as prescribed, to avoid severe side effects (if a dose is missed, it should be taken as soon as possible *without "doubling up"* on doses).

◆ Provide a list of side effects that should be reported immediately: palpitations, fainting, chest pains, wheezing, difficulty breathing, diarrhea.

◆ *Before administering, or for more information, see individual drugs.*

Diuretics

Prototypes: acetazolamide, furosemide, mannitol, triamterene, hydrochlorothiazide

Carbonic anhydrase inhibitors

acetazolamide (Diamox)	methazolamide (Neptazane)
dichlorphenamide (Daranide)	

Loop (high ceiling) diuretics

bumetanide (Bumex)	furosemide (Lasix)
ethacrynic acid (Edecrin)	

Osmotic diuretics

mannitol (Osmitrol)	urea (Ureaphil)

Potassium-sparing diuretics

amiloride hydrochloride (Midamor)	spironolactone (Aldactone)
	triamterene (Dyrenium)

Thiazide diuretics

benzthiazide (Exna, Aquatag)	methyclothiazide (Enduron)
chlorothiazide (Diuril)	polythiazide (Renese)
cyclothiazide (Anhydron)	trichlormethiazide (Aquazide)
hydrochlorothiazide (HydroDIURIL)	

Thiazide-like diuretics

chlorthalidone (Hygroton)	indapamide (Lozol)
metolazone (Diulo)	quinethazone (Hydromox)

Action Diuretics promote excretion of water, sodium, and (to a lesser extent) other electrolytes by enhancing the work of the kidney. These drugs cannot stimulate a failed kidney, but they can increase the output of a partially functioning or overtaxed kidney.

The kidney serves three major functions:

◆ **Elimination of excess fluid and reabsorption of useful metabolites.**

◆ **Maintenance of acid-base balance.**

◆ **Promotion of fluid and electrolyte balance.**

When kidney function is compromised, the individual is at risk for electrolyte imbalance and fluid retention.

Diuretics are categorized into five groups:

1 **Carbonic anhydrase inhibitors (CAIs)** are mild diuretics that have short-lived diuretic activity. In the eye, these drugs reduce intraocular pressure by decreasing formation of aqueous humor. In the kidney, they promote excretion of bicarbonate, sodium, potassium, and water by acting in the proximal tubule cells. The increased excretion of bicarbonate causes the urine to become more alkaline and tends to induce metabolic acidosis (which eventually counteracts the diuretic action). CAIs also have some anticonvulsant action, probably by inhibiting carbonic anhydrase in the CNS, which reduces abnormal paroxysmal or excessive nerve discharge.

2 **Loop (high-ceiling) diuretics** promote excretion of sodium, chloride, potassium, other electrolytes, and water by inhibiting sodium and chloride reabsorption in the ascending loop of Henle, and by decreasing their reabsorption but increasing potassium loss in the distal tubule.

3 **Osmotic diuretics** promote excretion of sodium, chloride, water, and (to a lesser extent) potassium by increasing the osmotic pressure of glomerular filtrate. Osmotic diuretics are filtered by the kidney but are poorly reabsorbed; osmotic pressure in the tubular fluid causes secretion of an osmotically equivalent amount of water. This osmotic effect also occurs in the bloodstream, where these drugs draw fluid from tissue spaces into the blood, thus decreasing intraocular and intracranial pressure.

4 **Potassium-sparing diuretics** promote excretion of sodium and water by inhibiting the sodium-potassium exchange mechanism in the distal tubule. They are usually used in combination with other agents.

5 **Thiazide and thiazide-like diuretics** promote excretion of sodium, chloride, potassium, and water by decreasing their reabsorption in the distal tubule.

Use/Therapeutic goal/Outcome

Diuretics have many uses, including the following: to enhance the kidney's work in regulating fluid and electrolyte balance when kidney function is compromised or overtaxed; to treat vascular fluid overload and edema associated with congestive heart failure (CHF), hepatic disease, pregnancy, and early kidney failure; and to reduce blood pressure, intraocu-

lar pressure, and brain swelling. ***Therapeutic goal:*** Promotion of sodium and water excretion and reduction of vascular volume and resulting edema. ***Outcome criteria:*** Increased urinary output, weight loss, absence of rales, and absence of peripheral and sacral edema; (for glaucoma) decreased intraocular pressure; (for brain swelling) decreased intracranial pressure (ICP).

Dose range/Administration

The dosage depends on the degree of cardiac and kidney function, route of administration, use of other drugs that may interact, and the individual's health, age, height, weight, and metabolic status. All diuretics are given PO, IM, or IV, with PO and IV being the most common routes. Sometimes these drugs are given in combination for best effects. CAIs have limited use as diuretics and are sometimes given on alternate days to reduce risk of metabolic acidosis.

☙ **Children have immature kidneys and require observation and careful dose calculation (some diuretics are contraindicated for children). The elderly are started on lower doses because of the risk of extreme diuresis and difficulty in adapting to the resulting hemodynamic changes. If response to the low dose is poor, dosage may be increased gradually.**

Contraindications/Precautions

Contraindicated if there is a known hypersensitivity to the drug (or to a drug that is closely related chemically) and hypovolemia, anuria, or hypokalemia (except for potassium-sparing diuretics).

☙ **Contraindicated for nursing mothers. Use with caution in children and the elderly.**

Side effects/Adverse reactions

Hypersensitivity: rash, urticaria, purpura. ***CV:*** orthostatic hypotension, dehydration. ***Hem:*** electrolyte imbalance (hypokalemia is common), hyperglycemia, hyperuricemia.

Nursing implications/Documentation

Possible nursing diagnoses: Fluid volume deficit; Altered patterns of urinary elimination; Potential for injury.

♦ Ascertain that baseline CBC, sodium, potassium, chloride, carbon dioxide, calcium, magnesium, BUN, creatinine, uric acid, and liver function studies have been obtained before giving first dose; report abnormalities, and monitor closely thereafter.

• Give doses in early morning and early afternoon (if possible) to avoid nocturnal diuresis.

• For bedridden patients, keep bedpan close at hand.

• Document and monitor blood pressure, daily weight, and intake and output; report significant discrepancies.

• Monitor for and report signs of fluid overload (auscultate lungs for rales; check feet, ankles, and sacrum for edema).

• Be aware that hypokalemia is often induced by diuretics and predisposes individuals to cardiac arrhythmias, cramping, and digoxin toxicity.

• Check with physician to determine dietary restrictions; if low-salt, high-potassium diet is recommended, consult with dietitian to plan a low-salt diet that includes foods and juices high in potassium (orange juice, bananas, leafy green vegetables).

• Observe the elderly for extreme diuresis (may require lower doses); monitor for orthostatic hypotension; supervise ambulation until response is determined.

Patient & family teaching/Home care

Possible nursing diagnoses: Knowledge deficit; Impaired home maintenance management.

• Before giving first dose, explain that the drug will increase the amount and frequency of urination.

• Explain the importance of taking these drugs exactly as prescribed, even when feeling well.

• Explain that diuretics enhance the work of the kidney and reduce the workload of the heart.

• Recommend taking doses in early morning and early afternoon to prevent the need to disturb sleep to void.

• Advise changing positions slowly to avoid dizziness.

• Stress the need to report dizziness, shortness of breath, swelling of hands and feet, or persistent sore throat; encourage daily monitoring of weight and reporting sudden weight gain (likely to be fluid retention).

• Provide a list of allowed foods and fluids; stress the need to stick to prescribed diet; explain the hazards of too much salt, too little

potassium, or (in renal failure) too much potassium.

• Explain that fatigue may be felt at first but should subside in time.

• Warn against driving or other activities that require alertness until response is determined.

◆ *Before administering, or for more information, see individual drug.*

Histamine₂ antagonists

Prototype: cimetidine
  cimetidine (Tagamet)   ranitidine hydrochloride
  famotidine (Pepcid)   (Zantac)
  nizatidine (Axid)

Action Histamine₂ antagonists decrease secretion of gastric acid by inhibiting the action of histamine at the H₂ receptors.

Use/Therapeutic goal/Outcome

Used to treat gastric and intestinal problems; active duodenal ulcers and benign gastric ulcers; gastroesophageal reflux; and gastric hypersecretion associated with Zollinger-Ellison syndrome, systemic mastocytosis, and multiple endocrine adenoma. Used prophylactically for duodenal ulcers and where the risk for gastric and intestinal ulcers is high (e.g., high-dose steroid treatment, extreme stress such as occurs with mechanical ventilation). **Therapeutic goal:** Reduction of acid secretion, prevention of ulcers, and promotion of healing. **Outcome criteria:** Report of decrease in or absence of nausea and pain, negative occult blood test of stools and gastric secretions, stabilization of hemoglobin and hematocrit, endoscopic evidence of healing.

Dose range/Administration

Dosage depends on the drug, indication, route of administration, age, height, weight, and health state. Histamine₂ antagonists may be given PO, IM, or IV. Although ulcer symptoms may subside within 1–2 weeks of therapy initiation, these drugs are given for 4–8 weeks to ensure healing.

Single PO doses are given at bedtime; bid doses are given with breakfast and at bedtime; qid doses are given with meals and at bedtime.

Interaction alert: Avoid giving these agents within 1 hr of antacids (which are frequently prescribed for ulcer pain but interfere with the absorption of histamine₂ antagonists). Cimetidine has multiple drug interactions that are not evident in other drugs in this class.

Contraindications/Precautions

Contraindicated in hypersensitivity to the specific agent. **Use with caution** in impaired kidney or liver function.

🖑 **Use with caution for children, pregnant or nursing mothers, and the elderly.**

Side effects/Adverse reactions

Hypersensitivity: pruritus, rashes. **CV:** hypotension and tachycardia with rapid infusion (less than 2 minutes). **CNS:** confusion (especially in the elderly). **GU:** gynecomastia or impotence (with use of cimetidine, which has antiandrogenic action).

Nursing implications/Documentation

Possible nursing diagnoses: Potential for injury; Sensory/perceptual alterations.

♦ Give PO doses with meals and at bedtime; if a single daily dose is ordered, give it at bedtime.

♦ Administer IV infusions slowly to prevent hypotension and arrhythmias.

♦ Assess for and report changes in mental status, especially in the elderly taking cimetidine; provide appropriate safety measures.

♦ Monitor results of tests for hepatic and renal function; report abnormalities (dose may need to be altered).

Patient & family teaching/Home care

Possible nursing diagnoses: Knowledge deficit; Impaired home maintenance management.

♦ Stress the need to take antacids as prescribed, especially in the presence of active ulcers; emphasize that antacid doses must be separated from histamine₂ antagonist doses by 1 hr.

♦ With treatment of active ulcers, point out that medication must be taken as prescribed for 4–8 weeks to insure healing, even though symptoms usually subside earlier.

♦ With active ulcer disease, stress the need to stop smoking and to avoid caffeine; after healing, advise against using these substances after the bedtime dose so that there can be optimal suppression of nocturnal gastric acid secretion.

♦ *Before administering, or for more information, see individual drugs.*

Immunosuppressants

Prototypes: azathioprine, cyclosporine
azathioprine (Imuran)   muromonab-CD3
cyclosporine (Sandimmune)   (Orthoclone OKT3)

Action Immunosuppressants reduce the immune response by interfering with the ability of lymphocytes to produce antibodies and killer T cells, which target foreign cells for destruction. Corticosteroids and antineoplastic agents also have immunosuppressant activity, but they act in a much different way (see overviews).

Use/Therapeutic goal/Outcome

Used in organ transplantation. **Therapeutic goal:** Prevent transplanted organ rejection. **Outcome criteria:** Measurable data indicating that the transplanted organ is functioning satisfactorily (for example, in a kidney transplant, a decrease in serum creatinine).

Azathioprine is also used to treat severe refractory rheumatoid arthritis (see azathioprine).

Dose range/Administration

Muromonab-CD3 is given for short-term treatment of acute rejections; azathioprine and cyclosporine are usually used in long-term therapy. Dose requirements for azathioprine and cyclosporine are usually higher immediately after the transplant; if there are no signs of rejection, doses are tapered to maintenance level. Additional factors that influence dosage include individual response, severity of side effects, health state, age, height, weight, nutritional status, and level of kidney and liver function. The route of administration also affects dosage (azathioprine and cyclosporine can be given PO or IV; muromonab-CD3 is given IV). Give these drugs at the same time every day to maintain satisfactory blood levels.

Contraindications/Precautions

Contraindicated in hypersensitivity to the drug and during active clinical infection. **Use with caution** in kidney or liver disease.

🖑 **Use with caution for children, the elderly, and pregnant women (benefits to the mother may outweigh the possible risk to the fetus).**

Side effects/Adverse reactions

The incidence of side effects and adverse reactions is high, especially during the early stages of treatment. **Hypersensitivity:** itching, rashes, chills, fever, headache, shortness of breath, anaphylaxis. *Misc:* increase in bone marrow toxicity when given in kidney insufficiency.

Nursing implications/Documentation

Possible nursing diagnoses: Potential for infection; Altered oral mucous membrane.

• Monitor for and report signs of infection (fever, sore throat, stomatitis, vaginal discharge); avoid assigning health care workers with respiratory symptoms.

• When giving drugs IV, watch closely for onset of side effects, which can be severe with early doses and must be treated promptly; check hospital protocol.

• Document on medication record the need to avoid giving IM injections to reduce risk of infection.

• Provide frequent mouth care.

Patient & family teaching/Home care

Possible nursing diagnoses: Knowledge deficit; Fear; Impaired home maintenance management.

• Point out the need to take drugs on time, exactly as prescribed, to maintain a therapeutic level.

• Explore fears and concerns; stress that the patient will be closely monitored for early detection and treatment of side effects.

• Teach that meticulous oral hygiene can help reduce incidence of oral inflammation.

• Advise avoiding contact with people with respiratory symptoms.

• Explain the importance of reporting signs and symptoms of infection early to initiate prompt treatment (point out the risk for opportunistic infections, such as herpes, cytomegalovirus).

◆ *Before administering, or for more information, see individual drug.*

Laxatives

Stimulant laxatives
bisacodyl (Dulcolax) senna (Senokot)
cascara sagrada (Cascara)

Hyperosmotic laxatives
lactulose (Cephulac) magnesium sulfate (Epsom
magnesium citrate (citrate of salts)
magnesia)

Stool softeners
docusate calcium (Surfak) docusate sodium (Colace)
docusate potassium (Dialose)

Bulk-forming laxatives
psyllium (Metamucil) methylcellulose (Citrucel)

Action Laxatives increase peristalsis and stimulate bowel elimination by directly stimulating the bowel, altering stool consistency, or increasing physical bulk within the bowel.

Laxatives are grouped into four categories according to how they achieve these actions:

1 **Stimulant laxatives** increase peristalsis by irritating the bowel mucosa and/or stimulating nerves that mediate motor activity of smooth muscle. They also interfere with the reabsorption of fluid and electrolytes by the mucosal lining of the small intestine (thereby increasing liquid content of the stool).

2 **Hyperosmotic (saline) laxatives** increase stool volume by withdrawing water from the capillaries of the intestine; the increase in volume stimulates stretch receptors, increasing peristalsis.

3 **Stool softeners** change the consistency of the stool by reducing the surface tension of fecal contents; the resulting penetration of liquid and fatty material forms a softer stool.

4 **Bulk-forming laxatives** (made from nondigestible materials) provide increased bulk and moisture content to the stool by absorbing water and expanding.

Use/Therapeutic goal/Outcome

Used to relieve or prevent constipation, especially in patients who are taking medications that constipate, who are on bed rest, or who must avoid straining to defecate (e.g., those with heart problems or hemorrhoids.) *Therapeutic goal:* Reduction in straining. *Outcome criteria:* Demonstration or report of passage of soft stool without straining.

Also used to evacuate the bowel before surgery or diagnostic procedures or during treatment for worm or parasite infestation. *Therapeutic goal:* Prompt and complete evacuation of stool. *Outcome criteria:* Prompt, complete, and watery passage of stool; absence of stool content in the bowel on X-ray or endoscopy studies.

Dose range/Administration

Choice of agent and dosage depend on the indication (prevention or treatment of constipation, or complete bowel evacuation), individual response, age, height, weight, and health state of the individual.

Laxatives are usually given PO but also can be given rectally as enemas or suppositories. They are frequently purchased OTC and self-prescribed.

Although more than one dose may be necessary to promote bowel elimination, laxatives are withheld and the physician notified if defecation does not occur after recommended dosage or if severe abdominal pain, nausea, or vomiting occurs after administration.

Contraindications/Precautions

Contraindicated in hypersensitivity to the specific agent; in nausea, vomiting, or diarrhea (because of risk of fluid and electrolyte imbalance); and in severe abdominal pain that might be due to GI obstruction or inflammation (because of risk of mechanical damage or perforation of the bowel).

✋ **Stimulant laxatives and hyperosmotic laxatives are contraindicated for pregnant or nursing mothers. Hyperosmotic and stimulant laxatives are contraindicated for the elderly unless the drug is given under the advice of a physician. All laxatives are used with caution for children (because of the risk of fluid and electrolyte imbalance) and are contraindicated for use on a continued basis without the approval of a physician.**

Side effects/Adverse reactions

Hypersensitivity: pruritus, rash, respiratory symptoms. **GI:** gas pains, pain with bowel movement, damage or perforation of the bowel; (with chronic use) inhibition of rhythmic bowel reflexes, resulting in laxative dependence; (with use of enemas) damage to rectum or lower bowel and loss of sphincter tone. **Hem:** fluid and electrolyte imbalance. **Misc:** interference with absorption of nutrients and oral medications.

Nursing implications/Documentation

Possible nursing diagnoses: Pain; Fluid volume deficit; Altered nutrition: less than body requirements.

♦ Determine usual bowel elimination pattern, and identify factors that may contribute to or put the person at risk for constipation.

♦ Determine whether there has been previous use of laxatives and identify usual response.

♦ Give laxatives at a time appropriate to their expected onset of action to reduce interference with sleep and activities.

♦ Assist and/or encourage participation in exercises consistent with health state.

♦ Monitor and record character of bowel sounds, stools, and results of laxatives and enemas.

♦ Provide water, fruit juices, and foods that promote normal bowel activity.

♦ If stools are excessively liquid, monitor for and report signs of electrolyte depletion (weakness, confusion, arrhythmias, muscle cramps).

Patient & family teaching/Home care

Possible nursing diagnoses: Knowledge deficit; Noncompliance.

♦ Stress that laxatives have no benefit when they are used for relief of the common cold or other maladies.

♦ Explain the relationship between constipation and inadequate exercise and fluid and fiber intake. Point out that infrequent constipation should be treated not by laxatives, but by a holistic approach incorporating the following measures: increasing fluid intake; increasing intake of fiber-rich food; reducing intake of constipating foods; increasing exercise; eliminating non-essential constipating drugs (e.g., calcium and aluminum antacids, calcium salts, and antidiarrheals); attending to sensation of fullness in the rectum, and providing uninterrupted time for toileting.

♦ Recommend bulk-forming laxatives for simple constipation that does not respond to a holistic approach.

♦ Instruct regarding onset of action of the specific laxative to avoid interference with sleep or daily activities.

♦ Caution about the hazards of laxative abuse. Warn patient not to use stimulant laxatives for initial treatment of constipation but for acute administration only; explain that frequent use of any laxative may cause laxative dependence. Stress that frequent use of enemas (even soap suds or tap water) can damage rectum and large bowel, inhibit bowel tone, and increase risk of fluid and electrolyte imbalance.

♦ Advise that using laxatives reduces the amount of time other medications remain in the intestine and therefore may reduce their absorption.

♦ *Before administering, or for more information, see individual drugs.*

Local anesthetics

Prototypes: lidocaine, procaine

bupivacaine hydrochloride
(Marcaine)
chloroprocaine
hydrochloride (Nesacaine)
etidocaine hydrochloride
(Duranest)
lidocaine hydrochloride
(Xylocaine)

mepivacaine hydrochloride
(Carbocaine)
procaine hydrochloride
(Novocain)
tetracaine hydrochloride
(Pontocaine)

Action Local anesthetics produce loss of sensation by inhibiting sodium influx across the cell membrane during depolarization, causing blockage of impulse generation and conduction.

Use/Therapeutic goal/Outcome

Used for surgical, dental, and obstetric procedures. *Therapeutic goal:* Abolish pain. *Outcome criteria:* Report of numbness and absence of pain in the anesthetized area, absence of guarding or withdrawal from pinprick.

Dose range/Administration

Doses are highly individual and vary with the type and duration of procedure, method of administration, area to be anesthetized, vascularity of tissues, condition of patient (age, height, weight, health state), and individual tolerance. These drugs must be administered only by clinicians well-versed in their use. Epinephrine, a potent sympathomimetic, is sometimes used in conjunction with local anesthetics to decrease systemic absorption and prolong duration of anesthesia.

Interaction alert: Local anesthetics containing epinephrine may interact with monoamine oxidase inhibitors (MAOIs), tricyclic antidepressants (TCAs), and phenothiazines to produce severe hypotension or hypertension. They may interact with oxytocic drugs to produce excessive hypertensive response and may cause an increased risk of cardiac dysrhythmias.

Extreme care must be taken to avoid inadvertent intravascular injection of local anesthetics—this may produce severe cardiovascular effects. The administration of regional intravenous nerve blocks, the only procedure in which these drugs are injected into a vessel, is done with the use of a tourniquet to avoid systemic absorption. Because of the possibility of severe adverse reactions, resuscitative drugs and equipment must always be readily available.

Local anesthetics are administered in five ways:

1 **Infiltration anesthesia** is the process of injecting diluted solutions of the drug first into the skin and then subcutaneously around the region to be anesthetized. This type of anesthesia is suitable for minor procedures, such as suturing of superficial wounds or incision and drainage of a wound.

2 **Peripheral nerve block** is a process in which the anesthetic is injected next to nerve fibers of the peripheral nervous system, near a nerve trunk that supplies the region of the operative site. A single nerve may be blocked, or the anesthetic may be injected where several nerve trunks emerge from the spinal cord. Because of the thickness of these nerve fibers, more concentrated solutions are used.

3 **Intravenous regional nerve blocks** are most commonly used to anesthetize an entire arm or leg. A tourniquet is applied to the proximal end of the patient's arm or leg to reduce blood supply to the extremity and to prevent systemic release of the anesthetic. A small amount of dilute anesthetic is then infused into the limb. After the procedure, the tourniquet is slowly deflated as the patient is carefully observed for systemic reactions. If these occur, the tourniquet is reinflated until the drug is absorbed into the tissue or the symptoms are managed medically.

4 **Spinal (subarachnoid) blocks** involve injection of small amounts of local anesthetic beneath the dura into the spinal fluid of the lower lumbar area, well below the tip of the spinal cord. The result is usually a loss of sensation and movement below the nipple area.

5 **Epidural and caudal (peridural) blocks** involve injection of small amounts of a local anesthetic into the epidural space (the dura mater is not penetrated), resulting in loss of sensation and movement below the abdomen.

All of these methods of anesthesia provide for good muscle relaxation, and none immediately affect cardiovascular function. These are advantages for the elderly, for those with heart and lung disease, and for those undergoing outpatient procedures.

Contraindications/Precautions

Contraindicated in hypersensitivity to the local anesthetic, to any of its components, or to similar drugs. Local anesthetics of the ester type may result in allergic reactions to the metabolite *p*-aminobenzoic acid (PABA); cross-sensitivity may occur in persons sensitive to sulfonamides or thiazide diuretics. Local anesthetics of the amide class are generally free of hypersensitivity potential. However, many of these solutions contain methylparaben as the preservative, and persons sensitive to PABA may be allergic to this preservative. Cross-sensitivity does not occur between the amide and ester classes of anesthetic. Some local anesthetics may be contraindicated in liver disease and kidney disease. Use with caution in the acutely ill.

👋 **Children, the acutely ill, and the elderly and debilitated often require lower doses of local anesthetic, as well as special considerations regarding choice of drugs, dosage, and administration.**

Side effects/Adverse reactions

Hypersensitivity: erythema, rash, pruritus, localized edema, hypotension, bronchospasm, anaphylactic responses. *CNS:* excitation with tremors, shivering, convulsions. *CV:* tachycardia, hypotension, intraventricular conduction defect, atrioventricular block (may lead to cardiac and respiratory arrest). *GI:* nausea, vomiting. *Misc:* Signs of intravascular injection that may precede seizure are tachycardia (especially with solutions containing epinephrine), light-headedness, dizziness, metallic taste in the mouth, numbness of the tongue or lips, slurred speech, tinnitus. Epinephrine in preparations of local anesthetic may result in anginal pain, tachycardia, tremors, headache, restlessness, palpitations, dizziness, hypertension.

Nursing implications/Documentation

Possible nursing diagnoses: Pain; Potential for injury.

♦ Record history of allergies and accurate height and weight before procedure.

♦ Recognize that epinephrine must not be used in tissues supplied by end arteries (fingers, toes, ears, nose, or penis) because blood supply can be compromised and tissue damaged.

♦ Document vital signs per protocol, and monitor for, and immediately report, signs of systemic or hypersensitivity reactions.

♦ Question anesthesiologist or anesthetist regarding any restrictions on patient movement (e.g., lowering or elevating the patient's head); post these at bedside.

♦ Monitor anesthetized area for level of sensation and motor function; watch for poor positioning, and protect area from injury.

♦ Give prescribed pain medication as sensation begins to return, before pain becomes severe.

♦ With pudendal block, monitor for hematoma formation or rectal puncture (blood flow through rectum) following block. Be aware that if block is ineffective, the patient may experience increased apprehension and fear.

♦ With epidural or caudal block, summon assistance immediately if the patient becomes hypotensive (hypotension requires immediate intervention, such as administering oxygen, elevating the legs, turning the patient on the left side, or increasing IV rate).

♦ With paracervical block, monitor fetal heart rate closely because of increased risk of fetal bradycardia and acidosis; report tachycardia or bradycardia immediately.

♦ With IV regional anesthesia, do not deflate the tourniquet sooner than 20 min after the injection, even if the procedure has been completed (allowing time for drug to be absorbed by tissues prevents inadvertent systemic bolus).

♦ With spinal anesthesia, do not use preparations containing preservatives. Keep the patient flat for 8 hrs following anesthesia. Encourage movement of legs as soon as motor function returns. Be sure that the patient is well hydrated to prevent hypotension and headache.

Patient & family teaching/Home care

Possible nursing diagnoses: Anxiety; Fear.

♦ Stress the need to protect areas of the body that have lost sensation.

♦ Explain rationale for taking prescribed pain medication before the pain becomes too severe.

♦ With rectal and anal anesthesia, advise using the lowest possible dose to minimize systemic toxicity.

♦ With oral or nasopharyngeal anesthesia, caution patient not to eat food or drink fluids for at least 1 hr after use of topical anesthetic (swallowing reflex may be depressed). Warn against chewing on affected side until sensation has returned (patient may inadvertently bite cheek).

♦ Additional guidelines for eye anesthesia

♦ Warn against rubbing or touching anesthetized eye.

- Teach the need to avoid touching the eyelid with dropper when self-administering drops; emphasize the need for good handwashing.

- Advise against using eye anesthetics longer than necessary (prolonged use may result in corneal epithelial erosion and delayed healing of corneal surface).

- *Before administering, or for more information, see individual drug.*

Narcotics and nonnarcotic analgesics

Narcotic prototype: morphine
Nonnarcotic prototypes: aspirin, acetaminophen
Narcotic analgesics

alfentanil hydrochloride (Alfenta)	morphine sulfate (Duramorph)
buprenorphine hydrochloride (Buprenex)	nalbuphine hydrochloride (Nubain)
codeine (♥Paveral)	oxycodone hydrochloride (Roxicodone)
fentanyl citrate (Sublimaze)	oxymorphone hydrochloride (Numorphan)
hydromorphone hydrochloride (Dilaudid)	pentazocine (Talwin)
levorphanol tartrate (Levo-Dromoran)	propoxyphene hydrochloride (Darvon)
meperidine hydrochloride (Demerol)	propoxyphene napsylate (Darvocet-N)
methadone hydrochloride (Methadose)	sufentanil citrate (Sufenta)
morphine hydrochloride (♥Morphitec)	

Nonnarcotic analgesics and antipyretics

Salicylates

aspirin (acetylsalicylic acid, ASA)	magnesium salicylate (Doan's)
choline magnesium trisalicylate (Trilisate)	salsalate (Mono-Gesic)
choline salicylate (Arthropan)	sodium salicylate (Uracel-5)
	sodium thiosalicylate (Asproject)

Miscellaneous agents

acetaminophen (Tylenol)	ibuprofen (Motrin)
diflunisal (Dolobid)	ketorolac (Toradol)

Urinary tract analgesics
phenazopyridine hydrochloride (Pyridium)

Action Narcotic and nonnarcotic analgesics alter pain perception through very different actions:

1 **Narcotic analgesics** decrease awareness of pain sensation by binding to opiate receptors at many sites in the CNS (cortex, brain stem, and spinal cord). Although the exact mechanism is not fully understood, it is believed that narcotics diminish transmission of pain impulses by decreasing the permeability of the cell membrane to sodium and altering the release of various neurotransmitters from afferent nerves sensitive to painful stimuli. Narcotic analgesics not only relieve moderate to severe pain but also may produce profound CNS effects: euphoria, drowsiness, somnolence, changes in mood, mental clouding, and narcosis (stupor). Respiratory depression and reduction in blood pressure are also common. Some narcotics (e.g., codeine) depress the cough reflex. Narcotics are known to cause *addiction* (the body develops a physical dependence on a drug) and *tolerance* (the body requires bigger and/or more frequent doses to achieve desired effects).

Narcotics have a high potential for abuse; strict regulations for dispensing these drugs are mandated by the Controlled Substance Act of 1970 and by state laws. The Controlled Substance Act bases the classification of narcotics on the potential for abuse and dependence. These classes, or schedules, are listed under Schedules of Controlled Substances on page xv.

2 **Nonnarcotic analgesics** (except phenazopyridine) act in the peripheral nervous system; they reduce pain sensation by inhibiting the formation or reactivity of prostaglandins (mediators of the inflammatory process that stimulate sensory nerves). Nonnarcotic analgesics relieve only mild to moderate pain and do not cause addiction or tolerance. Nonnarcotic analgesics (except phenazopyridine and acetaminophen) have additional anti-inflammatory actions (see Nonsteroidal Anti-inflammatory Drugs overview). Aspirin and acetaminophen are also antipyretics; it is thought that they stimulate the hypothalamus to produce vasodilation and promote heat loss from blood vessels to the surface of the skin. Salicylates also have antiplatelet actions.

Use/Therapeutic goal/Outcome

Narcotic analgesics: Treat pain that is not relieved by non-narcotic analgesics, e.g., in surgery, cancer, myocardial infarction, fractures, burns, childbirth, nerve injuries, and inflammatory bowel disease. **Therapeutic goal:** Promotion of comfort and reduction of the stress response. **Outcome criteria:** Report of relief of pain, normalization in pulse rate and blood pressure, demonstration of ability to perform necessary activities (e.g., turning, coughing, and breathing deeply).

Alfentanil, fentanyl, and sufentanil: also used as adjuncts to anesthesia. **Therapeutic goal:** Pain relief, reduced need for inhalation anesthetics. *Outcome criteria:* normalization of pulse and blood pressure, absence of guarding or muscle tension at operative site without increased need for inhalation anesthetics.

Methadone is also used for treatment of heroine withdrawal. *Therapeutic goal:* Prevention of withdrawal symptoms. *Outcome criteria:* Report of absence of withdrawal symptoms.

Nonnarcotic analgesics (except phenazopyridine): Treat mild to moderate musculoskeletal or nerve pain. *Therapeutic goal:* Promotion of comfort. *Outcome criteria:* Report of relief of pain, improved ability to perform daily activities.

Aspirin and acetaminophen: also used for control of fever. *Therapeutic goal:* Normalization of temperature. *Outcome criteria:* Temperature reading that demonstrates normalization of temperature (optimally, 37°C or 98.6°F)

♦ *For use of non-narcotic analgesics as anti-inflammatory agents, see Nonsteroidal anti-inflammatory drugs overview.*

Dose range/Administration

1 **Narcotic analgesics:** Dosage depends on drug potency, route of administration, severity of pain, individual responses, blood pressure and respirations, age, height, weight, and health status. Children and the elderly and debilitated require reduced dosage. Morphine, often the first choice for severe pain, remains the standard against which all analgesics are measured. Although many alkaloid and synthetic compounds produce similar analgesic effects, none have been proven to be clinically superior to morphine.

Depending on the drug and the indication, narcotic analgesics are given PO, SC, IM, or IV. For extremely severe pain, the most effective route is IV; however, only physicians and qualified nurses administer IV narcotics. Because of the risk of respiratory arrest, keep emergency drugs, including the narcotic antagonist naloxone hydrochloride (Narcan), and equipment for intubation nearby whenever narcotics are given IV.

As a rule, the least potent drug at the lowest dose that provides pain relief is given. For example, if a non-narcotic analgesic is ineffective, a narcotic analgesic may be required. Often, a combination of narcotic and non-narcotic analgesics—such as codeine with acetaminophen—enhances analgesic effects of both drugs, decreases the required narcotic

dose, reduces the risk of tolerance, dependence, and side effects, and allows the patient to remain more alert.

While it is important to remember to use the lowest dose necessary to provide pain relief, it is also important to remember that severe, unrelieved pain may require *higher* doses. If a narcotic analgesic is not given when needed, the pain may become so severe that the normal dose will be ineffective. For this reason, and because of the effectiveness of the intravenous route, severe postoperative pain is sometimes managed by *patient-controlled* analgesia (PCA), in which the patient pushes a button to deliver doses periodically as needed. The PCA pump limits the number and frequency of doses, preventing overdosage while still allowing patient control. You may also see cancer pain managed by *continuous* narcotic infusion. Continuous infusions, by contrast, are not patient-controlled; they are used to maintain a steady serum drug level. Some patients receive a combination of these two therapies. They get a basal rate of narcotic, with the ability to deliver additional doses as required. Morphine and meperidine are commonly used in PCA; morphine and hydromorphone are commonly used in continuous infusions. Individuals with terminal cancer often receive much higher than usual doses because they develop a tolerance to the medication.

2 **Nonnarcotic analgesics:** Dosage depends on the indication, drug, age, height, weight, and health status. These agents are usually given PO; aspirin and acetaminophen can also be given by suppository. For fever, aspirin and acetaminophen may be given alternately for optimal results.

Because ibuprofen, aspirin, and acetaminophen are available without a prescription, nurses should be aware of the need to question individuals about the use of these drugs. Many laymen are unaware of the risk of renal failure associated with high doses of ibuprofen, of the anticoagulant effect of aspirin, and of the severity of acetaminophen overdosage (may cause liver failure and death).

🖐 **Whenever possible, give salicylates and ibuprofen with food to prevent gastric irritation. Monitor those on long-term salicylate or ibuprofen therapy for signs of GI bleeding (nausea, black stools).**

Contraindications/Precautions

Narcotic analgesics: Contraindicated in hypersensitivity to the drug, CNS or respiratory depression, hypotension, acute alcohol withdrawal; when administration may hamper attempts to diagnose or monitor a problem (e.g., head trauma, cerebrovascular accident, abdominal pain). **Use with caution** in cholecystitis, biliary obstruction, respiratory problems, alcoholism, and diabetes.

✋ **Contraindicated during labor before rhythmic uterine contractions have been established.**

Nonnarcotic analgesics: Contraindicated in hypersensitivity to the drug or to a closely related drug. **Salicylates are contraindicated** in bleeding tendencies (e.g., hemophilia) and in history of peptic ulcers. **Use with caution** in hypertension and heart failure.

✋ **Salicylates are contraindicated during the last trimester of pregnancy and for children with chicken pox or flu-like symptoms (because of the risk of Reye's syndrome).**

Side effects/Adverse reactions

Narcotic analgesics: Hypersensitivity: pruritus, rash, wheezing, anaphylaxis. **CNS:** drowsiness, somnolence, euphoria, depression, dizziness, impaired coordination, ataxia. **Resp:** decreased rate and depth of respirations, bronchial constriction. **CV:** hypotension, bradycardia. **GI:** nausea, vomiting, constipation, paralytic ileus. **GU:** urinary retention, decreased uterine contractility and prolonged labor.

Nonnarcotic analgesics: Hypersensitivity: pruritus, rash, wheezing, anaphylaxis. **GI:** (except acetaminophen and phenazopyridine) nausea, gastric irritation and bleeding, constipation. **Hem:** (salicylates only) prolonged coagulation time.

Nursing implications/Documentation

Possible nursing diagnoses: Pain; Potential for injury; Anxiety; Fear; Sensory/perceptual alterations; Fatigue.

♦ Determine cause of pain; have patient describe pain and rate its intensity on a 1-to-10 scale before and after medication.

♦ Foster a feeling of trust that you are working with the patient to establish an effective regimen for pain relief; listen to patient and family concerns.

♦ For best results, give analgesics before pain becomes severe.

♦ **Additional guidelines for narcotic analgesics**

♦ Sign the narcotic control book for each dose, according to policy.

♦ Determine whether a less potent analgesic might effectively relieve pain; use narcotic only when non-narcotics are ineffective.

♦ To improve pain control and reduce narcotic requirements, discuss with physician the possibility of alternating or combining narcotics with non-narcotic analgesics or adding a tranquilizer to the regimen.

♦ For parenteral route, document pulse, respirations, and blood pressure immediately before and 1 hr after administration until response is determined; hold doses and report if hypotension or respiratory depression is present.

♦ Monitor mental status; keep side rails up when the person is in bed and supervise ambulation when out of bed.

♦ To enhance pain relief during movement and coughing, splint incisions, and support injured parts.

♦ Plan activities during periods of optimal pain relief and minimal drowsiness.

♦ Report excessive drowsiness or stupor to physician (who may decrease dose or change drug).

♦ If nausea, vomiting, dizziness, or hypotension is noted, keep head of the bed down to help relieve these symptoms.

♦ After prolonged use, monitor for and report signs of tolerance and dependence; discuss with physician whether attempt should be made to taper dosage (e.g., give lower dose during the day and a higher dose at bedtime). Recognize that sometimes the benefits of analgesics outweigh the risks of increasing dosage (e.g., with terminal illness, with burns).

Patient & family teaching/Home care

Possible nursing diagnoses: Knowledge deficit; Impaired home maintenance management; Anxiety; Fear; Pain; Social isolation.

♦ Stress the need for accurate diagnosis and treatment of cause of pain; advise against continuing to treat pain with OTC drugs without seeing a physician.

♦ Explain why analgesics are taken before pain becomes too severe.

♦ **Additional guidelines for narcotic analgesics**

• Before giving narcotics, openly discuss the issues of tolerance and addiction; stress that short-term use of narcotics for severe pain is unlikely to produce addiction.

• Explain that taking narcotics during the acute stages of illness reduces the stress response, which is especially important in cardiac patients, and enhances ability to perform activities (moving, coughing, deep breathing) that are essential to preventing complications of pain-related immobility. For people with terminal disease, stress that the need for pain control outweighs the concerns of addiction and that doses will be increased as necessary.

• Teach ways to minimize narcotic requirements while maintaining comfort: splinting incisions, combining or alternating non-narcotic analgesics with narcotics, using weaker medications during the day and stronger ones at night (when pain often seems worse), using relaxation techniques and guided imagery.

• To avoid dependence, tolerance, and abuse, stress the need to adhere to prescribed dose regimen; advise reporting unsatisfactory pain relief rather than increasing doses.

• Point out that narcotics are likely to cloud thinking and judgment; caution against driving or making important decisions while under the influence of narcotics.

• Warn that use with alcohol and other CNS depressants may cause excessive sedation.

• For chronic pain, provide phone numbers of pain control centers and support groups.

♦ *Before administering, or for more information, see individual drugs.*

Nonsteroidal anti-inflammatory drugs (NSAIDs)

Prototypes: aspirin, ibuprofen

aspirin (acetylsalicylic acid, ASA)
diclofenac sodium (Voltaren)
fenoprofen calcium (Nalfon)
flurbiprofen (Ansaid)
flurbiprofen sodium (Ocufen)
ibuprofen (Motrin)
indomethacin (Indocin)
indomethacin sodium trihydrate (Indometh)
ketoprofen (Orudis)

ketorolac (Toradol)
meclofenamate sodium (Meclomen)
mefenamic acid (Ponstel)
naproxen (Naprosyn)
naproxen sodium (Anaprox)
oxyphenbutazone (Oxalid)
phenylbutazone (Butazolidin)
piroxicam (Feldene)
sulindac (Clinoril)
tolmetin sodium (Tolectin)

Action Nonsteroidal anti-inflammatory drugs (NSAIDs) reduce inflammation and pain by decreasing the biosynthesis of prostaglandins. Prostaglandins are naturally occurring mediators of the inflammatory process that are found in tissues throughout the body. The reduction of prostaglandin biosynthesis affects local mediators of the inflammatory process and other substances that mediate pain, thereby reducing inflammation and pain.

NSAIDs also produce antipyretic effects, by stimulating the hypothalamus to produce vasodilation and promote heat loss from blood vessels to the surface of the skin.

Use/Therapeutic goal/Outcome

Prescribed by physicians to treat inflammation and pain associated with arthritic diseases, spondylitis, gout, tendonitis, bursitis, and muscle strains. *Self-prescribed* (ibuprofen and aspirin) to treat pain associated with headaches, backaches, toothaches, dysmenorrhea, and other aches and pains. *Therapeutic goal:* Reduction of inflammation and pain, increase in range of motion and ability to perform activities of daily living (ADLs). *Outcome criteria:* Reduced signs of inflammation (redness, swelling, pain) of the affected parts, report and demonstration of improved comfort, range of motion, and ability to perform ADLs.

Dose range/Administration

Dosage depends on the indications, drug, route of administration, individual response, age, height, weight, and health state. Lower doses are used in renal disease.

Give NSAIDs with food to reduce GI side effects, and administer regularly within a 24-hr period to maintain steady blood levels.

Clinical alert: Be aware of the potential for the abuse of OTC doses of ibuprofen—many people are unaware that high doses of ibuprofen may cause renal failure or that taking ibuprofen on an empty stomach may cause GI hemorrhage.

Interaction alert: Interactions with other drugs are significant, because these drugs become protein-bound in the body, displacing other drugs from binding sites, thus increasing effects and risk of toxicity. Use with anticoagulants may increase risk of bleeding. Refer to individual drugs for specific interactions.

OVERVIEW

Contraindications/Precautions

Contraindicated in hypersensitivity to the drug or a closely related drug (hypersensitivity to aspirin is usually considered a contraindication to the entire class) and possibly in renal or hepatic failure. **Use with caution** in GI problems, peptic ulcer, and hemophilia.

🖐 **Aspirin is contraindicated in children < 18 years with flu symptoms or chickenpox because of risk of Reye's syndrome. Safety of all NSAIDs for children < 6 months has not been established. Use in second trimester of pregnancy may cause premature closure of ductus arteriosis; use in third trimester decreases uterine contractility. Use with caution for the elderly.**

Side effects/Adverse reactions

Hypersensitivity: asthmatic symptoms, rhinitis, urticaria, rash, angioedema, bronchospasm. **GI:** irritation and bleeding, nausea, vomiting, constipation. **Hem:** prolonged coagulation time, elevated liver enzymes. **CNS:** dizziness, drowsiness. **Ear:** auditory disturbances, tinnitus. **Eye:** visual disturbances.

Nursing implications/Documentation

Possible nursing diagnoses: Pain; Impaired physical mobility.

◆ Before giving first dose, check baseline CBC, electrolytes, prothrombin time, BUN, creatinine, and liver function studies; monitor periodically thereafter if therapy is prolonged.

◆ Schedule drug administration so that doses are given at least 1 hr before maximum mobility is needed.

◆ Anticipate decreased dosage for the elderly and for patients with decreased kidney function.

◆ Monitor for and report GI symptoms that indicate possible peptic ulcer (nausea, pain, black stools).

◆ Document weight qod; report edema or sudden weight gain.

◆ Observe for and report visual and auditory changes (periodic auditory tests are recommended if therapy is prolonged).

◆ For diabetics, monitor blood sugar closely (requirements for insulin and oral agents may change).

Patient & family teaching/Home care

Possible nursing diagnoses: Knowledge deficit; Altered health maintenance.

◆ Point out the need to take this drug with food to reduce GI symptoms, and to watch for symptoms of GI bleeding (black stools, persistent GI distress).

◆ Instruct individuals to withhold drug and report if any of the following side effects are experienced: vertigo, rash, hematuria, hearing or visual changes, sudden weight gain, edema.

◆ Advise avoiding alcohol, aspirin, and other OTC drugs (unless they are approved by physician) because of increased risk of GI bleeding.

◆ Explain the importance of monitoring weight weekly (or, in some cases, more frequently) and reporting sudden weight gain or edema (teach how to check hands, ankles, feet).

◆ Warn against driving or other activities that require alertness until response is determined (drug may initially cause drowsiness and dizziness, but these effects are usually transient).

◆ Stress the importance of ongoing medical follow-up; explain that desired effects may not appear for 3–5 days and that the full effect may not appear for up to 2–4 weeks (if *no* difference is noted after 7 days, instruct patient to notify physician).

◆ Assist in planning daily schedule so that most activities are performed during periods of optimal pain relief.

◆ Explore life-style changes that may promote goal achievement (e.g., weight control, regular exercise); proceed with health teaching as indicated.

◆ For diabetics, explain the importance of monitoring blood sugars with a blood glucose monitor (e.g., Glucometer).

◆ *Before administering, or for more information, see individual drug.*

Skeletal muscle relaxants

Prototype: baclofen

baclofen (Lioresal)
carisoprodol (Soma)
chlorphenesin carbamate (Maolate)
chlorzoxazone (Paraflex)
cyclobenzaprine hydrochloride (Flexeril)

dantrolene sodium (Dantrium)
metaxalone (Skelaxin)
methocarbamol (Robaxin)
orphenadrine citrate (Norflex)

Action
Skeletal muscle relaxants depress the CNS and inhibit the transmission of impulses from the spinal cord to skeletal muscle. The exact mechanism is not fully understood. Generally, skeletal muscle relaxants do not depress neuronal conduction, neuromuscular transmission, or muscle excitability and cause no loss of voluntary motor function.

Use/Therapeutic goal/Outcome
Used to control muscle spasm and pain associated with acute and chronic musculoskeletal conditions. Use of these drugs in spasticity generated by cerebral or spinal cord condition is not always effective. **Therapeutic goal:** Promotion of comfort, range of motion, and mobility. **Outcome criteria:** Report of increase in comfort and ability to perform ADLs, demonstration of improved range of motion and ability to perform ADLs.

Dose range/Administration
The route of administration and dosage depend on the indication, health status, age, weight, height, and nutritional status. Dose increments vary according to patient response, desired outcome, and incidence of side effects. CNS depressants, alcohol, and narcotics may increase CNS effects.

● **Give PO doses with food to reduce GI symptoms.**

Contraindications/Precautions
Contraindicated in hypersensitivity to the drug or to a related drug and in kidney or hepatic impairment.

Side effects/Adverse reactions
Hypersensitivity: erythema, rash, pruritus, hives. **CNS:** drowsiness, dizziness, agitation. **GI:** nausea, vomiting, epigastric distress.

Nursing implications/Documentation
Possible nursing diagnoses: Constipation; Pain; Impaired physical mobility; Potential for injury.

♦ Monitor comfort level and range of motion before and after giving doses.

♦ Supervise ambulation until risk of drowsiness, dizziness, or loss of balance is determined.

♦ Monitor and document bowel elimination and food and fluid intake to prevent constipation.

♦ Be aware that stopping these drugs abruptly may cause withdrawal symptoms.

Patient & family teaching/Home care
Possible nursing diagnoses: Knowledge deficit; Impaired home maintenance management.

♦ Advise taking drug with milk or food to prevent gastric distress.

♦ Encourage increasing fluid and fiber intake to prevent constipation.

♦ Caution not to discontinue long-term therapy without consulting physician.

♦ Warn against driving or other activities requiring alertness because of possible drowsiness or dizziness.

♦ Explain the importance of following the individualized total plan of treatment, including rest, excercise, compliance with prescribed dosage, and other forms of therapy (e.g., relaxation techniques).

♦ Stress the importance of reporting abdominal discomfort, yellow skin or eyes, or signs of hypersensitivity reaction (e.g., rash).

♦ *Before administering, or for more information, see individual drug.*

Thyroid hormones

Prototype: levothyroxine
levothyroxine sodium (Synthroid)
liothyronine (Cytomel)
liotrix (Euthroid)
thyroglobulin (Proloid)
dessicated thyroid (Armour Thyroid)

Action
Thyroid hormones regulate DNA production of RNA (and eventually protein), which results in increased cellular metabolism, cardiac output, oxygen consumption, body temperature, and cholesterol metabolism. In children, thyroid hormones also promote growth and development. The exact mechanism of action is not fully understood.

Use/Therapeutic goal/Outcome
Used to replace or supplement natural thyroid hormones when the thyroid gland has been removed or is unable to secrete sufficient levels of the hormones; conditions include hypothyroidism, myxedema, cretinism in children, goiter, and postthyroidectomy. **Therapeutic goal:** Increased level of circulating thyroid hormones, promotion of normal metabolism. **Outcome criteria:** Increased T_3 and T_4 levels to normal levels; signs of normal metabolism

(normal heart rate, skin turgor, ability to sweat, bowel function, and growth and development; increased energy and alertness; weight loss).

Liothyronine is also used diagnostically (T_3 suppression test) to differentiate hyperthyroidism from euthyroidism in borderline situations.

Dose range/Administration

Dosage depends on the drug, individual's degree of thyroid function, response, age, height, weight, and health state. Because many people are very sensitive to thyroid hormones, very small dose changes can cause severe effects. The patient is started on the lowest dose possible and then monitored closely as the dose is gradually increased.

Contraindications/Precautions

Contraindicated in hypersensitivity to the drug and in untreated adrenal insufficiency, acute myocardial infarction, and thyrotoxicosis. **Use with caution** in angina, ischemia, hypertension, kidney or renal disease.

⇓ **Use with caution for the elderly (who usually require lower doses). Doses may need to be adjusted during pregnancy and after delivery. Use with caution for nursing mothers and for children.**

Side effects/Adverse reactions

Hypersensitivity: pruritus, rash. Other common side effects are usually dose-related. **CNS:** headache, nervousness, insomnia, tremors. **CV:** palpitations, tachycardia, arrhythmias, angina, hypertension, cardiac collapse. **GI:** increased appetite, nausea, diarrhea. **GU:** change in menstrual flow or cycle. **MS:** weight loss, increased rate of bone maturation in children.

Nursing implications/Documentation

Possible nursing diagnoses: Altered nutrition: less than body requirements; Altered nutrition: more than body requirements.

♦ Do not substitute different brands or generic brands for thyroid drugs without physician's approval (they may not be bioequivalent).

♦ Give these drugs at the same time every day to maintain stable blood levels.

♦ Monitor and document pulse, blood pressure, and weight at least daily during initial treatment.

♦ Monitor T_3 and T_4 levels (levels outside therapeutic range may necessitate a change in dose or drug).

♦ For patients over 40 years, monitor for and report symptoms of cardiovascular disease (chest pain, tachycardia, dyspnea).

♦ If radioactive iodine uptake tests are necessary, discontinue drug 1–4 weeks (depending on drug) before test.

♦ For children, monitor and document growth and development every 3–6 months.

Patient & family teaching/Home care

Possible nursing diagnoses: Knowledge deficit; Impaired home maintenance management.

♦ Emphasize the importance of taking thyroid daily as prescribed; advise not to use a different or generic brand and not to skip or "double up" doses.

♦ Teach the need to return for medical follow-up (stress that drug is likely to be needed for life).

♦ Advise reporting increased fatigue or nervousness, palpitations, tachycardia, or chest pain (dose may need to be changed).

♦ Stress that thyroid hormone is potentially dangerous and must not be used to lose weight or to combat fatigue.

♦ Explain that temporary hair loss may occur in children.

♦ *Before administering, or for more information, see individual drug.*

Thyroid hormone antagonists

Prototypes: propylthiouracil
methimazole (Tapazole)   sodium iodide I-131
propylthiouracil (PTU,   (Iodotope Therapeutic)
  ♣Propyl-Thyracil)

Action   Thyroid hormone antagonists reduce serum thyroid levels by interfering with the synthesis or release of thyroid hormones.

Use/Therapeutic goal/Outcome

Used to decrease the output of an overactive thyroid gland (hyperthyroidism, Graves' disease). **Therapeutic goal:** Reduction in circulating thyroid hormones, promotion of normal metabolism. **Outcome criteria:** Decrease in T_3 and T_4 levels to within normal limits, with signs of normal metabolism (normal heart rate, skin turgor, ability to sweat, bowel function, and growth and development; decreased nervousness; weight gain).

Radioactive iodine is used to destroy thyroid tissue (cancer, Graves' disease).

Dose range/Administration

Dosage depends on the drug; on the individual's response, age, height, weight, and health state; and on the underlying cause of the disease.

Contraindications/Precautions

Contraindicated in hypersensitivity to the drug.

🖐 **Contraindicated for nursing mothers. Monitor children, pregnant women, and the elderly carefully.**

Side effects/Adverse reactions

Hypersensitivity: pruritus, rash, drug fever, and (for iodides) eyelid swelling. Other common side effects are usually dose-related. *GI:* decreased appetite, loss of taste, salivary gland enlargement, hepatitis. *GU:* irregular menstruation.

Nursing implications/Documentation

Possible nursing diagnoses: Altered nutrition: less than body requirements; Altered nutrition: more than body requirements.

♦ Give these drugs at the same time every day to maintain stable blood levels.

♦ Monitor T_3 and T_4 levels (abnormal levels may indicate a need for change in dose or drug).

♦ Report fatigue, weight gain, or sluggishness (might indicate need to reduce dose).

♦ For children, monitor growth and development every 6 months.

Patient & family teaching/Home care

Possible nursing diagnoses: Knowledge deficit; Impaired home maintenance management.

♦ Warn against suddenly discontinuing antithyroid medications (may cause thyroid storm); teach that illness or infection may also cause thyroid storm.

♦ Stress the importance of taking drug exactly as prescribed at the same time every day and of returning for continuing medical follow-up.

♦ Advise reporting increased fatigue, nervousness, or weight changes (may be dose-related).

♦ *Before administering, or for more information, see individual drug.*

Section III

Drugs
Listed alphabetically by generic name

Generic name followed by phonetic pronunciation, listed alphabetically (brand name cross-reference in index).
Brands available in the U.S. ♣Canada only, ▲Australia only.

Class refers to chemical and functional class (classification list in Section II).
★ prototype drug identifies the drug as being one of those most commonly used.

Antidote lists the generic name of antidote.

Cautions grid Reminds you to check for key areas of concerns:
PEDS 🖐 Precautions for children (see below).
OK No documented problems for children.
PREG FDA assessment of safety for pregnant women (list in preface): **A** Generally considered safe; **B** No demonstrated risk; **C** Some risk possible, weigh advantages; **D** Risk shown, weigh advantages; **X** Generally contraindicated; **NR** No category assigned; 🖐 more than one pregnancy category.
GERI 🖐 Precautions for the elderly (see below).
OK No documented problems for the elderly.
Controlled substance risk of abuse (list in preface).

Action Gives a concise explanation of how the drug produces therapeutic effects.

Use Lists the uses and corresponding therapeutic goals and outcome criteria.
Outcome criteria are signs that demonstrate goal achievement.

Dose range/Administration
Interaction alert Interactions or incompatibilities that may affect drug action.
◆ 🍴 indicates the drug should be taken with or after food. 🍽 indicates the drug should be taken on an empty stomach. Be sure to read statements following symbols for clarification.
◆ Comprehensive information on dosage and administration.
Clinical alert on preparing or administering, available forms, and critical precautions.

Contraindications/Precautions Lets you know when doses should be withheld or given with caution.
🖐 Highlights concerns for children, pregnant or nursing mothers, and the elderly.

Side effects begin with **Hypersensitivity** to assist in early recognition of these responses, then lists other side effects by system in order of common occurrence (see preface for abbreviations).

Nursing implications Suggests possible **Nursing diagnoses** (see preface), then gives key nursing interventions and charting reminders.

Patient & family teaching/Home care
Suggests possible **Nursing diagnoses** for home care, then presents keys to safe and effective home administration and discusses supporting holistic measures.
◆ Cross-references direct you to overviews or other drugs for important additional information.

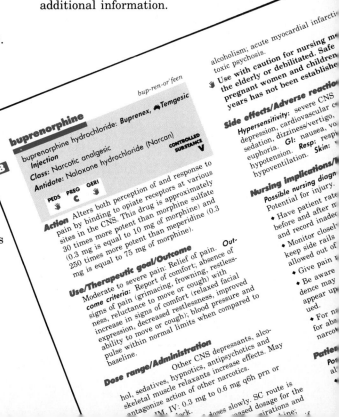

bup-ren-or'feen

buprenorphine
buprenorphine hydrochloride: Buprenex, ♣Temgesic
Injection
Class: Narcotic analgesic
Antidote: Naloxone hydrochloride (Narcan) **CONTROLLED SUBSTANCE V**

B PEDS PREG GERI
     🖐   C   🖐

Action Alters both perception of and response to pain by binding to opiate receptors at various sites in the CNS. This drug is approximately 30 times more potent than morphine sulfate (0.3 mg is equal to 10 mg of morphine) and 250 times more potent than meperidine (0.3 mg is equal to 75 mg of morphine).

Use/Therapeutic goal/Outcome Moderate to severe pain: Relief of pain. **Outcome criteria:** Report of comfort; absence of signs of pain (grimacing, frowning, restlessness, reluctance to move or cough) with increase in signs of comfort (relaxed facial expression, decreased restlessness, improved ability to move or cough); blood pressure and pulse within normal limits when compared to baseline.

Dose range/Administration Other CNS depressants, alcohol, sedatives, hypnotics, antipsychotics and skeletal muscle relaxants increase effects. May antagonize action of other narcotics.
IM, IV: 0.3 mg to 0.6 mg q6h prn or ... doses slowly. SC route is ...

alcoholism; acute myocardial infarctio...
toxic psychosis.
🖐 Use with caution for nursing me...
the elderly or debilitated. Safe...
pregnant women and children ...
years has not been establishe...

Side effects/Adverse reactio...
Hypersensitivity: severe CNS depression, cardiovascular c... sedation, dizziness/vertigo, euphoria. **GI:** nausea, vo... hypotension. **Resp:** respi... hypoventilation. **Skin:** ...

Nursing implications/...
Possible nursing diagn...
Potential for injury.
◆ Have patient rate ... before and after n... and record inadeq...
◆ Monitor closely ... keep side rails ... allowed out of ...
◆ Give pain m...
◆ Be aware ... dence may ... appear up... ued.
◆ For na... for abs... narco...

Patien...
Pos...
al...

acebutolol

aseh-byu'to-lol

Monitan, Sectral

Class: Selective beta-1 adrenergic blocking agent, Antihypertensive, antiarrhythmic

PEDS	PREG	GERI
✋	B	✋

Action Reduces blood pressure (precise mechanism is unclear), and controls arrhythmias by blocking beta-1 receptors in the myocardium, thereby reducing the response to catecholamines. Decreases cardiac output, peripheral resistance and renin release. Prolongs AV-node refractory period and slows atrial and AV-node conduction. Has mild to moderate intrinsic sympathomimetic activity (ISA).

Use/Therapeutic goal/Outcome

Hypertension: Reduction of blood pressure. ***Outcome criteria:*** Blood pressure within normal limits.

Arrhythmias: Resolution of arrhythmias. ***Outcome criteria:*** Absence of, or reduction in, ventricular premature beats.

Dose range/Administration

Interaction alert: Cardiac glycosides may cause profound bradycardia and may further depress the myocardium. Indomethacin may decrease the antihypertensive effect. May alter antidiabetic agent requirements.

Hypertension: Adult: PO: 400 mg/day in a single or divided doses (range 200–1200 mg/day).

Arrythmias: Adult: PO: 400 mg as single dose or in two divided doses (range 600–1200 mg/day). Maximum dose for the elderly is 800 mg/day.

Clinical alert: Be aware that patients taking this drug may not exhibit tachycardia with fever, hypoglycemia, or hyperthyroidism.

Contraindications/Precautions

PREG B

Contraindicated in hypersensitivity to acebutolol, and in cardiogenic shock, sinus bradycardia, second- or third-degree heart block (PR interval > 0.24 seconds), and overt CHF. ***Use with caution*** in patients with bronchospastic disease, thyrotoxicosis, renal or hepatic impairment, or diabetes.

✋ **Use with caution for pregnant women and the elderly. Safe use in children has not been established.**

Side effects/Adverse reactions

Hypersensitivity: rash, psoriasiform eruption. ***CV:*** chest pain, bradycardia, hypotension, CHF, edema, reduced peripheral circulation. ***GI:*** nausea, diarrhea, constipation, dyspepsia. ***CNS:*** mental depression, insomnia, nightmares, hallucinations, dizziness. ***GU:*** decreased sexual ability, frequent urination.

Nursing implications/Documentation

Possible nursing diagnoses: Activity intolerance; Fatigue; Potential for injury.

◆ Assess mental status and record pulse and blood pressure (if possible, lying, sitting, and standing, in both arms) before administration, and frequently thereafter until response is determined.

◆ Consult with physician to determine desired therapeutic range for blood pressure and heart rate (parameters for withholding the medication should be written by physician).

◆ Ascertain that baseline CBC, electrolytes, BUN, creatinine, and liver function studies have been obtained before giving first dose; report abnormalities and monitor closely thereafter.

◆ Monitor for allergic reactions, and signs of confusion, dizziness, bradycardia, CHF, and hypotension; hold drug and report immediately if these occur.

◆ Supervise ambulation until response is determined.

◆ Document and monitor daily weight, and intake and output; report significant negative or positive balance.

Patient & family teaching/Home care

Possible nursing diagnoses: Knowledge deficit; Impaired home maintenance management; Altered sexuality patterns.

◆ Explain the importance of taking this drug exactly as prescribed, even when feeling well; warn not to discontinue drug abruptly.

◆ Stress importance of medical follow-up; explain that this drug decreases "wear and tear" on blood vessels, reduces the workload of the heart, and improves longevity and health.

◆ Teach how to monitor pulse and blood pressure; stress that syncope, hypertension or hypotension, or persistent dizziness should be reported; provide pulse and blood pressure parameters for withholding medication.

▶

A

- Advise changing positions slowly to avoid dizziness.
- Encourage daily monitoring of weight and reporting sudden weight gain (frequently is fluid retention).
- Warn against drinking alcohol or taking *any* OTC drugs without physician approval (some interactions can cause severe reactions).
- Explain that this drug may alter sexual ability; explore concerns and seek consultation as needed.
- *See Beta Adrenergic Blockers, Antiarryhthmics, and Antihypertensives overviews for more information.*

acetaminophen
a-seat-a-mee'noe-fen

Acephen, Aceta, ♥Ace-Tabs, Acetaminophen Unicerts, Actamin, Actamin Extra, Anacin-3, Anacin-3 Maximum Strength, Anuphen, Apacet, Apacet Extra Strength, Apacet Oral Solution, APAP, ♥Apo-Acetaminophen, ♥Atasol, ♥Atasol Forte, Banesin, ♥Campain, ♠Ceetamol, Children's Anacin-3, Children's Apacet, Children's Geneapap, Children's Panadol, Children's Tylenol, Children's Ty-PAP, Children's Ty-Tabs, Dapa, Datril, Datril Extra Strength, Dolanex, ♠Dymadon, ♥Exdol, ♥Exdol Strong, Genapap, Genebs, Genebs Extra Strength, Gentabs, Halenol, Infant's Anacin-3, Infant's Apacet, Infant's Tylenol, Infant's Ty-PAP, ♠Junior Desprol, Liquiprin, Meda Cap, Meda Tab, Myapap, Neopap, Oraphen, PD, Panadol, Panadol Junior Strength, ♠Panamax, Panex, Paraphen, ♠Parmol, Pedric, Phenaphen, ♥Robigesic, ♥Rounox, Suppap, Tapanol, Tapanol Extra Strength, Tempra, Tenol, Ty Caplets, Ty Caps, Tylenol, Tylenol Extra Strength, Ty-Tabs, Valadol, Valorin.

Class: ★Analgesic and antipyretic prototype
Antidote: Acetylcysteine 20% solution

PEDS	PREG	GERI
🖐	B	🖐

Action Relieves pain by an unclear mechanism (probably through inhibition of prostaglandin synthesis, and synthesis or activity of other substances that sensitize pain receptors to mechanical or chemical stimulation). Reduces fever by acting on the hypothalamus heat-regulating center, causing peripheral vasodilation, perspiring, and heat dissipation. Acetaminophen does not have the antiplatelet activity of aspirin, does not cause gastric bleeding, and has limited anti-inflammatory, uricosuric, and antirheumatic properties.

Use/Therapeutic goal/Outcome
Mild to moderate pain: Relief of pain. **Outcome criteria:** Report of feeling more comfortable; absence of signs of discomfort (frowning, restlessness, crying).

Fever: Reduction of fever. **Outcome criteria:** Reduction of temperature on thermometer reading.

Dose range/Administration
Interaction alert: Do not give with diflunisal (increases acetaminophen blood levels). Cholestyramine decreases acetaminophen blood levels.

Adult: PO, Rectal: 325–650 mg q4-6h prn. *Maximum short-term dose:* 4 g/day. *Maximum long-term dose:* 2.6 g/day. **Child:** PO: 10–15 mg/kg q4h.

Clinical alert: Acetaminophen is available in tablet, chewable tablet, capsule, drops, oral solution, oral suspension, elixir, syrup, and rectal suppository. Tablet form may be crushed and taken with any fluid. Chewable tablets should be chewed thoroughly prior to swallowing.

Contraindications/Precautions
PREG B

Contraindicated in hypersensitivity to acetaminophen, and for prolonged use in anemia, chronic alcoholism, and cardiac, pulmonary, hepatic, or renal disease.

🖐 **Contraindicated for children under 3 years (unless directed by physician). Use with caution for pregnant or nursing mothers (excreted in breast milk) and the elderly.**

Side effects/Adverse reactions
Negligible with recommended dosage; severe liver damage may occur with toxic doses.

Acute toxicity: **GI:** anorexia, nausea, vomiting, diarrhea, epigastric or abdominal pain (2–24 hr post-ingestion); hepatotoxicity (often asymptomatic and indicated by increased serum transaminases and bilirubin 24–48 hrs after ingestion) hepatic coma, hepatic necrosis. **GU:** acute renal failure. **CNS:** dizziness, generalized weakness, lethargy, chills, diaphoresis. **CNS:** stimulation or depression, convulsions, coma, death. **Hem:** hypoprothrombinemia, elevated SGOT and LDH. **CV:** circulatory collapse, vascular collapse. **Misc:** hypoglycemia, metabolic acidosis, hyperthermia.

Chronic ingestion: **Hypersensitivity:** rash, urticaria. **Hem:** hemoglobinemia, neutropenia, leukopenia, thrombocytopenic purpura, agranulocytosis, hyper- or hypoglycemia. *GI:* acute pancreatitis, splenomegaly, liver damage. *GU:* kidney damage. *CNS:* psychologic changes.

Nursing implications/Documentation

Possible nursing diagnoses: Pain; Impaired physical mobility.

♦ Schedule doses so that drug is given *at least 1 hr* before maximum effect is needed; document and report inadequate pain control.

♦ Attempt to determine cause of fever before giving acetaminophen (may mask symptoms that should be treated more specifically; report persistent fever, and keep a record of temperature reading before and after administration).

♦ After long-term use, monitor for restlessness and excitement.

Patient & family teaching/Home care

Possible nursing diagnoses: Knowledge deficit; Impaired home maintenance management.

♦ Stress that overdose of acetaminophen is life threatening because it can destroy the liver; that dose regimen should be strictly monitored; and that suspected overdose should be reported to the emergency room immediately (antidote must be given within 16 hr).

♦ Warn that use of acetaminophen to reduce fever may mask serious illness; advise reporting fever that lasts longer than 2–3 days (for neonates, report immediately).

♦ Counsel families in management of fevers in children; stress that children under 6 years are more prone to febrile seizures.

♦ Advise that eating a high-carbohydrate diet may significantly retard acetaminophen absorption.

♦ Stress the need for medical follow-up if on high doses or on long-term therapy.

♦ *See Narcotic and non-narcotic analgesics overview for more information.*

acetazolamide
a-set-a-zole'a-mide

acetazolamide: ♣*Acetazolam, AK-zol, ♣Apo-Acetazolamide, Dazamide, Diamox, Diamox Sequels*

acetazolamide sodium: *Diamox Parenteral, ♣Diamox Sodium*

Class: Carbonic anhydrase inhibitor, Diuretic

PEDS	PREG	GERI
🖐	C	🖐

Action Inhibits the enzyme carbonic anhydrase: In the proximal tubule of the kidney, this results in diuresis of sodium, potassium, bicarbonate, and water. In the eye, this decreases intraocular pressure by reducing the rate of aqueous humor formation. In the CNS, this reduces seizure activity by an unclear mechanism.

Use/Therapeutic goal/Outcome

Adjunctive treatment of glaucoma: Reduction of intraocular pressure. *Outcome criteria:* Intraocular pressure within normal limits when measured with tonometer. *Seizures:* Prevention of seizures. *Outcome criteria:* Absence or reduction in seizures. *Acute mountain sickness:* Prevention, amelioration of attacks. *Outcome criteria:* Absence of headache, dizziness, shortness of breath.

Dose range/Administration

Interaction alert: Urinary alkalinization due to carbonic anhydrase inhibitors interferes with the action of methenamine. In addition, urinary alkalinization may increase quinidine, amphetamines, pseudoephedrine, and decrease serum levels of salicylates, methotrexate, primidone, lithium, chlorpropamide, digitalis, corticosteroids, and ACTH. Osteomalacia may occur with concomitant phenytoin.

🥄 **Give with food to minimize GI upset.**

Glaucoma: *Adult:* PO: 250–500 mg q4-6h. May be given IM or IV for short-term therapy. *Child:* PO: 5–10 mg/kg q6-8h.

Edema in CHF: *Adult:* PO, IM, or IV: 250 mg to 1 g/day in AM. *Child:* PO, IM, or IV: 5–10 mg/kg q6h.

Anticonvulsant: *Adult:* PO: 250 mg to 1 g/day in divided doses. *Child:* PO: 5–10 mg/kg q6h.

Acute mountain sickness: *Adult:* PO: 500 mg to 1 g/day, beginning 3 or 4 days before ascent and continuing during descent.

Contraindications/Precautions
PREG
C

Contraindicated in hypersensitivity to sulfonamides and derivatives (thiazide diuretics), and in hyponatremia, hypokalemia, other electrolyte imbalances, renal or hepatic dysfunction, adrenal insufficiency, obstructive pulmonary disease, hyperchloremic acidosis, and chronic noncongestive angle-closure glaucoma. Use with caution in diabetes mellitus.

🖐 **Contraindicated for pregnant women. Use with caution for children and the elderly. Safe use for nursing mothers has not been established.**

Side effects/Adverse reactions

Hypersensitivity: fever, rash. *CNS:* drowsiness, paresthesias, lethargy, convulsions, depression, fatigue, weakness, nervousness, confusion, ataxia, headache, tremor, fever. *Eye:* myopia. *GI:* nausea, vomiting, diarrhea, anorexia, taste alterations, melena, hepatic insufficiency. *Hem:* thrombocytopenia, aplastic anemia, hyponatremia, hemolytic anemia, leukopenia, pancytopenia, agranulocytosis, hypokalemia, hyperuricemia, hyperchloremic acidosis. *GU:* crystalluria, renal calculi, hematuria, polyuria, glycosuria. *Misc:* photosensitivity, tinnitus, flaccid paralysis.

Nursing implications/Documentation

Possible nursing diagnoses: Fluid volume deficit; Altered patterns of urinary elimination; Potential for injury.

◆ Ascertain that baseline CBC, sodium, potassium, chloride, carbon dioxide, calcium, magnesium, BUN, creatinine, uric acid, and liver function studies have been obtained before giving first dose; report abnormalities and monitor closely thereafter.

◆ Be aware that diuretics often induce hypokalemia, which predisposes individuals to cardiac arrhythmias, cramps, and digoxin toxicity.

◆ Supervise ambulation until response is determined.

◆ Check with physician to determine dietary restrictions; if a low-salt, high-potassium diet is recommended, consult with dietician to plan a low-salt diet that includes foods and juices high in potassium (orange juice, banana, green leafy vegetables).

Patient & family teaching/Home care

Possible nursing diagnoses: Knowledge deficit; Impaired home maintenance management.

◆ Before giving first dose, explain that the drug will increase the amount and frequency of urination.

◆ Stress the importance of returning for medical follow-up, and the importance of taking this drug exactly as prescribed, even when feeling well.

◆ For glaucoma, emphasize that vision damage can occur unnoticed; stress that ongoing follow-up for measurement of intraocular pressure is essential.

◆ Advise reporting dizziness or severe muscle weakness.

◆ Provide a list of allowed foods and fluids; stress the need to stick to prescribed diet (explain the hazards of too much salt, or too little potassium).

◆ Stress importance of adequate fluid intake to prevent kidney stones.

◆ Warn against driving and activities that require alertness until response has been determined.

◆ *See Diuretics overview for more information.*

acetohexamide   *a-seat-oh-hex'a-mide*

🍀*Dimelor, Dymelor*

Class: Antidiabetic (oral hypoglycemic), First-generation sulfonylurea

Antidote: D$_{50}$W, glucagon

PEDS	PREG	GERI
🖐	D	🖐

Action Reduces serum glucose and promotes cellular nutrition by stimulating insulin release in beta cells of the pancreas (not effective if beta cells have ceased to function). Onset of action occurs within 1 hour; peak action is in 2–4 hours, and duration of action is 12–24 hours.

Use/Therapeutic goal/Outcome

Type II diabetes mellitus (noninsulin-dependent) that is not controlled by meal plan and weight control alone: Normalization of blood glucose levels, glycemic control. *Outcome criteria:* Absence of clinical symptoms of hypoglycemia (confusion, shakiness, weakness, diaphoresis, apprehension) together with blood glucose studies that demonstrate glycemic control (fasting blood sugar: 100–140 mg/dl is good control; 140–200 mg/dl is fair control).

Dose range/Administration

Interaction alert: Anabolic steroids, chloramphenicol, clofibrate, guanethidine, oral anticoagulants, phenylbutazone, salicylates, sulfonamides, and MAO inhibitors increase hypoglycemic action. Corticosteroids, glucagon, rifampin, and thiazide diuretics decrease hypoglycemic response. Beta-blockers and clonidine may prolong hypoglycemic effect and mask symptoms of hypoglycemia. Alcohol may significantly alter hypoglycemic activity and cause a disulfiram-like reaction; use should be avoided.

Type II diabetes mellitus: *Adult:* PO: 250 mg/day, before the first meal; may increase q5-7 days by 250–500 mg/day. *Maximum dose:* 1.5 g/day in divided doses before evening and morning meals.

To replace insulin therapy: *Adult:* PO: 250 mg/day, before the first meal; slowly reduce insulin dose by 25–35% every other day while closely monitoring food intake and blood sugars.

Clinical alert: Acetohexamide is a first-generation sulfonylurea: assess for allergy to sulfa before giving first dose. Check blood glucose levels 3 times a day during transition from an insulin regimen to acetohexamide. Dose requirements vary with age, food intake, activity levels, and concurrent medical problems. Monitor the elderly closely for hypoglycemic reactions; they are likely to require slightly higher fasting blood sugars to prevent clinical symptoms of hypoglycemia.

Contraindications/Precautions

PREG
D

Contraindicated in hypersensitivity to acetohexamide and in Type I diabetes mellitus, uncontrolled diabetes mellitus, and severe renal, hepatic, or endocrine impairment. **Use with caution** in allergy to sulfa; and in Type II diabetics who require surgery, experience trauma, or are compromised by an infection (may require insulin).

⚠ **Contraindicated for children and pregnant or nursing mothers (require insulin). Use with caution for the elderly.**

Side effects/Adverse reactions

Hypersensitivity: itching, rashes. **Hem:** hypoglycemia, sodium loss. **GI:** heartburn, nausea, vomiting. **Skin:** facial flushing.

Nursing implications/Documentation

Possible nursing diagnoses: Potential for injury; Impaired skin integrity; Impaired tissue integrity; Altered nutrition: more than body requirements; Altered nutrition: less than body requirements.

◆ Keep a record of blood sugars taken upon rising in the morning, ½ hr before each meal, and before bedtime snack; report persistent

trends or significant episodes of hyperglycemia or hypoglycemia.

◆ Monitor food intake; notify physician when the patient is not eating.

◆ Monitor daily weights, especially during periods of illness.

◆ If signs of hypoglycemia (tremors, sweating, sudden weakness, pale skin, anxiety, confusion, agitation) are noted, confirm by a capillary blood glucose test first, then give 15 g of a fast-acting carbohydrate (4 oz of fruit juice, 4–6 pieces of hard candy, a tablespoon of sugar or honey). If blood glucose monitoring equipment is not immediately available, then give carbohydrate and check glucose level later.

◆ If signs of hyperglycemia (extreme thirst, frequent urination, fatigue, blurred vision) are noted, confirm by blood glucose meter and report immediately.

Patient & family teaching/Home care

Possible nursing diagnoses: Knowledge deficit; Impaired home maintenance management.

◆ Explain that oral hypoglycemics control blood sugars but do not cure diabetes; stress that regular exercise, careful regulation of diet and medication, close monitoring of blood sugars, and medical supervision help promote health and prevent the long-term complications of diabetes (heart, kidney, eyes).

◆ Advise taking doses in the earlier part of the day to avoid nighttime hypoglycemia.

◆ Point out that diet, activity, weight fluctuations, illness, and emotional stress can affect hypoglycemic medication requirements.

◆ Stress that everything on meal plan should be eaten, especially carbohydrates, but that concentrated sweets should be avoided.

◆ Teach the signs and symptoms of hypoglycemia and hyperglycemia; advise that a fast-acting carbohydrate (4 oz of fruit juice, 4–6 pieces of hard candy, 1 tablespoon of honey or sugar) should be taken for suspected *hypo*glycemia (suspected *hyper*glycemia should be reported immediately).

◆ Advise reporting weight fluctuations of over 10 pounds (5 kg) because it may affect dosage.

◆ Suggest carrying some form of fast-acting carbohydrate (e.g., small box of raisins) for treatment of hypoglycemia.

◆ Warn against use of alcohol and OTC drugs without physician's approval.

- ◆ Recommend wearing a medical alert bracelet to alert others to hypoglycemics use.
- ◆ *See Antidiabetics overview for more information.*

acetophenazine

a-set-oh-fen'a-zeen

acetophenazine maleate: ***Tindal***

Class: Phenothiazine antipsychotic

PEDS	PREG	GERI
🖐	C	🖐

Action Exact mechanism of action has not been determined. Believed to promote calmness and alleviate psychiatric symptoms (disorders of perception, thought, consciousness, mood, affect, and social interaction) by blocking dopamine receptors in the limbic system. Blocks peripheral muscarinic, adrenergic, and histamine receptors. Also has some effect on the hypothalamus and pituitary gland, causing changes in regulation of body temperature and endrocrine function. A 20 mg dose of acetophenazine is approximately equal to 100 mg of chlorpromazine.

Use/Therapeutic goal/Outcome

Schizophrenia, psychosis, agitated behavior, mania associated with bipolar disorders: Promotion of reality orientation, elimination of agitation and hyperactivity. ***Outcome criteria:*** Demonstration of reality orientation, and ability to problem solve and interact with others; absence of agitation/hyperactivity.

Dose range/Administration

Interaction alert: Antacids reduce absorption; separate doses of antacid and phenothiazines by at least 2 hr. Alcohol and other CNS depressants may cause excessive sedation.

Adult: PO: *For hospitalized patients:* Begin with 80–120 mg/day in divided doses. *Maximum dose (severe psychotic states):* 600 mg/day. *For outpatients:* 20 mg tid or qid. ***Child > 12 yrs:*** PO: 0.8–1.6 mg/kg/day in divided doses, to a maximum of 80 mg/day.

Clinical alert: When maintenance dose has been established, consider giving most or all of dose at bedtime to reduce daytime sedation (requires physician's order). Keep IV diphenhydramine available in case of side effect of acute dystonic reaction.

Contraindications/Precautions

Contraindicated in hypersensitivity to acetophenazine or phenothiazines, CNS depression, coma. ***Use with caution*** in hypertension and seizure disorders (may lower seizure threshold); parkinsonism, poorly controlled diabetes mellitus, bronchial asthma, emphysema, narrow-angle glaucoma, cardiac disease, history of hypotension, paralytic ileus, hepatic damage, and prostatic hypertrophy.

🖐 **Contraindicated for children under 12 years and for nursing mothers. Use with caution for the elderly or debilitated. Safe use for pregnant women has not been established.**

Side effects/Adverse reactions

Hypersensitivity: rash. ***CNS:*** high incidence of extrapyramidal reactions (pseudoparkinsonism, akathisia [restless need to keep moving], dystonia, tardive dykinesia), sedation, EEG changes, dizziness, neuroleptic malignant syndrome (fever, tachycardia, tachypnea, profuse sweating, muscle stiffness, pale skin, weakness). ***CV:*** orthostatic hypotension, palpitations, dysrhythmias, EKG changes. ***GI:*** appetite changes, dry mouth, constipation, abnormal liver function. ***GU:*** urinary retention or hesitancy, dark urine, impaired ejaculation, priapism, menstrual irregularities. ***Eye:*** blurred vision. ***Skin:*** photosensitivity. ***MS:*** weight gain. ***Hem:*** hyperglycemia, transient leukopenia, agranulocytosis. ***Misc:*** galactorrhea, gynecomastia.

Nursing implications/Documentation

Possible nursing diagnoses: Potential for injury; Altered thought processes; Constipation; Altered oral mucous membrane.

- ◆ Document baseline mental status and vital signs; record at least daily thereafter until response to therapy has been established, then periodically thereafter.

- ◆ Check CBC, liver function, BUN, and creatinine before giving first dose, and periodically thereafter.

- ◆ Be sure that doses are swallowed (not hoarded).

- ◆ Monitor for orthostatic hypotension, dizziness, and drowsiness; supervise ambulation until response is established.

- ◆ Record weights every 2 weeks; report significant weight gain.

- Prevent constipation by monitoring bowel movements and encouraging adequate fiber and fluid intake; offer laxatives or stool softeners before problem becomes severe.

- Report persistent sore throat, fever, and malaise, because these may indicate agranulocytosis (drug may have to be discontinued).

- Monitor for (and report immediately) signs of neuroleptic malignant syndrome (muscle rigidity, tremors, high fever, tachycardia); this is a rare, but potentially fatal, side effect.

Patient & family teaching/Home care

Possible nursing diagnoses: Sleep pattern disturbance; Impaired home maintenance management.

- Emphasize the need to continue medication, even when feeling well.

- Warn to change positions slowly to prevent dizziness.

- Stress that the effects of alcohol, sedatives and CNS depressants, and tranquilizers may be potentiated.

- Caution to consult with physician before using OTC drugs; stress the need for ongoing medical follow-up.

- Teach the need to report persistent sore throat, fever, and fatigue.

- Point out that doses should not be increased or stopped without checking with physician.

- Caution to wear a sunscreen (number 15), protective clothing, and sunglasses when out in the sun.

- Advise avoidance of driving and other potentially hazardous activities until response is established.

- Suggest using ice chips, hard candy, or gum to relieve side effect of dry mouth; stress the need for good mouth care.

- Warn women to report if pregnancy is planned or suspected.

- *See Antipsychotics overview for more information.*

acetylcysteine

a-se-til-sis'tay-een

A

❖*Airbron, Mucomyst, Mucosol,* ❖ ♠*Parvolex*

Class: Expectorant, Mucolytic, Acetaminophen overdose antidote

PEDS	PREG	GERI
⚘	B	✋

Action Liquifies thick respiratory secretions by breaking the disulfide links that bind mucoproteins within mucus. In acetaminophen poisoning, it lessens or prevents liver damage caused by a hepatotoxic metabolite of acetaminophen, and decreases the potential for fatal liver failure by replenishing hepatic glutathione, which inactivates the metabolite.

Use/Therapeutic goal/Outcome

Acute and chronic lung disease, postoperative lung congestion: Promotion of ability to bring forth mucus. *Outcome criteria:* Increased sputum production and expectoration; improvement in tidal volume; clearing of lung fields.

Antidote for acetaminophen overdose: Prevention of liver failure. *Outcome criteria:* Liver function studies within normal limits; serum acetaminophen levels within normal limits.

Dose range/Administration

Interaction alert: Do not use activated charcoal as an additional antidote to absorb acetaminophen, because it also absorbs acetylcysteine and decreases its effects. (If activated charcoal has been given, lavage before administering acetylcysteine.) Do not mix acetylcysteine with ampicillin, oxytetracycline, tetracycline, erthromycin lactobionate, amphotericin B, iodized oil (contrast medium), chymotrypsin, and trypsin because they are incompatible.

Acute and chronic lung disease, Postoperative lung congestion: *Adult and Child:* *Nebulization by face mask, mouthpiece, or tracheostomy:* 1–10 cc of 20% solution, or 2–20 cc of 10% solution q2-6h. *Nebulization by tent or croupette:* the volume necessary of the 10–20% solution to maintain a heavy mist—as much as 300 cc has been used during a single treatment. *Direct instillation:* 1–2 cc of 10–20% solution q1-4h.

Acetaminophen poisoning: *Adult and Child:* PO: 140 mg/kg initially, followed by 70 mg/kg q4h for 17 doses or until acetaminophen levels are within normal range. Contact the regional poison control center to verify dosage and protocol for use of acetylcysteine. The decision to give

▶

or continue acetylcysteine is based upon serum acetaminophen levels and specific nomograms.

Clinical alert: For inhalation therapy, the 20% solution should be diluted with Normal Saline or Sterile Water (for Injection or Inhalation) USP; the 10% solution may be used undiluted. Give inhalation doses upon arising in the morning and before meals for optimal effects and minimal incidence of nausea. Dilute oral doses with fruit juice, cola, or water.

Contraindications/Precautions

PREG **B**

Contraindicated in hypersensitivity to acetyl-cysteine. ***Use with caution*** for asthmatics, and the debilitated.

☙ **Use with caution for children and the elderly. Safe use for pregnant or nursing mothers has not been established, but benefit of use outweighs the risks.**

Side effects/Adverse reactions

Hypersensitivity: shortness of breath, tightness in chest, wheezing, skin rash, hives, anaphylaxis. ***GI:*** nausea, stomatitis. ***Resp:*** rhinorrhea, bronchospasm, burning sensation of the upper respiratory passages, hemoptysis.

Nursing implications/Documentation

Possible nursing diagnoses: Ineffective airway clearance; Altered oral mucous membrane.

◆ For expectorant use, document lung sounds and sputum production before and after dose.

◆ Encourage coughing and use suctioning for those with inadequate cough.

◆ Record intake and output, and monitor for dehydration; provide favorite fluids (intake should be at least 2 L/day).

◆ Provide special mouth care after each treatment.

Patient & family teaching/Home care

Possible nursing diagnoses: Knowledge deficit; Impaired home maintenance management.

◆ Stress that this drug is most effective when taken upon rising in the morning and before meals; teach to cough and clear lungs once before starting treatment.

◆ Stress the need to cough up secretions to prevent accumulation in airways.

◆ Warn that once opened, the vial or dropper should be refrigerated and used within 96 hr (4 days).

◆ Explain the importance of maintaining adequate hydration (at least 2 quarts/day).

◆ *See Antitussives, Expectorants, and Mucolytics overview for more information.*

acyclovir

ay-sye'kloe-ver

Zovirax

Class: ★Anti-infective (antiviral) prototype, Anti-rickettsial

PEDS	PREG	GERI
☙	C	☙

Action Limits multiplication of viruses by interfering with DNA synthesis. Has highly selective inhibitory activity against *Herpes simplex* types 1 and 2, *varicella zoster*, Epstein-Barr, and cytomegalovirus.

Use/Therapeutic goal/Outcome

Herpes simplex (HSV–1 and HSV–2), herpes zoster, and herpes varicella infections: Prevention or resolution of infection. ***Outcome criteria:*** Absence of growth of herpes virus on cultures, absence of clinical manifestations of herpetic infection (itching, fever, pain, swelling, redness, heat, drainage, lesions) normal WBC count.

Dose range/Administration

Adult/Child > ***12 yrs:*** PO: 1000 mg/day in 5 doses q4h for 7–10 days. *Recurrent episodes:* Treatment may last only 5 days. IV: 5 mg/kg q8h infused slowly over 1 hour, for 5 to 7 days. *For herpes zoster:* 800 mg 5 times a day for 7 days. *Topical:* Gently apply to cover all lesions q3h during waking hours. *Never apply to the eye.* ***Child 6 mos–12 yr:*** IV: 250 mg/m^2 q8h infused slowly over 1 hour.

Clinical alert: Never administer IV bolus or IM. Rapid IV infusion may result in precipitation of acyclovir crystals in renal tubules. Therapy should begin as soon as early symptoms (itching, tingling, pain) are noted.

Contraindications/Precautions

PREG **C**

Contraindicated in hypersensitivity to acyclovir or (for ointment) components of the topical ointment. Use with caution in renal impairment, dehydration, and neurological problems.

☙ **Use with caution for the elderly. Safe use for children under 12 years and pregnant or nursing mothers has not been established.**

Side effects/Adverse reactions

Hypersensitivity: itching, rash. *GI:* nausea, vomiting, diarrhea. *CNS:* headache, lethargy, hallucinations, agitation, seizures, coma. *CV:* (with IV route) hypotension, pain, redness, swelling, and thrombophlebitis at injection site. *GU:* (with IV route) transient elevation of serum creatinine, hematuria. *Skin:* (with ointment) mild burning or stinging. *Misc:* joint pain.

Nursing implications/Documentation

Possible nursing diagnoses: Potential for infection; Diarrhea; Pain; Impaired skin integrity.

♦ Encourage 2000–4000 ml of fluids per day to prevent renal toxicity; monitor and record intake and output.

♦ Weigh patient and obtain necessary baseline lab studies (CBC, BUN, creatinine, liver function studies) and necessary culture specimens, before administering first dose. (May not be necessary for routine prophylaxis).

Patient & family teaching/Home care

Possible nursing diagnoses: Knowledge deficit; Impaired home maintenance management; Potential sexual dysfunction.

♦ Teach the early signs and symptoms of infection (tingling, itching, pain) so that acyclovir can be started before infection fully develops.

♦ Explain the importance of preventing kidney side effects by drinking 2–4 quarts of fluid daily (not necessary with ointment).

♦ Explain that acyclovir is effective in managing the disease, but is not a cure, and neither eliminates the virus nor prevents its spread to others. (For genital herpes, encourage consistent use of a condom during sexual intercourse, even if lesions are not visible).

♦ Teach how to use disposable gloves when applying ointment, to prevent transmission and auto-inoculation.

♦ Point out the need to keep affected areas clean and dry, to avoid heat application to affected areas (e.g., hot liquids or baths), to avoid exposure to the sun, to not scratch or rub (which is likely to make lesions worse), and to wear loose-fitting clothes to prevent irritation of affected areas.

♦ Encourage females to have annual PAP tests (herpes is associated with increased risk of cervical cancer).

♦ See Anti-infectives overview for more information.

albumin
al-byou'min

> normal serum albumin 5% (human): **Albuminar 5%, Albutein 5%, Buminate 5%, Plasbumin 5%**
>
> normal serum albumin 25% (human): **Albuminar 25%, Albumisol 25%, Buminate 25%, Plasbumin 25%**
>
> *Class:* Blood volume expander
>
> | PEDS | PREG | GERI |
> |------|------|------|
> | 🤚 | C | 🤚 |

Action Replenishes plasma proteins and colloids (albumin) and expands circulating blood volume by exerting osmotic pull on tissue fluids. Reduces serum bilirubin in newborns by binding with circulating bilirubin; this complex is removed from circulation during exchange transfusion.

Use/Therapeutic goal/Outcome

Hypovolemic shock: Promotion of adequate circulatory volume and tissue perfusion until whole blood is available. *Outcome criteria:* Reversal in signs and symptoms of shock (e.g., systolic BP > 100 mm Hg; urine output > 25–30 ml/hr; heart rate < 100, with palpable peripheral pulses).

Hypoproteinemia: Replenishment of protein and albumin in the blood. *Outcome criteria:* Total serum protein within normal limits (5.7–7.9 g/dl); serum albumin within normal limits (3.4–4.8 g/dl).

Burns: Maintenance of normal plasma albumin levels. *Outcome criteria:* Plasma albumin level of 2–3 g/dl.

Newborn hyperbilirubinemia: Reduction in serum bilirubin. *Outcome criteria:* Total serum bilirubin within normal limits (0.2–1 mg/dl).

Dose range/Administration

Hypovolemic Shock: Adult and Child: IV: 500 ml 5% solution q 30 min prn.

Hypoproteinemia and Burns: Adult: IV: 1000–1500 ml/day 5% solution at 120–240 ml/hr (maximum rate 300–600 ml/hr), or 25–100 g/day 25% solution at 60 ml/hr (maximum rate 100 ml/hr). *Child:* IV: 25–50% of adult dose.

Hyperbilirubinemia and erythroblastosis fetalis: neonate: IV: 4 ml/kg of 25% solution 1–2 hr before transfusion. *Maximum dose:* 250 g/48 hr.

▶

A **Clinical alert:** Dosage is individualized based upon patient condition and response. Discard bottles that are not used within 4 hr of opening, and bottles that have cloudy solutions or sediment (solution should be clear amber).

Contraindications/Precautions
PREG C

Contraindicated in severe anemia and heart failure. **Use with caution** in low cardiac reserve, pulmonary disease, liver or kidney failure, dehydration, or sodium restrictions.

�™ **Use with caution for children and the elderly. Safe use for pregnant or nursing mothers has not been established.**

Side effects/Adverse reactions

Hypersensitivity: Fever, chills, itching, rashes. **CV:** (more likely with rapid infusion) circulatory overload with pulmonary edema, hypotension, altered pulse rate. **Resp:** dyspnea, tachypnea. **GI:** nausea, vomiting, increased salivation.

Nursing implications/Documentation

Possible nursing diagnosis: Potential for injury.

♦ Before infusing, record baseline assessment of lung and heart sounds, vital signs, and CVP or PAP (if available).

♦ Report presence of peripheral edema, sacral edema, or neck vein distension.

♦ During infusion, record vital signs every 15 min to every hr, depending on patient condition; record intake and output every 1 to 2 hours.

♦ Stop infusion if signs and symptoms of congestive heart failure or pulmonary edema (cough, dyspnea, rales, cyanosis) become evident; notify physician immediately.

♦ For use in hypovolemic shock due to hemorrhage, monitor for new bleeding sites: the increase in blood pressure may cause hemorrhage of severed vessel that failed to bleed at a lower blood pressure.

♦ Keep the patient in bed with side rails up.

Patient & family teaching/Home care

Possible nursing diagnoses: Anxiety; Fear; Knowledge deficit.

♦ Encourage voicing of questions and concerns; explain rationale for all actions.

♦ Explain that this solution replenishes deficient supplies of protein.

♦ Stress that vital signs will be monitored closely to ensure safety.

albuterol
al-byoo'ter-ole

albuterol (salbutamol): ♠*Respolin*

albuterol sulfate (salbutamol sulfate): *Proventil, Proventil Repetabs, Proventil Syrup,* ♠*Respolin, Ventolin,* ♠*Obstetric Injection*

Class: Sympathomimetic (adrenergic) bronchodilator

PEDS ☙   PREG C   GERI ☙

Action Produces bronchodilation by stimulating bronchial beta-2 adrenergic receptors, which relaxes the smooth muscle of the bronchial tree. Acts longer than isoproterenol and metaproterenol, and causes less cardiac stimulation.

Use/Therapeutic goal/Outcome

Bronchospasm in reversible obstructive airway disease: Reduction of airway resistance, improvement of air movement. **Outcome criteria:** Decreased wheezing, increased forced expiratory volume (FEV); clearing of lung fields; report of breathing easier and of fewer wheezing episodes.

Premature labor: Prevention of premature birth. **Outcome criteria:** Absence of uterine contractions.

Dose range/Administration

Interaction alert: Sympathomimetics, MAO inhibitors, and tricyclic antidepressants may increase cardiac stimulation. Albuterol and beta-blockers may inhibit the effects of each other.

Prevention of exercise-induced bronchospasm: Adult/Child > 13 yrs: Inhal: 1–2 inhalations q4-6h or 15 min before exercising prn.

Treatment of Bronchospasm: Adult/Child > 13 yrs: Inhal: 1–2 inhalations q4-6h (do not increase frequency). **Adult > 65 yrs:** PO(tablet, liquid): 2 mg tid or qid. **Adult/Child > 13 yrs:** PO: *Tablets, liquid:* 2–4 mg tid or qid; may gradually increase to a maximum of 8 mg qid. *Sustained-release tablets:* 4–8 mg q12h; may increase to a maximum of 16 mg q12h. **Child 6–13 yrs:** PO: 2 mg tid or qid. **Child 2–6 yrs:** PO: 0.1 mg/kg tid, not to exceed 2 mg tid.

Premature Labor: Adult: IV: Using a pump or controller, begin with 10 mg/min. Increase dose at 10-min intervals until contractions stop, then maintain drip rate for 1 hour. If there are no contractions for that hour, gradually taper dose by 50% increments at 6-hour intervals. Should not be used longer than 48 hours. PO: 4–8 mg.

Clinical alert: Schedule doses around the clock (q8h for tid, and q6h for qid) for optimal results.

Contraindications/Precautions

PREG
C

Contraindicated in hypersensitivity to albuterol. ***Use with caution*** in hypertension, cardiac disease, arrhythmias, convulsive disorders, diabetes mellitus, or hyperthyroidism.

🖐 **Use with caution for the elderly. Safe use for pregnant (except premature labor) or nursing mothers, or of inhalent for children under 12 years, or syrup for children under 2 years, has not been established.**

Side effects/Adverse reactions

Hypersensitivity: exaggeration of side effects. ***CNS:*** tremors, nervousness, dizziness, vertigo, headache, irritability, excitement, insomnia, weakness. ***CV:*** palpitations, hypertension, hypotension, tachycardia. ***GI:*** nausea, vomiting, heartburn. ***MS:*** muscle cramps.

Nursing implications/Documentation

Possible nursing diagnoses: Anxiety; Fear; Ineffective breathing pattern.

◆ **For respiratory use**

  ◆ Record lung sounds, respirations, pulse, and blood pressure, before and after dose administration, until response has been determined.

  ◆ Monitor for paradoxical bronchospasm; if this occurs, stop drug, report immediately, and support the patient.

  ◆ Provide favorite fluids, and monitor intake and output to ensure adequate hydration (at least 2 liters a day is recommended).

◆ **For use in premature labor**

  ◆ Monitor maternal heart rate and report tachycardia > 140.

Patient & family teaching/Home care

Possible nursing diagnoses: Knowledge deficit; Impaired home maintenance management.

  ◆ Explain that this drug is intended to prevent and relieve bronchospasm, and to make breathing easier.

◆ **For respiratory use**

  ◆ Point out that stress and exercise can aggravate wheezing and bronchospasm, and that

relaxation and controlled breathing techniques can help reduce severity and frequency of wheezing episodes.

  ◆ Teach the proper use of metered dose apparatus; warn that increasing dose or frequency is not recommended.

  ◆ Warn to withhold the drug and notify physician immediately if symptoms worsen after administration.

  ◆ Caution to avoid OTC drugs unless they are approved by the physician.

◆ **For use in premature labor**

  ◆ Reassure that both mother and infant will be closely monitored to ensure safe dosage.

◆ *See Bronchodilators and Adrenergics (Sympathomimetics) overviews for more information.*

alfentanil

al-phen'ta-nil

alfentanil hydrochloride: ***Alfenta, Rapifen***
Class: Narcotic analgesic
Antidote: Naloxone hydrochloride (Narcan)

PEDS	PREG	GERI	CONTROLLED SUBSTANCE
🖐	C	🖐	II

Action Alters both the perception of and response to pain through an unclear mechanism. Believed to act by binding with opiate receptor sites in the CNS.

Use/Therapeutic goal/Outcome

Primary anesthetic or analgesic adjunct to other anesthetics for induction or maintenance of anesthesia during surgical procedure lasting less than 1 hour: Promotion of relaxation, sedation, and comfort. ***Outcome criteria:*** Visible drowsiness or sleep; absence of observable signs of pain (grimacing, frowning, withdrawing from operative site, fighting endotracheal intubation); blood pressure and pulse within normal limits when compared to baseline.

Dose range/Administration

Interaction alert: Use cautiously and consider reduced alfentanil doses when given with diazepam or other CNS depressants (e.g., barbiturates, tranquilizers, opioids, or inhalation anesthetic agents).

Adjunct to anesthesia: Adult: IV: 8–75 mcg/kg, then 3–5 mcg/kg/min (stop 10–15 min before end of surgery).

Primary anesthetic: **Adult:** IV: 130–245 mcg/kg, then 0.5–1.5 mcg/kg/min (stop 10–15 min before end of surgery).

Clinical alert: This drug should be given only by those qualified to manage IV anesthetics. Expect reduced dosage for the elderly or debilitated. Keep narcotic antagonist (naloxone) and resuscitation equipment readily available.

Contraindications/Precautions
PREG C

Contraindicated in hypersensitivity to alfentanil. **Use with caution** in head injury, lung disease, and impaired respiratory, hepatic, or renal function.

Contraindicated for children under 12 years and pregnant women. Use with caution for nursing mothers and the elderly.

Side effects/Adverse reactions

Hypersensitivity: respiratory depression, skeletal muscle rigidity, bradycardia, asystole, arrhythmias. **CV:** hypotension, tachycardia. **GI:** nausea, vomiting. **CNS:** dizziness, sleepiness, postoperative sedation and confusion, headache. **Eye:** blurred vision. **Skin:** itching. **Resp:** laryngospasm, respiratory depression.

Nursing implications/Documentation

Possible nursing diagnoses: Potential for aspiration; Potential for injury; Pain.

• Be sure that history of allergies, weight, and baseline vital signs are posted on chart before procedure.

• Monitor airway and suction secretions as necessary.

• Watch closely for potential for injury; position extremities and head carefully; keep side rails up.

• Record vital signs every 5–15 min until recovered and stable, then per protocol or orders; monitor closely for delayed respiratory depression, bradycardia, arrhythmias, and hypotension.

• Give postoperative pain medication before pain is severe.

Patient & family teaching/Home care

Possible nursing diagnoses: Fear; Sensory/Perceptual alterations.

• Ascertain that necessary preoperative teaching has been done before giving afentanil.

• Explain procedures briefly and in simple terms (even if the patient is not awake, he may still be able to hear).

◆ *See Narcotic and non-narcotic analgesics overview for more information.*

allopurinol
al-oh-pure'i-nole

♠Alloremed, ♠Capurate, Lopurin, Zyloprim
Class: Antihyperuricemic, Antigout agent, Antiurolithic

PEDS	PREG	GERI
♨	C	♨

Action Reduces both urine and serum levels of uric acid by inhibiting the action of xanthine oxidase in the synthesis of uric acid.

Use/Therapeutic goal/Outcome

Gouty arthritis: Prevention or reduction of urate deposits in joints. **Outcome criteria:** Decreased joint deformities and reduced frequency of gout attacks.

Hyperuricemia: Prevention or reduction of gouty arthritis and/or renal damage from elevated uric acid levels due to disease or medication. **Outcome criteria:** Decrease in uric acid levels in serum and urine.

Dose range/Administration

Interaction alert: Antineoplastic agents increase the possibility of bone marrow suppression. May potentiate action of oral hypoglycemics and anticoagulants. Decreases excretion of phenytoin and theophylline.

Give with meals to reduce GI distress.
Adult: PO: 100–800 mg/day. *Maximum single dose:* 300 mg/day. **Child:** PO: 150–300 mg/day.

Clinical alert: Give doses over 300 mg in divided doses. During the first 3–6 months of treatment with allopurinol, colchicine may be administered prophylactically because of the increased possibility of acute attacks of gout.

Contraindications/Precautions
PREG C

Contraindicated in hypersensitivity to allopurinol. **Use with caution** in renal or hepatic impairment.

Use with caution for the elderly and pregnant or nursing mothers. Rarely indicated for children except in malignant diseases.

Side effects/Adverse reactions

Hypersensitivity: rash, fever, chills. *CNS:* drowsiness. *Eye:* cataracts. *Hem:* bone marrow suppression, leukopenia, leukocytosis, eosinophilia. *GI:* nausea, vomiting, diarrhea, hepatomegaly. *Skin:* pruritic maculopapular rash.

Nursing implications/Documentation

Possible nursing diagnoses: Potential for injury.

◆ Anticipate more frequent occurrence of adverse reaction in the elderly and those with decreased renal function.

◆ Assess for and report appearance of a rash which may be first indication of a hypersensitivity reaction.

◆ Encourage fluid intake to produce urinary output of at least 2 liters daily; monitor and record intake and output.

◆ Monitor results of liver and renal function studies to identify changes from pretreatment baseline.

Patient & family teaching/Home care

Possible nursing diagnoses: Knowledge deficit; Impaired home maintenance management; Impaired skin integrity.

◆ Advise to discontinue medication and report promptly the appearance of a rash, hives, or itching, especially if associated with chills, fever, muscle aches or pains, nausea, or vomiting.

◆ Caution that taking allopurinol may increase the frequency of acute attacks of gout during the first 6–12 months of therapy, but that attacks will become less severe and of shorter duration.

◆ Stress the need to continue taking allopurinol during acute attacks of gout as well as taking other medications to relieve pain and inflammation.

◆ With primary gout, advise that allopurinol may be taken at a decreased dose indefinitely to maintain low serum uric acid levels.

◆ Caution to avoid driving and operating dangerous machinery until response to allopurinol has been determined.

◆ Teach the importance of drinking at least 8–12 8-oz glasses of fluids daily.

◆ Encourage to have scheduled blood tests as ordered.

◆ Warn to avoid drinking alcohol which increases the amount of uric acid in the blood and lessens the effectiveness of allopurinol.

◆ Advise to minimize ultraviolet exposure which may increase risk of cataracts.

alprazolam

al-prey'zoe-lam

Xanax

Class: Antianxiety agent, benzodiazepine

PEDS	PREG	GERI
✋	**D**	✋

**CONTROLLED SUBSTANCE
IV**

Action Produces CNS depression and relaxation by potentiating the action of gamma-aminobuteric acid (GABA), which reduces neuronal activity in all regions of the CNS. Promotes muscle relaxation by inhibiting spinal motor reflex pathways. Decreases anxiety by inhibiting cortical and limbic arousal.

Use/Therapeutic goal/Outcome

Short-term treatment of anxiety (less than 4 months): Alleviation of symptoms of apprehension, muscle tension, and insomnia. *Outcome criteria:* Report of feeling more calm, sleeping better, and coping better; observable signs of decreased anxiety (decreased motor activity, reduced muscle tension, decrease in pulse and blood pressure).

Dose range/Administration

Interaction alert: Alcohol and other CNS depressants may cause excessive sedation. Cimetidine may increase blood levels. May increase serum levels of tricyclic antidepressants.

🥄 **Give with food or milk if GI upset is noted.**
Adult: PO: 0.25–0.5 mg tid. *Maximum dose:* 4 mg/day. *For the elderly:* 0.25 mg bid or tid.

Clinical alert: When discontinuing drug after long-term therapy (more than 1 month), doses should be tapered gradually, rather than withdrawn abruptly.

Contraindications/Precautions

**PREG
D**

Contraindicated in hypersensitivity or intolerance to alprazolam or other benzodiazepines, and in narrow-angle glaucoma. *Use with caution* in psychosis, depression, suicidal tendencies, or impaired liver or kidney function.

🖐 **Contraindicated for pregnant or nursing mothers. Use with caution for the elderly or debilitated. Safe use for children has not been established.**

A

Side effects/Adverse reactions

Hypersensitivity: rash, itching. *CNS:* lethargy, drowsiness, insomnia, tremors, dizziness, confusion, depression. *CV:* hypotension, transient tachycardia and bradycardia. *Resp:* respiratory depression. *GI:* anorexia, dry mouth, nausea, vomiting, constipation. *GU:* urinary retention. *Eye:* blurred vision, mydriasis. *Misc:* drug tolerance and dependence.

Nursing implications/Documentation

Possible nursing diagnoses: Potential for injury; Constipation.

♦ Record baseline blood pressure; monitor closely if dizziness is experienced. Supervise ambulation until response is determined.

♦ Be sure that doses are swallowed (not hoarded).

♦ Provide a quiet environment that is conducive to rest.

♦ Monitor bowel elimination and provide adequate fluids and fiber to prevent constipation; give laxatives before the problem is severe.

Patient & family teaching/Home care

Possible nursing diagnoses: Anxiety; Fear; Ineffective individual coping; Impaired home maintenance management.

♦ Advise taking this drug with milk or food if GI symptoms are noted.

♦ Help the individual identify stressors that contribute to anxiety and ways of coping effectively; stress that effective coping strategies can reduce the need for medication.

♦ Explain the importance of daily exercise in relieving stress, and encourage establishing a plan for getting enough exercise (e.g., daily walks).

♦ Point out that drug tolerance and dependence can occur, and that the drug should be used only when holistic measures (e.g., quiet music, relaxation techniques) are not effective.

♦ Emphasize that the effects of alcohol, other sedatives and CNS depressants, and tranquilizers may be potentiated (these should be avoided).

♦ Advise avoidance of driving and other potentially hazardous activities until response is established.

♦ *See Antianxiety agents/Sedatives/Hypnotics overview for more information.*

alteplase

all'ti-plaze

recombinant alteplase (tissue plasmingen activator [t-PA]): ♠*Actilyse, Activase*
Class: Thrombolytic enzyme (fibrinolytic)
Antidote: Aminocaproic acid

PEDS	PREG	GERI
🖑	C	🖑

Action Directly dissolves existing clots (thrombi) by selectively binding to clot fibrin and locally converting plasminogen to plasmin (the enzyme that degrades fibrin).

Use/Therapeutic goal/Outcome

Emergency treatment of acute myocardial infarction (not used more than 6 hr after onset of symptoms of coronary artery occlusion): Lysis of thrombi obstructing coronary arteries, reperfusion of ischemic cardiac tissue. *Outcome criteria:* Abrupt cessation of chest pain (often accompanied by sudden onset of hypotension and reperfusion arrhythmias); smaller Q waves, and return of ST segment to baseline on EKG; cardiac enzyme *washout* (cardiac enzymes peak faster than they do in untreated myocardial infarction); absence of coronary occlusion upon cardiac catheterization (may be performed hours or days later when risk of bleeding has diminished).

Dose range/Administration

Interaction alert: Do not mix any other IV drugs with alteplase solution. Risk of bleeding increases with concurrent oral anticoagulants, heparin, or drugs that affect platelet function (salicylates, dipyridamole, nonsteroidal antiinflammatory agents); however, concomitant IV heparin is common, as is therapy with aspirin and/or dipyridamole following heparin (check policy, because some physicians believe that these should be *avoided*).

Adult: IV infusion: As soon as possible after onset of symptoms, administer a total dose of 100 mg *over 3 hr:* Give a *lysis* dose of 60 mg, which consists of an initial 10 mg bolus injected over 2 min and then 50 mg infused over the remainder of the first hr. Give 20 mg/hr over the second and third hr. For smaller adults (weight less than 65 kg), total dose should be 1.25 mg/kg; 10 percent as a bolus, 50 percent over the remainder of the first hr and 20 percent per hr for the next 2 hr. *No more than a total of 150 mg of alteplase should be given because the risk of intracranial bleeding increases with higher doses.* Check package insert or hospital policy for method of reconstitution and administration. The following is suggested: *Reconstitution:* Slowly inject 1 cc of (*nonbacteriostatic*) sterile water for injection for each milligram of alteplase in vial. Do not use more than 1 cc of sterile water per 1 mg of altepase because it may cause precipitation. *Do not shake the mixture* (causes bubble formation and clumping of medication). *Do not use if vacuum is not present.* Reconstituted alteplase should be clear and colorless or pale yellow. Withdraw 100 mg of this alteplase solution (total volume should be 100 cc), and inject into 100 cc of D5W or N5, to make a concentration of 1 mg of alteplase per 2 cc of solution. *Administration:* Withdraw 20 cc of this solution (10 mg/20 cc bolus) and give over 1–2 min (do *not* use a filter). Follow this by administering remaining alteplase solution (90 mg in 180 cc) via IV pump or controller at 100 cc/hr *for the first hour* (to deliver 50 mg). *For the second and third hr,* set rate at 40 cc per hour (to deliver the remaining 40 mg at a rate of 20 mg/hr). To ensure that medication in tubing is given, remove the alteplase medication bag or bottle, attach a 50 cc bag of D5W to the same tubing, and infuse at 40 cc/hr. Once drug is infused, flush lock with saline or *change tubing* before next IV.

Clinical alert: This drug should be administered only by professionals who are well educated in all aspects of its administration. Be sure that three IV sites and any other invasive lines are established before administration of alteplase, and have the following at the patient's bedside:

- Electrocardiogram machine
- Emergency medications
- Advanced cardiac life support (ACLS) cart (with defibrillator)
- 100 cc bag of D5W
- IV tubing (*without* filter)
- 3 IV pumps or controllers.

Contraindications/Precautions

PREG
C

Contraindicated in hypersensitivity to alteplase, and in active internal bleeding or known source of potential bleeding (e.g., ulcer disease); cerebrovascular accident (CVA), intracranial neoplasm, arteriovenous malformation, intracranial aneurysm; known bleeding diathesis; diabetic retinopathy; cranial or spinal surgery (or trauma), organ biopsy, or cavity aspiration within less than 8 weeks; surgery, trauma, or CPR (especially with rib fractures) within 10 days; traumatic endotracheal intubation; persistent hypertension (with systolic blood pressure greater than 180 mm Hg, or diastolic greater than 110 mm Hg) after treatment; subacute bacterial endocarditis. *Use with caution* for patient with recent puncture (within 10 days) of a noncompressible vessel, prothrombin time greater than 15 seconds, aspirin consumption within 72 hours, known (or suspected) left heart thrombus.

☞ **Contraindicated in known or suspected pregnancy. Use with caution for those over 75 years (physician may deem to be contraindicated). Safety for children has not been established.**

Side effects/Adverse reactions

Hypersensitivity: itching, rashes. *CNS:* cerebral hemorrhage. *CV:* hypotension, dysrrhythmias. *GI:* nausea, vomiting, bleeding. *Misc:* bleeding of surgical or traumatic injury, bleeding from puncture sites, fever.

Nursing implications/Documentation

Possible nursing diagnoses: Potential for injury; Pain; Anxiety; Fear.

◆ Obtain a careful history of chest pain, and closely monitor level of chest pain, before, during, and after administration of alteplase.

◆ Expect SL and IV nitroglycerin to be given to rule out vasospasm before alteplase administration.

◆ Assess carefully for contraindications to alteplase.

◆ Attach patient to cardiac monitor and select the lead that shows the highest ST-segment elevation (also attach patient to a 12-lead EKG; periodic EKGs will be necessary during administration).

◆ *Check hospital policy and procedure to determine variations in the following interventions.*

◆ Be sure baseline and other "stat" lab studies are drawn before initiating alteplase (PT, PTT, CBC, fibrinogen level, renal lab studies, cardiac enzymes, type and crossmatch for 2 units of blood, and other routine coronary admission studies determined by hospital policy).

◆ Have the necessary equipment ready for three large-bore peripheral intravenous lines (one for administration of alteplase; another for administration of other drugs, such as heparin and lidocaine; and the third for drawing blood

A

samples; one of these may be needed for blood transfusion if hemorrhage occurs).

◆ Before, during, and after administration of alteplase, document and report presence of abnormal pulses, abnormal neurological findings, or skin lesions (may indicate coagulation defects).

◆ Document vital signs every 15 min during infusion and for 1–2 hr after infusion, then every 30 min until ordered otherwise; also document EKG strips to have a record of changes in ST segments.

◆ Document neurological signs on a flow sheet every 30 min for at least 2 hr (check policy).

◆ Be prepared to treat reperfusion dysrhythmias (ventricular tachycardia or fibrillation; atrial tachycardia or fibrillation) according to hospital protocol or individual physician orders; have emergency drugs and defibrillator readily available (some protocols will include starting a lidocaine drip and a heparin drip when alteplase is initiated).

◆ Keep all needle punctures to an absolute **minimum**, apply manual pressure for 10 min to all venous puncture sites, and for 30 min to arterial puncture sites; follow this with pressure dressing, and observe all intravenous and intra-arterial sites every 15 min for 1hr, every 30 min for 2 hr, every hr for 4 hr, then every 2 hr until removed.

◆ Place a sign on door and over bed to alert staff and phlebotomist of bleeding precautions.

◆ Maintain patient on complete bedrest until otherwise ordered, and monitor closely for bleeding: hemoptysis, CVA, hematuria, hematemesis, melena, pain or swelling from closed space bleeding, and signs and symptoms of cardiac tamponade (distended neck veins and significant pulsus paradoxus). Report immediately if these are observed.

◆ Keep aminocaproic acid available as antidote in case of hemorrhage.

◆ Check for the following lab orders post-infusion: CPK, CPK Isoenzymes (q4h × 3, then qd × 2); Hgb and Hct (q4h the first 24 hr, then once the next day); PTT (stat and q4h × 2, then daily throughout heparin therapy; should be maintained in the 80–120 second range.

Patient & family teaching/Home care

Possible nursing diagnoses: Anxiety; Fear; Knowledge deficit.

◆ Explain the rationale for prompt initiation of treatment, and for routine procedures that ensure patient safety.

◆ Encourage the person to voice questions and concerns, and to report development of new symptoms (headache, dizziness, chest discomfort, abdominal discomfort).

◆ Explain that symptoms associated with hypotension and dysrhythmias are likely to be transient.

◆ Emphasize the need to remain in bed.

◆ *See Anticoagulants and Thrombolytic Enzymes overview for more information.*

aluminum and magnesium

aluminum hydroxide and magnesium hydroxide: *Aludrox, Delcid, Gelusil II, Kudrox, Maalox, Mylanta, Rulox, WinGel*

Class: Antacid

PEDS	PREG	GERI
🤚	C	🤚

Action Neutralizes existing stomach acid; decreases pepsin activity by elevating gastric and esophageal pH.

Use/Therapeutic goal/Outcome

Hyperacidity and gastroesophageal reflux: Reduction of acid concentration within the esophagus and stomach. *Outcome criteria:* Report of decreased pain and upper GI irritation.

Dose range/Administration

Interaction alert: Do not give other oral medications for 2 hr after alumina and magnesia to ensure their absorption. Separate doses of alumina and magnesia from doses of enteric coated drugs by 1 hr (causes enteric coated drugs to be released while still in the stomach).

Adult: PO: *Liquid:* 5–20 ml 1 and 3 hr pc and hs. *Tablets or wafers:* 1–4 tablets 1 and 3 hr pc and hs. *Child:* PO: Individualize dose.

Clinical alert: For peptic ulcers, giving doses 1 and 3 hr after meals and at bedtime enhances therapeutic effects. Shake liquid form well before administration and follow with water or milk. After giving via nasogastric tube, flush with water. Combination of aluminum hydroxide and magnesium hydroxide reduces occurrence of constipation (seen with use of aluminum alone) and diarrhea (seen with use of magnesia alone). Different strength combinations of aluminum hydroxide and magnesium hydroxide are available in both liquid and tablet forms.

Contraindications/Precautions

PREG
C

Contraindicated in hypersensitivity to aluminum or magnesium products. **Use with caution** in renal impairment, decreased GI motility or obstruction, colostomies or ileostomies, and dehydration or fluid restriction.

✋ Use with caution for children and the elderly.

Side effects/Adverse reactions

Hypersensitivity: rare. **GI:** stomach cramps, constipation or diarrhea. **CNS:** neurotoxicity. **Misc:** phosphate depletion, osteomalacia, osteoporosis, hypermagnesemia.

Nursing implications/Documentation

Possible nursing diagnoses: Constipation; Diarrhea; Pain.

♦ Monitor bowel elimination pattern, especially in the elderly.

♦ Monitor serum phosphate levels and assess for symptoms of phosphate depletion, i.e., neurotoxicity, bone pain, swelling, anorexia, weakness, and weight loss.

Patient & family teaching/Home care

Possible nursing diagnoses: Knowledge deficit; Impaired home maintenance management.

♦ Advise that the liquid form of alumina and magnesia is more effective than tablet form; palatability may be increased by refrigeration.

♦ Teach the need to shake liquid preparations vigorously to achieve uniform suspension, and to follow with water to assure passage into stomach.

♦ Point out that chewable tablets should be chewed well before swallowing and followed with water for maximum effectiveness.

♦ Advise those with ulcers to take medication 1 and 3 hr after meals and at bedtime for best results.

♦ Stress the need to continue taking medication under medical supervision for 4 to 6 weeks after ulcer symptoms have subsided.

♦ Advise those who self-medicate with antacids to seek medical advice if symptoms recur frequently or persist longer than 2 weeks.

♦ Alert those on sodium-restricted diets to check label for sodium content.

aluminum hydroxide

ALternaGEL, Alu-Cap, Alu-Tab, Amphojel, ✦Amphotabs, Dialume, Nephrox
Class: Antacid, Antiurolithic, Antihyperphosphatemic

PEDS	PREG	GERI
✋	C	✋

Action Neutralizes existing stomach acid; decreases pepsin activity by binding pepsin and acid; reduces phosphate levels by forming insoluble aluminum-phosphate complexes in the intestine.

Use/Therapeutic goal/Outcome

Hyperacidity and gastroesophageal reflux: Reduction of acid concentration within the esophagus and stomach. **Outcome criteria:** Report of decreased pain and upper GI irritation.

Hyperphosphatemia: Control of elevated phosphate levels in renal disease. **Outcome criteria:** Decrease in serum phosphate levels.

Renal calculi: Prevention of phosphatic (struvite) urinary stones. **Outcome criteria:** Reduction of phosphates in urine.

Dose range/Administration

Interaction alert: Do not give other oral medications for 2 hr after aluminum hydroxide to ensure their absorption. Separate doses of aluminum hydroxide from doses of enteric coated drugs by 1 hr (causes enteric coated drugs to be released while still in the stomach).

Adult: PO: *Liquid:* 600 mg (5–10 ml) 1 and 3 hr pc and hs. *Tablets:* 300–600 mg pc and hs. **Child:** PO: Individualize dose.

Clinical alert: For peptic ulcers, giving doses 1 and 3 hr after meals and at bedtime enhances therapeutic effects. Shake liquid form well before giving and follow with water or milk. After giving via nasogastric tube, flush with water.

Contraindications/Precautions

PREG
C

Contraindicated in hypersensitivity to aluminum products. Use with caution in renal impairment, decreased GI motility or obstruction, and dehydration or fluid restriction.

A ✋ **Use with caution for children and the elderly.**

Side effects/Adverse reactions

Hypersensitivity: rare. *GI:* stomach cramps, constipation, fecal impaction. *CNS:* neurotoxicity. *Misc:* phosphate depletion, osteomalacia, osteoporosis, hypercalcemia.

Nursing implications/Documentation

Possible nursing diagnoses: Constipation; Pain.

♦ Monitor bowel elimination pattern, especially in the elderly, to prevent and detect constipation.

♦ Monitor serum phosphate levels and assess for symptoms of phosphate depletion, i.e., neurotoxicity, bone pain, swelling, anorexia, and weakness.

Patient & family teaching/Home care

Possible nursing diagnoses: Knowledge deficit; Impaired home maintenance management.

♦ Advise that the liquid form of aluminum hydroxide is more effective than tablet form; palatability may be increased by refrigeration.

♦ Stress the need to shake liquid preparation vigorously to achieve uniform suspension, and to follow with water to assure passage into stomach.

♦ Alert those on sodium restricted diet that liquid form may have high sodium content; advise to check labels.

♦ Point out that chewable tablets should be chewed well before swallowing and followed with water for maximum effectiveness.

♦ With ulcers, advise taking medication 1 and 3 hr after meals and at bedtime for best results.

♦ Stress the need to continue aluminum hydroxide under medical supervision for 4 to 6 weeks after ulcer symptoms have subsided.

♦ Advise those who self-medicate with antacids to seek medical advice if symptoms recur frequently or persist longer than 2 weeks.

♦ To prevent or treat constipation, suggest alternating aluminum and magnesium antacids.

♦ For urinary stones, advise drinking plenty of fluids and restricting dietary phosphate for best results.

amantadine

a-man′ta-deen

amantadine hydrochloride: ◆*Antadine, Symadine, Symmetrel*

Class: Antiparkinson agent, Antiviral

PEDS	PREG	GERI
✋	C	✋

Action Alleviates symptoms of parkinsonism, probably by releasing and delaying reuptake of dopamine in the CNS. Prevents influenza Type A virus respiratory illness by blocking assembly of the virus and release of its infectious RNA into the host cell.

Use/Therapeutic goal/Outcome

Treatment of parkinsonism or parkinsonian extrapyramidal drug reactions: Alleviation of symptoms. *Outcome criteria:* Demonstration of improved motor control.

Prophylaxis and treatment of influenza A viral respiratory illness: Prevention of influenza A respiratory illness. *Outcome criteria:* Absence of (or reduction in) influenza symptoms.

Dose range/Administration

Interaction alert: Anticholinergics increase CNS effects (may require reduced dose).

🖐 **Give after meals for best absorption.**

Parkinsonism: Adult: PO: 100 mg bid. If the patient is on other antiparkinsonian drugs, or if the patient is seriously ill, begin with 100 mg/day for 7–10 days, then may increase to 100 mg bid if necessary.

Extrapyramidal drug side effects: Adult: PO: 100 mg bid or tid (may give up to 400 mg/day in divided doses with close monitoring).

Prophylaxis and treatment of influenza A viral respiratory illness: Adult < 64 yrs/Child > 10 yrs: PO: 200 mg/day in a single dose or divided bid. *Adult > 64 yrs:* PO: 100 mg qd or divided into 2 doses bid (divided dose decreases risk of adverse neurological side effects). *Child 1–9 yrs:* PO: Give 4.4–8.8 mg/kg/day in divided bid or tid. *Maximum dose:* 150 mg/day.

Clinical alert: Be aware that prophylactic doses should begin as soon after exposure as possible, and should continue for 10 days after exposure (may continue for up to 90 days if exposure is repeated and vaccine is unavailable; if used with vaccine, continue for 2–3 weeks until immunity develops). For symptomatic treatment, dose should continue for 24–48 hr after symptoms disappear.

Contraindications/Precautions

PREG
C

Contraindicated in hypersensitivity to amantadine. **Use with caution** in history of seizure disorders, CHF, edema, orthostatic hypotension, psychosis, and kidney or liver disease.

👋 **Use with caution for the elderly. Safe use for infants under 1 year and pregnant or nursing mothers has not been established.**

Side effects/Adverse reactions

Hypersensitivity: itching, rashes. **CNS:** weakness, fatigue, depression, confusion, dizziness, irritability, anxiety, insomnia, hallucinations, psychosis, lightheadedness, headache, difficulty concentrating. **GI:** anorexia, nausea, vomiting, dry mouth, constipation. **GU:** urinary retention. **CV:** orthostatic hypotension, CHF, peripheral edema.

Nursing implications/Documentation

Possible nursing diagnoses: Potential for injury; Potential for infection.

◆ To avoid insomnia, give last dose several hours before bedtime.

◆ Monitor for and report orthostatic hypotension or increased neurological side effects.

◆ Monitor and document vital signs at least daily for the first 2–3 days of initial therapy or dosage increase.

◆ Report if clinical signs of improvement do not occur within 1–2 weeks, because drug should probably be discontinued.

Patient & family teaching/Home care

Possible nursing diagnoses: Knowledge deficit; Impaired home maintenance management.

◆ Stress the need to avoid alcohol and CNS stimulants.

◆ If taken for parkinsonism, stress not to abruptly discontinue drug (may precipitate parkinsonian crisis). Also explain that tolerance sometimes occurs, requiring an increase in dosage.

◆ Advise taking amatadine after meals, to reduce risk of dizziness by rising from sitting to standing position slowly, to report new or continued symptoms to the physician, and to return for periodical medical follow-up.

◆ *See Antiparkinsons and Anti-infectives overviews for more information.*

ambenonium

am-be-noe'nee-um

A

ambenonium chloride: *Mytelase*

Class: Cholinergic (parasympatholytic), Anticholinesterase

Antidote: Atropine

PEDS	PREG	GERI
👋	C	👋

Action When given in appropriate doses, promotes muscle tone and function by increasing the concentration of acetylcholine at the myoneural junction (inhibits acetylcholinesterase, the enzyme that destroys acetylcholine). Acetylcholine is responsible for facilitating impulse transmission from nerve cells to muscle cells. *Excessive or deficient* acetylcholine may cause *neuromuscular blockade.*

Use/Therapeutic goal/Outcome

Myasthenia gravis: Improvement of muscle strength and function. **Outcome criteria:** Respirations within normal range; normal vital capacity; improved ability to chew, swallow, talk, and perform activities of daily life; absence of ptosis; report of absence of double vision.

Dose range/Administration

Interaction alert: Increases the action of neuromuscular blockers. Corticosteroids, procainamide, quinidine, and magnesium may reduce effect of ambenonium chloride. Other cholinergics should be discontinued before giving ambenonium chloride.

👉 **Give with milk or food to reduce side effects.**

Adult: PO: Dose highly individualized. *Initial dose:* 5 mg tid to qid, then increase gradually q 1–2 days, closely monitoring response. Larger doses may be required before meals and afternoons. *Maintenance dose:* 5–25 mg tid to qid.

Clinical alert: Dosage is highly individualized. Give ambenonium chloride *exactly* on time to maintain a therapeutic level. Dosage may be varied according to activity level, with different dosages at different times of day. Severe muscle weakness may be caused by drug toxicity (generally within 30–60 min of dose) or exacerbation of myasthenia gravis. Report side effects (especially if dose > 200 mg/day) because they may indicate onset of toxicity. Keep atropine, suction, and resuscitative equipment readily available in case of cholinergic crisis.

▶

Contraindications/Precautions

Contraindicated in hypersensitivity to cholinergic agents, and in urinary tract or intestinal obstruction, bradycardia, and hypotension. **Use with caution** in arrhythmias, asthma, epilepsy, hyperthyroidism, peptic ulcer, megacolon, recent MI.

🖑 **Contraindicated for nursing mothers. Use with caution for the elderly. Safe use for children and pregnant women has not been established (fetal problems have not been documented, but transient muscle weakness has occurred in 20% of neonates).**

Side effects/Adverse reactions

Hypersensitivity: rash (may be acneiform). **CNS:** headache, confusion, dizziness, dysarthria, dysphagia, muscle weakness. **Eye:** lacrimation, diplopia. **Resp:** increased bronchial secretion, bronchospasm, paralysis of the muscles of respiration. **CV:** dysrhythmias (especially bradycardia), hypotension. **GI:** abdominal cramps, increased salivation, nausea, vomiting, diarrhea. **GU:** urinary frequency, incontinence. **Skin:** sweating. **Misc:** cholinergic crisis (characterized by increasing muscle weakness).

Nursing implications/Documentation

Possible nursing diagnoses: Activity intolerance; Potential for aspiration; Impaired swallowing; Fear.

♦ Closely monitor ability to chew, swallow, and talk, especially during periods of dose adjustment; document and report variations in strength and record pulse, respirations, and blood pressure every 4 hr.

♦ Once patient has demonstrated ability to manage dose regimen, check with physician to see if a supply of medication can be kept at the bedside for self-medication (those with long-standing disease often insist on this).

♦ With use during pregnancy, monitor neonate for transient muscle weakness.

Patient & family teaching/Home care

Possible nursing diagnoses: Knowledge deficit; Impaired home maintenance management.

♦ Explain that taking this drug is vital to promote normal muscle function, and that this may be a lifelong requirement; stress the need for ongoing medical follow-up, especially

because some individuals develop a resistance to this drug.

♦ Point out that taking ambenonium chloride with food helps reduce side effects; emphasize that doses must be taken on time exactly as prescribed, without missing doses.

♦ Advise reporting side effects or increased muscle weakness immediately, especially during periods of dose adjustment.

♦ Recommend wearing medical alert medal stating that the individual has myasthenia gravis and is taking this drug.

♦ *See Cholinergics overview for more information.*

amdinocillin

am-din-oe-sill'in

Coactin

Class: Anti-infective, Penicillin-like antibiotic

PEDS	PREG	GERI
🖑	B	🖑

Action Broad-spectrum, usually bacteriostatic antibiotic; limits bacterial growth by preventing the cell from elongating. High activity against gram-negative bacteria and low activity against gram-positive bacteria.

Use/Therapeutic goal/Outcome

Urinary tract infections (caused by susceptible strains of *Eschericia coli, Klebsiella*, and *Enterobacter*): Resolution of infection. **Outcome criteria:** Absence of pathogenic growth on cultures, absence of clinical manifestations of infection (dysuria, frequency, pain, swelling, redness, heat, odor, drainage), normal WBC count.

Dose range/Administration

Interaction alert: Probenecid inhibits excretion of amdinocillin; lower doses may be indicated.

Adult: IV, Deep IM: 60 mg/kg/day in divided doses. If used in conjunction with another antibiotic, reduce dose to 40 mg/kg/day, and give each drug separately.

Contraindications/Precautions

Contraindicated in allergy to penicillin. **Use with caution** in cephalosporin sensitivity, history of allergic responses (e.g., other drugs, hay fever, asthma).

🖑 **Use with caution for the elderly. Safe use for children under 12 years and pregnant or nursing mothers has not been established; use with caution.**

Side effects/Adverse reactions

Hypersensitivity: Itching, rashes, urticaria, fever, eosinophilia, difficulty breathing, anaphylaxis. **GI:** nausea, vomiting, anorexia, diarrhea. **Hem:** thrombocytosis, eosinophia; slight elevation in SGOT, SGPT, alkaline phosphatase. **CV:** pain, redness, thrombophlebitis at the injection site. **Misc:** superinfection.

Nursing implications/Documentation

Possible nursing diagnoses: Potential for infection; Diarrhea; Altered patterns of urinary elimination.

♦ Determine history of allergies, and (regardless of history) monitor closely for allergic reactions.

♦ Obtain baseline CBC and necessary cultures, before administering first dose; monitor closely thereafter if therapy is prolonged.

♦ Encourage fluids, and record and monitor intake and output, to ensure adequate hydration; report significant negative or positive balance.

♦ Monitor for and report signs of superinfection (sore throat, diarrhea, fever, fatigue, thrush, vaginal discharge).

♦ Administer IM doses deep into large muscle mass; document injection site.

Patient & family teaching/Home care

Possible nursing diagnoses: Knowledge deficit; Impaired home maintenance management.

♦ Teach importance of reporting allergic symptoms, diarrhea, signs and symptoms that do not abate, or *any* new signs and symptoms of discomfort that indicate superinfection (medication regimen may have to be changed).

♦ Stress the importance of adequate hydration in preventing and treating infection (at least 2 L per day).

♦ Point out the need to take antibiotics for the entire time prescribed, even if signs and symptoms abate.

♦ *See Anti-infectives overview for more information.*

amikacin

am-i-kay'sin

amikacin sulfate: *Amikin*

Class: Anti-infective, Aminoglycoside antibiotic

PEDS	PREG	GERI
🤚	C	✋

Action Kills bacteria (bactericidal) by binding to ribosomes, thereby disrupting bacterial protein synthesis.

Use/Therapeutic goal/Outcome

Serious infections (caused by *Pseudomonas aeruginosa, Escherichia coli, Proteus, Klebsiella, Serratia, Enterobacter, Acinetobacter, Providencia, Citrobacter, Staphylococcus*): Resolution of infection. **Outcome criteria:** Absence of pathogenic growth on cultures, absence of clinical manifestations of infection (fever, pain, swelling, redness, heat, odor, drainage, productive cough, dysuria, urinary frequency, increased WBC count, abnormal X rays).

Dose range/Administration

Interaction alert: Do not mix IV with any other drug. Loop diuretics (e.g., furosemide) increase risk of ototoxicity and nephrotoxicity. Dimenhydrinate may mask symptoms of ototoxicity. Use cautiously with other aminoglycosides, amphotericin B, methoxyflurane, and cisplatin (increased risk of toxicity).

Serious infections: Adult and Child: IM, IV: 15 mg/kg/day in divided doses q8-12h. Dilute IV dose in 100–200 cc D5W and infuse over 30–60 min. **Neonates:** IM, IV: *Loading dose:* 10 mg/kg diluted in D5W over 1–2 hr. *Maintenance dose:* 7.5 mg/kg q12h.

Meningitis: Adult and Child: *Intrathecal/intraventricular:* Additional 1–2 mg/day with regular therapy for serious infections.

Uncomplicated urinary tract infections: Adult: IM, IV: 250 mg q12h. *In the presence of impaired renal function:* 7.5 mg/kg initially, then determine dosage and frequency by blood amikacin levels and renal function studies.

Clinical alert: Doses are highly individualized, depending on weight, renal function, and peak and trough levels. Schedule blood drawing for peak levels 1 hour after IM dose, or 30–60 minutes after IV dose. Schedule blood drawing for trough levels just before next dose. Peak levels exceeding 30–35 mcg/ml, and trough levels exceeding 10 mcg/ml are associated with toxicity; monitoring of levels for ototoxicity is especially important if hearing ability is difficult to evaluate (e.g., in very young and elderly patients).

Contraindications/Precautions

PREG
C

Contraindicated in hypersensitivity to amikacin or other aminoglycoside antibiotics. **Use with caution** in impaired renal function, hearing loss or tinnitus, vertigo or dizziness, fever, and dehydration.

✋ **Use with caution for neonates, premature babies, infants, and the elderly. Safe use for infants (for more than 14 days) and pregnant or nursing mothers has not been established.**

Side effects/Adverse reactions

Hypersensitivity: rashes, eosinophilia, fever, blood dyscrasias, angioedema, exfoliative dermatitis, stomatitis, anaphylaxis. **CV:** hypotension. **Ear:** ototoxicity (hearing loss, tinnitus). **CNS:** headache, dizziness, weakness, lethargy, tremors, neuromuscular blockade with respiratory depression. **GI:** nausea, vomiting, stomatitis. **GU:** nephrotoxicity (oliguria, proteinuria, hematuria, decreased creatinine clearance, increased serum BUN and creatinine).

Nursing implications/Documentation

Possible nursing diagnoses: Potential for infection; Fluid volume deficit.

◆ Determine history of allergies, and (regardless of history), monitor closely for allergic reactions.

◆ Weigh patient, and obtain baseline renal function studies, hearing ability, and culture specimens before administering first dose.

◆ Monitor renal function (urine output, specific gravity, serum BUN and creatinine, creatinine clearance) and report signs of decreased function.

◆ Encourage fluid intake, and document and monitor intake and output, to ensure adequate hydration and prevent renal damage from chemical irritation of renal tubules.

◆ Monitor for and report symptoms of ototoxicity (hearing loss, tinnitus, vertigo) and superinfection (mouth lesions, thrush, vaginal irritation, diarrhea, respiratory symptoms).

◆ If there is no response within 3–5 days, consult with physician to determine whether drug regimen should be re-evaluated and new cultures drawn.

Patient & family teaching/Home care

Possible nursing diagnoses: Knowledge deficit; Impaired home maintenance management.

◆ Advise reporting ear symptoms (e.g., full feeling, difficulty hearing, ringing of the ears) immediately.

◆ Teach the need to report new signs and symptoms of illness (e.g., fever, mouth lesions, vaginal irritation, diarrhea, respiratory symptoms) since medication may have to be changed.

◆ Explain the importance of taking antibiotics for the entire time prescribed, regardless of absence of signs and symptoms, and of maintaining hydration (drinking at least 2 L per day is recommended).

◆ *See Anti-infectives overview for more information.*

amiloride
a-mill-oh'ride

amiloride hydrochloride: ♠*Kaluril, Midamor*
Class: Potassium-sparing diuretic, Antihypertensive

PEDS	PREG	GERI
✋	B	✋

Action Promotes excretion of sodium and water by inhibiting reabsorption of sodium in the distal tubule, inducing sodium excretion and promoting potassium retention.

Use/Therapeutic goal/Outcome

Adjunctive therapy (with other diuretic agents) for CHF: Reduction in blood pressure while maintaining serum potassium levels within normal range. **Outcome criteria:** Increased urine output; absence of rales; absence of peripheral and sacral edema; serum potassium within normal range.

Hypertension: Reduction in blood pressure while maintaining serum potassium levels within normal limits. **Outcome criteria:** Increased urinary output; blood pressure readings within acceptable range; serum potassium within normal range.

Dose range/Administration

Interaction alert: Monitor for hyperkalemia when given with other potassium-sparing diuretics, potassium products, ACI inhibiters, and salt substitutes.

🥄 **Give with meals to minimize GI upset.**

Adult: PO: 5 mg/day; may be increased to 10 mg/day. If necessary, 20 mg may be given with careful monitoring of electrolytes.

Clinical alert: Monitor serum potassium levels carefully; hold drug if value is greater than 5.5 mEq/L.

Contraindications/Precautions

Contraindicated in hypersensitivity to the drug, and in high serum potassium levels (greater than 5.5 mEq/L) or with other potassium-sparing agents; renal insufficiency, and diabetic nephropathy. **Use with caution** for the **elderly**.

✋ **Safe use for children and pregnant or nursing mothers has not been established.**

Side effects/Adverse reactions

Hypersensitivity: rash. **Hem:** hyperkalemia, hyponatremia, blood dyscrasias. **CNS:** headache, drowsiness, dizziness, weakness. **CV:** orthostatic hypotension, angina, palpations. **GI:** nausea, vomiting, diarrhea, anorexia, abdominal pain, constipation. **GU:** dysuria, bladder spasms, impotence, polyuria. **MS:** muscle cramps.

Nursing implications/Documentation

Possible nursing diagnoses: Fluid volume deficit; Altered patterns of urinary elimination; Potential for injury; Constipation.

♦ Ascertain that baseline CBC, sodium, potassium, chloride, carbon dioxide, calcium, magnesium, BUN, creatinine, uric acid, and liver function studies have been obtained before giving first dose; report abnormalities and monitor closely thereafter.

♦ Especially watch for hyperkalemia, since this is a potassium-sparing diuretic.

♦ Document and monitor blood pressure, pulse, daily weight, and intake and output; report significant discrepancies.

♦ Observe for and report signs of fluid overload (auscultate lungs for rales; check feet, ankles, and sacrum for edema).

♦ Check with physician to determine dietary restrictions; consult with dietician to plan diet.

♦ Observe the elderly for extreme diuresis (may require lower doses); monitor for orthostatic hypotension; supervise ambulation until response is determined.

Patient & family teaching/Home care

Possible nursing diagnoses: Knowledge deficits; Impaired home maintenance management.

♦ Before giving first dose, explain that the drug will increase the amount and frequency of urination.

♦ Advise taking this drug with food to prevent GI symptoms.

♦ Emphasize the importance of taking this drug exactly as prescribed, and the importance of returning for medical follow-up.

♦ Explain that diuretics enhance the work of the kidney and reduce the workload of the heart.

♦ Recommend taking doses in the early morning and early afternoon to prevent the need to disturb sleep to void.

♦ Explain that changing positions slowly helps prevent dizziness.

♦ Advise reporting dizziness, shortness of breath, muscle weakness or spasms, swelling of hands and feet, or persistent sore throat; encourage daily monitoring of weight and reporting sudden weight gain.

♦ Provide a list of allowed foods and fluids; stress the need to stick to prescribed diet (explain the hazards of too much salt and potassium).

♦ Warn against driving or activities that require alertness until response has been determined.

♦ Advise avoidance of OTC drugs, unless approved by physician.

♦ *See Diuretics and Antihypertensives overviews for more information.*

amino acid
ah-mee'no

amino acid solution: **Aminosyn, FreAmine III, Hepat-Amine, Novamine, NephrAmine, Travasol**

Class: Protein substrate, Nitrogen product, Caloric agent

PEDS	PREG	GERI
✋	C	OK

Action Promotes balanced nutritional state by supplying amino acids necessary for protein synthesis and conservation of existing body protein.

Use/Therapeutic goal/Outcome

Nutritional support: Improved nutritional state and maintenance of positive nitrogen balance. **Outcome criteria:** Weight gain; increase in serum albumin.

Dose range/Administration

Interaction alert: Tetracycline may reduce protein-sparing effects of amino acids infusions. **Adult:** IV: 1–1.5 gm/kg/day. **Child:** IV: 2–3 gm/kg/day.

A **Clinical alert:** Amino acid solution brands have different ratios of essential and nonessential amino acids, and varying concentrations of electrolytes. Specific preparations are available for use in renal and hepatic failure. Amino acids are usually combined with a nonprotein calorie source, such as dextrose, for peripheral and central parenteral nutrition (dextrose concentrations greater than 12.5% must be administered in a central vein). Vitamins and trace elements may also be added.

Contraindications/Precautions

PREG
C

Contraindicated in hypersensitivity to any component, and in severe liver disease with hyperammonemia, maple syrup urine disease, PKU, severe renal failure, uncorrected electrolyte or acid-base imbalance, or decreased blood volume. **Use with caution** in CHF, renal or hepatic disease, diabetes mellitus, and elevated BUN.

☝ **Use with caution for children and pregnant women.**

Side effects/Adverse reactions

Hypersensitivity: chills, flushing, rash, urticaria. **CNS:** dizziness, headache, confusion, unconsciousness. **CV:** phlebitis, hypertension, CHF, pulmonary edema. **GI:** nausea, vomiting, jaundice, elevated liver enzymes, hyperammonemia. **Skin:** extravasation, tissue necrosis. **Misc:** metabolic acidosis or alkalosis, electrolyte imbalances, hyperglycemia, glycosuria, rebound hypoglycemia, sepsis.

Nursing implications/Documentation

Possible nursing diagnoses: Altered nutrition; Potential for infection; Activity intolerance; Impaired tissue integrity.

♦ Administer only solutions that are freshly prepared in a laminar flow hood.

♦ Use aseptic technique when preparing and administering infusions; replace all bottles, tubing and filters every 24 hours as recommended by CDC.

♦ Maintain the single line, or one lumen of a multi-lumen catheter, exclusively for the nutritional infusion; do not use to draw or administer blood.

♦ Administer solutions through an in-line filter to remove particulate matter; use an infusion pump to maintain consistent flow rate and to avoid fluctuations in blood glucose levels; do not speed up or slow down established rates.

♦ Monitor fluid balance and document intake and output; weigh patient regularly at the same time of day and on the same scale.

♦ Check vital signs and auscultate lungs every 4 hours.

♦ Inspect infusion site for signs of extravasation, inflammation or infection.

♦ Monitor blood glucose to detect problems with glucose metabolism; if needed, supplementary insulin may be added directly to the infusion.

♦ Ascertain that laboratory studies are done as ordered; monitor results to determine therapeutic response.

♦ For patients with renal or liver impairment, and for infants, monitor blood ammonia levels closely (hyperammonemia can cause mental retardation in infants).

♦ Provide frequent mouth care to patients who are not eating.

♦ When discontinuing parenteral nutrition, reduce dextrose administration *gradually* to avoid rebound hypoglycemia.

Patient & family teaching/Home care

Possible nursing diagnoses: Impaired home maintenance management; Knowledge deficit; Potential for infection.

♦ Stress importance of maintaining aseptic technique when preparing and administering parenteral solutions.

♦ Teach how to use the infusion pump to ensure correct rate and administration over the prescribed time period.

♦ Teach proper method of discarding container, tubing, and needle.

♦ Advise reporting breathing difficulties, sudden weight gain, fever, or change in mental status.

♦ Emphasize importance of regularly scheduled laboratory tests to monitor effectiveness of therapy.

aminocaproic acid
a-mee-noe-ka-proe'ik

Amicar

Class: Systemic hemostatic, Antidote

PEDS	PREG	GERI
☝	C	☝

Action Promotes hemostatis by blocking plasminogen activators and, to a lesser degree, plasmin activity, thus inhibiting fibrinolysis (clot dissolution). Also serves as an antidote for overdose of alteplase, streptokinase, and urokinase.

Use/Therapeutic goal/Outcome

Bleeding secondary to hyperfibrinolysis: Promotion of clot formation, control of bleeding. *Outcome criteria:* Stable hemoglobin and hematocrit; coagulation studies within normal limits.

Dose range/Administration

Interaction alert: Oral contraceptives and estrogens may cause hypercoagulation.

Adult: PO, Slow IV: *Loading dose:* 4–5 g during first hr. *Maintenance dose:* 1 to 1.25 g/hr until bleeding is controlled. *Maximum dose:* 30 g/day. **Child:** PO, IV: *Loading dose:* 100 mg/kg (3 g/m^2) for first hr. *Continuous infusion:* 33.3 mg/kg/hr (1 g/m^2/hr) *Maximum dose:* 18 g/m^2/24 hr.

Clinical alert: Dilute IV preparation with Sterile Water for Injection, NS, D5W, or Ringer's Injection.

Contraindications/Precautions

PREG
C

Contraindicated in hypersensitivity to aminocaproic acid, and in severe renal impairment, and active disseminated intravascular clotting (DIC). **Use with caution** in kidney, heart, or liver disease, and with oral contraceptives.

✥ **Use with caution for children and the elderly. Safe use for pregnant or nursing mothers has not been established.**

Side effects/Adverse reactions

Hypersensitivity: itching, rashes. **CV:** thrombosis, rapid IV infusion may cause bradycardia, hypotension, and arrhythmias. **GI:** nausea, cramping, diarrhea. **CNS:** headache, dizziness. **Ear:** tinnitus. **Eye:** conjunctival suffusion (edema of the conjunctiva). **Resp:** nasal stuffiness. **GU:** renal failure. **Misc:** malaise.

Nursing implications/Documentation

Possible nursing diagnosis: Potential for injury.

◆ Document baseline vital signs before starting infusion and every 5–15 minutes during infusion.

◆ Monitor and record quality of peripheral pulses and circulation; protect patient from bumping.

◆ Report immediately symptoms of respiratory distress or chest or leg pain (may signify thrombosis).

Patient & family teaching/Home care

Possible nursing diagnoses: Anxiety; Fear; Knowledge deficit.

◆ Recognize that this drug is given only to hospitalized patients.

◆ Explain that this drug helps prevent bleeding.

◆ Stress the need to report new or unusual symptoms.

◆ Encourage voicing fears or concerns so that these issues can be addressed.

a-mean-no-gloo-teth'i-mide

aminoglutethimide

Cytadren
Class: Antineoplastic agent, Antihormone

PEDS	PREG	GERI
✥	D	✥

Action Inhibits cellular growth of adrenal-hormone–responsive malignant tumors by blocking the synthesis of glucocorticoids, mineralocorticoids, and estrogens that are needed to support tumor growth; blocks synthesis of adrenal steroids.

Use/Therapeutic goal/Outcome

Adrenal cancer, ACTH-producing tumors, advanced breast cancer in postmenopausal patients, metastatic prostate carcinoma, and suppression of adrenal function in Cushing's syndrome: Suppression of malignant cell proliferation; decreased synthesis of adrenal steroids. *Outcome criteria:* Tumor and disease regression or stabilization on radiologic and physical examination; reduction of circulating adrenal corticosteroids.

Dose range/Administration

Interaction alert: Alcohol increases the effects of aminoglutethimide. Aminoglutethimide increases metabolism of dexamethasone and decreases the effect of the following: coumadin, digitoxin, medroxyprogesterone, and theophylline.

Adult: PO: 250 mg q6h. May increase q 7–14 days by 250 mg/day if response is inadequate. *Maximum dose:* 2 g/day for Cushing's syndrome; 1 g/day for breast and prostatic cancer.

Clinical alert: Drug therapy should be initiated in a hospital setting until response is stable. Carefully monitor cortisol levels until desired level of suppression is achieved. Hold drug and

▶

report if platelets <100,000/mm³ and WBC <4000/mm³.

Contraindications/Precautions

PREG D

Contraindicated in hypersensitivity to aminoglutethimide or to glutethimide, and in chickenpox or herpes zoster. **Use with caution** in hypothyroidism, infection, or hepatic or renal impairment.

Contraindicated for children and pregnant or nursing mothers. Use with caution for the elderly.

Side effects/Adverse reactions

Hypersensitivity: morbilliform rash, pruritus, cholestatic jaundice. **CNS:** fever, headache, dizziness, lethargy. **GI:** anorexia; nausea, vomiting; hepatotoxicity. **Hem:** transient leukopenia, anemia; thrombocytopenia, pancytopenia, agranulocytosis, elevated SGOT, alkaline phosphatase, bilirubin. **CV:** hypotension, tachycardia. **Eye:** uncontrolled eye movements. **GU:** masculinization and hirsutism in females, precocious sexual development in males. **MS:** myalgia. **Misc:** adrenal insufficiency, hypothyroidism.

Nursing implications/Documentation

Possible nursing diagnoses: Fluid volume deficit; Self-esteem disturbance; Potential for injury; Altered nutrition: less than body requirements.

◆ See important Nursing implications in Antineoplastic agents overview.

♦ Monitor for orthostatic and persistent hypotension, which may result from suppression of aldosterone production.

♦ Check thyroid function studies periodically and monitor for signs of hypothyroidism (weight gain and lethargy).

♦ Monitor for adrenal insufficiency (weakness, fatigue, lethargy, darkening skin, diarrhea), especially if the patient suffers an acute illness or requires surgery (hydrocortisone and mineralocorticoid supplements may be required).

♦ Evaluate pulse rate, rhythm, and quality; report abnormalities.

♦ Report presence of rash that lasts longer than 5–8 days (may require discontinuing drug).

Patient & family teaching/Home care

Possible nursing diagnoses: Impaired home maintenance management; Knowledge deficit.

◆ See important Patient & family teaching in Antineoplastic agents overview.

♦ Teach the need to change position slowly and avoid standing for a long period of time; reduces incidence of dizziness from orthostatic hypotension.

♦ Advise taking special precautions to avoid injury or infection; report immediately if these occur.

♦ Teach how to evaluate pulse rate; stress the need to report abnormalities.

♦ Stress that most side effects decrease in incidence and severity within 2–6 weeks.

◆ See Antineoplastic agents overview for more information.

aminophylline

am-in-off'-i-lin

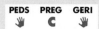

(also theophylline ethylenediamine): **Aminophyllin,** ♠**Cardophyllin,** ♣**Corophyllin, Phyllocontin, Somophyllin-DF**

Class: Antiasthmatic, smooth muscle relaxant, bronchodilator, CNS stimulant, respiratory stimulant, xanthine

PEDS 〰 **PREG** C **GERI** 〰

Action Causes bronchial smooth muscle relaxation and bronchodilation by increasing tissue concentration of AMP. Also causes cardiac and CNS stimulation, diuresis, and increased gastric secretions.

Use/Therapeutic goal/Outcome

Bronchospasm associated with asthma, bronchitis and COPD: Reduction in bronchiole obstruction with improved movement of air. **Outcome criteria:** Clearing of lung fields upon auscultation; forced expiratory volume (FEV) improved by 8%; patient report of breathing easier.

Dose range/Administration

Interaction alert: Don't mix IV aminophylline with any other medications. Simpathomimetics may increase CNS and cardiovascular side effects. Erythromycin, beta-blockers, cimetidine, and large doses of allopurinol decrease aminophylline metabolism (monitor for toxicity). Phenobarbital, rifampin, and carbamazepine increase aminophylline metabolism (may need higher doses). Smoking diminishes effect.

Give on an empty stomach with a full glass of water, unless GI symptoms are experi-

enced (then may give with food or antacids—absorption may be slower).

Adult: PO: *Loading dose:* 500 mg. *Maintenance dose:* 250–500 mg q6-8h. IV: *Loading dose:* 5.6 mg/kg over 30 min. *Maintenance dose:* Continuous infusion of 0.2–0.9 mg/kg/hr. Dilute in D5W or NS to avoid burning sensation; **rapid infusion may cause serious arrhythmias.** Do not use discolored or cloudy solution. Rectal: Give 250–500 mg suppository q6-8h. Be aware that rectal absorption is erratic and unpredictable. **Child:** PO: *Loading dose:* 5.6 mg/kg. *Maintenance dose:* 3–6 mg/kg q6-8h. IV: *Loading dose:* 5.6 mg/kg **slowly** over 20–30 min. *Maintenance dose:* Continuous infusion of 1 mg/kg/hr. Dilute in D5W to avoid burning sensation.

Clinical alert: Be aware that dosage is highly individualized depending upon patient response. Children need relatively high doses because of high rate of clearance. Determine whether the patient has been receiving any form of theophylline before administering aminophylline. Monitor theophylline levels closely; therapeutic levels are between 10–20 mcg/ml (hold dose and report if level is > 20 mcg/ml).

Contraindications/Precautions

PREG C

Contraindicated in hypersensitivity to the drug or to xanthine derivatives (caffeine, theobromine), and in pre-existing arrhythmias. **Use with caution** in CHF, cor pulmonale, and in kidney, liver, or ulcer disease.

✋ **Contraindicated for children < 6 months and (for long-acting forms) children < 6 years, as well as for nursing mothers. Use with caution during pregnancy and for children and the elderly.**

Side effects/Adverse reactions

Hypersensitivity: itching, rash, angioedema. **GI:** anorexia, nausea, vomiting, indigestion, cramping, bitter taste in mouth, diarrhea, anal irritation with suppository. **CV:** flushing, palpitations, hypotension, ventricular arrythmias, circulatory collapse; with IV route: pain, redness, swelling, thrombophlebitis at injection site. **Resp:** increased respiratory rate. **CNS:** headache, irritability, restlessness, nervousness, insomnia, dizziness, seizures, hyperexcitability.

Nursing implications/Documentation

A

Possible nursing diagnoses: Ineffective airway clearance; Potential for injury; Activity intolerance.

◆ During acute illness, record lung sounds and vital signs immediately before and 30 min after administration (a sudden, unexplained, sharp increase in pulse rate may indicate onset of toxicity; additional signs of toxicity include anorexia, nausea, vomiting, restlessness, tachycardia, seizures. Hold drug and report if these occur.

◆ Schedule doses around the clock.

◆ Monitor closely for tachycardia and ventricular arrythmias; hold drug and report if these are significant.

◆ Pace activity to allow for rest periods.

◆ Be aware that smokers are likely to need higher doses because of increased elimination of aminophylline.

◆ Monitor serum theophylline levels; report levels outside of therapeutic range.

◆ Observe for potential for injury related to restlessness and dizziness, and take appropriate precautions.

Patient & family teaching/Home care

Possible nursing diagnoses: Knowledge deficit; Impaired home maintenance management; Fear.

◆ Explain that this drug helps reduce wheezing and makes breathing easier.

◆ Reinforce the importance of taking doses exactly as prescribed, without missing or "doubling up" doses (if a dose is skipped, it should be taken as soon as possible).

◆ Stress that a different brand should not be substituted without physician approval.

◆ Explore factors that cause asthma attacks (environmental, emotional) and teach holistic measures for reducing stress and coping with wheezing.

◆ Instruct the patient to report palpitations or an increase in dyspnea.

◆ Emphasize the need for medical follow-up.

◆ Warn against taking OTC drugs without checking with physician, because there is a risk of drug interaction; advise to avoid caffeine.

◆ *See Bronchodilators overview for more information.*

A amiodarone

a-mee'oh-da-rone

amiodarone hydrochloride: *Cordarone*, ♠*Cord-arone X*

Class: Antiarrhythmic (Class III)

PEDS	PREG	GERI
♨	C	♨

Action Suppresses atrial and ventricular ectopy by prolonging the duration of the action potential and the refractory period of all cardiac tissues. Slows heart rate, decreases peripheral vascular resistance, increases coronary blood flow, and lengthens atrioventricular conduction time.

Use/Therapeutic goal/Outcome

Long-term prophylaxis of ventricular arrhythmias resistant to less toxic drugs (supraventricular arrhythmia, atrial fibrillation and flutter, and Wolff-Parkinson-White syndrome): Suppression of atrial and ventricular ectopy, promotion of effective heartbeat. *Outcome criteria:* Absence of or decrease in atrial and ventricular ectopy in EKG; regular palpable pulses.

Dose range/Administration

Interaction alert: Use cautiously with digoxin, warfarin, antihypertensives, phenytoin, and other antiarrhythmics; amiodarone increases blood levels of these drugs, and thus their effects. Concurrent use with beta-blockers and calcium channel blockers can cause bradycardia, sinus arrest, and AV block.

🖐 **Give with food to minimize GI upset.**

Adult: PO: *Loading dose:* 800–1600 mg/day in 3 divided doses for 1–3 weeks. *Maintenance dose:* 200–800 mg/day (bid for patients with GI intolerance). IV: *Loading dose:* 5–10 mg/kg (preferably via a central line) followed by an infusion of 10 mg/kg/day via IV pump for 3–5 days. (Note: IV amiodarone is investigational.)

Clinical alert: Place the patient on continuous cardiac monitoring when initiating amiodarone therapy, and continue monitoring until response is determined. Be aware that although amiodarone has been effective when other drugs have failed, it has a high incidence of side effects.

Contraindications/Precautions

PREG
C

Contraindicated in hypersensitivity to amiodarone, and in sinus-node dysfunction, sinus bradycardia that has resulted in syncope, second- and third-degree heart block. *Use with*

caution in impaired ventricular function or cardiomegaly.

🖐 **Use with caution for the elderly. Safe use for children and pregnant or nursing mothers has not been determined.**

Side effects/Adverse reactions

Hypersensitivity: skin rash, hepatitis. **Eye:** corneal microdeposits, blurred vision, blue-green halos around objects, sensitivity to light. **Resp:** pulmonary fibrosis. **CNS:** peripheral neuropathies, fatigue, tremor, poor coordination. **CV:** exacerbation of arrhythmia, bradycardia, CHF, hypotension. **GI:** malaise, altered liver-function tests, hepatic dysfunction, constipation, nausea, vomiting, anorexia. **Skin:** photosensitivity, slate-blue skin discoloration. **MS:** muscle weakness. **Misc:** thyroid imbalances.

Nursing implications/Documentation

Possible nursing diagnoses: Potential for injury; Activity intolerance.

♦ Be aware that before beginning amiodarone, an accurate history and examination is essential to rule out CHF, hepatic dysfunction, bradycardia, sinus-node disease, impaired ventricular function, and pulmonary disease.

♦ Be sure to check baseline chest X-ray, EKG, and laboratory studies (CBC, sodium, potassium, chloride, carbon dioxide, magnesium, BUN, creatinine, SGPT, and LDH) before giving first dose; monitor closely thereafter as indicated by clinical condition.

♦ Remember that oxygen requirements must be met, and that electrolyte imbalances (especially potassium and magnesium) and abnormal blood pH must be corrected, before expected antiarrhythmic effect can be seen; report abnormalities immediately.

♦ Document baseline vital signs, lung sounds, and cardiac monitor strip (measure and record PR and QRS segments) before giving first dose and at least every 8 hr; monitor closely until response is determined; report prolongation in PR or QRS segments.

♦ Keep patient in bed during IV administration; once allowed out of bed, supervise ambulation and observe for coordination problems.

♦ Coordinate care to provide frequent rest periods.

♦ Report visual disturbances (corneal microdeposits are common); may be minimized by instillation of methylcellulose ophthalmic solution.

Patient & family teaching/Home care

Possible nursing diagnoses: Fear; Knowledge deficit; Impaired home maintenance management.

◆ Explain that the purpose of this drug is to prevent arrhythmias and to promote an effective heartbeat.

◆ Stress the need to follow dose regimen closely and to return for medical follow-up for early detection of adverse reactions.

◆ Teach how to assess pulse for irregularities in rhythm and rate; stress that irregularities be reported.

◆ Stress that a cough accompanied by shortness of breath be reported immediately.

◆ Advise having an eye examination twice a year, and reporting to the eye physician that they are taking amiodarone.

◆ Emphasize the need to pace activities, avoid stress, and plan for rest periods.

◆ Caution to use a sunscreen and wear sunglasses when outside to avoid photosensitivity reaction.

◆ Encourage learning CPR; reinforce that survival rate of cardiac arrest is greatly increased when CPR is initiated immediately.

◆ *See Antiarrhythmics overview for more information.*

amitriptyline
a-mee-trip'ti-leen

amitriptyline hydrochloride: *Amitril, ✦Apo-Amitriptylene, Elavil, Emitrip, Endep, Enovil, ✦Laroxyl, ✦Levate, ✦Meravil, ✦Novo-Tripyn*

Class: Tricyclic antidepressant (TCA)

PEDS	PREG	GERI
👋	C	👋

Action Improves mood by increasing levels of the neurotransmitters norepinephrine and serotonin in the CNS. (Blocks neurotransmitter reuptake into presynaptic neurons by inhibiting the "amine pump." Reuptake normally terminates the action of neurotransmitters.) Produces more sedation than other TCAs. Has also been effective against intractable hiccups and chronic severe pain (exact mechanism action is unclear).

Use/Therapeutic goal/Outcome

Major depressive disorders: Promotion of sense of well-being, ability to cope with daily living. *Outcome criteria:* After 2–4 weeks, report of feeling less depressed, more energetic and able to cope; return of normal sleeping and eating habits; demonstration of improved ability to problem solve and perform activities of daily living.

Dose range/Administration

Interaction alert: Barbiturates may reduce antidepressant blood levels and effect. Cimetidine may increase levels. If given with epinephrine and norepinephrine, monitor for increased risk of hypertension. Avoid use with MAOIs (risk of excitation, hyperpyrexia, and seizures). Give cautiously with thyroid drugs because it may increase CNS stimulation and cardiac arrythmias.

🖐 **Give with (or immediately after) food to reduce GI symptoms.**

Adult: PO: Begin with 50–100 mg hs. *Maximum dose:* 300 mg/day. *For the elderly:* begin with 30 mg/day in divided doses or at hs, to a maximum of 150 mg/day. IM: (Use only when patient is unable to take tablet form) 20–30 mg qid *or* give entire dose at hs. *Child > 12 yrs:* PO: 30 mg/day in divided doses or at hs. *Maximum dose:* 150 mg/day.

Clinical alert: Monitor closely (especially the elderly) for oversedation until response is determined. Whenever possible give entire dose at bedtime.

Contraindications/Precautions
PREG C

Contraindicated in hypersensitivity to TCAs, for concomitant use with electroconvulsive therapy, and in elective surgery, or acute recovery period of myocardial infarction. *Use with caution* in renal or hepatic disease, hyperthyroidism, glaucoma, prostatic hypertrophy, urinary retention, hypomania, mania, and suicidal tendency.

🖐 **Contraindicated for children under 6 years and pregnant or nursing mothers. Use with caution for adolescents and the elderly or debilitated.**

Side effects/Adverse reactions

Hypersensitivity: rash, sensitivity to sunlight. **CNS:** drowsiness, dizziness, anxiety, headache, fatigue, agitation, extrapyramidal symptoms, sedation (especially the elderly). **CV:** orthostatic hypotension, palpitations, tachycardia,

EKG changes, hypertension. **GI:** anorexia, dry mouth, nausea, vomiting, constipation, paralytic ileus. **GU:** urinary retention, decreased libido. **Eye:** blurred vision. **Ear:** tinnitus. **Hem:** agranulocytosis.

Nursing implications/Documentation

Possible nursing diagnoses: Potential for injury; Constipation; Altered oral mucous membrane.

♦ Document mental status and vital signs at least bid until response to therapy has been established.

♦ Be sure that doses are swallowed (not hoarded).

♦ Monitor for orthostatic hypotension, dizziness, and drowsiness; supervise ambulation until response is established.

♦ Record intake and output, and observe for dehydration or urinary retention; provide special mouth care.

♦ Monitor for and report suicidal tendencies, increased depression, or excessive drowsiness (may require change in medication).

♦ Prevent constipation by monitoring bowel movements and encouraging adequate fiber and fluid intake; offer laxatives or stool softeners before the problem becomes severe.

Patient & family teaching/Home care

Possible nursing diagnoses: Ineffective coping (family and individual); Sleep pattern disturbance; Impaired home maintenance management.

♦ Stress that this medication helps reduce the depression that inhibits ability to make decisions and cope effectively (once the individual feels less depressed, it will be easier to take steps toward making healthy changes).

♦ Explain that side effects are often noted immediately, but usually diminish after a few weeks; on the other hand, it is likely to take 2–4 weeks before beneficial effects are noted (the patient may feel worse before feeling better).

♦ Warn to change positions slowly to prevent dizziness.

♦ Point out the role of adequate nutrition, exercise, and sleep in combating depression.

♦ Emphasize that the effects of alcohol, sedatives, and tranquilizers may be potentiated.

♦ Caution to consult physician before using OTC drugs; stress the need for ongoing medical follow-up.

♦ Recommend reporting continued depression; stress that doses should not be increased or stopped without checking with physician because this may cause severe problems.

♦ Advise avoidance of driving and other potentially hazardous activities until response is established.

♦ Suggest using ice chips, hard candy, or gum to relieve side effect of dry mouth; stress the need for good mouth care.

♦ Warn women to report immediately if pregnancy is planned or suspected.

♦ *See Antidepressants overview for more information.*

ammonium chloride   *a-moe'nee-um*

Class: Acidifier (systemic and urinary), Expectorant

PEDS	PREG	GERI
✋	B	✋

Action Decreases serum and urine pH (ammonium ions are converted in the liver to urea which liberates hydrogen ions, acidifies urine, induces diuresis, and decreases serum pH). Believed to have a mild expectorant effect by causing reflex stimulation of bronchial mucous glands.

Use/Therapeutic goal/Outcome

Metabolic alkalosis: Correction or prevention of metabolic alkalosis. **Outcome criteria:** Arterial pH within normal limits (7.35–7.45).

Urinary tract infections: Acidification of urine, promotion of an unfavorable environment for bacterial growth. **Outcome criteria:** Urine pH of 4.6–8.

Expectorant: Removal of excess respiratory secretions. **Outcome criteria:** Increased sputum production and expectoration; improvement in tidal volume.

Dose range/Administration

Interaction alert: Do not give with milk or antacids. Spironolactone may cause severe systemic acidosis (use caution). May increase excretion of antidepressants, ephedrine, methadone, pseudoephedrine, and sulfonyureas, and decrease effect. May decrease excretion of salicylates and increase their blood levels.

🥛 **Give PO doses after meals to reduce GI symptoms.**

Metabolic alkalosis: Adult and Child: IV: Dose is calculated by multiplying the serum chloride deficit (in mEq/ml) by the extracellular fluid volume (approximately 20% of body weight in kilograms). Half the dose is given immediately; the patient's condition evaluated; and, to prevent acidosis, the regimen is then individualized based upon CO_2 combining power and serum electrolytes. The concentrated (26.75%) solution should be diluted before administration: add 100 mEq ammonium chloride (20 cc) to 500 cc NS, or 200 mEq ammonium chloride (40 cc) to 1000 cc NS. An IV controller device should be used and the rate should not exceed 5 cc/min.

Urine acidifier: Adult: PO: 4–12 g/day in divided doses q4 to q6h. **Child:** PO: 75 mg/kg/day in divided doses q6h.

Expectorant: Adult: PO: 250–500 mg q2-4h with a full glass of water.

Clinical alert: The enteric-coated tablets are absorbed erratically.

Contraindications/Precautions

PREG B

Contraindicated in hypersensitivity to ammonium chloride, and in severe impaired liver or kidney function, and respiratory acidosis. **Use with caution** in edema resulting from CHF, pulmonary insufficiency.

❦ Use with caution for children and the elderly. Safe use for pregnant or nursing mothers has not been established.

Side effects/Adverse reactions

Hypersensitivity: rash. **Misc:** metabolic acidosis (nausea, vomiting, increased rate and depth of respirations), ammonia toxicity (headache, progressive drowsiness, confusion, convulsions, coma, pallor, vomiting, bradycardia, cardiac arrhythmias), pain at infusion site.

Nursing implications/Documentation

Possible nursing diagnoses: Sensory/perceptual alterations; Potential for aspiration; Potential for infection.

◆ For IV use, maintain a flow sheet of daily weights and critical lab values (electrolytes, ABGs, blood ammonia, BUN and creatinine) and keep it handy for quick reference.

◆ Monitor mental status and observe for risk of aspiration; position appropriately, keep side rails up, and keep suction equipment and airway at the bedside.

◆ Document and monitor vital signs frequently, depending on patient's condition (may be as frequent as every 15 minutes).

◆ Record lung sounds, rate and depth of respirations, and sputum production; document

intake and output, and monitor for significant negative or positive balance (expect diuresis for the first few days).

◆ When used as a urine acidifier, monitor urine pH.

Patient & family teaching/Home care

Possible nursing diagnoses: Knowledge deficit; Impaired home maintenance management.

◆ Stress the need to maintain dose schedule strictly, and to maintain ongoing medical follow-up.

◆ For use as an expectorant or urine acidifier, point out the importance of maintaining adequate hydration (at least 2 quarts/day).

◆ See Antitussives, Expectorants, and Mucolytics overview for more information.

amoxapine
a-mox'e-peen

Asendin

Class: Tricyclic antidepressant (TCA)

PEDS	PREG	GERI
❦	C	❦

Action Improves mood by increasing levels of the neurotransmitter norepinephrine in the CNS. (Blocks neurotransmitter reuptake into presynaptic neurons by inhibiting the "amine pump." Reuptake normally terminates the action of neurotransmitters.) Has anticholinergic and sedating effects similar to those of imipramine.

Use/Therapeutic goal/Outcome

Major depressive disorders, including those associated with anxiety and/or agitation: Promotion of sense of well-being, ability to cope with daily living. **Outcome criteria:** After 2–4 weeks, report of feeling less depressed, more energetic and able to cope; return of normal sleeping and eating habits; demonstration of improved ability to problem solve and perform activities of daily living.

Dose range/Administration

Interaction alert: Barbiturates may reduce antidepressant blood levels and effects. Cimetidine may increase blood levels. If given with epinephrine and norepinephrine, monitor for increased risk of hypertension. Avoid use with MAOIs (risk of excitation, hyperpyrexia, and seizures). Give cautiously with thyroid drugs because it may increase CNS stimulation and cardiac arrythmias.

▶

🍎 Give with (or immediately after) food to reduce GI symptoms.

Adult: PO: *Initial dose:* 50 mg tid. After 3 days, may increase to 100 mg tid (300 mg/day). Once stabilized, give entire dose at hs. *For hospitalized patients:* Maximum 600 mg/day.

Contraindications/Precautions

PREG
C

Contraindicated in hypersensitivity to TCAs for concomitant use with electroconvulsive therapy, in elective surgery, or acute recovery period of myocardial infarction. **Use with caution** in renal or hepatic disease, hyperthyroidism, glaucoma, prostatic hypertrophy, urinary retention, hypomania, mania, and suicidal tendency.

🖐 **Contraindicated for children under 16 years and pregnant or nursing mothers. Use with caution for adolescents and the elderly or debilitated.**

Side effects/Adverse reactions

Hypersensitivity: rash, sensitivity to sunlight. **CNS:** drowsiness, dizziness, anxiety, headache, fatigue, agitation, extrapyramidal symptoms, sedation (especially for the elderly). **CV:** orthostatic hypotension, palpitations, tachycardia, EKG changes, hypertension. **GI:** anorexia, dry mouth, nausea, vomiting, constipation, paralytic ileus. **GU:** urinary retention, decreased libido. **Eye:** blurred vision. **Ear:** tinnitus. **Hem:** agranulocytosis.

Nursing implications/Documentation

Possible nursing diagnoses: Potential for injury; Constipation; Altered oral mucous membrane.

♦ Document mental status and vital signs at least bid until response to therapy has been established.

♦ Be sure that doses are swallowed (not hoarded).

♦ Monitor for orthostatic hypotension, dizziness, and drowsiness; supervise ambulation until response is established.

♦ Record intake and output, and observe for dehydration or urinary retention; provide special mouth care.

♦ Monitor for and report suicidal tendencies, increased depression, or excessive drowsiness (may require change in medication).

♦ Prevent constipation by monitoring bowel movements and encouraging adequate fiber and fluid intake; offer laxatives or stool softeners before the problem becomes severe.

Patient & family teaching/Home care

Possible nursing diagnoses: Ineffective coping (family and individual); Sleep pattern disturbance; Impaired home maintenance management.

♦ Stress that this medication helps reduce the depression that inhibits ability to make decisions and cope effectively (once the individual feels less depressed, it will be easier to take steps toward making healthy changes).

♦ Explain that side effects are often noted immediately, but they usually diminish after a few weeks; on the other hand, it is likely to take 2–4 weeks before *beneficial* effects are noted (the patient may feel worse before feeling better).

♦ Warn to change positions slowly to prevent dizziness.

♦ Point out the role of adequate nutrition, exercise, and sleep in combating depression.

♦ Emphasize that the effects of alcohol, sedatives, and tranquilizers may be potentiated.

♦ Caution to consult with physician before using OTC drugs; stress the need for ongoing medical follow-up.

♦ Recommend reporting continued depression; stress that doses should not be increased or stopped without checking with physician because this may cause severe problems.

♦ Advise avoidance of driving and other potentially hazardous activities until response is established.

♦ Suggest using ice chips, hard candy, or gum to relieve side effect of dry mouth; stress the need for good mouth care.

♦ Warn women to report immediately if pregnancy is planned or suspected.

♦ *See Antidepressants overview for more information.*

amoxicillin

a-mox-i-sill'in

amoxicillin trihydrate: 🔺Alphamox, Amoxil, 🍁Apo-Amoxi, 🍁Axicillin, 🔺Cilamox, 🔺Ibiamox, 🔺Moxacin, 🍁Novamoxin, 🍁Polymox, Trimox, Utimox, Wymox

amoxicillin with potassium clavulanate: **Augmentin,** 🍁**Clavulin**

Class: Anti-infective, Antibiotic, Penicillin (potassium clavulanate is a beta-lactamase inhibitor)

PEDS	PREG	GERI
🖐	B	🖐

Action Broad-spectrum, usually bactericidal anti-biotic; amoxicillin kills bacteria by inhibiting cell wall synthesis. *Potassium clavulanate* potentiates its action by inactivating bacterial beta-lactamase, the enzyme that destroys amoxicillin.

Use/Therapeutic goal/Outcome

Amoxicillin trihydrate: Infection (systemic; acute and chronic urinary tract, respiratory tract, skin and soft tissue, sexually transmitted diseases): Prevention or resolution of infection. **Outcome criteria:** Absence of pathogenic growth on cultures, absence of clinical manifestations of infection (pain, swelling, redness, heat, odor, dysuria, drainage), normal X rays and WBC count.

Amoxicillin with potassium clavulanate: Infections (lower respiratory, ear, sinus, skin, urinary tract) caused by susceptible gram-negative and gram-positive organisms: Prevention or resolution of infection. **Outcome criteria:** Absence of pathogenic growth on cultures, absence of clinical manifestations of infection (pain, swelling, redness, heat, odor, drainage, productive cough, dysuria), normal WBC count, normal X rays.

Dose range/Administration

Interaction alert: Probenecid increases blood levels of amoxicillin (may be used for this purpose). Allopurinol increases incidence of rash.

🖐 **Give with meals to reduce GI distress.**

Adult/Child > 40 kg: PO: 250–500 mg amoxicillin q8h. *For gonorrhea:* 3 g amoxicillin with 1 g probenecid in a single dose. **Child < 40 kg:** PO: 20–40 mg/kg/day amoxicillin in divided doses q8h.

Clinical alert: Be aware that two 250 mg tablets of amoxicillin with potassium clavulanate are not equivalent to one 500 mg tablet of amoxicillin (each contains 125 mg of potassium clavulanate per tablet).

Contraindications/Precautions

PREG
B

Contraindicated in allergy to penicillin. **Use with caution** in cephalosporin sensitivity, in history of other allergic responses (e.g., other drugs, hay fever, asthma, etc.), or in mononucleosis (may cause a rash).

🖐 **Use with caution for children, the elderly, and pregnant or nursing mothers.**

Side effects/Adverse reactions

Hypersensitivity: itching, rashes, urticaria, fever, eosinophilia, difficulty breathing, ana-phylaxis. **GI:** nausea, vomiting, anorexia, diarrhea, pseudomembranous colitis. **Hem:** thrombocytosis, slight elevation in SGOT. (amoxicillin trihydrate) leukopenia or agranulocytosis. **Misc:** superinfection.

Nursing implications/Documentation

Possible nursing diagnoses: Potential for infection; Diarrhea.

◆ Determine history of allergies, and (regardless of history) monitor closely for allergic reactions.

◆ Obtain baseline CBC and necessary cultures before administering first dose; monitor closely thereafter if therapy is prolonged.

◆ Encourage fluids, and record and monitor intake and output, to ensure adequate hydration; report significant negative or positive balance.

◆ Monitor for and report signs of superinfection (sore throat, diarrhea, fever, fatigue, thrush, vaginal discharge).

Patient & family teaching/Home care

Possible nursing diagnoses: Knowledge deficit; Impaired home maintenance management.

◆ Explain that if GI symptoms are experienced, amoxicillin should be taken with food.

◆ Teach the importance of reporting allergic symptoms, diarrhea, signs and symptoms that do not abate, or *any* new signs and symptoms of discomfort that might indicate superinfection (medication regimen may have to be changed).

◆ Stress the importance of adequate hydration in preventing and treating infection (at least 2 L per day).

◆ Point out the need to take amoxicillin for the entire time prescribed, even if signs and symptoms abate.

◆ *See Anti-infectives overview for more information.*

amphetamine sulfate
am-fet'a-meen

Class: Cerebral stimulant, anorectic agent

PEDS	PREG	GERI	CONTROLLED
🖐	C	🖐	SUBSTANCE
			II

Action *In adults,* has a stimulant effect, *in hyperactive children,* a "paradoxical" calming effect. Probably stimulates the CNS by its action on the cerebral cortex and reticular activating system, where it promotes nerve impulse transmission by releasing stored norepinephrine from nerve terminals.

Use/Therapeutic goal/Outcome

Short-term appetite suppression: Reduction in desire for food. *Outcome criteria:* Report of lack of appetite.

Attention Deficit Disorders with Hyperactivity (ADDH): Promotion of ability to concentrate and pay attention. *Outcome criteria:* Demonstration of increased attention span and ability to sit quietly.

Narcolepsy: Promotion of alertness, reduction in sleep episodes. *Outcome criteria:* Report of feeling less fatigued or more alert; demonstration of ability to stay awake and pay attention.

Dose range/Administration

Interaction alert: Use within 14 days of MAO inhibitors may cause severe hypertensive crisis. May alter insulin requirements. Antacids, sodium bicarbonate, and acetazolamide may potentiate effect; ammonium chloride, ascorbic acid, phenothiazines, and haloperidol may reduce effect.

Narcolepsy: Adult: PO: 5–60 mg daily in divided doses. *Child > 12 yrs:* PO: 10 mg daily, with 10 mg weekly increments prn. *Child 6–12 yrs:* PO: : 5 mg daily, with weekly increments of 5 mg prn.

Appetite suppressant: Adult: PO: one or two 10- or 15-mg long-acting capsules daily (up to 30 mg/day); or 5–30 mg daily, or in divided doses 30–60 min before meals.

Attention Deficit Disorders with Hyperactivity (ADDH): Child 6 yrs and older: PO: 5 mg/day, with weekly increments of 5 mg prn. *Child 3–5 yrs:* PO: 2.5 mg daily, with weekly increments of 2.5 mg prn.

Clinical alert: Give doses at least 6 hr before bedtime to prevent insomnia. For treatment of ADDH in children, monitor for need to *decrease* dose; that is, watch for lessening effectiveness (this drug is usually stopped after puberty). For people with epilepsy, be aware that amphetamines may lower seizure threshhold.

Contraindications/Precautions

PREG
C

Contraindicated in hypersensitivity or intolerance to amphetamine, and in patients with glaucoma, symptomatic cardiac disease, angina, severe hypertension, hyperthyroidism, advanced arteriosclerosis, anxiety, agitation, history of mild hypertension, drug abuse, or within 14 days of taking MAO inhibitors. *Use with caution* in diabetes, parkinsonism, and depression.

✋ **Use with caution for the elderly and children with Tourette's disease. Safe use for pregnant or nursing mothers has not been established.**

Side effects/Adverse reactions

Hypersensitivity: itching, rashes. *CNS:* insomnia, restlessness, tremors, hyperactivity, talkativeness, irritability, headache, dizziness. *GI:* anorexia, metallic taste, nausea, vomiting, dry mouth, cramps, diarrhea, constipation. *CV:* tachycardia, hypertension, hypotension. *GU:* impotence, changes in libido. *Misc:* growth suppression in children.

Nursing implications/Documentation

Possible nursing diagnoses: Altered thought processes; Sleep pattern disturbance; Constipation; Altered nutrition: less than body requirements.

◆ Question about the use of beverages and OTC drugs that contain caffeine.

◆ Monitor attention span and ability to concentrate; report and document changes in status (dosage may need to be adjusted).

◆ Document blood pressure at least daily when beginning therapy, and periodically once stabilized.

◆ Document daily weights and keep a record of food intake to ensure adequate nutrition.

◆ Prevent side effect of constipation by monitoring bowel movements, ensuring adequate hydration, and providing fruits, juices, and vegetables (use laxatives only when necessary).

◆ Provide decaffeinated beverages.

Patient & family teaching/Home care

Possible nursing diagnoses: Knowledge deficit; Impaired home maintenance management.

◆ Explain that this drug has a high potential for abuse, and should only be taken as prescribed, and under continuous medical supervision.

◆ If used as an appetite suppressant, reinforce the importance of enrolling in a behavior modification weight-reduction program.

- Stress the importance of reading labels and realizing that caffeine may increase drug effects.

- Emphasize that side effect of constipation can be avoided by drinking plenty of fluids, eating fruits and fiber, ensuring adequate exercise, and using mild laxatives when necessary.

- *In addition to above, for use with children:* Teach the need to monitor physical and mental growth and to report growth failure and behavior extremes (dosage may have to be adjusted); explain that dosage will probably be reduced as child progresses to puberty, and that periodic "drug holidays" may be planned to determine if the drug is still necessary.

- *See Cerebral Stimulants overview for more information*

amphotericin B

am-foe-ter'i-sin

&Fungilin Oral, Fungizone

Class: ★Anti-infective (antifungal) prototype, Antibiotic

PEDS	PREG	GERI
✋	B	✋

Action Believed to act by binding to sterols in the cell membrane, altering cell permeability and allowing leakage of intracellular components. Can be fungicidal (kills fungi) or fungistatic (limits fungal growth), depending upon the concentration at the site of infection and susceptibility of the organisms.

Use/Therapeutic goal/Outcome

Fungal infections of the skin, or life-threatening confirmed systemic fungal infections: Resolution of infection. *Outcome criteria:* Absence of pathogenic growth on culture; absence of clinical manifestations of infection (redness, pain, swelling, fever, drainage, high WBC count).

Dose range/Administration

Interaction alert: Do not mix IV with any other drug or with solutions containing preservatives. *Use with caution* with other nephrotoxic drugs (monitor kidney function closely; damage is usually reversible if amphotericin B is discontinued at the first sign of dysfunction).

Adult and Child: IV: Begin with a test dose of 1 mg in 20 ml D5W, given over 20–30 min. If there is no reaction, infuse 0.25 mg/kg/day over 6 hrs (rapid infusion may cause cardiovas-

cular collapse). Then increase daily dose gradually depending upon patient response, up to 1 mg/kg/day (or may give 1.5 mg/kg qod). If therapy is interrupted for more than 1 week, begin again with initial dose and increase gradually. *Topical* (3% cream, lotion, ointment): Apply liberally to affected area bid to qid, rub in well. *Intrathecal:* 25 mcg/0.1 ml diluted in 10–20 ml of cerebrospinal fluid, given by barbotage 2–3 times/wk. *Maximum dose:* 100 mcg. *Into joint spaces (adults only):* 5–15 mg in a single dose.

Clinical alert: During IV administration of first dose, monitor vital signs every 15–30 minutes. Watch closely for fever and shaking chills (which may be reduced by premedication with aspirin, antihistamines, meparidine antiemetics, or low-dose corticosteroids; by adding phosphate buffer and heparin to the solution; and by alternate-day administration). To ensure safe administration dilute in 500 ml; give through an IV pump, preferably via a central line. If a peripheral line is used, change site with each dose to prevent phlebitis. Since preparation is a colloidal suspension, do not use an in-line filter of less than 1 micron; smaller filters will remove a significant amount of medication.

Contraindications/Precautions

PREG
B

Contraindicated in hypersensitivity to amphotericin and in severe bone marrow depression. *Use with caution* in renal function impairment.

✋ **Use with caution for children, pregnant and nursing mothers, and the elderly.**

Side effects/Adverse reactions

Hypersensitivity: (common) rashes, chills, fever; anaphylaxis. *Hem:* azotemia, hypokalemia, normochromic and normocytic anemia. *GI:* anorexia, nausea, vomiting, indigestion, epigastric cramping, diarrhea. *CNS:* headache, peripheral neuropathy, peripheral nerve pain and paresthesias. *CV:* hypotension, cardiac arrhythmias, cardiac arrest. *GU:* kidney dysfunction which may lead to permanent kidney damage, oliguria and anuria. *Misc:* weight loss; (with IV route) pain, burning at infusion site, tissue damage from extravasation.

Nursing implications/Documentation

Possible nursing diagnoses: Potential for infection; Altered nutrition: less than body requirements.

• Obtain necessary cultures before administering the first dose, and monitor periodically throughout treatment to detect organism resistance.

• Assess IV site carefully to avoid extravasation.

• Document and monitor intake and output, and ensure adequate hydration (report excessive negative or positive balance).

• Monitor weekly the serum drug level, CBC, electrolytes (especially potassium, sodium, calcium, magnesium), BUN, creatinine, alkaline phosphatase, and bilirubin; report abnormalities (may require dose adjustment or drug discontinuation).

• For topical use, rub preparation in gently; do not apply occlusive dressing (prompts yeast growth and toxin release).

Patient & family teaching/Home care

Possible nursing diagnosis: Knowledge deficit.

• Explain that long-term treatment, from 2 weeks to 3 months, may be required.

• Stress that unusual feelings or discomfort should be reported in case they are side effects that should be treated.

• For topical use, warn that amphotericin may stain clothing; caution to report itching, burning, or rashes.

• *See Anti-infectives overview for more information.*

ampicillin
am'pi-sill'in

ampicillin: *Amcill, ✦Ampicin, ✦Ampilean, ✦Apo-Ampi, ✦Novo Ampicillin, Omnipen, ✦Penbritin, Principen*

ampicillin sodium: *✦Ampicyn Injection, Omnipen-N, Polycillin-N, Totacillin-N*

ampicillin trihydrate: *Amcill, ✦Ampicyn Oral, D-Amp, Omnipen, Penamp-250, Penamp-500, ✦Penbritin, Polycillin, Principen-250, Principen-500, Totacillin*

ampicillin sodium with sulbactam sodium: *Unasyn*

Class: ★Anti-infective (aminopenicillin) proto-type, Antibiotic (sulbactam is beta-lactamase inhibitor)

PEDS	PREG	GERI
☝	B	☝

Action Broad-spectrum, usually bactericidal antibiotic; ampicillin kills bacteria by inhibiting cell wall synthesis. *Sulbactam* potentiates its action by inactivating bacterial beta-lactamase, the enzyme that destroys ampicillin.

Use/Therapeutic goal/Outcome

Ampicillin: Infection (urinary tract, respiratory, skin and soft tissue, sexually transmitted diseases): Prevention or resolution of infection. **Outcome criteria:** Absence of pathogenic growth on cultures, absence of clinical manifestations of infection (fever, pain, redness, heat, swelling, odor, drainage), normal WBC count, improvement of X rays.

Ampicillin with sulbactam: Intra-abdominal, gynecological, and skin and integument infections caused by susceptible bacteria: Resolution of infection. **Outcome criteria:** Absent or reduced pathogenic growth on cultures, absence of clinical manifestations of infection; (pain, swelling, redness, heat, odor, dysuria, drainage), normal WBC count, improvement of X rays.

Dose range/Administration

Interaction alert: Probenecid inhibits excretion of ampicillin and may be given to increase serum levels of the drug. Do not mix with aminoglycosides. Allopurinol may cause a rash.

🗋 **Give oral dose on an empty stomach 1 hour before or 2–3 hours after meals to maximize absorption.**

Ampicillin: Adult: PO: 250–500 mg q6h. *For gonorrhea:* 3.5 g ampicillin with 1 g probenecid in a single dose. IM, IV: (Use only for oral intolerance or severe infection) 2–12 g/day in divided doses q4-6h. **Child:** PO: 50–100 mg/kg/day in divided doses q4-6h. IM, IV: (Use only for oral intolerance or severe infection) 100–300 mg/kg/day in divided doses q4-6h.

Ampicillin with sulbactam: Preparation dose is based on combined dose of active components (1.5 g = 1 g ampicillin plus 0.5 g sulbactam). **Adult:** IM, IV: 1.5–3 g q6h. *Maximum dose:* 12 g/day (4 g sulbactam). Give IV doses slowly over 10–15 min (rapid infusion may induce seizures).

Clinical alert: Administer ampicillin with sulbactam at least 1 hour before bacteriostatic antibiotics; be aware that dosage should be decreased for patients with a creatinine clearance of less than 15–29 ml/min.

Contraindications/Precautions

PREG B

Contraindicated in allergy to penicillin, and in mononucleosis (causes a rash). *Use with caution* in cephalosporin sensitivity, in history of allergic responses (e.g., other drugs, hay fever, asthma) and in hepatic or renal insufficiency.

✋ **Use with caution for children, the elderly, and pregnant or nursing mothers. Safe use of sulbactam for children under 12 years has not been established.**

Side effects/Adverse reactions

Hypersensitivity: itching, rashes, urticaria, fever, eosinophilia, difficulty breathing, anaphylaxis, (with sulbactam) exfoliative dermatitis. *GI:* nausea, vomiting, anorexia, diarrhea, pseudomembranous colitis; (with sulbactam) flatulence and abdominal distension. *Hem:* anemia, granulocytopenia, agranulocytosis, thrombocytopenia, leukopenia, neutropenia, slight elevation in SGOT and SGPT. *GU:* nephrotoxicity with high doses, (with sulbactam) dysuria or urinary retention. *CNS:* neurotoxicity (with sulbactam) headache, chills, convulsions. *CV:* pain, redness, swelling, at injection site. *Skin:* (with sulbactam) erythema, edema. *Misc:* bone marrow depression, superinfection.

Nursing implications/Documentation

Possible nursing diagnoses: Potential for infection; Diarrhea; (with sulbactam) Urinary retention.

♦ Determine history of allergies, and (regardless of history) monitor closely for allergic reactions.

♦ Obtain baseline CBC and necessary cultures before administering first dose; monitor H & H and bleeding time, if therapy is prolonged. With sulbactam, obtain and monitor serum sodium and liver function studies.

♦ Encourage fluids, and document and monitor intake and output, to ensure adequate hydration; report significant negative or positive balance.

♦ Monitor for and report signs of superinfection (sore throat, diarrhea, fever, fatigue, thrush, vaginal discharge).

♦ Document and report diarrhea.

♦ With sulbactam, report unexplained bleeding (may be hypersensitivity reaction).

Patient & family teaching/Home care

Possible nursing diagnoses: Knowledge deficit; Impaired home maintenance management.

♦ Teach the importance of reporting allergic symptoms, diarrhea, signs and symptoms that do not abate, or *any* new signs and symptoms of discomfort that might indicate superinfection (medication regimen may have to be changed).

♦ Explain that ampicillin should be taken on an empty stomach (at least 1 hour before or 2 hours after meals) with a full glass of water for best absorption and effect.

♦ Advise drinking 2–3 L of fluids daily to maintain adequate hydration (especially important if fever exists).

♦ Stress the importance of taking ampicillin for the entire time prescribed, even if signs and symptoms abate.

♦ *See Anti-infectives overview for more information.*

amrinone lactate
am′ri-non

Inocor

Class: Positive inotrope, Cardiotonic

PEDS	PREG	GERI
✋	C	✋

Action Increases the force of ventricular contraction by inhibiting myocardial cyclic adenosine monophosphate (c-AMP) phosphodiesterase activity and increasing c-AMP at cellular level. Also has vasodilator properties.

Use/Therapeutic goal/Outcome

Acute congestive heart failure unresponsive to digoxin and diuretics: Reduction of afterload and preload, improved cardiac output. *Outcome criteria:* Respiratory rate and heart rate within normal limits; clearing of lung fields, improved urine output; pulmonary artery pressure (PAP), pulmonary capillary wedge pressure (PCWP), cardiac output (CO) and cardiac index (CI) within normal limits.

Dose range/Administration

Interaction alert: Do not dilute with solutions containing dextrose (although it may be injected through a Y-connector with running dextrose). **Do not mix with any other drug.**

Adult: IV: Initial bolus of 0.75 mg/kg given slowly over 2–3 min. Maintenance infusion of 5–10 mcg/kg/min is recommended. An additional 0.75 mg/kg bolus may be administered 30 min after initiation of therapy. The total daily dose (including bolus) should not exceed 10 mg/kg.

Clinical alert: May dilute with NS or 1/2 NS (0.45% NaCl) solution to a concentration of 1–3 mg/ml and infuse via pump. Adjust dose based on clinical response (measurement of PAP, PCWP, CO, CI). Be aware that cardiovascular effects begin within 2–5 min of initiating infusion and may last up to 30 min after infusion is stopped.

Contraindications/Precautions

PREG
C

Contraindicated in hypersensitivity to amrinone lactate or to bisulfites, and in severe aortic or pulmonic valvular disease. *Use with caution* in presence of hypertrophic subaortic stenosis.

✋ Use with caution for the elderly. Safe use for children and pregnant or nursing mothers has not been established.

Side effects/Adverse reactions

Hypersensitivity: pericarditis, pleuritis. *CV:* arrhythmias, hypotension, chest pain. *Hem:* thrombocytopenia. *GI:* nausea, vomiting, abdominal pain, anorexia, hepatic toxicity. *Misc:* fever, burning sensation at the infusion site.

Nursing implications/Documentation

Possible nursing diagnoses: Potential for injury; Activity intolerance; Fluid volume excess; Sleep pattern disturbance.

◆ Be sure to check baseline chest X ray, EKG, and laboratory studies (CBC, sodium, potassium, chloride, carbon dioxide, magnesium, BUN, creatinine, SGPT, and LDH) before giving first dose; monitor closely thereafter as indicated by clinical condition.

◆ Be aware that for optimal efficacy, electrolyte imbalances, serum pH imbalances, and decreased oxygen saturation should be corrected.

◆ Document and monitor PAP, PCWP, CO, CI, systemic vascular resistance, and mean arterial pressure every hr, or as ordered.

◆ Record pulse, respirations and blood pressure every 5–10 min until stabilized, then at least every hr thereafter; if hypotension occurs, decrease infusion rate (or stop IV) and report immediately.

◆ Measure urine output every hr; report urine output less than 25–30 cc/hr; monitor 8-hr intake and output closely for excessive imbalance.

◆ Monitor platelet count closely; report platelet count less than 150,000/mm^3 because dosage may need to be reduced.

◆ Keep patient in bed with side rails up.

◆ Coordinate care to provide uninterrupted rest whenever possible.

Patient & family teaching/Home care

Possible nursing diagnoses: Anxiety; Fear; Knowledge deficit.

◆ Explain that the purpose of this drug is to improve the pumping action of the heart.

◆ Reassure that frequent monitoring of hemodynamic parameters is needed to fine-tune dose for optimum effects.

◆ Stress that new symptoms of discomfort, difficulty breathing, or dizziness should be reported; these symptoms may mean that the dosage needs to be adjusted.

amsacrine

am'sa-kreen

amsacrine m-AMSA: *Amsidyl,* ✦*Amsidine*
Class: Antineoplastic agent

PEDS	PREG	GERI
✋	C	✋

Action Kills rapidly growing cells (cancer, hair follicles, bone marrow, GI lining, ova, and sperm) by inhibiting DNA synthesis through intercalation (it binds to DNA and produces chromosomal damage). Is cell-cycle–phase specific in the G_1- and S-phases.

Use/Therapeutic goal/Outcome

Myelogenous leukemia, lymphomas, T-cell lymphoma, malignant melanoma, adenocarcinoma of the lung and kidney, epidermoid carcinoma of esophagus, ovarian cancer, carcinoma of the breast and colon, Hodgkin's disease: Elimination or suppression of malignant cell proliferation. *Outcome criteria:* Tumor and disease regression or stabilization on radiologic and physical examination; for leukemias, absence of blasts in peripheral blood specimen.

Dose range/Administration

Interaction alert: Incompatible with heparin in solution. Use glass syringes for preparing solution (combining amsacrine and lactic acid); diluent may dissolve plastic syringes. Do not add to normal saline or to a chloride-containing solution (precipitate may form).

Leukemias: Adult: IV (or intra-arterial infusion): 90–120 mg/m^2 for 5–7 days.

Solid tumors: Adult: IV: 90–120 mg/m^2 every 21–28 days or 30–50 mg/m^2/day for 3 days.

Clinical alert: This drug should be given only by nurses who are knowledgeable in the comprehensive management of the administration of antineoplastic agents. Doses may vary at physician's discretion. Repeat doses are held until it is ascertained that the patient has recovered sufficiently from toxicities of previous doses. Established protocols/policies for drug preparation, administration, and accidental skin contamination *must be followed closely* (gloves or double gloves are worn when handling drug; if the drug touches the skin, the area is washed immediately with plenty of soap and water). Amsacrine is given *slowly* over 1–2 hr in 500 ml D5W (*not* saline) to minimize inflammation and pain along the vein.

Contraindications/Precautions

PREG
C

Contraindicated in hypersensitivity to amsacrine, and in hypokalemia. **Use with caution** in impaired hepatic and renal function (dosage reduction may be necessary).

🖐 **Contraindicated for pregnant or nursing mothers. Use with caution for children and the elderly.**

Side effects/Adverse reactions

Hypersensitivity: (rare) urticaria, anaphylaxis. **Hem:** granulocytopenia, thrombocytopenia, leukopenia (usually dose-limiting). **GI:** stomatitis; mucositis; mild nausea and vomiting; diarrhea (with high doses); hepatotoxicity. **Skin:** local sensitivity with direct drug contact; alopecia; pain, burning, and erythema at injection site; cellulitis, ulceration and sloughing if extravasation occurs. **CV:** CHF, dysrhythmias. **CNS:** headache, dizziness, peripheral neuropathy, CNS depression, grand mal seizures. **Ear:** ototoxicity.

Nursing implications/Documentation

Possible nursing diagnoses: Potential for infection; Potential for injury; Fatigue; Altered oral mucous membrane; Fluid volume deficit; Diarrhea; Altered nutrition: less than body requirements.

◆ *See important Nursing implications in Antineoplastic agents overview on page 72, which apply to all antineoplastics. The interventions that follow are additional and specific to this drug only.*

◆ Expect that platelet and WBC count will drop to the lowest point (nadir) at 7–10 days after therapy begins, with recovery in 21–23 days; blood transfusions and antibiotics may be required.

◆ Maintain a fluid intake of 2–3 L a day to prevent renal tubular damage from hyperuricemia secondary to cell lysis; record intake and output and report significant negative or positive balance.

◆ Establish a baseline for hearing capacity and monitor for ototoxicity thereafter.

Patient & family teaching/Home care

Possible nursing diagnoses: Knowledge deficit; Ineffective coping (individual and family); Hopelessness; Impaired home maintenance management.

◆ *See important Patient & family teaching in Antineoplastic agents overview on page 72, which apply to all antineoplastics. The teachings that follow are additional and specific to this drug only.*

◆ Stress the need to prevent kidney complications by drinking 2–3 L of fluid per day (if the patient can't keep fluids down, IV fluids may be necessary).

◆ Explain the need to report numbness or tingling of the feet and legs, weakness, or problems with coordination immediately.

◆ Advise that this drug may make urine orange.

◆ *See Antineoplastic agents overview for more information.*

amyl nitrite
am'il

Aspirole, Vaporoles

Class: Vasodilator, Organic nitrate, Antidote

PEDS	PREG	GERI
🖐	C	🖐

Action Decreases cardiac workload and myocardial oxygen demand by reducing left ventricular end-diastolic pressure (preload) and, to a

▶

lesser extent, by reducing systemic vascular resistance (afterload). Relaxes smooth muscle, particularly peripheral vascular smooth muscle, and has a systemic vasodilating effect on the large arteries and veins. Also enhances myocardial perfusion by promoting blood flow through collateral circulation. Acts as an antidote in cyanide poisoning by converting hemoglobin to methemoglobin, which binds with cyanide to form a nontoxic chemical. This drug has a rapid onset of action (30 seconds) and a short duration of action (3–5 min).

◆ *Action and adverse effects are similar to those of nitroglycerin. Amyl nitrite is rarely used for angina because of cost, odor, and side effects.*

Use/Therapeutic goal/Outcome

Angina: Improved perfusion of coronary tissue and relief of angina. *Outcome criteria:* Report of chest pain relief.

Cyanide poisoning: Neutralization of cyanide ion and prevention of death. *Outcome criteria:* Decrease in serum cyanide level, patient survival.

Dose range/Administration

Angina: Adult: Inhal: 0.2 to 0.3 cc (1 ampule crushed) prn.

Cyanide poisoning: Adult and Child: Inhal: 0.2 to 0.3 cc (1 ampule crushed) and vapor inhaled q1min until sodium nitrite infusion is started.

Clinical alert: Do not crush ampule near flame or intense heat. Seat or lay patient down before administering. Wrap ampule in towel, crush, and hold near patient's nose.

Contraindications/Precautions

PREG
C

Contraindicated in hypersensitivity to amyl nitrite and nitrates, and in head trauma, cerebral hemorrhage, hypotension, and glaucoma.

♨ **Use with caution for children and the elderly. Safe use for pregnant women has not been established.**

Side effects/Adverse reactions

Hypersensitivity: rash. **CNS:** headache, dizziness, weakness. **CV:** orthostatic hypotension, flushing, palpitations, and tachycardia. **Hem:** methemoglobinemia (which impairs oxygen-carrying capacity of RBCs) may occur with high doses.

Nursing implications/Documentation

Possible nursing diagnoses: Potential for injury; Pain.

◆ Keep a record of pulse and blood pressure, before and after drug administration.

◆ Observe for postural hypotension; when allowed up, supervise ambulation until response is determined.

◆ Be aware that this drug is inactivated when exposed to heat.

◆ Recognize that amyl nitrite is known as "poppers," "snappers," "Amy," and "whiffenpoppers" in street language, and is used illicitly to enhance intensity of sexual orgasm.

Patient & family teaching/Home care

Possible nursing diagnoses: Impaired home maintenance management.

◆ Stress that this drug should be used only under strict medical supervision.

◆ *See Antianginals overview for more information.*

anistreplase
a-niss'tre-plaze

anisoylated plasminogen-streptokinase activator complex (APSAC): *Eminase*

Class: Thrombolytic enzyme, Fibrinolytic

Antidote: Aminocaproic acid

PEDS	PREG	GERI
♨	C	♨

Action Degrades fibrin and directly dissolves clots (thrombi) by promoting conversion of plasminogen to plasmin (the enzyme that degrades fibrin). This drug is derived from lys-plasminogen and streptokinase; the active lys-plasminogen-streptokinase activator complex is formed in the bloodstream or within the thrombus.

Use/Therapeutic goal/Outcome

Emergency treatment of acute myocardial infarction (not used more than 6 hr after onset of symptoms of coronary artery occlusion): Lysis of thrombi obstructing coronary arteries, reperfusion of ischemic cardiac tissue. *Outcome criteria:* Abrupt cessation of chest pain (often accompanied by sudden onset of hypotension and reperfusion arrhythmias); smaller Q waves, and return of ST segment to baseline on EKG; cardiac enzyme washout (cardiac enzymes peak faster than they do in untreated myocardial infarction); absence of coronary occlusion upon cardiac catheterization (may be performed hours or days later when risk of bleeding has diminished).

Dose range/Administration

Interaction alert: Do not mix with any other IV drugs. Oral anticoagulants, heparin, or drugs that affect platelet function (salicylates, dipyridamole, nonsteroidal anti-inflammatory agents) increase risk of bleeding; concomitant IV heparin is common, as is therapy with aspirin or dipyridamole following heparin.

Adult: IV: As soon as possible after onset of symptoms, 30 units over 2–5 min by direct injection (do not dilute).

Clinical alert: To reconstitute, slowly add 5 ml sterile water for injection without preservatives (not bacteriostatic) by directing the stream against the side of the vial, rather than at the drug. Avoid foaming by gently rolling rather than shaking to mix the powder and solution. Observe for particles that have not dissolved; liquid should be colorless to pale yellow. If the solution is not used within 30 min of reconstitution, discard it. This drug should be administered only by professionals who are well educated in all aspects of its administration. Be sure that three IV sites and other invasive lines are established before administration of anistreplase, and have the following at the patient's bedside: electrocardiogram machine, emergency medications, advanced cardiac life support (ACLS) cart (with defibrillator), IV fluids. Be prepared to treat reperfusion arrhythmias, which are common.

Contraindications/Precautions

PREG
C

Contraindicated in hypersensitivity to anistreplase or streptokinase, and in active internal bleeding or known source of potential bleeding (e.g., ulcer disease), intracranial neoplasm, arteriovenous malformation, intracranial or abdominal aneurysm, bleeding diathesis, history of cerebrovascular accident, or within 2 months of cranial or spinal or thoracic surgery (or trauma), organ biopsy, or cavity aspiration. *Use with caution* in puncture of a noncompressible vessel within 10 days; prothrombin time > 15 sec; aspirin consumption within 72 hr; known or suspected left heart thrombus; surgery, trauma, or CPR (especially with rib fractures) within 10 days; traumatic endotracheal intubation; persistent hypertension (systolic pressure > 180 mm or diastolic pressure > 110 mm after treatment); subacute bacterial endocarditis; and diabetic retinopathy.

❦ **Use with caution if pregnancy is known or suspected, and for adults over 75 years.**

Safe use for children has not been established.

Side effects/Adverse reactions

Hypersensitivity: itching, rashes, fever, chills, rare anaphylaxis. *CNS:* cerebral hemorrhage. *CV:* hypotension, dysrhythmias. *GI:* nausea, vomiting, bleeding. *GU:* hematuria. *Skin:* delayed (2 weeks after therapy) purpuric rash. *Misc:* bleeding of surgical or traumatic injury, bleeding from puncture sites.

Nursing implications/Documentation

Possible nursing diagnoses: Potential for injury; Pain; Anxiety; Fear.

◆ Obtain a careful history of chest pain, and closely monitor level of chest pain before, during, and after administration of anistreplase.

◆ Expect SL and IV nitroglycerin to be given to rule out vasospasm before administration of anistreplase.

◆ Assess carefully for contraindications to anistreplase.

◆ Attach patient to cardiac monitor and select the lead that shows the highest ST-segment elevation (also attach patient to a 12-lead EKG; periodic EKGs will be necessary during administration).

◆ *Check policy and procedure to determine variations in the following interventions:*

◆ Be sure baseline and other "stat" lab studies are drawn before initiating anistreplase (PT, PTT, CBC, fibrinogen level, renal studies, cardiac enzymes, type and crossmatch for 2 units of blood, and other routine coronary admission studies determined by hospital policy).

◆ Have the necessary equipment ready for three large-bore peripheral intravenous lines (one for administration of anistreplase; another for administration of other drugs, such as continuous heparin and lidocaine; and the third for drawing blood samples; these may also be needed in case of hemorrhage).

◆ Before, during, and after administration of anistreplase, document and report presence of abnormal pulses, abnormal neurological findings, or skin lesions (may indicate coagulation defects).

◆ Record vital signs every 15 min for 1 hr after infusion, then every 30 min for 5 hr; also post EKG strips on chart to have a record of changes in ST segments.

▶

anistreplase   145

• Document neurological signs on a flow sheet every 30 min for at least 2 hr (check policy).

• Be prepared to treat reperfusion dysrhythmias (ventricular tachycardia or fibrillation, atrial tachycardia or fibrillation) according to hospital protocol or individual physician orders; have emergency drugs and defibrillator readily available (some protocols call for starting a lidocaine drip and heparin drip when anistreplase is initiated).

• Keep all needle punctures to an absolute minimum, apply manual pressure for 10 min to all venous puncture sites and for 30 min to arterial puncture sites; follow this with pressure dressing. Observe all intravenous and intra-arterial sites every 15 min for 1 hr, every 30 min for 2 hr, every hour for 4 hr, then every 2 hr until removed.

• Place a sign on door and over bed to alert staff and phlebotomist of bleeding precautions.

• Maintain patient on complete bedrest until otherwise ordered, and monitor closely for bleeding: hemoptysis, CVA, hematuria, hematemesis, melena, pain or swelling from closed space bleeding, and signs and symptoms of cardiac tamponade (distended neck veins and significant pulsus paradoxus). Report immediately if these are observed.

• Keep aminocaproic acid available in case of hemorrhage.

• Check physician's orders and policy for drawing lab work post infusion. This usually includes the following: CPK, CPK Isoenzymes (every 4 hr × 3, then daily × 2), Hgb and Hct (every 4 hr the first 24 hr, then once the next day), PTT (stat and every 4 hr × 2, then daily throughout heparin therapy; should be maintained in the 80–120 sec range).

Patient & family teaching/Home care

Possible nursing diagnoses: Anxiety; Fear; Knowledge deficit.

• Explain the rationale for prompt initiation of treatment and for routine procedures that ensure patient safety.

• Encourage voicing questions and concerns, and keeping nurses informed of new symptoms (headache, dizziness, chest discomfort, abdominal discomfort).

• Explain that symptoms associated with hypotension and dysrhythmias are likely to be transient.

• Stress the need to remain in bed.

◆ *See Anticoagulants and thrombolytic enzymes overview for more information.*

apraclonidine
ap-rah-kloe'ni-deen

apraclonidine hydrochloride: *Iopidine*
Class: Ocular alpha-adrenergic agonist

PEDS	PREG	GERI
🖐	C	🖐

Action Lowers intraocular pressure (IOP) by reducing production of intraocular aqueous humor. Onset of action is within 1 hour, with peak effectiveness at 4–5 hours after instillation.

Use/Therapeutic goal/Outcome

Ocular hypertension (after argon laser trabeculoplasty or iridotomy): Control of intraocular pressure. *Outcome criteria:* Pressure within normal limits measured by physician with tonometer.

Dose range/Administration

Adult: *Ophthalmic:* Instill 1 drop 1% solution into anterior segment of affected eye 1 hr before and 1 hr after surgery.

Clinical alert: Be sure that applicator tip does not touch the eyelid (may contaminate drops). To prevent *systemic absorption,* apply light finger pressure to lacrimal sac for 30–60 seconds after instilling drops.

Contraindications/Precautions
PREG C

Contraindicated in hypersensitivity to apraclonidine or clonidine. **Use with caution** in hypertension, severe cardiovascular disease, or history of vasovagal attacks.

🖐 **Contraindicated for children, adults under 21 years, and pregnant or nursing mothers. Use with caution for the elderly.**

Side effects/Adverse reactions

Hypersensitivity: pruritus, conjunctival hyperemia, eyelid swelling, tearing, exaggerated decrease in IOP. **Eye:** upper eyelid elevation, conjunctival blanching, mydriasis, foreign-body sensation, tired eyes, dryness, dimmed vision, hypotony.

The following systemic reactions are uncommon: **CV:** bradycardia, palpitations, hypotension. **GI:** dry mouth, nausea, vomiting, abdominal pain, diarrhea. **CNS:** insomnia, headache, fatigue, decreased libido.

Nursing implications/Documentation

Possible nursing diagnoses: Sensory/perceptual alterations (visual); Potential for injury.

◆ Wash hands thoroughly before and after administration.

◆ Ensure adequate light in the environment and monitor for risk of injury (blurred vision is common).

◆ Although incidence of systemic side effects is low, monitor patients with cardiovascular disease for hypotension, hypertension, bradycardia, or palpitations; document vital signs until response is determined.

Patient & family teaching/Home care

Possible nursing diagnoses: Knowledge deficit.

◆ Explain that this drug helps control pressure within the eye.

◆ Advise that systemic reactions are rare, but that dizziness or palpitations should be reported.

asparaginase

a-spare'a-ji-nase

l-asparaginase: **Elspar, ✦Kidrolase**

Class: Antineoplastic agent

PEDS	PREG	GERI
🖐	C	🖐

Action Kills rapidly growing cells (cancer, hair follicles, bone marrow, GI lining, ova, and sperm) by depriving cells of asparagine, which they require for protein synthesis. Drug is cell-cycle specific for the postmitotic G_1-phase.

Use/Therapeutic goal/Outcome

Lymphocytic leukemia and lymphomas: Elimination or suppression of malignant cell proliferation. **Outcome criteria:** Tumor and disease regression or stabilization on radiologic and physical examination; for leukemias, absence of blasts in peripheral blood specimen.

Dose range/Administration

Interaction alert: Monitor for increased toxicity when administered with vincristine and prednisone. Reduces effectiveness of methotrexate. Other cytotoxic agents can cause severe myelosuppression.

Adult and Child: IV: 1000 IU/kg/day for 2–20 days; or 200 IU/kg/day for 28 days when drug is sole induction agent. IM: 6000 IU/m², 3 times a week for 3 weeks as part of multiple-

agent induction. Do not give more than 2 ml in any single injection site.

Clinical alert: Recognize that hypersensitivity reactions, including anaphylaxis, are common. This drug should be given to hospitalized patients only by nurses who are knowledgeable in the comprehensive management of the administration of antineoplastic agents. Doses may vary at physician's discretion. Repeat doses are held until it is ascertained that the patient has recovered sufficiently from toxicities of previous doses. Established protocols/policies for drug preparation, administration, and accidental skin contamination *must be followed closely* (gloves or double gloves are worn when handling drug; if the drug touches the skin, the area is washed immediately with plenty of soap and water). Asparaginase is given *slowly* over 30–45 min in 50–100 ml fluid to minimize inflammation and pain along the vein. The solution should not be given if it is cloudy. The IV site should be monitored *closely* for infiltration. If infiltration occurs, the IV is stopped, and protocols for treatment are followed.

Contraindications/Precautions

PREG C

Contraindicated in hypersensitivity to asparaginase, and in preexisting pancreatitis. **Use with caution** in hepatic or renal dysfunction, diabetes mellitus, or bone marrow suppression.

🖐 **Contraindicated for pregnant or nursing mothers. Use with caution for children and the elderly.**

Side effects/Adverse reactions

Hypersensitivity: (common) urticaria, arthralgia, facial edema, hypotension, respiratory distress, acute anaphylaxis. **GI:** anorexia, nausea, vomiting, pancreatitis; hepatotoxicity. **MS:** weight loss. **GU:** azotemia, acute renal failure, renal insufficiency, uric acid nephropathy, polyuria. **CNS:** depression, drowsiness, confusion, agitation, hallucinations, Parkinson-like syndrome, headache, irritability. **Hem:** hypofibrinogenemia, depression of serum albumin and clotting factors, thrombocytopenia, hyperglycemia, transient bone marrow depression, anemia, leukopenia. **Skin:** hyperpigmentation along infusion site. **Misc:** fever, chills, and fatal hyperthermia.

Nursing implications/Documentation

Possible nursing diagnoses: Potential for infection; Potential for injury; Fatigue; Altered oral mucous membrane; Fluid volume deficit; Diarrhea; Altered nutrition: less than body requirements.

♦ *See important Nursing implications in Antineoplastic agents overview on page 72, which apply to all antineoplastics. The interventions that follow are additional and specific to this drug only.*

• Before administration, check that a hypersensitivity test with 2 IU L-asparaginase has been documented at least 1 hr before dose (the patient may require desensitization); monitor closely for anaphylaxis and have emergency drugs and equipment on hand.

• For combination therapy, give asparaginase after vincristine and prednisone to minimize toxicities, and after methotrexate for maximum effect.

• Maintain a fluid intake of 2–3 L a day to prevent renal tubular damage from hyperuricemia secondary to cell lysis; record intake and output and report significant positive or negative balance.

• Observe for and report signs of pancreatic toxicity (abdominal pain, increased amylase levels).

• Monitor for drug-induced hyperglycemia and for CNS side effects (confusion, drowsiness, hallucinations, depression, nervousness).

• Report low back or flank pain (may be hyperuricemia).

Patient & family teaching/Home care

Possible nursing diagnoses: Knowledge deficit; Ineffective coping (individual); Hopelessness; Impaired home maintenance management.

♦ *See important Patient & family teaching in Antineoplastic agents overview on page 72, which apply to all antineoplastics. The teachings that follow are additional and specific to this drug only.*

• Stress the need to prevent kidney complications by drinking 2–3 L of fluid per day (if the patient can't keep fluids down, IV fluids may be necessary).

• Point out the need to avoid immunizations and those who have recently taken oral polio vaccine.

♦ *See Antineoplastic agents overview for more information.*

aspirin

as'pir-in

acetylsalicylic acid: ♦*Ancasal*, ♦*Arthrinol*, *Artria SR, A.S.A., ASA Enseals, Aspergum,* ♠*Asprol,* ♦*Astrin, Bayer Aspirin,* ♠*Bex,* ♦*Coryphen, Easprin, Ecotrin, Empirin,* ♦*Entrophen, Measurin, Norwich Aspirin,* ♦*Novasen, Riphen-10,* ♦*Sal-Adult,* ♦*Sal-Infant,* ♠*Solprin,* ♦*Supasa, Triaphen-10,* ♠*Vincent's Powders,* ♠*Winsprin Capsules, Zorprin.*

Class: ★**Analgesic and antipyretic prototype,** ★**Nonsteroidal anti-inflammatory (NSAID) prototype,** Antiplatelet, Salicylate

PEDS	PREG	GERI
🤚	🤚	🤚

Action **Relieves pain** by blocking generation of pain impulses, possibly by inhibiting prostaglandin synthesis (peripheral action) and by effecting the hypothalamus (central action). **Reduces fever** by direct action on the hypothalamic heat-regulating center (causes peripheral vasodilation, which increases peripheral blood supply and promotes heat loss through sweating and cooling by evaporation). **Reduces inflammation** by inhibiting cyclooxygenase (an enzyme necessary for prostaglandin synthesis) and by interfering with other inflammatory-response mediators. **Impedes clotting**, probably by blocking prostaglandin synthesis (this prevents formation of the platelet-aggregating substance called thromoxane A_2, a prostaglandin derivative). Large doses have hypoglycemic and hypocholesterolemic effects. Recent preliminary research has shown evidence that aspirin may strengthen immunity and help fight off disease.

Use/Therapeutic goal/Outcome

Mild to moderate pain: Relief of pain. *Outcome criteria:* Report of greater comfort; absence of signs of discomfort (frowning, restlessness, crying).

Anti-inflammatory: Reduction of inflammation and promotion of mobility. *Outcome criteria:* Report of relief of pain, stiffness, and swelling of joints; improved mobility.

Fever: Reduction of fever. *Outcome criteria:* Reduction in temperature reading.

Thromboembolitic disorders: Prevention of thrombus and lengthening of clotting time (reduction in risk of stroke, heart attack). *Outcome criteria:* Prolonged clotting time.

Dose range/Administration

Interaction alert: Anticoagulants increase risk of bleeding. Ammonium chloride and other urine acidifiers increase risk of salicylate toxicity. High doses of antacids, urine alkalinizers, and corticosteroids decrease effects. Large doses (> 2 g/day) may decrease insulin requirements.

🖐 **Give with milk, food, or an antacid to reduce GI effects.**

Pain, fever: Adult: PO, Rectal: 325–650 mg q4h prn.

Arthritis: Adult: PO: 2.6–5.2 g/day in divided doses q4-6h. *Child:* PO: 90–130 mg/kg/day in divided doses q4-6h.

Acute rheumatic fever: Adult: PO: Dosage highly individualized. *Maximum dose:* 7.8 g/day in divided doses.

Thromboembolic disorders: Adult: PO: 325–650 mg qd to bid.

Transient ischemic attacks: Adult: PO: 650 mg bid or 325 mg qid.

Reduce risk of heart attack: Adult: PO: 80–325 mg qd.

Pain: Child: PO, Rectal: 65–100 mg/kg/day in divided doses q4-6h prn.

Fever: Child: PO, Rectal: 40–80 mg/kg/day in divided doses q6h prn.

Clinical alert: In prolonged therapy, consider use of enteric coated aspirin. Do not give salicylate to children under 18 years with chickenpox or influenza-like infections because of their association with Reye's syndrome. Observe the elderly for increased risk of toxicity.

Contraindications/Precautions
PREG
🖐

Contraindicated in hypersensitivity to salicylates, including methyl salicylate (oil of wintergreen), in GI bleeding or ulcer. *Use with caution* in hypoprothrombinemia; Vitamin K deficiency; bleeding disorders; "aspirin triad" (rhinitis, asthma, nasal polyps—because of risk of severe bronchospasm); and renal or hepatic impairment.

🖐 **Contraindicated for children under 18 years with influenza-like illness or chickenpox and pregnant women (first 2 trimesters, preg C; in third trimester, preg D). Use with caution for the elderly.**

Side effects/Adverse reactions

Hypersensitivity: rashes, shortness of breath, bronchospasm (wheezing), tightness in chest, severe rhinitis, anaphylaxis. *GI:* nausea, vomiting, bleeding. *Hem:* prolonged bleeding time. *Ear:* ringing of the ears. *Misc:* Salicylism (tinnitus, reversible hearing loss, dizziness, confusion, nausea, vomiting, GI distress and irritation, prolonged bleeding time, rash, bruising, abnormal liver function tests, hepatitis).

Nursing implications/Documentation

Possible nursing diagnoses: Pain; Impaired physical mobility.

◆ Schedule doses so that drug is given *at least 1 hr* before maximum effect is needed; report and record inadequate pain control.

◆ Attempt to determine cause of fever before giving aspirin (may mask symptoms that should be treated more specifically; report persistent fever, and keep a record of temperature reading before and after administration).

◆ Monitor for and report GI symptoms that may indicate peptic ulcer (nausea, pain, black stools).

◆ Observe the elderly for increased susceptibility to toxicity.

◆ Do not give aspirin if surgery is anticipated within 1 week.

Patient & family teaching/Home care

Possible nursing diagnoses: Knowledge deficit; Impaired home maintenance management.

◆ Stress the need to take aspirin with food to reduce GI symptoms; explain the importance of watching for symptoms of GI bleeding (black stools, persistent GI distress).

◆ Advise taking aspirin 1 hr before maximum effect is needed.

◆ Point out that long-term use of aspirin (or use in high doses) is likely to increase risk of bleeding and that those taking aspirin on a long-term basis should be followed by a physician.

◆ Advise telling physician and dentist if aspirin is taken on a regular basis.

◆ Warn that using aspirin to reduce fever may mask serious illness; advise reporting fever that lasts longer than 2–3 days.

◆ Stress that those under 18 years with flu-like symptoms or chicken pox should not receive aspirin (risk of developing Reye's Syndrome).

◆ *See Narcotic and non-narcotic analgesics and Nonsteroidal anti-inflammatory drugs overviews for more information.*

A astemizole

as-tem'i-zole

Hismanal

Class: Nonsedating antihistamine (H₁ receptor antagonist)

PEDS	PREG	GERI
✋	C	✋

Action Prevents but does not reverse histamine-mediated allergic responses by competing with histamine for H_1 receptors on effector cells. Does not affect CNS at therapeutic doses, and is not sedating.

Use/Therapeutic goal/Outcome

Seasonal allergic rhinitis and chronic idiopathic urticaria, decrease in allergic response. *Outcome criteria:* Report and demonstration of decreased or absent allergic symptoms (sneezing, nasal stuffiness and secretions, itching).

Dose range/Administration

▣ **Give on an empty stomach and hold food for 1 hr after dose.**

Adult/Child > 12 yrs: PO: 10 mg/day. To obtain rapid therapeutic levels, a loading dose of 30 mg may be administered on the first day, 20 mg on the second day, and 10 mg/day thereafter.

Contraindications/Precautions

PREG
C

Contraindicated in hypersensitivity to astemizole (rare). *Use with caution* in liver or kidney disease.

✋ **Use with caution for the elderly. Safe use for pregnant or nursing mothers and for children under 12 years has not been established.**

Side effects/Adverse reactions

Hypersensitivity: (rare) angioedema, bronchospasm, pruritis, rash. *CNS:* drowsiness, headache, fatigue, nervousness, dizziness. *GI:* appetite increase, weight increase, dry mouth, nausea, diarrhea, abdominal pain, pharyngitis. *Eye:* conjunctivitis. *MS:* arthralgia.

Nursing implications/Documentation

Possible nursing diagnoses: Potential for injury; Fluid volume deficit.

♦ Determine and record known allergies; provide an environment that is free from allergens (especially sleeping areas).

♦ Provide favorite fluids and ensure adequate hydration (2 liters/day).

Patient & family teaching/Home care

Possible nursing diagnoses: Knowledge deficit; Impaired home maintenance management.

♦ Stress the need to take this drug on an empty stomach and to avoid eating for 1 hr after dose.

♦ Point out that avoiding pollens and staying in an air-conditioned environment may help reduce seasonal rhinitis.

♦ Emphasize that dose should not be increased without the approval of physician.

♦ Explain the need to stop antihistamines for 4 days before allergy testing to ensure accurate results.

♦ *See Antihistamines overview for more information.*

atenolol

a-ten'oh-lole

Tenormin, ♠Noten

Class: Selective beta-1 adrenergic blocking agent, Antihypertensive, Antianginal

PEDS	PREG	GERI
✋	C	✋

Action Reduces blood pressure (precise mechanism is unclear), and relieves angina by blocking beta-1 receptors in the myocardium, thereby reducing response to catecholamines. Decreases cardiac output, myocardial oxygen demand, peripheral resistance, and renin release. Slows SA- and AV-node conduction.

Use/Therapeutic goal/Outcome

Hypertension: Reduction of blood pressure. *Outcome criteria:* Blood pressure within normal limits.

Myocardial reinfarction prophylaxis: Prevention of reinfarction. *Outcome criteria:* Lack of enzymatic or cardiographic evidence of reinfarction.

Angina: Resolution or prevention of angina. *Outcome criteria:* Report of decreased anginal attacks, with increase in activity tolerance.

Dose range/Administration

Interaction alert: With cardiac glycosides, monitor for excessive bradycardia. Other antihypertensives increase hypotensive effects. Indomethacin may decrease antihypertensive effects. May alter antidiabetic agent requirements.

Hypertension: *Adult:* PO: 25–50 mg/day; increase to 50–100 mg/day; after 2 weeks if needed and tolerated.

Myocardial reinfarction prophylaxis: IV: 5 mg over 5 min, another 5 mg after 10 min, then 50 mg PO after another 10 min.

Antianginal: *Adult:* PO: 50 mg/day. Increase to 100 mg after 7 days.

Clinical alert: Be aware that patients taking atenolol may not demonstrate tachycardia as a symptom of fever, hypoglycemia, or hyperthyroidism. Oral doses should begin 10 minutes after last IV dose.

Contraindications/Precautions

PREG
C

Contraindicated in hypersensitivity to the drug, and in cardiogenic shock, sinus bradycardia, second- or third- degree heart block (PR interval > 0.24 seconds), overt CHF. **Use with caution** in pulmonary disease, diabetes, impaired renal function.

🖐 **Use with caution for the elderly. Safe use for children and pregnant women has not been established.**

Side effects/Adverse reactions

Hypersensitivity: rash, psoriasiform eruption. **CV:** hypotension, CHF, bradycardia, edema, peripheral vascular disease. **CNS:** fatigue, mental depression, nightmares, dizziness, hallucinations, lethargy. **GI:** nausea, vomiting, diarrhea. **Misc:** fever. **GU:** decreased sexual ability.

Nursing implications/Documentation

Possible nursing diagnoses: Activity intolerance; Fatigue; Potential for injury.

◆ Assess mental status, and record pulse and blood pressure (if possible, lying, sitting, and standing, in both arms) before administering drug, and frequently thereafter until response is determined.

◆ Consult with physician to determine desired therapeutic range for blood pressure and heart rate (parameters for withholding the medication should be written by physician).

◆ Ascertain that baseline CBC, electrolytes, BUN, creatinine, and liver function studies have been obtained before giving first dose; report abnormalities and monitor closely thereafter.

◆ Monitor for allergic reactions and signs of confusion, dizziness, bradycardia, CHF, and hypotension; hold drug and report immediately if these occur.

◆ Supervise ambulation until response is determined.

◆ Document and monitor daily weight, and intake and output; report significant negative or positive balance.

Patient & family teaching/Home care

Possible nursing diagnoses: Knowledge deficit; Impaired home maintenance management; Altered sexuality patterns.

◆ Explain the importance of taking this drug exactly as prescribed, even when feeling well; warn not to discontinue drug abruptly.

◆ Stress the importance of good medical follow-up, explain that this drug reduces "wear and tear" on blood vessels, reduces the workload of the heart, and improves longevity and health.

◆ Teach how to monitor pulse and blood pressure; stress that syncope, hypertension or hypotension, or persistent dizziness should be reported; provide pulse and blood pressure parameters for withholding medication.

◆ Advise changing positions slowly, to avoid dizziness.

◆ Encourage monitoring weight daily and reporting sudden weight gain (frequently is fluid retention).

◆ Warn against drinking alcohol or taking *any* OTC drugs without physician approval (some interactions can cause severe reactions).

◆ Explain that this drug may alter sexual ability; explore concerns and seek consultation as needed.

◆ *See Beta Adrenergic Blockers, Antihypertensives, and Antianginals overviews for more information.*

atracurium

a-tra-kyoor'ee-um

atracurium besylate: **Tracrium**

Class: Skeletal-muscle relaxant, Nondepolarizing neuromuscular blocker

Antidote: Neostigmine methylsulfate

PEDS	PREG	GERI
🖐	C	🖐

Action Relaxes or paralyzes (depending on dose) skeletal muscles by competing with acetylcholine for cholinergic receptor sites, thereby inhibiting neuromuscular transmission. Does not alter consciousness or thought processes or relieve pain.

Use/Therapeutic goal/Outcome

Endotracheal intubation, adjunct to general anesthesia, mechanical ventilation: Facilitation of endotracheal tube and mechanical ventilation tolerance; relaxation of skeletal muscle. *Outcome criteria:* Tolerance of endotracheal intubation and mechanical ventilation; diminished or absent voluntary and reflexive movement.

Dose range/Administration

Interaction alert: Enflurane, isoflurane, halothane, certain antibiotics (aminoglycosides and polymyxins), lithium, magnesium salts, procainamide, thiazide diuretics, and quinidine may increase the action of this drug. Succinylcholine increases onset and depth of neuromuscular blockade of atracurium.

Adult/Child > 2 yrs: IV: *Initial dose:* 0.4–0.5 mg/kg. *Maintenance dose:* 0.08–0.1 mg/kg; begin 20–45 min after initial dose, then repeat q 15–25 min prn. *After succinylcholine:* 0.3–0.4 mg/kg.

Clinical alert: Atracurium should be given only by physicians and nurses who are familiar with its use, and in the presence of a physician, nurse anesthetist, or respiratory therapist who is qualified to manage endotracheal intubation.

Contraindications/Precautions

PREG C

Contraindicated in hypersensitivity to atracurium bysylate. *Use with caution* in myasthenia gravis, Eaton-Lambert syndrome, electrolyte or acid-base imbalance, cardiovascular disease, severe anaphylactic reactions, asthma, and carcinomatosis.

✋ **Use with caution for pregnant women and the elderly. Safe use for children under 2 years and nursing mothers has not been established.**

Side effects/Adverse reactions

Hypersensitivity: flushing, erythema, itching, wheezing, urticaria, increased bronchial secretion. *CV:* transient hypotension or tachycardia. *Resp:* respiratory depression.

Nursing implications/Documentation

Possible nursing diagnoses: Impaired communication; Pain; Potential for aspiration; Potential for injury.

◆ Ascertain that baseline CBC, electrolytes, BUN, creatinine, liver function, chest X ray, and EKG studies are posted on chart before drug administration (report abnormalities).

◆ Protect airway, position for drainage of oropharyngeal secretions (if possible), and keep suction at bedside until the patient is fully alert; have emergency equipment and drugs available.

◆ Monitor and record vital signs every 15 min until stable; report abnormalities that might indicate potential complications.

◆ Recognize that this drug may *paralyze*, but does not relieve pain (provide analgesic if pain is suspected, anticipate human needs).

◆ Monitor for potential for injury: protect eyes if there is no blink reflex (tape shut); watch positioning of all extremities (provide range of motion exercises if therapy is prolonged).

Patient & family teaching/Home care

Possible nursing diagnoses: Anxiety; Fear.

◆ Explain all procedures, even if the person seems unconscious (the ability to hear may be present).

◆ Reassure individual that muscle paralysis, weakness, or stiffness will subside.

◆ For use with mechanical ventilation, stress that you are aware that the patient cannot move, and that this drug is being given to control breathing; reassure that breathing is being closely monitored to be sure that the lungs are being adequately oxygenated, and that ability to move will return as soon as drug is stopped. Also reassure that medication for pain and anxiety will be given to help tolerate the endotracheal tube.

atropine

a'troe-peen

atropine sulfate: *Atropisol, ♠Atropt, BufOpto Atropine, Isopto-Atropine (for optic use only)*

Class: ★**Anticholinergic, (cholinergic blocker) prototype,** Antiarrhythmic, Mydriatic

Antidote: Physostigmine

PEDS	PREG	GERI
🖐	C	🖐

Action Relaxes smooth muscles, inhibits salivary and bronchial secretions and dilates pupils by acting selectively on parasympathetic postganglionic receptor sites and by blocking the muscarinic effects of acetylcholine through competitive inhibition. Increases heart rate by counteracting vagal effects on the SA node.

Use/Therapeutic goal/Outcome

Preoperative: Suppression of saliva and respiratory secretions, dilatation of bronchial passages. **Outcome criteria:** Report of feeling dry or thirsty, visible dry mouth.

Antiarrhythmic: Counteraction of bradycardia, increase in heart rate. **Outcome criteria:** Heart rate more than 60 beats/min, return of normal sinus rhythm on EKG; increase in blood pressure; increase in femoral, carotid, and peripheral pulse rate and quality.

Ophthalmic: Pupillary dilatation (mydriasis) for eye exam or suppression of inflammatory response of inflamed or infected eyes. **Outcome criteria:** Enlarged, nonreactive pupil(s), decreased tearing and redness, patient report of less discomfort and blurry vision.

Dose range/Administration

Interaction alert: Methotrimeprazine may produce extrapyramidal side effects. Potentiates action of antidepressants, MAOIs, and other anticholinergics. Do not mix in a syringe with any other drug except analgesics.

Pre-operative: Adult: IM: 0.4–0.6 mg, 45–60 min before anesthesia. **Child:** IM: 0.1–0.4 mg/kg, 45–60 min before anesthesia.

Bradycardia: Adult: IV: 0.5–1 mg IV push. May repeat in 5 min. *Maximum dose:* 2 mg. **Child:** IV: 0.01 mg/kg IV push. *Maximum dose:* 0.4 mg. May repeat q4-6h.

Ophthalmic: Adult: 1–2 gtt 0.5–1% solution or a small amount of ointment applied to eye(s) bid to tid. **Child:** 1–2 gtt 0.5% solution or 3 cm 0.5% ointment tid.

Clinical alert: Expect small doses for the elderly, because they are especially prone to "atropine fever" (high temperature caused by suppression of perspiration). They also are more prone to the side effect of confusion.

Contraindications/Precautions

PREG C

Contraindicated in hypersensitivity to belladonna alkaloids, and in narrow-angle glaucoma (increases intraocular pressure), obstructive diseases of GI or urinary tract, and myasthenia gravis. **Use with caution** in cardiac disease, hypertension, and renal or hepatic impairment.

🖐 **Contraindicated for nursing mothers. Use with caution for children under 6 years and the elderly. Safe use for pregnant women has not been established.**

Side effects/Adverse reactions

Hypersensitivity: rash of the face and upper trunk, urticaria, conjunctivitis. **GI:** dry mouth, constipation. **Eye:** pupillary dilation (may be desired effect for eye exam), blurred vision. **CNS:** mental confusion, excitement, dizziness, headache. **CV:** palpitations, tachycardia. **GU:** urinary hesitancy and retention. **Skin:** decreased sweating.

Nursing implications/Documentation

Possible nursing diagnoses: Urinary retention; Potential for injury; Altered oral mucous membrane; Sensory-perceptual alteration: visual.

♦ Document vital signs, especially blood pressure, and quality and rate of pulses and respirations before and after administration of atropine. Be aware that IV administration may cause initial bradycardia, which usually lasts 1–2 min, and may be followed by tachycardia.

♦ Provide frequent mouth care to help relieve dry mouth.

♦ Have the patient void before doses (if possible) and document urinary output, because this drug may contribute to urinary retention.

♦ Keep patient in bed with side rails up until response is determined, then supervise ambulation until stable.

Patient & family teaching/Home care

Possible nursing diagnoses: Knowledge deficit; Impaired home maintenance management.

♦ Explain that dry mouth is a transient side effect.

- Point out that because of pupillary dilation, there may be blurring of vision, light sensitivity, and inability to judge distance.

- Ophthalmic use

  - Teach the procedure for administering eye medications and observe return demonstration.

  - Warn against driving while vision is affected; suggest wearing sunglasses to minimize light sensitivity.

  - Advise holding dose and reporting immediately if eye pain, palpitations, or dizziness is experienced.

- *See Anticholinergics and Antiarrhythmics overviews for more information.*

auranofin

aur-an-oh'fin

Ridaura

Class: Antirheumatic, Gold compound, Disease modifying agent

PEDS	PREG	GERI
🖐	C	🖐

Action Suppresses joint inflammation by inhibiting the release of lysosomal enzymes, decreasing phagocytosis and modifying the immune response.

Use/Therapeutic goal/Outcome

Rheumatoid arthritis: Modification or suppression of disease; prevention of damage to affected joints. *Outcome criteria:* (After 3–6 months) Reduction in swelling of affected joints; decreased sedimentation rate; improved grip strength; decreased use of analgesics; report of decreased morning stiffness, increased ability to ambulate, and decreased fatigue.

Dose range/Administration

Interaction alert: Immunosuppressants and cytotoxic drugs increase the risk of blood dyscrasias. May produce phenytoin toxicity.

Adult: PO: 6 mg qd or 3 mg bid. *Maximum dose:* 3 mg tid.

Contraindications/Precautions

PREG C

Contraindicated in hypersensitivity to gold or other heavy metals; systemic lupus erythematosus. *Use with caution* in blood dyscrasias, diabetes mellitus, hepatic or renal disease, eczema, inflammatory bowel disease, and with medications known to cause blood dyscrasias.

🖐 Use with caution for pregnant women and the elderly. Safe use for children or nursing mothers has not been established.

Side effects/Adverse reactions

Hypersensitivity: rash, itching. *GI:* diarrhea, abdominal cramps, nausea, vomiting, anorexia, ulcers or white spots in mouth or throat, metallic taste, hepatotoxicity. *Eye:* conjunctivitis. *Hem:* thrombocytopenia. *GU:* albumin, protein, or RBCs in urine. *Skin:* painful, pruritic rash.

Nursing implications/Documentation

Possible nursing diagnoses: Diarrhea; Altered oral mucous membrane.

- Monitor bowel activity; document and report diarrhea. Diarrhea may respond to a reduction in dosage and use of psyllium hydrophilic mucilloid (Metamucil).

- Assess for mouth ulcers and skin rashes to detect early signs of toxicity.

- Monitor results of blood and platelet counts and hepatic and renal function tests.

- For mild reactions, expect therapy to be temporarily discontinued and restarted at a lower dose; for severe reactions or with evidence of hypersensitivity or thrombocytopenia, therapy will be permanently discontinued.

- Recognize that gold salts will not reverse *existing* joint damage.

Patient & family teaching/Home care

Possible nursing diagnoses: Knowledge deficit; Impaired home maintenance management; Impaired skin integrity.

- Advise that response to therapy does not usually occur for at least 3–6 months.

- Warn against taking more than prescribed amount and doubling doses to make up missed doses.

- Stress the need to remain under close medical supervision and have blood and urine testing done as frequently as recommended (usually every 2 weeks initially and then once monthly).

- Teach that diarrhea is the most common adverse reaction to oral gold and should be reported; any episodes of bloody diarrhea must be reported promptly.

- Point out that itching, hives, dermatitis, and mouth ulcers should be reported. Advise that a metallic taste may precede mouth ulcers.

• Inform that dermatitis and mouth ulcers may occur for many months after discontinuing the medication; their development is often associated with marked improvement of the arthritis.

• Warn to avoid exposure to sunlight to prevent photosensitivity reaction or skin rash.

aurothioglucose
aur-oh-thye-oh-gloo'cose

♣Gold-50, Solganal

Class: Antirheumatic, Gold compound, Disease modifying agent

PEDS	PREG	GERI
✋	C	✋

Action Suppresses joint inflammation by inhibiting the release of lysosomal enzymes, decreasing phagocytosis, and modifying the immune response.

Use/Therapeutic goal/Outcome

Rheumatoid arthritis: Modification or suppression of disease; prevention of damage to affected joints. *Outcome criteria:* (After 8–12 weeks) Reduction in swelling of affected joints; decreased sedimentation rate; improved grip strength; decreased use of analgesics; report of decreased morning stiffness, increased ability to ambulate, and decreased fatigue.

Dose range/Administration

Interaction alert: Immunosuppressants and cytotoxic drugs may increase the risk of blood dyscrasias.

Adult: IM: *Loading dose:* 10 mg wk 1, then 25 mg wk 2 and 3, then 25–50 mg/wk to total of 1000 mg. *Maintenance dose:* 25–50 mg q 2–6 wk. **Child:** IM: *Loading dose:* 200–250 mg total in divided doses: 2.5 mg wk 1, then 6.25 mg wk 2 and 3, then 12.5 mg/wk to total of 200–250 mg. *Maintenance dose:* 6.25–12.5 q 3–4 wk.

Clinical alert: Immerse vial in warm water to facilitate withdrawing suspension; shake well to obtain uniform suspension. Administer deep IM *only* into the upper outer quadrant of the gluteal region, using an 18–gauge, 1 1/2–inch needle. Observe immediately after injection for possibility of nitritoid reaction (flushing, dizziness, sweating, and hypotension) or anaphylaxis. Have epinephrine readily available to treat life-threatening reactions.

Contraindications/Precautions

Contraindicated in hypersensitivity to gold, other heavy metals, and sesame oil (used in suspension), and in thrombocytopenia with previous gold therapy and systemic lupus erythematosus. **Use with caution** in blood dyscrasias, diabetes mellitus, hepatic or renal disease, eczema, and with medications known to cause blood dyscrasias.

🐾 **Contraindicated for nursing mothers. Use with caution for children, pregnant women, and the elderly.**

Side effects/Adverse reactions

Hypersensitivity: itching; difficulty breathing or swallowing; swelling of face, lips, or eyelids; bradycardia; syncope; anaphylactic shock. **Skin:** painful, pruritic skin rashes. **CV:** nitritoid reaction (flushing, dizziness, sweating, and hypotension) immediately after injection. **Hem:** thrombocytopenia; aplastic anemia. **GI:** soreness of tongue, gums, or throat; metallic taste; mouth ulcers; hepatotoxicity. **GU:** albumin, protein, or RBCs in urine; nephrotic syndrome.

Nursing implications/Documentation

Possible nursing diagnoses: Impaired skin integrity; Altered oral mucous membrane.

• Assess for mouth ulcers, easy bruising or bleeding, and rashes prior to each subsequent injection to detect early signs of toxicity.

• Monitor results of blood and platelet counts and hepatic and renal function tests.

• For mild reactions, expect that therapy will be temporarily discontinued and restarted at a lower dose; for severe reactions or with evidence of blood dyscrasias or renal dysfunction, therapy will be discontinued permanently.

• Recognize that gold injections will not reverse *existing* joint damage.

Patient & family teaching/Home care

Possible nursing diagnoses: Knowledge deficit; Home maintenance management.

• Advise that response to therapy does not usually occur for at least 8–12 weeks.

• Explain that joint pain may occur for 1 or 2 days after the first few injections.

• Stress the need to remain under close medical supervision and to have blood and urine testing done as frequently as recommended, usually before every other dose.

• Teach that dermatitis is the most common adverse reaction to gold therapy and is frequently preceded by itching and hives; mouth ulcers are the second most common reaction and may be preceded by a metallic taste. These early symptoms should be reported promptly.

• Inform that dermatitis or mouth ulcers may occur for many months after discontinuing the medication; their development is usually accompanied by marked improvement in the arthritis.

• Warn to avoid exposure to sunlight to prevent photosensitivity reaction or rash.

azatadine

a-za'ta-deen

azatadine maleate: *Optimine, ♠Zadine*

Class: Antihistamine (H₁ receptor antagonist)

PEDS	PREG	GERI
🖐	B	🖐

Action Prevents but does not reverse histamine-mediated allergic responses by competing with histamine for H_1 receptors on smooth muscle of blood vessels, bronchioles, and GI tract.

Use/Therapeutic goal/Outcome

Allergic conditions: Decrease in allergic response. *Outcome criteria:* Report and demonstration of absence or decrease in allergic symptoms (nasal secretions, sneezing, itching).

Dose range/Administration

Interaction alert: CNS depressants and alcohol may cause excessive sedation. Do not give with MAOIs or anticholinergics.

🖐 **Give with milk or food to avoid GI upset.**

Adult: PO: 1–2 mg bid to a maximum of 4 mg/day.

Clinical alert: Expect reduced dosage for the elderly, and monitor for excessive drowsiness and dizziness.

Contraindications/Precautions

PREG B

Contraindicated in hypersensitivity to azatadine, and with MAOIs. *Use with caution* in increased intraocular pressure, narrow-angle glaucoma, pyloroduodenal obstruction, stenosing peptic ulcer, prostatic hypertrophy, bladder neck obstruction, history of bronchial asthma, hyperthyroidism, hypertension, cardiovascular disease, and convulsive disorders.

🖐 **Not recommended for children under 12 years or for nursing mothers; and should be used in pregnancy only when clearly necessary. Use with caution for the elderly.**

Side effects/Adverse reactions

Hypersensitivity: urticaria, rash, photosensitivity, anaphylaxis. *CNS:* drowsiness, dizziness, disturbed coordination, fatigue, confusion, paresthesias, neuritis, excitation, nervousness, euphoria, restlessness, hysteria, insomnia, tremor, headache, chills, irritability, convulsions. *CV:* hypotension, palpitation, tachycardia, extrasystole. *Resp:* nasal stuffiness, dry nose, mouth and throat, thickening of bronchial secretions, chest tightness, wheezing. *Ear:* tinnitus, vertigo. *GI:* epigastric distress, nausea, vomiting, anorexia, diarrhea, constipation. *GU:* urinary frequency, dysuria, urinary retention, early menses. *Hem:* hemolytic anemia, thrombocytopenia, agranulocytosis. *Eye:* blurred vision, diplopia, dilated pupils. *Skin:* excessive perspiration.

Nursing implications/Documentation

Possible nursing diagnoses: Potential for injury; Fluid volume deficit.

• Determine and record known allergies; provide an environment that is free from allergens (especially sleeping areas).

• Provide favorite fluids and ensure adequate hydration (2 liters/day).

• If therapy is prolonged, monitor CBC for blood dyscrasias.

Patient & family teaching/Home care

Possible nursing diagnoses: Knowledge deficit; Impaired home maintenance management.

• Advise taking this drug with food if GI symptoms are experienced.

• Point out that avoiding pollens and staying in an air-conditioned environment may help reduce symptoms of seasonal rhinitis.

• Emphasize that dose should not be increased without physician's approval; explain that tolerance may occur, requiring a change in medication.

• Warn that alcohol and other CNS depressants may cause excessive drowsiness; advise against driving until response is determined.

• Suggest that coffee or tea may reduce drowsiness, and that sugarless gum or hard candy may relieve dry mouth.

• Explain the need to stop antihistamines for 4 days before allergy testing to ensure accurate results.

◆ *See Antihistamines overview for more information.*

azathioprine

ay-za-thye'oh-preen

Imuran, ♠*Thioprine*

Class: ★**Cytotoxic immunosuppressant prototype,** Purine antagonist, Antirheumatic

PEDS	PREG	GERI
♨	**D**	♨

Action Suppresses immune response by inhibiting purine synthesis and suppressing T-cell activity (occurs during the early stages of antibody response).

Use/Therapeutic goal/Outcome

Organ transplantation: Prevention of rejection. *Outcome criteria:* Absence of signs of rejection; evidence of satisfactory organ function.

Severe refractory rheumatoid arthritis: Reduction of autoimmune response, reduction of joint inflammation. *Outcome criteria:* Report of decreased pain; decreased swelling with increased mobility.

Dose range/Administration

Interaction alert: Allopurinol inhibits azathioprine metabolism (azathioprine dose should be reduced).

🖐 **Give with food or in divided doses (must be prescribed) if GI distress is noted.**

Prevention of organ rejection: Adult and Child: PO, IV: Begin on the first day of transplantation with 3–5 mg/kg/day (homotransplants, begin 1–5 days before surgery). *Maintenance dose:* 1–3 mg/kg/day, highly variable, depending upon individual response.

Severe refractory rheumatoid arthritis: Adult: PO: Begin with 1 mg/kg/day in a single dose, or in two divided doses. If desired response is not achieved in 6–8 wk, increase 0.5 mg/kg/day at 4-wk intervals. *Maximum dose:* 2.5 mg/kg/day.

Clinical alert: Monitor hemoglobin, WBC, and platelet count at least every month; *hold drug* and report if leukocytes < 3000 mm³. Wear gloves when handling and preparing doses.

Contraindications/Precautions

PREG D **A**

Contraindicated in hypersensitivity to azathioprine or metacaptoprine, and during active clinical infection. Use with caution in liver or kidney transplants (especially if a cadaver kidney is used), and with herpes zoster.

🖐 **Contraindicated for pregnant or nursing mothers. Use with caution for children and the elderly.**

Side effects/Adverse reactions

Hypersensitivity: rashes, formication (sensations of creeping ants), joint pain, interstitial pneumonitis, polyarthritis, serum sickness, hepatitis, polyneuritis, pancreatitis. *GI:* nausea, vomiting, stomatitis, anorexia, esophagitis, hepatotoxicity. *Hem:* leukopenia, thrombocytopenia, megaloblastic anemia. *MS:* muscle wasting. *Skin:* jaundice, hair loss. *Misc:* increased susceptibility to infection (cytomegalovirus, herpes, Pneumocystis carinii, Serratia, Cryptococcus, Legionella, and gram-negative bacteria); increased prevalence of malignancy.

Nursing implications/Documentation

Possible nursing diagnoses: Potential for infection; Altered oral mucous membrane; Social isolation.

◆ Avoid giving IM injections to reduce risk of infection (document on medication record).

◆ Monitor for and report signs and symptoms of liver side effects (jaundice, itching, clay colored stools; increased alkaline phosphatase, bilirubin, SGOT, SGPT).

◆ Record and monitor intake and output and daily weights; report positive balance or weight gain.

◆ Report signs and symptoms of infection immediately; avoid assigning health care workers with respiratory symptoms.

◆ Provide frequent mouth care.

Patient & family teaching/Home care

Possible nursing diagnoses: Knowledge deficit, Impaired home maintenance management.

◆ Teach that meticulous oral hygiene can help reduce oral inflammation.

◆ Advise to report signs and symptoms of infection early to ensure prompt treatment.

◆ For rheumatoid arthritis, explain that it may take 3–4 months to see effects.

◆ Point out the need to avoid people with bacterial or viral infections.

▶

♦ Warn women to use contraceptives during treatment, and for 12 weeks after completing therapy.

♦ *See Immunosuppressants overview for more information.*

azlocillin
az-loe-sill'in

azlocillin sodium: *Azlin,* **♠***Securopen*

Class: Anti-infective, Antibiotic, Extended–spectrum penicillin

PEDS	PREG	GERI
♨	B	♨

Action Extended-spectrum, usually bactericidal antibiotic; kills bacteria by inhibiting cell wall synthesis.

Use/Therapeutic goal/Outcome

Infections (respiratory, urinary tract, skin, septicemia): Prevention or resolution of infection. *Outcome criteria:* Absence of pathogenic growth on cultures, absence of clinical manifestations of infection (pain, swelling, redness, heat, odor, dysuria, drainage), normal WBC count, improvement of X rays.

Dose range/Administration

Interaction alert: Inactivates aminoglycosides (e.g., gentamicin, tobramycin); do not mix together in solution. Probenecid inhibits excretion of azlocillin and may be given to increase serum levels of the drug. Because of antiplatelet effect, concurrent use with oral anticoagulants may increase risk of bleeding. Azlocillin may reduce the effect of oral contraceptives.

Adult: IV: 100–300 mg/kg/day in 4–6 divided doses. Give slowly, over at least 5 min. *Maximum dose: 24 g/day. Child > 1 wk: For acute pulmonary exacerbation of cystic fibrosis:* IV: 75 mg/kg q4h. Give slowly, over at least 30 min. *Maximum dose: 24 g/day.*

Clinical alert: Rapid IV infusion may cause chest pain. Almost always given together with other antibiotics. Should be administered 1 hour after aminoglycosides.

Contraindications/Precautions

PREG
B

Contraindicated in allergy to penicillin. *Use with caution* in cephalosporin sensitivity, in history of allergic responses (e.g., other drugs, hay fever, asthma) or hepatic or renal dysfunction.

♨ Use with caution for chilren, the elderly, and pregnant or nursing mothers. Safe use for neonates has not been established.

Side effects/Adverse reactions

Hypersensitivity: itching, rashes, urticaria, fever, eosinophilia, arthalgia, myalagia, difficulty breathing, anaphylaxis. *GI:* nausea, vomiting, anorexia, disturbances of taste and smell, stomatitis, flatulence, diarrhea, epigastric distension. *Hem:* thrombocytopenia, slight elevation in SGOT, SGPT, LDH, bilirubin, alkaline phosphatase, creatinine. *CV:* pain, redness, swelling, thrombophlebitis at injection site. *CNS:* neuromuscular excitability, convulsions.

Nursing implications/Documentation

Possible nursing diagnoses: Potential for infection; Diarrhea.

♦ Determine history of allergies, and (regardless of history) monitor closely for allergic reactions.

♦ Obtain baseline CBC, serum sodium, liver function studies, and necessary cultures before administering first dose; monitor closely thereafter if therapy is prolonged.

♦ Encourage fluids, and record and monitor intake and output, to ensure adequate hydration; report significant negative or positive balance.

♦ Monitor for and report signs of superinfection (sore throat, fever, fatigue, thrush, vaginal discharge, diarrhea).

Patient & family teaching/Home care

Possible nursing diagnoses: Knowledge deficit; Impaired home maintenance management.

♦ Teach the importance of reporting allergic symptoms, diarrhea, signs and symptoms that do not abate, or *any* new signs and symptoms of discomfort that might indicate superinfection (medication regimen may have to be changed).

♦ Advise drinking 2–3 L of fluids daily to maintain adequate hydration (especially important if fever exists).

♦ Stress the importance of taking antibiotics for the entire time prescribed, even if signs and symptoms abate.

♦ *See Anti-infectives overview for more information.*

aztreonam

aze-tree'owe-nam

Azactam

Class: Anti-infective, Narrow-spectrum antibiotic, Antimicrobial

PEDS	PREG	GERI
⍓	B	⍓

Action Narrow-spectrum, bactericidal antibiotic; kills bacteria by inhibiting cell wall synthesis. (Specifically for gram-negative aerobic pathogens only.)

Use/Therapeutic goal/Outcome

Severe gram-negative infections: Resolution of infection. *Outcome criteria:* Absence of pathogenic growth on cultures, absence of clinical manifestations of infection (fever, pain, swelling, redness, heat, odor, drainage, productive cough, dysuria), normal WBC count, normal X rays.

Dose range/Administration

Adult: IV, Deep IM: 500 mg to 2 g q6-12h, depending upon severity of infection. *Maximum dose:* 8 g/day. IV infusions should be completed within 20–60 min. Give single doses > 1 g IV, not IM.

Clinical alert: When reconstituting, shake container *vigorously, immediately after adding diluent.* Discard unused solution. Mixed solution may be clear, straw yellow, or light pink. For IV infusion, mix with a minimum of 50 ml per gram. For IV bolus, give slowly over 3–5 minutes.

Contraindications/Precautions

PREG B

Contraindicated in hypersensitivity to aztreonam. *Use with caution* in the presence of impaired renal function.

⍓ **Safe use for the elderly depends on creatinine clearance. Safe use for children and pregnant or nursing mothers has not been established.**

Side effects/Adverse reactions

Hypersensitivity: itching, rashes, drug fever, difficulty breathing, anaphylaxis (rare). *GI:* nausea, vomiting, diarrhea. *Although this drug is very safe, the following rare reactions have occurred: GI:* abdominal cramping, mouth ulcers, altered taste, numb tongue, halitosis, diarrhea, GI bleeding. *CNS:* headache, dizziness, weakness, fatigue, seizures, confusion, insomnia. *CV:* hypotension, transient PVCs.

Ear: tinnitus. *Eye:* double vision. *Resp:* sneezing, nasal congestion. *Skin:* diaphoresis. *Hem:* pancytopenia, thrombocytopenia, neutropenia, anemia, leukocytosis, eosinophilia, and pain, redness, thrombophlebitis at injection site; slight elevation in serum creatinine, SGOT, SGPT, alkaline phosphatase, prothrombin and partial thromboplastin times; positive direct Coomb's test. *Misc:* breast tenderness; superinfection.

Nursing implications/Documentation

Possible nursing diagnoses: Potential for infection; Diarrhea.

♦ Be aware that since aztreonam has a very narrow spectrum, it usually is given in conjunction with another antibiotic.

♦ Determine history of allergies, and (regardless of history) monitor closely for allergic reactions.

♦ Obtain baseline CBC, creatinine, liver function studies, and necessary cultures before administering first dose; monitor closely thereafter if therapy is prolonged.

♦ Encourage fluids, and record and monitor intake and output, to ensure adequate hydration; report significant negative or positive balance.

♦ Monitor for and report signs of superinfection (sore throat, fever, fatigue, thrush, vaginal discharge).

♦ Give IM doses deep into large muscle mass.

Patient & family teaching/Home care

Possible nursing diagnoses: Knowledge deficit; Impaired home maintenance management.

♦ Teach importance of reporting allergic symptoms, signs and symptoms that do not abate, or *any* new signs and symptoms of discomfort that might indicate superinfection (medication regimen may have to be changed).

♦ Advise drinking 2–3 L of fluids daily to maintain adequate hydration (especially important if fever exists).

♦ Stress the importance of taking antibiotics for the entire time prescribed, even if signs and symptoms abate.

♦ *See Anti-infectives overview for more information.*

bacampicillin

ba-kam-pi-sill'in

B

bacampicillin hydrochloride: ✤*Penglobe, Spectrobid*

Class: Anti-infective, Antibiotic, Aminopenicillin

PEDS	PREG	GERI
OK	B	OK

Action Broad-spectrum, usually bactericidal antibiotic; kills bacteria by inhibiting cell wall synthesis.

Use/Therapeutic goal/Outcome

Systemic Infections (respiratory tract, urinary tract, skin, gonorrhea): Prevention or resolution of infection. *Outcome criteria:* Absence of pathogenic growth on cultures, absence of clinical manifestations of infection (fever, pain, redness, heat, swelling, odor, drainage, dysuria), normal WBC count, improvement of X rays.

Dose range/Administration

Interaction alert: Probenecid inhibits excretion of bacampicillin and may be given to increase serum levels of the drug. Do not mix with aminoglycosides. Allopurinol may cause a rash. Avoid use with disulfiram (Antabuse).

🍂 **Give with food if GI distress occurs.**

🗄 **Give oral suspension on an empty stomach.**

Hemophilus influenzae, and respiratory, urinary, and skin infections: **Adult:** PO: 400–800 mg q12h. **Child:** PO: *Suspension:* 25–50 mg/kg/day, in divided doses q12h. Under 25 kg, use suspension, over 25 kg use tablets.

Gonorrhea: **Adult:** PO: 1.6 g bacampicillin with 1 g probenecid in a single dose.

Contraindications/Precautions

PREG B

Contraindicated in allergy to penicillin, and in patients with mononucleosis (may cause skin rash). *Use with caution* in cephalosporin sensitivity, history of allergic responses (e.g., other drugs, hay fever, asthma), and renal insufficiency.

🖐 **Use with caution for children, the elderly, and pregnant or nursing mothers.**

Side effects/Adverse reactions

Hypersensitivity: itching, rashes, hives, fever, difficulty breathing, anaphylaxis. *GI:* nausea, vomiting, diarrhea, gastritis, stomatitis, black "hairy" tongue, pseudomembranous colitis. *Hem:* slight elevation in SGOT. *CNS:* coma, convulsions. *Misc:* superinfection, bone marrow depression.

Nursing implications/Documentation

Possible nursing diagnoses: Potential for infection; Diarrhea.

♦ Determine history of allergies, and (regardless of history) monitor closely for allergic reactions.

♦ Obtain baseline CBC, and necessary cultures before administering first dose; monitor closely thereafter if therapy is prolonged.

♦ Encourage fluids, and record and monitor intake and output, to ensure adequate hydration; report significant negative or positive balance.

♦ Monitor for and report signs of superinfection (sore throat, fever, fatigue, thrush, vaginal discharge, diarrhea).

Patient & family teaching/Home care

Possible nursing diagnoses: Knowledge deficit; Impaired home maintenance management.

♦ If GI distress is experienced with *tablet*, suggest taking it with food (*suspension* should be taken on an *empty* stomach).

♦ Teach the importance of reporting allergic symptoms, diarrhea, signs and symptoms that do not abate, or *any* new signs and symptoms of discomfort that might indicate superinfection (medication regimen may have to be changed).

♦ Advise drinking 2–3 L of fluids daily to maintain adequate hydration (especially important if fever exists).

♦ Stress the importance of taking antibiotics for the entire time prescribed, even if signs and symptoms abate.

♦ See *Anti-infectives overview* for more information.

baclofen

bak'loe-fen

Lioresal, Lioresal DS

Class: Skeletal-muscle relaxant (centrally acting), Antispasmodic

PEDS	PREG	GERI
🖐	C	🖐

Action Produces skeletal muscle relaxation by an uncertain mechanism of action. Inhibits both mono- and polysynaptic spinal reflexes. May also act at certain supraspinal sites. Relaxes external sphincter of hyperreflexic urinary bladder and appears to control involuntary bladder spasms.

Use/Therapeutic goal/Outcome

Multiple sclerosis and diseases or injuries of the spinal cord: Relaxation of skeletal muscle spasticity; promotion of comfort. ***Outcome criteria:*** Decreased involuntary movement and muscle tonicity; report of relief of pain, anxiety, and tension; increased range of motion.

Hyperreflexive urinary incontinence: Relaxation of urinary sphincter; prevention of involuntary bladder spasms. ***Outcome criteria:*** Absence of incontinence; normal patterns of urinary elimination.

Dose range/Administration

Interaction alert: May increase CNS effects of other CNS depressants and alcohol. May alter insulin requirements.

🦶 **Give with food or milk to prevent gastric distress.**

Adult: PO: Dosage individualized. *Initial dose:* 5 mg tid, then increase gradually until optimal response achieved. *Maximum dose:* 80 mg/day.

Clinical alert: Do not exceed maximum dosage. If therapeutic effect is not observed in 1–2 months, the drug should be withdrawn (over a period of 1–2 weeks).

Contraindications/Precautions

PREG
C

Contraindicated in hypersensitivity to baclofen, and for use in rheumatic disorders. ***Use with caution*** in impaired renal function, epilepsy, and when spasticity is used to maintain motor function.

✋ **Use with caution for pregnant women and the elderly. Safe use for children and nursing mothers has not been established.**

Side effects/Adverse reactions

Hypersensitivity: rash. ***CNS:*** drowsiness, dizziness, confusion, headache, insomnia. ***GI:*** nausea, constipation. ***Hem:*** increased SGOT and alkaline phosphatase. ***CV:*** ankle edema, weight gain, hypotension. ***MS:*** weakness, fatigue. ***GU:*** urinary frequency. ***Resp:*** nasal congestion. ***Misc:*** hyperglycemia. Some CNS and GU symptoms may be related to underlying disease process.

Nursing implications/Documentation

Possible nursing diagnoses: Impaired physical mobility; Potential for injury; Pain; Altered patterns of urinary elimination.

♦ Do not withdraw drug abruptly, except in cases of severe adverse reaction (may cause hallucinations, severe tachycardia, and seizures).

♦ Check blood pressure, weight, blood sugar, urine, and hepatic function periodically to detect adverse effects.

♦ Supervise out-of-bed activities because transient drowsiness and loss of balance may occur.

♦ In epileptics, observe for increased seizure activity.

♦ For incontinence, consult with incontinence specialist to develop a plan to establish an effective urine elimination pattern.

♦ Monitor diabetics for altered insulin requirements.

Patient & family teaching/Home care

Possible nursing diagnoses: Impaired home maintenance management; Knowledge deficit.

♦ Advise taking doses with milk or food to prevent gastric distress.

♦ Caution not to operate dangerous machinery or drive, especially during initial phase of therapy.

♦ Stress the importance of holding medication and reporting adverse reactions immediately.

♦ Explain the need to refrain from alcohol.

♦ Warn not to discontinue drug without consulting a physician.

♦ Advise diabetics that this drug may alter insulin requirements.

♦ *See Skeletal-muscle relaxants overview for more information.*

beclomethasone
be-kloe-meth′a-sone

beclomethasone dipropionate: **⇒Aldecin Aqueous Nasal Spray, ⇒Aldecin Inhaler, ⇒Becloforte Inhaler, Beclovent, ♥Beclovent Rotocaps, Beconase AQ Nasal Spray, Beconase Nasal Inhaler, Vancenase AQ Nasal Spray, Vancenase Nasal Inhaler, Vanceril**

Class: Synthetic adrenocorticosteroid, Glucocorticoid, Steroidal anti-inflammatory, Immunosuppressant, Antiasthmatic

PEDS	PREG	GERI
✋	C	OK

Action Suppresses inflammation by inhibiting accumulation of inflammatory cells, reducing dilatation and permeability of capillaries, and inhibiting release of chemical mediators of inflammation. Modifies immune response by

▶

suppressing cell-mediated immune reactions. Inhibits bronchoconstriction and enhances effects of bronchodilators.

Use/Therapeutic goal/Outcome

Chronic bronchial asthma, allergic rhinitis: Symptomatic relief. *Outcome criteria:* Improved forced expiratory volume (FEV); decreased wheezing, coughing, and dyspnea; decreased nasal secretions and sneezing.

Dose range/Administration

Adult: *Inhalation:* 2–4 puffs tid or qid. *Maximum dose:* 20/day. *Intranasal:* 1 spray bid to qid. **Child:** *Inhalation:* 1–2 puffs tid or qid. *Maximum dose:* 10 puffs/day.

Clinical alert: In chronic asthma, switch from *systemic* corticosteroids to inhalation preparation is not usually made until symptoms are under control; then systemic dose is gradually reduced. Give prescribed bronchodilator inhalations 5 minutes before beclomethasone to increase bronchial penetration.

Contraindications/Precautions

PREG
C

Contraindicated in hypersensitivity to corticosteroids or fluorocarbon propellants, and in status asthmaticus, asthma adequately controlled by bronchodilators or nonsteroidal medication, and nonasthmatic bronchitis. **Use with caution** in active bacterial, fungal, or viral infections of mouth, throat, or lung; and (for intranasal route) recent nasal septal ulcers, trauma, or surgery.

✋ Use with caution for children over 6 years and pregnant or nursing mothers. Safe use for children under 6 years has not been established.

Side effects/Adverse reactions

Hypersensitivity: rash, bronchospasm. **GI:** fungal infection of mouth or throat. **Resp:** hoarseness; sore throat; bloody mucus, nose bleeds, nasal crusting.

Nursing implications/Documentation

Possible nursing diagnoses: Altered oral mucous membrane.

♦ Assess for proper use of inhalation therapy.

♦ Monitor oral mucous membrane for signs of fungal infection; document and report abnormal findings.

♦ During transfer from systemic therapy, monitor for symptoms of adrenal insufficiency (e.g.,

hypotension, hypoglycemia, nausea, anorexia, depression, mood swings).

Patient & family teaching/Home care

Possible nursing diagnoses: Altered oral mucous membrane; Knowledge deficit; Impaired home maintenance management.

♦ Instruct to shake container well before each inhalation or nasal spray.

♦ With intranasal use, instruct to clear nasal passages of secretions before administration; nasal decongestant may be used prior to administration if excessive secretions or edema are present.

♦ Teach proper inhalation techniques; suggest using a spacer device if there is difficulty coordinating inhalation with activation of the inhaler.

♦ Advise gargling and rinsing mouth (without swallowing) after inhalation to help prevent fungal infection in mouth and throat.

♦ Stress the need to assess oral mucosa for creamy white patches indicating fungal infection; advise reporting suspicion of infection.

♦ Point out that beclomethasone should be used *regularly* for prevention of asthma attacks and will not provide relief of *acute* asthmatic attacks.

♦ Warn against increasing doses or frequency of use without consulting physician.

♦ Advise reporting stress (infection, trauma, surgery, or emotional crisis) or severe asthma attack during transfer from systemic to local therapy; supplemental steroids may be required.

♦ Reinforce the importance of medical follow-up for evaluation of therapy.

♦ *See Adrenocorticosteroids overview for more information.*

benzonatate

ben-zoe'na-tate

Tessalon

Class: Nonnarcotic antitussive

PEDS   PREG   GERI
✋   C   ✋

Action Suppresses cough by an anesthetic effect on stretch receptors of the respiratory tract. Has a greater effect on nonproductive dry cough than a cough that produces copious amounts of sputum.

Use/Therapeutic goal/Outcome

Nonproductive cough: Prevention, reduction of coughing episodes. *Outcome criteria:* Patient reports and demonstrates decreased coughing.

Dose range/Administration

Adult/Child > 10 yrs: PO: 100–200 mg tid, to a maximum of 600 mg/day. *Child < 10 yrs:* PO: 8 mg/kg/day in 3–6 divided doses.

Clinical alert: Warn not to chew capsules or dissolve them in mouth because they will anesthetize the mouth and may cause choking.

Contraindications/Precautions
PREG C

Contraindicated in hypersensitivity to benzonatate or related compounds (local anesthetics).

🖑 Use with caution for children and the elderly. Safe use for pregnant or nursing mothers has not been established.

Side effects/Adverse reactions

Hypersensitivity: itching, rash. *CNS:* drowsiness, dizziness, headache, chills. *GI:* nausea, constipation. *Resp:* nasal congestion. *Eye:* burning sensation.

Nursing implications/Documentation

Possible nursing diagnoses: Ineffective airway clearance; Fluid volume deficit.

◆ Record lung sounds and sputum production to monitor effectiveness; report cough that lasts longer than a week.

◆ Provide preferred fluids to promote hydration.

Patient & family teaching/Home care

Possible nursing diagnoses: Knowledge deficit; Impaired home maintenance management.

◆ Warn not to chew capsule (see Clinical alert). Advise reporting a rash or an increase in breathing problems, because it may indicate a need to stop this drug.

◆ Stress the importance of adequate hydration; advise taking doses with a full glass of water.

◆ Point out that increased environmental humidity with decreased environmental irritants (e.g., smoke) can minimize aggravating factors.

◆ Advise reporting a cough that persists longer than a week.

◆ *See Antitussives, Expectorants, and Mucolytics overview for more information.*

benzthiazide
bens-thye'a-zide

B

Aquatag, Exna, Hydrex, Proaqua
Class: Thiazide diuretic, Antihypertensive

PEDS	PREG	GERI
🖑	D	🖑

Action Promotes excretion of sodium chloride, potassium, and water by inhibiting sodium reabsorption in the early portion of the distal tubule. Lowers blood pressure by reducing plasma and extra-cellular volume.

Use/Therapeutic goal/Outcome

Hypertension: Promotion of diuresis, reduction of blood pressure. *Outcome criteria:* After 3–4 days, blood pressure within normal limits.
Edema: Promotion of diuresis, resolution of edema. *Outcome criteria:* Increased urinary output; weight loss; absence of peripheral and sacral edema.
CHF: Promotion of diuresis, resolution of CHF. *Outcome criteria:* Absence of rales; non-distended neck veins; CVP/PAP within normal limits; urine output > 30 cc/hr.

Dose range/Administration

Interaction alert: Cholestyramine and colestipol decrease intestinal absorption. Diazoxide potentiates the hyperglycemic, hyperuricemic, and hypotensive effects. Nonsteroidal anti-inflammatory drugs may decrease effects. Give cautiously with corticosteroids, antidiabetics, lanoxin, and skeletal muscle relaxants. Do not give with lithium.

Adult: PO: 50–200 mg/day. Dose may be divided. *Child:* PO: 1–4 mg/kg/day in 3 divided doses.

Clinical alert: Give in morning to prevent nocturnal diuresis. Antihypertensive response may be delayed for several days.

Contraindications/Precautions
PREG D

Contraindicated in hypersensitivity to thiazides or sulfonamides, and anuria. *Use with caution* in history of renal or hepatic disease, gout, diabetes, electrolyte imbalance, pancreatitis, arteriosclerosis, systemic lupus erythematosus, asthma, bronchitis, and multiple allergies.

🖑 Contraindicated for nursing mothers. Not safe for pregnant woman. Use with caution for the elderly. Safe use in children has not been established, but benzthiazide has been used.

▶

Side effects/Adverse reactions

Hypersensitivity: anaphylaxis, rash, dermatitis with photosensitivity, urticaria, purpura, vasculitis, respiratory difficulty, fever. **CV:** volume depletion, orthostatic hypotension, dehydration. **Hem:** aplastic anemia, agranulocytosis, thrombocytopenia, hypokalemia, asymptomatic hyperuricemia, hyperglycemia, impaired glucose tolerance, leukopenia, lipid abnormalities, fluid and electrolyte imbalances, metabolic alkalosis, hypercalcemia. **GI:** anorexia, nausea, pancreatitis, hepatic encephalopathy. **Misc:** gout.

Nursing implications/Documentation

Possible nursing diagnoses: Fluid volume deficit; Altered patterns of urinary elimination; Potential for injury.

◆ Ascertain that baseline CBC, sodium, potassium, chloride, carbon dioxide, calcium, magnesium, BUN, creatinine, uric acid, and liver function studies have been obtained before giving first dose; report abnormalities and monitor closely thereafter.

◆ Document and monitor blood pressure, pulse, daily weight, and intake and output; report significant discrepancies.

◆ Monitor for hyperglycemia because of risk of thiazide-induced diabetes.

◆ Observe for and report signs of fluid overload (auscultate lungs for rales; check feet, ankles, and sacrum for edema).

◆ Be aware that diuretics often induce hypokalemia, which predisposes individuals to cardiac arrhythmias, cramping, and digoxin toxicity.

◆ Check with physician to determine dietary restrictions; if low-salt, high-potassium diet is recommended, consult with dietician to plan a low-salt diet that includes foods and juices high in potassium (orange juice; banana; green leafy vegetables).

◆ Observe the elderly for extreme diuresis; monitor for orthostatic hypotension; supervise ambulation until response is determined.

Patient & family teaching/Home care

Possible nursing diagnoses: Knowledge deficit; Impaired home maintenance management.

◆ Before giving first dose, explain that the drug will increase the amount and frequency of urination.

◆ Emphasize the importance of taking this drug exactly as prescribed, and the importance of returning for medical follow-up.

◆ Explain that diuretics enhance the work of the kidney and reduce the workload of the heart.

◆ Recommend taking doses in early morning and early afternoon to prevent the need to disturb sleep to void.

◆ Explain that changing positions slowly helps prevent dizziness.

◆ Advise reporting dizziness, shortness of breath, swelling of hands and feet, or persistent sore throat; encourage daily monitoring of weight and reporting sudden weight gain.

◆ Provide a list of allowed foods and fluids; stress the need to stick to prescribed diet (explain the hazards of too much salt, or too little potassium).

◆ Warn against driving and activities that require alertness until response has been determined.

◆ Advise avoidance of OTC drugs unless approved by physician; stress need to wear a sunscreen.

◆ Warn that hyperglycemia may occur; advise reporting thirst, fatigue, and weight loss.

◆ *See Diuretics and Antihypertensives overviews for more information.*

benztropine

benz'troe-peen

benztropine mesylate: ✚*Apo-Benzotropine,* ✚*Bensylate, Cogentin,* ✚*PMS Benzotropine*

Class: Anticholinergic, Cholinergic blocker (parasympatholytic)

Antidote: Physostigmine

PEDS	PREG	GERI
🖐	C	🖐

Action Reduces extrapyramidal muscle movements by blocking excess CNS cholinergic activity associated with dopamine deficiency in basal ganglia. Also has some peripheral anticholinergic action.

Use/Therapeutic goal/Outcome

Extrapyramidal reactions: Control of extrapyramidal side effects of antipsychotic drugs (e.g., haloperidol, phenothiazines, thiothixene). **Outcome criteria:** After 2–3 days, absence of or decrease in abnormal muscle movement and rigidity.

Parkinsonism: Control of symptoms; promotion of mobility. *Outcome criteria:* After 2–3 days, absence of or decrease in tremors, rigidity, akinesia, and drooling; improvement in gait, balance, posture, and speech.

Dose range/Administration

Interaction alert: Reduce dosage if administering with amantadine. Alcohol, antihistamines, narcotics, sedative, hypnotics, phenothiazines, and antidepressants may increase CNS depression and anticholinergic effects. Enhances effect of levodopa and Sinemet.

🖐 **Give with food or after meals to reduce GI symptoms.**

Extrapyramidal reactions: Adult: PO, IM, IV: 1–2 mg, then 1–2 mg PO bid to prevent recurrence.

Parkinsonism: Adult: PO: 0.5–1 mg, increase gradually prn as tolerated. *Maximum dose:* 6 mg/day.

Clinical alert: This drug should not be discontinued abruptly (dose should be gradually tapered). Single daily dose at bedtime often provides maximum effect.

Contraindications/Precautions

PREG
C

Contraindicated in hypersensitivity to benztropine and in narrow-angle glaucoma and obstructive diseases of GI or urinary tract. *Use with caution* in tachycardia and prostatic hypertrophy.

🖐 **Use with caution for the elderly or debilitated. Safe use for pregnant or nursing mothers has not been established.**

Side effects/Adverse reactions

Hypersensitivity: rash. *GI:* constipation, dry mouth, nausea, vomiting, epigastric distress. *CNS:* dizziness, restlessness, irritability, hallucinations, confusion, muscle weakness. *Eye:* blurred vision, photophobia. *CV:* tachycardia, palpitations. *GU:* urinary retention. *Misc:* anhidrosis (diminished sweating).

Nursing implications/Documentation

Possible nursing diagnoses: Potential for injury; Urinary retention.

♦ Document vital signs, especially pulse rate; report tachycardia.

♦ Monitor the elderly or debilitated for increased incidence of side effects.

♦ Observe and record response to drug, indicating improvement or deterioration in symptoms.

♦ Have the patient void before doses and monitor intake and output because this drug may cause voiding difficulties.

♦ Relieve dry mouth with ice chips, gum, or hard candy and increased unsweetened fluids.

Patient & family teaching/Home care

Possible nursing diagnoses: Knowledge deficit; Impaired home maintenance management.

♦ Teach that taking doses with food helps reduce GI side effects.

♦ Warn that other CNS depressants and alcohol may cause drowsiness.

♦ Explain that mouth dryness is a common side effect.

♦ Point out the need to avoid strenuous work in hot environment because anhidrosis (diminished sweating) may cause heat stroke (especially in the elderly).

♦ Caution not to discontinue drug abruptly because dosage must be reduced gradually; advise avoidance of OTC cold preparations.

♦ Warn that drowsiness, dizziness, or blurred vision may occur; advise against driving until response is determined.

♦ *See Anticholinergics overview for more information.*

bethanechol

be-than'e-kole

bethanechol chloride: *Duvoid, Urabeth, Urecholine,* 🍁*Urocarb Liquid,* 🍁*Urocarb Tablets*
Class: Cholinergic (parasympatholytic)
Antidote: Atropine

PEDS	PREG	GERI
🖐	C	🖐

Action Increases the tone of smooth muscles in the urinary bladder and the gastrointestinal tract by enhancing action of cholinergic receptor cells.

Use/Therapeutic goal/Outcome

Nonobstructive urinary retention or neurogenic bladder: Promotion of normal patterns of urinary elimination. *Outcome criteria:* Ability to void in amounts of 150 ml or greater.

Abdominal distention: Stimulation of gastrointestinal tract motility. *Outcome criteria:* Increase in bowel sounds, passage of flatus or stool.

Dose range/Administration

Interaction alert: Procainamide, quinidine, and anticholinergics may reverse cholinergic effects. Other cholinergic drugs should be stopped before giving bethanechol chloride. Ganglionic blocking agents may cause severe hypotension.

Give on empty stomach to reduce incidence of nausea and vomiting.

Adult: PO: 10–30 mg tid to qid. *For urinary retention:* up to 50–100 mg per dose. Use minimum effective dose. SC: 2.5 to 10 mg, tid to qid.

Clinical alert: Never give IM or IV (may cause circulatory collapse). To determine minimal effective dose, give 2.5 mg SC as a test dose and repeat every 15–30 min for a total of 4 doses. Have atropine 0.5 mg readily available for use as an antidote.

Contraindications/Precautions

PREG C

Contraindicated in hypersensitivity to bethanechol chloride, and in mechanical obstructions of GI or urinary tract, asthma, hyperthyroidism, peptic ulcer, cardiac disease, epilepsy, parkinsonism, COPD, and hypotension. *Use with caution* in hypertension, vasomotor instability, bradycardia, recent bowel or bladder surgery, and acute inflammatory conditions of GI tract.

Contraindicated for pregnant or nursing mothers. Use with caution for the elderly. Safe use for children has not been established.

Side effects/Adverse reactions

Hypersensitivity: rashes, exaggeration of side effects. *GI:* abdominal cramps, diarrhea, nausea, vomiting, belching. *CNS:* headache, sweating, malaise. *CV:* bradycardia, hypotension, flushing, cardiac arrest. *Resp:* bronchoconstriction. *GU:* urinary urgency. *Eye:* lacrimation, miosis.

Nursing implications/Documentation

Possible nursing diagnoses: Altered patterns of urinary elimination; Diarrhea; Potential for injury.

♦ Monitor and record respiratory status and vital signs frequently, especially with SC administration.

♦ Document time and amount of voiding to monitor for voiding difficulties; keep bedpan readily available.

♦ Observe for side effects for at least 1 hr following SC administration.

♦ Supervise ambulation until response is determined.

Patient & family teaching/Home care

Possible nursing diagnoses: Knowledge deficit; Impaired home maintenance management.

♦ Explain that this drug is likely to cause the urge to void and pass flatus.

♦ Stress the need to report side effects, especially shortness of breath, wheezing, or chest tightness.

♦ Advise changing positions slowly because of risk of orthostatic hypotension.

♦ *See Cholinergics overview for more information.*

biperiden

bye-per'i-den

biperiden hydrochloride: *Akineton*
biperiden lactate: *Akineton Lactate*
Class: Anticholinergic, Cholinergic blocker (parasympatholytic)
Antidote: Physostigmine

PEDS 🖐 **PREG** C **GERI** 🖐

Action Prevents abnormal muscle movements by blocking excess CNS cholinergic activity associated with dopamine deficiency in basal ganglia. Also has some peripheral anticholinergic action.

Use/Therapeutic goal/Outcome

Parkinsonism: Control of symptoms; promotion of mobility. *Outcome criteria:* Absence of or decrease in tremors, rigidity, akinesia, and drooling; improvement in gait, balance, posture, and speech.

Extrapyramidal reactions: Control of extrapyramidal side effects associated with reserpine and phenothiazines. *Outcome criteria:* Absence or decrease in abnormal muscle movements and rigidity.

Dose range/Administration

Interaction alert: Alcohol, antihistamines, narcotics, phenothiazines, antidepressants, and hypnotics may cause increased CNS depression.

Give oral doses after food to reduce GI side effects.

Parkinsonism: *Adult:* PO: 2 mg tid to qid.

Extrapyramidal reactions: **Adult:** PO: 2 mg bid to tid, depending on severity of symptoms. IM, IV: 2 mg injected slowly. May repeat in 30 min. *Maximum dose:* 8 mg/24 hr.

Clinical alert: After parenteral administration, keep patient supine in bed (because of risk of postural hypotension). Monitor blood pressure as head of bed is raised. Keep in mind that some patients develop a resistance to this drug, requiring an increase in dosage.

Contraindications/Precautions

Contraindicated in hypersensitivity to biperiden hydrochloride or lactate. **Use with caution** in narrow-angle glaucoma, cardiac dysrhythmias, and prostatic hypertrophy.

🖐 **Use with caution for the elderly or debilitated. Safe use for children and pregnant or nursing mothers has not been established.**

Side effects/Adverse reactions

Hypersensitivity: rash, exaggeration of side effects. *GI:* dry mouth, constipation, nausea, vomiting. *Eye:* blurred vision. *CNS:* drowsiness, disorientation, restlessness, euphoria. *CV:* postural hypotension. *GU:* urinary hesitancy or retention.

Nursing implications/Documentation

Possible nursing diagnoses: Potential for injury; Urinary retention; Constipation.

• Record vital signs, monitor for postural hypotension, and supervise ambulation until response is determined.

• Have patient void before doses; monitor intake and output because this drug can cause voiding difficulties.

• Monitor the elderly or debilitated for increased incidence of side effects.

• Relieve dry mouth by providing frequent mouth care and keeping ice chips at the bedside.

• Monitor for constipation; provide adequate fluids and fiber (laxatives and/or stool softeners should be given before problem is severe).

Patient & family teaching/Home care

Possible nursing diagnoses: Knowledge deficit; Impaired home maintenance management.

• Point out that taking this drug with food helps reduce GI side effects.

• Explain that dry mouth is a transient side effect.

• Warn that this drug may cause drowsiness and dizziness; caution to change position slowly.

• Advise against driving until response is determined.

• Stress the need to avoid OTC cold medications.

• Emphasize that this drug should not be discontinued abruptly, because this may precipitate adverse reactions.

◆ *See Anticholinergics overview for more information.*

bisacodyl

bis-a-koe'dill

> ✦Bisacolax, 🍁Bisalax, Bisco-Lax, Dacodyl, Deficol, Dulcolax, 🍁Durolax, Fleet Bisacodyl, Laxit, Thera-lax
>
> **Class:** Stimulant laxative
>
> | PEDS | PREG | GERI |
> |------|------|------|
> | 🖐 | C | 🖐 |

Action Increases peristalsis by direct effect on the nerve supply of the smooth muscles of the intestine; promotes fluid and ion accumulation in colon.

Use/Therapeutic goal/Outcome

Constipation and preparation for surgery or diagnostic studies: Evacuation of fecal material from colon. **Outcome criteria:** Forceful bowel evacuation (within 6–12 hr with tablet form and within 15 min to 1 hr after suppository or enema).

Dose range/Administration

Interaction alert: Do not give within 1 hr of antacids or milk (may cause enteric coating to dissolve too rapidly, causing irritation of stomach or duodenum). May interfere with the effectiveness of potassium-sparing diuretics or potassium supplements by promoting potassium loss through intestinal tract.

Adult: PO: 10–15 mg, up to 30 mg for thorough evacuation before surgery or diagnostic studies. RECT: 10 mg suppository, 1.25 oz enema. **Child:** PO: 5–10 mg. RECT: 5–10 mg suppository, 1/2 of micro enema.

Contraindications/Precautions

Contraindicated in hypersensitivity to stimulant laxatives, and in symptoms of appendicitis
or intestinal obstruction, undiagnosed rectal
bleeding, and those with colostomy or ileostomy.

🖐 **Contraindicated for infants under two
years. Use with caution for children 2–6
years, pregnant or nursing mothers, and
the elderly.**

Side effects/Adverse reactions

Hypersensitivity: skin rash, difficulty breathing.
GI: nausea, abdominal cramping, diarrhea.
MS: muscle weakness. *Skin:* irritation around
rectal area. *Misc:* hypokalemia, fluid and
electrolyte imbalance, laxative dependence.

Nursing implications/Documentation

Possible nursing diagnoses: Impaired skin integrity; Diarrhea; Pain.

◆ Give tablets with a full glass of water at
bedtime (unless otherwise ordered); do not
crush tablet.

◆ Administer suppository and enema forms at
the time evacuation is desired; encourage
patient to retain both forms for 15–30 min.

◆ Assess for abdominal distention and bowel
sounds.

◆ Monitor and document frequency, appearance,
and amount of stool evacuated.

◆ Assess perianal area and provide appropriate
measures for cleansing.

◆ Expect side effects and laxative dependence
to be more common and/or severe in elderly
patients.

Patient & family teaching/Home care

Possible nursing diagnoses: Knowledge deficit;
Impaired home maintenance management.

◆ Warn not to chew or crush tablet or not to
take milk or antacids within 1 hour to pre-
serve enteric coating.

◆ Teach proper method of administering suppository or enema.

◆ Stress the importance of following directions
and precautions printed on packaging.

◆ Caution that regular use of bisacodyl can
cause laxative dependence and loss of essential
electrolytes, especially in the elderly.

◆ Stress the importance of regular toileting
routine, dietary bulk, fluids, and exercise in
preventing constipation.

◆ *See Laxatives overview for more information.*

bitolterol
bi-tol-ter'ol

bitolterol mesylate: *Tornalate*

Class: Sympathomimetic (adrenergic) bronchodilator

PEDS	PREG	GERI
🖐	C	🖐

Action After conversion by esterases to active
drug (colterol) produces bronchial dilation by
stimulating beta-2 adrenergic receptors.

Use/Therapeutic goal/Outcome

Bronchospasm from respiratory diseases:
Reduction of airway resistance, improvement
in air movement. *Outcome criteria:* Decreased
wheezing, increased forced expiratory volume
(FEV); clearing of lung fields; report of breathing easier, and of fewer wheezing episodes.

Dose range/Administration

*Prevention of bronchospasm: Adult/Child > 12
yrs: Inhal:* 2 inhalations q8h.

*Treatment of bronchospasm: Adult/Child > 12
yrs: Inhal:* 2 inhalations (1–2 min apart); followed by a third inhalation prn.

Clinical alert: If needed, may increase dose cautiously, but do not exceed 3 inhalations q6h or
2 inhalations q4h. Action onset is 3–4 minutes,
peak is in 30–60 minutes, and duration is up
to 8 hr.

Contraindications/Precautions

Contraindicated in hypersensitivity to beta-
adrenergic agonists. *Use with caution* in
hypertension, ischemic heart disease, hyperthyroidism, diabetes mellitus, arrhythmias, seizure disorders.

🖐 **Use with caution for the elderly. Safe use
for pregnant or nursing mothers and for
children under 12 years has not been
established.**

Side effects/Adverse reactions

Hypersensitivity: exaggeration of side effects.
CV: palpitations, tachycardia, transient
increase in PVCs. *CNS:* tremors, nervousness,
headache, insomnia, dizziness. *Resp:* cough,
tightness in chest, bronchospasm, irritated
throat. *GI:* nausea.

Nursing implications/Documentation

Possible nursing diagnoses: Anxiety; Fear; Ineffective breathing pattern.

♦ Record lung sounds, respirations, pulse, and blood pressure, before and after dose administration, until response is determined.

♦ Provide favorite fluids, and monitor intake and output to ensure adequate hydration (at least 2 liters a day is recommended).

♦ Hold drug and report if persistent tachycardia is noted.

Patient & family teaching/Home care

Possible nursing diagnoses: Knowledge deficit; Impaired home maintenance management.

♦ Explain that this drug is intended to prevent and relieve bronchospasm and make breathing easier, and that effects should be noted within 2–4 min (with peak effects at 30–60 min, and duration of effects up to 8hr).

♦ Point out that stress and exercise can aggravate wheezing and bronchospasm, and that relaxation and controlled breathing techniques can help reduce severity and frequency of wheezing episodes.

♦ Teach the proper use of metered inhaler (exhale completely, hold mouthpiece to mouth, inhale deeply while pressing canister down, remove mouthpiece from mouth, hold breath for 10 seconds, then slowly exhale).

♦ Warn that increasing dose or frequency is not recommended (may cause tachycardia).

♦ Caution to avoid using OTC drugs unless they are approved by the physician.

♦ *See Bronchodilators and Adrenergics overviews for more information.*

bleomycin

blee-oh-mye'sin

bleomycin sulfate: *Blenoxane*

Class: Antineoplastic (antibiotic) agent

PEDS ♥   **PREG** D   **GERI** ♥

Action Kills rapidly growing cells (cancer, hair follicles, bone marrow, GI lining, ova, and sperm) by interfering with DNA, RNA, and protein synthesis and disrupting nucleic acid function. Is cell-cycle specific in the G_2- and M-phases.

Use/Therapeutic goal/Outcome

Squamous cell carcinoma of the head, neck, penis, cervix, and vulva; Hodgkin's disease; reticulum cell sarcoma; lymphosarcoma; testicular carcinoma: Elimination or suppression of malignant cell proliferation. *Outcome criteria:* Tumor and disease regression, or stabilization on radiologic and physical examination (changes are noted within 2 weeks for Hodgkin's disease and testicular cancer).

Dose range/Administration

Interaction alert: Radiation therapy and other antineoplastic agents (vincristine, vinblastine) may cause increased toxicity. Cisplatin decreases bleomycin clearance.

Squamous cell carcinoma, lymphosarcoma, reticulum cell sarcoma, testicular carcinoma: **Adult:** IV, IM, SC: 0.25 to 0.5 units/kg (10–20 units/m²) once or twice weekly.

Hodgkin's disease: **Adult:** IV, IM, SC: *Initial dose:* 0.25 to 0.5 units/kg (10–20 units/m²) once or twice weekly. *Maintenance dose:* After 50% response, 1 unit/day or 5 units/wk; do not give SC.

Lymphomas: **Adult:** IM, IV: 2 units or less in first 2 doses, then, with no allergic reaction, after 2 hr, use Hodgkin's disease dose.

Clinical alert: This drug should be given only by nurses who are knowledgeable in the comprehensive management of the administration of antineoplastic agents. Doses may vary at physician's discretion. Repeat doses are held until it is ascertained that the patient has recovered sufficiently from toxicities of previous doses. Established protocols/policies for drug preparation, administration, and accidental skin contamination *must be followed closely* (gloves or double gloves are worn when handling drug; if the drug touches the skin, the area is washed immediately with plenty of soap and water). Bleomycin sulfate is diluted in 50–100 ml fluid and infused over 15–30 min to minimize pain and inflammation. Bleomycin may be given as a regional arterial perfusion or as an intracavitary instillation in the treatment of malignant effusions. Hold drug and report if platelets <100,000/mm³ and WBC <4000/mm³.

Contraindications/Precautions

PREG D

Contraindicated in hypersensitivity to bleomycin and idiosyncratic reactions (similar to anaphylaxis). *Use with caution* in renal, hepatic, or pulmonary impairment.

♨ **Use with caution for the elderly. Safe use for children and pregnant or nursing mothers has not been established.**

Side effects/Adverse reactions

Hypersensitivity: rash, pruritus, flushing, fever up to 41°C, hypotension, chills, anaphylaxis. **CNS:** chills and fever (60% occurrence) 4–10 hr after drug is given (may last 48 hr). **Skin:** erythema, rash, hyperpigmentation, vesiculation, hyperkeratosis on palms and fingers, nail changes, acne, and alopecia, pain and burning at injection site. **GI:** anorexia (13%), nausea, vomiting, diarrhea, stomatitis. **Resp:** pneumonitis, pulmonary fibrosis (10%), pulmonary toxicity, persistent cough. **Hem:** myelosuppression (rare).

Nursing implications/Documentation

Possible nursing diagnoses: Potential for infection; Potential for injury; Fatigue; Altered oral mucous membrane; Fluid volume deficit; Diarrhea; Altered nutrition: less than body requirements.

◆ *See important Nursing implications in Antineoplastic agents overview on page 72, which apply to all neoplastics. The interventions that follow are additional and specific to this drug only.*

◆ Check for preadministration pulmonary function tests and monitor for and report early signs of pulmonary toxicity (shortness of breath, persistent cough); the risk is increased with age and when cumulative doses exceed 400 units.

◆ Expect the common reaction of fever to occur within 3–6 hr of administration (usually treated with antipyretics).

◆ Record and monitor intake and output; prevent kidney complications by maintaining adequate hydration.

◆ When changing dressings, do not use adhesive on the skin because this drug accumulates in keratin of squamous epithelium and may cause streaking.

Patient & family teaching/Home care

Possible nursing diagnoses: Knowledge deficit; Ineffective coping (individual and family); Hopelessness; Impaired home maintenance management.

◆ *See important Patient & family teaching in Antineoplastic agents overview on page 72, which apply to all neoplastics. The interventions*

that follow are additional and specific to this drug only.

◆ Stress that shortness of breath, persistent cough, or chest pain should be reported; they may indicate pulmonary toxicity.

◆ Explain that drinking 2–3 L per day can help prevent kidney complications.

◆ *See Antineoplastic agents overview for more information.*

bretylium tosylate

bre-til'ee-um

♥🍁**Bretylate, Bretylol**

Class: Antiarrhythmic (Class III)

PEDS	PREG	GERI
✋	C	✋

Action A specific mechanism of action has not been established. It is known to suppress ventricular tachycardia and fibrillation by inhibiting release of norepinephrine in postganglionic nerve endings.

Use/Therapeutic goal/Outcome

Ventricular arrhythmias (tachycardia and fibrillation) that have not responded to first-line antiarrhythmics, such as lidocaine or procainamide: Prevention or resolution of ventricular tachycardia and fibrillation, promotion of effective heartbeat. **Outcome criteria:** Absence of ventricular tachycardia or fibrillation on EKG; regular palpable pulses.

Dose range/Administration

Interaction alert: Monitor for additive hypotensive effects if given with antihypertensives. May initially aggravate digitalis toxicity.

Adult: IV: Undiluted bolus of 5 mg/kg by rapid injection; may repeat with 10 mg/kg q15-30min until 30 mg/kg has been administered. If ventricular tachycardia persists, dilute one ampule of 500 mg bretylium tosylate in 50 cc DSW or NS, and either infuse continuously at a rate of 1–2 mg/min (with IV pump), or inject 5–10 mg/kg q6h (injection time should be longer than 8 min). IM: 5–10 mg/kg undiluted at 1–2 hr intervals. For maintenance give the same dose q6-8h. The IM route should be used only if an IV cannot be established.

Clinical alert: When administering by IV, keep patient supine and document blood pressure q2-5min, monitoring hypotensive effects. Transient *hyper*tension may precede hypotension. Once dose is infused and blood pressure is stable, monitor for orthostatic hypotension while raising the head of the bed slowly. Keep resuscitative drugs and equipment readily available.

Contraindications/Precautions

Contraindicated in hypersensitivity to bretylium and in digitalis-induced arrhythmias. **Use with caution** in pulmonary hypertension, and aortic stenosis.

🖐 **Use with caution for the elderly. Safe use for children and pregnant or nursing mothers has not been established.**

Side effects/Adverse reactions

Hypersensitivity: allergic reactions are not listed. **CV:** hypotension (especially orthostatic), transient worsening of arrhythmias, bradycardia, angina. **CNS:** vertigo, dizziness, lightheadedness, syncope. **GI:** nausea and vomiting with rapid infusion. **Resp:** stuffy nose, shortness of breath.

Nursing implications/Documentation

Possible nursing diagnoses: Potential for injury; Sleep pattern disturbance; Activity intolerance.

◆ Be sure to check baseline chest X-ray, EKG, and laboratory studies (CBC, sodium, potassium, chloride, carbon dioxide, magnesium, BUN, creatinine, SGPT, and LDH) before giving first dose; monitor closely thereafter as indicated by clinical condition.

◆ Remember that oxygen requirements must be met, and that electrolyte imbalances (especially potassium and magnesium) and abnormal blood pH must be corrected, before expected antiarrhythmic effect can be seen; report abnormalities immediately.

◆ Document baseline vital signs, lung sounds, and cardiac monitor strip (measure and record PR and QRS segments) before giving first dose and at least every 8 hr; monitor closely until response is determined; report prolonged PR or QRS segments.

◆ Monitor closely for risk of injury; keep patient in bed with side rails up.

◆ Coordinate care to provide frequent rest periods.

Patient & family teaching/Home care

Possible nursing diagnoses: Anxiety; Fear.

◆ Explain that the purpose of this drug is to prevent arrhythmias and promote an effective heartbeat.

◆ Reassure that close monitoring of vital signs helps to fine-tune dosage and prevent adverse effects.

◆ Advise to avoid sudden changes in position; stress the need to remain in bed.

◆ *See Antiarrhythmics overview for more information.*

bromocriptine

broe-moe-crip'teen

bromocriptine mesylate: **Parlodel**

Class: Antiparkinsonian, Dopaminergic agent, Ovulatory stimulant

PEDS	PREG	GERI
🖐	C	🖐

Action controls parkinsonian symptoms by directly stimulating and activating postsynaptic dopamine receptors in the CNS. Blocks the release of prolactin from the anterior pituitary by stimulating secretion of prolactin inhibitory factor (PIF) from the hypothalmus.

Use/Therapeutic goal/Outcome

Parkinsonism (after prolonged levodopa therapy with deterioration in symptoms): Control of parkinsonian symptoms and promotion of mobility. **Outcome criteria:** Absence of (or decrease in) tremors, rigidity, akinesia, and drooling; improvement in gait, balance, posture, and speech.
Hyperprolactinemia: Restoration of normal ovulatory and menstrual cycle after 8 weeks of therapy. **Outcome criteria:** Establishment of regular menses.
Postpartum lactation: Prevention of postpartum lactation (secretion, congestion, engorgement). **Outcome criteria:** Absence of lactation, engorgement.

Dose range/Administration

Interaction alert: May potentiate antihypertensive agents. Enhances action of levodopa. Tricyclic antidepressants may decrease the effectiveness of bromocriptine. Oral contraceptives, estrogens, and progestins inhibit bromocriptine (do not use together). Alcohol may cause disulfiram-like reaction.

🖐 **Give with meals.**

Parkinsonism: Adult: PO: 1.25 mg bid; dosage may be increased slowly every 14–28 days to a maximum of 100 mg/day.

Hyperprolactinemia: Adult: PO: 2.5 mg bid or tid for 14 days (maximum length of therapy is 6 months).

Suppression of postpartum lactation: Adult: PO: 2.5 mg bid for 14–21 days.

Clinical alert: Dose should be titrated to minimal effective dose because the incidence of side effects is high, especially during beginning of treatment. Patients receiving the very high doses needed for treatment of Parkinson's disease may be severely disabled during early treatment because of side effects.

Contraindications/Precautions

PREG
C

Contraindicated in hypersensitivity to bromocriptine or other ergot derivatives, and in severe ischemic heart disease, hypertension, or peripheral vascular disease. **Use with caution** in hypotension, epilepsy, psychosis, arrhythmias, and impaired hepatic or renal function.

🖑 **Contraindicated for pregnant or nursing mothers. Use with caution for the elderly. Safe use in children under 15 years has not been established.**

Side effects/Adverse reactions

Hypersensitivity: skin rash and ergotism (numbness and tingling in extremities, cold feet, muscle cramping, and Raynaud's phenomenon). **GI:** nausea (most common reaction), vomiting, abdominal discomfort, diarrhea, anorexia, dry mouth, dysphagia. **CNS:** headache, dizziness, nervousness, drowsiness, fatigue, depression, insomnia, nightmares, lightheadedness, confusion, abnormal involuntary movements. **Eye:** visual disturbances, blepharospasm. **Resp:** nasal congestion, pulmonary infiltration and effusion, shortness of breath. **CV:** hypotension. **Skin:** foot and ankle edema, mottling. **GU:** urinary frequency.

Nursing implications/Documentation

Possible nursing diagnoses: Potential for injury; Impaired physical mobility.

♦ For use in Parkinson's disease, establish a baseline profile of patient's abilities and disabilities to differentiate between desired responses and drug-induced side effects (keep in mind that side effects may be severe at first, but should diminish).

♦ Have patient dangle legs before ambulating; supervise ambulation until response is determined.

♦ Report changes in mental status (psychotic symptoms have been reported).

Patient & family teaching/Home care

Possible nursing diagnoses: Self-care deficit; Impaired home maintenance management; Altered patterns of sexuality.

♦ Stress that taking this drug with food helps reduce GI symptoms; suggest taking close to bedtime to better tolerate nausea and dizziness.

♦ Caution that there is a high incidence of side effects, especially at beginning of therapy (lifestyle may have to change until side effects subside); advise reporting persistent adverse reactions.

♦ Warn that dizziness is common at beginning of treatment and that position changes should be made slowly; advise to avoid driving until response is determined.

♦ Explain to those with Parkinson's disease that they are likely to require more help with self-care during initial treatment.

♦ Advise women (especially postpartum) that fertility is likely to increase, and that to avoid pregnancy; birth control methods other than oral contraceptives should be used.

♦ *See Antiparkinsons overview for more information.*

brompheniramine

brome-fen-ir'a-meen

brompheniramine maleate: **Brombay, Bromphen, Chlorphed, Codimal-A, Conjec-B, Cophene-B, Dehist, Diamine T.D., Dimetane, Dimetane Extentabs, Dimetane-Ten, Histaject Modified, Nasahist B, ND-Stat Revised, Oraminic II, Sinusol B, Veltane**

Class: Antihistamine (H₁ receptor antagonist)

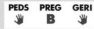

PEDS	PREG	GERI
🖑	B	🖑

Action Prevents but does not reverse histamine-mediated allergic responses by competing with histamine for H_1 receptors on effector cells. Has anticholinergic action.

Use/Therapeutic goal/Outcome

Allergic conditions: Decrease in allergic response. **Outcome criteria:** Report and demonstration of relief of allergic symptoms (sneezing, nasal secretions, itching).

Dose range/Administration

Interaction alert: Alcohol and other CNS depressants may cause excessive drowsiness. Do not give with MAOIs or anticholinergics.

🖐 **Give with food or milk to avoid GI upset.**

Self medication (OTC): Adult/Child > 12 yrs:
PO: *Tablet:* 4 mg q4-6h, to a maximum of 24 mg in 24 hr. *Extended-release tablet:* 8 or 12 mg q8-12h for adult, q12h for child. *Child 6–12 yrs:* PO: 2 mg q4-6h, to a maximum of 12 mg in 24 hr.

Under physician's direction: Adult: SC, IM, IV: 5–20 mg q6-12h, to a maximum of 40 mg in 24 hr. *Child < 12 yrs:* SC, IM, IV: 0.5 mg/kg/24 hr divided into 3 or 4 doses. *Child 6–12 yrs:* PO: *Extended-release tablet:* 8 or 12 mg q12h. *Child 2–6 yrs:* PO: 1 mg q4-6h, to a maximum of 6 mg in 24 hr.

Clinical alert: Expect reduced dosage for the elderly, and monitor closely for excessive drowsiness and dizziness. Give IM and SC without dilution. Give IV doses slowly, undiluted or diluted in DSW or NS (unless otherwise specified by manufacturer).

Contraindications/Precautions

PREG
B

Contraindicated in hypersensitivity to brompheniramine or chemically related antihistamines, in acute asthma, and within 14 days of treatment with MAO inhibitors. *Use with caution* in prostatic hypertrophy, bladder obstruction, urinary retention, narrow-angle glaucoma, hypertension, cardiovascular or renal disease, or hyperthyroidism.

🖐 **Contraindicated for newborns and nursing mothers. Use with caution for children and the elderly. Safe use in pregnancy has not been established.**

Side effects/Adverse reactions

Hypersensitivity: high fever, chills, urticaria, rash. *CNS:* sedation, drowsiness, dizziness, headache, disturbed coordination. *GI:* dry mouth, stomach upset. *Hem:* thrombocytopenia, agranulocytosis.

Nursing implications/Documentation

Possible nursing diagnoses: Potential for injury; Fluid volume deficit.

◆ Determine and record known allergies; provide an environment that is free from allergens (especially sleeping areas).

◆ Provide favorite fluids and ensure adequate hydration (2 liters/day).

◆ If therapy is prolonged, monitor CBC for blood dyscrasias.

◆ For IV route, keep patient flat in bed, with side rails up, until response is determined

(may cause transient hypotension, drowsiness, dizziness, or syncope).

Patient & family teaching/Home care

Possible nursing diagnoses: Knowledge deficit; Impaired home maintenance management.

◆ Advise taking this drug with food or milk if GI symptoms are experienced.

◆ Point out that avoiding pollens and staying in an air-conditioned environment may help reduce symptoms of seasonal rhinitis.

◆ Emphasize that dose should not be increased without physician's approval; explain that tolerance may occur, requiring a change in medication.

◆ Warn that alcohol and other CNS depressants may cause excessive drowsiness; advise against driving until response is determined.

◆ Suggest that coffee or tea may reduce drowsiness, and that sugarless gum or hard candy may relieve dry mouth.

◆ Explain the need to stop antihistamines 4 days before allergy testing to ensure accuracy of results.

◆ *See Antihistamines overview for more information.*

bumetanide

byoo-met'a-nide

Bumex, 🔺Burinex

Class: Loop (high-ceiling) diuretic

PEDS	PREG	GERI
🖐	C	🖐

Action Promotes diuresis by inhibiting the reabsorption of sodium and chloride in the ascending limb of the loop of Henle.

Use/Therapeutic goal/Outcome

Edema associated with CHF, hepatic or renal disease: Promotion of diuresis, resolution of edema. *Outcome criteria:* Increased urinary output; weight loss; absence of rales and peripheral and sacral edema.

Dose range/Administration

Interaction alert: Aminoglycosides and other ototoxic drugs may potentiate ototoxicity. Probenecid and indomethacin may inhibit the diuretic effect.

Adult: PO: 0.5–2 mg/day; may repeat q4-5h. *Maximum dose:* 10 mg/day. IM, IV: 0.5–1 mg slowly over 1–2 min; may repeat q2-3h. *Maximum dose:* 10 mg/day.

▶

B

Clinical alert: Give in morning (if possible) to avoid nocturnal diuresis. Be aware that 1 mg of bumetanide is approximately equivalent to 40 mg of furosemide. When administered IV, diuresis begins within minutes, and peaks at 15–30 min. IM, IV, and PO route produce approximately equivalent diuretic responses.

Contraindications/Precautions

PREG
C

Contraindicated in hypersensitivity to bumetanide or sulfonamides, and in anuria, electrolyte imbalance, hepatic coma, and elevated BUN. **Use with caution** in decreased renal function, cirrhosis, and ascites.

🖐 **Use with caution for the elderly. Safe use for children and pregnant or nursing mothers has not been established.**

Side effects/Adverse reactions

Hypersensitivity: rash, urticaria. **CV:** orthostatic hypotension, volume depletion, EKG changes. **Hem:** hypokalemia, hypochloremic alkalosis, hyperuricemia, fluid and electrolyte imbalance, hyperglycemia, azotemia. **CNS:** dizziness, headaches. **Ear:** impaired hearing. **GI:** nausea, vomiting, diarrhea, constipation. **Misc:** hypochloremic alkalosis.

Nursing implications/Documentation

Possible nursing diagnoses: Fluid volume deficit; Altered patterns of urinary elimination; Potential for injury.

◆ Ascertain that baseline CBC, sodium, potassium, chloride, carbon dioxide, calcium, magnesium, BUN, creatinine, uric acid, and liver function studies have been obtained before giving first dose; report abnormalities and monitor closely thereafter.

◆ Give doses in early morning and early afternoon (if possible) to avoid nocturnal diuresis.

◆ Document and monitor blood pressure, daily weight, and intake and output; report significant discrepancies.

◆ Monitor for and report signs of fluid overload (auscultate lungs for rales; check feet, ankles, and sacrum for edema).

◆ Be aware that diuretics often induce hypokalemia, which predisposes individuals to cardiac arrhythmias, cramping, and digoxin toxicity.

◆ Check with physician to determine dietary restrictions; if a low-salt, high-potassium diet is recommended, consult with dietician to plan a low-salt diet that includes foods and juices high in potassium (orange juice; banana; green leafy vegetables).

◆ Observe the elderly for extreme diuresis (may require lower doses); monitor for orthostatic hypotension; supervise ambulation until response is determined.

Patient & family teaching/Home care

Possible nursing diagnoses: Knowledge deficit; Impaired home maintenance management.

◆ Before giving first dose, explain that the drug will increase the amount and frequency of urination.

◆ Emphasize the importance of taking this drug exactly as prescribed, and the importance of returning for medical follow-up.

◆ Explain that diuretics enhance the work of the kidney and reduce the workload of the heart.

◆ Recommend taking doses in early morning and early afternoon to prevent the need to disturb sleep to void.

◆ Explain that changing positions slowly helps prevent dizziness.

◆ Advise reporting dizziness, shortness of breath, swelling of hands and feet, or persistent sore throat; encourage daily monitoring of weight and reporting sudden weight gain.

◆ Provide a list of allowed foods and fluids; stress the need to stick to prescribed diet (explain the hazards of too much salt, or too little potassium).

◆ Warn against driving and activities that require alertness until response determined.

◆ Explain that fatigue may occur at first, but that this should diminish with time.

◆ *See Diuretics overview for more information.*

bupivacaine

byoo-piv'e-kane

bupivacaine hydrochloride: ◢*Marcain, Marcaine, Sensorcaine*

Class: Local anesthetic (amide type)

PEDS	PREG	GERI
🖐	C	🖐

Action Produces local anesthesia by inhibiting sodium flux across the nerve cell membrane, thus preventing depolarization and generation and conduction of nerve impulses. Bupivacaine has high potency and toxicity; and slow onset

(4–17 min) and long duration (3–6 hr), especially when combined with epinephrine.

Use/Therapeutic goal/Outcome

All types of local and regional anesthesia when a prolonged duration is desired: Prevention of pain during and after surgical, dental, or obstetric procedures. *Outcome criteria:* Report of numbness and absence of pain in anesthetized area; patients receiving epidural or spinal anesthesia will also demonstrate loss of motor function below the level of the block.

Dose range/Administration

Clinical alert: These drugs should only be administered by clinicians who are well versed in their use. Dose is highly individualized, depending on the procedure, method of administration, area to be anesthetized, vascularity of tissue, and on patient condition, tolerance, and response. **Inadvertent intravascular injection may result in cardiac arrest** that is resistant to therapy; women in labor may be more susceptible. Preparations with epinephrine may result in angina, tachycardia, tremors, headache, restlessness, palpitations, dizziness, and hypertension. Have oxygen and resuscitative drugs and equipment readily available. Dosages listed are for use *without* epinephrine.

Adult: Epidural: After test doses to verify position of catheter. 50–100 mg 0.5% solution (10–20 cc); or 25–50 mg 0.25% solution (10–20 cc). *Caudal*: 75–150 mg 0.5% solution (15–30 cc); or 37.5–75 mg 0.25% solution (15–30 cc). *Peripheral nerve block:* 25–175 mg maximum (5–37.5 cc of 0.5% solution). *Doses should not be repeated* in less than 3 hr; maximum 400 mg/24 hr.

Contraindications/Precautions

PREG C

Contraindicated in hypersensitivity to bupivacaine and amide-type anesthetics, PABA and derivatives, and metabisulfites; also in acidosis, heart block, severe hemorrhage, severe liver disease, hypotension, hypertension, cerebrospinal disease, and obstetrical paracervical block. *Use with caution* for the debilitated, in liver or kidney disease, and dysrhythmias.

✋ **Contraindicated for children under 12 years. Use with caution for the elderly.**

Side effects/Adverse reactions

Hypersensitivity: rashes, cutaneous lesions, urticaria, sneezing, diaphoresis, syncope, hyperthermia, angioneurotic edema (including laryngeal edema), anaphylaxis. *CNS:* nervousness, anxiety, excitement, dizziness, drowsiness, tremors, convulsions, unconsciousness. *Resp:* respiratory arrest. *CV:* hypotension, ventricular arrhythmias, myocardial depression, decreased cardiac output, bradycardia, cardiac arrest. *Eye:* pupillary constriction; blurred or double vision. *GI:* nausea, vomiting. *Ear:* tinnitus. *Misc:* inflammation and/or sepsis at injection site, chills; (for epidural anesthesia) total spinal block, urinary retention, fecal incontinence, loss of perineal sensation and sexual function; persistent analgesia, paresthesia, slowing of labor, increased incidence of forceps delivery, cranial nerve palsies.

Nursing implications/Documentation

Possible nursing diagnoses: Pain; Potential for injury.

♦ Be sure that allergy history and accurate height and weight are recorded before procedure.

♦ Record vital signs according to protocol; monitor for and report immediately signs of systemic or hypersensitivity reactions.

♦ Determine from anesthesiologist or anesthetist whether there are any restrictions on patient positioning; post these at bedside.

♦ Monitor anesthetized area for level of sensation and motor function; watch for poor positioning, and protect area from injury.

♦ Be aware that the duration of action of bupivacaine may be as long as 12 hr, especially with the preparations containing epinephrine.

♦ Give prescribed pain medication as sensation begins to return, **before pain is severe**.

Patient & family teaching/Home care

Possible nursing diagnoses: Anxiety; Fear.

♦ Stress the need to protect areas of the body that have lost sensation.

♦ Explain rationale for taking prescribed pain medication before pain becomes too uncomfortable.

♦ *See Local anesthetics overview for more information.*

buprenorphine

bup-ren-or'feen

buprenorphine hydrochloride: *Buprenex,* ◆*Temgesic Injection*

Class: Narcotic analgesic

Antidote: Naloxone hydrochloride (Narcan)

PEDS	PREG	GERI	CONTROLLED SUBSTANCE
♨	C	♨	V

Action Alters both perception of and response to pain by binding to opiate receptors at various sites in the CNS. This drug is approximately 30 times more potent than morphine sulfate (0.3 mg is equal to 10 mg of morphine) and 250 times more potent than meperidine (0.3 mg is equal to 75 mg of morphine).

Use/Therapeutic goal/Outcome

Moderate to severe pain: Relief of pain. *Outcome criteria:* Report of comfort; absence of signs of pain (grimacing, frowning, restlessness, reluctance to move or cough) with increase in signs of comfort (relaxed facial expression, decreased restlessness, improved ability to move or cough); blood pressure and pulse within normal limits when compared to baseline.

Dose range/Administration

Interaction alert: Other CNS depressants, alcohol, sedatives, hypnotics, antipsychotics and skeletal muscle relaxants increase effects. May antagonize action of other narcotics.

Adult: IM, IV: 0.3 mg to 0.6 mg q6h prn or around the clock.

Clinical alert: Give IV doses slowly. SC route is not recommended. Use decreased dosage for the elderly and debilitated. Check respirations and blood pressure before giving buprenorphine; hold drug and report if respirations < 10, or if there is hypotension. Be aware that naloxone alone is unlikely to reverse drug-induced respiratory depression; it may require large naloxone doses (more than 0.4 mg), administration of dioxapram, and mechanical ventilation.

Contraindications/Precautions

PREG
C

Contraindicated in hypersensitivity to buprenorphine hydrochloride, and in narcotics addiction, and respirations less than 12/min. *Use with caution* in head injury; increased intracranial pressure; severe hepatic, pulmonary, or renal impairment; CNS depression; prostatic hypertrophy; hypothyroidism; acute alcoholism; acute myocardial infarction; and toxic psychosis.

♨ **Use with caution for nursing mothers and the elderly or debilitated. Safe use for pregnant women and children under 13 years has not been established.**

Side effects/Adverse reactions

Hypersensitivity: severe CNS and respiratory depression, cardiovascular collapse. *CNS:* sedation, dizziness/vertigo, sweating, headache, euphoria. *GI:* nausea, vomiting. *CV:* hypotension. *Resp:* respiratory depression, hypoventilation. *Skin:* pruritus.

Nursing implications/Documentation

Possible nursing diagnoses: Pain; Anxiety; Potential for injury.

◆ Have patient rate pain on a scale of 1–10 before and after medication is given; report and record inadequate pain control.

◆ Monitor closely for risk factors for injury; keep side rails up and supervise ambulation if allowed out of bed.

◆ Give pain medication before pain is severe.

◆ Be aware that psychic and physical dependence may develop; withdrawal symptoms may appear up to 14 days after drug is discontinued.

◆ For narcotic-dependent individuals, monitor for abstinence syndrome because this drug has narcotic antagonist properties.

Patient & family teaching/Home care

Possible nursing diagnoses: Sensory/perceptual alterations; Knowledge deficit.

◆ Stress the need to report pain or discomfort before it is severe.

◆ Advise those who are ambulatory to refrain from activities that require alertness and to seek assistance if there is any question about ability to get out of bed (e.g., if there is weakness or light headedness).

◆ Explain procedures briefly and in simple terms.

◆ Warn not to exceed prescribed dose because of risk of overdose, dependence, and abuse (instead of increasing dose regimen, unsatisfactory pain relief should be reported).

◆ *See Narcotic and non-narcotic analgesics overview for more information.*

bupropion

bu-pro'pee-un

bupropion hydrochloride: **Wellbutrin**

Class: Antidepressant (atypical)

PEDS	PREG	GERI
🖐	B	🖐

Action Exact mechanism of action has not been determined. Believed to improve mood by increasing levels of the neurotransmitters norepinephrine, serotonin, and, to some extent, dopamine in the CNS.

Use/Therapeutic goal/Outcome

Major depression lasting longer than 6 weeks: Promotion of sense of well-being, ability to cope with daily living. **Outcome criteria:** After 2–4 weeks, report of feeling less depressed, less anxious, more energetic and able to cope; return of normal sleeping and eating habits; demonstration of improved ability to problem solve and perform activities of daily living.

Dose range/Administration

Interaction alert: Concurrent use with alcohol may lower seizure threshold; antidepressants, haloperidol, lithium, loxapine, molindone, phenothiazines or thioxanthenes may lower seizure threshold and increase risk of major motor seizures. Avoid use with MAOIs because of increased risk of acute toxicity, hyperpyrexia, and seizures.

🖐 **Give with (or immediately after) food to reduce GI symptoms.**

Adult: PO: 100 mg bid for the first 3 days. On day 4, may increase to 300 mg/day in 3 divided doses. May increase after several weeks to 450 mg/day in divided doses. A single dose should not exceed 150 mg. The lowest dose that maintains remission should be used.

Clinical alert: Monitor for and report excessive CNS side effects: this drug has been associated with seizures in some patients.

Contraindications/Precautions

**PREG
B**

Contraindicated in hypersensitivity to buprion hydrochloride and in CNS tumors or history of seizures. **Use with caution** in impaired kidney or liver function, and in recent MI, schizophrenia, and history of bulemia or anorexia nervosa.

🖐 **Contraindicated for children and nursing mothers. Use with caution for pregnant women and the elderly or debilitated.**

Side effects/Adverse reactions

Hypersensitivity: rash. **CNS:** drowsiness, dizziness, anxiety, headache, ataxia, agitation, extrapyramidal symptoms, sedation, insomnia, tremors, seizures. **CV:** orthostatic hypotension, palpitations, tachycardia, hypertension. **GI:** disturbances in taste, dry mouth, nausea, constipation, paralytic ileus. **GU:** urinary retention, decreased libido. **Eye:** blurred vision. **Ear:** auditory disturbances. **Skin:** excessive sweating.

Nursing implications/Documentation

Possible nursing diagnoses: Potential for injury; Constipation; Altered oral mucous membrane.

◆ Document mental status and vital signs at least twice a day until response to therapy has been established.

◆ Be sure that doses are swallowed (not hoarded).

◆ Monitor for orthostatic hypotension, dizziness, and drowsiness; supervise ambulation until response is established.

◆ Record intake and output, and observe for dehydration or urinary retention; provide special mouth care.

◆ Monitor for and report suicidal tendencies, increased depression, or excessive drowsiness (may require change in medication).

◆ Prevent constipation by monitoring bowel movements and encouraging adequate fiber and fluid intake; offer laxatives or stool softeners before the problem becomes severe.

Patient & family teaching/Home care

Possible nursing diagnoses: Ineffective coping (family and individual); Sleep pattern disturbance; Impaired home maintenance management.

◆ Advise to take with food to reduce GI irritation.

◆ Stress that this medication helps reduce the depression that inhibits ability to make decisions and cope effectively (once the individual feels less depressed, it will be easier to take steps toward making healthy changes).

◆ Explain that side effects are often noted immediately, but they usually diminish after a few weeks; on the other hand, it is likely to take 2–4 weeks before *beneficial* effects are noted (the patient may feel worse before feeling better).

- Warn to change positions slowly to prevent dizziness.

- Point out the role of adequate nutrition, exercise, and sleep in combating depression.

- Emphasize that the effects of alcohol, sedatives, and tranquilizers may be potentiated.

- Caution to consult with physician before using OTC drugs; stress the need for ongoing medical follow-up.

- Recommend reporting continued depression; stress that doses should not be increased or stopped without checking with physician because this may cause severe problems.

- Advise avoidance of driving and other potentially hazardous activities until response is established.

- Suggest using ice chips, hard candy, or gum to relieve side effect of dry mouth; stress the need for good mouth care.

- Warn women to report immediately if pregnancy is planned or suspected.

- *See Antidepressants overview for more information.*

buspirone

byoo-spear'own

buspirone hydrochloride: *BuSpar*

Class: Antianxiety agent

PEDS PREG GERI
 ✋   B   ✋

Action Exact mechanism of action has not been determined. Appears to produce relaxation by having a high affinity for serotonin receptors and a moderate affinity for dopamine receptors. Does not have anticonvulsant or muscle relaxant properties. Less sedating than other anxiolytics, but sedative effect is dependent on the individual.

Use/Therapeutic goal/Outcome

Short-term treatment of anxiety: Alleviation of symptoms of apprehension and insomnia. *Outcome criteria:* After 1–2 weeks, report of feeling calmer, sleeping better, and coping better; observable signs of decreased anxiety (decreased motor activity, decrease in pulse and blood pressure).

Dose range/Administration

Interaction alert: Alcohol and other CNS depressants may cause excessive sedation. Should *not* be used with MAOIs.

🍲 **Give with food to reduce GI symptoms.**

Adult: PO: 5 mg tid; may increase daily dose by 5 mg every 2–3 days. *Maximum dose:* 60 mg/day.

Contraindications/Precautions

PREG
B

Contraindicated in hypersensitivity or intolerance to buspirone hydrochloride, and with concurrent MAOI therapy, impaired liver or kidney function, or other psychotropic drug therapy. *Use with caution* in suicidal tendencies.

🖐 **Contraindicated for pregnant or nursing mothers. Use with caution for the elderly or debilitated. Safe use for children has not been established.**

Side effects/Adverse reactions

Hypersensitivity: itching, rash, exaggeration of side effects. *CNS:* dizziness, headache, drowsiness, paresthesia, ataxia, fatigue, insomnia, tremors; paradoxical excitement, confusion, tremors, depression, decreased concentration. *CV:* tachycardia, chest pain, palpitations. *GI:* nausea, vomiting, diarrhea, constipation. *Eye:* blurred vision. *Ear:* tinnitus. *MS:* pain, tingling, weakness, cramps. *Misc:* sore throat, sweating, fever.

Nursing implications/Documentation

Possible nursing diagnoses: Potential for injury; Constipation.

- Record baseline blood pressure; monitor closely if dizziness is experienced. Supervise ambulation until response is determined.

- Be sure that doses are swallowed (not hoarded).

- Provide a quiet environment that is conducive to rest.

- Monitor bowel elimination and provide adequate fluids and fiber to prevent constipation; offer laxatives before the problem is severe.

Patient & family teaching/Home care

Possible nursing diagnoses: Anxiety; Fear; Ineffective individual coping; Impaired home maintenance management.

- Advise taking this drug with food to reduce GI symptoms.

- Help the individual identify stressors that contribute to anxiety and ways of coping effectively; stress that effective coping strategies can reduce the need for medication.

◆ Explain the importance of daily exercise in relieving stress, and encourage establishing a plan for getting enough exercise (e.g., daily walks).

◆ Point out that although this drug has not been known to produce tolerance and dependence, it should be used only when holistic measures (e.g., quiet music, relaxation techniques) are not effective.

◆ Emphasize that the effects of alcohol, other sedatives, and tranquilizers may not be predictable (these should be avoided).

◆ Advise avoidance of driving and other potentially hazardous activities until response is established.

- *See Antianxiety agents/Sedatives/Hypnotics overview for more information.*

busulfan

byoo-sul'fan

Myleran

Class: Antineoplastic (alkylating) agent

PEDS ✋ PREG D GERI ✋

Action Kills rapidly growing cells (cancer, hair follicles, bone marrow, GI lining, ova, and sperm) by interfering with DNA replication and RNA transcription through alkylation (cross-linking of DNA occurs). Is cell-cycle–phase nonspecific, affecting both actively dividing cells and dormant (resting) cells.

Use/Therapeutic goal/Outcome

Chronic myelogenous leukemia: Elimination or suppression of malignant cell proliferation. ***Outcome criteria:*** Tumor and disease regression or stabilization on radiologic and physical examination, reduction in spleen size; for leukemias, absence of blasts in peripheral blood specimen.

Dose range/Administration

Adult: PO: 4–8 mg daily until WBC falls to 15,000/mm^3. Discontinue until WBC rises to 50,000/mm^3. *Maintenance dose:* 1–3 mg daily. ***Child:*** PO: 0.06 to 0.12 mg/kg or 1.8 to 4.6 mg/m^2/day. Titrate to maintain WBC at 20,000/mm^3.

Clinical alert: Hold dose and report when WBC falls below 20,000/mm^3. WBC, platelets, and erythrocytes should nadir (drop to the lowest point) in 1 mo; recovery may take 1 month to 5 years.

Contraindications/Precautions

PREG D

Contraindicated in hypersensitivity to busulfan, and pre-existing pulmonary disease. ***Use with caution*** in previous radiation therapy, myelosuppressive drug therapy, or depressed neutrophil/platelet counts.

✋ **Contraindicated for pregnant or nursing mothers. Use with caution for children and the elderly.**

Side effects/Adverse reactions

Hypersensitivity: urticaria, fever, chills, tachycardia, hypotension. ***Hem:*** severe bone marrow depression, leukopenia (WBC falls in 2–3 wk), anemia, thrombocytopenia; agranulocytosis; hyperuricemia. ***GI:*** nausea, vomiting, diarrhea, cheilosis, glossitis, hepatic dysfunction and jaundice. ***GU:*** testicular atrophy, impotence, sterility, amenorrhea, and gynecomastia. ***Resp:*** pneumonitis, pulmonary fibrosis, or "busulfan lung" (rales, fever, persistent cough, and dyspnea). ***Skin:*** transient hyperpigmentation, alopecia. ***Misc:*** Addison-like wasting syndrome (melanoderma, apathy, confusion).

Nursing implications/Documentation

Possible nursing diagnoses: Potential for infection; Potential for injury; Fatigue; Altered oral mucous membrane; Fluid volume deficit; Diarrhea; Altered nutrition: less than body requirements.

- *See important nursing implications in Antineoplastic agents overview on page 72, which apply to all antineoplastics. The interventions that follow are additional and specific to this drug only.*

◆ Monitor for and report persistent cough, fever, rales, dyspnea, or chest pain (pulmonary fibrosis or "busulfan lung" may occur 4–6 months to 10 years after therapy begins).

◆ Maintain a fluid intake of 2–3 L per day to prevent renal tubular damage from hyperuricemia secondary to cell lysis.

Patient & family teaching/Home care

Possible nursing diagnoses: Knowledge deficit; Ineffective coping (individual and family); Hopelessness; Impaired home maintenance management.

- *See important Patient & family teaching in Antineoplastic agents overview on page 72, which apply to all antineoplastics. The* teachings that follow are additional and specific to this drug only.

♦ Advise that therapeutic response is usually seen in 1–2 weeks.

♦ Point out that drinking 2–3 L helps prevent kidney complications.

♦ Stress that persistent cough, dyspnea, or chest pain should be reported immediately.

♦ *See Antineoplastic agents overview for more information.*

butorphanol tartrate
byoo-tor'fa-nole

Stadol

Class: Narcotic analgesic

Antidote: Naloxone hydrochloride (Narcan)

PEDS	PREG	GERI
🤚	🤚	🤚

Action Alters both perception of and response to pain by binding with opiate receptor sites at numerous CNS sites. Its potent analgesic action is believed to be subcortical, possibly in the limbic system. Inhibits release of antidiuretic hormone (ADH) from hypothalamus. Has both narcotic agonist and antagonist potential.

Use/Therapeutic goal/Outcome

Moderate to severe pain: Relief of pain. **Outcome criteria:** Report of comfort; absence of observable signs of pain (grimacing, frowning, restlessness, reluctance to move or cough) with increase in signs of comfort (relaxed facial expression, decreased restlessness, improved ability to move or cough); blood pressure and pulse within normal limits when compared to baseline.

Preoperative medication: Promotion of relaxation, comfort. **Outcome criteria:** Report of feeling relaxed and comfortable; observable drowsiness or sleep.

Dose range/Administration

Interaction alert: Other narcotic analgesics may *decrease* analgesic effect. Alcohol, sedatives, hypnotics, other CNS depressants, antipsychotics, narcotics, and skeletal-muscle relaxants may increase effects.

Adult: IM: 1–4 mg q3-4h. IV: 0.5–2 mg q3-4h.

Clinical alert: Give IV doses slowly. SC route is not recommended. Use decreased dosage for the elderly and debilitated. Check respirations and blood pressure before giving butorphanol tar-

trate. Hold drug and report if respirations < 12, or if there is hypotension.

Contraindications/Precautions   PREG ⇊

Contraindicated in hypersensitivity to butorphanol tartrate and in narcotic-dependency. **Use with caution** in head injury, increased intracranial pressure, acute MI, coronary insufficiency, ventricular dysfunction, respiratory depression or disease, and hepatic or renal dysfunction.

⇊ **Use with caution for the elderly. Safe use for children and pregnant or nursing mothers has not been established (first 2 trimesters, preg B; in third trimester, preg D).**

Side effects/Adverse reactions

Hypersensitivity: itching, rash, anaphylaxis. **CNS:** sedation, headache, vertigo, lethargy, agitation, unusual dreams, euphoria, hallucinations. **Eye:** blurred vision. **CV:** increase or decrease in blood pressure. **Skin:** clamminess. **GI:** nausea.

Nursing implications/Documentation

Possible nursing diagnoses: Pain; Anxiety; Potential for injury.

♦ Have patient rate pain on a scale of 1–10 before and after medication is given; report and record inadequate pain control.

♦ Monitor closely for risk factors for injury; keep side rails up and supervise ambulation if allowed out of bed.

♦ Give pain medication before pain is severe.

♦ Be aware that psychic and physical dependence may develop; monitor emotionally unstable patients for anticipation of pain, rather that actual discomfort (providing reassurance may be all that is required).

♦ If side effect of nausea is experienced, place the individual in a recumbent position.

♦ For those who are narcotic-dependent, monitor for abstinence syndrome (withdrawal symptoms) because this drug has narcotic antagonist properties.

♦ For obstetrical use, place mother on fetal monitor and monitor mother and neonate for signs of respiratory depression.

Patient & family teaching/Home care

Possible nursing diagnoses: Sensory/perceptual alterations; Knowledge deficit.

- Explain the rationale for reporting pain or discomfort before it is severe.
- Stress the need to remain in bed until given permission to ambulate.
- Explain procedures briefly and in simple terms.
- Teach that lying down can prevent side effect of nausea.
- Warn that exceeding prescribed dose may cause overdose, dependence, and increased potential for abuse (instead of increasing dose regimen, unsatisfactory pain relief should be reported).
- *See Narcotic and non-narcotic analgesics overview for more information.*

caffeine

kaf-feen'

Caffedrine, Dexitac, No Doz, Quick Pep, Tirend, Vivarin

Class: Cerebral stimulant

PEDS	PREG	GERI
✋	B	✋

Action Produces central nervous system stimulation (causing respiratory stimulation, vasoconstriction, pupillary dilation, mental alertness, constriction of the urinary sphincter) by inhibiting phosphodiesterase, the enzyme that degrades c-AMP.

Use/Therapeutic goal/Outcome

Temporary relief of drowsiness and fatigue: Promotion of mental alertness. *Outcome criteria:* Report of feeling less drowsy or more alert; demonstration of ability to stay awake.

Neonatal apnea: Prevention of apnea episodes. *Outcome criteria:* Absence of periods of apnea; serum caffeine levels within therapeutic range (5–20 mg/l).

Dose range/Administration

Interaction alert: Use with theophylline or beta-adrenergic agonists may cause excessive CNS stimulation.

Cerebral Stimulant: **Adult:** PO: 100–200 mg anhydrous caffeine q4h prn. Daily dosage should not exceed 1 g.

Neonatal Apnea: **Neonate:** PO, IM, IV: loading dose of 5–10 mg/kg, followed by daily maintenance dose of 2.5–5 mg, depending upon infant tolerance and serum caffeine levels.

Clinical alert: Be aware that large doses may intensify severe drug-induced depression.

Contraindications/Precautions

Contraindicated in hypersensitivity or intolerance to caffeine or other xanthines, and in deep respiratory depression, ulcer disease, acute myocardial infarction, and fibrocystic breast disease.

✋ **Not recommended for children (except neonates, for apnea), or for pregnant or nursing mothers. Use with caution for the elderly.**

Side effects/Adverse reactions

Hypersensitivity: itching, rashes. *CNS:* insomnia, restlessness, hyperactivity, nervousness, headache, tremors, twitches. *CV:* palpitations, tachycardia. *GU:* diuresis. *GI:* nausea, vomiting, diarrhea.

Nursing implications/Documentation

Possible nursing diagnoses: Sleep pattern disturbance; Altered thought processes; Ineffective breathing pattern.

- Question about the use of beverages and OTC drugs that contain caffeine.
- Document if patient has a history of large amounts of caffeine intake (may explain other signs and symptoms).
- For neonates, monitor serum caffeine levels for therapeutic range 24 hours after loading dose, then 1–2 times per week; maintain on apnea monitor.

Patient & family teaching/Home care

Possible nursing diagnoses: Knowledge deficit; Impaired home maintenance management.

- Explain that caffeine has a high potential for psychological dependence and tolerance, and should be taken only occasionally when sleep is highly undesirable.
- Reinforce the benefits of sticking to a schedule for sleeping and staying awake, and of using holistic measures to promote alertness (e.g., exercise, cold water on face).
- Warn that when caffeine is withdrawn, headache may be experienced, but will subside in a few days.
- For neonate, explain to parents that caffeine stimulates respiration; ensure that the parents can demonstrate CPR before child goes home.
- *See Cerebral Stimulants overview for more information.*

calcifediol

kal-si-fe-dye'ole

Calderol

Class: Vitamin D analog, Parathyroid-like agent

PEDS	PREG	GERI
🖐	C	OK

Action Regulates serum calcium by stimulating GI absorption of calcium and by promoting reabsorption of calcium from bone to blood. Decreases parathyroid hormone production.

Use/Therapeutic goal/Outcome

Hypocalcemia/management of metabolic bone disease associated with chronic renal failure: Regulation of serum calcium levels. **Outcome criteria:** In the presence of normal albumin levels, normal serum calcium levels (8.5–10.5 mg/dl).

Dose range/Administration

Interaction alert: Do not give any preparations containing Vitamin D to anyone taking calcifediol (calcifediol is a metabolite of Vitamin D, so there is an increased risk of Vitamin D toxicity). Thiazide diuretics increase risk of hypercalcemia. Cholestyramine, colestipol, mineral oil, and corticosteroids may inhibit therapeutic effect.

Adult: PO: 300–350 mcg/wk in divided doses given daily or every other day; may increase dose q 4 wks; individualize depending on response. *Maintenance dose:* 50–100 mcg/day or 100–200 mcg qod.

Clinical alert: Effectiveness of therapy is dependent upon adequate daily intake of calcium (RDA 1000 mg; often a calcium supplement will be prescribed).

Contraindications/Precautions
PREG C

Contraindicated in hypersensitivity to calcifediol or to Vitamin D, and in hypercalcemia, hyperphosphatemia, and Vitamin D toxicity.

Use with caution in concurrent use of digitalis preparations, hypoparathyroidism, sarcoidosis, and renal and cardiac impairment.

🖐 **Use with caution for pregnant or nursing mothers and young children.**

Side effects/Adverse reactions

Hypersensitivity: rare. **Hem:** hypercalcemia, anemia. **GU:** proteinuria. **CNS:** ataxia. **Misc:** Vitamin D intoxication (drowsiness, dizziness, vertigo, weakness, headache, anorexia, nausea, vomiting, thirst, dry mouth, diarrhea, constipation, abdominal cramping, metallic taste, blurred vision, photophobia, conjunctivitis, bone or muscle pain, hypercalciuria, hyperphosphatemia, fever, nephrocalcinosis, weight loss).

Nursing implications/Documentation

Possible nursing diagnoses: Altered nutrition: less than body requirements; Potential for injury.

♦ Monitor serum calcium, phosphorus, magnesium, and alkaline phosphatase; BUN; creatinine; and 24-hr urinary calcium and phosphorus levels at least weekly during initial treatment because toxicity can occur rapidly (serum calcium times serum phosphate should not be greater than 70; a drop in serum alkaline phosphatase usually signals onset of hypercalcemia).

♦ Document and monitor daily weights and intake and output; report weight gain and positive balance.

♦ Be aware that patient is likely to be on fluid restrictions, sodium restrictions, and potassium restrictions because of renal failure.

♦ Assess environment for hazards to ambulation (because of risk of bone injury).

Patient & family teaching/Home care

Possible nursing diagnoses: Knowledge deficit; Impaired home maintenance management.

♦ Stress the importance of maintaining adequate calcium intake (RDA is 1000 mg/day; encourage dairy products, broccoli, nuts, whole grains, and legumes as good sources of calcium).

♦ Stress that symptoms of hypercalcemia (metallic taste, dry mouth, excessive thirst, anorexia, nausea, vomiting, cramps, diarrhea, constipation, bone pain, muscle weakness, headache, fatigue, ringing of the ears, changes in mental status, irregular pulse, increased respirations, light sensitivity of the eyes, or eye irritation) should be reported.

♦ Caution to take extra care with ambulating because of increased risk of bone injury.

♦ Warn that Vitamin D should be taken exactly as prescribed (because of seriousness of toxicity).

calcitonin

kal-si-toe'nin

human calcitonin: *Cibacalcin*

salmon calcitonin: *Calcimar, Miacalcin*

Class: Bone metabolism regulator, Parathyroid hormone antagonist

PEDS	PREG	GERI
✋	C	✋

Action Regulates bone metabolism by decreasing bone reabsorption and blood calcium levels and increasing deposits of calcium in the bones.

Use/Therapeutic goal/Outcome

Paget's disease, hypercalcemia, and postmenopausal osteoporosis: Promotion of formation of bone; reduction in serum calcium levels. *Outcome criteria:* After 6 months of treatment, normal serum calcium levels (8.5–10.5 mg/dl); report of decreased bone pain with X-ray evidence of decreased osteoporosis.

Dose range/Administration

Interaction alert: Vitamin D may antagonize calcitonin effects.

Hypercalcemia: *Adult:* SC, IM: 4 IU/kg salmon calcitonin q12h (rapidly absorbed; many patients achieve normal calcium levels in only a few days).

Postmenopausal osteoporosis: *Adult:* SC, IM: 100 IU/day salmon calcitonin.

Paget's disease of the bone: *Adult:* SC: 0.5 mg/day human calcitonin; if improvement achieved, reduce to 0.25 mg day or 2–3 times a week; some patients require up to 1 mg/day; or 100 IU/day salmon calcitonin. *Maintenance dose:* 50–100 IU qd or qod.

Clinical alert: Administer at bedtime to reduce nausea. Be aware that a skin test to test for hypersensitivity is usually given before first dose. If a red wheal appears within 15 minutes of administration, the drug should not be given (keep epinephrine handy). Human calcitonin is given when the patient has developed a resistance to salmon calcitonin; however, human calcitonin may have less efficacy because of antibody formation or hypersensitivity reactions.

Contraindications/Precautions

PREG C

Contraindicated in hypersensitivity to calcitonin or to the diluent used for reconstitution, or to fish proteins.

✋ **Contraindicated for children and nursing mothers. Use with caution for pregnant women and the elderly.**

Side effects/Adverse reactions

Hypersensitivity: rashes, dyspnea, anaphylaxis. **Skin:** facial and hand flushing (common, and usually passes after 1 hr); swelling, tingling, and tenderness of hands. **Hem:** hypercalcemia, hyperglycemia. **CNS:** headaches. **GI:** unusual taste in mouth; transient nausea, vomiting, anorexia, diarrhea. **GU:** transient diuresis.

Nursing implications/Documentation

Possible nursing diagnoses: Altered nutrition: more than body requirement; Potential for injury.

♦ Establish a baseline for urinary hydroxyproline excretion levels and for serum calcium, phosphorus, magnesium, and alkaline phosphatase; monitor every 3–6 months thereafter.

♦ Monitor for and report signs of hypocalcemia (muscle twitching and tetany may precede seizures) and for signs of hypercalcemic relapse (bone pain, renal calculi, nausea, vomiting, changes in mental status).

♦ Assess environment for hazards to ambulation (because of risk of bone injury).

Patient & family teaching/Home care

Possible nursing diagnoses: Knowledge deficit; Impaired home maintenance management.

♦ For women with osteoporosis, stress the importance of maintaining adequate calcium intake (RDA for calcium is 1000 mg/day, for Vitamin D, 400 IU; encourage dairy products as a good source of calcium and Vitamin D).

♦ Stress that symptoms of hypercalcemia (metallic taste, dry mouth, bone pain, muscle weakness, headache, fatigue, ringing of the ears, changes in mental status, irregular pulse, increased respirations, anorexia, nausea, vomiting, cramps, diarrhea, constipation) or hypocalcemia (muscle twitching, nervousness, changes in mental status) should be reported.

♦ Caution to take extra care with ambulating because of increased risk of bone injury.

calcitriol

kal-si-tree'ole

(1,25-dihydroxycholecalciferol): *Rocaltrol*

Class: Parathyroid-like agent, Calcium regulator, Vitamin D hormone

PEDS   PREG   GERI

Action Regulates serum calcium levels by increasing GI absorption of calcium and by promoting reabsorption of calcium from bone to blood.

Use/Therapeutic goal/Outcome

Hypocalcemia associated with chronic renal dialysis, hypoparathyroidism, and pseudohypoparathyroidism: Regulation of serum calcium. *Outcome criteria:* Normal serum calcium levels (8.5–10.5 mg/dl).

Dose range/Administration

Interaction alert: Do not give any preparations containing Vitamin D to anyone taking calcitriol (calcitriol is a metabolite of Vitamin D, so there is an increased risk of Vitamin D toxicity). Thiazide diuretics increase risk of hypercalcemia. Cholestyramine, colestipol HCL, mineral oil, and corticosteroids may inhibit therapeutic effect. Do not give concurrently with sucralfate or magnesium-containing antacids.

Hypocalcemia associated with chronic renal dialysis: **Adult:** PO: 0.25 mcg/day, increase 0.25 mcg/day at 2–8 wk intervals prn. *Maintenance dose:* 0.25 mcg qod. *Maximum dose:* 0.5–1.25 mcg/day. **Child:** PO: 0.25–2 mcg/day.

Hypoparathyroidism and pseudohypoparathyroidism: **Adult:** PO: 0.25 mcg/day, increase at 4–8 wk intervals prn. *Maintenance dose:* 0.25 mcg qod. *Maximum dose:* 2 mcg/day. **Child > 1 yr:** PO: 0.04–0.08 mcg/kg/day.

Clinical alert: Effectiveness of therapy is dependent upon adequate daily intake of calcium (RDA 1000 mg; often a calcium supplement will be prescribed).

Contraindications/Precautions

PREG

Contraindicated in hypersensitivity to calcitriol and in Vitamin D toxicity, hypercalcemia, and hyperphosphatemia. *Use with caution* in renal calculi or dysrhythmias.

Contraindicated for nursing mothers. Use with caution for pregnant women (low doses preg A; high doses preg D) and the elderly. Safe use for infants under 1 year has not been established.

Side effects/Adverse reactions

Hypersensitivity: rare. *Hem:* hypercalcemia. *Misc:* Vitamin D intoxication (drowsiness, dizziness, vertigo, weakness, headache, anorexia, nausea, vomiting, thirst, dry mouth, diarrhea, constipation, abdominal cramping, metallic taste, blurred vision, photophobia, conjunctivitis, bone or muscle pain, decreased bone development, hypercalciuria, hyperphosphatemia, polyuria, hematuria, fever).

Nursing implications/Documentation

Possible nursing diagnoses: Potential for injury; Altered nutrition: less than body requirements.

♦ Establish a baseline serum calcium, phosphorus, magnesium and alkaline phosphatase, and 24-hour urinary calcium and phosphorus; monitor at least weekly during initial treatment because toxicity can occur rapidly.

♦ Document and monitor daily weights and intake and output; report weight gain over 2 pounds or positive balance.

♦ Assess environment for hazards to ambulation (because of increased risk of bone injury).

Patient & family teaching/Home care

Possible nursing diagnoses: Knowledge deficit; Impaired home maintenance management.

♦ Emphasize the importance of maintaining adequate calcium intake (RDA is 1000 mg/day; encourage dairy products as a good source of calcium).

♦ Stress that symptoms of hypercalcemia (metallic taste, dry mouth, bone pain, muscle weakness, headache, fatigue, ringing of the ears, changes in mental status, irregular pulse, increased respirations, anorexia, nausea, vomiting, cramps, diarrhea, constipation) should be reported.

♦ Warn that this is the most potent form of Vitamin D available and that it should be taken exactly as prescribed (because of seriousness of toxicity).

♦ Advise taking care ambulating because of increased risk of bone injury.

calcium carbonate

Alka-Mints, Amitone, Calcilac, ♠Calcimax, Calglycine, ♣Cal-Sup, Chooz, Dicarbosil, ♠Effercal-600, Equilet, Genalac, Glycate, Gustalac, Mallamint, Os-Cal, Pama No.1, Rolaids Calcium Rich, Titracid, Titralac, Tums

Class: Antacid, Calcium supplement

PEDS	PREG	GERI
🖐	C	🖐

Action Neutralizes existing stomach acid; provides elemental calcium essential for bone and tooth mineralization, blood clotting, nerve impulse transmission, and muscle contraction.

Use/Therapeutic goal/Outcome

Hyperacidity: Reduction of acid concentration in stomach. **Outcome criteria:** Report of decreased pain and upper GI irritation.

Hypocalcemia: Maintenance or restoration of optimal calcium levels. **Outcome criteria:** Serum calcium levels within normal range and absence of signs and symptoms of hypocalcemia.

Dose range/Administration

Interaction alert: Do not give other oral medications for 2 hr after calcium carbonate to ensure their absorption. Separate doses of calcium carbonate from doses of enteric coated drugs by 1 hr (causes enteric coated drugs to be released while still in the stomach).

Adult: PO: 500 mg–2 g qid. **Child:** PO: Individualize dose.

Clinical alert: For antacid use, giving doses 1 hr after meals and at bedtime enhances therapeutic effects. Shake liquid form well before giving and follow with water or milk. After giving via nasogastric tube, flush with water.

Contraindications/Precautions

PREG C

Contraindicated in hypersensitivity to calcium products and in hypercalcemia, ventricular fibrillation, hypochlorhydria or history of renal calculi. **Use with caution** in renal impairment, decreased GI motility or obstruction, and dehydration or fluid restriction.

🖐 **Use with caution for children and the elderly.**

Side effects/Adverse reactions

Hypersensitivity: rare. **GI:** constipation, fecal impaction, abdominal cramping or pain;

rebound hyperacidity. **GU:** renal calculi. **Misc:** hypercalcemia, milk-alkali syndrome.

Nursing implications/Documentation

Possible nursing diagnoses: Constipation; Pain.

♦ For calcium supplementation, give with meals.

♦ Monitor bowel elimination pattern, especially in the elderly, to prevent and detect constipation.

♦ With high dose therapy, assess for symptoms of hypercalcemia (irritability, depression, weakness, increased urination) and renal calculi (difficult or painful urination).

Patient & family teaching/Home care

Possible nursing diagnoses: Knowledge deficit; Impaired home maintenance management.

♦ Teach the need to shake liquid form vigorously to achieve uniform suspension.

♦ Alert those on sodium restricted diet that some liquid forms may have high sodium content.

♦ Caution against taking calcium carbonate within 1 to 2 hr of taking other medicines by mouth.

♦ Point out that chewable tablets should be chewed well before swallowing and followed with water for maximum effectiveness.

♦ For ulcers, advise taking medication 1 to 3 hr after eating and at bedtime for best results.

♦ Advise to continue taking calcium carbonate under medical supervision for 4 to 6 weeks after ulcer symptoms have subsided.

♦ Inform those who self-medicate with antacids to seek medical advice if symptoms recur frequently or persist longer than 2 weeks.

♦ Warn not to exceed 1,500 mg calcium carbonate per day without specific medical direction.

♦ Caution those with history of kidney stones not to increase dietary or supplementary calcium without consulting physician.

♦ Teach post-menopausal women to decrease risk of osteoporosis by increasing dietary intake of calcium, avoiding smoking, limiting alcoholic beverages, and performing weight-bearing exercises regularly.

♦ Teach that spinach, rhubarb, bran and whole-grain cereals may interfere with the absorption of calcium.

* To avoid constipation, advise ample fluid intake, foods high in fiber, and regular exercise.

capreomycin
kap-ree-oh-mye'sin

capreomycin sulfate: **Capastat**

Class: Anti-infective, antibiotic (polypeptide), Antitubercular

PEDS	PREG	GERI
🖐	C	🖐

Action Limits tubercle bacilli and mycobacterial growth (bacteriostatic action); exact mechanism of action is unknown.

Use/Therapeutic goal/Outcome

Clinical tuberculosis (in combination with other drugs): Resolution of infection. *Outcome criteria:* Absence of acid-fast bacilli on sputum culture; improvement of X rays; decreased productive cough; temperature within normal range.

Dose range/Administration

Interaction alert: Aminoglycosides, colistin, or vancomycin may increase nephrotoxicity and ototoxicity; use together cautiously and monitor (should not be given with streptomycin, viomycin).

Adult: IM: 15 mg/kg/day (up to 1 g/day; to a maximum of 20 mg/kg/day) into a large muscle mass for 2–4 months, then 1 g 2–3 times a week for 12–24 months. Lower doses are used in kidney impairment.

Clinical alert: Wait 2–3 min after reconstituting to allow for complete dissolution of the drug, then draw up dose. Give **deep IM** only.

Contraindications/Precautions
PREG
C

Contraindicated in hypersensitivity to capreomycin. *Use with caution* in kidney, liver, or hearing impairment, multiple allergies, myasthenia gravis, and parkinsonism.

🖐 **Use with caution for the elderly. Safe use in children, infants, lactation, and pregnancy has not been established.**

Side effects/Adverse reactions

Hypersensitivity: itching, rash, fever. *Ear:* ototoxicity (tinnitis, hearing loss, dizziness). *GU:* nephrotoxicity (elevated BUN, decreased creatinine clearance, proteinuria, tubular necrosis; red and white blood cells and casts in urine). *GI:* hepatotoxicity. *CNS:* headache. *Hem:* eosinophilia, leukocytosis, leukopenia, hypokalemia, alkalosis. *Misc:* pain, bleeding, and sterile abscess at injection site.

Nursing implications/Documentation

Possible nursing diagnoses: Potential for infection; Fatigue; Activity intolerance; Fluid volume deficit.

* Ascertain that baseline CBC, BUN, creatinine, and liver function studies are obtained, and that necessary culture specimens are collected, before starting capreomycin; monitor periodically thereafter, depending on condition.

* Be aware of the risk of hypokalemia, and of kidney and liver toxicity (monitor lab studies closely and report abnormalities).

* Monitor and record intake and output and provide favorite fluids to ensure adequate hydration.

* Allow for a balance between rest and activity.

* Monitor for and report ear symptoms (tinnitis, dizziness, hearing loss).

Patient & family teaching/Home care

Possible nursing diagnoses: Knowledge deficit; Impaired home maintenance management.

* Stress the importance of taking this drug as prescribed without missing doses, and the importance of long-term medical follow-up to avoid relapses or complications.

* Warn to avoid alcohol to prevent liver toxicity.

* Encourage drinking at least 2 L of fluid a day to maintain adequate hydration.

* *See Anti-infectives overview for more information.*

captopril
kap'toe-pril

Capoten

Class: ★**Antihypertensive prototype**, Angiotensin converting enzyme (ACE) inhibitor

PEDS	PREG	GERI
🖐	C	🖐

Action Reduces blood pressure by acting on the renin-angiotensin system: Inhibits angiotensin converting enzyme (ACE), thereby blocking the conversion of angiotensin I to angiotensin II, which is a very potent vasoconstrictor that also stimulates aldosterone secretion (causing kidney to reabsorb sodium and water). Captopril thus prevents vasoconstriction and retention of sodium and water; and reduces peripheral vascular resistance (afterload), central venous pressure, and pulmonary capillary wedge pressure (preload).

Use/Therapeutic goal/Outcome

Moderate to severe hypertension not responsive to other drug therapies: Reduction of blood pressure. **Outcome criteria:** Blood pressure within normal range.

Congestive heart failure: Resolution of CHF. **Outcome criteria:** Clear lungs; absence of edema; improved exercise tolerance; reduction of CVP and PCWP; urine output > 30 cc/hr.

Dose range/Administration

Interaction alert: Antacids decrease captopril effects. Salicylates, indomethacin and other nonsteroidal anti-inflammatory agents may reduce antihypertensive effect. Nitrates, and ganglionic agents, may cause excessive hypotension. Avoid potassium supplements unless hypokalemia is proven.

Administer one hour before meals (food reduces absorption).

Hypertension: PO: 25 mg bid or tid; may increase after 1–2 weeks to 50 mg bid or tid if necessary. If desired effect in not seen, a diuretic is added; *maximum dose* 450 mg/day.

Congestive Heart Failure: Adult: PO: 6.25–12.5 mg tid; may increase daily as needed. *Maintenance dose:* 50–100 mg tid. Maximum dose is 450 mg/day.

Clinical alert: Patients with impaired renal function may require lower dosage (drug is excreted by the kidneys). Monitor closely for hyperkalemia.

Contraindications/Precautions

PREG
C

Contraindicated in hypersensitivity to any ACE inhibitor. **Use with caution** in impaired renal status, autoimmune disease, coronary or cerebrovascular disease, with drugs that cause leukopenia or agranulocytosis.

Contraindicated for pregnant women. Use with caution for the elderly. Safe use for children and nursing mothers has not been established. Captopril is excreted in breast milk.

Side effects/Adverse reactions

Hypersensitivity: urticaria, rash, maculopapular rash, angioedema of the face and extremities. **CV:** tachycardia, hypotension, angina pectoris,

CHF, pericarditis. **Hem:** leukopenia, pancytopenia, agranulocytosis, hyperkalemia. **CNS:** dizziness, fainting. **GU:** proteinuria, nephrotic syndrome, renal failure, membranous glomerulopathy. **GI:** loss of taste, anorexia. **Skin:** pruritis. **MS:** joint pain. **Misc:** fever.

Nursing implications/Documentation

Possible nursing diagnoses: Activity intolerance; Fatigue; Potential for injury.

◆ Assess mental status, and record pulse and blood pressure (lying, sitting, and standing, in both arms) before administration, and frequently thereafter until response is determined.

◆ Consult with physician to determine desired therapeutic range for blood pressure (be aware that some patients may require a slightly elevated blood pressure to perfuse vital organs).

◆ Ascertain that baseline CBC, electrolytes, BUN, creatinine, and liver function studies have been obtained before giving first dose; report abnormalities and monitor closely thereafter. WBC count should be performed every 2–3 weeks for the first 3 months, and periodically thereafter.

◆ Monitor for confusion, dizziness, tachycardia, or hypotension; hold drug and report immediately if these occur.

◆ Supervise ambulation until response is determined.

◆ Document and monitor daily weight and intake and output; report significant negative or positive balance.

Patient & family teaching/Home care

Possible nursing diagnoses: Knowledge deficit; Impaired home maintenance management.

◆ Explain the importance of taking medication exactly as prescribed, even when feeling well.

◆ Stress the importance of good medical follow-up, explain that this drug reduces "wear and tear" on blood vessels and improves longevity and health.

◆ Teach how to monitor pulse and blood pressure; emphasize that syncope, hypertension or hypotension, or persistent dizziness should be reported.

◆ Advise changing positions slowly to avoid dizziness.

◆ Encourage daily monitoring of weight and reporting sudden weight gain (frequently is fluid retention).

♦ Point out the need to report symptoms of sore throat, fever, or malaise, because they may indicate an abnormal WBC count.

♦ Warn against taking *any* OTC drugs without physician approval (some interactions can cause severe reactions).

♦ *See Antihypertensives overview for more information.*

carbamazepine

kar-ba-maz'e-pine

♣Apo-Carbazepine, Epitol, ♣Mazepine, Tegretol, ♣Tegretol CR, ♠Teril

Class: Anticonvulsant

PEDS	PREG	GERI
🖑	C	🖑

Action Limits seizure activity through an unclear mechanism: may inhibit high-frequency discharges near epileptic foci by altering the flux of sodium ions across neuronal cell membranes. Decreases pain of trigeminal neuralgia by reducing synaptic transmission within trigeminal nucleus. Is chemically related to the tricyclic antidepressants. Produces mild sedative, anticholinergic, muscle relaxant, and analgesic effects.

Use/Therapeutic goal/Outcome

Grand mal seizures, psychomotor seizures, temporal lobe epilepsy, seizure disorders unresponsive to other agents: Limitation of seizure activity. *Outcome criteria:* Marked decrease or absence of seizure activity.

Trigeminal neuralgia, glossopharyngeal neuralgia: Relief of pain. *Outcome criteria:* Report of improved comfort.

(Unlabeled use) Bipolar disorders, schizoaffective disorders, resistant schizophrenia: Promotion of reality orientation. *Outcome criteria:* Improved reality orientation and ability to perform self-care and interact appropriately.

Dose range/Administration

Interaction alert: Phenytoin, primidone, phenobarbital, and nicotinic acid may decrease carbamazepine blood levels and effect. MAO inhibitors may increase side effects. Propoxyphene, erythromycin, cimetidine, isoniazid, and calcium channel blockers may increase plasma levels and toxic effects of carbamazepine. May decrease blood levels and effects of phenytoin, oral anticoagulants, doxycycline, theophylline, haloperidol and oral anticoagulants. Give cau-

tiously with troleandomycin, which increases carbamazepine levels.

🌱 **Give with meals if GI distress is noted.**

Seizure: Adult/Child > 12 yrs: PO: 200 mg bid; may increase by 200 mg/day in divided doses given q6-8h. *Maximum dose:* 1 g daily for child 12–15 yrs old; 1200 mg daily for adult and child > 15 yrs old (usual range is 800–1200 mg/day). *Child 6–12 yrs:* PO: 10–20 mg/kg in 2–4 divided doses.

Trigeminal neuralgia: Adult: PO: 100 mg bid; increase by 100 mg increments q12h prn, to a maximum of 1200 mg/day (usual range is 200–400 mg bid).

Clinical alert: Available in chewable tablets and suspension; for suspension, expect lower and more frequent doses because it produces higher serum levels. Monitor serum carbamazepine levels closely (therapeutic range is 3–9 mcg/ml). Hematological and liver side effects can be severe: monitor for and report abnormal lab studies that may indicate bone marrow depression. Check CBC, platelet and reticulocyte count, and iron level weekly for the first 3 months, then every 3 months thereafter. Check urinalysis, BUN, and other liver function tests at least every 3 months.

Contraindications/Precautions

PREG C

Contraindicated in hypersensitivity to carbamazepine or tricyclic antidepressants, and in history of bone marrow depression. *Use with caution* in liver, kidney, or cardiovascular disease.

🖑 **Use with caution for the elderly. Safe use for children under 6 years and pregnant or nursing mothers has not been established.**

Side effects/Adverse reactions

Hypersensitivity: rash, urticaria. *Skin:* petechiae, exfoliative dermatitis, photosensitivity, alopecia, aggravated disseminated lupus erythematosus, Stevens-Johnson syndrome. *Hem:* aplastic anemia, agranulocytosis, thrombocytopenia. *CNS:* confusion, incoordination, speech disturbances, involuntary movement, visual hallucinations, depression, peripheral neuritis, paresthesia. *CV:* edema, congestive heart failure.

Nursing implications/Documentation

Possible nursing diagnoses: Potential for injury; Potential for aspiration.

♦ Document history of seizures (type, frequency, duration, usual time they occur, precipitating factors, presence of an aura); initiate seizure precautions as indicated.

- Keep an oral airway readily available.
- Monitor for and report signs of bone marrow depression (frequent infections, opportunistic infections, mouth ulcers, sore throat, fever).

Patient & family teaching/Home care

Possible nursing diagnoses: Fear; Self-esteem disturbance; Knowledge deficit; Impaired home maintenance management.

- Advise taking drug with meals if GI symptoms are noted.
- Stress the need for close medical follow-up; emphasize that anorexia, persistent fever, sore throat, mouth ulcers, infections, or easy bruising may be signs of side effects or excessive dosage that should be reported.
- Warn that stopping anticonvulsants suddenly can cause an increase in severity and frequency of seizures.
- Determine caregiver's ability to protect patient during a seizure; proceed with necessary teaching.
- Caution against driving until response is determined (may cause drowsiness at first).
- *If used for trigeminal neuralgia,* advise that attempts to stop or decrease drug should be tried every 3 months.
- *See Anticonvulsants overview for more information.*

carbenicillin
kar-ben-i-sill'in

carbenicillin disodium: ✦*Carbapen, Geopen, Pyopen*

carbenicillin indanyl sodium: *Geocillin,* ✦*Geopen Oral*

Class: ★Anti-infective (extended–spectrum penicillin) prototype, Antibiotic

PEDS	PREG	GERI
♨	B	♨

Action Extended-spectrum, usually bactericidal antibiotic; kills bacteria by inhibiting cell wall synthesis. Carbenicillin indanyl sodium is especially effective against *Pseudomonas* urinary tract infections.

Use/Therapeutic goal/Outcome

Carbenicillin disodium: Systemic infections caused by susceptible gram-positive and gram-negative organisms: Resolution of infection.

Outcome criteria: Absence of pathogenic growth on cultures, absence of clinical manifestations of infection (pain, redness, swelling, fever, odor, dysuria, drainage), normal WBC count, normal X rays.

Carbenicillin indanyl sodium: Urinary tract infections and prostatitis (indanyl sodium preparations not used for systemic infections because adequate blood levels are not achieved): Resolution of infection. **Outcome criteria:** Absence of pathogenic growth on cultures, absence of clinical manifestations of infection (pain, fever, odor, dysuria, frequency), normal WBC count, patient report of normal urination without pain.

Dose range/Administration

Interaction alert: Probenecid inhibits excretion of carbenicillin and may be given to increase serum levels of this drug. Inactivates aminoglycosides (e.g., gentamicin, tobramycin); do not mix together in solution; give carbenicillin 1 hour before aminoglycosides, preferably in a separate site. May potentiate action of anticoagulants because of antiplatelet effect.

- Give carbenicillin indanyl sodium 1–2 hours before or 2–3 hours after meals; food may inhibit absorption.

Carbenicillin disodium: Systemic infections: Adult: IM, IV: 4–5 g q6h. *Maximum dose:* 40 g/day. **Child:** IV: 50–500 mg/kg/day in divided doses q4-6h.

Gonorrhea: Adult: IM, IV: 4 g (IM, divide and administer at 2 injection sites). Give 30 min after oral administration of 1 g probenecid.

Carbenicillin indanyl sodium: Adult: PO: 382–764 mg q6h.

Clinical alert: With indanyl sodium form, report to physician if creatinine clearance ≤ 10 ml/min (drug may be discontinued).

Contraindications/Precautions
PREG B

Contraindicated in allergy to penicillin. **Use with caution** in cephalosporin sensitivity, history of allergic responses (e.g., other drugs, hay fever, asthma), hepatic or renal dysfunction, and sodium restriction.

- Use with caution for children, the elderly, and pregnant or nursing mothers. Safe use of indanyl sodium form for children has not been established.

Side effects/Adverse reactions

Hypersensitivity: itching, rashes, urticaria, fever, difficulty breathing, anaphylaxis. **GI:** nausea, vomiting, diarrhea, (indanyl sodium form) flatulence, cramps, unpleasant taste. **Hem:** anemia, thrombocytopenia, eosinophilia, leukopenia, hypernatremia, hyperkalemia (with indanyl sodium form, hypokalemia), slight elevation in SGOT and SGPT. **CV:** pain, redness, swelling, sterile abscess at injection site, thrombophlebitis. **GU:** (indanyl sodium form) vaginitis. **Misc:** superinfection, bone marrow depression.

Nursing implications/Documentation

Possible nursing diagnoses: Potential for infection; Diarrhea.

◆ Determine history of allergies, and (regardless of history) monitor closely for allergic reactions.

◆ Obtain baseline CBC, serum sodium, liver function studies, and necessary cultures before administering first dose; monitor closely thereafter if therapy is prolonged.

◆ Encourage fluids, and document and monitor intake and output, to ensure adequate hydration; report significant negative or positive balance.

◆ Monitor for and report signs of superinfection (sore throat, fever, fatigue, thrush, vaginal discharge, diarrhea).

◆ Report unusual bruising or bleeding (may be due to antiplatelet effect).

Patient & family teaching/Home care

Possible nursing diagnoses: Knowledge deficit; Impaired home maintenance management.

◆ Teach the importance of reporting allergic symptoms, diarrhea, signs and symptoms that do not abate, or *any* new signs and symptoms of discomfort that might indicate superinfection (medication regimen may have to be changed).

◆ Advise drinking 2–3 L of fluids daily to maintain adequate hydration (especially important if fever exists).

◆ Stress the importance of taking carbenicillin for the entire time prescribed, even if signs and symptoms abate.

◆ *See Anti-infectives overview for more information.*

carbidopa-levodopa

kar-bi-doe'pa

Sinemet

Class: Antiparkinsons, Dopaminergic agent

PEDS	PREG	GERI
✋	C	✋

Action Levodopa converts to dopamine (a neurotransmitter) in the extrapyramidal centers of the brain, restoring the depleted dopamine levels thought to cause Parkinsonian symptoms. Carbidopa prevents peripheral metabolism (decarboxylation) of levodopa, which makes more levodopa available to the brain. Addition of carbidopa decreases the required amount of levodopa by approximately 75 percent, and reduces the inhibitory effect of pyridoxine (Vitamin B6) on levodopa.

Use/Therapeutic goal/Outcome

Parkinsonism: Control of parkinsonian symptoms, promotion of mobility. **Outcome criteria:** Absence of or decrease in tremors, rigidity, akinesia and drooling; improvement in gait, balance, posture, speech, and handwriting.

Dose range/Administration

Interaction alert: If the patient has been taking levodopa, it should be discontinued for at least 8 hr before starting carbidopa-levodopa. Effects of this drug may be decreased by antipsychotics, benzodiazepines, phenytoin, Vitamin B6 (pyridoxine) and reserpine. Levodopa may enhance the effects of antihypertensive drugs, and the cardiovascular effects of sympathomimetic drugs such as amphetamine, ephedrine, and epinephrine (monitor for dysrhythmias). The therapeutic effects of levodopa may be potentiated by propranolol, methyldopa, and anticholinergic agents. Do not give concurrently with MAO inhibitors because of risk of tachycardia and hypertension. Monitor glucose levels of those taking oral hypoglycemics for hyperglycemia.

🖤 **Give shortly before meals to reduce GI side effects and enhance absorption.**

Adult: (The first number in dose refers to carbidopa; the second, to levodopa.) PO: 3–6 tablets daily of 25/100 carefully titrated; may increase to a maximum of 3–8 tablets of 25/250 mixture.

Clinical alert: Double-check Sinemet label for correct dose (available in ratios of 10/100, 25/100, and 25/250; some patients respond better to one ratio than another). Dosage is highly individualized, depending on clinical response and incidence of side effects (dose should be carefully titrated to lowest effective dose). Report muscle twitching and eyelid twitching immediately (may indicate toxicity).

Contraindications/Precautions

PREG
C

Contraindicated in hypersensitivity to carbidopa or levodopa, and in narrow angle glaucoma, melanoma, undiagnosed skin lesions, and psychosis. *Use with caution* in cardiovascular disease, renal disease, liver disease, respiratory disorders, asthma, seizures, diabetes, endocrine disorders.

☝ **Use with caution for the elderly (monitor closely for side effects). Safe use for pregnant or nursing mothers and for children has not been established.**

Side effects/Adverse reactions

No adverse reactions have been reported for carbidopa (side effects are due to levodopa). **Hypersensitivity:** rash, flushing. **CV:** orthostatic hypotension, tachycardia, hypertension. **GI:** anorexia, nausea, vomiting, abdominal pain, dry mouth, bitter taste, constipation, diarrhea, hepatotoxicity. **CNS:** involuntary movements, ataxia, muscle twitching, weakness, confusion, behavioral changes, insomnia, nightmares, depression. **Eye:** blurred vision, spasm or closing of eyelids. **GU:** urinary retention, incontinence, dark urine. **Skin:** dark-colored sweat. **Misc:** increased sexual drive.

Nursing implications/Documentation

Possible nursing diagnoses: Potential for injury; Impaired physical mobility; Fluid volume deficit.

◆ Establish a baseline profile of patient's abilities and disabilities to differentiate between desired responses and drug-induced side effects (keep in mind that side effects may be severe at first, but then should diminish).

◆ Recognize that the addition of carbidopa to levodopa is likely to decrease the required dose of levodopa by 75 percent, which also reduces the incidence of side effects.

◆ Monitor vital signs closely during periods of dose adjustment; record at least bid.

◆ For those on long-term therapy, check blood sugar, and liver and kidney function studies periodically.

◆ Have patient dangle legs before ambulating (because of risk of postural hypotension); supervise ambulation until response is determined.

Patient & family teaching/Home care

Possible nursing diagnoses: Self-care deficit; Impaired home maintenance management.

◆ Point out the need to take this drug shortly before meals to reduce GI side effects and enhance absorption; advise avoidance of high-protein foods.

◆ Caution not to increase or decrease doses without the physician's approval; stress the need for ongoing medical follow-up.

◆ Explain that more help with self-care may be needed until stabilized on dose regimen.

◆ Advise reporting muscle twitching or eyelid twitching, because this may indicate drug toxicity.

◆ Point out that multivitamins containing Vitamin B6 (pyridoxine) reverse the effects of Levodopa (check vitamin labels).

◆ *See Antiparkinsons overview for more information.*

carbinoxamine

kar-bin-nox'a-meen

carbinoxamine maleate: *Clistin*

Class: Antihistamine (H₁ receptor antagonist)

PEDS	PREG	GERI
☝	C	☝

Action Prevents but does not reverse histamine-mediated allergic responses by competing with histamine for H₁ receptors on effector cells. Has anticholinergic action.

Use/Therapeutic goal/Outcome

Allergic conditions: Decrease in allergic response. *Outcome criteria:* Report and demonstration of relief of allergic symptoms (sneezing, nasal secretions, itching).

Dose range/Administration

◆ **Dose should be individualized according to patient response and tolerance.**

Interaction alert: CNS depressants and alcohol may cause excessive sedation. Do not give with MAOIs or anticholinergics.

🖐 **Give with food or milk to avoid GI upset.**

Adult/Child > 12 yrs: PO: *Tablet, elixir:* 4–8 mg tid or qid. *Sustained-release tablet:* 8 or 12 mg

▶

q12h. ***Child 6–12 yrs:*** PO: *Tablets, elixir:* 4–6 mg tid or qid. ***Child 3–6 yrs:*** PO: *Tablets, elixir:* 2–4 mg tid or qid. ***Child 1–3 yrs:*** PO: *Elixir:* 2 mg tid or qid.

Clinical alert: Sustained-release tablets are not recommended for children. Expect reduced dosage for the elderly, and monitor for excessive sedation.

Contraindications/Precautions

PREG
C

Contraindicated in hypersensitivity to carbinoxamine or chemically related antihistamines, and within 14 days of treatment with MAOIs, in acute asthma, narrow-angle glaucoma, and obstructive prostatic hypertrophy. ***Use with caution*** in increased intraocular pressure, cardiovascular or renal disease, hypertension, history of asthma, hyperthyroidism, urinary retention, prostatic hypertrophy, and stenosing peptic ulcer.

🖑 **Contraindicated for children under 1 year and for nursing mothers. Avoid use for pregnant women. Use with caution for older children and the elderly.**

Side effects/Adverse reactions

Hypersensitivity: rash. ***CNS:*** sedation, stimulation, dizziness. ***Resp:*** thickening of bronchial secretions. ***GI:*** dry mouth, anorexia, GI distress, nausea. ***GU:*** urinary retention. ***Eye:*** blurred vision.

Nursing implications/Documentation

Possible nursing diagnoses: Potential for injury; Fluid volume deficit.

♦ Determine and record known allergies; provide an environment that is free from allergens (especially sleeping areas).

♦ Provide favorite fluids and ensure adequate hydration (2 liters/day).

Patient & family teaching/Home care

Possible nursing diagnoses: Knowledge deficit; Impaired home maintenance management.

♦ Advise taking this drug with food or milk if GI symptoms are experienced.

♦ Point out that avoiding pollens and staying in an air-conditioned environment may help reduce seasonal rhinitis.

♦ Emphasize that dose should not be increased without physician's approval; explain that tolerance may occur, requiring a change in medication.

♦ Warn that alcohol and other CNS depressants may cause excessive drowsiness; advise against driving until response is determined.

♦ Suggest that coffee or tea may reduce drowsiness, and that sugarless gum or hard candy may relieve dry mouth.

◆ *See Antihistamines overview for more information.*

carboplatin

car-bo-pla'tin

Paraplatin

Class: Antineoplastic (alkylating) agent

PEDS	PREG	GERI
🖑	D	🖑

Action Kills rapidly growing cells (cancer, hair follicles, bone marrow, GI lining, ova, and sperm) by interfering with DNA replication and RNA transcription through alkylation (cross-linking of DNA occurs). Is cell-cycle–phase nonspecific, affecting both actively dividing cells and dormant (resting) cells.

Use/Therapeutic goal/Outcome

Ovarian carcinoma (recurrent after chemotherapy with cisplatin), head and neck tumors, small-cell lung cancer, and seminoma: Elimination or suppression of malignant cell proliferation. ***Outcome criteria:*** Tumor and disease regression or stabilization on radiologic and physical examination.

Dose range/Administration

Interaction alert: Aminoglycosides increase the risk of nephrotoxicity and ototoxicity. Radiation therapy or other cytotoxic agents can cause severe myelosuppression.

Adult: IV: 360 mg/m² q 4 wk. Do not repeat if platelets <100,000/mm³.

Clinical alert: This drug should be given only by nurses who are knowledgeable in the comprehensive management of the administration of antineoplastic agents. Doses may vary at physician's discretion and are held until the patient sufficiently recovers from toxicities of previous doses. Protocols for drug preparation, administration, and accidental skin contamination must be followed. Gloves or double gloves must be worn when handling carboplatin (skin contamination may cause a local reaction). Contaminated areas should be washed with large amounts of soap and water. Carboplatin is a platinum-containing compound that causes less reactions than cisplatin. Needles or IV sets containing aluminum parts should not be used because interactions reduce carboplatin potency. This drug should be diluted in 50–100 ml D5W and given over 15–60 min.

Contraindications/Precautions

PREG
D

Contraindicated in hypersensitivity to carboplatin, cisplatin, mannitol (included in carboplatin preparation), or other platinum-containing compounds, and in preexisting renal or bone marrow damage (increased hematotoxicity). *Use with caution* in previous radiation or cytotoxic drug therapy.

✋ **Contraindicated for pregnant or nursing mothers. Use with caution for the elderly. Safe use for children has not been established.**

Side effects/Adverse reactions

Hypersensitivity: rash, urticaria, erythema, pruritus, bronchospasm, and hypotension. *GI:* nausea and vomiting (most severe for the first 24 hr); gastrointestinal pain; diarrhea and constipation; hepatotoxicity. *Hem:* delayed and cumulative anemia; leukopenia, neutropenia, and thrombocytopenia; significant bone marrow depression for those with impaired renal function (creatinine clearance <60 ml/min); decreased serum electrolyte values (Na+, K+, Ca+, and Mg+). *GU:* nephrotoxicity. *CNS:* peripheral neuropathies. *Ear:* ototoxicity. *Skin:* alopecia. *Misc:* pain and asthenia (related to tumor and anemia).

Nursing implications/Documentation

Possible nursing diagnoses: Potential for infection; Potential for injury; Fatigue; Altered oral mucous membrane; Fluid volume deficit; Diarrhea; Altered nutrition: less than body requirements.

◆ *See important Nursing implications in Antineoplastic agents overview on page 72, which apply to all antineoplastics. The interventions that follow are additional and specific to this drug only.*

◆ Have emergency drugs and equipment readily available to treat anaphylactic reactions.

◆ Monitor for and report early signs of peripheral neuropathy (numbness or tingling of extremities, muscle weakness, wristdrop, footdrop).

◆ Increase fluid intake to 2–3 L a day to prevent renal tubular damage from hyperuricemia secondary to cell lysis.

◆ Obtain baseline and periodic audiometric testing and neurologic function studies.

◆ Expect WBC and platelet count to drop to the lowest point after 21 days, with recovery in 30 days after dose; granulocyte nadir occurs at 21–28 days with recovery by day 35.

◆ Be aware that therapeutic response is often accompanied by toxicity.

Patient & family teaching/Home care

Possible nursing diagnoses: Knowledge deficit; Ineffective coping (individual and family); Hopelessness; Impaired home maintenance management.

◆ *See important Patient & family teaching in Antineoplastic agents overview on page 72, which apply to all antineoplastics. The teachings that follow are additional and specific to this drug only.*

◆ Point out that drinking 2–3 L a day helps prevent kidney complications.

◆ Explain that numbness or tingling of extremities, muscle weakness, wristdrop, footdrop, or problems with balance should be reported.

◆ *See Antineoplastic agents overview for more information.*

carisoprodol

kar-eye-soe-proe'dole

Rela, Sodol, Soma, Soprodol, Soridol
Class: Skeletal-muscle relaxant (centrally acting), Analgesic, Antispasmodic

PEDS	PREG	GERI
✋	C	✋

Action Relaxes skeletal muscle without loss of voluntary muscle function by inhibiting synaptic reflexes centrally in the descending reticular formation and in the spinal cord.

Use/Therapeutic goal/Outcome

Muscle spasm associated with bursitis, low back disorders, contusions, fibrositis, spondylitis, sprains, muscle strains and cerebral palsy: Promotion of mobility; improved comfort. *Outcome criteria:* Increased range of motion and ability to perform activities of daily life; report of relief of pain, anxiety, and tension.

Dose range/Administration

Interaction alert: CNS depressants, psychotropic drugs, and alcohol increase CNS effects.

🖤 **Give with food to reduce GI symptoms.**

Adult: PO: 350 mg tid and at bedtime.

Clinical alert: Monitor for allergic reactions, especially between first and fourth doses. Give last dose at bedtime to reduce GI symptoms.

Contraindications/Precautions

PREG C

Contraindicated in hypersensitivity to carisoprodol, meprobamate, tybamate, and tartrazine, and in acute intermittent porphyria or suspected porphyria. **Use with caution** in impaired liver or kidney function and addiction-prone individuals.

ᘒ Use with caution for the elderly. Safe use for children and pregnant or nursing mothers has not been established.

Side effects/Adverse reactions

Hypersensitivity: itching, rashes, fever, angioedema, anaphylaxis. **CNS:** drowsiness, dizziness, ataxia, visual disturbances, agitation, tremor, transient quadriplegia, confusion. **GI:** nausea, vomiting, hiccups, epigastric distress. **CV:** orthostatic hypotension, facial flushing, tachycardia. **Resp:** asthmatic reaction.

Nursing implications/Documentation

Possible nursing diagnoses: Impaired physical mobility; Potential for injury; Pain.

♦ Monitor comfort level and range of motion before and after dose is given.

♦ Document physiologic and psychologic response because psychologic dependence may develop.

♦ If therapy is prolonged, do not stop carisoprodol abruptly because withdrawal symptoms (headache, abdominal cramps, or insomnia) may occur.

♦ Supervise out-of-bed activities, especially if drowsiness is present.

Patient & family teaching/Home care

Possible nursing diagnoses: Impaired home maintenance management; Knowledge deficit.

♦ Advise taking doses with food and last dose at bedtime to avoid GI upset.

♦ Warn against activities requiring alertness, although drowsiness may be transient.

♦ Stress avoidance of alcohol and other depressants.

♦ Advise to stop drug and contact physician if side effects develop (rash, blurred vision, dizziness).

♦ Explain the importance of following total plan of treatment, including rest, other forms of therapy, and prescribed dose of drug.

♦ Caution to change position slowly to avoid hypotensive episode and resulting dizziness.

♦ *See Skeletal-muscle relaxants overview for more information.*

carmustine

kar-mus'teen

BCNU: *BiCNU*

Class: Antineoplastic (nitrosourea alkylating) agent

PEDS	PREG	GERI
ᘒ	D	ᘒ

Action Kills rapidly growing cells (cancer, hair follicles, bone marrow, GI lining, ova, and sperm) by interfering with DNA replication and RNA transcription through alkylation (cross-linking of DNA occurs). Is cell-cycle–phase nonspecific, affecting both actively dividing cells and dormant (resting) cells.

Use/Therapeutic goal/Outcome

Primary and metastatic brain tumors; lung, colon, and stomach cancers; Hodgkin's disease and non-Hodgkin's lymphomas; hepatomas; multiple myeloma (in combination with prednisone); and melanomas: Elimination or suppression of malignant cell proliferation. **Outcome criteria:** Tumor and disease regression or stabilization on radiologic and physical examination.

Dose range/Administration

Interaction alert: Aminoglycosides increase the risk of nephrotoxicity and ototoxicity. Cimetidine, radiation therapy, or other cytotoxic agents can cause severe myelosuppression. Vitamin A or caffeine enhances the drug's cellular uptake.

Adult: IV: 75–100 mg/m^2/day (over 1–2 hr) for 2 days; or 200 mg/m^2 as a single dose q 6–8 wk; or 40 mg/m^2/day for 5 days q 6 wk while platelets >100,000/mm^3 and WBC >4000/mm^3. Dosage reduced 50% if platelets <75,000–100,000/mm^3 or WBC <3,000–4,000/mm^3.

Clinical alert: This drug should be given only by nurses who are knowledgeable in the comprehensive management of the administration of antineoplastic agents. Doses may vary at physician's discretion and are held until the patient has recovered sufficiently from toxicities of previous doses. Protocols for drug preparation, administration, and accidental skin contamination must be followed. Gloves or double gloves must be worn when handling carmustine (skin contamination may cause a local reaction). Contaminated areas should be washed with large amounts of soap and water. Carmustine should be diluted in 150–500 ml D5W in a *glass* bottle only and given over 1–2 hr. Do not use a powder that is oily (indicates drug decomposition).

Contraindications/Precautions

PREG D

Contraindicated in hypersensitivity to carmustine and in pulmonary fibrosis (pulmonary toxicity can be fatal), and severe leukopenia or thrombocytopenia (hematologic toxicity is cumulative). ***Use with caution*** in preexisting liver/kidney disorders (increased incidence of hepatic and renal toxicity).

Contraindicated for pregnant or nursing mothers. Use with caution for the elderly. Safe use for children has not been established.

Side effects/Adverse reactions

Hypersensitivity: urticaria, hypotension, anaphylaxis. ***Hem:*** delayed and cumulative myelosuppression 4–5 weeks after dose (thrombocytopenia, leukopenia, anemia). ***GI:*** nausea and vomiting 2–4 hr after giving (dose related, may last for 6 hr); stomatitis; hepatotoxicity. ***GU:*** nephrotoxicity; hyperuricemia in lymphoma patients (rapid cell lysis). ***Resp:*** pulmonary fibrosis with prolonged therapy. ***Eye:*** ophthalmic infarctions and retinal hemorrhage with high doses. ***Skin:*** transient hyperpigmentation of skin with accidental contact of drug solution; pain, burning, and inflammation at injection site.

Nursing implications/Documentation

Possible nursing diagnoses: Potential for infection; Potential for injury; Fatigue; Altered oral mucous membrane; Fluid volume deficit; Diarrhea; Altered nutrition: less than body requirements.

- *See important Nursing implications in Antineoplastic agents overview on page 72, which apply to all antineoplastics. The interventions that follow are additional and specific to this drug only.*
  - Monitor for and report early signs of pulmonary toxicity (persistent cough, dyspnea, chest pain).
  - Increase fluid intake to 2–3 L a day to prevent renal tubular damage from hyperuricemia secondary to cell lysis.
  - Expect WBC and platelets to drop to the nadir (lowest point) at 4–6 weeks.
  - Be aware that therapeutic response is often accompanied by toxicity.

Patient & family teaching/Home care

Possible nursing diagnoses: Knowledge deficit; Ineffective coping (individual and family); Hopelessness; Impaired home maintenance management.

- *See important Patient & family teaching in Antineoplastic agents overview on page 72, which apply to all antineoplastics. The teachings that follow are additional and specific to this drug only.*
  - Point out that drinking 2–3 L a day helps prevent kidney complications.
  - Instruct to report nonproductive cough, dyspnea, or chest pain.
- *See Antineoplastic agents overview for more information.*

carteolol

cart-te-o'lole

Cartrol

Class: Nonselective beta-adrenergic blocking agent, Antihypertensive

PEDS	PREG	GERI
✋	C	✋

Action Reduces blood pressure and heart rate by blocking beta-1 (cardiac) and beta-2 adrenergic receptors. Also reduces effect of adrenergic stimulation of myocardial excitability and AV-node conduction velocity. Has intrinsic sympathomimetic activity, but no significant membrane-stabilizing activity.

Use/Therapeutic goal/Outcome

Hypertension: Reduction of blood pressure. ***Outcome criteria:*** Blood pressure within normal limits.

Dose range/Administration

Interaction alert: Other antihypertensives may potentiate hypotensive effects. General anesthetics may exaggerate hypotension, bradycardia; nonsteroidal antiinflammatory agents, especially indomethacin, can decrease antihypertensive effects.

Hypertension: Adult: PO: 2.5 mg/day; gradually increase to 5–10 mg/day. *Maintenance dose:* 2.5–5 mg/day.

Clinical alert: When discontinuing, wean over a 1–2 week period to avoid precipitating thyroid storm, angina, or myocardial infarction. Be aware that patients taking this drug may not exhibit tachycardia as a symptom of fever, hypoglycemia, or hyperthyroidism.

Contraindications/Precautions

PREG
C

Contraindicated in hypersensitivity to carteolol, and in cardiogenic shock, sinus bradycardia, second- or third-degree heart block (PR interval > 0.24 seconds), CHF, COPD, bronchial asthma. **Use with caution** in patients with diabetes, hyperthyroidism, and renal impairment.

✋ Use with caution for the elderly. Safe use for children and pregnant and nursing mothers has not been established.

Side effects/Adverse reactions

Hypersensitivity: rash, pruritis. **CV:** bradycardia, hypotension, CHF, peripheral vascular disease. **CNS:** weakness; dizziness; fatigue; insomnia; paresthesia; abdominal, back, and chest pain. **Resp:** increased airway resistance. **GI:** nausea, vomiting, diarrhea. **GU:** decreased sexual ability. **MS:** arthralgia, muscle cramps, cold hands and feet. **Hem:** hypoglycemia. **Misc:** fever.

Nursing implications/Documentation

Possible nursing diagnoses: Activity intolerance; Fatigue; Potential for injury.

◆ Assess mental status and record pulse and blood pressure (if possible, lying, sitting, and standing, in both arms) prior to administration, and frequently thereafter until response is determined.

◆ Consult with physician to determine desired therapeutic range for blood pressure and heart rate (parameters for withholding the medication should be written by physician).

◆ Ascertain that baseline CBC, electrolytes, BUN, creatinine, and liver function studies are obtained before giving first dose; report abnormalities and monitor closely thereafter.

◆ Monitor for allergic reactions and signs of confusion, dizziness, bradycardia, CHF, and or hypotension; hold drug and report immediately if these occur.

◆ Supervise ambulation until response is determined.

◆ Document and monitor daily weight, and intake and output; report significant negative or positive balance.

Patient & family teaching/Home care

Possible nursing diagnoses: Knowledge deficit; Impaired home maintenance management; Altered sexuality patterns.

◆ Explain the importance of taking this drug exactly as prescribed, even when feeling well; warn not to discontinue drug abruptly (may precipitate angina).

◆ Stress importance of medical follow-up; explain that this drug decreases "wear and tear" on blood vessels, reduces the workload of the heart, and improves longevity and health.

◆ Teach how to monitor pulse and blood pressure; emphasize that syncope, hypertension or hypotension, or persistent dizziness should be reported; provide pulse and blood pressure parameters for withholding medication.

◆ Advise changing positions slowly to avoid dizziness.

◆ Encourage daily monitoring of weight, and reporting sudden weight gain (frequently is fluid retention).

◆ Warn against drinking alcohol or taking *any* OTC drugs without physician approval (some interactions can cause severe reactions).

◆ Advise against excessive exposure to cold; point out that persistent cold feet or hands should be reported.

◆ Explain that this drug may alter sexual activity; counsel about concerns.

◆ *See Beta Adrenergic Blockers and Antihypertensives overviews for more information.*

cascara sagrada

kas-kar'a

cascara sagrada
cascara sagrada aromatic fluid extract
cascara sagrada fluid extract
Class: Stimulant laxative

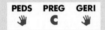

PEDS	PREG	GERI
✋	C	✋

Action Increases peristalsis by direct effect on the nerve supply of the smooth muscles of the intestine; promotes fluid and ion accumulation in colon.

Use/Therapeutic goal/Outcome

Constipation and preparation for surgery or diagnostic studies: Evacuation of fecal material from colon. *Outcome criteria:* Forceful bowel evacuation (within 6–12 hr).

Dose range/Administration

Interaction alert: May interfere with the effectiveness of potassium-sparing diuretics or potassium supplements by promoting potassium loss through intestinal tract.

Adult: PO: *Tablets:* 325 mg. *Fluid extract:* 1 ml. *Aromatic fluid extract:* 5 ml. *Child > 2 yrs:* PO: 1/2 adult dose. *Child < 2 yrs:* PO: 1/4 adult dose.

Contraindications/Precautions
PREG C

Contraindicated in hypersensitivity to stimulant laxatives, and in symptoms of appendicitis or intestinal obstruction, undiagnosed rectal bleeding, and those with a colostomy or ileostomy.

Use with caution for children under 6 years, pregnant or nursing mothers, and the elderly.

Side effects/Adverse reactions

Hypersensitivity: rash, difficulty breathing. *GI:* nausea, abdominal cramping, diarrhea. *MS:* muscle weakness. *Skin:* irritation around rectal area. *Misc:* hypokalemia, fluid and electrolyte imbalance, laxative dependence.

Nursing implications/Documentation

Possible nursing diagnoses: Impaired skin integrity; Diarrhea; Pain.

◆ Give cascara sagrada with a full glass of water at bedtime, unless otherwise instructed.

◆ Assess for abdominal distention and bowel sounds.

◆ Monitor and document frequency, appearance, and amount of stool evacuated.

◆ Monitor perianal area and provide appropriate measures for good hygiene.

◆ Expect side effects to be more frequent or severe in the elderly.

Patient & family teaching/Home care

Possible nursing diagnoses: Knowledge deficit; Impaired home maintenance management.

◆ Caution to follow directions and precautions printed on packaging.

◆ Advise that liquid preparations are more reliable than tablets and that the aromatic fluid is less active, but more palatable, than nonaromatic.

◆ Inform that urine and feces may become yellowish or reddish–brown in color.

◆ For nursing mothers, point out that brown discoloration of breast milk may be seen and that diarrhea may occur in infant.

◆ Teach that regular use of cascara sagrada can cause laxative dependence and loss of essential electrolytes, especially in the elderly.

◆ Stress the importance of regular toileting routine, dietary bulk, fluids, and exercise in preventing constipation.

◆ *See Laxatives overview for more information.*

cefaclor
sef'a-klor

Ceclor

Class: Anti-infective, Antibiotic, Cephalosporin (second generation)

PEDS 🖐 **PREG B** **GERI** 🖐

Action Broad-spectrum bactericidal antibiotic; kills bacteria by inhibiting cell wall synthesis.

Use/Therapeutic goal/Outcome

Infections (respiratory, skin, soft tissue, ear): Prevention or resolution of infection. *Outcome criteria:* Absence of pathogenic growth on cultures, absence of clinical manifestations of infection (fever, pain, swelling, redness, heat, odor, drainage, productive cough, dysuria), normal X rays, normal WBC count.

Dose range/Administration

Interaction alert: Probenecid inhibits excretion; lower doses may be indicated.

Give with meals if GI distress occurs.

Contraindications/Precautions
PREG B

Contraindicated in hypersensitivity to cefaclor or to other cephalosporins. *Use with caution* in penicillin allergy and impaired renal function.

Use with caution for pregnant or nursing mothers and the elderly. Safe use for infants under 1 month has not been established.

Side effects/Adverse reactions

Hypersensitivity: Itching, rashes, eosinophilia, joint pain or swelling, fever, angioedema, difficulty breathing, anaphylaxis, serum sickness-like reactions. **GI:** nausea, vomiting, anorexia, diarrhea, pseudomembranous colitis. **CNS:** Dizziness, headache. **GU:** vaginitis, nephrotoxicity (increased BUN and creatinine). **Hem:** thrombocytopenia, positive direct Coombs' test, slight elevation in SGOT, SGPT. **Misc:** superinfection.

Nursing implications/Documentation

Possible nursing diagnoses: Potential for infection; Fluid volume deficit.

♦ Determine history of allergies, and (regardless of history) monitor closely for allergic reactions.

♦ Obtain baseline CBC, creatinine, liver function studies, and necessary cultures before administering first dose; monitor closely thereafter if therapy is prolonged.

♦ Encourage fluids, and monitor and document intake and output, to ensure adequate hydration; report significant negative or positive balance.

♦ Monitor for and report signs of superinfection (sore throat, fever, fatigue, thrush, persistent diarrhea, vaginal discharge).

Patient & family teaching/Home care

Possible nursing diagnoses: Knowledge deficit; Impaired home maintenance management.

♦ Teach the importance of reporting allergic symptoms, persistent diarrhea, signs and symptoms that do not abate, or *any* new signs and symptoms of discomfort that might indicate superinfection (medication regimen may have to be changed).

♦ Advise drinking 2–3 L of fluids daily to maintain adequate hydration (especially important if fever exists).

♦ Stress the importance of taking antibiotics for the entire time prescribed, even if signs and symptoms abate.

♦ If GI distress occurs, advise taking drug with food.

♦ *See Anti-infectives overview for more information.*

cefadroxil
sef-a-drox'ill

cefadroxil monohydrate: **Duricef, Ultracef**

Class: Anti-infective, Antibiotic, Cephalosporin (first generation)

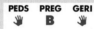

PEDS	PREG	GERI
✋	B	✋

Action Broad-spectrum, usually bactericidal, antibiotic; kills bacteria by inhibiting cell wall synthesis.

Use/Therapeutic goal/Outcome

Infections (urinary, skin and soft tissue, throat): Prevention or resolution of infection. **Outcome criteria:** Absence of pathogenic growth on cultures, absence of clinical manifestations of infection (fever, pain, swelling, redness, heat, odor, drainage, productive cough, dysuria), normal chest X rays, normal WBC count.

Dose range/Administration

Interaction alert: Probenecid decreases excretion; cefadroxil dosage may be decreased. Monitor for increased toxicity if given with aminoglycocides.

🍴 **Give with meals if GI distress occurs.**

Adult: PO: 1–2 g/day in a single dose or bid, depending on severity of infection. **Child:** PO: 30 mg/kg/day in divided doses q12h.

Clinical alert: Dosage in impaired renal function should be adjusted according to creatinine clearance to prevent drug accumulation.

Contraindications/Precautions
PREG B

Contraindicated in hypersensitivity to cefadroxil or to cephalosporins. **Use with caution** in penicillin sensitivity and impaired renal function.

✋ **Use with caution for children, pregnant women, and the elderly. Safe use for nursing mothers has not been established.**

Side effects/Adverse reactions

Hypersensitivity: itching, rashes, eosinophilia, joint pain or swelling, fever, angioedema, difficulty breathing, anaphylaxis, serum sickness-like reactions. **GI:** nausea, vomiting, diarrhea, pseudomembranous colitis. **CNS:** dizziness, headache, fatigue. **GU:** vaginitis, nephrotoxicity (increased BUN and creatinine). **Hem:** thrombocytopenia, eosinophilia, positive direct Coombs' test, slight elevation in SGOT, SGPT. *Misc:* superinfection.

Nursing implications/Documentation

Possible nursing diagnoses: Potential for infection; Fluid volume deficit.

♦ Determine history of allergies, and (regardless of history) monitor closely for allergic reactions.

♦ Obtain baseline CBC, creatinine, liver function studies, and necessary cultures before administering first dose; monitor closely thereafter if therapy is prolonged.

♦ Encourage fluids, and record and monitor intake and output, to ensure adequate hydration; report significant negative or positive balance.

♦ Monitor for and report signs of superinfection (sore throat, fever, persistent diarrhea, fatigue, thrush, vaginal discharge).

Patient & family teaching/Home care

Possible nursing diagnoses: Knowledge deficit; Impaired home maintenance management.

♦ Teach the importance of reporting allergic symptoms, persistent diarrhea, signs and symptoms that do not abate, or *any* new signs and symptoms of discomfort that might indicate superinfection (medication regimen may have to be changed).

♦ Advise drinking 2–3 L of fluids daily to maintain adequate hydration (especially important if fever exists).

♦ Stress the importance of taking antibiotics for the entire time prescribed, even if signs and symptoms abate.

♦ If GI distress occurs, advise taking drug with food.

♦ *See Anti-infectives overview for more information.*

cefamandole
sef'a-man'dole

cefamandole nafate: *Mandol*

Class: Anti-infective, Antibiotic, Cephalosporin (second generation)

PEDS	PREG	GERI
⍦	B	⍦

Action Broad-spectrum, usually bactericidal, antibiotic; kills bacteria by inhibiting cell wall synthesis.

Use/Therapeutic goal/Outcome

Severe infections (respiratory, GU, skin and soft tissue, bone and joint, blood, peritoneum): Prevention or resolution of infection. *Outcome criteria:* Absence of pathogenic growth on cultures, absence of clinical manifestations of infection (fever, pain, swelling, redness, heat, odor, drainage, productive cough, dysuria), normal X rays, normal WBC count.

Dose range/Administration

Interaction alert: Do not mix IV with aminoglycosides or vancomycin. Probenecid inhibits excretion of cefamandole; lower doses may be indicated. Alcohol may cause nausea, vomiting, flushing, throbbing headache, hypotension.

Adult: IV, Deep IM: 250 mg–1 g q6-8h. *Maximum dose:* 12 g/day for severe infections.

Child > 1 mo: IV, Deep IM: 50–100 mg/kg in divided doses. *Maximum dose:* 150 mg/kg/day.

Contraindications/Precautions
PREG
B

Contraindicated in hypersensitivity to cefamandole or to cephalosporins. *Use with caution* in penicillin allergy and impaired renal function.

⍦ Use with caution for pregnant women and the elderly. Safe use for infants under 1 month and nursing mothers has not been established.

Side effects/Adverse reactions

Hypersensitivity: itching, rashes, eosinophilia, joint pain or swelling, fever, angioedema, difficulty breathing, anaphylaxis, serum sickness-like reactions. *GI:* anorexia, nausea, vomiting, diarrhea, pseudomembranous colitis. *CV:* pain, redness, swelling, thrombophlebitis at injection site. *CNS:* dizziness, headache, fatigue. *GU:* vaginitis, nephrotoxicity (increased BUN and creatinine). *Hem:* thrombocytopenia, positive direct Coombs' test, slight elevation in SGOT, SGPT. *Misc:* superinfection.

Nursing implications/Documentation

Possible nursing diagnoses: Potential for infection; Fluid volume deficit.

♦ Determine history of allergies, and (regardless of history) monitor closely for allergic reactions.

♦ Obtain baseline CBC, creatinine, liver function studies, and necessary cultures before administering first dose; monitor closely thereafter if therapy is prolonged.

• Encourage fluids, and record and monitor intake and output, to ensure adequate hydration; report significant negative or positive balance.

• Monitor for and report signs of superinfection (sore throat, fever, persistent diarrhea, fatigue, thrush, vaginal discharge).

Patient & family teaching/Home care

Possible nursing diagnoses: Knowledge deficit; Impaired home maintenance management.

• Teach the importance of reporting allergic symptoms, persistent diarrhea, signs and symptoms that do not abate, or *any* new signs and symptoms of discomfort that might indicate superinfection (medication regimen may have to be changed).

• Advise drinking 2–3 L of fluids daily to maintain adequate hydration (especially important if fever exists).

• Stress the importance of taking antibiotics for the entire time prescribed, even if signs and symptoms abate.

• Caution that drinking alcohol may cause severe nausea, vomiting, headache, palpitations.

• *See Anti-infectives overview for more information.*

cefazolin

sef'a-zoe-lin

cefazolin sodium: *Ancef, Kefzol*

Class: ★Anti-infective first-generation cephalosporin prototype, Antibiotic

PEDS	PREG	GERI
⚘	**B**	⚘

Action Broad-spectrum, usually bactericidal, antibiotic; kills bacteria by inhibiting cell wall synthesis.

Use/Therapeutic goal/Outcome

Serious infections (respiratory, GU, skin and soft tissue, bone and joint, blood, heart): Prevention or resolution of infection. *Outcome criteria:* Absence of pathogenic growth on cultures, absence of clinical manifestations of infection (fever, pain, swelling, redness, heat, odor, drainage, productive cough, dysuria), normal X rays, normal WBC count.

Dose range/Administration

Interaction alert: Do not mix IV with aminoglycosides or vancomycin. Probenecid inhibits

excretion of cefazolin; lower doses may be indicated. Alcohol may cause nausea, vomiting, flushing, throbbing headache, hypotension.

Adult: IV, Deep IM: 250 mg–1 g q6-8h. *Maximum dose:* 12 g/day for severe infections.
Child > 1 mo: IV, Deep IM: 25–50 mg/kg in divided doses. *Maximum dose:* 100 mg/kg/day.

Contraindications/Precautions

PREG
B

Contraindicated in allergy to the drug or to cephalosporins. **Use with caution** in penicillin allergy and impaired renal function.

⚘ **Use with caution for pregnant women and the elderly. Safe use for infants under 1 month and nursing mothers has not been established.**

Side effects/Adverse reactions

Hypersensitivity: itching, rashes, eosinophilia, joint pain or swelling, fever, angioedema, difficulty breathing, anaphylaxis, serum sickness-like reactions. **GI:** anorexia, nausea, vomiting, diarrhea, pseudomembranous colitis. **CV:** pain, redness, swelling, thrombophlebitis at injection site. **CNS:** dizziness, headache, fatigue. **GU:** vaginitis. **Hem:** positive direct Coombs' test, slight elevation in SGOT, SGPT, and BUN. **Misc:** superinfection.

Nursing implications/Documentation

Possible nursing diagnoses: Potential for infection; Fluid volume deficit.

• Determine history of allergies, and (regardless of history) monitor closely for allergic reactions.

• Obtain baseline CBC, creatinine, liver function, and necessary cultures before administering first dose; monitor closely thereafter if therapy is prolonged.

• Encourage fluids, and record and monitor intake and output, to ensure adequate hydration; report significant negative or positive balance.

• Monitor for and report signs of superinfection (sore throat, fever, persistent diarrhea, fatigue, thrush, vaginal discharge).

• Give IM doses deep into large muscle mass.

Patient & family teaching/Home care

Possible nursing diagnoses: Knowledge deficit; Impaired home maintenance management.

• Teach the importance of reporting allergic symptoms, persistent diarrhea, signs and symptoms that do not abate, or *any* new signs and symptoms of discomfort that might indicate superinfection (medication regimen may have to be changed).

♦ Advise drinking 2–3 L of fluids daily to maintain adequate hydration (especially important if fever exists).

♦ Stress the importance of taking antibiotics for the entire time prescribed, even if signs and symptoms abate.

♦ Warn about adverse reactions if taken with alcohol.

◆ *See Anti-infectives overview for more information.*

cefonicid
se-fon'i-sid

cefonicid sodium: *Monocid*

Class: Anti-infective, Antibiotic, Cephalosporin (second generation)

PEDS	PREG	GERI
♨	B	♨

Action Broad-spectrum, usually bactericidal, antibiotic; kills bacteria by inhibiting cell wall synthesis.

Use/Therapeutic goal/Outcome

Serious infections (lower respiratory and urinary tract, skin, bone and joint): Prevention or resolution of infection. *Outcome criteria:* Absence of pathogenic growth on cultures, absence of clinical manifestations of infection (fever, pain, swelling, redness, heat, odor, drainage, productive cough, dysuria), normal X rays, normal WBC count.

Dose range/Administration

Interaction alert: Probenecid inhibits excretion of cefonicid; lower doses may be indicated.

Adult: IV, Deep IM: 0.5 g to 2 g/d. *For surgical prophylaxis:* 1 g one hour prior to surgery, may be repeated bid if indicated.

Clinical alert: If given by IV bolus, give slowly over 3–5 minutes.

Contraindications/Precautions
PREG B

Contraindicated in allergy to cefonicid or to cephalosporins. **Use with caution** in penicillin allergy and impaired renal function.

♨ **Use with caution for pregnant or nursing mothers and the elderly. Safe use for children has not been established.**

Side effects/Adverse reactions

Hypersensitivity: itching, rashes, eosinophilia, myalagia, fever, angioedema, difficulty breathing, anaphylaxis, serum sickness-like reactions. **GI:** anorexia, nausea, vomiting, diarrhea, pseudomembranous colitis. **CV:** pain, redness, swelling, thrombophlebitis at injection site. **GU:** vaginitis, nephrotoxicity (increased BUN and creatinine). **CNS:** dizziness, headache, malaise. **Hem:** positive direct Coombs' test, slight elevation in SGOT and SGPT. **Misc:** superinfection.

Nursing implications/Documentation

Possible nursing diagnoses: Potential for infection; Fluid volume deficit.

♦ Determine history of allergies and (regardless of history) monitor closely for allergic reactions.

♦ Obtain baseline CBC, creatinine, liver function, and necessary cultures before giving first dose; monitor closely thereafter if therapy is prolonged.

♦ Encourage fluids, and record and monitor intake and output, to ensure adequate hydration; report significant negative or positive balance.

♦ Monitor for and report signs of superinfection (sore throat, fever, persistent diarrhea, fatigue, thrush, vaginal discharge).

♦ Give IM doses deep into large muscle mass.

Patient & family teaching/Home care

Possible nursing diagnoses: Knowledge deficit; Impaired home maintenance management.

♦ Teach importance of reporting allergic symptoms, persistent diarrhea, signs and symptoms that do not abate, or *any* new signs and symptoms of discomfort that might indicate superinfection (medication regimen may have to be changed).

♦ Advise drinking 2–3 L of fluids daily to maintain adequate hydration (especially important if fever exists).

♦ Stress the importance of taking antibiotics for the entire time prescribed, even if signs and symptoms abate.

◆ *See Anti-infectives overview for more information.*

cefoperazone

sef-oh-per'a-zone

cefoperazone sodium: *Cefobid*

Class: Anti-infective, Antibiotic, Cephalosporin (third generation)

PEDS	PREG	GERI
☝	B	☝

Action Broad-spectrum, usually bactericidal, antibiotic; kills bacteria by inhibiting cell wall synthesis.

Use/Therapeutic goal/Outcome

Serious infections (respiratory, intraabdominal, GYN, skin, blood): Prevention or resolution of infection. ***Outcome criteria:*** Absence of pathogenic growth on cultures, absence of clinical manifestations of infection (fever, pain, swelling, redness, heat, odor, drainage, productive cough, dysuria), normal X rays, normal WBC count.

Dose range/Administration

Interaction alert: Consumption of alcohol within 72 hours of administration may cause nausea, vomiting, flushing, throbbing headache, and hypotension. Aspirin and alcohol increases risk of bleeding.

Adult: IV, Deep IM: 2–4 g in divided doses q12h. *Maximum dose:* 12–16 g/day for severe infections or resistant organisms.

Clinical alert: Infuse IV doses over 15–30 min; never give via bolus.

Contraindications/Precautions

**PREG
B**

Contraindicated in allergy to cefoperazone or to cephalosporins. ***Use with caution*** in penicillin allergy, impaired hepatic or renal function, and biliary obstruction.

☝ **Use with caution for pregnant or nursing mothers and the elderly. Safe use for children has not been established.**

Side effects/Adverse reactions

Hypersensitivity: itching, rashes, eosinophilia, joint pain or swelling, fever, angioedema, difficulty breathing, anaphylaxis, serum sickness-like reactions. ***GI:*** anorexia, nausea, vomiting, glossitis, indigestion, abdominal cramps, diarrhea, pseudomembranous colitis, oral thrush. ***CV:*** pain, redness, swelling, thrombophlebitis at injection site. ***CNS:*** dizziness, headache, fatigue. ***GU:*** vaginitis, nephrotoxicity (increased BUN and creatinine). ***Hem:*** transient neutropenia, eosinophilia, hypopro-

thrombinemia, hemolytic anemia, positive direct Coombs' test, slight elevation in SGOT, SGPT. ***Misc:*** superinfection.

Nursing implications/Documentation

Possible nursing diagnoses: Potential for infection; Fluid volume deficit.

◆ Determine history of allergies, and (regardless of history) monitor closely for allergic reactions.

◆ Obtain baseline CBC, creatinine, liver function studies, prothrombin time, and necessary cultures before administering first dose; monitor closely thereafter if therapy is prolonged.

◆ Encourage fluids, and record and monitor intake and output, to ensure adequate hydration; report significant negative or positive balance.

◆ Monitor for and report signs of superinfection (sore throat, fever, persistent diarrhea, fatigue, thrush, vaginal discharge).

◆ Give IM doses deep into large muscle mass.

Patient & family teaching/Home care

Possible nursing diagnoses: Knowledge deficit; Impaired home maintenance management.

◆ Teach the importance of reporting allergic symptoms, persistent diarrhea, signs and symptoms that do not abate, or *any* new signs and symptoms of discomfort that might indicate superinfection (medication regimen may have to be changed).

◆ Advise drinking 2–3 L of fluids daily to maintain adequate hydration (especially important if fever exists).

◆ Stress the importance of taking the antibiotic for the entire time prescribed, even if signs and symptoms abate.

◆ Warn that drinking alcohol within 72 hours of taking cefoperazone may cause violent nausea, vomiting, and a throbbing headache.

◆ *See Anti-infectives overview for more information.*

ceforanide

sef'or-a-nide

Precef

Class: Anti-infective, Antibiotic, Cephalosporin (second generation)

PEDS	PREG	GERI
☝	B	☝

Action Broad-spectrum, usually bactericidal, antibiotic; kills bacteria by inhibiting cell wall synthesis.

Use/Therapeutic goal/Outcome

Serious infections (lower respiratory and urinary tract, skin, bone and joint, blood, heart): Prevention or resolution of infection. *Outcome criteria:* Absence of pathogenic growth on cultures, absence of clinical manifestations of infection (fever, pain, swelling, redness, heat, odor, drainage, productive cough, dysuria), normal X rays, normal WBC count.

Dose range/Administration

Interaction alert: If given with furosemide, aminoglycosides, or vancomycin, monitor for increased risk of toxicity.

Adult: IV, Deep IM: 0.5 g to 1 g/day in divided doses q12h. *Child > 1 yr:* IV, Deep IM: 20–40 mg/kg/day in divided doses q12h.

Contraindications/Precautions

PREG
B

Contraindicated in allergy to ceforanide or to cephalosporins. *Use with caution* in penicillin allergy and impaired renal function.

☙ **Use with caution for pregnant or nursing mothers and the elderly. Safe use for infants under 1 year has not been established.**

Side effects/Adverse reactions

Hypersensitivity: itching, rashes, eosinophilia, fever, angioedema, difficulty breathing, anaphylaxis, serum sickness-like reactions. *GI:* anorexia, nausea, vomiting, diarrhea, pseudomembranous colitis. *CV:* pain, redness, swelling, thrombophlebitis at injection site. *GU:* vaginitis, nephrotoxicity (increased BUN and creatinine). *CNS:* confusion, lethargy, headache. *Hem:* thrombocytopenia, positive direct Coombs' test. *Misc:* superinfection.

Nursing implications/Documentation

Possible nursing diagnoses: Potential for infection; Fluid volume deficit.

♦ Determine history of allergies, and (regardless of history) monitor closely for allergic reactions.

♦ Obtain baseline CBC, creatinine, liver function studies, and necessary cultures before administering first dose; monitor closely thereafter if therapy is prolonged.

♦ Encourage fluids, and record and monitor intake and output, to ensure adequate hydra-

tion; report significant negative or positive balance.

♦ Monitor for and report signs of superinfection (sore throat, fever, persistent diarrhea, fatigue, thrush, vaginal discharge).

♦ Give IM dose deep into large muscle mass.

Patient & family teaching/Home care

Possible nursing diagnoses: Knowledge deficit; Impaired home maintenance management.

♦ Teach the importance of reporting allergic symptoms, persistent diarrhea, signs and symptoms that do not abate, or *any* new signs and symptoms of discomfort that might indicate superinfection (medication regimen may have to be changed).

♦ Advise drinking 2–3 L of fluids daily to maintain adequate hydration (especially important if fever exists).

♦ Stress the importance of taking antibiotics for the entire time prescribed, even if signs and symptoms abate.

♦ *See Anti-infectives overview for more information.*

cefotaxime

sef-oh-taks'eem

Claforan

Class: ★Anti-infective third-generation cephalosporin prototype, Antibiotic

PEDS	PREG	GERI
OK	B	☙

Action Broad-spectrum, usually bactericidal, antibiotic; kills bacteria by inhibiting cell wall synthesis.

Use/Therapeutic goal/Outcome

Serious infection (lower respiratory and urinary tract, CNS, GYN, skin, blood): Prevention or resolution of infection. *Outcome criteria:* Absence of pathogenic growth on cultures, absence of clinical manifestations of infection (fever, pain, swelling, redness, heat, odor, drainage, productive cough, dysuria), normal X rays, normal WBC count.

Dose range/Administration

Interaction alert: Probenecid inhibits excretion of cefotaxamine; lower doses may be indicated.

Adult/Child over 50 kg: IV, Deep IM: 1 g/day in divided doses q6-8h. *Maximum dose:* 12 g/day, depending on severity of infection. *Child 4 wk to 12 yrs, < 50 kg:* IV, Deep IM: 50–180 mg/kg/

▶

day divided q4-6h. *Infant 1–4 wk:* IV: 25–50 mg/kg q8h. *Infant < 1 wk:* IV: 25–50 mg/kg q12h.

Contraindications/Precautions

PREG B

Contraindicated in allergy to cefotaxime or to cephalosporins. *Use with caution* in penicillin allergy and impaired renal function.

꙳ **Use with caution for pregnant or nursing mothers and the elderly.**

Side effects/Adverse reactions

Hypersensitivity: itching, erythema, rashes, urticaria, fever, difficulty breathing, anaphylaxis. *GI:* nausea, vomiting, anorexia, diarrhea, pseudomembranous colitis. *CV:* pain, redness, swelling, thrombophlebitis at injection site. *Hem:* positive direct Coombs' test, slight elevation in SGOT, SGPT, BUN, and alkaline phophatase. *GU:* vaginitis. *CNS:* headache, dizziness, fatigue. *Misc:* superinfection.

Nursing implications/Documentation

Possible nursing diagnoses: Potential for infection; Fluid volume deficit.

◆ Determine history of allergies, and (regardless of history) monitor closely for allergic reactions.

◆ Obtain baseline CBC, creatinine, liver function studies, and necessary cultures before administering first dose; monitor closely thereafter if therapy is prolonged.

◆ Encourage fluids, and record and monitor intake and output, to ensure adequate hydration; report significant negative or positive balance.

◆ Monitor for and report signs of superinfection (sore throat, fever, persistent diarrhea, fatigue, thrush, vaginal discharge).

◆ Give IM doses deep into large muscle mass.

Patient & family teaching/Home care

Possible nursing diagnoses: Knowledge deficit; Impaired home maintenance management.

◆ Teach the importance of reporting allergic symptoms, persistent diarrhea, signs and symptoms that do not abate, or *any* new signs and symptoms of discomfort that might indicate superinfection (medication regimen may have to be changed).

◆ Advise drinking 2–3 L of fluids daily to maintain adequate hydration (especially important if fever exists).

◆ Stress the importance of taking antibiotics for the entire time prescribed, even if signs and symptoms abate.

◆ *See Anti-infectives overview for more information.*

cefotetan

sef'oh-tee-tan

cefotetan disodium: *Cefotan*

Class: Anti-infective, Antibiotic, Cephalosporin (second generation)

PEDS	PREG	GERI
꙳	B	꙳

Action Broad-spectrum, usually bactericidal, antibiotic; kills bacteria by inhibiting cell wall synthesis.

Use/Therapeutic goal/Outcome

Serious infections (urinary and lower respiratory, GYN, skin, intraabdominal, bone and joint): Prevention or resolution of infection. *Outcome criteria:* Absence of pathogenic growth on cultures, absence of clinical manifestations of infection (fever, pain, swelling, redness, heat, odor, drainage, productive cough, dysuria), normal WBC count, normal X rays.

Dose range/Administration

Interaction alert: Probenecid inhibits excretion of cefotetan; lower doses may be indicated. Consumption of alcohol within 72 hours of administration may cause nausea, vomiting, tachycardia, flushing, throbbing headache, and hypotension.

Adult: IV, Deep IM: 1–2 g q12h. *Maximum dose:* 6 g/day, depending on severity of infection. *For perioperative prophylaxis:* 1 g 30–60 min prior to surgery.

Contraindications/Precautions

PREG B

Contraindicated in allergy to cefotetan or to cephalosporins. *Use with caution* in penicillin allergy and impaired renal function.

꙳ **Use with caution for pregnant or nursing mothers and the elderly. Safe use for children has not been established.**

Side effects/Adverse reactions

Hypersensitivity: itching, erythema, rashes, urticaria, difficulty breathing, anaphylaxis. *GI:* nausea, vomiting, anorexia, diarrhea, pseudomembranous colitis. *CV:* pain, redness, swelling, thrombophlebitis at injection site. *Hem:* thrombocytopenia, positive direct

Coombs' test, slight elevation in SGOT, SGPT, LDH, and alkaline phosphatase. *GU:* vaginitis. *CNS:* headache, dizziness, fatigue. *Misc:* superinfection.

Nursing implications/Documentation

Possible nursing diagnoses: Potential for infection; Fluid volume deficit.

♦ Determine history of allergies, and (regardless of history) monitor closely for allergic reactions.

♦ Obtain baseline CBC, creatinine, liver function studies, and necessary cultures before administering first dose; monitor closely thereafter if therapy is prolonged.

♦ Encourage fluids, and record and monitor intake and output, to ensure adequate hydration; report significant negative or positive balance.

♦ Monitor for and report signs of superinfection (sore throat, fever, persistent diarrhea, fatigue, thrush, vaginal discharge).

♦ Give IM doses deep into large muscle mass.

Patient & family teaching/Home care

Possible nursing diagnoses: Knowledge deficit; Impaired home maintenance management.

♦ Teach the importance of reporting allergic symptoms, signs and symptoms that do not abate, or *any* new signs and symptoms of discomfort that might indicate superinfection (medication regimen may have to be changed).

♦ Advise drinking 2–3 L of fluids daily to maintain adequate hydration (especially important if fever exists).

♦ Stress the importance of taking antibiotics for the entire time prescribed, even if signs and symptoms abate.

♦ Warn to avoid alcohol for at least 72 hours after administration (may cause severe nausea, vomiting, headache).

♦ *See Anti-infectives overview for more information.*

cefoxitin

se-fox'i-tin

cefoxitin sodium: *Mefoxin*

Class: ★Anti-infective second-generation cephalosporin prototype, Antibiotic

PEDS	PREG	GERI
♄	**B**	♄

Action Broad-spectrum, usually bactericidal, antibiotic; kills bacteria by inhibiting cell wall synthesis.

Use/Therapeutic goal/Outcome

Serious infections (respiratory and GU tract, skin and soft tissue, bone and joint, intraabdominal, blood): Prevention or resolution of infection. *Outcome criteria:* Absence of pathogenic growth on cultures, absence of clinical manifestations of infection (fever, pain, swelling, redness, heat, odor, drainage, productive cough, dysuria), normal chest X rays, normal WBC count.

Dose range/Administration

Interaction alert: Probenecid inhibits excretion of cefoxitin; lower doses may be indicated. Monitor for toxicity if given with aminoglycocides.

Adult: IV, Deep IM: 1–2 g q6-8h. *Maximum dose:* 12 g/day depending on severity of infection. *For perioperative prophylaxis:* 2 g 30–60 min prior to surgery, followed by 2 g q6h for 24 hours. *Child > 3 mos:* IV, Deep IM: 80–160 mg/kg/day divided q4-6h. *Maximum dose:* 12 g/day.

Contraindications/Precautions

PREG
B

Contraindicated in allergy to cefoxitin or to cephalosporins. *Use with caution* in penicillin allergy and impaired renal function.

♄ **Use with caution for pregnant or nursing mothers and the elderly. Safe use for infants under 3 months has not been established.**

Side effects/Adverse reactions

Hypersensitivity: itching, erythema, rashes, urticaria, fever, eosinophilia, difficulty breathing, anaphylaxis. *GI:* nausea, vomiting, anorexia, diarrhea, pseudomembranous colitis. *CV:* pain, redness, swelling, thrombophlebitis at injection site. *Hem:* positive direct Coombs' test, slight elevation in SGOT, SGPT, BUN, and alkaline phosphatase. *GU:* vaginitis. *CNS:* headache, dizziness, fatigue. *Misc:* superinfection.

Nursing implications/Documentation

Possible nursing diagnoses: Potential for infection; Fluid volume deficit.

♦ Determine history of allergies, and (regardless of history) monitor closely for allergic reactions.

- Obtain baseline CBC, creatinine, liver function studies, and necessary cultures before administering first dose; monitor closely thereafter if therapy is prolonged.
- Encourage fluids, and record and monitor intake and output, to ensure adequate hydration; report significant negative or positive balance.
- Monitor for and report signs of superinfection (sore throat, fever, persistent diarrhea, fatigue, thrush, vaginal discharge).
- Give IM doses deep into large muscle mass.

Patient & family teaching/Home care

Possible nursing diagnoses: Knowledge deficit; Impaired home maintenance management.

- Teach the importance of reporting allergic symptoms, persistent diarrhea, signs and symptoms that do not abate, or *any* new signs and symptoms of discomfort that might indicate superinfection (medication regimen may have to be changed).
- Advise drinking 2–3 L of fluids daily to maintain adequate hydration (especially important if fever exists).
- Stress the importance of taking antibiotics for the entire time prescribed, even if signs and symptoms abate.
- *See Anti-infectives overview for more information.*

ceftazidime
sef´tah-zye-deem

Fortaz, ✦Magnacef, Tazicef, Tazidime

Class: Anti-infective, Antibiotic, Cephalosporin (third generation)

PEDS	PREG	GERI
✋	B	✋

Action Broad-spectrum, usually bactericidal, antibiotic; kills bacteria by inhibiting cell wall synthesis.

Use/Therapeutic goal/Outcome

Serious infection (lower respiratory and urinary tract, GYN, CNS, intraabdominal, blood): Prevention or resolution of infection. *Outcome criteria:* Absence of pathogenic growth on cultures, absence of clinical manifestations of infection (fever, pain, swelling, redness, heat, odor, drainage, productive cough, dysuria), normal X rays, normal WBC count.

Dose range/Administration

Interaction alert: Do not mix in solution with sodium bicarbonate (causes instability of ceftazidime).

Adult: IV, Deep IM: 1 g q8-12h. *Maximum dose:* 6 g/day. **Child < 4 wk:** IV, Deep IM: 30–50 mg/kg q12h. **Child 1 mo to 12 yr:** IV, Deep IM: 30–50 mg/kg q8h. *Maximum dose:* 6 g/day.

Contraindications/Precautions
PREG B

Contraindicated in hypersensitivity to ceftazidime or to cephalosporins. *Use with caution* in penicillin allergy and impaired renal function.

- Use with caution for pregnant or nursing mothers and the elderly.

Side effects/Adverse reactions

Hypersensitivity: itching, erythema, rashes, urticaria, fever, eosinophilia, difficulty breathing, anaphylaxis. *GI:* nausea, vomiting, anorexia, abdominal pain, diarrhea, pseudomembranous colitis. *CV:* pain, redness, swelling, thrombophlebitis at injection site. *Hem:* positive direct Coombs' test, slight elevation in SGOT, SGPT, BUN, and creatinine. *GU:* vaginitis. *CNS:* headache, dizziness, fatigue. *Misc:* superinfection.

Nursing implications/Documentation

Possible nursing diagnoses: Potential for infection; Fluid volume deficit.

- Determine history of allergies, and (regardless of history) monitor closely for allergic reactions.
- Obtain baseline CBC, creatinine, liver function studies, and necessary cultures before administering first dose; monitor closely thereafter if therapy is prolonged.
- Encourage fluids, and record and monitor intake and output, to ensure adequate hydration; report significant negative or positive balance.
- Monitor for and report signs of superinfection (sore throat, fever, persistent diarrhea, fatigue, thrush, vaginal discharge).
- Give IM doses deep into large muscle mass.

Patient & family teaching/Home care

Possible nursing diagnoses: Knowledge deficit; Impaired home maintenance management.

- Teach the importance of reporting allergic symptoms, signs and symptoms that do not abate, or *any* new signs and symptoms of discomfort that might indicate superinfection (medication regimen may have to be changed).

◆ Advise drinking 2–3 L of fluids daily to maintain adequate hydration (especially important if fever exists).

◆ Stress the importance of taking antibiotics for the entire time prescribed, even if signs and symptoms abate.

◆ *See Anti-infectives overview for more information.*

ceftizoxime

sef'ti-zox-eem

ceftizoxime sodium: **Cefizox**

Class: Anti-infective, Antibiotic, Cephalosporin (third-generation)

PEDS	PREG	GERI
🖐	**B**	🖐

Action Broad-spectrum, usually bactericidal, antibiotic; kills bacteria by inhibiting cell wall synthesis.

Use/Therapeutic goal/Outcome

Serious infection (lower respiratory and urinary tract, GYN, intraabdominal, bone and joint, meningitis, blood): Prevention or resolution of infection. *Outcome criteria:* Absence of pathogenic growth on cultures, absence of clinical manifestations of infection (fever, pain, swelling, redness, heat, odor, drainage, productive cough, dysuria), normal X rays, normal WBC count.

Dose range/Administration

Interaction alert: Probenecid inhibits excretion; lower doses may be indicated.

Adult: IV, Deep IM: 1–2 g q8-12h. *Maximum dose:* 2 g q4h for life-threatening infections. *Child > 6 mos:* IV, Deep IM: 50 mg/kg q6-8h. *Maximum dose:* 200 mg/kg/day.

Contraindications/Precautions

PREG B

Contraindicated in allergy to ceftizoxime or to cephalosporins. **Use with caution** in penicillin allergy and impaired renal function.

🖑 **Use with caution for pregnant or nursing mothers and the elderly. Safe use for infants under 6 months has not been established.**

Side effects/Adverse reactions

Hypersensitivity: itching, erythema, rashes, urticaria, fever, eosinophilia, difficulty breathing, anaphylaxis. **GI:** nausea, vomiting, diarrhea, pseudomembranous colitis. **CV:** pain, redness, swelling, thrombophlebitis at injection site. **Hem:** thrombocytopenia, positive direct Coombs' test, slight elevation in SGOT, SGPT, BUN, and alkaline phosphatase. **GU:** vaginitis. **CNS:** headache, dizziness, fatigue. **Misc:** superinfection.

Nursing implications/Documentation

Possible nursing diagnoses: Potential for infection; Diarrhea.

◆ Determine history of allergies, and (regardless of history) monitor closely for allergic reactions.

◆ Obtain baseline CBC, creatinine, liver function studies, and necessary cultures before administering first dose; monitor closely thereafter if therapy is prolonged.

◆ Encourage fluids, and record and monitor intake and output, to ensure adequate hydration; report significant negative or positive balance.

◆ Monitor for and report signs of superinfection (sore throat, fever, persistent diarrhea, fatigue, thrush, vaginal discharge).

◆ Give IM doses deep into large muscle mass.

Patient & family teaching/Home care

Possible nursing diagnoses: Knowledge deficit; Impaired home maintenance management.

◆ Teach the importance of reporting allergic symptoms, persistent diarrhea, signs and symptoms that do not abate, or *any* new signs and symptoms of discomfort that might indicate superinfection (medication regimen may have to be changed).

◆ Advise drinking 2–3 L of fluids daily to maintain adequate hydration (especially important if fever exists).

◆ Stress the importance of taking the antibiotic for the entire time prescribed, even if signs and symptoms abate.

◆ *See Anti-infectives overview for more information.*

ceftriaxone

sef-tree-axe'own

ceftriaxone sodium: **Rocephin**

Class: Anti-infective, Antibiotic, Cephalosporin (third-generation)

PEDS	PREG	GERI
🤚	B	🤚

Action Broad-spectrum, usually bactericidal, antibiotic; kills bacteria by inhibiting cell wall synthesis.

Use/Therapeutic goal/Outcome

Serious infection (lower respiratory and urinary tract, GYN, skin, blood, meningitis, Lyme's): Prevention or resolution of infection. **Outcome criteria:** Absence of pathogenic growth on cultures, absence of clinical manifestations of infection (fever, pain, swelling, redness, heat, odor, drainage, productive cough, dysuria), normal X rays, normal WBC count.

Dose range/Administration

Interaction alert: If given with aminoglycosides, furosemide, colistin, or sulfinpyrazone, monitor for increased risk of toxicity.

Adult: IV, Deep IM: 1–2 g qd or bid. *Maximum dose: 4 g/day. For surgical prophylaxis:* 1 g 30 min to 2 hr prior to surgery. **Child:** IV, Deep IM: 50–75 mg/kg/day in divided doses q12h. *Maximum dose:* 2 g/day; for meningitis, 4 g/day.

Contraindications/Precautions

PREG B

Contraindicated in allergy to ceftriaxone or to cephalosporins. **Use with caution** in penicillin allergy, and impaired renal and hepatic function.

🤚 **Contraindicated for hyperbilirubinemic neonates. Use with caution for pregnant or nursing mothers and the elderly.**

Side effects/Adverse reactions

Hypersensitivity: itching, erythema, rashes, urticaria, fever, eosinophilia, difficulty breathing, anaphylaxis. **GI:** nausea, vomiting, anorexia, diarrhea, pseudomembranous colitis. **CV:** pain, redness, swelling, thrombophlebitis at injection site. **Hem:** thrombocytopenia, positive direct Coombs' test, slight elevation in SGOT, SGPT, BUN, and alkaline phosphatase. **GU:** vaginitis. **CNS:** headache, dizziness, fatigue. **Misc:** superinfection.

Nursing implications/Documentation

Possible nursing diagnoses: Potential for infection; Fluid volume deficit.

♦ Determine history of allergies, and (regardless of history) monitor closely for allergic reactions.

♦ Obtain baseline CBC, creatinine, liver function studies, and necessary cultures before administering first dose; monitor closely thereafter if therapy is prolonged.

♦ Encourage fluids, and record and monitor intake and output, to ensure adequate hydration; report significant negative or positive balance.

♦ Monitor for and report signs of superinfection (sore throat, fever, persistent diarrhea, fatigue, thrush, vaginal discharge).

♦ Give IM doses deep into large muscle mass.

Patient & family teaching/Home care

Possible nursing diagnoses: Knowledge deficit; Impaired home maintenance management.

♦ Teach the importance of reporting allergic symptoms, persistent diarrhea, signs and symptoms that do not abate, or *any* new signs and symptoms of discomfort that might indicate superinfection (medication regimen may have to be changed).

♦ Advise drinking 2–3 L of fluids daily to maintain adequate hydration (especially important if fever exists).

♦ Stress the importance of taking antibiotics for the entire time prescribed, even if signs and symptoms abate.

♦ *See Anti-infectives overview for more information.*

cefuroxime

se-fyoor-ox'eem

cefuroxime axetil: **Ceftin**

cefuroxime sodium: **Kefurox, Zinacef**

Class: Anti-infective, Antibiotic, Cephalosporin (second generation)

PEDS	PREG	GERI
🤚	B	🤚

Action Broad-spectrum, usually bactericidal, antibiotic; kills bacteria by inhibiting cell wall synthesis.

Use/Therapeutic goal/Outcome

Serious infection (lower respiratory and urinary tract, skin, blood, meningitis, gonorrhea): Prevention or resolution of infection. **Outcome criteria:** Absence of pathogenic growth on cultures, absence of clinical manifestations of infection (fever, pain, swelling, redness, heat, odor, drainage, productive cough, dysuria), normal X rays, normal WBC count.

Dose range/Administration

Interaction alert: Probenecid inhibits excretion of cefuroxime; lower doses may be indicated.

🍃 **Give oral doses with food to enhance absorption.**

Adult: IV, Deep IM: 750 mg to 1.5 g q8h. *Maximum dose:* 3 g q6h. **Adult:** PO: 250–500 mg q12h. **Child < 12 yrs:** PO: 125 mg q12h. **Child > 3 mos:** IV, Deep IM: 50–100 mg/kg/day.

Contraindications/Precautions

PREG
B

Contraindicated in allergy to cefuroxime or to cephalosporins. **Use with caution** in penicillin allergy and impaired renal function.

✋ **Use with caution for pregnant or nursing mothers and the elderly. Safe use for infants under 3 months has not been established.**

Side effects/Adverse reactions

Hypersensitivity: itching, erythema, rashes, urticaria, fever, eosinophilia, difficulty breathing, anaphylaxis. **GI:** nausea, vomiting, anorexia, diarrhea, pseudomembranous colitis. **CV:** pain, redness, swelling, thrombophlebitis at injection site. **Hem:** positive direct Coombs' test, slight elevation in SGOT, SGPT, BUN, and alkaline phosphatase. **GU:** vaginitis. **CNS:** headache, dizziness, fatigue. **Misc:** superinfection.

Nursing implications/Documentation

Possible nursing diagnoses: Potential for infection; Diarrhea.

◆ Determine history of allergies, and (regardless of history) monitor closely for allergic reactions.

◆ Obtain baseline CBC, creatinine, liver function studies, and necessary cultures before administering first dose; monitor closely thereafter if therapy is prolonged.

◆ Encourage fluids, and record and monitor intake and output, to ensure adequate hydration; report significant negative or positive balance.

◆ Monitor for and report signs of superinfection (sore throat, fever, persistent diarrhea, fatigue, thrush, vaginal discharge).

◆ Give IM doses deep into large muscle mass.

Patient & family teaching/Home care

Possible nursing diagnoses: Knowledge deficit; Impaired home maintenance management.

◆ Teach the importance of reporting allergic symptoms, persistent diarrhea, signs and symptoms that do not abate, or *any* new signs and symptoms of discomfort that might indicate superinfection (medication regimen may have to be changed).

◆ Advise drinking 2–3 L of fluids daily to maintain adequate hydration (especially important if fever exists).

◆ Stress the importance of taking the antibiotic for the entire time prescribed, even if signs and symptoms abate.

◆ *See Anti-infectives overview for more information.*

cephalexin

sef-a-lex'in

cephalexin monohydrate: 🍃 🍁 *Ceporex, Keflet, Keflex, Keftab,* 🍁 *Novolexin*

Class: ★Anti-infective first-generation cephalosporin prototype, Antibiotic

PEDS PREG GERI
✋   B   ✋

Action Broad-spectrum, usually bactericidal, antibiotic; kills bacteria by inhibiting cell wall synthesis.

Use/Therapeutic goal/Outcome

Infections (ear, GU, respiratory, skin and soft tissue, bone and joint): Prevention or resolution of infection. **Outcome criteria:** Absence of pathogenic growth on cultures, absence of clinical manifestations of infection (fever, pain, swelling, redness, heat, odor, drainage, productive cough, dysuria), normal chest X rays, normal WBC count.

Dose range/Administration

Interaction alert: Probenecid inhibits excretion of cephalexin; lower doses may be indicated.

🍃 **Give with meals if GI upset occurs.**

Adult: PO: 250 mg q6h (1–4 g/day, depending on severity of infection). **Child:** PO: 25–50 mg/kg/day in divided doses.

Contraindications/Precautions

PREG B

Contraindicated in allergy to cephalexin or to cephalosporins. **Use with caution** in penicillin allergy and impaired renal function.

🖑 **Use with caution for pregnant or nursing mothers, children, and the elderly.**

Side effects/Adverse reactions

Hypersensitivity: itching, erythema, rashes, urticaria, angioedema, eosinophilia, difficulty breathing, anaphylaxis. **GI:** nausea, vomiting, abdominal pain, diarrhea, pseudomembranous colitis. **Hem:** slight elevation in SGOT and SGPT. **GU:** vaginitis. **CNS:** headache, dizziness, fatigue. **Misc:** superinfection.

Nursing implications/Documentation

Possible nursing diagnoses: Potential for infection; Fluid volume deficit.

◆ Determine history of allergies, and (regardless of history) monitor closely for allergic reactions.

◆ Obtain baseline CBC, creatinine, liver function studies, and necessary cultures before administering first dose; monitor closely thereafter if therapy is prolonged.

◆ Encourage fluids, and record and monitor intake and output, to ensure adequate hydration; report significant negative or positive balance.

◆ Monitor for and report signs of superinfection (sore throat, fever, persistent diarrhea, fatigue, thrush, vaginal discharge).

Patient & family teaching/Home care

Possible nursing diagnoses: Knowledge deficit; Impaired home maintenance management.

◆ If GI distress is experienced, advise taking cephalexin with food.

◆ Teach the importance of reporting allergic symptoms, persistent diarrhea, signs and symptoms that do not abate, or *any* new signs and symptoms of discomfort that might indicate superinfection (medication regimen may have to be changed).

◆ Advise drinking 2–3 L of fluids daily to maintain adequate hydration (especially important if fever exists).

◆ Stress the importance of taking antibiotics for the entire time prescribed, even if signs and symptoms abate.

◆ *See Anti-infectives overview for more information.*

cephalothin

sef-a'loe-thin

cephalothin sodium: ✤ ♠*Ceporacin, Keflin*

Class: Anti-infective, Antibiotic, Cephalosporin (first-generation)

PEDS	PREG	GERI
OK	B	🖑

Action Broad-spectrum antibiotic; kills bacteria (bactericidal) or inhibits their growth (bacteriostatic) by inhibiting cell wall synthesis.

Use/Therapeutic goal/Outcome

Serious infection (respiratory, GU, or GI tract; skin, bone and joint, peritoneal, blood, heart): Prevention or resolution of infection. **Outcome criteria:** Absence of pathogenic growth on cultures, absence of clinical manifestations of infection (fever, pain, swelling, redness, heat, odor, drainage, productive cough, dysuria), normal X rays, normal WBC count.

Dose range/Administration

Interaction alert: Probenecid inhibits excretion of cephalothin; lower doses may be indicated.

Adult: IV, Deep IM: 500 mg to 1 g q4-6h. *Maximum dose:* 12 g/day in divided doses. *For perioperative prophylaxis:* 1–2 g 30–60 min prior to surgery, then 1–2 g during surgery, then 1–2 g q6h for 24 hr after surgery. **Child:** IV, Deep IM: 80–160 mg/kg/day in divided doses.

Contraindications/Precautions

PREG B

Contraindicated in allergy to cephalothin or to cephalosporins. **Use with caution** in penicillin allergy and impaired renal function.

🖑 **Use with caution for pregnant or nursing mothers and the elderly.**

Side effects/Adverse reactions

Hypersensitivity: itching, erythema, rashes, urticaria, fever, difficulty breathing, eosinophilia, anaphylaxis. **GI:** nausea, vomiting, diarrhea, pseudomembranous colitis. **CV:** pain, redness, swelling, thrombophlebitis at injection site. **Hem:** thrombocytopenia, neutropenia, hemolytic anemia, positive direct Coombs' test, slight elevation in SGOT, BUN, alkaline phosphatase, creatinine. **GU:** vaginitis. **CNS:** headache, dizziness, fatigue. **Misc:** superinfection.

Nursing implications/Documentation

Possible nursing diagnoses: Potential for infection; Fluid volume deficit.

♦ Determine history of allergies and (regardless of history) monitor closely for allergic reactions.

♦ Obtain baseline CBC, creatinine, liver function studies, and necessary cultures before administering first dose; monitor closely thereafter if therapy is prolonged.

♦ Encourage fluids, and record and monitor intake and output, to ensure adequate hydration; report significant negative or positive balance.

♦ Monitor for and report signs of superinfection (sore throat, fever, diarrhea, fatigue, thrush, vaginal discharge).

♦ Avoid IM administration, which is painful (if IM administration is necessary, give deep into large muscle mass).

Patient & family teaching/Home care

Possible nursing diagnoses: Knowledge deficit; Impaired home maintenance management.

♦ Teach the importance of reporting allergic symptoms, persistent diarrhea, signs and symptoms that do not abate, or *any* new signs and symptoms of discomfort that might indicate superinfection (medication regimen may have to be changed).

♦ Advise drinking 2–3 L of fluids daily to maintain adequate hydration (especially important if fever exists).

♦ Stress the importance of taking antibiotics for the entire time prescribed, even if signs and symptoms abate.

♦ *See Anti-infectives overview for more information.*

cephapirin
sef-a-pye'rin

cephapirin sodium: **Cefadyl**

Class: Anti-infective, Antibiotic, Cephalosporin (first-generation)

PEDS	PREG	GERI
♨	B	♨

Action Broad-spectrum, usually bactericidal, antibiotic; kills bacteria by inhibiting cell wall synthesis.

Use/Therapeutic goal/Outcome

Serious infection (respiratory, GI, or GU tract; skin and soft tissue, bone and joint, blood, heart): Prevention or resolution of infection. **Outcome criteria:** Absence of pathogenic growth on cultures, absence of clinical manifestations of infection (fever, pain, swelling, redness, heat, odor, drainage, productive cough, dysuria), normal chest X rays, normal WBC count.

Dose range/Administration

Interaction alert: Probenecid inhibits excretion of cephapirin; lower doses may be indicated.

Adult: IV, Deep IM: 500 mg to 1 g q4-6h. *Maximum dose:* 12 g/day in divided doses. **Child > 3 mos:** IV, Deep IM: 40–80 mg/kg/day divided q6h.

Contraindications/Precautions
PREG
B

Contraindicated in allergy to cephapirin or to cephalosporins. **Use with caution** in penicillin allergy and impaired renal function.

♨ **Use with caution for pregnant or nursing mothers and the elderly. Safe use for infants under 3 months has not been established.**

Side effects/Adverse reactions

Hypersensitivity: itching, erythema, rashes, urticaria, fever, eosinophilia, difficulty breathing, anaphylaxis. **GI:** nausea, vomiting, anorexia, abdominal pain, diarrhea, pseudomembranous colitis. **CV:** pain, redness, swelling, thrombophlebitis at injection site. **Hem:** thrombocytopenia, neutropenia, anemia, positive direct Coombs' test, slight elevation in bilirubin, SGOT, BUN, and alkaline phosphatase. **GU:** vaginitis. **CNS:** headache, dizziness, fatigue. **Misc:** superinfection.

Nursing implications/Documentation

Possible nursing diagnoses: Potential for infection; Fluid volume deficit.

♦ Determine history of allergies, and (regardless of history) monitor closely for allergic reactions.

♦ Obtain baseline CBC, creatinine, liver function studies, and necessary cultures before administering first dose; monitor closely thereafter if therapy is prolonged.

♦ Encourage fluids, and record and monitor intake and output, to ensure adequate hydration; report significant negative or positive balance.

* Monitor for and report signs of superinfection (sore throat, fever, persistent diarrhea, fatigue, thrush, vaginal discharge).
* Give IM doses deep into large muscle mass.

Patient & family teaching/Home care

Possible nursing diagnoses: Knowledge deficit; Impaired home maintenance management.

* Teach the importance of reporting allergic symptoms, persistent diarrhea, signs and symptoms that do not abate, or *any* new signs and symptoms of discomfort that might indicate superinfection (medication regimen may have to be changed).
* Advise drinking 2–3 L of fluids daily to maintain adequate hydration (especially important if fever exists).
* Stress the importance of taking antibiotics for the entire time prescribed, even if signs and symptoms abate.

♦ *See Anti-infectives overview for more information.*

cephradine

sef'ra-deen

Anspor, Velosef

Class: Anti-infective, Antibiotic, Cephalosporin (first-generation)

PEDS	PREG	GERI
♨	B	♨

Action Broad-spectrum, usually bactericidal, antibiotic; kills bacteria by inhibiting cell wall synthesis.

Use/Therapeutic goal/Outcome

Serious infection: Prevention or resolution of infection. **Outcome criteria:** Absence of pathogenic growth on cultures, absence of clinical manifestations of infection (fever, pain, swelling, redness, heat, odor, drainage, productive cough, dysuria), normal WBC count, normal X rays.

Dose range/Administration

Interaction alert: Probenecid inhibits excretion of cephradine; lower doses may be indicated. Physically incompatible with Lactated Ringer's Injection.

🖐 **Give with food to reduce GI symptoms.**

Adult: PO: 250–500 mg q6h. *Maximum dose:* 4 g/day. IV, Deep IM: 500 mg to 1 g q6-12h. *Maximum dose:* 8 g/day in divided doses. **Child > 1 yr:** PO: 6–25 mg/kg q6h. *Maximum dose:* 4 g/day. IV, Deep IM: 12–25 mg/kg q6h. *Maximum dose:* 8 g/day.

Contraindications/Precautions

PREG B

Contraindicated in allergy to cephradine or to cephalosporins. **Use with caution** in penicillin allergy and impaired renal function.

🖐 **Use with caution for infants over 1 month, pregnant or nursing mothers, and the elderly. Safe use for infants under 1 month has not been established.**

Side effects/Adverse reactions

Hypersensitivity: itching, erythema, rash, urticaria, fever, eosinophilia, difficulty breathing, anaphylaxis. **GI:** nausea, vomiting, diarrhea, pseudomembranous colitis, hepatomegaly. **CV:** pain, redness, swelling, thrombophlebitis at injection site. **Hem:** thrombocytopenia, positive direct Coombs' test, slight elevation in SGOT, SGPT, BUN, bilirubin, and alkaline phosphatase. **GU:** vaginitis. **CNS:** headache, dizziness, fatigue. **Misc:** superinfection.

Nursing implications/Documentation

Possible nursing diagnoses: Potential for infection; Fluid volume deficit.

* Determine history of allergies, and (regardless of history) monitor closely for allergic reactions.
* Obtain baseline CBC, creatinine, liver function studies, and necessary cultures before administering first dose; monitor closely thereafter if therapy is prolonged.
* Encourage fluids, and record and monitor intake and output, to ensure adequate hydration; report significant negative or positive balance.
* Monitor for and report signs of superinfection (sore throat, fever, persistent diarrhea, fatigue, thrush, vaginal discharge).
* Give IM doses deep into large muscle mass.

Patient & family teaching/Home care

Possible nursing diagnoses: Knowledge deficit; Impaired home maintenance management.

* Explain that taking drug with food will reduce GI symptoms.
* Teach the importance of reporting allergic symptoms, persistent diarrhea, signs and symptoms that do not abate, or *any* new signs and symptoms of discomfort that might indicate superinfection (medication regimen may have to be changed).

- Advise drinking 2–3 L of fluids daily to maintain adequate hydration (especially important if fever exists).
- Stress the importance of taking the antibiotic for the entire time prescribed, even if signs and symptoms abate.
- *See Anti-infectives overview for more information.*

chenodiol

kee-noe-dye'ole

Chenix

Class: Anticholelithic

PEDS	PREG	GERI
✋	X	OK

Action Gradually dissolves gallstones by increasing the ratio of bile acids to cholesterol in biliary pool, thereby promoting removal of cholesterol from uncalcified gallstones.

Use/Therapeutic goal/Outcome

Gallstones: Dissolution of radiolucent cholesterol gallstones in patients who are poor surgical risks. *Outcome criteria:* Evidence of dissolution of stone by cholecystogram or ultrasound.

Dose range/Administration

Interaction alert: Aluminum-containing antacids, sucralfate, cholestyramine, and colestipol may interfere with absorption of chenodiol. Concurrent use of estrogens may decrease effectiveness.

🖐 **Give with milk or food for better absorption.**

Adult: PO: *Initial dose:* 250 mg bid, increase to 13–16 mg/kg/day in two doses.

Clinical alert: Diarrhea occurs in 30–50 percent of patients; dosage may be reduced if diarrhea becomes persistent and antidiarrheal agents may be ordered. Return to therapeutic dose of chenodiol will be done gradually, since lower than recommended doses are associated with increased cholecystectomy rates. Expect higher dose for obese patients.

Contraindications/Precautions

PREG
X

Contraindicated in intolerance to bile acid products, liver dysfunction, non-functioning gallbladder, bile duct abnormalities, gallstone complications or radiopaque stones, and disorders of pancreas. *Use with caution* in atherosclerosis, or inflammatory bowel disease.

🖐 **Contraindicated for pregnant women. Use with caution for nursing mothers. Safe use for children has not been established.**

Side effects/Adverse reactions

Hypersensitivity: rare. **GI:** diarrhea, abdominal cramps, indigestion, flatulence, nausea or vomiting, constipation, liver damage.

Nursing implications/Documentation

Possible nursing diagnoses: Diarrhea; Pain.
- Monitor and document bowel elimination pattern; assess for occurrence of diarrhea.
- Monitor results of liver function studies.
- Expect therapy to be discontinued if dissolution of stone is not demonstrated by ultrasound or cholecystogram within 18 months.

Patient & family teaching/Home care

Possible nursing diagnoses: Knowledge deficit; Impaired home maintenance management.
- Advise taking doses with food or milk for best results.
- Stress that restricting dietary cholesterol, increasing dietary bran, and losing weight may improve response to chenodiol.
- Reassure that gas or indigestion usually disappear after 2–4 weeks.
- Caution to have scheduled blood tests done as ordered to detect early evidence of liver damage.
- Inform that medication must be taken over long period of time to dissolve gallstones; advise reporting diarrhea (may require dose alteration).
- Warn women of childbearing years to practice contraception during treatment with chenodiol, and to inform physician if pregnancy is planned or suspected.
- Teach patient signs of acute gallbladder disease (severe upper right quadrant pain with severe nausea and vomiting) and emphasize the need to report these to physician promptly.

chloral hydrate

klor'al hye'drate

Aquachloral Supprettes, Noctec, ♣Novochlorhydrate

Class: Sedative-hypnotic

PEDS	PREG	GERI
✋	C	✋

CONTROLLED
SUBSTANCE
IV

Action Produces relaxation or sleep (mild cerebral depression) by inhibiting transmission of impulses in the reticular activating system.

Use/Therapeutic goal/Outcome

Sedation and sleep: Promotion of relaxation and sleep. *Outcome criteria:* Report of feeling less anxious and more relaxed, having slept well; observable signs of drowsiness or sleep.

Dose range/Administration

Interaction alert: Alcohol, narcotics, analgesics, and other CNS depressants intensify respiratory and CNS depression. Avoid use with IV furosemide (may cause flushing, sweating, and unstable blood pressure).

Give PO doses after meals. Have the patient swallow capsules whole with a full glass of water. Dilute liquid form in half a glass of liquid.

Sedation: *Adult:* PO or R: 250 mg tid. *Child:* PO or R: 8 mg/kg tid (maximum of 500 mg).

Insomnia (hypnotic use): *Adult:* PO or R: 500 mg to 1 g at bedtime. *Child:* PO or R: 50 mg/kg at bedtime (maximum of 1 g).

Premedication for EEG: *Child:* PO or R: 25 mg/kg in a single dose (maximum dose of 1 g).

Clinical alert: Hold dose and report if signs of respiratory depression or overdosage (constricted pupils, somnolence, hypotension, clammy skin, cyanosis) are present.

Contraindications/Precautions

PREG C

Contraindicated in hypersensitivity or intolerance to chloral hydrate, and in marked renal or hepatic impairment, and severe cardiac disease. *Avoid rectal administration* for patients with proctitis or new myocardial infarction. *Avoid oral administration* in presence of GI tract irritation or ulcers. *Use with caution* for patients with history of porphyria, asthma, drug dependence, depression, or suicidal tendencies.

Use with caution for children and the elderly. Safe use for pregnant or nursing mothers has not been established.

Side effects/Adverse reactions

Hypersensitivity: itching, rashes, hives.
GI: nausea, vomiting, diarrhea, flatulence, unpleasant taste, gastritis, breath odor.
CNS: drowsiness, lethargy, hangover, headache, nightmares, disorientation, confu-

sion, paradoxical excitement (most often in the elderly), ataxia.

Nursing implications/Documentation

Possible nursing diagnoses: Sensory, perceptual alterations (visual and auditory); Potential for injury.

♦ Document mental status before administration, monitor patient activity closely following administration, and employ appropriate measures to ensure safety (i.e., side rails up, call bell within reach, and no unsupervised smoking).

♦ If given to a patient with unrelieved pain, be aware that paradoxical excitement may occur.

♦ Monitor for symptoms of GI irritation, including those of the anal area if given rectally.

♦ For suppository lubrication, use water only.

♦ Monitor for and report signs of overdosage (slurred speech, continued somnolence, respiratory depression, confusion) and tolerance (increased anxiety or wakefulness).

♦ Be sure doses are swallowed, not hoarded.

Patient & family teaching/Home care

Possible nursing diagnoses: Sleep pattern disturbance; Ineffective coping (individual and family); Impaired home maintenance management.

♦ Explore problems that may contribute to insomnia or anxiety, and ways of coping effectively with these problems (stress the fact that effective coping can promote restful sleep).

♦ Explain the importance of daily exercise in promoting rest.

♦ Stress that drug tolerance and dependence can occur, and that the drug should be used only when holistic measures (e.g., quiet music, relaxation techniques) don't work.

♦ Emphasize that the effects of alcohol, other sedatives, and tranquilizers may be potentiated, and that these should be avoided.

♦ Reinforce the importance of consulting with physician before using OTC drugs, and of returning for medical follow up.

♦ Teach the person to avoid driving and other potentially hazardous activities while under the effects of the medication.

♦ *See Antianxiety Agents, Sedatives, and Hypnotics overview for more information.*

chlorambucil

klor-am'byoo-sil

Leukeran

Class: Antineoplastic (alkylating) agent

PEDS	PREG	GERI
🖐	D	🖐

Action Kills rapidly growing cells (cancer, hair follicles, bone marrow, GI lining, ova, and sperm) by interfering with DNA, RNA and protein synthesis through alkylation (cross-linking of DNA occurs). Is cell-cycle–phase nonspecific, affecting both actively dividing cells and dormant (resting) cells.

Use/Therapeutic goal/Outcome

Chronic lymphocytic leukemia; malignant lymphomas; Hodgkin's disease; ovarian and testicular neoplasms: Elimination or suppression of malignant cell proliferation. **Outcome criteria:** Tumor and disease regression or stabilization on radiologic and physical examination; for leukemias, absence of blasts in peripheral blood specimen.

Dose range/Administration

Adult: PO: 0.1 to 0.2 mg/kg or 4–8 mg/m^2/day for 3–6 weeks. *Maintenance dose:* 2 mg/day.
Child: PO: 0.1 to 0.2 mg/kg or 4.5 mg/m^2/day in single or divided doses.

Clinical alert: WBC, platelets, and erythrocytes should nadir (drop to the lowest point) in 10–14 days, and recovery begins 10 days after last dose. Hold drug and report if platelets are <100,000/mm^3 or WBC is <4000/mm^3.

Contraindications/Precautions

PREG D

Contraindicated in hypersensitivity or resistance to chlorambucil; within 4 weeks of radiation, chemotherapy (additive bone marrow depression), or live virus vaccination.

🖐 **Do not use during first trimester of pregnancy. Contraindicated for nursing mothers. Use with caution for children and the elderly.**

Side effects/Adverse reactions

Hypersensitivity: rash, dermatitis, fever, tachycardia, hypotension. **Hem:** hyperuricemia, moderate to severe, dose-dependent and rapidly reversible myelosuppression (1–3 week onset); leukopenia (usually after 3 weeks, lasting for 10 days after last dose); anemia; thrombocytopenia; and permanent bone marrow depression. **GI:** nausea, vomiting, and diarrhea. **CNS:** nervousness, confusion, seizures. **Resp:** pneumonia and pulmonary fibrosis. **Skin:** exfoliative dermatitis.

Nursing implications/Documentation

Possible nursing diagnoses: Potential for infection; Potential for injury; Fatigue; Altered oral mucous membrane; Fluid volume deficit; Diarrhea; Altered nutrition: less than body requirements.

◆ *See important Nursing implications in Antineoplastic agents overview on page 72, which apply to all antineoplastics. The interventions that follow are additional and specific to this drug only.*

♦ Monitor for and report persistent cough, dyspnea, or chest pain (pulmonary fibrosis may occur 4–6 months after therapy begins).

♦ Maintain a fluid intake of 2–3 L per day to prevent renal tubular damage from hyperuricemia secondary to cell lysis.

♦ Be aware that therapeutic response is often accompanied by toxicity.

Patient & family teaching/Home care

Possible nursing diagnoses: Knowledge deficit; Ineffective coping (individual and family); Hopelessness; Impaired home maintenance management.

◆ *See important Patient & family teaching in Antineoplastic agents overview on page 72, which apply to all antineoplastics. The teachings that follow are additional and specific to this drug only.*

♦ Point out that drinking 2–3 L helps prevent kidney complications.

♦ Stress that persistent cough, dyspnea, or chest pain should be reported immediately.

◆ *See Antineoplastic agents overview for more information.*

chloramphenicol

klor-am-fen'i-kole

chloramphenicol: **Ak-Chlor,Chloromycetin, Chloromycetin Ophthalmic, Chloromycetin Otic, Chloroptic, Chloroptic SOP, ♠Chlorsig, ♣Fenicol, ♣Isopto Fenicol, ♣Novochlorocap, Ophthoclor Ophthalmic, ♣Pentamycetin, ♣Sopamycetin**

chloramphenicol palmitate: **Chloromycetin Palmitate**

chloramphenicol sodium succinate: **Chloromycetin, ♣Pentamycetin**

Class: Anti-infective, Antibiotic, Antirickettsial

PEDS	PREG	GERI
🖐	C	🖐

Action Broad-spectrum antibiotic that kills bacteria (bactericidal) or limits bacterial growth (bacteriostatic) probably by binding to 50S ribosomal unit and inhibiting bacterial metabolism.

Use/Therapeutic goal/Outcome

Severe infection (*Salmonella typhi, Haemophilus influenzae* meningitis, bacteremia, and other infections caused by sensitive *Salmonella* species, *Rickettsia,* lymphogranuloma, psittacosis, or various gram-negative organisms): Resolution of infection. **Outcome criteria:** Absence of pathogenic growth on cultures, absence of clinical manifestations of infection (fever, pain, swelling, redness, heat, odor, drainage), normal WBC count.

Dose range/Administration

Interaction alert: Incompatible with many drugs (check package insert). If given with acetaminophen, monitor for chloramphenicol toxicity. Decreases action of penicillin, iron, folic acid and Vitamin B_{12}.

Give oral doses with a full glass of water on an empty stomach, 1 hour before or 2 hours after meals for optimal blood levels. *Adult/Child > 2 wk:* PO, IV: 50 mg/kg/day, in doses divided q6h. *Maximum dose:* 100 mg/kg/day. (May be injected directly as a 100 mg/ml solution over at least 1 min, or by slow infusion). *Topical:* Gently rub into cleansed affected area tid or qid. *Ophthalmic ointment:* Apply a small strip of 1% ointment to lower conjunctival sac q3-4h. *Ophthalmic solution:* 1–2 drops 0.16%, 0.25%, or 0.5% solution q1-6h. *Otic solution:* 2–3 drops 0.5% solution tid (q8h). *Infant < 2 wk:* PO, IV: 25 mg/kg/day in divided doses q6h. *Topical/ophthalmic:* Use adult dose.

Clinical alert: Serious adverse reactions, including bone marrow depression, blood dyscrasias, neurotoxicity and gray syndrome (abdominal distention, vomiting, pallor with cyanosis, skin blotches, irregular respirations, vasomotor collapse, hypothermia, and death), have occurred in infants with systemic or ophthalmic treatment; report early signs of abdominal distention, pallor, failure to feed, and changes in vital signs.

Contraindications/Precautions

PREG
C

Contraindicated in hypersensitivity or toxic reactions to chloramphenicol or to any ingredients in the formulation, for prophylaxis or treatment of minor infections, in bone marrow depression, and for use in conjunction with drugs that produce bone marrow depression. **Use with caution** in impaired hepatic or renal function, and for premenopausal women.

❧ **Contraindicated for pregnant or nursing mothers. Use with caution for children and the elderly.**

Side effects/Adverse reactions

Hypersensitivity: itching, burning, stinging, rashes, angioedema, vesicular or maculopapular dermatitis. **GI:** nausea, vomiting, diarrhea. **Hem:** hypoprothrombinemia, bone marrow depression, aplastic anemia, anemia, blood dyscrasias. **CNS:** neurotoxicity (headache, confusion, depression, digital paresthesias, peripheral neuritis). **Eye:** (with ophthalmic use) conjunctivitis; visual difficulties; optic neuritis; optic nerve atrophy. **Misc:** superinfection, gray syndrome (abdominal distention, vomiting, pallor with cyanosis, skin blotches, irregular respirations, vasomotor collapse, hypothermia, and death).

Nursing implications/Documentation

Possible nursing diagnoses: Potential for infection; Diarrhea.

◆ Determine history of allergies, and (regardless of history) monitor closely for allergic reactions.

◆ Obtain baseline CBC, creatinine, liver function studies, and necessary cultures before administering first dose; monitor closely thereafter if therapy is prolonged.

◆ Encourage fluids, and record and monitor intake and output, to ensure adequate hydration; report significant negative or positive balance.

◆ Record temperature every 4 hours, and report to physician if temperature has been normal for 48 hours (drug may be discontinued).

◆ Be aware that systemic absorption and toxicity can occur with frequent or prolonged use of topical, ophthalmic, and otic preparations.

◆ Do not warm ear drops above body temperature (loses potency).

◆ Monitor for and report signs of superinfection (sore throat, fever, fatigue, thrush, vaginal discharge).

◆ Document and report diarrhea.

Patient & family teaching/Home care

Possible nursing diagnoses: Knowledge deficit; Impaired home maintenance management.

♦ Explain importance of taking the medication on an empty stomach.

♦ Teach importance of reporting allergic symptoms, signs and symptoms that do not abate, or *any* new signs and symptoms of discomfort that might indicate superinfection (medication regimen may have to be changed).

♦ Advise drinking 2–3 L of fluids daily to maintain adequate hydration (especially important if fever exists).

♦ Stress the importance of taking antibiotics for the entire time prescribed, even if signs and symptoms abate.

♦ With IV administration, explain that a transient bitter taste may occur, but will disappear in 1–2 min.

♦ For topical use, teach patient (or significant other) and have them demonstrate proper cleansing of affected area and application of drug; explain that topical preparations are not interchangeable; stress the importance of following the dosage and application regimen closely.

♦ *See Anti-infectives overview for more information.*

chlordiazepoxide

klor-dye-a-ze-pox'ide

chlordiazepoxide: *Libritabs*

chlordiazepoxide hydrochloride: ♣*Apo-Chlordiazepoxide, Librium, Lipoxide,* ♣*Medilium, Mitran,* ♣*Novopoxide, Reposans, Sereen,* ♣*Solium*

Class: Antianxiety agent, Benzodiazepine

PEDS	PREG	GERI	CONTROLLED SUBSTANCE
৬	D	৬	IV

Action Produces CNS depression and relaxation by potentiating the action of gamma-aminobuteric acid (GABA), which reduces neuronal activity in all regions of the CNS. Promotes muscle relaxation by inhibiting spinal motor reflex pathways. Decreases anxiety by inhibiting cortical and limbic arousal.

Use/Therapeutic goal/Outcome

Short-term treatment of anxiety: Alleviation of symptoms of apprehension, muscle tension, and insomnia. **Outcome criteria:** Report of feeling more calm, sleeping better, and coping better; observable signs of decreased anxiety (decreased motor activity, reduced muscle tension, decrease in pulse and blood pressure).

Acute alcohol withdrawal: Prevention or management of delirium tremens. **Outcome criteria:** Reduction in, or absence of agitation, tremors, hallucinations; improved reality orientation.

Dose range/Administration

Interaction alert: Alcohol and other CNS depressants may cause excessive sedation. Cimetidine increases blood levels. If given with anticoagulants, monitor prothrombin times. Do not mix parenteral form in a syringe with any other drug.

🖐 **Give with food or milk if GI upset is noted.**

Moderate anxiety: **Adult:** PO: 5–10 mg tid or qid. **Child > 6 yrs:** PO: 5 mg bid or qid. *Maximum dose:* 30 mg/day.

Severe anxiety: **Adult:** PO: 10–25 mg tid or qid.

Acute alcohol withdrawal: **Adult:** PO, IM. IV: 50–100 mg prn. *Maximum dose:* 300 mg/day.

Clinical alert: IM route is not recommended since absorption may be slow and erratic. Check package insert directions for reconstitution of powder (usually, add 2 ml of diluent to powder and mix till clear; use immediately). When using IV route, dilute powder with 5 ml of NS instead of packaged diluent, and give over 1 min. If this drug has been taken for over a month, dosage should be tapered gradually, rather than withdrawn abruptly. Chlordiazepoxide accumulates in the body, and elimination after discontinuation may take weeks.

Contraindications/Precautions

PREG
D

Contraindicated in hypersensitivity or intolerance to chlordiazepoxide or other benzodiazepines, and in narrow-angle glaucoma. **Use with caution** in blood dyscrasias, psychosis, depression, suicidal tendencies, or impaired liver or kidney function.

🖐 **Contraindicated for pregnant or nursing mothers. Use with caution for children over 6 years and the elderly or debilitated. Safe use for children under 6 years has not been established.**

Side effects/Adverse reactions

Hypersensitivity: itching, rash, exaggeration of side effects. **CNS:** headache, lethargy, drowsiness, dizziness, syncope, tremors, confusion, depression. **CV:** hypotension, transient tachycardia and bradycardia. **Resp:** respiratory depression. **GI:** dry mouth, nausea, vomiting, constipation, diarrhea, liver dysfunction. **GU:** urinary retention. **Eye:** blurred vision, mydriasis. **Hem:** agranulocytosis, leukopenia. **Misc:** drug tolerance and dependence.

Nursing implications/Documentation

Possible nursing diagnoses: Potential for injury; Constipation.

♦ Record baseline blood pressure; monitor closely if dizziness is experienced. Supervise ambulation until response is determined.

♦ Keep those who have received parenteral drug in bed with side rails up.

♦ Be sure that doses are swallowed (not hoarded).

♦ Provide a quiet environment that is conducive to rest.

♦ Monitor bowel movements and provide adequate fluids and fiber; offer laxatives before the problem is severe.

Patient & family teaching/Home care

Possible nursing diagnoses: Anxiety; Fear; Ineffective individual coping; Impaired home maintenance management.

♦ Advise taking this drug with milk or food if GI symptoms are noted.

♦ Help the individual identify stressors that contribute to anxiety and ways of coping effectively; stress that effective coping strategies can reduce the need for medication.

♦ Explain the importance of daily exercise in relieving stress, and encourage establishing a plan for getting enough exercise (e.g., daily walks).

♦ Point out that drug tolerance and dependence can occur, and that the drug should be used on a short-term basis.

♦ Warn that abrupt withdrawal of chlordiazepoxide may cause severe problems (doses should be tapered under medical supervision).

♦ Emphasize that the effects of alcohol, other sedatives and CNS depressants, and tranquilizers may be potentiated (these should be avoided).

♦ Advise avoidance of driving and other potentially hazardous activities until response is established.

♦ *See Antianxiety agents/Sedatives/Hypnotics overview for more information.*

chloroprocaine
klor-oh-proe′kane

chloroprocaine hydrochloride: **Nesacaine**
Nesacaine-MPF
Class: Local anesthetic (ester-type)

PEDS	PREG	GERI
✋	C	✋

Action Produces local anesthesia by inhibiting sodium flux across the nerve-cell membrane, thus preventing depolarization and generation and conduction of nerve impulses. Chloroprocaine has a rapid onset (2–8 min), is short-acting (30–60 min), and has low potency and toxicity. When combined with epinephrine, action is prolonged.

Use/Therapeutic goal/Outcome

Local anesthesia (local infiltration, nerve blocks, and epidural anesthesia): Prevention of pain during surgical or obstetric procedures. **Outcome criteria:** Report of numbness and absence of pain in anesthetized area. Patients receiving epidural anesthesia will also demonstrate loss of motor function in the anesthetized area.

Dose range/Administration

Interaction alert: Incompatible with iodine, iodides, silver salts. Do not use these agents to disinfect the skin or mucous membrane before chloroprocaine administration.

Adult: *Infiltrate and nerve block:* 30–200 mg 1% solution (3–20 cc), *or* 40–800 mg 2% solution (2–40 cc). *Maximum dose:* 11 mg/kg (14 mg/kg with epinephrine). *Caudal and epidural*: 300–750 mg 2–3% solution (15–25 cc); may repeat with smaller doses q40-60min. With epinephrine, dose and interval between additional doses may increase. *Maximum dose:* 800 mg (or 1 g with epinephrine).

Clinical alert: These drugs should be administered only by clinicians thoroughly familiar with their use. Doses are highly individualized and vary with the procedure, method of administration, area to be anesthetized, and vascularity of tissue. For epidural route, a test dose must be given to verify position of catheter or needle. Epinephrine used in local anesthesia may result in angina, tachycardia, tremors, headache, restlessness, palpitations, dizziness, and hypertension. Have oxygen and resuscitative drugs and equipment readily available.

Contraindications/Precautions

PREG C

Contraindicated in hypersensitivity to chloroprocaine, ester-type anesthetics, PABA and its derivates, or bisulfites; concurrent use of bupivacaine. Not recommended for topical, spinal, or IV regional anesthesia. *Use with caution* in history of drug hypersensitivity, dysrhythmias, cardiac or liver disease, and for the debilitated or acutely ill patient.

🖐 **Safe use for pregnant and nursing mothers or for children under 12 years has not been established. Use with caution for the elderly.**

Side effects/Adverse reactions

Hypersensitivity: rashes, cutaneous lesions of delayed onset; urticaria, sneezing, anaphylaxis. *CNS:* anxiety, nervousness, tremors, sedation, circumoral paresthesia, convulsions followed by drowsiness, respiratory arrest. *CV:* myocardial depression, hypotension, arrhythmias, bradycardia, cardiac arrest. *Eye:* blurred or double vision. *Ear:* tinnitus. *GI:* nausea, vomiting. *Misc:* (with caudal or epidural anesthesia) urinary retention, fecal or urinary incontinence, slowing of labor or increased incidence of forceps delivery, headache, backache, edema, status asthmaticus.

Nursing implications/Documentation

Possible nursing diagnoses: Pain; Potential for injury.

♦ Be sure that history of allergies and accurate height and weight are recorded before procedure.

♦ Be aware that Nesacaine contains methylparaben (preservative) and sodium bisulfite, both of which may cause allergic reactions.

♦ Record vital signs according to protocol, and monitor for and report immediately signs of systemic or hypersensitivity reactions.

♦ Determine from anesthesiologist or anesthetist whether there are any restrictions on patient positioning; post these at bedside.

♦ Monitor anesthetized area for level of sensation and motor function; watch for poor positioning and protect area from injury.

♦ Give prescribed pain medication as sensation begins to return, **before pain is severe**.

Patient & family teaching/Home care

Possible nursing diagnoses: Anxiety; Fear.

♦ Stress the need to protect areas of the body that have lost sensation.

♦ Explain rationale for taking prescribed pain medication before pain becomes too uncomfortable.

♦ *See Local anesthetics overview for more information.*

chlorothiazide
klor-oh-thy'a-zide

chlorothiazide: **🞂Azide, 🞂Chlotride, Diachlor, 🞂Diuret, Diuril**

chlorothiazide sodium: *Diuri Sodium*

Class: Thiazide diuretic, Antihypertensive

PEDS	PREG	GERI
🖐	D	🖐

Action Promotes excretion of sodium chloride, potassium, and water by inhibiting sodium reabsorption in the early portion of the distal tubule. Lowers blood pressure by reducing plasma and extra-cellular volume.

Use/Therapeutic goal/Outcome

Edema: Resolution of edema. *Outcome criteria:* Increased urine output; weight loss; absence of rales and peripheral and sacral edema. *Hypertension:* Reduction of blood pressure. *Outcome criteria:* After 3–4 days blood pressure within normal limits.

Dose range/Administration

Interaction alert: Cholestyramine and colestipol decrease intestinal absorption. Diazoxide potentiates the hyperglycemic, hyperuricemic, and hypotensive effects. Do not give concomitantly with lithium. Give cautiously with corticosteroids, antidiabetics, lanoxin, and skeletal muscle relaxants. Nonsteroidal anti-inflammatory drugs may decrease effects.

Adult: PO or IV: 500 mg to 2 g/day, in divided doses. *Child < 6 mos:* PO, IV: Up to 30 mg/kg/day in 2 divided doses. *Child > 6 mos:* PO, IV: 20 mg/kg/day in 2 doses.

Clinical alert: Do not administer IV to infants and children. Avoid extravasation. Give in morning to prevent nocturnal diuresis. Antihypertensive response may not occur for several days.

Contraindications/Precautions

Contraindicated in hypersensitivity to sulfonamides or thiazides, and in oliguria, anuria, hypokalemia, and renal insufficiency. **Use with caution** in patients with allergic history, bronchial asthma, renal or hepatic dysfunction, gout, diabetes, pancreatitis, systemic lupus erythematosus, and debilitation, and for jaundiced children.

☝ **Contraindicated for pregnant women. Use with caution for children and the elderly.**

Side effects/Adverse reactions

Hypersensitivity: anaphylaxis, rash, urticaria, purpura, dermatitis with photosensitivity, fever, pneumonitis, respiratory distress. **Hem:** hypokalemia, hyperglycemia, impaired glucose tolerance, asymptomatic hyperuricemia, fluid and electrolyte imbalances, metabolic alkalosis, hypercalcemia, lipid abnormalities, aplastic anemia, agranulocytosis, leukopenia, thrombocytopenia. **CV:** volume depletion, orthostatic hypotension, dehydration. **GI:** anorexia, nausea, pancreatitis, hepatic encephalopathy. **Skin:** necrosis with extravasation. **Misc:** gout.

Nursing implications/Documentation

Possible nursing diagnoses: Fluid volume deficit; Altered patterns of urinary elimination; Potential for injury.

◆ Ascertain that baseline CBC, sodium, potassium, chloride, carbon dioxide, calcium, magnesium, BUN, creatinine, uric acid, and liver function studies have been obtained before giving first dose; report abnormalities and monitor closely thereafter.

◆ Document and monitor blood pressure, pulse, daily weight, and intake and output; report significant discrepancies.

◆ Monitor for hyperglycemia because of risk of thiazide diabetes.

◆ Observe for and report signs of fluid overload (auscultate lungs for rales; check feet, ankles, and sacrum for edema).

◆ Be aware that diuretics often induce hypokalemia, which predisposes individuals to cardiac arrhythmias, cramping, and digoxin toxicity.

◆ Check with physician to determine dietary restrictions; if a low-salt, high-potassium diet is recommended, consult with dietician to plan a low-salt diet that includes foods and juices high in potassium (orange juice; banana; green leafy vegetables).

◆ Observe the elderly for extreme diuresis (may require lower doses); monitor for orthostatic hypotension; supervise ambulation until response is determined.

Patient & family teaching/Home care

Possible nursing diagnoses: Knowledge deficit; Impaired home maintenance management.

◆ Before giving first dose, explain that the drug will increase the amount and frequency of urination.

◆ Emphasize the importance of taking this drug exactly as prescribed, and the importance of returning for medical follow-up.

◆ Explain that diuretics enhance the work of the kidney and reduce the workload of the heart.

◆ Recommend taking doses in early morning and early afternoon to prevent the need to disturb sleep to void.

◆ Explain that changing positions slowly helps prevent dizziness.

◆ Advise reporting dizziness, shortness of breath, swelling of hands and feet, or persistent sore throat; encourage daily monitoring of weight and reporting sudden weight gain.

◆ Warn that hyperglycemia is common; advise reporting thirst, fatigue, or weight loss.

◆ Provide a list of allowed foods and fluids; stress the need to stick to prescribed diet (explain the hazards of too much salt, or too little potassium).

◆ Warn against driving or activities that require alertness until response has been determined.

◆ Advise avoidance of OTC drugs unless approved by physician; stress need to wear a sunscreen.

◆ *See Diuretics and Antihypertensives overviews for more information.*

chlorphenesin

klor-fen'e-sin

chlorphenesin carbamate: *Maolate*
Class: Skeletal-muscle relaxant (centrally acting)

PEDS	PREG	GERI
☝	C	☝

Action Relaxes skeletal musles by depressing polysynaptic spinal reflexes and CNS. Has no direct effect on striated muscle.

Use/Therapeutic goal/Outcome

Muscle spasms associated with sprains, trauma, and inflammation: Relaxation of skeletal muscle; relief of spasm and pain. ***Outcome criteria:*** Increased range of motion and ability to perform activities of daily life; report of decreased pain, spasm, and associated anxiety and tension.

Trigeminal neuralgia (investigational use): Promotion of comfort. ***Outcome criteria:*** Report of decreased facial pain.

Dose range/Administration

Interaction alert: May increase CNS effects of other CNS depressants and alcohol.

🥄 **Give with food or milk to prevent gastric distress.**

Adult: PO: *Initial dose:* 800 mg tid, until desired effect is obtained. *Maintenance dose:* 400 mg tid.

Clinical alert: Therapy should not exceed 8 weeks duration.

Contraindications/Precautions

PREG
C

Contraindicated in hypersensitivity to chlorphenesin, and tartrazine, and in severe hepatic impairment. ***Use with caution*** in renal or hepatic impairment.

Side effects/Adverse reactions

Hypersensitivity: rash, itching, drug fever, anaphylaxis. ***CNS:*** drowsiness, dizziness, confusion, headache, weakness, agitation, insomnia. ***GI:*** nausea, epigastric distress, sore mouth and throat. ***Hem:*** thrombocytopenia, leukopenia, agranulocytosis.

Nursing implications/Documentation

Possible nursing diagnoses: Impaired physical mobility; Potential for injury; Pain.

♦ Monitor comfort level and range of motion before and after dose is taken.

♦ Monitor for and report abnormal blood studies (CBC, liver function) and sensitivity reactions (excessive fatigue, easy bruising or bleeding, sore throat).

♦ Supervise out-of-bed activities, especially if drowsiness is present.

Patient & family teaching/Home care

Possible nursing diagnoses: Impaired home maintenance management; Knowledge deficit.

♦ Advise taking doses with food to reduce GI symptoms.

♦ Warn against combining with other depressants or alcohol and against driving or operating machinery if drowsiness is present.

♦ Stress the importance of following total treatment plan, including rest and other forms of therapy (e.g., relaxation techniques).

♦ *See Skeletal-muscle relaxants overview for more information.*

chlorpheniramine   *klor-fen-eer'a-meen*

chlorpheniramine maleate: ***Aller-Chlor,*** 🍁***Allergex, Chlo-Amine, Chlorate, Chlor-100, Chlor-Niramine, Chlor-Pro, Chlor-Pro 10, Chlorspan-12, Chlortab-4, Chlortab-8, Chlor-Trimeton, Chlor-Trimeton Repetabs, Chlor-Tripolon, Genallerate,*** 🍁***Novopheniram, Pfeffer's Allergy, Phenetron,*** 🍁***Piriton, Pyranistan, Telachlor, Teldrin, Trymegan***

Class: Antihistamine (H$_1$ receptor antagonist)

PEDS	PREG	GERI
🖐	B	🖐

Action Prevents but does not reverse histamine-mediated allergic responses by competing with histamine for H$_1$ receptors on effector cells. Has anticholinergic action.

Use/Therapeutic goal/Outcome

Allergic conditions: Decrease in allergic response. ***Outcome criteria:*** Report and demonstration of relief of allergic symptoms (sneezing, nasal secretions, itching).

Dose range/Administration

Interaction alert: CNS depressants and alcohol may cause excessive sedation. Do not give with MAOIs or anticholinergics.

🥄 **Give with food or milk to avoid GI upset.**

Self-medication: Adult/Child > 12 yrs: PO: *Tablets, syrup:* 4 mg q4-6h, to a maximum of 24 mg in 24 hr. *Sustained-release tablet:* 8 or 12 mg q12h, to a maximum of 24 mg in 24 hr.

Under physician's direction: Adult: SC, IM, IV: 5–20 mg as a single dose, to a maximum of 40 mg/day. For IV use, inject over 1 min, and use the preservative-free preparation. ***Child 6–12 yrs:*** PO: *Tablets, syrup:* 2 mg q4-6h, to a maximum of 12 mg in 24 hr. *Sustained-release tablet:* 8 mg hs. ***Child 2–6 yrs:*** PO: 1 mg q4-6h, to a maximum of 6 mg in 24 hr.

Clinical alert: Do not crush sustained-release tablets. Expect reduced dosage for the elderly, and monitor for excessive drowsiness and dizziness.

▶

This drug should be given to children under 12 years only as directed by a physician.

Contraindications/Precautions

Contraindicated in hypersensitivity to chlorpheniramine or to chemically related antihistamines, and within 14 days of treatment with MAOIs, in acute asthma, narrow-angle glaucoma, obstructive prostatic hypertrophy, and GI obstruction or stenosis. ***Use with caution*** in convulsive disorders, increased intraocular pressure, hyperthyroidism, cardiovascular disease, hypertension, diabetes mellitus, history of asthma.

✋ **Contraindicated for children under 6 years. Avoid use for pregnant or nursing mothers.Use with caution for older children and the elderly.**

Side effects/Adverse reactions

Hypersensitivity: skin rash, urticaria, photosensitivity, anaphylaxis. ***CNS:*** sedation, stimulation, dizziness, vertigo, headache, disturbed coordination, tingling, insomnia. ***CV:*** palpitations, tachycardia, mild hypotension. ***Resp:*** dry nose and throat, thickened bronchial secretions, wheezing, sensation of chest tightness. ***Ear:*** tinnitus. ***GI:*** dry mouth, epigastric distress. ***GU:*** urinary frequency or retention. ***Eye:*** blurred vision, diplopia. (following parenteral administration: transitory stinging or burning at injection site, sweating, pallor, transient hypotension.)

Nursing implications/Documentation

Possible nursing diagnoses: Potential for injury; Fluid volume deficit.

♦ Determine and record known allergies; provide an environment that is free from allergens (especially sleeping areas).

♦ Provide favorite fluids and ensure adequate hydration (2 liters/day).

♦ For parenteral route, keep patient flat in bed until response is determined (may cause transient hypotension, drowsiness, dizziness).

Patient & family teaching/Home care

Possible nursing diagnoses: Knowledge deficit; Impaired home maintenance management.

♦ Advise taking this drug with food or milk if GI symptoms are experienced; warn not to crush or chew sustained-release tablets.

♦ Point out that avoiding pollens and staying in an air-conditioned environment may help reduce seasonal rhinitis.

♦ Emphasize that dose should not be increased without physician's approval; explain that tolerance may occur, requiring a change in medication.

♦ Warn that alcohol and other CNS depressants may cause excessive drowsiness; advise against driving until response is determined.

♦ Suggest that coffee or tea may reduce drowsiness, and that sugarless gum or hard candy may relieve dry mouth.

♦ *See Antihistamines overview for more information.*

chlorpromazine

klor-pro'ma-zeen

chlorpromazine hydrochloride: ✦***Chlorpromanyl,*** ✦ ♠***Largactil,*** ✦***Novo-Chlorpromaine,*** ♠***Protran, Thorazine, Thor-Pram***

Class: ★**Phenothiazine antipsychotic prototype,** Antiemetic

PEDS ✋   PREG C   GERI ✋

Action Exact mechanism of action has not been determined. Believed to promote calmness and alleviate psychiatric symptoms (disorders of perception, thought, consciousness, mood, affect, and social interaction) by blocking dopamine receptors in the limbic system. Acts as an antiemetic by inhibiting the medullary chemoreceptor trigger zone. Produces sedative or tranquilizing effect within 60 min of oral or rectal administration, and within 10 min of injection; antipsychotic effect take much longer. Blocks peripheral muscarinic, adrenergic, and histamine receptors. Also has some effect on the hypothalamus and pituitary gland, causing changes in regulation of body temperature and endocrine function.

Use/Therapeutic goal/Outcome

Schizophrenia, psychosis, agitated behavior, mania associated with bipolar disorders: Promotion of reality orientation, elimination of agitation and hyperactivity. ***Outcome criteria:*** Demonstration of reality orientation, and ability to problem solve and interact with others; absence of agitation or hyperactivity.

Severe behavioral disturbances in children: Elimination of explosive and combative behavior. ***Outcome criteria:*** Absence of explosive and combative behavior.

Severe anxiety or agitation: Promotion of calmness or relaxation. **Outcome criteria:** Report of feeling more calm and relaxed; demonstration of decreased restlessness or agitation.

Nausea and vomiting: Relief of nausea and vomiting. **Outcome criteria:** Report and demonstration of absence of nausea and vomiting.

Intractable hiccups: Elimination of hiccups. **Outcome criteria:** Absence of hiccups.

Acute intermittent porphyria: Elimination of symptoms associated with porphyria. **Outcome criteria:** Report of absence of abdominal discomfort and neurological symptoms associated with porphyria.

Dose range/Administration

Interaction alert: Antacids reduce absorption; separate doses of antacid and phenothiazines by at least 2 hr. Alcohol and other CNS depressants may cause excessive sedation. Barbiturates and lithium may decrease phenothiazine effects. May decrease antihypertensive effects of centrally-acting antihypertensives. Use with propranolol may increase levels of both drugs. May decrease the effect of anticoagulants.

🖐 **Give PO doses with food to avoid GI upset.**

Psychiatric disorders: Adult: PO: 500 mg daily in divided doses to a maximum of 2 g/day in divided doses, depending upon severity of symptoms. Once symptoms are controlled, more than 1 g/day is rarely useful. IM: 25–50 mg q1-4h prn for severe disturbances. Change to oral route as soon as possible. **Child:** PO: 0.25 mg/kg q4-6h. *Maximum dose:* 40 mg for child < 5 yrs, 75 mg for child 5–12 yrs. IM: 0.25 mg/kg q6-8h. *Maximum dose:* 40 mg for child < 5 yrs, 75 mg for child 5–12 yrs. Change to oral route as soon as possible. RECT: 0.5 mg/kg q6-8h. *Maximum dose:* 40 mg for child < 5 yrs, 75 mg for child 5–12 yrs.

Severe anxiety/agitation: Adult: PO: 200–800 mg/day in divided doses. IM: Use psychiatric disorders dose.

Nausea and vomiting: Adult: PO: 10–20 mg q4-6h prn. IM: 25–50 mg q3-4h prn. RECT: 50–100 mg q6-8h prn. **Child:** PO: 0.25 mg/kg q4-6h prn. IM: 0.25 mg/kg q6-8h prn. *Maximum dose:* 40 mg for child < 5 yrs, 75 mg for child 5–12 yrs. RECT: 0.5 mg/kg q6-8h prn.

Intractable hiccups: Adult: PO: 25–50 mg tid or qid. IM: (only if oral route fails) 25–50 mg q4h. IV: (only if oral and IM routes fail and hiccups are severe) 25–50 mg diluted in 500–1000 cc NS, infused at a rate of 1–2 mg/min (monitor blood pressure).

Acute intermittent porphyria: Adult: PO: 25–50 mg tid or qid. IM: 25 mg tid or qid. Change to oral route as soon as possible.

Clinical alert: Before administering by parenteral route, count respirations and check blood pressure; hold dose and report if respirations are less than 12 per minute, or if the patient is hypotensive. After administering, keep patient lying down for 1 hour and have IV diphenhydramine available in case of side effect of acute dystonic reaction. If compliance is a problem with oral form, consider using liquid form, which must be diluted in a beverage just before administration.

Contraindications/Precautions

PREG
C

Contraindicated in hypersensitivity to phenothiazines, and in coma, in patients who have taken large doses of CNS depressants, in liver damage, in withdrawal from alcohol, barbiturates, or other nonbarbiturate sedatives, and in respiratory depression, parkinsonism, poorly controlled diabetes mellitus, asthma, emphysema, narrow-angle glaucoma, cardiac disease, hypotension, paralytic ileus, liver disease, prostatic hypertrophy, bone marrow depression, and Reye's syndrome.

🖐 **Contraindicated for nursing mothers. Use only in life-saving emergencies for infants under 6 months. Use with caution for children and the elderly or debilitated. Safe use for pregnant women and children under 6 months has not been established.**

Side effects/Adverse reactions

Hypersensitivity: blood dyscrasias, jaundice, anaphylaxis, contact dermatitis, rash. **CNS:** sedation, high incidence of extrapyramidal reactions (pseudoparkinsonism, akathisia [restless need to keep moving], dystonia, tardive dykinesia), EEG changes, dizziness, neuroleptic malignant syndrome (fever, tachycardia, tachypnea, profuse diaphoresis). **CV:** orthostatic hypotension, palpitations, dysrhythmias, EKG changes. **GI:** appetite changes, dry mouth, susceptibility to oral thrush, constipation, abnormal liver function. **GU:** urinary retention or hesitancy, dark urine, priapism, impaired ejaculation, amenorrhea. **Eye:** blurred vision, photophobia. **Skin:** photosensitivity. **MS:** weight gain. **Hem:** hyperglycemia, transient leukopenia, agranulocytosis. **Misc:** galactorrhea, gynecomastia, fever. **After abrupt withdrawal of long-term therapy:** gastritis, nausea, vomiting, lightheadedness, tremors, feeling of warmth or cold, diaphoresis, tachycardia, headache, insomnia.

Nursing implications/Documentation

Possible nursing diagnoses: Potential for injury; Constipation; Altered oral mucous membrane.

♦ Record mental status and vital signs before and 1 hr after administration during initial phase of treatment, then bid until response to therapy has been established, then periodically thereafter.

♦ Check CBC, liver function, BUN, and creatinine before giving first dose and periodically thereafter.

♦ Be sure that doses are swallowed (not hoarded).

♦ Monitor for orthostatic hypotension, dizziness, and drowsiness; supervise ambulation until response is established.

♦ Record weight every 2 weeks; report significant weight gain. Provide special mouth care and observe for signs of oral candidiasis (may require medication).

♦ Prevent constipation by monitoring bowel movements and encouraging adequate fiber and fluid intake; offer laxatives or stool softeners before problem becomes severe.

♦ Report persistent sore throat, fever, and malaise, because these may indicate agranulocytosis (drug may have to be discontinued).

♦ Monitor for (and report immediately) signs of neuroleptic malignant syndrome (muscle rigidity, tremors, high fever, tachycardia); this is a rare, but potentially fatal, side effect.

♦ *For antiemetic use, see Nursing implications and Patient & family teaching in Antiemetics overview.*

Patient & family teaching/Home care

Possible nursing diagnoses: Sleep pattern disturbance; Impaired home maintenance management.

♦ Emphasize the need to continue medication, even when feeling well.

♦ Warn to change positions slowly to prevent dizziness.

♦ Explain that meticulous brushing and flossing can help prevent side effect of oral infection.

♦ Stress that the sedative effect of alcohol, sedatives, and tranquilizers may be potentiated.

♦ Caution to consult with physician before using OTC drugs; stress the need for ongoing medical follow-up.

♦ Teach the need to report persistent sore throat, fever, and fatigue.

♦ Point out that doses should not be increased or stopped without checking with physician.

♦ Caution to wear a sunscreen (number 15), protective clothing, and sunglasses when out in the sun.

♦ Advise avoidance of driving and other potentially hazardous activities until response is established.

♦ Suggest using ice chips, hard candy, or gum to relieve side effect of dry mouth; stress the need for good mouth care.

♦ Teach that this drug may cause urine to be red or brown (due to a metabolite, not blood).

♦ Warn women to report if pregnancy is planned or suspected.

♦ *See Antipsychotics and Antiemetics overviews for more information.*

chlorpropamide

klor-proe'pa-mide

♦*Apo-Chlorpropamide, Diabinese, Glucamide,* ♦*Novo-propamide*

Class: Antidiabetic (oral hypoglycemic), First-generation sulfonylurea

Antidote: $D_{50}W$, glucagon

PEDS	PREG	GERI
🤚	**D**	🤚

Action Reduces serum glucose and promotes cellular nutrition by stimulating insulin release in beta cells of the pancreas and by reducing glucose output by the liver (not effective if beta cells have ceased to function). Exerts an antidiuretic effect in pituitary-deficient diabetes insipidus. Onset of action occurs in 60 minutes; peak action is in 3–6 hours, and duration of action is 36–60 hours.

Use/Therapeutic goal/Outcome

Mild to moderately severe, stable, Type II (noninsulin-dependent) diabetes mellitus; for those not controlled by meal plan or weight control alone: Normalization of blood glucose levels, glycemic control. **Outcome criteria:** Absence of clinical symptoms of hypoglycemia (confusion, shakiness, weakness, diaphoresis, apprehension) together with blood glucose studies that demonstrate glycemic control (fasting blood sugar: 100–140 mg/dl is good control; 140–200 mg/dl is fair control).

Dose range/Administration

Interaction alert: Alcohol, anabolic steroids, insulin, chloramphenicol, oral anticoagulants, salicylates, NSAIDs, MAOIs, phenylbutazone, sulfonamides, and clofibrate may *increase* hypoglycemic activity. Corticosteroids, glucagon, calcium channel blockers, thyroid preparation, rifampin, and thiazide diuretics may *decrease* hypoglycemic activity and exacerbate diabetic symptoms. Alcohol ingestion may cause a disulfiram-like reaction (facial reddening, headache, nausea, vomiting) known as chlorpropamide-alcohol flush (CPAF). Beta-blockers and clonidine may mask and prolong hypoglycemic reactions.

Adult: PO: 250–500 mg/day, with the first meal or in divided doses with morning and evening meals; may increase by 50–125 mg/day q3-5 days. *For the elderly:* 100–125 mg in divided doses with meals.

Clinical alert: Because chlorpropamide is a first-generation sulfonylurea, assess for allergy to sulfa before giving first dose. Check blood glucose levels 3 times a day during transition from an insulin regimen to chlorpropamide. Recognize that dose requirements vary with age, food intake, activity levels, and concurrent medical problems. Monitor the elderly closely for hypoglycemic reactions. They are likely to require slightly higher fasting blood sugars to prevent clinical symptoms of hypoglycemia. Individuals who have had a hypoglycemic episode should be monitored for repeated episodes because duration of action may be as long as 60 hours.

Contraindications/Precautions

PREG
D

Contraindicated in hypersensitivity to chlorpropamide and in Type I diabetes mellitus, uncontrolled diabetes mellitus, and severe renal, hepatic, or endocrine impairment. *Use with caution* in allergy to sulfa, in Type II diabetics who require surgery, experience trauma, or are compromised by an infection (may require insulin); and in heart disease.

✋ **Contraindicated for children and pregnant or nursing mothers. Use with caution for the elderly.**

Side effects/Adverse reactions

Hypersensitivity: skin eruptions, rash, blood dyscrasias, jaundice, low-grade fever, eosino-

philia. *Hem:* prolonged hypoglycemia, leukopenia, thrombocytopenia, anemia; dilutional hyponatremia. *GI:* nausea, vomiting, diarrhea, abdominal cramping, hepatitis. *CNS:* headache, dizziness. *GU:* tea-colored urine. *CV:* increase in signs of CHF.

Nursing implications/Documentation

Possible nursing diagnoses: Potential for injury; Impaired skin integrity; Impaired tissue integrity; Altered nutrition: more than body requirements; Altered nutrition: less than body requirements.

◆ Keep a record of blood sugars taken upon rising in the morning, ½ hr before each meal, and before bedtime snack; report persistent trends or significant episodes of hyperglycemia or hypoglycemia.

◆ Monitor food intake; notify physician when the patient is not eating.

◆ Monitor daily weights, especially during periods of illness.

◆ If signs of hypoglycemia (tremors, sweating, sudden weakness, pale skin, anxiety, confusion, agitation) are noted, confirm by a capillary blood glucose test first, then give 15 g of a fast acting carbohydrate (4 oz of fruit juice, 4–6 pieces of hard candy, a tablespoon of sugar or honey). If blood glucose monitoring equipment is not immediately available, give carbohydrate and check glucose level later.

◆ If signs of hyperglycemia (extreme thirst, frequent urination, fatigue, blurred vision) are noted, confirm by blood glucose meter and report immediately.

Patient & family teaching/Home care

Possible nursing diagnoses: Knowledge deficit; Impaired home maintenance management.

◆ Explain that oral hypoglycemics control blood sugars but do not cure diabetes; stress that regular exercise, careful regulation of diet and medication, close monitoring of blood sugars, and medical supervision help promote health and prevent the long-term complications of diabetes (heart, kidney, eyes).

◆ Advise taking doses in the earlier part of the day to avoid nighttime hypoglycemia.

◆ Point out that diet, activity, weight fluctuations, illness, and emotional stress can affect hypoglycemic medication requirements.

- Stress that everything on meal plan should be eaten, especially carbohydrates, but that concentrated sweets should be avoided.

- Teach the signs and symptoms of hypoglycemia and hyperglycemia; advise that a fast-acting carbohydrate (4 oz of fruit juice, 4–6 pieces of hard candy, 1 tablespoon of honey or sugar) should be taken for suspected hypoglycemia (suspected hyperglycemia should be reported immediately).

- Advise reporting weight fluctuations of over 10 pounds (5 kg) because it may affect dosage.

- Suggest carrying some form of fast-acting carbohydrate (e.g., small box of raisins) for treatment of hypoglycemia.

- Warn against use of alcohol and OTC drugs without physician's approval.

- Recommend wearing a medical alert bracelet to alert others to hypoglycemics use.

- *See Antidiabetics overview for more information.*

chlorprothixene

klor-proe-thix'een

Taractan, ♣Tarasan

Class: Thioxanthene antipsychotic

PEDS	PREG	GERI
🖐	C	🖐

Action Exact mechanism of action has not been determined. Believed to produce calmness and alleviate psychiatric symptoms (disorders of perception, thought, consciousness, mood, affect, and social interaction) by blocking dopamine receptors in the limbic system. Blocks peripheral muscarinic, adrenergic, and histamine receptors. Also has some effect on the hypothalamus and pituitary gland, causing changes in regulation of body temperature and endocrine function. A dose of 100 mg of chlorprothixene is therapeutically equivalent to 100 mg of chlorpromazine.

Use/Therapeutic goal/Outcome

Schizophrenia, psychotic disorders and associated agitation: Promotion of reality orientation, reduction in agitation. *Outcome criteria:* Demonstration of reality orientation, and ability to problem solve and interact with others, with decrease in signs of agitation (pacing, hyperactivity).

Dose range/Administration

Interaction alert: Alcohol and other CNS depressants may cause excessive sedation. May reduce effects of centrally acting antihypertensives. May potentiate effects of anticholinergics. May block effects of epinephrine.

🥄 **Give with milk or food to avoid GI upset.**
Adult: PO: 25–50 mg tid to qid; may increase gradually until desired response, or to a maximum of 600 mg/day. IM: 25–50 mg tid to qid. *Child > 6 yrs:* PO: 10–25 mg tid to qid. IM: Not recommended for children.

Clinical alert: Avoid skin contact with liquid and parenteral forms because it may cause contact dermatitis. Before IM doses, count respirations and check blood pressure; hold dose and report if respirations are less than 12/min or if the patient is hypotensive. Keep patient lying down for 1 hr after injection. Keep IV diphenhydramine available in case of side effect of acute dystonic reaction.

Contraindications/Precautions

PREG
C

Contraindicated in hypersensitivity to chlorprothixene or to thioxanthenes, and in CNS depression, comatose states, Reye's syndrome, parkinsonism, poorly controlled diabetes mellitus, asthma, emphysema, narrow-angle glaucoma, cardiac disease, hypotension, paralytic ileus, liver disease, prostatic hypertrophy, and bone marrow depression. *Use with caution* in seizure disorders, alcoholism, peptic ulcer, and hypertension.

🖐 **Contraindicated for nursing mothers. Use with caution for children and the elderly or debilitated. Safe use for children under 6 years and pregnant women has not been established.**

Side effects/Adverse reactions

Hypersensitivity: rash, contact dermatitis. *CNS:* extrapyramidal reactions (pseudoparkinsonism, akathisia [restless need to keep moving], dystonia, tardive dykinesia), sedation, EEG changes, dizziness, neuroleptic malignant syndrome (fever, tachycardia, tachypnea, profuse diaphoresis). *CV:* orthostatic hypotension, palpitations, tachycardia, EKG changes. *GI:* appetite changes, dry mouth, constipation, abnormal liver function. *GU:* urinary retention or hesitancy, dark urine, impaired ejaculation, priapism, amenorrhea. *Eye:* blurred vision. *Skin:* photosensitivity. *Hem:* hyperglycemia, transient leukopenia, agranulocytosis. *Misc:* weight gain, gynecomastia, galactorrhea.

After abrupt withdrawal of long-term therapy: gastritis, nausea, vomiting, lightheadedness, tremors, feeling of warmth or cold, diaphoresis, tachycardia, headache, insomnia.

Nursing implications/Documentation

Possible nursing diagnoses: Potential for injury; Constipation; Altered oral mucous membrane.

♦ Record mental status and vital signs before and 1–2 hr after administration during initial phase of treatment, then bid until response to therapy has been established, then periodically thereafter.

♦ Check CBC, liver function, BUN, and creatinine before giving first dose, and periodically thereafter.

♦ Be sure that doses are swallowed (not hoarded).

♦ Monitor for orthostatic hypotension, dizziness, and drowsiness; supervise ambulation until response is established.

♦ Provide special mouth care; observe for and report oral ulcers.

♦ Prevent constipation by monitoring bowel movements and encouraging adequate fiber and fluid intake; offer laxatives or stool softeners before problem becomes severe.

♦ Report persistent sore throat, fever, and malaise, because these may indicate agranulocytosis.

♦ Monitor for (and report immediately) signs of neuroleptic malignant syndrome (muscle rigidity, tremors, high fever, tachycardia); this is a rare, but potentially fatal, side effect.

Patient & family teaching/Home care

Possible nursing diagnoses: Sleep pattern disturbance; Impaired home maintenance management.

♦ Emphasize the need to continue medication, even when feeling well.

♦ Warn to change positions slowly to prevent dizziness.

♦ Stress that the effects of alcohol, sedatives and CNS depressants, and tranquilizers may be potentiated.

♦ Caution to consult with physician before using OTC drugs; stress the need for ongoing medical follow-up.

♦ Teach the need to report persistent sore throat, fever, and fatigue.

♦ Point out that doses should not be increased or stopped without checking with physician.

♦ Caution to wear a sunscreen (number 15), protective clothing, and sunglasses when out in the sun.

♦ Advise avoidance of driving and other potentially hazardous activities until response is determined.

♦ Suggest using ice chips, hard candy, or gum to relieve side effect of dry mouth; stress the need for good mouth care.

♦ Warn women to report if pregnancy is planned or suspected.

♦ *See Antipsychotics overview for more information.*

chlorthalidone

klor-thal'-i-dohn

♣**Apo-Chlorthalidone, Hygroton,** ♣**Novothalidone, Thalitone,** ♣**Uridon**

Class: Thiazide-like diuretic, Antihypertensive

PEDS	PREG	GERI
✋	**D**	✋

Action Promotes excretion of sodium chloride, potassium, and water by inhibiting sodium reabsorption in the early portion of the distal tubule. Lowers blood pressure by reducing plasma and extra-cellular volume.

Use/Therapeutic goal/Outcome

Hypertension: Reduction of blood pressure. **Outcome criteria:** After 3–4 days, blood pressure within normal limits.

Edema: Resolution of edema. **Outcome criteria:** Increased urine output; weight loss; absence of rales and peripheral and sacral edema.

Dose range/Administration

Interaction alert: Chloestyramine and colestipol decrease intestinal absorption. Diazoxide potentiates the antihypertensive, hyperglycemic, and hyperuricemic effects. Nonsteroidal anti-inflammatory drugs may decrease effects.

Adult: PO: 25–100 mg/day or 3 times a week.
Child: PO: 2 mg/kg 3 times per week.

Clinical alert: Give in morning to avoid nocturnal diuresis. Antihypertensive response may not occur for 3–4 days.

Contraindications/Precautions

Contraindicated in hypersensitivity to chlorthalidone, sulfonamides, thiazides, and in anuria and hypokalemia. *Use with caution* in the presence of gout, systemic lupus erythematosus, diabetes, and history of hepatic or renal failure, allergies or bronchial asthma.

✋ **Contraindicated for pregnant or nursing mothers. Use with caution for children and the elderly.**

Side effects/Adverse reactions

Hypersensitivity: rash, urticaria, vasculitis, dermatitis with photosensitivity. *Hem:* hypokalemia, hyperglycemia, impaired glucose tolerance, asymptomatic hyperuricemia, fluid and electrolyte imbalances, metabolic alkalosis, hypercalcemia, aplastic anemia, agranulocytosis, leukopenia, thrombocytopenia. *CV:* volume depletion, orthostatic hypotension, dehydration. *GI:* anorexia, nausea, pancreatitis, hepatic encephalopathy. *Misc:* gout, impotence.

Nursing implications/Documentation

Possible nursing diagnoses: Fluid volume deficit; Altered patterns of urinary elimination; Potential for injury.

◆ Ascertain that baseline CBC, sodium, potassium, chloride, carbon dioxide, calcium, magnesium, BUN, creatinine, uric acid, and liver function studies have been obtained before giving first dose; report abnormalities and monitor closely thereafter.

◆ Document and monitor blood pressure, pulse, daily weight, and intake and output; report significant discrepancies.

◆ Monitor for hyperglycemia because of risk of thiazide diabetes.

◆ Observe for and report signs of fluid overload (auscultate lungs for rales; check feet, ankles, and sacrum for edema).

◆ Be aware that diuretics often induce hypokalemia, which predisposes individuals to cardiac arrhythmias, cramping, and digoxin toxicity.

◆ Check with physician to determine dietary restrictions; if a low-salt, high-potassium diet is recommended, consult with dietician to plan a low-salt diet that includes foods and juices high in potassium (orange juice; banana; green leafy vegetables).

◆ Observe the elderly for extreme diuresis (may require lower doses); monitor for orthostatic hypotension; supervise ambulation until response is determined.

Patient & family teaching/Home care

Possible nursing diagnoses: Impaired home maintenance management; Altered patterns of sexuality.

◆ Before giving first dose, explain that the drug will increase the amount and frequency of urination.

◆ Emphasize the importance of taking this drug exactly as prescribed, and the importance of returning for medical follow-up.

◆ Explain that diuretics enhance the work of the kidney and reduce the workload of the heart.

◆ Recommend taking doses in early morning and early afternoon to prevent the need to disturb sleep to void.

◆ Explain that changing positions slowly helps prevent dizziness.

◆ Advise reporting dizziness, shortness of breath, swelling of hands and feet, or persistent sore throat; encourage daily monitoring of weight and reporting sudden weight gain.

◆ Warn that hyperglycemia is common; advise reporting thirst, fatigue, or weight loss.

◆ Provide a list of allowed foods and fluids; stress the need to stick to prescribed diet (explain the hazards of too much salt, or too little potassium).

◆ Warn against driving and activities that require alertness until response has been determined.

◆ Advise avoidance of OTC drugs unless approved by physician.

◆ Suggest using a (Number 15) sunscreen when outside because of photosensitivity (avoid products with PABA).

◆ Be aware that this drug may affect sexuality; explore concerns with patient and spouse.

◆ *See Diuretics and Antihypertensives overviews for more information.*

chlorzoxazone

klor-zox'a-zone

Paraflex, Parafon Forte DSC, Strifon Forte DSC

Class: Skeletal-muscle relaxant (centrally acting), Antispasmodic

PEDS	PREG	GERI
OK	C	🖐

Action Relaxes skeletal muscle by inhibiting polysynaptic reflexes in spinal cord, subcortical areas, and brainstem, and by its sedative action. Not effective for spastic or dyskinetic CNS disorders.

Use/Therapeutic goal/Outcome

Muscle spasm associated with acute musculoskeletal conditions: Relief of muscle spasm; improved comfort. **Outcome criteria:** Increased range of motion and ability to perform activities of daily life; report of relief of pain, anxiety, and tension.

Dose range/Administration

Interaction alert: CNS depressants and alcohol increase CNS effects.

🍎 **Give with food to prevent gastric irritation.** **Adult:** PO: 250–750 mg tid or qid. Dose may be reduced as improvement occurs. **Child:** PO: 20 mg/kg/day in divided doses.

Contraindications/Precautions

PREG C

Contraindicated in hypersensitivity to chlorzoxazone and severe liver dysfunction. **Use with caution** in history of impaired liver or renal function.

🖐 Use with caution for children and the elderly. Safe use for pregnant or nursing mothers has not been established.

Side effects/Adverse reactions

Hypersensitivity: rash, hives, redness, pruritus, petechiae, bruising, angioneurotic edema, anaphylaxis. **CNS:** drowsiness, headache, paresthesias, agitation, insomnia, nervousness. **GI:** nausea, vomiting, diarrhea, constipation, GI bleeding, hepatotoxicity. **Hem:** hematologic changes (anemia, granulocytopenia). **GU:** urine discoloration (orange or purple-red).

Nursing implications/Documentation

Possible nursing diagnoses: Impaired physical mobility; Potential for injury; Pain.

♦ Monitor comfort level and range of motion before and after dose is taken.

♦ Supervise out-of-bed activities if drowsiness is present.

♦ Monitor for and report abnormal hepatic laboratory studies and skin color (jaundice).

Patient & family teaching/Home care

Possible nursing diagnoses: Knowledge deficit; Impaired home maintenance management.

♦ Advise taking doses with food to prevent gastric distress.

♦ Warn against operating machinery, driving, or combining with other CNS depressants or alcohol—especially if drowsiness develops.

♦ Explain that this drug may cause urine discoloration (orange or purple-red).

♦ Encourage following treatment plan, including rest and other forms of therapy (e.g., use of relaxation techniques).

♦ Stress the importance of consulting physician prior to taking OTC drugs.

♦ *See Skeletal-muscle relaxants overview for more information.*

cholestyramine

koe-less-tir'a-mean

Cholybar, Questran

Class: ★**Antilipemic prototype**, Antipruritic, Ion-exchange resin, Bile acid sequestrant

PEDS	PREG	GERI
🖐	C	🖐

Action Reduces total serum cholesterol by binding with bile acids to form a nonabsorbable compound that is excreted in feces, thus increasing cholesterol clearance. May produce a modest increase in high-density lipoprotein (HDL) with long-term use.

Use/Therapeutic goal/Outcome

Primary hypercholesterolemia (types IIA and IIB): Reduction of serum cholesterol levels. **Outcome criteria:** Decreased plasma levels of cholesterol and low-density lipoproteins (LDL).

Pruritus from partial biliary obstruction: Reduction of bile acid deposits on the skin. **Outcome criteria:** Patient report of relief from itching.

Dose range/Administration

Interaction alert: Give all PO drugs with narrow therapeutic range 1 hour before or 4 hours after giving cholestyramine, because drug absorption may be substantially decreased by cholestyramine. Monitor digoxin level closely

▶

in patients receiving both drugs; digoxin toxicity may result when cholestyramine is stopped (dose adjustment probably will be needed).

🥛 **Give 30 min before meals.**

Adult: PO: 4 g tid, not to exceed 32 g/day; *or* 1 chewable bar bid. *Maintenance dose:* 1–3 bars/day. *Child > 6 yrs:* PO: 80 mg/kg tid. *Maintenance dose:* 1–3 chewable bars/day.

Clinical alert: Available in powder or chewable bar form. Do not give powder in dry form; sprinkle on surface of beverage of choice or wet food. Let stand a few minutes before mixing to obtain a uniform suspension. Use a large glass (and at least 2–6 ounces of fluid), and avoid carbonated beverages, which cause excessive foaming. After mixture is taken, swish a small amount of fluid in glass and have patient swallow this to ensure that the entire dose is taken.

Contraindications/Precautions

PREG
C

Contraindicated in hypersensitivity to cholestyramine, and in complete biliary obstruction. *Use with caution* in the presence of bleeding disorders, gallstones, constipation, hemorrhoids, steatorrhea, peptic ulcers, or renal impairment.

✋ **Contraindicated in children under 6 years. Use with caution for pregnant or nursing mothers and the elderly (because of GI effects).**

Side effects/Adverse reactions

Hypersensitivity: rash or soreness of skin, tongue, or perianal area; asthma. *GI:* constipation in 20–50 percent of patients (may be mild to severe), indigestion, flatulence, anorexia, cholecystitis, pancreatitis, bloating, stomach pain, nausea, vomiting, diarrhea, bleeding from gums, tarry stools. *CNS:* headache. *Hem:* hyperchloremic acidosis. *Skin:* bruising. *GU:* hematuria. *Misc:* Vitamin A, D, and K deficiency.

Nursing implications/Documentation

Possible nursing diagnoses: Constipation; Altered nutrition: more than body requirements.

♦ Monitor and document bowel function to detect constipation; provide adequate fluids and fiber; give laxatives before constipation becomes severe (consult with physician about using stool softener).

♦ Monitor for and report symptoms of bleeding (bruising, petechiae, tarry stools).

Patient & family teaching/Home care

Possible nursing diagnoses: Altered health maintenance; Knowledge deficit; Impaired home maintenance management.

♦ Explain that the purpose of this drug is to reduce serum cholesterol and to decrease the risk of cardiovascular disease.

♦ Stress the need to take this drug before meals and the need for a 2-hour interval between the dose of cholestyramine and doses of other drugs.

♦ Teach the proper method of mixing (see clinical alert); warn that this medication should *never* be taken in dry form, because this may cause choking.

♦ Emphasize the need to reduce other cardiac risk factors (obesity, smoking, high cholesterol diet, sedentary lifestyle), and help develop a plan to reduce these.

♦ Discuss the role of adequate hydration, fiber intake, and exercise in preventing constipation; help develop a plan to prevent constipation.

♦ Stress that persistent GI symptoms and bruising or bleeding tendencies should be reported.

♦ Reinforce that this drug will have to be taken for a long time, and that ongoing medical follow-up of cholesterol level is essential.

♦ *See Antilipemics overview for more information.*

choline magnesium trisalicylate

Trilisate

Class: Non-narcotic analgesic, Nonsteroidal anti-inflammatory drug (NSAID), Salicylate

PEDS	PREG	GERI
✋	C	✋

Action Relieves pain by an ill-defined effect on the hypothalamus (central action) and by blocking generation of pain impulses (peripheral action, which may involve inhibition of prostaglandin synthesis). Reduces inflammation, probably by inhibiting prostaglandin synthesis and synthesis or action of other mediators of the inflammatory response. Reduces fever by acting on the hypothalamic heat-regulating center to cause peripheral vasodilation, which increases peripheral blood supply and promotes heat loss through sweating and cooling by evaporation.

Use/Therapeutic goal/Outcome

Analgesic: Relief of pain. **Outcome criteria:** Report of greater comfort; absence of signs of discomfort (frowning, restlessness, crying).

Anti-inflammatory: Reduction of inflammation. **Outcome criteria:** Report of reduced stiffness, swelling, and increased mobility.

Antipyretic: Reduction of fever. **Outcome criteria:** Reduced temperature.

Dose range/Administration

Interaction alert: Anticoagulants increase risk of bleeding (use together cautiously). Ammonium chloride and other urine acidifiers may increase risk of salicylate toxicity. Antacids (high doses), other urine alkalinizers, and corticosteroids may decrease effects. Large doses may decrease insulin and oral hypoglycemics requirements.

🍎 **Give with milk or food to reduce GI symptoms.**

Anti-inflammatory: Adult: PO: 1–2 tablets or tsp bid or qd (each 500-mg tablet or tsp has salicylate content of 650 mg aspirin). **Child 12–37 kg:** PO: 50 mg/kg/day in divided doses bid. **Child > 37 kg:** 2250 mg in divided doses. Cherry-flavored liquid provides 500 mg salicylate per tsp (5 ml).

Analgesic or antipyretic: Adult: PO: 2–3 g/day in divided doses.

Clinical alert: If liquid is needed, consider using choline salicylate. Monitor the elderly for increased risk of toxicity.

Contraindications/Precautions

PREG C

Contraindicated in hypersensitivity to salicylates, and in GI bleeding. **Use with caution** in Vitamin K deficiency, hypoprothrombinemia, bleeding disorders, and for asthmatics with nasal polyps (possible severe bronchospasms).

✋ **Contraindicated for pregnant or nursing mothers. Use with caution for the elderly. Safe use for children is not established.**

Side effects/Adverse reactions

Hypersensitivity: rashes, anaphylaxis, asthma. **Ear:** (high doses) tinnitus, deafness (first signs of toxicity). **CNS:** dizziness, sweating, mental confusion. **GI:** nausea, vomiting, GI distress, hepatitis, hepatotoxicity. **Resp:** hyperventilation.

Nursing implications/Documentation

Possible nursing diagnoses: Pain; Impaired physical mobility.

◆ Schedule drug administration so that drug is given *at least 1 hr* before maximum effect is needed; document and report inadequate pain control.

◆ Attempt to determine cause of fever before giving choline; (may mask symptoms that should be treated more specifically; report persistent fever and keep a record of temperature reading before and after administration).

◆ Monitor for and report GI symptoms that may indicate peptic ulcer (nausea, pain, black stools).

◆ Observe the elderly for toxicity.

Patient & family teaching/Home care

Possible nursing diagnoses: Knowledge deficit; Impaired home maintenance management.

◆ Explain the importance of watching for symptoms of GI bleeding (black stools, persistent GI distress).

◆ Point out that long-term use of salicylates (or use in high doses) is likely to increase risk of bleeding and that those taking this drug on a long-term basis should be followed by a physician.

◆ Advise telling physician and dentist if choline is taken on a regular basis.

◆ Warn not to take drugs containing aspirin or salicylates while taking this drug.

◆ *See Narcotic and non-narcotic analgesics and Nonsteroidal anti-inflammatory drugs overviews for more information.*

choline salicylate   *koe'leen sah-lis'i-late*

Arthropan, ✦*Teejel*

Class: Analgesic, Nonsteroidal anti-inflammatory drug (NSAID), Antipyretic, Salicylate

PEDS	PREG	GERI
✋	C	✋

Action Relieves pain through an ill-defined effect on the hypothalamus (central action) and by blocking generation of pain impulses (peripheral action, which may involve inhibition of prostaglandin synthesis). Reduces inflammation, probably by inhibiting prostaglandin synthesis and synthesis or action of other mediators of the inflammatory response. Reduces fever by acting on the hypothalamic heat-

▶

regulating center to cause peripheral vasodilation, which increases peripheral blood supply and promotes heat loss through sweating and cooling by evaporation. Causes less GI distress and bleeding than aspirin.

Use/Therapeutic goal/Outcome

Antipyretic: Reduction of fever. **Outcome criteria:** Reduced temperature.

Anti-inflammatory: Reduction of inflammation. **Outcome criteria:** Report of reduced pain, stiffness, and swelling of joints; with increased mobility.

Analgesic: Relief of pain. **Outcome criteria:** Report of increased comfort; absence of signs of discomfort (frowning, restlessness, crying).

Dose range/Administration

Interaction alert: Separate doses of antacids from choline by at least 2 hr. Avoid use with oral anticoagulants (increases risk of bleeding). PABA, ammonium chloride, and other urine acidifiers increase risk of toxicity. Antacids (high doses), other urine alkalinizers, and corticosteroids may decrease effects.

🍃 Give with food (not milk) to reduce GI symptoms.

Adult: PO: 5 ml (870 mg) q3-4h prn, not over 6 doses/day. **Child 3–6 yrs:** PO: 105–210 mg liquid solution q4h prn. **Child 6–12 yrs:** 210–420 mg liquid solution q4h prn.

Clinical alert: Each 870 mg (5 ml) is equal to 650 mg aspirin. Do not give salicylates to children under 18 years with chickenpox or influenza-like symptoms because of the association with Reye's syndrome. Monitor the elderly for increased risk of toxicity.

Contraindications/Precautions
PREG C

Contraindicated in hypersensitivity to salicylates, and in GI bleeding. **Use with caution** in Vitamin K deficiency, hypoprothrombinemia, bleeding disorders, and asthmatics with nasal polyps (possible severe bronchospasms).

✋ Contraindicated for pregnant or nursing mothers and for children under 18 years with chickenpox or influenza-like symptoms. Use with caution for children and the elderly (increased risk of toxicity).

Side effects/Adverse reactions

Hypersensitivity: rash, hives, itching, asthma, anaphylaxis. **GI:** nausea, vomiting, GI distress, abnormal liver-function studies, hepatitis, hepatotoxicity. **Ear:** at high doses, tinnitus

and deafness (first signs of toxicity). **CNS:** dizziness, mental confusion. **Resp:** hyperventilation. **Skin:** sweating.

Nursing implications/Documentation

Possible nursing diagnoses: Pain; Impaired physical mobility.

◆ Schedule doses so that drug is given at least one hour before maximum effect is needed; report and record inadequate pain control.

◆ Attempt to determine cause of fever before giving choline; (may mask symptoms that should be treated more specifically; report persistent fever, and keep a record of temperature reading before and after administration).

◆ Monitor for and report GI symptoms that may indicate peptic ulcer (nausea, pain, black stools).

◆ Observe the elderly for toxicity.

Patient & family teaching/Home care

Possible nursing diagnoses: Knowledge deficit; Impaired home maintenance management.

◆ Explain the importance of watching for symptoms of GI bleeding (black stools, persistent GI distress).

◆ Point out that long-term use of salycilates (or use in high doses) is likely to increase risk of bleeding and that those taking this drug on a long-term basis should be followed by a physician.

◆ Advise telling physician and dentist if choline is taken on a regular basis.

◆ Warn not to use other drugs containing aspirin at the same time.

◆ For children, stress that those under 18 years with flu-like symptoms or chickenpox should not receive aspirin or this drug (because of risk of developing Reye's syndrome).

◆ *See Narcotic and non-narcotic analgesics and Nonsteroidal anti-inflammatory drugs overviews for more information.*

chymopapain
kye'moe-pa-pane

Chymodiactin, Discase
Class: Proteolytic enzyme

PEDS	PREG	GERI
✋	C	✋

Action Reduces intradisc pressure by breaking down mucopolysaccharide-protein complexes when injected into intravertebral disc. Also reduces osmotic activity within the nucleus pulposus and decreases fluid absorption.

Use/Therapeutic goal/Outcome

Nonsurgical approach for herniated lumbar disc: Reduction of herniation. *Outcome criteria:* After several days, report of less pain, with increased range of motion and increased ability to perform ADLs; demonstration of improved muscle strength and X-ray study.

Dose range/Administration

Interaction alert: Halothane or epinephrine increases the risk of dysrhythmias.

Adult: Intradiscally: Chymodiactin: 2000–3000 pKat U/disc. Reconstitute with sterile water only; use within 2 hr. *Maximum total dose for more than one disc:* 8000 pKat U. Discase: 5 nKat/disc. Use reconstituted solution within 30 minutes. *Maximum total dose for more than one disc:* 10 nKat/U.

Clinical alert: This drug is administered in the hospital only by physicians trained in the diagnosis and treatment of lumbar disc disease. Be aware that incidence of anaphylaxis is higher in females, especially black females (may occur immediately or up to 2 hr after injection; patients having more than 2 injections are at greater risk). Maintain at least one IV line in place prior to and during administration, and have steroids, epinephrine, and resuscitative equipment and medications readily available.

Contraindications/Precautions

PREG
C

Contraindicated in hypersensitivity to chymopapain, papaya or papaya derivatives (such as those in contact lens cleaners and meat tenderizers), and in severe spondylolisthesis, spinal stenosis, progressive paralysis, spinal cord tumor, other lesions producing spinal motor or sensory dysfunction, and previous injection with chymopapain (may produce allergic response). *Use with caution* in history of hypertension, cardiovascular anomaly, CVA, and family history of CVA.

✋ Use with caution for the elderly. Safe use for children and pregnant women has not been established.

Side effects/Adverse reactions

Hypersensitivity: rash, urticaria, and pruritus up to 15 days after injection; anaphylaxis (mild to severe, including hypotension, bronchospasm, laryngeal edema, cardiac dysrhythmia, and cardiac arrest). *CNS:* paraplegia, para-

paresis, subarachnoid or intracerebral hemorrhage, seizures, sacral or leg pain, tingling, numbness, and leg weakness. *MS:* muscle spasms, back pain and stiffness for up to 2 weeks after injection.

Nursing implications/Documentation

Possible nursing diagnoses: Impaired physical mobility; Pain; Potential for injury.

◆ Monitor closely for and report signs and symptoms of hypersensitivity (rash, itching, hypotension) or adverse neurologic reactions.

◆ Record and monitor vital signs, respiratory status, and neurological status (level of consciousness and ability to move extremities every 15 min for 2 hr; longer if indicated).

◆ Observe for risk factors for injury (dizziness, weakness); supervise ambulation until response is determined.

Patient & family teaching/Home care

Possible nursing diagnoses: Anxiety; Fear.

◆ Warn that pain and involuntary muscle spasm of the lower back may be experienced for several days after injection; residual stiffness or soreness may persist for several months.

◆ Emphasize the role of holistic measures (e.g., relaxation techniques, approved back exercise program) in reducing back pain.

◆ Stress the need to contact the physician immediately if side effects such as rash or itching develop; this may occur up to 2 weeks after procedure.

◆ If patient develops a hypersensitive reaction to this drug, advise checking labels of contact lens cleaners and meat tenderizers as they contain papaya preparations (papain) which may enhance reaction.

cimetidine

sye-met'ih-deen

♠*Doractin, Tagamet*

Class: ★Histamine$_2$ receptor antagonist prototype, Antiulcer agent, Gastric acid secretion inhibitor

PEDS	PREG	GERI
✋	B	✋

Action Decreases basal and nocturnal gastric acid secretion by inhibiting the action of histamine at the H$_2$ receptors in the gastric parietal cells; decreases gastric acid secretion in response to food or chemical stimulus.

Use/Therapeutic goal/Outcome

Peptic ulcers: Promotion of healing and relief of pain. **Outcome criteria:** Report of absence of pain; hemoglobin and hematocrit within normal range; vital signs stable; stools negative for occult blood; endoscopic evidence of healing.

Prophylaxis of ulcer recurrence and stress-induced ulcers: Prevention. **Outcome criteria:** Report of absence of gastric pain; stable hemoglobin and hematocrit; stool and gastric secretions free of blood.

Hypersecretory conditions (e.g., Zollinger-Ellison syndrome): Control of hypersecretion of acid. **Outcome criteria:** Report of relief of epigastric pain; decreased diarrhea or steatorrhea; decreased acidity of gastric secretions.

Dose range/Administration

Interaction alert: Give antacids 1 hr before or after cimetidine to avoid interference with absorption. May increase serum levels of oral anticoagulants, metoprolol, phenytoin, cyclosporine, disulfiram, oral contraceptives, isoniazid, procainamide, benzodiazepines, antidepressants, propranolol, theophylline, bone marrow depressants, calcium channel blocking agents, lidocaine, and mexiletine.

🖐 **Administer oral doses with meals to maximize effects.**

Adult: PO: 300 mg qid with meals and at bedtime; or 400–600 mg bid with breakfast and at bedtime; or 400–800 mg at bedtime. IV: Continuous infusion—900 mg/24 hr. IM, IV: 300 mg q6-8h. *Maintenance dose:* 400 mg at bedtime. *Maximum dose:* 2400 mg/day (may be greater for treatment of hypersecretion). **Child:** PO: 5–10 mg/kg qid with meals and at bedtime. IM, IV: 5–10 mg/kg q6-8h.

Clinical alert: In moderate to severe renal function, reduced doses should be used.

Contraindications/Precautions

PREG
B

Contraindicated in hypersensitivity to histamine (H_2) receptor antagonists. **Use with caution** in renal and hepatic impairment, and chronic inflammatory diseases.

🖐 **Contraindicated for nursing mothers. Use with caution for children under 16 years, pregnant women, and the elderly.**

Side effects/Adverse reactions

Hypersensitivity: fever, skin rash, vasculitis. **CNS:** dizziness, somnolence, headache; confu-sional states (especially in the elderly with renal or hepatic disease). **CV:** hypotension, arrhythmias after rapid IV bolus. **Hem:** neutropenia. **GI:** diarrhea. **GU:** gynecomastia, impotence.

Nursing implications/Documentation

Possible nursing diagnoses: Diarrhea; Potential for infection; Sensory/perceptual alterations; Potential for injury.

◆ Use liquid form when administering by NG tube.

◆ Avoid rapid IV administration to prevent cardiac arrhythmias and hypotension.

◆ For continuous infusion, dose may be diluted in 100 to 1000 ml of most commonly used intravenous solutions; use infusion controller to maintain consistent rate and to protect patient from cardiovascular reactions.

◆ Assess for and record changes in mental state, especially in the elderly.

◆ Monitor for elevated blood levels or signs of toxicity of drugs whose metabolism may be decreased by cimetidine (e.g., theophylline, phenytoin, warfarin, and beta blockers).

Patient & family teaching/Home care

Possible nursing diagnoses: Knowledge deficit; Potential for injury; Impaired home maintenance management.

◆ Point out that for best effects cimetidine should be taken with meals and at bedtime; single daily dose should be taken at bedtime.

◆ Explain the need to avoid taking antacids within 1 hr of cimetidine.

◆ Advise smokers not to smoke after the bedtime dose to provide optimal suppression of nocturnal gastric acid secretion.

◆ Inform those being treated for active ulcer disease that this medication should be taken as prescribed for 4 to 8 weeks, to ensure healing of the ulcer, even though symptoms usually subside earlier.

◆ Counsel smokers with active ulcer disease to stop smoking and to avoid the use of caffeine.

◆ Stress the need to advise primary physician if diarrhea, dizziness, somnolence, rash, or hallucinations develop or if "coffee grounds" vomitus or tarry stools occur.

◆ *See Histamine$_2$ Antagonists overview for more information.*

cinoxacin

sin-ox'a-sin

Cinobac

Class: Urinary tract anti-infective

Action Kills bacteria (bactericidal) by inhibiting DNA replication and synthesis.

Use/Therapeutic goal/Outcome

Urinary tract infection caused by *Escherichia coli, Klebsiella, Enterobacter, Proteus mirabilis, Proteus vulgaris, Proteus morgani, Serratia,* and *Citrobacter:* Prevention/resolution of infection. **Outcome criteria:** Absence of growth on urine culture; report of absence of dysuria, frequency.

Dose range/Administration

Interaction alert: Probenecid decreases urinary excretion of cinoxacin, thus decreasing its urine concentration and effectiveness, and increasing its risk of toxicity.

🖎 **Give with meals to reduce GI distress.**

Adult/Child > 12 yrs: PO: 1 g/day in 2–4 divided doses with food for 7–14 days. *For prophylaxis:* 250 mg at bedtime for 5 mos.

Clinical alert: Monitor for and report persistent or increasing CNS side effects (may indicate serious toxicity, requiring discontinuation of medication). Observe the elderly for signs of septic shock.

Contraindications/Precautions

PREG B

Contraindicated in hypersensitivity to cinoxacin or naladixic acid. **Use with caution** in kidney or liver disease.

🖎 **Use with caution for pregnant women and the elderly. Safe use for children under 12 years and nursing mothers has not been established.**

Side effects/Adverse reactions

Hypersensitivity: itching, rashes, edema. **GI:** nausea, vomiting, abdominal pain, diarrhea. **CNS:** drowsiness, headache, dizziness, convulsions. **Skin:** tendency to sunburn, photosensitivity.

Nursing implications/Documentation

Possible nursing diagnoses: Altered patterns of urinary elimination; Fluid volume deficit.

◆ Obtain urine for culture and sensitivity, and ensure that necessary lab studies (e.g., CBC, BUN, creatinine, liver function studies) are done before administering first dose. Monitor closely thereafter if therapy is prolonged.

◆ Provide acidic juices (cranberry, plum, prune), and document and monitor intake and output, to maintain adequate hydration (at least 2 L daily; not more, or urine will be too dilute).

◆ Report joint pain in adolescents immediately.

Patient & family teaching/Home care

Possible nursing diagnoses: Knowledge deficit; Impaired home maintenance management.

◆ Advise taking doses with food to reduce GI symptoms.

◆ Explain that acidic juices (cranberry, plum, prune) enhance drug action, that the patient should drink 2 L of fluid daily (not more), and that intake of alkaline food (vegetables, milk, peanuts) should be limited.

◆ Advise reporting immediately any symptoms that do not abate after 3 days, excessive CNS side effects, new symptoms of illness (fever, sore throat), symptoms of allergy (itching, rashes).

◆ Stress the importance of taking cinoxacin without missing doses for the entire time prescribed, even if symptoms disappear.

◆ Advise against exposure to the sun (number 15 sunscreen should be worn).

◆ *See Anti-infectives overview for more information.*

ciprofloxacin

si-pro-flox'a-sin

Cipro, ✦Ciproxin

Class: Anti-infective, Antibiotic, Quinolone

Action Broad-spectrum, bactericidal antibiotic; kills bacteria, probably by inhibiting microbial DNA synthesis in susceptible bacteria.

Use/Therapeutic goal/Outcome

Infections (urinary tract, bone and joint, respiratory, skin, intestines): Resolution of infection. **Outcome criteria:** Absence of pathogenic growth on cultures, absence of clinical manifestations of infection (fever, pain, redness, heat, swelling, odor, drainage, dysuria, urinary frequency).

Dose range/Administration

Interaction alert: Antacids containing magnesium hydroxide or aluminum hydroxide decrease absorption; separate doses of these from ciprofloxacin doses by at least 2 hours. Probenecid inhibits excretion and increases blood levels of ciprofloxacin. Ciprofloxacin may increase theophylline half-life and plasma concentration.

Give 2 hours before meals for best absorption.

Adult: PO: 250–750 mg q12h (higher dose for more severe infections). IV: 400 mg diluted in 250 cc of fluid and given over 60 min.

Clinical alert: Be aware that patients with renal dysfunction may need adjustment in dosage.

Contraindications/Precautions

PREG
C

Contraindicated in hypersensitivity to ciprofloxacin or to quinolone antibiotics. ***Use with caution*** in CNS disorders and history of seizures.

Contraindicated for children and pregnant or nursing mothers. Use with caution for the elderly.

Side effects/Adverse reactions

Hypersensitivity: rashes. ***GI:*** nausea, vomiting, diarrhea, abdominal discomfort, oral candidiasis. ***CNS:*** headache, restlessness, tremors, dizziness, confusion, seizures, hallucinations. ***GU:*** crytalluria.

Nursing implications/Documentation

Possible nursing diagnoses: Potential for infection; Diarrhea.

◆ Be aware that this new antibiotic has the effectiveness of many parenteral antibiotics; prolonged use may result in overgrowth of ciprofloxacin-resistant bacteria.

◆ Determine history of allergies, and (regardless of history) monitor closely for allergic reactions.

◆ Weigh patient and obtain baseline CBC, BUN, creatinine, liver function studies, and necessary culture specimens before administering first dose; monitor closely thereafter if therapy is prolonged.

◆ Encourage fluids (at least 2 L per day), and record and monitor intake and output, to maintain adequate hydration (helps reduce crystalluria).

◆ Monitor for and report symptoms of superinfection (mouth lesions, thrush, vaginal irritation, diarrhea, respiratory symptoms).

Patient & family teaching/Home care

Possible nursing diagnoses: Knowledge deficit, Impaired home maintenance management.

◆ Stress that taking ciprofloxacin 2 hours before meals enhances drug absorption; caution against ingesting milk or dairy products within 2 hours of doses.

◆ Explain that drinking at least 2 L of fluid daily helps prevent kidney complications.

◆ Teach the need to report persistent or new signs and symptoms of illness (e.g., fever, mouth lesions, vaginal irritation, respiratory symptoms, diarrhea) medication change may be necessary.

◆ Point out the importance of taking antibiotics for the entire time prescribed, even if symptoms abate.

◆ *See Anti-infectives overview for more information.*

cisplatin

sis'pla-tin

Platinol, ◆Platamine
Class: Antineoplastic (alkylating) agent

PEDS	PREG	GERI
🖐	D	🖐

Action Kills rapidly growing cells (cancer, hair follicles, bone marrow, GI lining, ova, and sperm) by interfering with DNA and RNA synthesis through alkylation (cross-linking of DNA occurs) and disrupting nucleic acid function and protein synthesis. Is cell-cycle–phase nonspecific, affecting both actively dividing cells and dormant (resting) cells.

Use/Therapeutic goal/Outcome

Testicular and ovarian neoplasms; cervical carcinoma; bladder and lung cancer (non-small cell carcinoma); squamous cell carcinoma of the head and neck; cancer of the bladder, prostate, and cervix; renal cell carcinoma: Elimination or suppression of malignant cell proliferation.
Outcome criteria: Tumor and disease regression or stabilization on radiologic and physical examination.

Dose range/Administration

Interaction alert: Do not give with aminoglycoside antibiotics (nephrotoxicity is cumulative). Decreases plasma levels of phenytoin. Use with loop diuretics has caused increased ototoxicity (monitor hearing); cyclophosphamide increases cytotoxic effects.

Testicular cancer: ***Adult and Child:*** IV: 15–20 mg/m^2/day for 5 days, q 3–4 wk for 3 cycles.

Ovarian cancer: ***Adult and Child:*** IV: 100 mg/m^2 q 4 wk, or 50 mg/m^2 q 3 wk with doxorubicin.

Advanced bladder cancer: ***Adult and Child:*** IV: 50–70 mg/m^2 q 3–4 wk.

Clinical alert: This drug should be given only by nurses who are knowledgeable in the comprehensive management of the administration of antineoplastic agents. Doses may vary at physician's discretion and are held until the patient has sufficiently recovered from toxicities of previous doses. Protocols for drug preparation, administration, and accidental skin contamination must be followed. Gloves or double gloves must be worn when handling cisplatin (skin contamination may cause a local reaction). Contaminated areas should be washed with large amounts of soap and water. Cisplatin is given slowly over 6–8 hr diluted in 1–2 L of diluent (solution may contain mannitol or furosimide). Aluminum needles should not be used in administration.

Contraindications/Precautions

PREG D

Contraindicated in hypersensitivity to cisplatin, platinum compounds, renal or hearing impairment, or in preexisting drug or radiation-induced bone marrow suppression.

✋ **Contraindicated for pregnant or nursing mothers. Use with caution for children (has increased ototoxicity) and the elderly.**

Side effects/Adverse reactions

Hypersensitivity: urticaria, facial edema, bronchoconstriction, hypotension, anaphylaxis. ***GU:*** severe, cumulative renal toxicity. ***Ear & Eye:*** cumulative ototoxicity (tinnitus, hearing loss); blurred vision, and optic neuritis. ***Hem:*** reversible myelosuppression (leukopenia, thrombocytopenia, and anemia), which occurs in 25–30% of patients; and electrolyte disturbances (decreased magnesium, calcium, potassium, phosphate). ***CV:*** cardiac abnormalities. ***GI:*** severe nausea and vomiting (beginning within 4 hr after dose and lasting for 24 hr);

diarrhea. ***CNS:*** peripheral neuropathies (may occur 4–7 months after therapy), seizures. ***Resp:*** fibrosis. ***Skin:*** dermatitis; pain and erythema at injection site.

Nursing implications/Documentation

Possible nursing diagnoses: Potential for infection; Potential for injury; Fatigue; Altered oral mucous membrane; Fluid volume deficit; Diarrhea; Altered nutrition: less than body requirements.

♦ *See important Nursing implications in Antineoplastic agents overview on page 72, which apply to all antineoplastics. The interventions that follow are additional and specific to this drug only.*

♦ Have emergency drugs and equipment readily available to treat anaphylactic reactions.

♦ Prehydrate with 1–2 L of IV fluid 8–12 hr before giving drug to reduce renal toxicity and ototoxicity (mannitol may be prescribed before and during drug infusion to maintain output).

♦ Document and monitor urinary output for 4 hr before and 24 hr after giving drug. Do not give drug if urinary output is less than 100–200 ml/hr.

♦ Do not repeat dose if serum creatinine >1.5 mg/100 ml or BUN >25 mg/100ml, if platelets <100,000/mm^3 WBC < 4,000/mm^3, or if hearing impairment occurs.

♦ Monitor for and report early signs of CNS toxicity (muscle weakness, tingling or numbness of legs and feet, balance problems).

♦ Expect that blood counts should drop to the nadir (lowest point) in 2–3 weeks, with recovery in 5–6 weeks.

♦ Be aware that therapeutic response is often accompanied by toxicity.

Patient & family teaching/Home care

Possible nursing diagnoses: Knowledge deficit; Ineffective coping (individual and family); Hopelessness; Impaired home maintenance management.

♦ *See important Patient & family teaching in Antineoplastic agents overview on page 72, which apply to all antineoplastics. The teachings that follow are additional and specific to this drug only.*

♦ Point out that drinking 2–3 L helps prevent kidney complications.

- Stress that numbness or tingling of the legs and feet, or balance problems should be reported immediately.

- *See Antineoplastic agents overview for more information.*

clemastine fumarate
klem'as-teen

Tavist, Tavist-1

Class: Antihistamine (H$_1$ receptor antagonist)

PEDS	PREG	GERI
🤚	C	🤚

Action Prevents but does not reverse histamine-mediated allergic responses by competing with histamine for H$_1$ receptor sites on effector cells. Has anticholinergic action.

Use/Therapeutic goal/Outcome

Allergic conditions: Relief of allergic symptoms. **Outcome criteria:** Patient demonstrates and reports relief of allergic symptoms (sneezing, nasal secretions, itching, angioedema).

Dose range/Administration

Interaction alert: CNS depressants and alcohol may cause excessive drowsiness. Do not give with MAOIs or anticholinergics.

�*/ Give with food or milk to avoid GI upset.** **Adult/Child > 12 yrs:** PO: 1.34 mg bid to 2.68 mg tid; not to exceed 8.04 mg/24 hr. **Child 6–12 yrs:** PO: 0.5–3 mg/day in divided doses.

Clinical alert: Expect reduced dosage for the elderly and monitor for increased drowsiness, dizziness.

Contraindications/Precautions
PREG C

Contraindicated in hypersensitivity to clemastine, or to chemically related antihistamines, in acute asthma, and within 14 days of treatment with MAOIs. **Use with caution** in bladder-neck obstruction, urinary retention, prostatic hypertrophy, stenosing peptic ulcer, history of asthma, hypertension, hyperthyroidism, increased intraocular pressure, and cardiovascular or kidney disease.

🖐 **Contraindicated for infants and nursing mothers. Use with caution for older children and the elderly. Safe use in pregnancy and in children less than 6 years has not been established.**

Side effects/Adverse reactions

Hypersensitivity: urticaria, rash, photosensitivity, anaphylaxis. **CNS:** drowsiness (most common), dizziness, headache, weakness, disturbed coordination; confusion, restlessness, nervousness, hysteria, convulsions, tremors, chills, irritability, euphoria, insomnia, paresthesias, neuritis. **CV:** hypotension, palpitations, tachycardia, extrasystoles. **Resp:** dry nose and throat, thickening of bronchial secretions, tight feeling in chest, wheezing, nasal stuffiness. **GI:** dry mouth, anorexia, epigastric distress, nausea, vomiting, diarrhea, constipation. **GU:** dysuria, urinary frequency or retention, early menses. **Hem:** hemolytic anemia, thrombocytopenia, agranulocytosis. **Skin:** excessive perspiration.

Nursing implications/Documentation

Possible nursing diagnoses: Potential for injury; Fluid volume deficit.

- Determine and record known allergies; provide an environment that is free from allergens (especially sleeping areas).

- Provide favorite fluids and ensure adequate hydration (2 liters/day).

- If therapy is prolonged, monitor CBC for blood dyscrasias.

Patient & family teaching/Home care

Possible nursing diagnoses: Knowledge deficit; Impaired home maintenance management.

- Advise taking this drug with food or milk if GI symptoms are experienced.

- Point out that avoiding pollens and staying in an air-conditioned environment may help reduce seasonal rhinitis.

- Emphasize that dose should not be increased without physician's approval; explain that tolerance may occur, requiring a change in medication.

- Warn that alcohol and other CNS depressants may cause excessive drowsiness; advise against driving until response is determined.

- Suggest that coffee or tea may reduce drowsiness, and that sugarless gum or hard candy may relieve dry mouth.

- Explain that antihistamines should be stopped for 4 days before allergy testing to ensure accurate results.

- *See Antihistamines overview for more information.*

clindamycin

klin-da-mye'sin

clindamycin hydrochloride: *Cleocin HCl,* ✦🍁*Dalacin C*

clindamycin palmitate hydrochloride: *Cleocin Pediatric,* ✦🍁*Dalacin C Palmitate*

clindamycin phosphate: *Cleocin, Cleocin Phosphate,* ✦🍁*Dalacin C, Dalacin C Phosophate*

Class: Anti-infective, Antibiotic

PEDS	PREG	GERI
✋	C	✋

Action Kills bacteria (bactericidal) by binding to the 50S ribosomal subunit, which inhibits protein synthesis.

Use/Therapeutic goal/Outcome

Serious infections (when less toxic alternatives are contraindicated) caused primarily by anaerobic bacteria: Resolution of infection. **Outcome criteria:** Absence of pathogenic growth on culture; absence of clinical manifestations of infection (redness, pain, swelling, fever, drainage, increased WBC count, productive cough); improvement of X rays.

Dose range/Administration

Interaction alert: Chloramphenicol and erythromycins may block action of clindamycin.

📋 **Give capsules with a full glass of water or with food to avoid ulceration of the esophagus.**

Adult: PO: 150–450 mg q6h (give capsule with a full glass of water to prevent dysphagia). IM, IV: 600–900 mg q6h, q8h, or q12h. *Maximum dose:* 8 g/day. *Topical for acne:* Apply to affected area bid. **Child > 1 mo:** PO: 30–60 mg/kg/day, in divided doses q6-8h. IM, IV: 15–40 mg/kg/day, in divided doses q6h.

Clinical alert: Do not exceed IV rate of 1200 mg/hr (never give by bolus) or the patient may experience cardiac arrhythmias. Clindamycin phosphate injection contains benzyl alcohol which has been associated with a fatal gasping syndrome in infants.

Contraindications/Precautions

PREG
C

Contraindicated in hypersensitivity to clindamycin, lincomycin, or doxorubicin, and in history of colitis, regional enteritis, and antibiotic-associated diarrhea. **Use with caution** in history of GI disease, kidney disease, liver disease, asthma, eczema, drug allergies, or multiple allergies.

✋ **Contraindicated for infants under 1 month. Use with caution for the elderly. Safe use for pregnant or nursing mothers has not been established.**

Side effects/Adverse reactions

Hypersensitivity: itching, rashes, serum sickness, wheezing, dyspnea, generalized edema, anaphylaxis. **GI:** anorexia, nausea, vomiting, abdominal pain, flatulence, esophagitis, dysphagia, diarrhea, pseudomembranous colitis, bloody or tarry stools. **CV:** cardiac arrhythmias, hypotension (with rapid IV infusion), pain at injection site, phlebitis (with IV route). **Hem:** elevated SGOT, alkaline phosphatase, bilirubin. **Misc:** superinfection.

Nursing implications/Documentation

Possible nursing diagnoses: Potential for infection; Diarrhea; Fluid volume deficit.

◆ Determine history of allergies, and (regardless of negative history) monitor closely for allergic reactions.

◆ Weigh patient and obtain baseline CBC, BUN, creatinine, liver function studies, and necessary culture specimens before administering first dose; monitor closely thereafter if therapy is prolonged.

◆ Encourage fluids, and record and monitor intake and output, to ensure adequate hydration and urine output.

◆ Monitor for and report symptoms of superinfection (mouth lesions, thrush, vaginal irritation, diarrhea, respiratory symptoms).

◆ Be aware that diphenoxylate compound (Lomotil) should not be given if side effect of diarrhea occurs (may prolong and worsen diarrhea).

◆ If there is no improvement within 3–5 days, consult with physician to determine if antibiotic regimen should be re-evaluated (and new cultures drawn).

Patient & family teaching/Home care

Possible nursing diagnoses: Knowledge deficit; Impaired home maintenance management.

◆ Teach the patient and family to report persistent or new symptoms of illness (e.g., rashes, fever, mouth lesions, vaginal irritation, respiratory symptoms, diarrhea); medication change may be necessary.

- Explain the importance of taking antibiotics for the entire time prescribed, even if symptoms abate.
- For patients using topical form, explain that some of the drug is absorbed and that systemic side effects or reactions should be reported.

◆ *See Anti-infectives overview for more information.*

clofibrate
kloe-fye'brate

♠Arterioflexin, Atromid-S, ♦Claripe, ♦Novo-fiborat

Class: Antilipemic

PEDS	PREG	GERI
☵	C	☵

Action Exact mechanism of action is unclear. Interferes with triglyceride synthesis, and/or increases catabolism of very-low-density lipoproteins (VLDL) to low-density lipoproteins (LDL). Believed to reduce serum cholesterol by inhibiting early stages of cholesterol formation. Also has platelet-inhibiting action.

Use/Therapeutic goal/Outcome

Hyperlipidemias (type III): Reduction of serum triglyceride and VLDL levels to within normal range. **Outcome criteria:** Plasma lipid levels within normal limits.

Dose range/Administration

Interaction alert: Oral contraceptives and rifampin may interfere with clofibrate's lipid-lowering effect. Probenecid may increase drug effect by decreasing its elimination. Anticoagulant dosage may need to be decreased with clofibrate use, because bleeding time may be prolonged. May potentiate the effect of oral hypoglycemics, furosemide, and sulfonamides.

🍴 **Give with meals to prevent gastrointestinal distress.**

Adult: PO: 2 g/day in 4 divided doses.

Contraindications/Precautions

PREG C

Contraindicated in hypersensitivity to the drug, and in primary biliary cirrhosis, significant hepatic or renal dysfunction. **Use with caution** with peptic ulcer disease and diabetes mellitus.

☵ **Contraindicated for pregnant or nursing mothers. Use with caution for the elderly because of antiplatelet effect. Safe use for children has not been established.**

Side effects/Adverse reactions

Hypersensitivity: rash, urticaria, pruritus. **GI:** polyphagia, nausea, diarrhea, vomiting, dyspepsia, increased liver function enzyme levels, flatulence, gallstones. **CNS:** fatigue, weakness. **CV:** arrhythmias. **MS:** myalgias, arthralgias. **Hem:** leukopenia. **Skin:** alopecia, dry skin and hair. **Misc:** weight gain, flu-like symptoms, fever, decreased libido, impotence.

Nursing implications/Documentation

Possible nursing diagnoses: Diarrhea; Altered nutrition: more than body requirements.

- Check baseline CBC, electrolytes, blood sugar, and renal and hepatic profiles before giving first dose; monitor periodically thereafter.
- Be aware that the safety of clofibrate is in question; therefore, it should be discontinued if serum cholesterol is not reduced. (This drug has been associated with a increased risk of tumors and gallstones.)
- Monitor for and report diarrhea.

Patient & family teaching/Home care

Possible nursing diagnoses: Altered health maintenance; Knowledge deficit; Impaired home maintenance management.

- Explain that the purpose of this drug is to reduce serum cholesterol and to decrease the risk of cardiovascular disease.
- Emphasize the need to reduce other cardiac risk factors (obesity, smoking, high cholesterol diet, sedentary lifestyle); and help develop a plan to reduce these.
- Reinforce that this drug will have to be taken for a long time and that ongoing medical follow-up of cholesterol level is essential.

◆ *See Antilipemics overview for more information.*

clomiphene
kloe'mi-feen

clomiphene citrate: **Clomid**

Class: Ovarian stimulant

PEDS	PREG	GERI
☵	X	☵

Action Promotes ovarian follicle maturation, ovulation, and maturation of the corpus luteum by stimulating the release of the pituitary gonadotropins, follicle-stimulating hormone (FSH), and leuteinizing hormone (LH).

Use/Therapeutic goal/Outcome

Female infertility: Induction of ovulation. *Outcome criteria:* Regular menses with characteristic changes in basal body temperature (slight decrease, followed by a sharp increase the next day usually signifies ovulation; this usually occurs 4–10 days after last treatment).

Dose range/Administration

Adult: PO: 50–100 mg/day, for any 5 consecutive days or beginning on day 3 or day 5 of menstrual cycle. Repeat until conception occurs or for 3 courses.

Contraindications/Precautions

PREG
X

Contraindicated in hypersensitivity to clomiphene, and in hepatic dysfunction, abnormal uterine bleeding of undetermined cause, and ovarian cysts. *Use with caution* in hypertension, depression, visual abnormalities, seizures, diabetes mellitus, thrombophlebitis, or sensitivity to pituitary gonadotropins.

✋ **Contraindicated for children, pregnant or nursing mothers, and the elderly.**

Side effects/Adverse reactions

Hypersensitivity: urticaria, rash, allergic dermatitis. *CNS:* headache, restlessness, hot flashes, depression, fatigue, insomnia. *Eye:* diplopia, photophobia, transient blurring of vision. *GI:* nausea, vomiting, increased appetite, weight gain, abdominal distention, bloating. *GU:* ovarian enlargement/cyst formation, heavier menses. *Skin:* reversible alopecia. *Misc:* breast tenderness, hot flashes.

Nursing implications/Documentation

Possible nursing diagnoses: Pain.

♦ Report visual disturbance immediately.

♦ Monitor for and report signs and symptoms of ovarian overstimulation (pelvic pain, bloating, abdominal distention); drug may need to be discontinued.

Patient & family teaching/Home care

Possible nursing diagnoses: Altered sexuality patterns; Self-esteem disturbance; Coping, ineffective (family and individual); Knowledge deficit.

♦ Explain that this drug will stimulate ovulation, usually with the first course of therapy (if pregnancy doesn't occur, 2 subsequent courses may be given; if there is no pregnancy after 2 courses of therapy, further studies should be done).

♦ Caution that multiple births have occurred after taking clomiphene citrate.

♦ Stress that doses should be taken at the same time every day.

♦ Reinforce procedure for taking daily basal temperature upon rising in the morning; explain that a slight decrease in temperature, followed by a sharp increase usually indicates ovulation; stress that coitus should occur around the time of ovulation.

♦ Caution to stop drug and report immediately if pregnancy is suspected (may harm fetus), if visual disturbances are experienced, or if abdominal discomfort or vaginal bleeding is noted.

♦ Point out that infertility is a common problem today (statistics report 1:7 couples struggle with infertility).

♦ Explore feelings concerning self-esteem, sexual patterns, and ability to cope with prescribed regimen; encourage counseling as needed.

♦ If dizziness is noted; stress the need to avoid driving or activities that require alertness.

clomipramine

clom-ip'ra-meen

clomipramine hydrochloride: *Anafranil*
Class: Tricyclic antidepressant (TCA), Antiobsessional

PEDS	PREG	GERI
✋	C	✋

Action Improves mood and reduces obsessive-compulsive tendencies through an unclear mechanism, possibly by selectively inhibiting the reuptake of the neurotransmitter serotonin in the CNS. Has anticholinergic action.

Use/Therapeutic goal/Outcome

Obsessive-compulsive disorders: Elimination of obsessive-compulsive behaviors. *Outcome criteria:* After 2–4 weeks, report and demonstration of elimination of persistent ideas, thoughts, images, or impulses that interfere with social or occupational functioning.

Dose range/Administration

Interaction alert: Alcohol and CNS depressants may cause excessive sedation. If given with antihypertensives, monitor for increased hypotensive effects. Avoid use with MAOIs. If given with thyroid medications, monitor for

▶

increased risk of cardiac dysrhythmias and increased CNS stimulation.

🖐 **Give with (or immediately after) food to reduce GI symptoms.**

Adult: PO: Begin with 25 mg/day in divided doses, may gradually increase during the first 14 days to 100 mg/day. *Maximum dose:* 250 mg/day for outpatients and 300 mg/day for those who are hospitalized. *Child > 10 yrs:* PO: Begin with 25 mg/day in divided doses, may gradually increase during the first 14 days to 100 mg/day. *Maximum dose:* 3 mg/kg/day or 100 mg/day, whichever is smaller.

Clinical alert: Once on maintenance, give entire dose at bedtime to reduce daytime sedation. This is a new drug and information may change with additional clinical use.

Contraindications/Precautions

PREG
C

Contraindicated in hypersensitivity to TCAs, and for concomitant use with electroconvulsive therapy, and during acute recovery period of myocardial infarction. *Use with caution* in renal or hepatic disease, hyperthyroidism, glaucoma, prostatic hypertrophy, urinary retention, hypomania, mania, suicidal tendency, and for the debilitated.

🖐 **Contraindicated for children under 10 years and nursing mothers. Use with caution for children over 10 years. Safe use for pregnant women and the elderly has not been established.**

Side effects/Adverse reactions

Hypersensitivity: rash, sensitivity to sunlight. *CNS:* drowsiness, dizziness, anxiety, headache, sedation, fatigue, agitation, extrapyramidal symptoms, seizures, hallucinations, disorientation. *CV:* orthostatic hypotension, palpitations, tachycardia, hypertension. *GI:* changes in appetite, dry mouth, nausea, vomiting, constipation, paralytic ileus. *GU:* urinary retention, decreased libido. *Eye:* blurred vision. *Ear:* tinnitus. *Hem:* agranulocytosis.

Nursing implications/Documentation

Possible nursing diagnoses: Potential for injury; Constipation; Altered oral mucous membrane.

◆ Document mental status and vital signs at least bid until response to therapy has been established.

◆ Be sure that doses are swallowed (not hoarded).

◆ Record intake and output, and observe for dehydration or urinary retention; provide special mouth care.

◆ Prevent constipation by monitoring bowel movements and encouraging adequate fiber and fluid intake; offer laxatives or stool softeners before the problem becomes severe.

Patient & family teaching/Home care

Possible nursing diagnoses: Ineffective coping (family and individual); Sleep pattern disturbance; Impaired home maintenance management.

◆ Explain that side effects are often noted immediately, but they usually diminish after a few weeks; on the other hand, it is likely to take 2–4 weeks before *beneficial* effects are noted (the patient may feel worse before feeling better).

◆ Warn to change positions slowly to prevent dizziness.

◆ Emphasize that the effects of alcohol, sedatives, and tranquilizers may be potentiated.

◆ Caution to consult physician before using OTC drugs; stress the need for ongoing medical follow-up.

◆ Reinforce that doses should not be increased or stopped without checking with physician because this may cause severe problems.

◆ Advise avoidance of driving and other potentially hazardous activities until response is established.

◆ Suggest using ice chips, hard candy, or gum to relieve side effect of dry mouth; stress the need for good mouth care.

◆ Warn women to report immediately if pregnancy is planned or suspected.

◆ *See Antidepressants overview for more information.*

clonazepam

kloe-na′ze-pam

Klonopin, Rivotril

Class: Anticonvulsant, Benzodiazepine

PEDS	PREG	GERI
🖐	C	🖐

Action Suppresses spike and wave discharge in absence (petit mal) seizures, and decreases the frequency, amplitude, spread, and duration of discharge in minor motor seizures. Suppression of the spread of activity appears to occur near foci in the cortex, lymbic system, and thalamus.

Use/Therapeutic goal/Outcome

Absence seizures, epileptic states, infantile spasms, restless legs, photosensitivity epilepsy: Limitation of seizure activity. *Outcome criteria:* Marked decrease or absence of seizures.

Dose range/Administration

Interaction alert: Other anticonvulsants and drugs with CNS-depressant effects increase the depressant effects of clonazepam. Can precipitate grand mal seizures in patients with multiple seizure disorders: dosage of phenobarbital and phenytoin may need to be increased. Use with valproic acid may produce prolonged absence seizures.

Adult/Child > 10 yrs: PO: Initially do not exceed 1.5 mg/day in 3 divided doses. Daily dosage may be increased every 3 days by 0.5 to 1 mg increments prn, to a maximum of 20 mg/day. *Child < 10 yrs:* PO: Initially do not exceed 0.01–0.03 mg/kg/day in divided doses q8h (initial maximum is 0.5 mg/day). Daily dosage may be increased every 3 days by 0.25 to 0.5 mg prn, to a maximum daily dose of 0.1–0.2 mg/kg.

Clinical alert: Dose is highly individualized. Monitor the elderly closely for CNS depression.

Contraindications/Precautions

PREG
C

Contraindicated in hypersensitivity to benzodiazepines, and in severe liver disease, acute narrow angle glaucoma, breast feeding.

ψ **Use with caution for children and the elderly. Safe use for pregnant women has not been established.**

Side effects/Adverse reactions

Hypersensitivity: rash. *CNS:* drowsiness, ataxia, abnormal behavior, confusion, insomnia, depression, hysteria, hallucinations, headache, involuntary movements, vertigo. *Eye:* nystagmus, diplopia. *GI:* anorexia, constipation, dry mouth, gastritis, sore gums, coated tongue, enlarged liver. *CV:* shortness of breath, ankle edema. *GU:* dysuria, urinary retention, enuresis, nocturia, impotence. *Hem:* leukopenia, thrombocytopenia, eosinophilia.

Nursing implications/Documentation

Possible nursing diagnoses: Potential for injury; Potential for aspiration.

◆ Document history of seizures (type, frequency, duration, usual time they occur, precipitating factors, presence of an aura); initiate seizure precautions as indicated.

◆ Keep an oral airway readily available.

◆ Monitor CBC and liver function studies periodically.

Patient & family teaching/Home care

Possible nursing diagnoses: Fear; Self-esteem disturbance; Knowledge deficit; Impaired home maintenance management.

◆ Warn that stopping anticonvulsants suddenly can cause an increase in severity and frequency of seizures.

◆ Determine caregiver's ability to protect patient during a seizure; proceed with necessary teaching.

◆ Caution against driving until response is determined (may cause drowsiness at first).

◆ *See Anticonvulsants overview for more information.*

clonidine

kloe'ni-deen

Catapres, ✦ ♠*Dixarit, Catapres-TTS*
Class: ★**Antihypertensive prototype,** Alpha-adrenergic agonist

PEDS	PREG	GERI
ψ	C	ψ

Action Reduces systolic and diastolic blood pressure, and heart rate, by activating alpha receptors in the CNS, which decreases sympathetic outflow to the heart, kidneys, and peripheral vasculature.

Use/Therapeutic goal/Outcome

Hypertension: Reduction of blood pressure. *Outcome criteria:* Blood pressure readings within normal limits.

Dose range/Administration

Interaction alert: Beta-adrenergic blockers may cause paradoxical hypertension. CNS depressants may enhance clonidine CNS depression. Drugs that decrease heart rate may cause enhanced bradycardia. Tricyclic antidepressants and MAO inhibitors may decrease antihypertensive effect.

Adult: PO: 0.1 mg bid; may increase daily dosage by increments of 0.1–0.2 mg. *Maintenance dose:* 0.2–0.8 mg/day in divided doses. *Maximum dose:* 2.4 mg/day (very rare). *For uncon-*

▶

trolled accelerated hypertension: PO: 0.1 mg q10h to a maximum of 0.6 mg. Transdermal: Apply 1 patch weekly to hairless area of torso or upper arm.

Clinical alert: Be aware that drug effect begins within 30–60 minutes of oral administration. Administer last dose at bedtime for overnight blood pressure control.

Contraindications/Precautions

PREG C

Contraindicated in hypersensitivity to clonidine. **Use with caution** in cerebrovascular disease, coronary insufficiency, diabetes, chronic renal failure, recent myocardial infarction, history of mental depression, Raynaud's disease and thromboangiitis obliterans.

👋 **Use with caution in the elderly. Safe use for children and pregnant women has not been established.**

Side effects/Adverse reactions

Hypersensitivity: pruritis, dermatitis. **CV:** severe rebound hypertension, orthostatic hypotension, bradycardia. **CNS:** fatigue, depression, drowsiness, sedation, nervousness, headache. **GI:** constipation, mouth dryness. **Hem:** glucose intolerance. **GU:** impotence, urinary retention. **Misc:** sodium and fluid retention.

Nursing implications/Documentation

Possible nursing diagnoses: Activity intolerance; Fatigue; Potential for injury; Constipation.

♦ Assess mental status, and record pulse and blood pressure (lying, sitting, and standing, in both arms) before administration, and frequently thereafter until response is determined.

♦ Consult with physician to determine desired therapeutic range for blood pressure (be aware that some patients may require a slightly elevated blood pressure to perfuse vital organs).

♦ Ascertain that baseline CBC, electrolytes, BUN, creatinine, and liver function studies have been obtained before giving first dose; report abnormalities and monitor closely thereafter.

♦ Monitor for allergic reactions, confusion, dizziness, bradycardia, hypotension, depression, visual changes; hold drug and report immediately if these occur.

♦ Supervise ambulation until response is determined.

♦ Document and monitor daily weight, and intake and output; report significant negative or positive balance.

♦ Be aware that this drug should not be discontinued abruptly (may cause palpitations, tremors, anxiety, muscle pain).

Patient & family teaching/Home care

Possible nursing diagnoses: Altered sexuality patterns; Knowledge deficit; Impaired home maintenance management.

♦ Explain the importance of taking medication exactly as prescribed, even when feeling well.

♦ Stress the importance of good medical follow-up, explain that this drug reduces "wear and tear" on blood vessels and improves longevity and health.

♦ Teach how to monitor pulse and blood pressure; emphasize that syncope, hypertension or hypotension, depression, visual changes, or persistent dizziness should be reported.

♦ Advise changing positions slowly to avoid dizziness.

♦ Encourage daily monitoring of weight and reporting sudden weight gain (frequently is fluid retention).

♦ Explain that driving should be avoided until response is determined (may cause drowsiness).

♦ Warn against discontinuing drug abruptly or taking *any* OTC drugs without physician approval (some interactions can cause severe reactions).

♦ Caution that drinking alcohol may cause excessive drowsiness.

♦ *See Antihypertensives overview for more information.*

clorazepate

klor-az'e-pate

Gen-Xene, ✚Novoclopate, Tranxene, Tranxene-SD, Tranxene-T-Tab

Class: Antianxiety agent, Sedative-hypnotic, Anticonvulsant

PEDS 👋 **PREG D** **GERI** 👋

CONTROLLED SUBSTANCE IV

Action Produces CNS depression and relaxation, and increases seizure threshold by potentiating the action of gamma-aminobuteric acid (GABA), which reduces neuronal activity in all regions of the CNS. Promotes muscle relaxation by inhibiting spinal motor reflex pathways. Decreases anxiety by inhibiting cortical and limbic arousal.

Use/Therapeutic goal/Outcome

Short-term treatment of anxiety: Alleviation of symptoms of apprehension, muscle tension, and insomnia. **Outcome criteria:** Report of feeling more calm, sleeping better, and coping better; observable signs of decreased anxiety (decreased motor activity, reduced muscle tension, decrease in pulse and blood pressure).

Acute alcohol withdrawal: Prevention or management of delirium tremens. **Outcome criteria:** Reduction in, or absence of, agitation, tremors, hallucinations; improved reality orientation.

Adjunct to anticonvulsive therapy: Prevention/elimination of seizures. **Outcome criteria:** Absence of seizures.

Dose range/Administration

Interaction alert: Alcohol and other CNS depressants may cause excessive sedation. Cimetidine increases blood levels.

🖐 **Give with food or milk if GI distress is noted.**

Anxiety: Adult: PO: 15–60 mg/day in divided doses.

Acute alcohol withdrawal: Adult: PO: *Day 1:* 30 mg, then 30–60 mg in divided doses. *Day 2:* 45–90 mg in divided doses. *Day 3:* 22.5–45 mg in divided doses. *Day 4–15:* 30 mg in divided doses. Then gradually taper dose to 7.5–15 mg/day.

Seizures (adjunctive treatment): Adult/Child > 12 yrs: PO: 7.5 mg bid to tid, may increase as needed by 7.5 mg/week. *Maximum dose:* 90 mg/day. **Child 9–12 yrs:** PO: 7.5 mg bid, may increase by 7.5 mg/week. *Maximum dose:* 60 mg/day.

Clinical alert: Do not withdraw drug abruptly (may cause severe problems). Clorazepate accumulates in the body, and elimination after discontinuation may take weeks.

Contraindications/Precautions
PREG **D**

Contraindicated in hypersensitivity or intolerance to clorazepate or other benzodiazepines, and in narrow-angle glaucoma. **Use with caution** in psychosis, depression, suicidal tendencies, or impaired liver or kidney function.

🖐 **Contraindicated for children under 9 years and pregnant or nursing mothers. Use with caution for children over 9 years and the elderly or debilitated.**

Side effects/Adverse reactions

Hypersensitivity: itching, rash, exaggeration of side effects. **CNS:** lethargy, drowsiness, dizziness, syncope, confusion, ataxia, insomnia, tremors, depression. **CV:** hypotension, transient tachycardia and bradycardia. **Resp:** respiratory depression. **GI:** dry mouth, nausea, vomiting, constipation, diarrhea. **Eye:** blurred vision, mydriasis. **Misc:** drug tolerance and dependence.

Nursing implications/Documentation

Possible nursing diagnoses: Potential for injury; Constipation.

♦ Record baseline blood pressure; monitor closely if dizziness is experienced. Supervise ambulation until response is determined.

♦ Be sure that doses are swallowed (not hoarded).

♦ Provide a quiet environment that is conducive to rest.

♦ Monitor bowel elimination and provide adequate fluids and fiber to prevent constipation; offer laxative before the problem is severe.

♦ *For use as adjunct in anticonvulsant, see Nursing implications and Patient & family teaching in Anticonvulsants overview.*

Patient & family teaching/Home care

Possible nursing diagnoses: Anxiety; Fear; Ineffective individual coping; Impaired home maintenance management.

♦ Advise taking this drug with milk or food if GI symptoms are noted.

♦ Help the individual identify stressors that contribute to anxiety and ways of coping effectively; stress that effective coping strategies can reduce the need for medication.

♦ Explain the importance of daily exercise in relieving stress, and encourage establishing a plan for getting enough exercise (e.g., daily walks).

♦ For use in anxiety, point out that drug tolerance and dependence can occur, and that the drug should be used only on a short-term basis.

♦ Emphasize that the effects of alcohol, other sedatives and CNS depressants, and tranquilizers may be potentiated (these should be avoided).

- Advise avoidance of driving and other potentially hazardous activities until response is established.
- *See Antianxiety agents/Sedatives/Hypnotics and Anticonvulsants overviews for more information.*

clotrimazole

klo-trim'a-zole

♣*Canesten, Gyne-Lotrimin, Lotrimin (1% clotrimazole), Mycelex, Mycelex-G*

Class: Local anti-infective, Topical antifungal

PEDS	PREG	GERI
🖐	B	🖐

Action Inhibits fungal growth by altering cell wall permeability, causing the loss of potassium and cellular contents.

Use/Therapeutic goal/Outcome

Fungal infections [tinea pedis, tinea cruris, tinea corporis (ringworm), tinea versicolor, cutaneous, oropharyngeal, and vulvovaginal candidiasis (moniliasis)]: Suppression or elimination of fungal growth, resolution of infection. *Outcome criteria:* After 1–4 weeks, absence of fungal growth on culture and absence of manifestations of infection (pain, redness, swelling, drainage).

Dose range/Administration

Oropharyngeal candidiasis: **Adult and Child:** PO: 1 lozenge (10 mg) dissolved in mouth 5 times daily for 2 wk.
Superficial fungal infections: **Adult and Child:** *Topical:* Apply a thin layer of 1% cream, solution, or lotion bid for 1–8 weeks. Gently massage into affected area and surrounding skin until medication disappears.
Candidal vulvovaginitis: **Adult:** *Vaginal:* 1 applicator (5 g) or 1 vaginal tablet (100 mg) hs for 7–14 days, or 2 tablets (200 mg) at bedtime for 3 days, or 1 tablet (500 mg) hs once only.
Clinical alert: Keep ointment away from eyes, nose, and mouth. For oral troches, teach the need to keep dose in mouth and allow it to dissolve slowly over 15–20 minutes before swallowing (should not be chewed or swallowed whole).

Contraindications/Precautions

PREG B

Contraindicated in hypersensitivity to clotrimazole. **Use with caution** in liver impairment.

Use with caution for pregnant or nursing mothers and the elderly. Safe use for children under 3 years has not been established.

Side effects/Adverse reactions

Hypersensitivity: itching, burning, redness, stinging, peeling, urticaria, fissures, irritation, rash. **GU:** vaginal soreness during intercourse, dyspareunia, urinary frequency, cystitis. **GI:** lower abdominal cramping and bloating.

Nursing implications/Documentation

Possible nursing diagnoses: Potential for infection: Impaired skin integrity; Altered oral mucous membrane.

- Record appearance of lesions daily.
- Report increased inflammation or lack of improvement after 4 weeks of therapy.
- For oral use, provide special mouth care.

Patient & family teaching/Home care

Possible nursing diagnoses: Knowledge deficit; Impaired home maintenance management.

- Caution to keep ointment away from mouth, eyes, and nose (local irritation can be severe).
- Demonstrate procedure for cleansing and applying medication; observe return demonstration.
- Warn not to cover area with an occlusive dressing (tight underwear or pants should be avoided).
- Point out that this medication must be applied for full course of treatment, even after clinical manifestations have disappeared.
- Advise reporting an increase in inflammation or failure to improve after 4 weeks.
- During vaginal therapy, caution women that this drug may cause skin irritation in sexual partner (restraint from sexual intercourse or use of a condom is recommended). Stress the need to continue medication even with menstruation.
- For use for tinea corporis (ringworm), advise washing clothes separately from those of other family members.
- *See Anti-infectives overview for more information.*

cloxacillin

klox-a-sill'in

cloxacillin sodium: ♠Alclox, ♣Apo-Cloxi, ♠Austra-staph, ♣Bactopen, Cloxapen, ♣Novocloxin, ♣Or-benin, ♠Orbenin Injection, Tegopen

Class: Anti-infective, Antibiotic, Penicillin (penicillinase—resistant)

PEDS	PREG	GERI
☝	B	☝

Action Broad-spectrum, usually bactericidal antibiotic; kills bacteria by inhibiting cell wall synthesis. Resistant to bacterial penicillinases (enzymes that degrade some penicillins).

Use/Therapeutic goal/Outcome

Systemic infections (caused by penicillinase-producing staphylococci): Resolution of infection. *Outcome criteria:* Absence of pathogenic growth on cultures, absence of clinical manifestations of infection (fever, pain, redness, heat, swelling, odor, drainage, dysuria), normal WBC count.

Dose range/Administration

Interaction alert: Probenecid inhibits excretion of cloxacillin and may be given to increase serum levels of the drug.

🥤 **Give with a full glass of water on an empty stomach (drug is inactivated by acids) 1–2 hours before or 2–3 hours after meals. Acid in fruit juices and carbonated beverages will inactivate the drug; food may inhibit absorption.**

Adult: PO: 2–4 g/day in divided doses q6h. *Child > 20 kg:* PO: 50–100 mg/kg/day, in divided q6h. *Child < 20 kg:* PO: 12.5–25 mg/kg q6h.

Clinical alert: Give at least 1 hour before bacteriostatic antibiotics for optimum effect.

Contraindications/Precautions

Contraindicated in allergy to penicillin. *Use with caution* in cephalosporin sensitivity, history of allergic responses (e.g., other drugs, hay fever, asthma), renal dysfunction, and sodium restriction.

☝ Use with caution for children, the elderly, and pregnant or nursing mothers. Safe use for neonates has not been established.

Side effects/Adverse reactions

Hypersensitivity: itching, rashes, urticaria, fever, difficulty breathing, anaphylaxis. *GI:* nausea, vomiting, diarrhea, furry tongue. *CNS:* neurotoxicity. *Hem:* slight elevation in SGOT. *Misc:* superinfection.

Nursing implications/Documentation

Possible nursing diagnoses: Potential for infection; Diarrhea.

♦ Determine history of allergies, and (regardless of history) monitor closely for allergic reactions.

♦ Obtain baseline CBC, serum sodium, liver function studies, and necessary cultures before administering first dose; monitor closely thereafter if therapy is prolonged.

♦ Encourage fluids, and record and monitor intake and output, to ensure adequate hydration; report significant negative or positive balance.

♦ Monitor for and report signs of superinfection (sore throat, fever, fatigue, thrush, vaginal discharge, diarrhea).

Patient & family teaching/Home care

Possible nursing diagnoses: Knowledge deficit; Impaired home maintenance management.

♦ Teach importance of reporting allergic symptoms, diarrhea, signs and symptoms that do not abate, or *any* new signs and symptoms of discomfort that might indicate superinfection (medication regimen may have to be changed).

♦ Advise drinking 2–3 L of fluids daily to maintain adequate hydration (especially important if fever exists).

♦ Stress the importance of taking antibiotics for the entire time prescribed, even if signs and symptoms abate.

♦ See Anti-infectives overview for more information.

clozapine

klos'a-peen

Clozaril

Class: Dibenzodiazapine antipsychotic

PEDS	PREG	GERI
☝	B	☝

Action Produces calmness and alleviates psychiatric symptoms (disorders of perception, thought, consciousness, mood, affect, and social interaction) by interfering with the binding of dopamine at D_1 and D_2 receptors in the limbic system. Acts as an antagonist at adrenergic, cholinergic, histaminergic, and serotonergic receptors.

Use/Therapeutic goal/Outcome

Severely ill schizophrenic persons who are not well controlled with other antipsychotic agents, or who are not able to tolerate the extrapyramidal symptoms of other antipsychotic agents (even with administration of an antiparkinson agent), or those in whom adverse reactions preclude attainment of a standard dose of other antipsychotics: Promotion of reality orientation, reduction in agitation. *Outcome criteria:* Demonstration of reality orientation, and ability to problem solve and interact with others, with decrease in signs of agitation (pacing, hyperactivity).

Dose range/Administration

Interaction alert: May potentiate the hypotensive effects of antihypertensive drugs and the anticholinergic effects of atropine-type drugs. May increase plasma concentrations of oral anticoagulants, heparin, phenytoin, and digoxin. Because of the primary CNS effects of clozapine, use with caution with other CNS-active drugs.

Adult: PO: 25–50 mg on the first day. If well tolerated, increase daily dose by 25–50 mg increments for 2 weeks to 300–450 mg. *Therapeutic range:* 300–500 mg/day in divided doses. *Maximum dose:* 900 mg/day.

Clinical alert: This is a new drug which has shown significant improvement in certain patients who have previously failed to respond to other antipsychotics. All individuals receiving clozapine should have weekly blood studies to limit the risk of agranulocytosis.

Contraindications/Precautions

PREG
B

Contraindicated in hypersensitivity to clozapine, concurrent use of agents that suppress bone marrow function, myeloproliferative disorders, granulocytopenia, agranulocytosis or history of agranulocytosis, CNS depression, and coma. *Use with caution* in fever, prostatic enlargement, narrow-angle glaucoma, seizure disorders, and cardiac, kidney, or liver disease.

Contraindicated for nursing mothers. Give with caution for the elderly or debilitated. Safe use in children under 16 years has not been established.

Side effects/Adverse reactions

Hypersensitivity: blood dyscrasias, rash. *CNS:* sedation, headache, confusion, syncope, sei-

zures, tardive dykinesia, dizziness, extrapyramidal reactions (pseudoparkinsonism, akathisia, (inability to sit down, need to keep moving) dystonia, neuroleptic malignant syndrome (muscular rigidity, tremors, high fever, respiratory distress, tachycardia). *CV:* orthostatic hypotension, hypertension, angina, tachycardia. *Hem:* leukopenia, agranulocytosis. *GI:* appetite changes, hypersalivation, dry mouth, constipation, diarrhea, abnormal liver function. *GU:* urinary retention or hesitancy, impaired ejaculation, priapism. *Misc:* fever (usually in first 3 weeks of therapy); unusual weight gain.

Nursing implications/Documentation

Possible nursing diagnoses: Potential for injury; Constipation; Altered oral mucous membranes.

◆ Record mental status and vital signs before and 1–2 hr after administration during initial phase of treatment, then bid until response to therapy has been established, then periodically thereafter.

◆ Check CBC, liver function, BUN, and creatinine before giving first dose and periodically thereafter; check WBC and granulocyte count weekly, and for 4 weeks after therapy is discontinued.

◆ Be sure that doses are swallowed (not hoarded).

◆ Monitor for orthostatic hypotension, dizziness, and drowsiness; supervise ambulation until response is established.

◆ Provide special mouth care; observe for and report oral ulcers.

◆ Prevent constipation by monitoring bowel movements and encouraging adequate fiber and fluid intake; offer laxatives or stool softeners before problem becomes severe.

◆ Report persistent sore throat, fever, and malaise, because these may indicate agranulocytosis, for which there is a significant risk.

◆ Monitor for (and report immediately) signs of neuroleptic malignant syndrome (muscle rigidity, tremors, high fever, tachycardia); this is a rare, but potentially fatal, side effect.

Patient & family teaching/Home care

Possible nursing diagnoses: Sleep pattern disturbance; Impaired home maintenance management.

- ◆ Emphasize the need to continue medication, even when feeling well; explain the need for weekly blood tests.
- ◆ Warn to change positions slowly to avoid dizziness.
- ◆ Stress that the effects of alcohol, sedatives and CNS depressants, and tranquilizers may be potentiated.
- ◆ Caution to consult with physician before using OTC drugs; stress the need for ongoing medical follow-up.
- ◆ Teach the need to report persistent sore throat, fever, and fatigue.
- ◆ Point out that doses should not be increased or stopped without checking with physician.
- ◆ Advise avoidance of driving and other potentially hazardous activities until response is determined.
- ◆ Suggest using ice chips, hard candy, or gum to relieve side effect of dry mouth; stress the need for good mouth care.
- ◆ Warn women to report if pregnancy is planned or suspected.
- ◆ *See Antipsychotics overview for more information.*

codeine

koe'deen

codeine: *Methylmorphine*

codeine phosphate: ❧*Paveral*

codeine sulfate

Class: Narcotic analgesic, Opiate agonist, Antitussive

Antidote: naloxone hydrochloride (Narcan)

PEDS	PREG	GERI	CONTROLLED SUBSTANCE
✋	C	✋	II

Action Alters the perception of and response to pain by an unclear mechanism. Believed to act by binding with opiate receptors at numerous CNS sites. Suppresses cough reflex by a direct central action on the cough center in the medulla. Not as potent or as long-lasting as morphine. Reported to be less effective than prostaglandin inhibitors, such as aspirin, for uterine or dental pain.

Use/Therapeutic goal/Outcome

Mild to moderate pain: Relief of pain. *Outcome criteria:* Report of comfort; absence of observable signs of pain (grimacing, frowning, restlessness, reluctance to move or cough),

decreased restlessness; blood pressure and pulse within normal limits when compared to baseline.

Nonproductive or hyperactive cough: Suppression of cough. *Outcome criteria:* Decreased frequency and intensity of coughing.

Dose range/Administration

Interaction alert: Other CNS depressants, alcohol, narcotics, sedative/hypnotics, antipsychotic drugs, tranquilizers, and skeletal-muscle relaxants increase effects.

🖢 **Give PO doses with milk or food to decrease GI distress.**

Pain: Adult: PO, SC, IM: 15–60 mg q4h prn or around the clock. *Child:* PO: 3 mg/kg/day in divided doses q4h prn or around the clock.

Cough: Adult: PO: 8–20 mg q4-6h. *Maximum dose:* 120 mg in 24 hr. *Child:* PO: 1–1.5 mg/kg/day in 4 divided doses. *Maximum dose:* 60 mg in 24 hr.

Clinical alert: Be aware that codeine is frequently given together with aspirin or acetaminophen for best effects (they are synergistic).

PREG
C

Contraindications/Precautions

Contraindicated in hypersensitivity to codeine or other morphine derivatives. *Use with caution* in increased intracranial pressure, head injury, history of drug abuse, renal or hepatic dysfunction, hypothyroidism, Addison's disease, acute alcoholism, seizures, respiratory depression, and shock.

✋ **Use with caution for children, nursing mothers, and the elderly or debilitated. Safe use for pregnant women has not been established.**

Side effects/Adverse reactions

Hypersensitivity: itching, rashes, excessive perspiration, shortness of breath, facial flushing, respiratory depression, extreme somnolence, skeletal-muscle flaccidity, anaphylaxis. *GI:* nausea, vomiting, constipation, dry mouth. *CNS:* sedation, euphoria, (high doses) convulsions. *GU:* urinary retention. *CV:* hypotension. *Resp:* respiratory depression.

Nursing implications/Documentation

Possible nursing diagnoses: Pain; Constipation; Potential for injury.

- ◆ Have patient rate pain on a scale of 1–10 before and after medication is given; report and record inadequate pain control.

- Give codeine before pain is severe.
- Monitor closely for risk factors for injury until response is determined.
- Document and monitor bowel function to detect constipation; provide adequate fluids and fiber; give laxatives before problem is severe.
- Be aware that psychic and physical dependence may develop; monitor the emotionally unstable for anticipation of pain, rather than actual discomfort (providing reassurance may be all that is required).
- If given for cough suppressant, document frequency and character of sputum production; report increase in sputum production.

Patient & family teaching/Home care

Possible nursing diagnoses: Sensory/perceptual alterations; Knowledge deficit.

- Explain the rationale for taking codeine before pain is severe.
- Stress the need to avoid activities requiring alertness while taking codeine.
- Warn that exceeding prescribed dose may cause overdose, dependence, and increased potential for abuse (instead, unsatisfactory pain relief should be reported).
- Warn to avoid constipation by eating adequate fiber, drinking plenty of fluids, and (if necessary) using a mild laxative before problem is severe.
- Advise changing positions slowly to avoid dizziness.
- Explain that lying down will alleviate light-headedness, dizziness, or nausea (persistent symptoms should be reported).
- For coughs, teach that coughing can be diminished by providing adequate humidity, reducing irritants, and maintaining adequate hydration (at least 2 L/day); advise use of hard candy to prevent throat dryness.
- Warn that alcohol and other CNS depressants may cause increased sedation.
- *See Narcotic and non-narcotic analgesics overview for more information.*

colchicine

kol'chi-seen

♠Colchicine MR, ♠Colgout, Colsalide, ♣Novo-colchicine

Class: ★Antigout prototype, Anti-inflammatory agent

PEDS	PREG	GERI
🖐	D	🖐

Action Reduces inflammatory response to urate crystals by decreasing leukocyte motility, phagocytosis, and lactic acid formation.

Use/Therapeutic goal/Outcome

Gouty arthritis: Symptomatic relief of acute attacks and prophylaxis of recurrence. **Outcome criteria:** Reduction or absence of inflammation, pain, and swelling in affected joint.

Dose range/Administration

Interaction alert: Vitamin B_{12} malabsorption occurs with colchicine. Use with antidepressants, antihistamines, narcotics, and sedatives may cause oversedation.

🖐 **Give oral doses with food.**

Acute attack: Adult: PO: 0.6–1.2 mg, then 0.6–1.2 mg q1-2h until pain is relieved. *Maximum dose:* 10 mg. IV: 2 mg, then 0.5 mg q6h for 2 days. *Maximum dose:* 4 mg/day.

Prophylactic: Adult: PO: 0.6 mg daily to tid.

Clinical alert: First dose should be given as soon as possible after onset of pain and inflammation. Dilute IV doses in NS or sterile water for injection; do not give if solution is turbid. After ascertaining that needle is in the vein, administer dose over 2–5 minutes. Monitor closely for extravasation; never give IM because it can cause severe tissue irritation.

Contraindications/Precautions

PREG
D

Contraindicated in hypersensitivity to colchicine. **Use with caution** in history of peptic ulcer or ulcerative colitis; in heart, liver, or renal disease and blood dyscrasias.

🖐 **Contraindicated for children and pregnant or nursing mothers. Use with caution for the elderly.**

Side effects/Adverse reactions

Hypersensitivity: hives, rash, itching, and fainting. **GI:** diarrhea, nausea, vomiting, abdominal pain. **Hem:** agranulocytosis, aplastic anemia. **CNS:** peripheral neuritis, mental confusion. **CV:** phlebitis at IV site.

Nursing implications/Documentation

Possible nursing diagnoses: Diarrhea; Pain.

• Encourage fluid intake to maintain urinary output of 2000 ml daily to promote urate excretion and to prevent renal crystals from forming; record intake and output.

• Assess comfort level before administering each dose during acute episodes; record level of pain.

• Hold dose and report if signs of toxicity (weakness, nausea, vomiting, diarrhea) become evident; this is more common in the elderly or debilitated.

• Be aware that acute attacks of gout may be precipitated by surgical procedures; colchicine may be given for several days before and after procedures.

Patient & family teaching/Home care

Possible nursing diagnoses: Knowledge deficit; Impaired home maintenance management; Diarrhea; Activity intolerance.

• Caution women of childbearing age not to take colchicine during pregnancy because of the possibility of fetal harm.

• Point out the need to continue taking other medications that have been prescribed for gout; colchicine is for relief of acute symptoms.

• Suggest keeping a supply of colchicine on hand and to begin taking prescribed dose at first signs of an acute attack.

• Teach the need to maintain high daily water intake to prevent renal damage, and to report flank pain or bloody or darkened urine.

• Caution to stop taking colchicine at therapeutic dose level as soon as acute pain is relieved; explain the maximum dosage (10 mg) that should be taken for each attack and stress the importance of not exceeding it.

• Advise that simple diarrhea may be managed with antidiarrheal drugs; bloody or profuse diarrhea should be reported.

• Caution to report the development of sore throat, fever, bleeding, or unusual bruising.

• Encourage to maintain medical supervision for safe regulation of long-term treatment.

• Teach to reduce acute episodes by avoiding aspirin, alcohol, and foods high in purines.

• Advise to discuss with physician the need for colchicine before surgical and dental procedures.

colestipol hydrochloride *koe-les'ti-pole*

colestipol hydrochloride: *Colestid, ◄Clalalap*
Class: Antilipemic

PEDS	PREG	GERI
✋	C	✋

Action Reduces serum cholesterol by binding with bile salts to form an insoluble compound that is then excreted in feces.

Use/Therapeutic goal/Outcome

Hypercholesterolemia (type IIA): Reduction of serum cholesterol levels to within normal range. **Outcome criteria:** Serum cholesterol levels within normal range.

Dose range/Administration

Interaction alert: To avoid impairing absorption of other drugs, do not give cholestipol within 1 hour before or 4–6 hours after other medication. Oral hypoglycemics may impair colestipol absorption.

▣ **Give 30 min before meals.**

Adult: PO: 15–30 g/day in divided doses (bid or qid).

Clinical alert: Do not give powder in dry form; mix in at least 3 ounces of beverage of choice. After dose is taken, swish a small amount of fluid in glass and have the patient swallow this to ensure that entire dose is taken. To improve palatability, mix the evening before and store in refrigerator.

Contraindications/Precautions
_{PREG C}

Contraindicated in hypersensitivity to the drug and in complete biliary obstruction or hypertriglyceridemia.

✋ **Use with caution for the elderly. Safe use for children and pregnant or nursing mothers has not been established.**

Side effects/Adverse reactions

Hypersensitivity: Allergic reactions are not listed. *GI:* constipation, fecal impaction, hemorrhoids, flatulence, nausea, vomiting, steatorrhea, bloating, rashes of tongue and perianal area. *CNS:* headache, dizziness, weakness, fatigue. *Skin:* skin irritation. *Misc:* Vitamin A, D, and K deficiencies.

Nursing implications/Documentation

Possible nursing diagnoses: Constipation; Altered nutrition: more than body requirements.

♦ Monitor and document bowel elimination to detect constipation; provide adequate fluids and fiber; give laxatives before constipation becomes severe (consult with physician about using stool softener).

♦ Monitor for and report persistent GI symptoms.

Patient & family teaching/Home care

Possible nursing diagnoses: Altered health maintenance; Knowledge deficit; Impaired home maintenance management.

♦ Explain that the purpose of this drug is to reduce serum cholesterol and to decrease the risk of cardiovascular disease.

♦ Stress the need to take this drug before meals, and 1 hour before or 4–6 hours after other medications.

♦ Teach the proper method of mixing (see clinical alert); warn never to take dose in dry form, because this may cause choking.

♦ Emphasize the need to reduce other cardiac risk factors (obesity, smoking, high cholesterol diet, sedentary lifestyle), and help develop a plan to reduce these.

♦ Discuss the role of adequate hydration, fiber intake, and exercise in preventing constipation; help develop a plan to prevent constipation.

♦ Reinforce that this drug will have to be taken for a long time, and that ongoing medical follow-up of cholesterol level is essential.

♦ Warn against taking other drugs without physician's approval.

♦ *See Antilipemics overview for more information.*

colisceril

koe-liss'ir-ill

colisceril palmitate: **Exosurf Neonatal**

Class: Synthetic surfactant

PEDS	PREG	GERI
✋	NR	✋

Action Reduces surface tension at the air-alveolar interface and prevents alveoli from collapsing by providing an exogenous source of surfactant. Surfactant is a lipoprotein (made up of phospholipids, neutral lipids, and highly saturated lecithins) that is naturally synthesized during gestation by pneumocytes.

Use/Therapeutic goal/Outcome

Hyaline membrane disease (HMD), infant respiratory distress syndrome (IRDS): Prevention of alveolar collapse, atelectasis, and lung collapse; improvement in lung compliance and gas exchange. **Outcome criteria:** Arterial blood gases and oxygen saturation within normal range; decreased need for high levels of supplemental oxygen and ventilator therapy.

Dose range/Administration

Infants: *Endotracheal tube: Prophylaxis:* 60–200 mg/kg in a single dose as soon as possible after delivery; may give second and third dose in 12 and 24 hr. *Rescue:* First dose as soon as clinical or radiographic signs of IRDS are noted; then second dose in 12 hr, then third dose prn in 24 hr.

Clinical alert: This drug should be administered only in the delivery room or intensive care nursery by nurses and physicians who are qualified in the comprehensive management of its administration. Hospital protocols should be followed for reconstitution and administration. A common procedure for its administration follows: Before administration, confirm the placement of the endotracheal tube (ETT) and suction the infant. Attach appropriately sized endotracheal tube adaptor supplied by the manufacturer. Place the ventilator on the intermittent mandatory ventilation (IMV) mode. With the ETT in midline position, connect the syringe to the side port of the ETT adapter. Inject 1/2 the dose into the tube in short bursts during inspiration slowly over 1–2 min (30–50 mechanical breaths); if the heart rate decreases or if the oxygen saturation decreases by 15%, further slow the rate of dosing. After 1/2 the dose has been given, roll the infant 45 degrees to the right for 30 sec, then return to midline (allow gravity to assist in the distribution of the drug). At this point administer the second half of the dose over a period of 1–2 min (30–50 mechanical breaths), roll the infant 45 degrees to the left for 30 sec, then return to midline. Monitor respiratory status closely for 30 min after dosing; compliance changes may occur rapidly, requiring immediate changes in ventilator settings. The infant should not be suctioned for 2 hr after dosing.

Contraindications/Precautions

⚕ Contraindicated for use after 48 hr of life. This drug is given only to neonates who are intubated.

Side effects/Adverse reactions

Hypersensitivity: None reported. **CV:** bradycardia. **Resp:** pulmonary hemorrhage, mucus plugging of ETT.

Nursing implications/Documentation

Possible nursing diagnoses: Impaired gas exchange; Activity intolerance; Potential for aspiration.

◆ Recognize that risk factors for IRDS include prematurity, pregnancy-related stress, prenatal medical treatment, perinatal asphyxia, male sex, maternal history of premature infants with IRDS, and possibly maternal diabetes.

◆ Monitor infants with these risk factors closely for early signs of respiratory distress (cyanosis, grunting, chest retractions, and tachypnea).

◆ Review hospital policies, procedures, and protocols to be sure that you have all the necessary equipment on standby, ready for use.

◆ Record baseline vital signs, lung sounds, arterial blood gases, and oxygen saturation; keep a flow sheet with this information readily available, recording data as frequently as required by clinical status, physician's orders, and unit protocols.

◆ Recognize that there is often a need for rapid adjustment of oxygen concentration and ventilator settings, requiring astute, constant observations and assessments.

◆ Allow the infant to rest as much as possible (handle or disturb child as little as possible).

Patient & family teaching/Home care

Possible nursing diagnoses: Fear; Anxiety; Knowledge deficit; Altered parenting.

◆ Reassure significant others that this drug has been very successful in reducing the incidence of lung problems and promoting survival of neonates.

◆ Encourage parents to voice fears and concerns so that these issues may be addressed.

◆ Support parents in interacting with their infant; stress that while the child should be *disturbed as little as possible*, hand-holding may be soothing.

corticotropin

kor-ti-koe-troe'pin

ACTH, Acthar, ✦Acthar Gel (H.P.), ACTH Gel, Cortigel-40, Cortigel-80, Cortrophin Gel, Cortrophin Zinc, Cortropic Gel-40, Cortropic Gel-80, H.P. Acthar Gel

Class: Anterior pituitary hormone, Adrenocorticotropic hormone

PEDS	PREG	GERI
⚕	C	⚕

Action Stimulates cortex of functional adrenal glands to secrete cortisol, cortisone, and other adrenal steroids by activating endogenous synthesis.

Use/Therapeutic goal/Outcome

Diagnostic testing of adrenal cortex function: Determination of ability of adrenal cortex to respond to stimulation. **Outcome criteria:** Increase in cortisol blood levels indicates functioning adrenal glands.

Inflammatory or immune disease: Symptomatic relief. **Outcome criteria:** Decrease in presenting signs and symptoms of disorder being treated.

Dose range/Administration

Interaction alert: May decrease effectiveness of oral anticoagulants and antidiabetics. May diminish antibody response to vaccines and toxoids and cause neurologic complications. Potassium-depleting diuretics may cause severe hypokalemia. Increases renal clearance of salicylates. Medications known to cause gastric irritation may cause gastric bleeding.

Diagnostic testing: Adult: IV: 10–25 U in 500 ml 5% glucose solution over 8 hr.

Therapeutic: Adult: IM, SC: *Aqueous solution:* 40–80 U/day. *Repository gel:* 40–80 U q24-72h. IM: *Zinc suspension:* 40 U q12-48h. **Child:** IV, SC: 1.6 U/kg/day in 3–4 divided doses. IM: 1.6 U/kg/day in 1–2 divided doses.

Exacerbation of multiple sclerosis: Adult: IM: 80–120 U/day for 2–3 wks.

Clinical alert: In suspicion of sensitivity to pork products, skin testing is recommended prior to administration. Repository gel form may be administered by IM (preferred) or SC routes; zinc suspension should be administered only by IM route. For repository gel form, warm to room temperature and administer deeply with 22-gauge needle; advise patient that injection may be painful. For zinc suspension, shake well and administer by deep intramuscular

▶

injection. Observe closely during intravenous administration and immediately after administration by any injection route for signs of sensitivity reaction; prolonged use increases risk of such reactions.

Contraindications/Precautions

PREG C

Contraindicated in hypersensitivity to corticotropin or to pork protein, and in active peptic ulcer disease, scleroderma, recent surgery, active tuberculosis; fungal infections, and herpes of eyes, lips, or genitals. **Use with caution** in acquired immunodeficiency syndrome (AIDS), hypertension, congestive heart failure, diabetes mellitus, glaucoma, seizure disorders, renal insufficiency, hypothyroidism, osteoporosis, mysathenia gravis, thrombophlebitis, and history of bleeding ulcers or mental illness.

🖐 **Use with caution for children, women of childbearing age, pregnant or nursing mothers, and the elderly.**

Side effects/Adverse reactions

Hypersensitivity: rash, hives, itching, fever, dizziness, nausea, vomiting, wheezing, anaphylaxis. **CNS:** euphoria, restlessness, insomnia, hallucinations, depression, or psychosis. **Eye:** glaucoma, cataracts. **MS:** impaired growth in children. **CV:** thrombophlebitis, embolism, irregular heartbeat. **GI:** increased appetite, oral candidiasis. **Hem:** hyperglycemia. **Misc:** withdrawal syndrome.

With prolonged use: Skin: acne; increased hair growth; thin, shiny skin; ecchymosis, petechiae; delayed wound healing. **GI:** ulcerative esophagitis, pancreatitis, nausea, vomiting, GI bleeding. **MS:** muscle wasting; osteoporosis; pain in hips, back, ribs, arms, or legs. **CV:** hypertension, edema, hypokalemia. **GU:** menstrual irregularity. **Misc:** increased susceptibility to infection, Cushingoid appearance (moon-face and buffalo hump), withdrawal syndrome, or acute adrenal insufficiency.

Nursing implications/Documentation

Possible nursing diagnoses: Fluid volume excess; Impaired skin integrity; Altered growth and development.

♦ Record baseline weight, blood pressure, and electrolyte levels.

♦ Obtain history of allergic reaction to pork or pork products.

♦ Monitor injection site for pain, redness, or swelling.

♦ Monitor intake and output and record twice weekly weights to identify need for salt and fluid restriction.

♦ Assess for signs of infection or delayed wound healing.

♦ With long-term therapy, monitor and record growth and development of infants and children.

♦ Do not administer vaccines or immunization during corticotropin therapy.

♦ Assess and document improvement in condition being treated, so dosage can be decreased as early as possible.

♦ Be aware that drug must be withdrawn gradually following long-term therapy.

♦ Be aware that supplemental doses of rapidly acting corticosteroids may be required during times of physical and emotional stress.

♦ Monitor neonates of mothers who received corticotropin during pregnancy for hypoadrenalism.

Patient & family teaching/Home care

Possible nursing diagnoses: Knowledge deficit; Impaired home maintenance management; Potential for infection.

♦ Point out the need to inform other physicians and dentist of corticotropin therapy.

♦ Stress the importance of salt restriction and potassium supplementation; advise reporting development of edema.

♦ Caution to avoid drinking alcohol.

♦ Teach the symptoms of adrenal insufficiency (hypotension, hypoglycemia, nausea, anorexia, depression, mood swings).

♦ In long-term therapy, advise reporting signs of infection during therapy and for 1 year after corticotropin has been discontinued.

♦ *See Adrenocorticosteroids overview for more information.*

cortisone

kor'ti-sone

cortisone acetate: ♠*Cortate, Cortone Acetate*

Class: Naturally occurring adrenocorticosteroid, Short-acting glucocorticoid, Steroidal anti-inflammatory, Immunosuppressant

PEDS	PREG	GERI
🖐	C	🖐

Action Provides physiologic glucocorticoid and mineralocorticoid activity when endogenous hormones are diminished.

Use/Therapeutic goal/Outcome

Adrenal insufficiency: Replacement of deficient endogenous hormones. *Outcome criteria:* Improved appetite, decreased fatigue, normal blood pressure, normal skin color and turgor, report of improved sense of well-being.

Dose range/Administration

Interaction alert: May decrease effectiveness of anticoagulants and antidiabetics. Vaccines may lead to diminished antibody response and serious infection. Potassium-depleting diuretics may cause severe hypokalemia. Alcohol or medications known to cause gastric irritation may lead to gastric bleeding. Drugs that increase metabolism of corticosteroids (e.g., phenytoin, barbiturates, ephedrine, and rifampin), and those that decrease its absorption (e.g., cholestyramine, colestipol, and antacids) may decrease cortisone levels, requiring an increase in cortisone dosage.

🖐 **Give oral doses with food or milk to reduce gastric irritation.**

Adult: PO, IM: 25–300 mg/day. *Child:* PO, IM: 0.7–10 mg/kg/day.

Clinical alert: For replacement therapy, give 2/3 of daily dose in the mornings and 1/3 in the evening to simulate endogenous secretion. For IM doses, shake suspension well and give deeply into gluteal muscle.

Contraindications/Precautions
PREG
C

Contraindicated in hypersensitivity to corticosteroids, and in active peptic ulcer disease, active tuberculosis or fungus infections, and herpes of eyes, lips or genitals. *Use with caution* in acquired immunodeficiency syndrome (AIDS), hypertension, thrombophlebitis, congestive heart failure, diabetes mellitus, hypothyroidism, glaucoma, osteoporosis, myasthenia gravis, and history of bleeding ulcers, seizure disorder, or mental illness.

🖐 **Use with caution for children, pregnant or nursing mothers, and the elderly.**

Side effects/Adverse reactions

Physiologic doses of cortisone administered for treatment of adrenocortical insufficiency rarely cause side effects.

Nursing implications/Documentation

Possible nursing diagnoses: Impaired tissue integrity; Fluid volume excess.

◆ Record baseline weight, blood pressure, and electrolyte levels.

◆ Assess for physical and psychological stress which may create need for additional cortisone.

◆ Monitor electrolyte levels to detect sodium retention and potassium loss; assess for edema and/or muscle weakness and report and record abnormal findings.

◆ During dose reduction, monitor for symptoms of adrenal insufficiency (hypotension, hypoglycemia, weight loss, vomiting, and diarrhea).

◆ Recognize that this drug has little use in inflammatory and allergic conditions because it causes sodium retention and potassium loss when given in pharmacologic (rather than physiologic) doses.

Patient & family teaching/Home care

Possible nursing diagnoses: Knowledge deficit; Impaired home maintenance management; Fatigue.

◆ Stress the need to take oral doses with food or milk.

◆ Advise wearing medical alert identification stating that cortisone is being taken for adrenal insufficiency.

◆ Explain that this drug will probably be needed life–long.

◆ Advise against taking OTC or prescription drugs without consulting primary physician.

◆ Emphasize importance of medical follow-up for evaluation of therapy.

◆ *See Adrenocorticosteroid overview for more information.*

co-trimoxazole
coe-trye-mox'a-zole

sulfamethoxazole-trimethoprim: ♥*Apo-Sulfatrim*, ♥*Apo-Sulfatrim DS, Bactrim, Bactrim DS, Bactrim I.V. Infusion, Cotrim, Cotrim DS,* ♥*Novotrimel,* ♥*Novotrimel DS,* ♥*Protrin,* ♥*Protrin DF,* ♠*Resprim,* ♥*Roubac,* ♥*Roubac DS, Septra, Septra DS, Septra I.V. Infusion,* ♠*Septrin, SMZ-TNP, Sulfamethoprim, Sulfamethoprim DS, Sulmeprim,* ♠*Trib, Uroplus DS, Uroplus SS*

Class: Anti-infective, Sulfonamide

PEDS	PREG	GERI
🖐	🖐	**OK**

Action Usually bacteriostatic, limits bacterial growth by blocking the biosynthesis of folic acid. Combining sulphamethoxazole and trimethoprim produces synergistic effect.

Use/Therapeutic goal/Outcome

Infections (urinary tract, shigellosis, ear, systemic, pnemocystis carinii pneumonia): Resolution of infection. *Outcome criteria:* Absence of pathogenic growth on cultures, absence of clinical manifestations of infection (fever, pain, swelling, redness, heat, odor, drainage, productive cough, dysuria), normal chest X rays, normal WBC count.

Dose range/Administration

Interaction alert: Increases the effect of methotrexate, phenytoin, oral hypoglycemics, and anticoagulants. Ammonium chloride or ascorbic acid may cause precipitation of sulfonamide with resultant crystalluria. Decreases effectiveness of oral contraceptives and increases risk of breakthrough bleeding. Thiazide diuretics may increase incidence of thrombocytopenia with purpura in the elderly.

Give oral doses with a full glass of water.

Trimethoprim content is always ⅕ of sulfamethoxazole content. *Adult:* PO, IV: 80–160 mg trimethoprim with 400–800 mg sulfamethoxazole q6-12h. *Child > 2 mos:* PO, IV: 8 mg/kg/day trimethoprim with 40 mg/kg/day sulfamethoxazole, divided q6-12h.

Clinical alert: Monitor those with AIDS for increased side effects.

Contraindications/Precautions

Contraindicated in allergy to trimethoprim or sulfonamides, and in porphyria, and megaloblastic anemia due to folate deficiency. *Use with caution* in alcoholism, in conjunction with anticonvulsant therapy, in impaired renal or hepatic function, malabsorption syndrome or malnutrition, and history of other allergic responses (e.g., other drugs, hay fever, asthma).

Contraindicated for infants under 2 months and pregnant or nursing mothers (preg C; preg D if near term).

Side effects/Adverse reactions

Hypersensitivity: itching, rashes, exfoliative dermatitis, fever, Stevens-Johnson syndrome, angioedema, difficulty breathing, anaphylaxis. *GI:* abdominal pain, stomatitis, nausea, vomiting, diarrhea, pseudomembranous colitis, hepatitis. *GU:* nephrotoxicity (oliguria, anuria, crystalluria, hematuria). *CV:* pain, redness, swelling, thrombophlebitis at injection site, tissue damage with extravasation. *CNS:* headache, dizziness, mental depression, fatigue, hallucinations, seizures. *Hem:* agranulocytosis, aplastic anemia, eosinophilia, thrombocytopenia, leukopenia, hemolytic anemia, hypoglycemia, bleeding disorders. *Ear:* tinnitus. *Skin:* photosensitivity. *Misc:* superinfections.

Nursing implications/Documentation

Possible nursing diagnoses: Potential for infection; Potential fluid volume deficit; Diarrhea.

♦ Determine history of allergies, and (regardless of history) monitor closely for allergic reactions (higher incidence of adverse reactions in patients with AIDS).

♦ Weigh patient and obtain baseline CBC, BUN, creatinine, liver function studies, and necessary culture specimens before administering first dose; monitor closely thereafter if therapy is prolonged.

♦ Monitor for bleeding tendencies (check gums, urine).

♦ Encourage fluids, record and monitor input and output; 3000–4000 ml/day is advised (for urine output of 1500 ml/day).

♦ Document and report diarrhea.

♦ If there is no improvement within 3–5 days, consult with physician to determine if antibiotic regimen should be re-evaluated (and new cultures drawn).

Patient & family teaching/Home care

Possible nursing diagnoses: Knowledge deficit; Impaired home maintenance management.

♦ Stress the importance of drinking 3 to 4 quarts of fluids daily to optimize drug action and minimize side effects.

♦ Teach the need to report persistent diarrhea, or new symptoms of illness (e.g., fever, mouth lesions, vaginal irritation, respiratory symptoms, diarrhea); medication change may be necessary.

♦ Explain the importance of taking antibiotics for the entire time prescribed, even if symptoms abate.

♦ Caution that this drug may cause increased sensitivity to the sun; warn women that effectiveness of oral contraceptives may be reduced.

♦ *See Anti-infectives overview for more information.*

cromolyn
kroe'moe-lin

cromolyn sodium: *Gastrocrom, Intal, Intal Inhaler,*
♣*Intal Spincaps, Nalcrom, Nasalcrom, Opticrom*
4% Opthalmic, ♣*Rynacrom*

Class: Antiasthmatic, antiallergic, Mast cell stabilizer

PEDS	PREG	GERI
🖐	B	🖐

Action Prevents allergic responses by inhibiting the release of allergy mediators (such as histamine and slow-reacting substance of anaphylaxis [SRS-A]) from mast cells and other cells.

Use/Therapeutic goal/Outcome

Severe perennial bronchial asthma, Exercise-induced asthma: Prevention of bronchospasm. ***Outcome criteria:*** Report and demonstration of absence of (or decrease in) episodes of wheezing or asthma, with increased exercise tolerance.

Allergic conditions (rhinitis, food allergies, occular disorders): Prevention of symptoms. ***Outcome criteria:*** Report and demonstration of absence of (or decrease in) allergy symptoms (runny nose, sneezing, itching, rashes, tearing and redness of the eyes).

Mastocytosis: Control of symptoms. ***Outcome criteria:*** Decreased symptoms (diarrhea, flushing, headache, vomiting, hives, abdominal pain, nausea, and itching).

Inflammatory bowel disease: Reduction in inflammation. ***Outcome criteria:*** Absence of (or decrease in) diarrhea; report of increased comfort.

Dose range/Administration

Interaction alert: May reduce corticosteroid requirements.

🥄 **Give PO doses 15–20 min before meals, especially if given for food allergies.**

Bronchial asthma: Adult/Child > 5 yrs: Inhal: 2 aerosol inhalations q6h. Alteratively, may inhale the contents of a 20-mg capsule q6h. (Also available in solution for a nebulizer).

Exercise-induced asthma: Adult/Child > 5 yrs: Inhal: 2 aerosol inhalations, or inhalation of the contents of a 20-mg capsule no more than 1 hr before anticipated exercise.

Allergic occular disorders: Adult/Child > 4 yrs: *Ophthalmic:* 1–2 drops in each eye q4-6h.

Allergic rhinitis: Adult/Child > 5 yrs: *Nasal:* 1 spray into each nostril q6-8h, up to 6 times daily.

Mastocytosis: Adult: 100–200 mg qid.

Food allergies: Adults/Child > 13 yrs: PO: 200 mg qid taken 15–20 min before meals. Dose may be doubled in 2–3 weeks if necessary. ***Child 2–13 yrs:*** PO: 100 mg qid taken 15–20 min before meals. Dose may be doubled in 2–3 weeks if necessary, to a maximum of 40 mg/kg/day. ***Child < 2 yrs:*** PO: Up to 20 mg/kg/day, taken 15–20 min before meals.

Inflammatory bowel disease: Adults/Child > 14 yrs: PO: 200 mg qid, taken 15–20 min before meals. ***Child 2–14 yrs:*** PO: 100 mg qid, taken 15–20 min before meals.

Clinical alert: Assess for lactose intolerance before giving cromolyn sodium capsules for inhalation, because they contain lactose. Do not give cromolyn during an acute asthmatic attack (wait until patient can inhale without wheezing). For oral use, contents of a capsule should be dissolved in warm water and taken as a solution.

Contraindications/Precautions
PREG B

Contraindicated in hypersensitivity to cromolyn (and for capsules for inhalation, to lactose), and in acute asthma, and status asthmaticus. ***Use with caution*** in liver or kidney impairment, and for long-term use.

🖐 **Use with caution for children, pregnant or nursing women, and the elderly. Safety of capsules for inhalation and nebulizer in children under 2 years, and of aerosol inhaler in children under 5 years, has not been established.**

Side effects/Adverse reactions

Generally well tolerated. ***Hypersensitivity:*** erythema, urticaria, rash, contact or exfoliative dermatitis, photodermatitis, eosinophilic pneumonia, bronchospasm, anaphylaxis (rare). ***CNS:*** headache, dizziness, vertigo. ***Resp:*** coughing, wheezing, sneezing, nasal stinging, burning, and congestion, postnasal drip, irritation of throat and trachea, hoarseness, hemoptysis. ***GI:*** dry mouth, slightly bitter aftertaste, nausea, vomiting. ***GU:*** dysuria, frequency. ***CV:*** periarteritis vasculitis, pericarditis. ***Hem:*** anemia. ***MS:*** joint swelling and pain, polymyositis. ***Misc:*** fever, swelling of parotid glands. For ophthalmic solution: ***Eye:*** itching, burning, stinging, lacrimation.

Nursing implications/Documentation

Possible nursing diagnoses: Activity intolerance; Ineffective breathing pattern; Altered nutrition: less than body requirements.

▶

- Determine and record known allergies; provide an environment that is free from allergens (e.g. use air conditioning).
- Monitor for dehydration and malnutrition, especially when given for food allergies; consult with dietician to plan meals.

Patient & family teaching/Home care

Possible nursing diagnoses: Knowledge deficit; Impaired home maintenance management.

- Advise taking PO doses with food or milk if GI symptoms are experienced (unless used for food allergies).
- For asthmatics, stress that cromolyn therapy is preventative. It should be used even if asthma attacks stop. Point out that use during an acute attack may be an aggravating factor.
- Assess for environmental allergens at home (mold is common), and help identify ways to diminish them (e.g., air conditioning, dehumidifiers.
- Point out that controlled breathing and relaxation techniques can reduce severity and frequency of asthma attacks.
- For capsule inhalation, teach patient and have them demonstrate the use of the Spinhaler (insert capsule, exhale completely, place mouthpiece in mouth, inhale deeply and rapidly with a steady breath, remove inhaler, hold breath a few seconds, then exhale); repeat until all the powder has been inhaled.
- For opthalmic and nasal preparations instruct patients and have them demonstrate the use of eye drops or nose spray.

cyanocobalamin
sye-an-oh-koe-bal'a-min

Anacobin, Bedoce, ♦Bedoz, Betalin 12, ♠Bioglan B₁₂ Plus, Crystamine, ♦Cyanabin, Cyanocobalamin, Cyano-Gel, Dodex, Kaybovite, Poyamin, Redisol, Rubesol-1000, ♦Rubion, Rubramin, Sigamine

Class: Vitamin B$_{12}$, Antianemic, Water-soluble vitamin

PEDS	PREG	GERI
OK	❦	OK

Action Promotes fat and carbohydrate metabolism and protein synthesis by acting as a coenzyme; promotes normal growth, cell reproduction, maturation of RBCs and synthesis of nucleoprotein and myelin by metabolism of methionine, folic acid, and malonic acid.

Use/Therapeutic goal/Outcome

Vitamin B$_{12}$ deficiency or malabsorption, pernicious anemia: Adequate Vitamin B$_{12}$ blood levels. *Outcome criteria:* Increased reticulocyte and RBC count, absence or improvement in symptoms of deficiency (paresthesias, anorexia, fatigue, and red, sore tongue).

Dose range/Administration

Decreased absorption may occur with neomycin, colchicine, para-aminosalicylic acid, timed-release potassium preparations, or excessive use of alcohol. Chloramphenicol may inhibit the hematopoietic activity of cyanocobalamin.

❦ **Administer oral doses with food to maximize absorption.**

Nutritional supplement: Adult: PO: 1–25 mcg/day. *Child:* PO: 0.3 to 1 mcg/day.

Deficiency/Anemia: Adult: IM, SC: *Loading dose:* 100 mcg/day for 6–7 days, then 100 mcg qod for 14 days (7 doses), then 100 mcg q3-4d for 2–3 wk. *Maintenance dose:* 100–200 mcg/month. *Child:* IM, SC: *Loading dose:* 30–50 mcg/day for 2 wk. *Maintenance dose:* 100 mcg/month.

Parenteral preparations containing benzyl alcohol are not to be used for newborn and immature infants.

Contraindications/Precautions
PREG
❦

Contraindicated in hypersensitivity to Vitamin B$_{12}$ or to cobalt, and in optic nerve atrophy. *Use with caution* in history of gout.

❦ **May be used safely in recommended daily allowances (RDA) for pregnant women (preg A); safe use for pregnant women in doses greater than RDA has not been established (preg C).**

Side effects/Adverse reactions

Hypersensitivity: Rash, hives, wheezing, anaphylaxis. *GI:* transient diarrhea. *CV:* peripheral vascular thrombosis, CHF, pulmonary edema. *Hem:* hypokalemia. *Misc:* pain at injection site.

Nursing implications/Documentation

Possible nursing diagnoses: Diarrhea; Activity intolerance; Altered peripheral tissue perfusion.

- For patients with history of sensitivities, administer intradermal test dose before beginning parenteral therapy.

• Do not mix in syringe with other medications or solutions.

• Administer parenteral doses IM or deep SC to avoid local irritation; not used IV, except for small amounts in parenteral nutrition solutions.

• Monitor potassium level, reticulocyte and RBC count, hemoglobin, and Vitamin B_{12} level.

• Assess for CHF and pulmonary edema in cardiac patients.

Patient & family teaching/Home care

Possible nursing diagnoses: Knowledge deficit; Impaired home maintenance management.

• For dietary deficiency, identify foods high in Vitamin B_{12} (meats, fish, egg yolk, aged cheeses).

• With strict vegetarian diets, advise of need to supplement, but caution not to exceed recommended daily allowance.

• For pernicious anemia or noncorrectable malabsorption, explain that Vitamin B_{12} injections must be continued throughout life to prevent irreversible neurological damage.

• Explain that the stinging, burning sensation that may occur after injection is transient.

cyclacillin
sye-kla-sill'in

Cyclapen-W

Class: Anti-infective, Antibiotic, Aminopenicillin

PEDS	PREG	GERI
∭	B	∭

Action Broad-spectrum, usually bactericidal antibiotic; kills bacteria by inhibiting cell wall synthesis.

Use/Therapeutic goal/Outcome

Systemic and urinary tract infections (caused by penicillinase-producing staphylococci): Resolution of infection. *Outcome criteria:* Absence of pathogenic growth on cultures, absence of clinical manifestations of infection (fever, pain, redness, heat, swelling, odor, drainage, dysuria, frequency), normal WBC count.

Dose range/Administration

Interaction alert: Probenecid inhibits excretion of cyclacillin and may be given to increase serum levels of the drug.

Give with a full glass of water 1–2 hours before or 2–3 hours after meals; food may inhibit absorption.

Adult: PO: 250–500 mg q6h. *Child:* PO: 50–100 mg/kg/day, in divided doses q6h.

Clinical alert: Give cyclacillin at least 1 hour before bacteriostatic antibiotics for optimum effect. Dosage in renal insufficiency should be adjusted according to creatinine clearance.

Contraindications/Precautions
PREG
B

Contraindicated in allergy to penicillin. *Use with caution* in cephalosporin sensitivity, history of allergic responses (e.g., other drugs, hay fever, asthma), and in renal insufficiency.

∭ Use with caution for children, the elderly, and pregnant or nursing mothers.

Side effects/Adverse reactions

Hypersensitivity: itching, rashes, urticaria, fever, difficulty breathing, anaphylaxis. *GI:* nausea, vomiting, diarrhea, pseudomembranous colitis. *CNS:* dizziness, headache. *Hem:* anemia, thrombocytopenia purpura, leukopenia, neutropenia, eosinophilia, slight elevation in SGOT. *Misc:* superinfection.

Nursing implications/Documentation

Possible nursing diagnoses: Potential for infection; Diarrhea.

• Determine history of allergies, and (regardless of history) monitor closely for allergic reactions.

• Obtain baseline CBC, liver function studies, and necessary cultures before administering first dose; monitor closely thereafter if therapy is prolonged.

• Encourage fluids, and record and monitor intake and output, to ensure adequate hydration; report significant negative or positive balance.

• Monitor for and report signs of superinfection (sore throat, fever, fatigue, thrush, vaginal discharge, diarrhea).

Patient & family teaching/Home care

Possible nursing diagnoses: Knowledge deficit; Impaired home maintenance management.

• Explain the need to take cyclacillin with a full glass of water 1–2 hours before meals or 2–3 hours after meals.

• Teach the importance of reporting allergic symptoms, diarrhea, signs and symptoms that do not abate, or *any* new signs and symptoms of discomfort that might indicate superinfection (medication regimen may have to be changed).

♦ Advise drinking 2–3 L of fluids daily to maintain adequate hydration (especially important if fever exists).

♦ Stress the importance of taking antibiotics for the entire time prescribed, even if signs and symptoms abate.

♦ *See Anti-infectives overview for more information.*

cyclandelate
sye-klan'de-late

Cyclan, Cyclospasmol, Cydel

Class: Vasodilator, peripheral

PEDS	PREG	GERI
♨	C	♨

Action Dilates blood vessels by producing a direct papaverine-like relaxation of smooth muscle. There is no significant effect upon blood pressure and heart rate.

Use/Therapeutic goal/Outcome
Occlusive vascular disease and vasospastic conditions (artherosclerosis obliterans, intermittent claudication, nocturnal leg cramps, and Raynaud's disease): Promotion of circulation and increased activity tolerance. *Outcome criteria:* Improvement of pulse volume, skin color and temperature; report of decreased pain; evidence of increased activity tolerance.

Dose range/Administration
🍎 Give with food or milk to reduce GI distress.

Adult: PO: Initially, 200–400 mg qid. After clinical response, reduce by 200 mg increments to 400–800 mg/day in 2–4 divided doses.

Contraindications/Precautions
PREG
C

Contraindicated in hypersensitivity to cyclandelate. *Use with caution* in obliterative coronary artery or cerebrovascular disease, bleeding disorders, hypertension, or glaucoma.

♨ Use with caution for the elderly. Safe use for children and pregnant or nursing mothers has not been established.

Side effects/Adverse reactions
Hypersensitivity: rash. *CV:* facial flushing, tachycardia. *CNS:* tingling of the extremities, dizziness. *GI:* nausea, heartburn. *Hem:* High doses may prolong bleeding time. *Skin:* sweating.

Nursing implications/Documentation
Possible nursing diagnoses: Activity intolerance; Pain.

♦ Document baseline circulatory status (presence and quality of peripheral pulses, skin color, and temperature) and activity tolerance; monitor periodically thereafter.

♦ Monitor for dizziness, and supervise ambulation until response is determined.

Patient & family teaching/Home care
Possible nursing diagnoses: Knowledge deficit; Impaired home maintenance management.

♦ Advise taking cyclandelate with food or milk to reduce GI symptoms.

♦ Stress that improvement in symptoms is usually gradual with cyclandelate; long-term therapy is necessary for optimal effects.

♦ Explain the need to change positions slowly to reduce dizziness; point out that side effects usually subside after a few weeks of therapy.

♦ *See Antianginals overview for more information.*

cyclobenzaprine
sye-kloe-ben'za-preen

cyclobenzaprine hydrochloride: *Flexeril*

Class: Skeletal-muscle relaxant (centrally acting), Antispasmodic

PEDS	PREG	GERI
♨	B	♨

Action Relaxes skeletal muscle by depressing tonic and somatic motor activity at the brain stem. Not effective for spasticity due to cerebral or spinal cord diseases. Structurally and functionally resembles tricyclic antidepressants.

Use/Therapeutic goal/Outcome
Muscle spasms associated with acute musculoskeletal conditions: Relief of muscle spasms without loss of voluntary motor function; improved comfort. *Outcome criteria:* Increased range of motion and ability to perform activities of daily life; report of decreased pain.

Dose range/Administration

Interaction alert: CNS effects may be additive to those of alcohol, barbiturates, and other CNS depressants. Use cautiously with anticholinergics and MAO inhibitors, or within 14 days after discontinuation of MAO inhibitors.

Adult: PO: 10–20 mg tid.

Clinical alert: Not to exceed 60 mg/day or 2–3 weeks of therapy.

Contraindications/Precautions

PREG
B

Contraindicated in hypersensitivity to cyclobenzaprine, and in acute recovery-phase myocardial infarction, dysrhythmias, heart block, conduction disturbances, congestive heart failure, or hyperthyroidism. *Use with caution* in history of urinary retention, angle closure glaucoma, increased intraocular pressure, seizures, hepatic impairment, and history of psychiatric disturbance.

✋ **Use with caution for the elderly or debilitated. Safe use for children under 15 years and pregnant or nursing mothers has not been determined.**

Side effects/Adverse reactions

Hypersensitivity: pruritus, hives, rash, edema of face and tongue. *CNS:* drowsiness, blurred vision, dizziness, weakness, insomnia, ataxia, tremors, sweating, fatigue. *GI:* nausea, dry mouth, constipation, hepatitis. *GU:* urinary retention. *CV:* tachycardia.

Nursing implications/Documentation

Possible nursing diagnoses: Impaired physical mobility; Constipation; Pain; Potential for injury.

♦ Monitor comfort level and range of motion before and after dose is taken.

♦ Monitor and document bowel pattern and food and fluid intake as constipation may develop.

♦ Observe for and report signs of toxicity and cardiac changes (dysrhythmia, prolonged conduction time).

♦ Supervise out-of-bed activities if drowsiness is present.

Patient & family teaching/Home care

Possible nursing diagnoses: Knowledge deficit; Impaired home maintenance management.

♦ Advise against operating machinery, driving, or combining with CNS depressants or alcohol, especially if drowsiness is present.

♦ Warn that dry mouth may occur; suggest using ice chips, sugarless gum, or hard candy for relief.

♦ Explain the importance of contacting physician before taking OTC medications or if side effects develop.

♦ Point out the importance of increasing fluids and high-fiber foods to prevent constipation.

♦ Stress the importance of continuing with treatment plan, including rest and other forms of therapy (e.g., relaxation techniques).

♦ *See Skeletal-muscle relaxant overview for more information.*

cyclophosphamide
sye-kloh-fos'fah-mide

♠Cycoblastin, Cytoxan, Cytoxan Lyophilized, ♠Endoxan-Asta, Neosar, ♥Procytox

Class: ★Antineoplastic (alkylating) agent prototype

PEDS PREG GERI
✋   D   ✋

Action Kills rapidly growing cells (cancer, hair follicles, bone marrow, GI lining, ova, and sperm) by interfering with DNA, RNA, and protein synthesis through alkylation (cross-linking of DNA occurs). Is cell-cycle–phase nonspecific, affecting both actively dividing cells and dormant (resting) cells.

Use/Therapeutic goal/Outcome

Hodgkin's disease and malignant lymphomas; multiple myeloma; leukemias; mycosis fungoides; neuroblastoma; ovarian carcinoma; retinoblastoma; and cancers of the breast, testes, lung, head, and neck: Elimination or suppression of malignant cell proliferation. *Outcome criteria:* Tumor and disease regression or stabilization on radiologic and physical examination for leukemias, absence of blasts in peripheral blood specimen.

Dose range/Administration

Interaction alert: Increased toxicity may occur if used with aminoglycosides and thiazide diuretics. Phenobarbital may increase drug metabolism. Insulin requirements may be altered. May decrease digoxin levels. Corticosteroids and chloramphenicol may reduce drug activity. When cyclophosphamide is combined with

▶

allopurinol, doxorubicin, vincristine, or phenothiazines cytotoxic effects may be potentiated.

🖥 **Give drug on an empty stomach; if GI
upset occurs, give with food.**

Adult: IV: 40–50 mg/kg or 1.5 to 1.8 g/m^2/day
in divided doses over 2–5 days. *Other regimens
include:* 10–15 mg/kg every 7–10 days or 3–5
mg/kg twice weekly. PO: 1–5 mg/kg/day,
depending on tolerance. *Child:* IV, PO: 2–8
mg/kg or 60–250 mg/m^2/day for 6 days. *Other
regimens include:* 2–5 mg/kg or 50–150 mg/m^2
twice weekly.

Clinical alert: This drug should be given only by
nurses who are knowledgeable in the comprehensive management of the administration of
antineoplastic agents. Doses may vary at physician's discretion and are held until the
patient has sufficiently recovered from toxicities of previous doses. Protocols for drug preparation, administration, and accidental skin contamination must be followed. Gloves or double
gloves must be worn when handling cyclophosphamide (skin contamination may cause a local
reaction). Contaminated areas should be
washed with large amounts of soap and water.
Cyclophosphamide is given over 1 min IV push
or in 50–100 ml fluid.

Contraindications/Precautions

PREG
D

Contraindicated in hypersensitivity to cyclophosphamide and during viral illnesses such as
chicken pox and herpes (this drug is a potent
immunosuppressant). *Use with caution* in
impaired renal or hepatic function.

✋ **Contraindicated for pregnant or nursing
mothers. Use with caution for children and
the elderly.**

Side effects/Adverse reactions

Hypersensitivity: urticaria, tachycardia,
hypotension, anaphylaxis. *Hem:* leukopenia,
thrombocytopenia, anemia, hyponatremia,
hyperuricemia. *GI:* anorexia; nausea and
vomiting (within 6 hr); diarrhea; stomatitis;
jaundice; hepatotoxicity. *GU:* hematuria, hemorrhagic cystitis (infrequent yet dose-related).
Skin: alopecia (50% occurrence within 3
weeks); dermatitis; hyperpigmentation of skin
and fingernails. *Resp:* pulmonary fibrosis
(high doses). *CV:* cardiotoxicity. *CNS:* headache, dizziness. *Misc:* secondary malignancies,
SIADH with high doses.

Nursing implications/Documentation

Possible nursing diagnoses: Potential for infection; Potential for injury; Fatigue; Altered oral
mucous membrane; Fluid volume deficit; Diarrhea, Altered nutrition: less than body requirements.

◆ *See important Nursing implications in
Antineoplastic agents overview on page 72,
which apply to all antineoplastics. The
interventions that follow are additional and
specific to this drug only.*

◆ Expect that the patient will be hydrated with
300–400 ml normal saline prior to dose and
100–200 ml after dose when a single dose is
greater than 500 mg.

◆ Hold drug and report if hemorrhagic cystitis
is noted; maintain a fluid intake of at least
3 L and encourage voiding every 1–2 hr to prevent this.

◆ Expect that leukocytes and erythrocytes
should drop to the nadir (lowest point) in 1–2
weeks, with recovery in 3 weeks (drug is
"platelet sparing").

◆ Be aware that therapeutic response is often
accompanied by toxicity.

Patient & family teaching/Home care

Possible nursing diagnoses: Knowledge deficit;
Ineffective coping (individual and family);
Hopelessness; Impaired home maintenance
management.

◆ *See important Patient & family teaching in
Antineoplastic agents overview on page 72,
which apply to all antineoplastics. The
teachings that follow are additional and specific
to this drug only.*

◆ Point out that drinking 3 L a day and voiding hourly helps prevent hemorrhagic cystitis
and that voiding frequently (at least once during the night) helps prevent prolonged contact
of metabolites with bladder mucosa.

◆ Stress the need to use nonhormonal birth
control and to report suspected pregnancy
immediately.

◆ *See Antineoplastic agents overview for more
information.*

cycloserine

sye-kloe-ser'een

Seromycin

Class: Anti-infective, Antitubercular

PEDS	PREG	GERI
🖐	C	🖐

Action Limits bacterial growth (bacteriostatic action) by inhibiting cell wall biosynthesis (interferes with the utilization of amino acids).

Use/Therapeutic goal/Outcome

Active tuberculosis (in combination with other antitubercular drugs): Resolution of infection. *Outcome criteria:* Absence of acid-fast bacilli on sputum culture, decreased productive cough, normal temperature, improvement of X rays.

Dose range/Administration

Interaction alert: Isoniazid and ethionamide increase CNS toxicity; monitor for dizziness and drowsiness. Concurrent alcohol ingestion causes seizures.

Adult: PO: Begin with 250 mg q12h for 2 weeks; if there are no signs of toxicity (see side effects) and if blood levels are < 25–30 mcg/ml (therapeutic range), increase dose to 250 mg q8h for 2 weeks. If blood levels remain low and there are no signs of toxicity, increase dose to 250 mg q6h, to a maximum of 1 g/day. If CNS toxicity occurs, discontinue drug for 1 week, then resume at 250 mg daily for 2 weeks; if no serious toxic effects are noted, increase daily dose by 250 mg every 10 days until therapeutic serum drug levels are achieved.

Clinical alert: In the presence of kidney impairment, expect decreased dosage.

Contraindications/Precautions

PREG C

Contraindicated in hypersensitivity to cycloserine, and in seizures, depression, severe anxiety, severe kidney disease, or chronic alcoholism. *Use with caution* in mild-to-moderate kidney disease.

🖐 **Contraindicated for nursing mothers. Use with caution for the elderly. Safe use for children and during pregnancy has not been established.**

Side effects/Adverse reactions

Hypersensitivity: dermatitis, itching, rashes. *CNS:* drowsiness, dizziness, headache, seizures, confusion, memory loss, nervousness, tremor, hyperreflexia, hyperirritability, paresthesias,

depression, suicidal tendencies, psychosis. *CV:* arrhythmias, CHF.

Nursing implications/Documentation

Possible nursing diagnoses: Potential for infection; Fatigue; Activity intolerance; Fluid volume deficit.

◆ Ascertain that baseline CBC, BUN, creatinine, and liver function studies are obtained, and that necessary culture specimens are collected, before starting cycloserine; monitor periodically thereafter (sputum specimens should be obtained to detect organism resistance).

◆ Report serum drug levels above 30 mg/ml (serious toxic reactions may occur).

◆ Allow for a balance between rest and activity.

◆ Monitor for and report psychotic reactions.

◆ Monitor and record intake and output and provide favorite fluids to ensure adequate hydration.

Patient & family teaching/Home care

Possible nursing diagnoses: Knowledge deficit; Impaired home maintenance management.

◆ Stress the importance of taking this drug as prescribed without missing doses, and the importance of long-term medical follow-up to avoid relapses or complications.

◆ Explain the need to report drowsiness, dizziness, tremors, depression, hyperirritability, or tingling of extremities.

◆ Warn that drinking alcohol can precipitate seizures.

◆ Encourage drinking at least 2 L of fluid a day to maintain adequate hydration.

◆ *See Anti-infectives overview for more information.*

cyclosporine

sye'kloe-spor-een

🍁*Sandimmun, Sandimmune*

Class: ★Immunosuppressant (T-cell suppressor) prototype

PEDS	PREG	GERI
🖐	C	🖐

Action Suppresses immune response by inhibiting T-lymphocytic action, thus preventing rejection of transplanted bone marrow and organs (kidney, heart, liver, lung, pancreas).

Use/Therapeutic goal/Outcome

Organ transplantation: Prevention of rejection. **Outcome criteria:** Laboratory studies indicating improved function of transplanted organ (e.g., decreased serum creatinine, in the case of a kidney transplant).

Dose range/Administration

Interaction alert: Avoid giving with potassium-sparing diuretics, because of risk of hyperkalemia. Ketoconazole, amphotericin B, cimetidine, erythromycin, doxycycline, corticosteroids, calcium channel blockers, and oral contraceptives increase cyclosporin blood levels; monitor for cyclosporin toxicity. Anticonvulsants (phenytoin and others), metamizole, nafcillin, and rifampin, decrease immunosuppressive effects of cyclosporine. If given with gentamycin, tobramycin, amphotericin B, melphalan, trimethoprim, monitor for nephrotoxicity.

For best absorption, and to prevent nausea, give 1 hour after meals (use a glass to minimize adherence of drug to container walls; mix with whole milk, chocolate milk, or juice to increase palatability).

Adult and Child: PO: 15 mg/kg 4–12 hr before transplantation, and daily after surgery for 1–2 wks. Gradually reduce dose by 5%/wk. *Maintenance dose:* 5–10 mg/kg/ qAM. IV: 4–5 mg 4–12 hr before transplantation, and qd. Change to PO route as soon as possible.

Clinical alert: Measure liquid oral doses carefully, using oral syringe. For parenteral administration, keep emergency drugs and equipment available in case of anaphylaxis. Oral cyclosporine absorption is erratic, especially for diabetics (give at the *same time* every day to ensure adequate drug levels over a 24-hour period).

Contraindications/Precautions

PREG C

Contraindicated in hypersensitivity to cyclosporine, or with herpes zoster or recent exposure to chickenpox. **Use with caution** in kidney or liver disease.

Use with caution for children, pregnant or nursing mothers, and the elderly.

Side effects/Adverse reactions

Hypersensitivity: (with IV solution) wheezing, dyspnea, hypotension, anaphylaxis. **CNS:** headache, tremors (common, even on maintenance dose). **GI:** nausea, vomiting, stomatitis, oral thrush, gum hyperplasia, hepatotoxicity. **CV:** hypertension. **Hem:** hyperkalemia. **GU:** renal failure (from toxicity), albuminuria, proteinuria, hematuria. **Skin:** itching, rashes, hirsuitism (common, even on maintenance dose). **Misc:** increased susceptibility to infection (cytomegalovirus, herpes, Pneumocystis carini, Serratia, Cryptococcus, Legionella, and gram-negative bacteria).

Nursing implications/Documentation

Possible nursing diagnoses: Potential for infection; Altered oral mucous membrane.

♦ Be aware that cyclosporine should always be given concomitantly with corticosteroids; expect oral nystatin to be ordered to prevent thrush.

♦ Monitor cyclosporine levels closely (insufficient drug levels could result in rejection of transplanted organ; excessive amounts could result in nephrotoxicity).

♦ Monitor for and report abnormalities in kidney function studies (BUN and creatinine) and abnormalities in liver function studies (alkaline phosphatase, AST, ALT, SGOT, bilirubin).

♦ Monitor and document blood pressure, intake and output, and daily weights; report hypertension, positive balance, or weight gain.

♦ Monitor hemoglobin, WBC, and platelet count at least every month; hold drug and report if leukocytes are < 3000 mm^3.

♦ Avoid giving IM injections to reduce risk of infection (document on medication record).

♦ Report signs and symptoms of infection immediately; avoid assigning health care workers with respiratory symptoms.

♦ Provide frequent mouth care.

Patient & family teaching/Home care

Possible nursing diagnoses: Knowledge deficit; Impaired home maintenance management.

♦ Teach that meticulous oral hygiene can help reduce incidence of oral inflammation.

♦ Stress that cyclosporine should be taken exactly as prescribed: dose should be measured carefully and taken at the same time every day to maintain adequate blood levels and reduce the risk of organ rejection or nephrotoxicity.

♦ Point out the need to report signs and symptoms of infection early to ensure prompt treatment (explain that there is risk for opportunistic infections, such as herpes and cytomegalovirus).

- Warn women to use contraceptives during treatment, and for 12 weeks after completing therapy; if hirsuitism is bothersome, encourage use of a depilatory.

- *See Immunosuppressants overview for more information.*

cyclothiazide

sye-kloe-thye'a-zide

Anhydron, Fluidil

Class: Thiazide diuretic, Antihypertensive

PEDS	PREG	GERI
✋	**D**	✋

Action Increases excretion of sodium chloride, potassium, and water by inhibiting sodium reabsorption in the early portion of the distal tubule. Lowers blood pressure by reducing plasma and extra-cellular volume.

Use/Therapeutic goal/Outcome

Hypertension: Promotion of diuresis, reduction of blood pressure. **Outcome criteria:** Increased urinary output; after 3–4 days, blood pressure within normal limits.

Edema: Promotion of diuresis, resolution of edema. **Outcome criteria:** Increased urinary output; weight loss; absence of rales and peripheral and sacral edema.

Dose range/Administration

Interaction alert: Cholestyramine and colestipol decrease intestinal absorption. Diazoxide potentiates the hyperglycemic, hyperuricemic, and hypotensive effects. Do not give concomitantly with lithium. Give cautiously with corticosteroids, antidiabetics, lanoxin, and skeletal muscle relaxants. Nonsteroidal anti-inflammatory drugs may decrease effects.

🖐 **Administer with food to decrease GI upset.**

Hypertension: Adult: PO: 2 mg/day; may increase up to 2 mg bid or tid.

Edema: Adult: PO: 1–2 mg/day. *Maintenance dose:* 1–2 mg 2–3 times/week. **Child:** PO: 0.02–0.04 mg/kg/day.

Clinical alert: Give in morning to prevent nocturnal diuresis. Antihypertensive response may not occur for 3–4 days.

Contraindications/Precautions

PREG D

Contraindicated in hypersensitivity to sulfonamides or thiazides, and in anuria, hypokalemia, and renal decompensation. **Use with caution** in diabetes, gout, systemic lupus erythematosus, pancreatitis, arteriosclerosis, renal or hepatic disease, debilitated patients, and patients with allergies or bronchial asthma.

🖐 **Contraindicated for pregnant or nursing mothers. Use with caution for children and the elderly.**

Side effects/Adverse reactions

Hypersensitivity: rash, urticaria, dermatitis with photosensitivity, pneumonitis, vasculitis. **Hem:** hypokalemia, hyperglycemia, impaired glucose tolerance, azotemia, asymptomatic azotemia, electrolyte imbalances, metabolic alkalosis, hypercalcemia, lipid abnormalities, aplastic anemia, agranulocytosis, leukopenia, thrombocytopenia. **CV:** volume depletion, dehydration, orthostatic hypotension. **GI:** anorexia, nausea, pancreatitis, hepatic encephalopathy. **Misc:** gout.

Nursing implications/Documentation

Possible nursing diagnoses: Fluid volume deficit; Altered patterns of urinary elimination; Potential for injury.

- Ascertain that baseline CBC, sodium, potassium, chloride, carbon dioxide, calcium, magnesium, BUN, creatinine, uric acid, and liver function studies have been obtained before giving first dose; report abnormalities and monitor closely thereafter.

- Document and monitor blood pressure, pulse, daily weight, and intake and output; report significant discrepancies.

- Monitor for hyperglycemia and for weight gain, because of risk of thiazide diabetes.

- Observe for and report signs of fluid overload (auscultate lungs for rales; check feet, ankles, and sacrum for edema).

- Be aware that diuretics often induce hypokalemia, which predisposes individuals to cardiac arrhythmias, cramping, and digoxin toxicity.

- Check with physician to determine dietary restrictions; if a low-salt, high-potassium diet is recommended, consult with dietician to plan a low-salt diet that includes foods and juices high in potassium (orange juice; banana; green leafy vegetables).

- Observe the elderly for extreme diuresis (may require lower doses); monitor for orthostatic hypotension; supervise ambulation until response is determined.

▶

Patient & family teaching/Home care

Possible nursing diagnoses: Knowledge deficit; Impaired home maintenance management.

♦ Advise taking this drug with food to reduce GI symptoms.

♦ Before giving first dose, explain that the drug will increase the amount and frequency of urination.

♦ Emphasize the importance of taking this drug exactly as prescribed, and the importance of returning for medical follow-up.

♦ Explain that diuretics enhance the work of the kidney and reduce the workload of the heart.

♦ Recommend taking doses in early morning and early afternoon to prevent the need to disturb sleep to void.

♦ Explain that changing positions slowly helps prevent dizziness.

♦ Advise reporting dizziness, shortness of breath, swelling of hands and feet, or persistent sore throat; encourage daily monitoring of weight and reporting sudden weight gain.

♦ Warn that hyperglycemia is common; advise reporting thirst, fatigue, or weight loss.

♦ Provide a list of allowed foods and fluids; stress the need to stick to prescribed diet (explain the hazards of too much salt, or too little potassium).

♦ Warn against driving or activities that require alertness until response has been determined.

♦ Advise avoidance of OTC drugs unless approved by physician; stress need to wear a sunscreen.

♦ *See Diuretics and Antihypertensives overviews for more information.*

cyproheptadine
si-proe-hep'ta-deen

cyproheptadine hydrochloride: *Periactin*

Class: Antihistamine (H$_1$ receptor antagonist), Antipruritic, Serotonin antagonist

PEDS	PREG	GERI
☡	B	☡

Action Prevents but does not reverse histamine- and serotonin-mediated allergic responses by competing with histamine for H$_1$ receptors, and with serotonin for its receptors, on effector cells. Has anticholinergic action.

Use/Therapeutic goal/Outcome

Allergic conditions: Decrease in allergic response. **Outcome criteria:** Report and demonstration of decrease in allergic symptoms (sneezing, nasal secretions, itching).

Dose range/Administration

Interaction alert: CNS depressants and alcohol may cause excessive drowsiness. Do not give with MAOIs or anticholinergics.

🖐 **Give with food or milk to avoid GI upset.**

Adult/Child > 14 yrs: PO: 4 mg bid to tid, to a maximum of 0.5 mg/kg/day. Therapeutic dose range is 4–20 mg/day. **Child < 14 yrs:** PO: 0.25 mg/kg/day, divided into 2 or 3 equal doses. **Child 2–6 yrs:** Do not exceed 12 mg/day. **Child 7–14 yrs:** Do not exceed 16 mg/day.

Clinical alert: Expect reduced dosage for the elderly and monitor for increased drowsiness, dizziness.

Contraindications/Precautions
PREG B

Contraindicated in hypersensitivity to cyproheptadine or other antihistamines, in acute asthma, and with MAOI therapy, bladder-neck obstruction, symptomatic prostatic hypertrophy, stenosing peptic ulcer. **Use with caution** in urinary retention, history of asthma, hypertension, hyperthyroidism, increased intraocular pressure, and cardiovascular or kidney disease.

☝ **Contraindicated for premature infants, newborns, nursing mothers, and debilitated elderly. Use with caution for children and the healthy elderly. Safe use during pregnancy has not been established.**

Side effects/Adverse reactions

Hypersensitivity: skin rash, pruritis. **CNS:** drowsiness, dizziness, faintness, headache, agitation, confusion, ataxia, tremors (especially in children), insomnia, convulsions, hallucinations, hysteria. **Resp:** dry nose and throat, thickened bronchial secretions. **GU:** urinary frequency or retention, dysuria. **GI:** dry mouth, nausea, epigastric distress, anorexia, cholestatic jaundice (abdominal discomfort, dark urine, clay-colored stools, abnormal liver function tests).

Nursing implications/Documentation

Possible nursing diagnoses: Potential for injury; Fluid volume deficit.

- ◆ Determine and record known allergies; provide an environment that is free from allergens (especially sleeping areas).
- ◆ Provide favorite fluids and ensure adequate hydration (2 liters/day).

Patient & family teaching/Home care

Possible nursing diagnoses: Knowledge deficit; Impaired home maintenance management.

- ◆ Advise taking this drug with food or milk if GI symptoms are experienced.
- ◆ Point out that avoiding pollens and staying in an air-conditioned environment may help reduce seasonal rhinitis.
- ◆ Emphasize that dose should not be increased without physician's approval; explain that tolerance may occur, requiring a change in medication.
- ◆ Warn that alcohol and other CNS depressants may cause excessive drowsiness; advise against driving until response is determined.
- ◆ Suggest that coffee or tea may reduce drowsiness, and that sugarless gum or hard candy may relieve dry mouth.
- ◆ Explain that antihistamines should be stopped for 4 days before allergy testing to ensure accurate results.
- ◆ Warn parents that children may exhibit CNS side effects, such as agitation, tremors, or hallucinations (may require dose reduction; and should be reported).
- ◆ *See Antihistamines overview for more information.*

cytarabine
sye-tare'a-been

ara-C, cytosine arabinoside: **♠Alexan, Cytosar-U**

Class: Antineoplastic (antimetabolite) agent

PEDS	PREG	GERI
⍟	**D**	⍟

Action Kills rapidly growing cells (cancer, hair follicles, bone marrow, GI lining, ova, and sperm) by inhibiting DNA, RNA, and protein synthesis (pyrimidine antagonist). Drug is cell cycle specific in the S-phase.

Use/Therapeutic goal/Outcome

Acute and chronic myelogenous and lymphocytic leukemias, erythroleukemia, sarcomas, Hodgkin's disease, non-Hodgkin's lymphoma in children, and cancers of the head and neck (used mainly in combination therapy): Elimina-

tion or suppression of malignant cell proliferation. **Outcome criteria:** Tumor and disease regression or stabilization on radiologic and physical examination; for leukemias, absence of blasts in peripheral blood specimen.

Dose range/Administration

Interaction alert: Use with L-Asparaginase may cause acute pancreatitis. Nausea and vomiting may be severe if given with methotrexate. Radiation therapy or other cytotoxic agents may cause severe myelosuppression.

Adult and Child: IV: 200 mg/m²/day by continuous infusion for 5 days at 2-wk intervals, or 100 mg/m²/day for 10 days (induction / remission). IV, SC: 1 to 1.5 mg/kg q 1–4 wk (maintenance therapy). *Intrathecal:* 10–30 mg/m² q 4 days in 10 ml of preservative-free sterile saline.

Clinical alert: Dose may vary depending on concurrent therapies and clinical status. Follow protocol for drug preparation, administration, and accidental skin contamination. Use gloves or double gloves (check institution policy) when handling cytarabine (skin contact can cause a local reaction). Wash contaminated skin areas with large amounts of soap and water.

Contraindications/Precautions
PREG D

Contraindicated in hypersensitivity to cytarabine, and in preexisting renal or liver disease or preexisting drug- or radiation-induced bone marrow suppression. **Use with caution** in active infections, chronic debilitating disease, or decreased bone marrow reserve (myelosuppression can be fatal with preexisting disease complications).

⍟ **Contraindicated for pregnant or nursing mothers. Use with caution for children and the elderly.**

Side effects/Adverse reactions

Hypersensitivity: urticaria, eczema, bradycardia, anaphylaxis. **Hem:** hyperuricemia, anemia, thrombocytopenia, leukopenia, myelosuppression. **GI:** anorexia; nausea and vomiting (in 50% of patients), diarrhea and abdominal pain; hematemesis, GI hemorrhage, and oral inflammation/ulceration (in 5–10 days); mild hepatotoxicity. **Eye:** conjunctivitis. **GU:** urinary retention, renal failure. **CNS:** headache, dizziness, neuritis, ataxia. **Skin:** cellulitis; skin ulceration and peeling (if given with radiation); alopecia; pain and inflammation at injection site. **Resp:** dyspnea and pneumonia.

CV: chest pain; cardiopathy; thrombophlebitis at injection site. **Misc:** flulike syndrome and "cytarabine syndrome" (fever, myalgia, bone pain, rash, malaise, conjunctivitis) 6–12 hr after treatment.

Nursing implications/Documentation

Possible nursing diagnoses: Potential for infection; Potential for injury; Fatigue; Altered oral mucous membrane; Fluid volume deficit; Diarrhea; Altered nutrition: less than body requirements.

◆ *See important Nursing implications in Antineoplastic agents overview on page 72, which apply to all antineoplastics. The interventions that follow are additional and specific to this drug only.*

◆ Monitor for and report early signs of pulmonary toxicity (persistent cough, dyspnea, chest pain) or CNS toxicity (numbness or tingling of extremities, muscle weakness, balance problems).

◆ Increase fluid intake to 2–3 L a day to prevent renal tubular damage from hyperuricemia secondary to cell lysis.

◆ Observe for and report eye inflammation (may be treated with steroid eye drops).

◆ Expect WBC nadir (lowest point) at 1 week (then a brief rise until day 12, then a deeper nadir at days 15–24, then back to baseline 10 days later); platelet nadir is at 10 days, with recovery over the next 10 days.

Patient & family teaching/Home care

Possible nursing diagnoses: Knowledge deficit; Ineffective coping (individual and family); Hopelessness; Impaired home maintenance management.

◆ *See important Patient & family teaching in Antineoplastic agents overview on page 72, which apply to all antineoplastics. The teachings that follow are additional and specific to this drug only.*

◆ Point out that drinking 2–3 L a day helps prevent kidney complications.

◆ Teach the need to report persistent cough, dyspnea, chest pain, balance problems, muscle weakness, numbness or tingling of extremities.

◆ *See Antineoplastic agents overview for more information.*

dacarbazine

da-kar'ba-zeen

DTIC–Dome

Class: Antineoplastic (alkylating) agent

PEDS	PREG	GERI
🖐	C	🖐

Action Kills rapidly growing cells (cancer, hair follicles, bone marrow, GI lining, ova, and sperm) by interfering with DNA replication and RNA transcription by alkylation (crosslinking of DNA occurs). Is cell-cycle–phase nonspecific, affecting both actively dividing and dormant (resting) cells.

Use/Therapeutic goal/Outcome

Malignant melanoma, Hodgkin's disease, sarcomas, and neuroblastomas: Elimination or suppression of malignant cell proliferation. **Outcome criteria:** Tumor and disease regression or stabilization on radiologic and physical examination.

Dose range/Administration

Interaction alert: Phenytoin and phenobarbital decrease effectiveness. Radiation therapy or other cytotoxic agents can cause severe myelosuppression.

Malignant melanoma: Adult: IV: 2–4.5 mg/kg/day or 70–160 mg/m^2/day for 10 days, repeat q 4 wk; or 150–250 mg/m^2/day for 5 days q 3 wk.

Hodgkin's disease: Adult: IV: 150 mg/m^2/day for 5 days q 4 wk (with other agents); or 375 mg/m^2 once, repeated every 15 days (with other agents).

Clinical alert: This drug should be given only by nurses who are knowledgeable in the comprehensive management of the administration of antineoplastic agents. Doses may vary at physician's discretion and are held until the patient has sufficiently recovered from toxicities of previous doses. Protocols for drug preparation, administration, and accidental skin contamination must be followed. Gloves or double gloves must be worn when handling dacarbazine (skin contamination may cause a local reaction). Contaminated areas should be washed with large amounts of soap and water. Dacarbazine is given via bolus over 1 min or diluted in 50–100 ml D5W over 15–30 min. This drug is a vesicant: Careful assessment of the IV is necessary to prevent extravasation. If extravasation is suspected, the IV should be stopped immediately, the physician notified, and protocols for treatment followed.

Contraindications/Precautions

Contraindicated in hypersensitivity to dacarbazine and in severe leukopenia and thrombocytopenia (hematologic toxicity is cumulative). **Use with caution** in infection and renal or hepatic failure.

✋ **Contraindicated for nursing mothers. Use with caution for pregnant women and the elderly. Safe use for children has not been established.**

Side effects/Adverse reactions

Hypersensitivity: urticaria, hypotension, anaphylaxis. **Hem:** delayed and cumulative myelosuppression 2–4 weeks after last dose (leukopenia, thrombocytopenia, and anemia). **GI:** moderate to severe nausea and vomiting 1–3 hr after dosage (may last 12 hr) in over 90 percent of people; hepatotoxicity. **Skin:** dermatitis; photosensitivity; alopecia; severe pain and burning at injection site. **Eye:** photosensitivity and blurred vision. **Misc:** flulike syndrome (myalgias, headache, sinus congestion, malaise) beginning 1 week after treatment and lasting up to 3 weeks.

Nursing implications/Documentation

Possible nursing diagnoses: Potential for infection; Potential for injury; Fatigue; Altered oral mucous membrane; Fluid volume deficit; Diarrhea; Altered nutrition: less than body requirements.

◆ *See important Nursing implications in Antineoplastic agents overview on page 72, which apply to all antineoplastics. The interventions that follow are additional and specific to this drug only.*

  ◆ Limit PO fluids and food several hours before treatment.

  ◆ Expect that WBC, platelet, and erythrocyte counts will drop to the nadir (lowest point) in 16 days and recover 3–5 days after.

  ◆ Consult for use of antipyretics and mild analgesics for flulike symptoms (usually noted 7 days after treatment is stopped, and may last up to 21 days).

  ◆ Be aware that therapeutic response is often accompanied by toxicity.

Patient & family teaching/Home care

Possible nursing diagnoses: Knowledge deficit; Ineffective coping (individual and family); Hopelessness; Impaired home maintenance management.

◆ *See important Patient & family teaching in Antineoplastic agents overview on page 72, which apply to all antineoplastics. The teachings that follow are additional and specific to this drug only.*

  ◆ Advise that nausea may subside after several doses.

  ◆ Explain the need to avoid sunlight for 48 hr after treatment.

◆ *See Antineoplastic agents overview for more information.*

dactinomycin
dak-ti-noe-mye'sin

actinomycin D: **Cosmegen**

Class: Antineoplastic (antibiotic) agent

PEDS	PREG	GERI
✋	C	✋

Action Kills rapidly growing cells (cancer, hair follicles, bone marrow, GI lining, ova, and sperm) by interfering with the synthesis of DNA, RNA, and protein, causing disruption of nucleic acid function. Is cell-cycle–phase nonspecific.

Use/Therapeutic goal/Outcome

Wilms' Tumor, rhabdomyosarcoma, Ewing's sarcoma, choriocarcinoma, testicular cancer, and Kaposi's sarcoma, mainly in combination chemotherapy in conjunction with surgery/radiation: Elimination or suppression of malignant cell proliferation. **Outcome criteria:** Tumor and disease regression or stabilization on radiologic and physical examination.

Dose range/Administration

Interaction alert: If used with radiation, expect reduced dosage; may cause "radiation recall" skin reactions. Methotrexate and chlorambucil can cause severe hematological toxicities.

Adult: IV: 500 mcg/day for 5 days (do not exceed 15 mg/kg/day); wait for bone marrow recovery, then repeat every q 2–4 wk. *Alternate dose:* 2 mg as a single dose; wait for bone marrow recovery and then repeat dose q 3–4 wk. **Child > 6 mos:** IV: 15 mcg/kg/day for 5 days; wait for bone marrow recovery, then repeat q 2–4 wk.

Clinical alert: This drug should be given only by nurses who are knowledgeable in the comprehensive management of the administration of antineoplastic agents. Dose may vary at physician's discretion. Repeat doses are held until it is ascertained that the patient has recovered sufficiently from toxicities of previous doses. Established protocols/policies for drug preparation, administration, and accidental skin contamination *must be followed closely* (gloves or double gloves are worn when handling drug; if the drug touches the skin, the area is washed immediately with plenty of soap and water). Dactinomycin is given *slowly* over at least 1 min or in 50–100 ml fluid to minimize inflammation and pain along the vein. This drug is a *potent* vesicant (can cause severe damage to tissues). *Prevention* of extravasation is essential. The drug is given by administering only when it is clear that the needle is in the vein (good blood return), and the infusion site is monitored *closely* for early signs of extravasation (pain and swelling at infusion site). If extravasation is suspected, the infusion is stopped *immediately,* the physician is notified, and protocols and policies for treatment are followed.

Contraindications/Precautions

PREG C

Contraindicated in hypersensitivity to dactinomycin, severe myelosuppression, impaired renal or hepatic function, or concurrent infection with chickenpox or herpes zoster. **Use with caution** in impaired bone marrow function, chronic debilitating disease, active infections, and previous radiation treatment.

☝ **Contraindicated for infants under 6 months and pregnant or nursing mothers. Use with caution for older children and the elderly.**

Side effects/Adverse reactions

Hypersensitivity: rash, fever, tachycardia, hypotension, and anaphylaxis. **Skin:** alopecia; erythema; hyperpigmentation (especially in previously irradiated areas); vesiculation; pain and erythema at injection site; cellulitis; ulceration and sloughing if extravasation occurs (drug is extremely damaging to soft tissues). **Hem:** anemia, leukopenia, thrombocytopenia, myelosuppression, hypocalcemia. **GI:** anorexia; nausea and vomiting (may be severe, lasting up to 20 hr); stomatitis; dysphagia; oral ulcerations; abdominal pain; diarrhea; hepatotoxicity. **CNS:** malaise, fatigue, lethargy, fever.

Nursing implications/Documentation

Possible nursing diagnoses: Potential for infection; Potential for injury; Fatigue; Altered oral mucous membrane; Fluid volume deficit; Diarrhea; Altered nutrition: less than body requirements.

◆ *See important Nursing implications in Antineoplastic agents overview on page 72, which apply to all antineoplastics. The interventions that follow are additional and specific to this drug only.*

  ◆ Report stomatitis or persistent diarrhea (may require dose adjustment).

  ◆ Document and monitor intake and output to detect dehydration; maintain fluid intake of 2–3 L per day, and report significant positive or negative balance.

Patient & family teaching/Home care

Possible nursing diagnoses: Knowledge deficit; Ineffective coping (individual and family); Hopelessness; Impaired home maintenance management.

◆ *See important Patient & family teaching in Antineoplastic agents overview on page 72, which apply to all antineoplastics. The teachings that follow are additional and specific to this drug only.*

  ◆ Stress that oral ulcers or persistent diarrhea should be reported.

◆ *See Antineoplastics overview for more information.*

danazol

da'na-zole

♣*Cyclomen, Danocrine*

Class: Synthetic androgen, Gonadotropin inhibitor, Angioedema prophylactic

PEDS	PREG	GERI
☝	C	☝

Action Produces amenorrhea/anovulation and atrophy of endometrial tissue by inhibiting release of follicle-stimulating hormone (FSH) and luteinizing hormone (LH) by pituitary gland; reduces stimulation of breast tissue by decreasing ovarian production of estrogen; increases serum levels of complement system components.

Use/Therapeutic goal/Outcome

Endometriosis: Involution of ectopic endometrial tissue. **Outcome criteria:** Amenorrhea, report of pain relief, resolution of endometrial lesions as seen by laparoscopy.

Fibrocystic breast disease: Suppression of hormonal stimulation of breast tissue. **Outcome**

criteria: Relief of pain and tenderness after 2–3 months; decreased nodularity after 4–6 months.

Hereditary angioedema: Prophylaxis. *Outcome criteria:* Decreased frequency or severity of episodes of cutaneous, abdominal, and laryngeal edema.

Dose range/Administration

Interaction alert: Increases effect of oral anticoagulants; decreases response to oral hypoglycemics and insulin; cyclosporine increases risk of nephrotoxicity.

🖐 **Give with food or milk to minimize GI symptoms.**
Endometriosis: Adult: PO: 100–400 mg bid for 3–9 mos.
Fibrocystic breast disease: Adult: PO: 50–200 mg bid for 2–6 mos.
Hereditary angioedema: Adult: PO: 200 mg bid or tid, then titrate to lowest effective dose.

Clinical alert: For endometriosis and fibrocystic breast disease, administration of danazol should begin on day 1 of menstruation or with negative result of pregnancy test. Pediatric dosage has not been established.

Contraindications/Precautions

PREG C

Contraindicated in hypersensitivity to danazol, lactose, or parabens preservative. *Use with caution* in severe cardiac, hepatic, or renal impairment; epilepsy; migraine headaches; diabetes mellitus; undiagnosed abnormal vaginal bleeding; in fibrocystic breast disease, rule out breast cancer before beginning danazol.

✋ **Contraindicated for pregnant or nursing mothers. Use with caution for children and the elderly.**

Side effects/Adverse reactions

Hypersensitivity: rashes, nasal congestion. *GU:* amenorrhea; anovulation; breakthrough bleeding; spotting; decreased breast size; irregular menstrual periods; vaginal burning, dryness, or itching; clitoral hypertrophy; testicular atrophy; blood in urine. *Skin:* acne, oily skin or hair, hirsutism. *CNS:* dizziness, headaches, nervousness, emotional lability, tremors, paresthesias. *Eye:* blurring or loss of vision, cataracts. *CV:* increased blood pressure. *Hem:* thrombocytopenia. *GI:* nausea, vomiting, diarrhea, jaundice. *MS:* muscle cramps or spasms, carpal tunnel syndrome, premature epiphyseal closure in children. *Skin:* edema. *Misc:* deep-

ening of voice, weight gain, androgenic effects on female fetus.

Nursing implications/Documentation

Possible nursing diagnoses: Body image disturbance; Fluid volume excess.

♦ Obtain negative results of pregnancy test before administering danazol, unless therapy begins during menstruation.

♦ Record baseline blood pressure and weight.

♦ Assess for and report edema, increased blood pressure, weight gain, and congestive failure.

♦ Monitor results of liver function tests.

♦ For diabetics, monitor glucose levels closely for hyperglycemia.

Patient & family teaching/Home care

Possible nursing diagnoses: Knowledge deficit; Impaired home maintenance management; Sexual dysfunction.

♦ Stress the need to continue taking danazol as prescribed for full time of therapy.

♦ Caution women to use reliable nonhormonal birth control measures and to stop drug and report immediately if pregnancy is suspected.

♦ For women, stress the importance of reporting occurrence of masculinizing effects (abnormal growth of facial hair, deepening of voice, enlarged clitoris); androgenic effects may not be reversible.

♦ For treatment of endometriosis, advise that normal menstrual cycles will not occur, but that ovulation and cyclic bleeding will return within 2–3 months after danazol is discontinued.

♦ For treatment of fibrocystic breast disease, advise that menstrual cycles may become irregular or stop, but that normal cycles should return after danazol is discontinued.

♦ For fibrocystic breast disease, teach breast self-exam (BSE) and stress the need to report any new nodules, or enlargement or hardening of existing nodules.

♦ For diabetics, caution about possible elevation of blood sugar levels and need for adjustment of doses of hypoglycemics.

♦ For adolescent males, advise that periodic evaluation of semen volume, sperm count, and motility are necessary.

♦ Point out the need to maintain close medical supervision for early detection of adverse reactions.

D

dantrolene

dan'troe-leen

dantrolene sodium: ***Dantrium, Dantrium Intravenous***

Class: Skeletal-muscle relaxant (centrally acting), Antispasmodic

PEDS	PREG	GERI
🤚	C	🤚

Action Decreases force of muscle contraction and reduces hyperreflexia, spasticity, involuntary movements, and clonus by inhibiting Ca^{++} ion release from sarcoplasmic reticulum, preventing contraction of skeletal muscle.

Use/Therapeutic goal/Outcome

Chronic spasticity secondary to upper motor neuron disorders (cerebral palsy, spinal cord injury, stroke (CVA) and multiple sclerosis): Control of spasticity; relief of pain. ***Outcome criteria:*** Observable decrease in muscle spasticity; self-report of increased comfort.

Malignant hyperthermia: Prevention of hypermetabolism of skeletal muscle. ***Outcome criteria:*** Absence of signs of malignant hyperthermia (fever, muscle rigidity, and cardiac dysrhythmias).

Exercise-induced muscle pain (investigational use): Relief of pain. ***Outcome criteria:*** Report of relief of pain.

Dose range/Administration

Interaction alert: The CNS effects may be additive to those of tranquilizers and alcohol.

🥄 **Give with food to prevent gastric distress.**
Chronic spasticity: Adult: PO: *Initial dose:* 25 mg/day, then increase gradually by 25 mg q 4–7 days until maximum effect achieved. *Maximum dose:* 100 mg bid to qid (400 mg/day).
Child > 5 yrs: PO: *Initial dose:* 0.5 mg/kg bid, then increase by 0.5 mg/kg q 4–7 days prn. *Maximum dose:* 3 mg/kg bid to qid (100 mg/day).

Malignant hyperthermia: Adult and Child: PO: *To prevent recurrence:* 4–8 mg/kg/day in divided doses for 1–3 days. *Preoperative:* 4–8 mg/kg/day in divided doses for 1–2 days. IV: 1 mg/kg push, repeat prn to cumulative dose of 10 mg/kg.

Clinical alert: Use IV solution within 6 hours; avoid extravasation because this solution is extremely irritating.

Contraindications/Precautions

Contraindicated in hypersensitivity to dantrolene, and in hepatitis or cirrhosis. ***Use with caution*** when spasticity is used to maintain motor function, in severely impaired cardiac function, and in women over 35 years receiving estrogen therapy.

🤚 **Use with caution for children over 5 years and the elderly. Safe use for children under 5 years and pregnant or nursing mothers has not been determined.**

Side effects/Adverse reactions

Untoward reactions are related to oral therapy. No reactions have been reported in short-term IV therapy. ***Hypersensitivity:*** pruritus, urticaria, eczema, rash, photosensitivity, pleural effusion with pericarditis. ***CNS:*** drowsiness, dizziness, headache, nervousness, confusion, sweating, chills, fever. ***MS:*** weakness, fatigue. ***Resp:*** respiratory depression. ***GI:*** constipation, diarrhea, hepatitis, gastric distress, anorexia. ***CV:*** tachycardia. ***Eye:*** visual disturbances. ***GU:*** urinary frequency, impotence.

Nursing implications/Documentation

Possible nursing diagnoses: Impaired physical mobility; Potential for injury; Pain.

♦ Explain the need to take doses with food to reduce GI symptoms.

♦ Supervise out-of-bed activities, especially if weakness or drowsiness are present.

♦ Monitor bowel function; report severe diarrhea as drug may need to be discontinued. Long-term use may cause severe constipation and bowel obstruction.

♦ Observe for signs of hepatitis or hepatotoxicity (dark urine, jaundice, fever).

Patient & family teaching/Home care

Possible nursing diagnoses: Knowledge deficit; Impaired home maintenance management.

♦ Stress that taking doses with food will reduce GI symptoms.

♦ Warn against operating machinery, driving, or taking alcohol or other CNS depressants, especially if drowsiness or dizziness is present (early therapy response should be determined).

♦ Teach to avoid OTC drugs without physician approval.

♦ Provide a list of things that should be reported to the physician: signs of hepatitis (yellow skin or eyes, dark urine, clay-colored stools); itching; abdominal discomfort; side effects such as diarrhea, vision changes, or skin eruptions; return of spasticity.

♦ With malignant hyperthermia, stress that a medical alert bracelet should be worn.

♦ *See Skeletal-muscle relaxants overview for more information.*

daunorubicin
daw-noe-roo'bi-sin

daunorubicin hydrochloride (DNR): ♠*Cerubidin, Cerubidine*

Class: Antineoplastic (antibiotic) agent

PEDS	PREG	GERI
🖑	**D**	🖐

Action Kills rapidly growing cells (cancer, hair follicles, bone marrow, GI lining, ova, and sperm) by interfering with the synthesis of DNA, RNA, and protein, causing disruption of nucleic acid function. Is cell-cycle specific for the S-phase.

Use/Therapeutic goal/Outcome

Acute nonlymphocytic leukemia in adults (myelogenous, erythroid, nomocytic), non-Hodgkin's lymphomas, and acute lymphocytic leukemia in children: Suppression of malignant cell proliferation. *Outcome criteria:* Tumor/disease regression or stabilization on radiologic and physical examination; for leukemias, absence of blasts in peripheral blood specimen.

Dose range/Administration

Interaction alert: Radiation therapy or other antineoplastic agents may cause increased toxicity (expect decreased dosage). Combined cumulative dose of daunorubicin and adriamycin should not exceed 550 mg/m² (400 mg/m² if patient has been radiated near the heart or is taking cyclophosphamide, a cardiotoxic agent). Do not mix IV with any other drug.

Adult: IV: *As a single agent:* 60 mg/m²/day for 3 days q 3–4 wk. *In combination:* 45 mg/m²/day for 3 days, then for 2 days with cytosine arabinoside infusions. *Child > 2 yr:* IV: 25 mg/m²/wk with vincristine and oral prednisone.

Clinical alert: This drug should be given only by nurses who are knowledgeable in the comprehensive management of the administration of antineoplastic agents. Doses may vary at physician's discretion. Repeat doses are held until it is ascertained that the patient has recovered sufficiently from toxicities of previous doses. Established protocols/policies for drug preparation, administration, and accidental skin con-

tamination *must be followed closely* (gloves or double gloves are worn when handling drug; if the drug touches the skin, the area is washed immediately with plenty of soap and water). Daunorubicin is given *slowly* over 1–3 min or diluted to minimize inflammation and pain along the vein. This drug is a *potent* vesicant (can cause severe damage to tissues). *Prevention* of extravasation is essential. The drug is given by administering only when it is clear that the needle is in the vein (good blood return), and the infusion site is monitored *closely* for early signs of extravasation (pain and swelling at infusion site). If extravasation is suspected, the infusion is stopped *immediately,* the physician is notified, and protocols/policies for treatment are followed.

Contraindications/Precautions
PREG
D

Contraindicated in hypersensitivity to daunorubicin, and in the presence of cardiac disease, myelosuppression, and severe systemic infection. *Use with caution* in liver/kidney dysfunction, history of urate calculi or gout, those who have recently received myelosuppressive cytotoxic agents, cardiotoxic drugs, or previous radiation to the cardiac area.

🖑 **Contraindicated for infants under two years and pregnant or nursing mothers. Use with caution for older children and the elderly.**

Side effects/Adverse reactions

Hypersensitivity: fever, chills, rash. *Hem:* myelosuppression (leukopenia, anemia, thrombocytopenia), hyperuricemia. *CV:* cardiomyopathy (irreversible and potentially fatal CHF with cumulative doses> 550 mg/m² for adults, 300 mg/m² for children > 2 yr, and 10 mg/kg for children < 2 yr), pericarditis, myocarditis, dysrhythmias, transient EKG changes. *GI:* nausea, vomiting, anorexia, diarrhea, abdominal pain, stomatitis, esophagitis, hepatotoxicity. *GU:* hyperuricemia, transient red-colored urine, nephrotoxicity, gonadal suppression. *Skin:* alopecia; pain and erythema at injection site; cellulitis; ulceration and sloughing if extravasation occurs.

Nursing implications/Documentation

Possible nursing diagnoses: Potential for infection; Potential for injury; Fatigue; Altered oral mucous membrane; Fluid volume deficit; Diarrhea; Altered nutrition: less than body requirements.

♦ See important Nursing implications in *Antineoplastic agents overview* on page 72, which apply to all antineoplastics. The interventions that follow are additional and specific to this drug only.

◆ Record and monitor bilirubin and creatinine closely (dose adjustments are made for increased levels).

◆ Observe for and report early signs of cardiac toxicity (resting pulse > 100, difficulty breathing); stop drug and report immediately if these are noted.

◆ Expect WBC, platelet, and erythrocyte counts to drop to the nadir (lowest point) at 10–14 days with recovery in about 3 weeks.

Patient & family teaching/Home care

Possible nursing diagnoses: Knowledge deficit; Ineffective coping (individual and family); Hopelessness; Impaired home maintenance management.

♦ See important Patient & family teaching in *Antineoplastic agents overview* on page 72, which apply to all neoplastics. The teachings that follow are additional and specific to this drug only.

◆ Stress that difficulty breathing, rapid pulse, or swelling of the ankles and feet should be reported immediately; they may require treatment.

◆ Warn that urine may have a reddish color for several days after treatment (stress that this is not blood).

◆ Explain that although nausea and vomiting may be severe, it should subside within 24–48 hr.

♦ See Antineoplastic agents overview for more information.

demeclocycline

dem-e-kloe-sye'kleen

demeclocycline hydrochloride: *Declomycin,* ♠*Ledermycin*

Class: Anti-infective, Broad-spectrum tetracycline antibiotic

PEDS	PREG	GERI
✋	D	✋

Action Limits bacterial growth (bateriostatic) by binding to the 30S ribosomal subunit and inhibiting protein synthesis. Promotes diuresis by inhibiting ADH-induced water reabsorption in the renal distal convoluted tubules and collecting tubules.

Use/Therapeutic goal/Outcome

Infections (caused by susceptible gram-negative and gram-positive pathogens, trachoma, rickettsia): Resolution of infection. ***Outcome criteria:*** Absence of pathogenic growth on cultures, absence of clinical manifestations of infection (fever, pain, swelling, redness, heat, odor, drainage, productive cough, dysuria, frequency), normal WBC count, normal X rays.

Syndrome of inappropriate antidiuretic hormone (SIADH): Inhibition of excessive antidiuretic hormone. ***Outcome criteria:*** Serum sodium within normal limits.

Dose range/Administration

Interaction alert: To prevent interference with antibiotic absorption, give 1 hour before or 2 hours after food, milk or other dairy products, antacids (including sodium bicarbonate), or laxatives containing aluminum, magnesium, or calcium. *Decreases* effects of penicillin and *increases* effect of anticoagulants. Give 2 hours before or 3 hours after iron products or zinc. Methoxyflurane increases risk of nephrotoxicity. May decrease effectiveness of oral contraceptives and increase breakthrough bleeding.

🥄 **Give with a full glass of water on an empty stomach 1 hour before or 2 hours after meals for best absorption.**

Infections (caused by susceptible gram-negative and gram-positive pathogens, trachoma, rickettsia): **Adult:** PO: 150 mg q6h, or 300 mg q12h. **Child > 8 yrs:** PO: 6–12 mg/kg/day in divided doses q6-12h.

Gonorrhea: **Adult:** PO: 600 mg initially, then 300 mg q12h for 4 days (total of 3 g).

Uncomplicated endocervical, urethral, or rectal infections: **Adult:** PO: 300 mg qid for at least 7 days.

SIADH: **Adult:** PO: 600–1200 mg/day in divided doses.

Clinical alert: Prevent esophageal irritation by giving doses with a full glass of water and having the patient remain in a vertical position for at least 90 seconds after swallowing demeclocycline. To prevent esophagitis, avoid giving demeclocycline within 1 hour of bedtime. Recognize that taking outdated tetracyclines has been associated with fatal nephrotoxicity.

Contraindications/Precautions

PREG
D

Contraindicated in allergy to demeclocycline or other tetracycline antibiotics, and in cirrhosis, common bile duct obstruction, and immunosuppression; contraindicated in esophageal obstruction. **Use with caution** in diabetes insipidus and impaired renal or liver function.

ξ **Contraindicated for children under 8 years (causes tooth discoloration and retards bone growth) and pregnant or nursing mothers. Use with caution for the elderly.**

Side effects/Adverse reactions

Hypersensitivity: (rare) itching, rashes, fever, anaphylaxis. **GI:** sore throat, dysphagia, glossitis, stomatitis, epigastric discomfort, nausea, cramps, diarrhea, enterocolitis, anogenital inflammation, abdominal pain. **CNS:** dizziness, lightheadedness, headache, intracranial hypertension. **CV:** pericarditis. **Hem:** blood dyscrasias. **Skin:** photosensitivity. **Misc:** diabetes insipidus syndrome (weakness, polyuria, polydipsia).

Nursing implications/Documentation

Possible nursing diagnoses: Potential for infection; Potential fluid volume deficit.

♦ Determine history of allergies, and (regardless of history) monitor closely for allergic reactions.

♦ Weigh patient and obtain baseline CBC, BUN, creatinine, liver function studies, and necessary culture specimens before administering first dose; monitor closely thereafter if therapy is prolonged.

♦ Encourage fluids, and record and monitor intake and output, to ensure adequate hydration and urine output.

♦ Monitor for and report symptoms of superinfection (mouth lesions, thrush, vaginal irritation, diarrhea, respiratory symptoms).

♦ If there is no improvement within 3–5 days, consult with physician to determine if antibiotic regimen should be re-evaluated (and new cultures drawn).

Patient & family teaching/Home care

Possible nursing diagnoses: Knowledge deficit, Impaired home maintenance management.

♦ Advise taking demeclocycline on an empty stomach with a full glass of water 1 hour before or 2 hours after milk or food, and avoiding taking it within 1 hour of bedtime or within 1–2 hours of taking antacids.

♦ Stress the need to avoid iron-containing products; point out that this drug decreases effects of oral contraceptives.

♦ Advise avoiding exposure to sunlight and warn that photosensitivity may continue for

weeks after demeclocycline has been discontinued.

♦ Teach the importance of reporting persistent or new symptoms of illness (e.g., fever, mouth lesions, vaginal irritation, respiratory symptoms, diarrhea); medication change may be necessary.

♦ Explain the need to take antibiotics for the entire time prescribed, even if symptoms abate.

♦ *See Anti-infectives overview for more information.*

desipramine

dess-ip'ra-meen

desipramine hydrochloride: **Norpramin, Pertofrane, ♠Pertofran**

Class: Tricyclic antidepressant (TCA)

PEDS	PREG	GERI
ξ	C	ξ

Action Improves mood by increasing levels of the neurotransmitter norepinephrine in the CNS. (Blocks neurotransmitter reuptake into presynaptic neurons by inhibiting the "amine pump." Reuptake normally terminates the action of neurotransmitters.) Has less anticholinergic, cardiovascular, and sedating effects than imipramine.

Use/Therapeutic goal/Outcome

Major depressive disorders: Promotion of sense of well-being, ability to cope with daily living. **Outcome criteria:** Patient report of feeling less depressed, more energetic and able to cope; return of normal sleeping and eating habits; demonstration of improved ability to problem solve and perform activities of daily living.

Dose range/Administration

Interaction alert: Barbiturates may reduce antidepressant blood levels and effects. Cimetidine and methylpenidate may increase levels. If given with epinephrine and norepinephrine, monitor for increased risk of hypertension. Avoid use with MAOIs (risk of excitation, hyperpyrexia, and seizures). Give cautiously with thyroid drugs because it may increase CNS stimulation and cardiac arrythmias.

ϸ **Give with (or immediately after) food to reduce GI symptoms.**

Adult: PO: Begin with 75–100 mg/day in divided doses, may gradually increase to a maximum of 300 mg/day. Once stabilized give entire dose at hs. *For the elderly:* Begin with 25–50 mg/day in divided doses, may increase

▶

desipramine   275

gradually to a maximum of 150 mg/day.
Child > 12 yrs: PO: Use elderly dose.

Clinical alert: This drug contains tartrazine (FD&C Yellow No. 5), which has caused allergic responses in some patients.

Contraindications/Precautions

PREG
C

Contraindicated in hypersensitivity to TCAs, for concomitant use with electroconvulsive therapy, in elective surgery, and acute recovery period of myocardial infarction. ***Use with caution*** in renal or hepatic disease, hyperthyroidism, glaucoma, prostatic hypertrophy, urinary retention, hypomania, mania, and suicidal tendency.

Contraindicated for children under 6 years and pregnant or nursing mothers. Use with caution for adolescents and the elderly or debilitated.

Side effects/Adverse reactions

Hypersensitivity: rash, sensitivity to sunlight. ***CNS:*** drowsiness, dizziness, anxiety, headache, fatigue, agitation, extrapyramidal symptoms, sedation (especially the elderly). ***CV:*** orthostatic hypotension, palpitations, tachycardia, EKG changes, hypertension. ***GI:*** anorexia, dry mouth, nausea, vomiting, constipation, paralytic ileus. ***GU:*** urinary retention, decreased libido. ***Eye:*** blurred vision. ***Ear:*** tinnitus. ***Hem:*** agranulocytosis.

Nursing implications/Documentation

Possible nursing diagnoses: Potential for injury; Constipation; Altered oral mucous membrane.

◆ Document mental status and vital signs at least bid until response to therapy has been established.

◆ Be sure that doses are swallowed (not hoarded).

◆ Monitor for orthostatic hypotension, dizziness, and drowsiness; supervise ambulation until response is established.

◆ Record intake and output, and observe for dehydration or urinary retention; provide special mouth care.

◆ Monitor for and report suicidal tendencies, increased depression, or excessive drowsiness (may require change in medication).

◆ Prevent constipation by monitoring bowel movements and encouraging adequate fiber and fluid intake; offer laxatives or stool softeners before the problem becomes severe.

Patient & family teaching/Home care

Possible nursing diagnoses: Ineffective coping (family and individual); Sleep pattern disturbance; Impaired home maintenance management.

◆ Stress that this medication helps reduce the depression that inhibits ability to make decisions and cope effectively (once the individual feels less depressed, it will be easier to take steps toward making healthy changes).

◆ Explain that side effects are often noted immediately, but they usually diminish after a few weeks; on the other hand, it is likely to take 2–4 weeks before *beneficial* effects are noted (the patient may feel worse before feeling better).

◆ Warn to change positions slowly to prevent dizziness.

◆ Point out the role of adequate nutrition, exercise, and sleep in combating depression.

◆ Emphasize that the effects of alcohol, sedatives, and tranquilizers may be potentiated.

◆ Caution to consult with physician before using OTC drugs; stress the need for ongoing medical follow-up.

◆ Recommend reporting continued depression; stress that doses should not be increased or stopped without checking with physician because this may cause severe problems.

◆ Advise avoidance of driving and other potentially hazardous activities until response is established.

◆ Suggest using ice chips, hard candy, or gum to relieve side effect of dry mouth; stress the need for good mouth care.

◆ Warn women to report immediately if pregnancy is planned or suspected.

◆ *See Antidepressants overview for more information.*

desmopressin

des-moe-press'in

DDAVP, ♠Minirin, Stimate

Class: Posterior pituitary hormone, Antidiuretic hormone, Hemostatic

PEDS	PREG	GERI
🖐	B	🖐

Action Decreases urine output by increasing water reabsorption in kidneys; controls bleeding by releasing endogenous factor VIII from plasma storage sites and increasing clotting activity.

Use/Therapeutic goal/Outcome

Neurogenic diabetes insipidus: Prevention or control of dehydration. **Outcome criteria:** Reduction in volume and frequency of urination, especially during sleeping hours; decreased thirst; increased urine osmolality and specific gravity.

Hemophilia A, von Willebrand's disease: Prevention or control of spontaneous, trauma-related, or surgical bleeding. **Outcome criteria:** Improved factor VIII levels and partial thromboplastin times (PTT); absence of evidence of bleeding.

Nocturnal enuresis: Prevention of bed-wetting. **Outcome criteria:** Absence or decrease in bed-wetting.

Dose range/Administration

Interaction alert: Demeclocycline, lithium, or norepinephrine may *decrease* antidiuretic effect; carbamazepine, chlorpropamide, or clofibrate may *increase* antidiuretic effect.

Antidiuretic: Adult: *Intranasal:* 10 mcg hs, increase 2.5 mcg/night until satisfactory sleep obtained; 10 mcg qAM if required to keep urine output < 2 L/day. IV, SC: 2–4 mcg/day, in divided doses qAM and qhs. **Child:** *Intranasal:* 5 mcg hs, increase 2.5 mcg/night until satisfactory sleep obtained; 5 mcg qAM if required to keep urine output < 1.5–2 L/day.

Antihemorrhagic: Adult and Child: IV: 0.3 mcg/kg, diluted in NSS over 15–30 min.

Nocturnal enuresis: Child: Intranasal: 10 mcg in each nostril hs; adjust according to response. *Maximum dose:* 40 mcg.

Clinical alert: Separate intravenous doses by 24–48 hr to avoid decreased response. Single doses of desmopressin may be infused 30 min before cardiac surgery to reduce blood loss.

Contraindications/Precautions

PREG
B

Contraindicated in hypersensitivity to desmopressin, and in nephrogencic diabetes insipidus; and intranasal route in upper respiratory infections, nasal congestion, or allergic rhinitis. **Use with caution** in hypertension and coronary artery disease.

Contraindicated for children under 3 months and nursing mothers. Use with caution for other young children, pregnant women, and the elderly.

Side effects/Adverse reactions

Hypersensitivity: bronchoconstriction, dyspnea, anaphylaxis. **CV:** elevated blood pressure; hypotension with rapid intravenous infusion. **CNS:** headache. **Resp:** runny or stuffy nose. **GI:** nausea, abdominal cramps. **GU:** pain in vulva. **Skin:** flushing; pain, redness, or swelling at injection site. **Misc:** water intoxication, hyponatremia.

Nursing implications/Documentation

Possible nursing diagnoses: Fluid volume excess; Fluid volume deficit; Pain; Impaired tissue integrity.

♦ For nocturia, administer single daily dose at bedtime.

♦ For intranasal solution, use special catheter supplied to measure dose; insert tip of catheter into nose and assist patient to blow on other end to deliver dose deep into nasal cavity; air-filled syringe may be used to deliver dose to small children or unconscious patients.

♦ With intranasal metered spray container, do not use beyond the labeled number of sprays.

♦ With IV administration, run infusion slowly over 15–30 min; monitor blood pressure during infusion.

♦ Assess injection site for redness, pain, or swelling.

♦ Record intake and output; assess for return of polyuria and nocturia, which may indicate need for more frequent administration.

♦ Record blood pressure twice daily and weight daily.

♦ Adjust fluid intake to decrease potential for water intoxication and hyponatremia; assess for signs of these side effects (headache, drowsiness, listlessness, or confusion).

♦ Be aware that children and the elderly are at greater risk for water intoxication and hyponatremia.

Patient & family teaching/Home care

Possible nursing diagnoses: Knowledge deficit; Impaired home maintenance management.

♦ Stress the importance of not using more medication than the prescribed amount.

♦ Teach intranasal administration technique, provide package insert with complete instructions, and observe return demonstration.

♦ Caution that nasal congestion may decrease absorption of drug and increase urine output;

point out that this should be reported so dose can be adjusted.

♦ Advise that tolerance may develop with long-term use, and response may decrease.

♦ Teach to measure and record fluid intake and output to identify increased or decreased response to drug; significant discrepancies in fluid balance should be reported.

♦ Stress the need to report signs of water intoxication and hyponatremia (drowsiness, listlessness, headache, confusion, weight gain).

♦ Advise refrigerating desmopressin and protecting drug from excessive heat when traveling.

dexamethasone
dex-a-meth'a-sone

dexamethasone: *Aeroseb-Dex, Decadron, Decadron Respihaler, Decaderm, Decaspray, Deronil, ♦Dexasone, Dexone, Hexadrol, Maxidex Ophthalmic Suspension, Mymethasone, Maxidex*

dexamethasone acetate: *Dalalone D.P., Dalalone L.A., Decadron L.A., Decaject-L.A., Decameth L.A., Dexacen LA, Dexasone-LA, Dexone LA, Dexon LA, Solurex-LA*

dexamethasone sodium phosphate: *AK-Dex, Dalalone, Decadrol, Decadron Phosphate, Decadron Phosphate Opthalmic, Decaject, Decameth, Dex, Dexacen, Dexasone, Dexon, Dexone, Hexadrol Phosphate, Maxidex, Maxidex Ophthalmic, Ocu-Dex, Solurex, Turbinaire*

Class: Synthetic adrenocorticosteroid, Long-acting glucocorticoid, Steroidal anti-inflammatory, Immunosuppressant

PEDS	PREG	GERI
🖐	C	🖐

Action Suppresses inflammation by inhibiting accumulation of inflammatory cells, reducing dilatation and permeability of capillaries, and inhibiting release of chemical mediators of inflammation. Modifies immune response by suppressing cell-mediated immune reactions. Inhibits bronchoconstriction and enhances effects of bronchodilators.

Use/Therapeutic goal/Outcome

Bronchial asthma: Improved air movement. **Outcome criteria:** Improved forced expiratory volume (FEV); decreased wheezing, coughing, and dyspnea.

Allergic and inflammatory reactions: Symptomatic relief. **Outcome criteria:** Decreased

symptoms associated with condition being treated.

Cerebral edema: Prevention or reduction of brain swelling. **Outcome criteria:** Improved responsiveness, vital signs within normal range, normal pupillary response, decreased headache and vomiting, reduction of increased intracranial pressure (ICP).

Shock: Promotion of tissue perfusion. **Outcome criteria:** Improvement in vital signs and increased urinary output.

Dose range/Administration

Interaction alert: May decrease effectiveness of anticoagulants and antidiabetics. Vaccines may lead to diminished antibody response and serious infection. Potassium-depleting diuretics may cause severe hypokalemia. Alcohol or medications known to cause gastric irritation may lead to gastric bleeding. Drugs that increase metabolism of corticosteroids (e.g., phenytoin, barbiturates, ephedrine, and rifampin) and those that decrease its absorption (e.g., cholestyramine, colestipol, and antacids) may decrease dexamethasone levels, requiring an increase in dexamethasone dosage.

💊 **Give oral doses with food to reduce gastric irritation.**

Asthma: **Adult:** *Inhalation:* 3 puffs tid or qid. *Maximum dose:* 12 puffs/day. **Child:** *Inhalation:* 2 puffs tid or qid. *Maximum dose:* 8 puffs/day.

Allergy, inflammation: **Adult:** PO: 0.75–9 mg/day. IV: 0.5–24 mg/day. IM: 8–16 mg in single dose; repeat in 1–3 weeks prn. *Nasal Spray:* 2 sprays each nostril bid to tid. **Child:** PO: 0.024–0.34 mg/kg/day. IM: 0.02–0.16 mg/kg qd to bid. **Adult and Child:** *Ophthalmic:* 1 drop or thin strip tid to qid. *Otic:* 3–4 drops bid to tid. *Topical:* Apply sparingly qd to tid.

Shock: **Adult:** IV: 40 mg, repeat q2-6h prn.

Cerebral edema: **Adult:** IV: *Initial dose:* 10 mg. IM: 4 mg q6h.

Clinical alert: Dexamethasone may be injected directly into joints, soft tissues, or lesions. Rapid IV injection or large doses may cause sudden and acute (but transient) peri-anal itching. For inhalation route, give prescribed bronchodilator 5 minutes before dexamethasone to increase bronchial penetration.

Contraindications/Precautions

PREG
C

Contraindicated in hypersensitivity to corticosteroids, parabens, sulfites, or fluorocarbon propellants present in some preparations; and in active peptic ulcer disease, active tuberculosis, viral or fungal infections, and herpes of eyes, lips, or genitals. *Use with caution* in acquired immunodeficiency syndrome (AIDS), hypertension, thrombophlebitis, congestive heart failure, diabetes mellitus, hypothyroidism, glaucoma, osteoporosis, myasthenia gravis, and history of bleeding ulcers, seizure disorder, or mental illness.

✋ **Use with caution for children, pregnant or nursing mothers, and the elderly.**

Side effects/Adverse reactions

Hypersensitivity: rash, hives, hypotension, respiratory distress, anaphylaxis. *CNS:* euphoria, restlessness, insomnia, hallucinations, depression, psychosis. *Eye:* glaucoma, cataracts. *MS:* impaired growth in children. *CV:* thrombophlebitis, embolism, irregular heartbeat. *GI:* increased appetite, oral candidiasis (with rapid IV injection or large doses), peri-anal itching. *Misc:* hyperglycemia, withdrawal syndrome.

With prolonged use: Skin: acne; increased hair growth; thin, shiny skin; ecchymosis or petechiae; delayed wound healing. *GI:* nausea, vomiting, GI bleeding, pancreatitis. *MS:* osteoporosis; pain in hip, back, ribs, arms, or legs; muscle wasting. *CV:* hypertension, edema, hypokalemia. *GU:* menstrual irregularity. *Misc:* increased susceptibility to infection; Cushingoid appearance (moon-face and buffalo hump); withdrawal syndrome or acute adrenal insufficiency.

Nursing implications/Documentation

Possible nursing diagnoses: Impaired skin integrity; Fluid volume excess; Altered oral mucous membrane.

◆ Monitor for hypersensitivity reactions, especially with parenteral administration.

◆ Record baseline weight, blood pressure, and electrolyte levels.

◆ Give single daily dose in morning to lessen adrenal suppression.

◆ Administer IM doses deep into gluteal muscle to lessen muscle atrophy.

◆ Apply topical cream sparingly to clean, moist skin; occlusive dressing will increase absorption.

◆ Assess for proper use of inhalation therapy; suggest use of spacer device if unable to coordinate inhalation with activation of inhaler.

◆ With oral inhalation, assess oral mucous membrane for signs of fungal infection and record and report abnormal findings.

◆ With non-systemic routes of administration, be aware that systemic effects *may* occur.

◆ Assess, document, and report improvement in condition being treated, so dosage can be decreased as early as possible.

◆ Monitor for signs of infection and slowed wound healing.

◆ With prolonged use or high-dose therapy, monitor for withdrawal symptoms (hypotension, hypoglycemia, weight loss, vomiting, and diarrhea), while tapering or discontinuing drug.

Patient & family teaching/Home care

Possible nursing diagnoses: Knowledge deficit; Impaired home maintenance management; Potential for infection; Impaired physical mobility; Body image disturbance.

◆ Explain the need to take oral doses with food or milk.

◆ Advise against taking OTC medications without consulting physician.

◆ Counsel to adhere to prescribed dose schedule and not to discontinue medication against medical advice.

◆ For long-term therapy, advise wearing a medical alert medal indicating the need for supplemental systemic glucocorticoids in case of trauma or surgery.

◆ During withdrawal from long-term systemic therapy, stress the need to follow prescribed schedule for gradual reduction of medication.

◆ Advise reporting symptoms of adrenal insufficiency (fatigue, anorexia, nausea, vomiting, diarrhea, weight loss, weakness, dizziness, depression, and mood swings).

◆ Teach proper inhalation techniques; advise to use prescribed bronchodilator inhalations 5 minutes before dexamethasone to increase bronchial penetration.

◆ With oral inhalation, advise gargling and rinsing mouth (without swallowing) after inhalation to help prevent fungal infection in mouth or throat.

- Teach how to assess oral mucosa for creamy white patches indicating fungal infection; stress that these findings should be reported.

- With intranasal use, instruct to clear nasal passages of secretions before administration; nasal decongestant may be used prior to administration if excessive secretions or edema are present.

- Emphasize importance of medical follow-up for evaluation of therapy.

- *See Adrenocorticosteroids overview for more information.*

dex-klor-fen-eer'a-meen

dexchlorpheniramine

Dexchlor, Poladex TD, Polaramine, Polaramine Repetabs, Polargen

Class: Antihistamine (H_1 receptor antagonist)

PEDS	PREG	GERI
🖐	B	🖐

Action Prevents but does not reverse histamine-mediated allergic responses by competing with histamine for H_1 receptors on effector cells. Has anticholinergic action. This drug is the more active form of chlorpheniramine, and has similar actions, uses, contraindications, and precautions; however, it is more potent, and required dosage is smaller.

Use/Therapeutic goal/Outcome

Allergic conditions: Decrease in allergic responses. *Outcome criteria:* Report and demonstration of relief of allergy symptoms (sneezing, runny nose, itching).

Dose range/Administration

Interaction alert: CNS depressants and alcohol cause increased sedation. Do not give with MAOIs or anticholinergics.

🖐 **Give with food or milk to avoid GI upset.**

Adult/Child > 12 yrs: PO: *Tablets, syrup:* 2 mg q4-6h. *Sustained-release tablets:* 4 or 6 mg hs, or q8-10h. *Child 6–12 yrs:* PO: *Tablets, syrup:* 1 mg q4-6h. *Sustained-release tablet:* 4 mg hs. *Child 2–6 yrs:* PO: *Tablet, syrup:* 0.5 mg q4-6h.

Clinical alert: The 6 mg sustained-release tablets are not recommended for children less than 12 years, and the 4 mg in children less than 6 years. They should not be chewed or crushed. Expect reduced dosage for the elderly and monitor for increased drowsiness, dizziness.

Contraindications/Precautions

PREG
B

Contraindicated in hypersensitivity to dexchlorpheniramine or chemically related antihistamines, with MAOI therapy, and for acute asthma. *Use with caution* in narrow-angle glaucoma, increased intraocular pressure, stenosing peptic ulcer, pyeloduodenal obstruction, symptomatic prostatic hypertrophy, urinary retention, bladder-neck obstruction, hyperthyroidism, and renal or cardiovascular disease.

🖐 **Contraindicated for premature infants, newborns, children under 2 years, and nursing mothers. Use with caution for older children and the elderly. Safe use in pregnancy has not been established.**

Side effects/Adverse reactions

Hypersensitivity: rash. *CNS:* drowsiness, dizziness, weakness, headache, excitation, neuritis, disturbed coordination, insomnia, euphoria, paresthesias. *Ear:* vertigo, tinnitus, acute labyrinthitis. *Eye:* blurred vision. *CV:* palpitations, tachycardia, hypotension, extrasystoles. *GI:* nausea and vomiting, anorexia, dry mouth, constipation, diarrhea. *GU:* dysuria, urinary retention or frequency, early menses. *Skin:* skin eruptions.

Nursing implications/Documentation

Possible nursing diagnoses: Potential for injury; Fluid volume deficit.

- Determine and record known allergies; provide an environment that is free from allergens (especially sleeping areas).

- Provide favorite fluids and ensure adequate hydration (2 liters/day).

Patient & family teaching/Home care

Possible nursing diagnoses: Knowledge deficit; Impaired home maintenance management.

- Stress that sustained-release tablets should not be crushed or chewed.

- Point out that avoiding pollens and staying in an air-conditioned environment may help reduce seasonal rhinitis.

- Emphasize that dose should not be increased without physician's approval; explain that tolerance may occur, requiring a change in medication.

- Warn that alcohol and other CNS depressants may cause excessive drowsiness; advise against driving until response is determined.

- Suggest that coffee or tea may reduce drowsiness, and that sugarless gum or hard candy may relieve dry mouth.

- Explain that antihistamines should be stopped for 4 days before allergy testing to ensure accurate results.

- *See Antihistamines overview for more information.*

dextroamphetamine *dex-troe-am-fet'a-meen*

dextroamphetamine sulfate: *Dexedrine, Ferndex, Oxydess II, Robese, Spancap #1*

Class: ★Cerebral stimulant prototype, sympathomimetic, amphetamine, anorectic agent

PEDS	PREG	GERI	CONTROLLED SUBSTANCE
✋	C	✋	II

Action *In adults,* has a stimulant effect, *in hyperactive children,* a "paradoxical" calming effect. Probably stimulates the CNS by its action upon the cerebral cortex and reticular activating system, where it promotes nerve impulse transmission by releasing stored norepinephrine from nerve terminals.

Use/Therapeutic goal/Outcome

Narcolepsy: Promotion of mental alertness, reduction in sleep episodes. *Outcome criteria:* Report of feeling less fatigued or more alert; demonstration of ability to stay awake.
Short-term appetite suppression: Reduction in desire for food. *Outcome criteria:* Report of lack of appetite.
Attention Deficit Disorders with Hyperactivity (ADDH): Promotion of ability to concentrate or pay attention. *Outcome criteria:* Demonstration of increased attention span; increased ability to sit quietly.

Dose range/Administration

Interaction alert: MAO inhibitors may cause severe hypertensive crisis. May alter insulin requirements. Antacids, sodium bicarbonate, and acetazolamide may potentiate amphetamine effect; ammonium chloride, ascorbic acid, phenotiazines, and haloperidol may reduce amphetamine effect.

Narcolepsy: *Adult:* PO: 5–60 mg daily in divided doses. *Child > 12 yrs:* PO: 10 mg daily, with weekly increments of 10 mg prn. *Child 6–12 yrs:* PO: 5 mg daily, with weekly increments of 5 mg prn.

Appetite suppressant: *Adult:* PO: one or two 10- or 15-mg long-acting capsule daily (up to 30 mg/day); or 5–30 mg daily, or in divided doses taken 30 min before meals.

Attention Deficit Disorders with Hyperactivity (ADDH): *Child 6 yrs and older:* PO: 5 mg once or twice daily, with weekly increments of 5 mg prn. *Child 3–5 yrs:* PO: 2.5 mg daily, with weekly increments of 2.5 mg prn.

Clinical alert: Give doses at least 6 hr before bedtime to prevent insomnia. For treatment of ADDH in children, monitor for need to *decrease* dose; that is, watch for lessening effectiveness (this drug is usually stopped after puberty). For people with epilepsy, be aware that amphetamines may decrease seizure threshhold.

Contraindications/Precautions

PREG
C

Contraindicated in hypersensitivity or intolerance to dextroamphetamine, (for spansules and 5 mg tablets) allergy to tartrazine, and in patients with glaucoma, symptomatic cardiac disease, angina, moderate to severe hypertension, hyperthyroidism, advanced arteriosclerosis, agitation, or history of drug abuse. *Use with caution* in diabetics.

✋ Use with caution for the elderly, and for children with Tourette's disease. Safe use for pregnant or nursing mothers has not been established.

Side effects/Adverse reactions

Hypersensitivity: Itching, rashes. *CNS:* insomnia, restlessness, tremors, hyperactivity, talkativeness, irritability, headache, dizziness, tachycardia. *GI:* anorexia, metallic taste, nausea, vomiting, dry mouth, cramps, diarrhea, constipation. *CV:* hypertension, hypotension. *GU:* impotence, changes in libido. *Misc:* growth supression in children.

Nursing implications/Documentation

Possible nursing diagnoses: Altered thought processes; Sleep pattern disturbance; Constipation; Altered nutrition: less than body requirements.

- Question about the use of beverages and OTC drugs that contain caffeine.

- Monitor attention span and ability to concentrate, and report and document changes in status (dosage may need to be adjusted).

- Document blood pressure at least daily when beginning therapy, and periodically once stabilized.

- Document daily weights and keep a record of food intake to ensure adequate nutrition.

- Provide decaffeinated beverages.

• Prevent side effect of constipation by monitoring bowel movements, ensuring adequate hydration, and providing fruits, juices, and vegetables (use laxatives only when necessary).

Patient & family teaching/Home care

Possible nursing diagnoses: Knowledge deficit; Impaired home maintenance management.

• Explain that this drug has a high potential for abuse, and should only be taken as prescribed, and under continuous medical supervision.

• If used as an appetite suppressant, reinforce the importance of enrolling in a behavior modification weight-reduction program.

• Stress the importance of checking labels for caffeine content and avoiding caffeine (may increase drug effects).

• Emphasize that side effect of constipation can be avoided by drinking plenty of fluids, eating fruits and fiber, ensuring adequate exercise, and using mild laxatives when necessary.

• **For use with children**
Teach the need to monitor physical and mental growth, and to report growth failure and behavior extremes (dosage may have to be adjusted); explain that dosage will probably be reduced as child progresses to puberty, and that periodic "drug holidays" may be planned to determine if the drug is still necessary.

• *See Cerebral Stimulants overview for more information.*

dextromethorphan *dex-troe-meth-or'fan*

dextromethorphan hydrobromide: *Balminil DM, Benylin DM, ♣Broncho-Grippol-DM, Congespirin For Children, Cremacoat 1, DM Cough, Hold, Koffex, Mediquell, ♣Neo-DM, Pediacare 1, Pertussin 8 Hour Cough Formula, ♣Robidex, ♣Sedatuss, St. Joseph for Children, Sucrets Cough Control Formula. In combination: Contac Cough Formula, Contac Cough and Sore Throat Formula, Contac Jr. Children's Cold Medicine, Contac Nighttime, Cold Medicine, Contac Severe Cold Formula Caplets, Novahistine DMX Liquid, Phenergan with Dextromethorphan, Robitussin-DM, Rondec-DM, Triaminicol Multi-Symptom Cold, Trind-DM Liquid, Tussi-Organidin-DM Liquid*

Class: Nonnarcotic antitussive

PEDS	PREG	GERI
♥	C	♥

Action Suppresses cough reflex (without depressing respiration) by direct action on the cough center of the medulla. A dose of 15–30 mg of dextromethorphan is equal to 8–15 mg of codeine in antitussive effect.

Use/Therapeutic goal/Outcome

Nonproductive cough: Prevention, reduction of coughing episodes. **Outcome criteria:** Patient reports and demonstrates decreased coughing.

Dose range/Administration

Interaction alert: Hold dose and report if the patient has taken MAO inhibitors within 14 days (see Contraindications).

Adult/Child > 12 yrs: PO: 10–20 mg q4h, *or* 30 mg q6-8h, to a maximum of 120 mg/day. *Controlled-release liquid:* 60 mg bid. **Child 6–12 yrs:** PO: 5–10 mg q4h, *or* 15 mg q6-8h, to a maximum of 60 mg/day. *Controlled-release liquid:* 30 mg bid. **Child 2–6 yrs:** PO: 2.5–5 mg q4h, *or* 7.5 mg q6-8h, to a maximum of 30 mg/day. *Controlled release liquid:* 15 mg bid.

Clinical alert: This drug is a component of most OTC cough medications (check OTC drug labels).

Contraindications/Precautions PREG C

Contraindicated in hypersensitivity to dextromethorphan, in persistent or chronic cough, and for use within 14 days of MAO inhibitors. **Use with caution** in nausea, vomiting, high fever, rash, or persistent headache.

✋ Use with caution for children and the elderly. Safe use for children under 2 years, and for pregnant or nursing mothers, has not been established.

Side effects/Adverse reactions

Hypersensitivity: itching, rash. **CNS:** dizziness, drowsiness. **GI:** gastric and intestinal upset.

Nursing implications/Documentation

Possible nursing diagnoses: Ineffective airway clearance; Fluid volume deficit.

• Record lung sounds and sputum production to monitor effectiveness; report cough that lasts longer than a week.

• Provide preferred fluids to promote hydration.

Patient & family teaching/Home care

Possible nursing diagnoses: Knowledge deficit; Impaired home maintenance management.

- Advise reporting a rash or an increase in breathing problems, because it may indicate a need to change the medication.

- Stress the importance of adequate hydration; advise taking doses with a full glass of water.

- Point out that increased environmental humidity with decreased environmental irritants (e.g., smoke) can minimize aggravating factors.

- Advise reporting a cough that persists longer than a week.

- See *Antitussives, Expectorants, and Mucolytics* overview for more information.

dextrothyroxine

dex-tro-thy-rox'seen

dextrothyroxine sodium: *Choloxin*

Class: Antilipemic (Thyroid hormone)

PEDS	PREG	GERI
✋	C	✋

Action Reduces serum cholesterol by stimulating the liver to increase cholesterol catabolism and to promote its excretion.

Use/Therapeutic goal/Outcome

Hypercholesterolemia (type IIA) and elevated low-density lipoprotein levels (LDL) in hyperlipidemic euthyroid patients: Reduction of serum lipid levels. *Outcome criteria:* Serum lipid levels within normal limits.

Dose range/Administration

Interaction alert: May enhance the action of oral anticoagulants, and prothrombin time may increase. May increase blood sugar when used with insulin, oral hypoglycemics, digitalis preparations, epinephrine, antidepressants, or betablockers.

Adult: PO: 1–2 mg/day. May be increased by 1–2 mg/month. Give minimum effective dose. *Maintenance dose:* 4–8 mg/day. *Maximum dose:* 8 mg/day. *Child:* PO: Initially 0.05 mg/kg/day; may increase by 0.05 mg/kg/day each month. *Maintenance dose:* 0.1 mg/kg/day. *Maximum dose:* 4 mg/day.

Clinical alert: Accurate health history and physical examination are essential before giving dextrothyroxine sodium to rule out heart disease or thyroid disorder.

Contraindications/Precautions

Contraindicated in hypersensitivity to this drug or (for 2 mg and 6 mg tablets) to tartrazine, and in organic heart disease, angina pectoris, history of myocardial infarction, history of arrhythmias, rheumatic heart disease, congestive heart failure, hypertension, liver or kidney disease, history of iodism.

✋ **Contraindicated for pregnant and nursing mothers. Use with caution for children and the elderly.**

Side effects/Adverse reactions

Hypersensitivity: itching. *CV:* angina pectoris, arrhythmias, enlarged heart, myocardial ischemia, pulmonary edema, palpitations. *MS:* weight loss, muscle pain. *CNS:* insomnia, tremors, headache, dizziness, nervousness, paresthesias, psychic changes. *GI:* nausea, vomiting, constipation, diarrhea, anorexia, gallstones. *Skin:* alopecia, flushing, sweating. *GU:* diuresis, menstrual irregularities. *Eye:* visual disturbances, exophthalmos. *Ear:* tinnitus. *Misc:* malaise, altered libido, hyperthermia, hoarseness.

Nursing implications/Documentation

Possible nursing diagnoses: Constipation; Diarrhea; Altered nutrition: more than body requirements.

- Monitor and document bowel elimination to detect constipation or diarrhea; establish a plan to prevent constipation; report diarrhea to physician.

- Monitor for signs of increased metabolism (tachycardia, palpitations, weight loss), which may have adverse effects, especially on the heart.

- Do not give for 2 weeks before surgery to reduce risk of cardiac arrhythmias.

Patient & family teaching/Home care

Possible nursing diagnoses: Altered health maintenance; Knowledge deficit; Impaired home maintenance management.

- Explain that the purpose of this drug is to reduce serum cholesterol and to decrease the risk of cardiovascular disease.

- Emphasize the need to reduce other cardiac risk factors (obesity, smoking, high cholesterol diet, sedentary lifestyle), and help develop a plan to reduce these.

- ♦ Caution that chest pain, palpitations, sweating, diarrhea, headache, or skin rash must be reported immediately to the physician.
- ♦ Stress the need for ongoing medical follow-up.
- ♦ *See Antilipemic overview for more information.*

diazepam

dye-az'e-pam

♣Apo-Diazepam, ♣Diazemuls, Diazepam Intensol, ♣E-Pam, ♣Meval, ♣Novodipam, Q-Pam, ♣Rival, Valium, Valrelease, Vasepam, ♣Vivol, Zetran

Class: ★Benzodiazepine prototype, Antianxiety agent

PEDS	PREG	GERI	CONTROLLED SUBSTANCE
🖐	D	🖐	IV

Action Produces CNS depression and relaxation, and increases seizure threshold by potentiating the action of gamma-aminobuteric acid (GABA), which reduces neuronal activity in all regions of the CNS. Promotes muscle relaxation by inhibiting spinal motor reflex pathways. Decreases anxiety by inhibiting cortical and limbic arousal.

Use/Therapeutic goal/Outcome

Short-term treatment of anxiety agitation: Alleviation of symptoms of apprehension, agitation, muscle tension, and insomnia. *Outcome criteria:* Report of feeling more calm, sleeping better, and coping better; observable signs of decreased anxiety or agitation (decreased motor activity, reduced muscle tension, decrease in pulse and blood pressure).

Seizures: Elimination of seizure activity. *Outcome criteria:* Absence of seizure activity.

Skeletal muscle spasms: Relief of muscle spasms. *Outcome criteria:* Report of absence of pain and demonstration of improved range of motion.

Sedation (pre-procedure, during procedure, ventilator phasing): Promotion of relaxation, amnesia of procedure, promotion of toleration of mechanical ventilation. *Outcome criteria:* Report of feeling relaxed or not remembering discomfort; (for mechanical ventilation) respirations synchronized with ventilator.

Dose range/Administration

Interaction alert: Alcohol and other CNS depressants may cause excessive sedation. Cimetidine increases blood levels. Do not mix IV in syringe or tubing with any other drug (is incompatible with most drugs, NS and Lac-

tated Ringer's). Do not store diazepam in plastic syringes.

💗 **Give with food or milk if GI upset is noted.**

Anxiety/agitation, skeletal muscle spasm, adjunct in seizure disorders: **Adult:** PO: *Tablet:* 2–10 mg tid or qid. *Sustained-release capsule:* 15–30 mg once daily. **Child > 6 mos:** PO: 1–2.5 mg tid or qid.

Status epilepticus: **Adult:** IV: 2–5 mg q1min. *Maximum dose:* 60 mg. **Child:** IV: 0.1–0.3 mg/kg, at 1 mg/min. May repeat q15min for 2 doses. *Maximum dose, child < 5 yrs:* 5 mg. *Maximum dose, child > 5 yrs:* 10 mg at a time.

Sedation: **Adult:** PO: 5–10 mg 1 hr before procedure (use IV route for ventilator phasing). IV: 1–10 mg initially; may repeat prn to a maximum of 30 mg in the first hr, then 1–5 mg/hr prn. **Child > 5 yrs:** IV: 1 mg q2-5min to a maximum of 10 mg. Repeat q2-4h prn. **Child 1 mo–5 yrs:** 0.2–0.5 mg q2-5min to a maximum of 5 mg. Repeat q2-4h prn.

Clinical alert: IM route is not recommended because of erratic absorption; in addition, the alkalinity of the solution makes it painful. Give IV doses *slowly*, no faster than 5 mg/min; inject directly into the vein (or into IV tubing as close to the vein as possible, because of incompatibilities). For IV administration, have resuscitative drugs and equipment nearby. When discontinuing diazepam, taper doses gradually to avoid withdrawal symptoms. Diazepam accumulates in the body, and elimination after discontinuation may take weeks.

Contraindications/Precautions

PREG D

Contraindicated in hypersensitivity or intolerance to diazepam or other benzodiazepines, and in narrow-angle glaucoma, shock, respiratory depression (unless mechanical ventilation is used), acute alcohol intoxication, and myasthenia gravis. *Use with caution* in psychosis, depression, suicidal tendencies, or impaired liver or kidney function.

🖐 **Contraindicated for pregnant or nursing mothers and (oral form) for children under 6 months. Use with caution for older children and the elderly or debilitated.**

Side effects/Adverse reactions

Hypersensitivity: itching, rash, exaggeration of side effects. *CNS:* lethargy, drowsiness, headache, dizziness, confusion, ataxia, tremors, depression. *CV:* hypotension, transient tachycardia and bradycardia, cardiovascular collapse. **Resp:** respiratory depression, (with IV route) respiratory arrest. **GI:** dry mouth, anorexia, nausea, vomiting, constipation, diarrhea. **GU:** urinary retention. **Eye:** blurred vision, mydriasis. **Misc:** drug tolerance and dependence.

Nursing implications/Documentation

Possible nursing diagnoses: Potential for injury; Constipation.

◆ Record baseline blood pressure; monitor closely if dizziness is experienced.

◆ Supervise ambulation until response is determined; monitor the elderly for prolonged effects.

◆ Keep those who have received parenteral drug in bed with side rails up.

◆ Be sure that doses are swallowed (not hoarded).

◆ Monitor bowel elimination and provide adequate fluids and fiber to prevent constipation; offer laxatives before the problem is severe.

◆ Provide a quiet environment that is conducive to rest.

◆ For long-term use, monitor CBC and liver function studies periodically.

Patient & family teaching/Home care

Possible nursing diagnoses: Anxiety; Fear; Ineffective individual coping; Impaired home maintenance management.

◆ Advise taking this drug with milk or food if GI symptoms are noted.

◆ Help the individual identify stressors that contribute to anxiety and ways of coping effectively; stress that effective coping strategies can reduce the need for medication.

◆ Explain the importance of daily exercise in relieving stress, and encourage establishing a plan for getting enough exercise (e.g., daily walks).

◆ Point out that drug tolerance and dependence can occur, and that the drug should be used only on a short-term basis.

◆ Emphasize that the effects of alcohol, other sedatives and CNS depressants, and tranquilizers may be potentiated (these should be avoided).

◆ Advise avoidance of driving and other potentially hazardous activities until response is established.

◆ See *Antianxiety agents/Sedatives/Hypnotics and Anticonvulsants overviews* for more information.

diazoxide
dye-as-ox'ide

Hyperstat (parenteral), **Proglycem** (oral)

Class: Antihypertensive (parenteral), Antihypoglycemic (oral)

PEDS	PREG	GERI
🖐	**D**	🖐

Action When given parenterally, reduces blood pressure by directly dilating peripheral arteriolar smooth muscle. (Antihypertensive effect counteracted somewhat by increased heart rate, cardiac output, renin secretion.) When given orally, inhibits release of insulin from the pancreas and stimulates release of endogenous catecholamines causing hyperglycemia. (Oral doses do not significantly lower blood pressure.) Increases reabsorption of sodium in proximal tubules and decreases glomerular filtration rate, which leads to sodium and water retention.

Use/Therapeutic goal/Outcome

Hypertensive emergencies: Reduction of blood pressure. **Outcome criteria:** Blood pressure within normal limits.

Hypoglycemia: Rise in serum blood glucose. **Outcome criteria:** Blood glucose within normal limits (80–140).

Dose range/Administration

Interaction alert: Antihypertensives, phenothiazines, thiazides, diuretics, and vasodilators may potentiate the antihypertensive effect of diazoxide. Corticosteroids, oral contraceptives, phenothiazines, thiazide and other diuretics may potentiate the hyperglycemic effects of diazoxide. Alpha-adrenergic blockers may antagonize hyperglycemic effect. Increases blood level of anticoagulants. May increase metabolism of phenytoin. Use with oral hypoglycemics may reduce the hyperglycemic effects of diazoxide.

Hypertension: Adult and Child: IV: 1–3 mg/kg (to a maximum single dose of 150 mg), undiluted, over 30 sec every 5–15 min. Repeat in 4–24 hr prn until appropriate oral antihypertensive therapy can be initiated. *Maximum dose:* 1.2 g/day.

Hypoglycemia: Adult: PO: 3–8 mg/kg/day in divided doses q8-12h. **Child:** PO: 3–8 mg/kg/day in divided doses q8-12h. **Infants:** PO: 8–15 mg/kg/day in divided doses q8-12h.

Clinical alert: Administer IV doses with patient lying flat; keep flat for 30 minutes after infusion. Monitor closely for extravasation (drug is highly irritating). Never give IM or SC. Keep norepinephrine ready to treat severe hypotension. This drug should not be used by IV route for longer than 10 days. Oral doses should be stopped if there is no response in 2–3 weeks.

Contraindications/Precautions

PREG C

Contraindicated in hypersensitivity to diazoxide, thiazides, or sulfonamides, and in compensatory hypertension, coronary artery disease, dissecting aortic aneurysm, eclampsia.

👋 **Contraindicated for pregnant women. Use with caution for children and the elderly.**

Side effects/Adverse reactions

Hypersensitivity: rash, urticaria, fever. **CV:** EKG changes, myocardial ischemia, arrhythmias, orthostatic hypotension, angina. **CNS:** dizziness, lightheadedness, flushing, headache, euphoria. **GI:** abdominal discomfort, nausea, vomiting. **Hem:** leukopenia, hyperuricemia, hyperglycemia. **Skin:** warmth, inflammation and pain from extravasation, increased hair growth on forehead, back, arms, and legs. **Misc:** fever, sodium and water retention.

Nursing implications/Documentation

Possible nursing diagnoses: Activity intolerance; Fatigue; Potential for injury.

- **For IV route**

  ◆ Assess mental status, and record pulse and blood pressure (if possible, lying, sitting, and standing in both arms) before administration, and frequently thereafter until response is determined.

  ◆ Consult with physician to determine desired therapeutic range for blood pressure (be aware that some patients may require a slightly elevated blood pressure to perfuse vital organs).

  ◆ Ascertain that baseline blood sugar, CBC, electrolytes, BUN, creatinine, uric acid, and liver function studies have been obtained before giving first dose; report abnormalities and monitor closely thereafter.

  ◆ Monitor for allergic reactions, and for confusion, dizziness, rales, arrhythmias, angina, hypotension; hold drug (or decrease IV rate) and report immediately if these occur.

  ◆ Supervise ambulation until response is determined (patients on IV route should remain in bed).

  ◆ Document and monitor daily weight, and intake and output; report significant negative or positive balance.

- **For oral route**

  ◆ Monitor blood glucose levels closely until response is determined; then periodically thereafter.

Patient & family teaching/Home care

Possible nursing diagnoses: Knowledge deficit; Impaired home maintenance management.

- **For IV route**

  ◆ Explain the importance of taking antihypertensive medications exactly as prescribed, even when feeling well.

  ◆ Stress the importance of good medical follow-up, explain that this drug reduces "wear and tear" on blood vessels and improves longevity and health.

  ◆ Teach how to monitor pulse and blood pressure; emphasize that syncope, hypertension or hypotension, or persistent dizziness should be reported.

  ◆ Advise changing positions slowly to avoid dizziness.

  ◆ Encourage daily monitoring of weight and reporting sudden weight gain (likely to be water weight gain).

  ◆ Warn against taking *any* OTC drugs without physician approval (some interactions can cause severe reactions).

  ◆ Explain that increased hair growth may occur as a side effect.

- **For oral route**

  ◆ Stress the need to follow dietary restrictions for successful treatment.

  ◆ Teach how to monitor blood sugar; stress the need for medical supervision.

- *See Antihypertensives overview for more information.*

dichlorphenamide
dye-klor-fen′a-mide

Daranide

Class: Carbonic anhydrase inhibitor

PEDS	PREG	GERI
👋	C	👋

Action Lowers intraocular pressure by inhibiting carbonic anhydrase, thus reducing the rate of aqueous humor formation.

Use/Therapeutic goal/Outcome

Adjunctive treatment of chronic simple (open-angle) and secondary glaucoma, and preoperatively for acute angle-closure glaucoma: Reduction of intraocular pressure. *Outcome criteria:* Intraocular pressure within normal limits when measured with tonometer.

Dose range/Administration

🌰 **Give with food to minimize GI upset.**

Adult: PO: *Loading dose:* 100–200 mg, followed by 100 mg q12h. *Maintenance dose:* 25–50 mg 1–3 times a day (in conjunction with a miotic).

Contraindications/Precautions

PREG C

Contraindicated in hypersensitivity to sulfonamides and derivatives (thiazide diuretics), and in hyponatremia, hypokalemia, other electrolyte imbalances, renal or hepatic dysfunction, adrenal insufficiency, obstructive pulmonary disease, hyperchloremic acidosis, and chronic noncongestive angle-closure glaucoma. *Use with caution* in diabetes mellitus.

🖐 **Contraindicated for pregnant women. Use with caution for children and the elderly. Safe use for nursing mothers has not been established.**

Side effects/Adverse reactions

Hypersensitivity: rash, fever. *CNS:* drowsiness, paresthesias, lethargy, malaise. *GI:* nausea, vomiting, diarrhea, anorexia, weight loss. *Hem:* aplastic anemia, hemolytic anemia, leukopenia, hypokalemia, hyperuricemia. *Eye:* myopia. *GU:* crystalluria, renal calculi. *Misc:* hyperchloremic acidosis, photosensitivity.

Nursing implications/Documentation

Possible nursing diagnoses: Fluid volume deficit; Altered patterns of urinary elimination; Potential for injury.

◆ Ascertain that baseline CBC, sodium, potassium, chloride, carbon dioxide, calcium, magnesium, BUN, creatinine, uric acid, and liver function studies have been obtained before giving first dose; report abnormalities and monitor closely thereafter.

◆ Question about eye symptoms.

◆ Supervise ambulation until response is determined.

Patient & family teaching/Home care

Possible nursing diagnoses: Knowledge deficit; Impaired home maintenance management.

◆ Before giving first dose, explain that the drug will increase the amount and frequency of urination.

◆ Advise taking this drug with food to reduce GI symptoms.

◆ Emphasize that vision damage can occur unnoticed; stress that ongoing follow-up for measurement of intraocular pressure is essential.

◆ Stress that eye pain, muscle cramping, and edema should be reported, and that hypokalemia is common.

D

diclofenac

dik'loe-fen-ak

diclofenac sodium: *Voltaren,* 🍁*Voltaren SR*
Class: Nonsteroidal anti-inflammatory drug (NSAID), Analgesic, Antipyretic

PEDS	PREG	GERI
🖐	**B**	🖐

Action Although the mechanism of action is unclear, diclofenac sodium is believed to reduce inflammation by inhibiting prostaglandin synthesis. Prostaglandin is found throughout the body tissues and is a naturally occurring mediator of the inflammatory process.

Use/Therapeutic goal/Outcome

Pain and inflammation: Promotion of comfort and mobility; suppression of inflammation. *Outcome criteria:* Report of increased comfort with increased range of motion and ability to perform activities of daily life; reduction in or absence of joint stiffness, swelling, redness, and warmth.

Dose range/Administration

Interaction alert: May enhance the effect of digoxin, methotrexate, cyclosporin, and lithium. May inhibit diuretics. Aspirin may decrease therapeutic effect of NSAID and increase risk of bleeding. May alter response to antidiabetis agents.

🌰 **Give with milk or food to decrease GI irritation.**

Osteoarthritis: Adult: PO: 100–150 mg/day in divided doses bid or tid.

Rheumatoid arthritis: Adult: PO: 150–200 mg/day in divided doses bid, tid, or qid. *Rectal:* (where available) 50–100 mg suppository at bedtime (substitute for last oral dose of the day).

Ankylosing spondylitis: Adult: PO: 100–125 mg/day in divided doses; an extra 25 mg hs prn.

Clinical alert: Do not exceed 200 mg/day. Expect reduced dosage for the elderly and those with decreased renal function.

D

Contraindications/Precautions

PREG
B

Contraindicated in hypersensitivity to diclofenac, other NSAIDs, or aspirin. *Use with caution* in history of renal or hepatic impairment, GI bleeding, and coagulation defects.

✋ **Use with caution for pregnant women and the elderly. Safe use for children under 14 years has not been established.**

Side effects/Adverse reactions

Hypersensitivity: swelling of eyelids, lips, pharynx, larynx, anaphylaxis, urticaria, asthma, and bronchospasm, sometimes with concomitant hypotension. *CV:* fluid retention and edema, hypertension. *GI:* ulceration and bleeding, constipation, nausea, heartburn, diarrhea, elevated liver enzymes. *CNS:* headache. *GU:* oliguria. *Skin:* photosensitivity.

Nursing implications/Documentation

Possible nursing diagnoses: Pain; Impaired physical mobility.

♦ Establish a baseline for CBC, electrolytes, prothrombin time, BUN, creatinine, and liver function studies; monitor periodically thereafter if therapy is prolonged.

♦ Schedule drug administration so that drug is given at least 1 hr before maximum mobility is needed.

♦ Monitor for and report GI symptoms that may indicate peptic ulcer (nausea, pain, black stools).

♦ Record weight every other day; report edema or sudden weight gain.

♦ For diabetics, monitor blood sugar closely since insulin requirements may change.

Patient & family teaching/Home care

Possible nursing diagnoses: Anxiety; Knowledge deficit.

♦ Advise taking doses with food to reduce GI symptoms; explain the importance of watching for symptoms of GI bleeding (black stools, persistent GI distress).

♦ Stress the need to avoid aspirin, alcohol, and other OTC drugs (unless approved by physician) because of increased risk of GI bleeding.

♦ Instruct individuals to hold drug and report if any of the following side effects are experienced: vertigo, rashes, blood in urine, hearing or visual changes, sudden weight gain, edema.

♦ Explain the importance of limiting sodium intake.

♦ Stress the need for medical supervision; advise telling dentist that diclofenac is being taken.

♦ For diabetics, explain the importance of monitoring blood sugars with a blood glucose meter.

♦ *See Nonsteroidal anti-inflammatory drugs overview for more information.*

dicloxacillin

dye-klox-a-sill'in

dicloxacillin sodium: *Dycill, Dynapen, Pathocil*

Class: Anti-infective, Antibiotic, Penicillin (penicillinase-resistant)

PEDS	PREG	GERI
✋	B	✋

Action Broad-spectrum, usually bactericidal antibiotic; kills bacteria by inhibiting cell wall synthesis. Resistant to bacterial penicillinases (enzymes that degrade some penicillins).

Use/Therapeutic goal/Outcome

Systemic infections (caused by penicillinase-producing staphylococci): Resolution of infection. *Outcome criteria:* Absence of pathogenic growth on cultures, absence of clinical manifestations of infection (fever, pain, redness, heat, swelling, odor, drainage), normal WBC count, improvement of X rays.

Dose range/Administration

Interaction alert: Probenecid inhibits excretion of dicloxacillin and may be given to increase serum levels of the drug.

🥤 **Give with a full glass of water 1–2 hours before or 2–3 hours after meals; food may inhibit absorption.**

Adult: PO: 125–250 mg q6h. *Child:* PO: 12.5–25 mg/kg/day, in divided doses q6h.

Clinical alert: Give at least 1 hour before bacteriostatic antibiotics for optimum effect.

Contraindications/Precautions

Contraindicated in allergy to penicillin. **Use with caution** in cephalosporin sensitivity, history of allergic responses (e.g., other drugs, hay fever, asthma), and renal insufficiency.

👋 Use with caution for children, the elderly, and pregnant or nursing mothers.

Side effects/Adverse reactions

Hypersensitivity: itching, rashes, urticaria, fever, difficulty breathing, anaphylaxis. **GI:** nausea, vomiting, diarrhea, flatulence. **GU:** bleeding. **Hem:** eosinophilia, slight elevation in SGOT and SGPT. **CNS:** seizures. **Misc:** bone marrow depression, superinfection.

Nursing implications/Documentation

Possible nursing diagnoses: Potential for infection; Diarrhea.

♦ Determine history of allergies, and (regardless of history) monitor closely for allergic reactions.

♦ Obtain baseline CBC, serum sodium, liver function studies, and necessary cultures before administering first dose; monitor closely thereafter if therapy is prolonged.

♦ Encourage fluids, and record and monitor intake and output, to ensure adequate hydration; report significant negative or positive balance.

♦ Monitor for and report signs of superinfection (sore throat, fever, fatigue, thrush, vaginal discharge, diarrhea).

Patient & family teaching/Home care

Possible nursing diagnoses: Knowledge deficit; Impaired home maintenance management.

♦ Advise taking dicloxacillin with a full glass of water 1–2 hours before meals or 2–3 hours after meals.

♦ Teach the importance of reporting allergic symptoms, diarrhea, signs and symptoms that do not abate, or *any* new signs and symptoms of discomfort that might indicate superinfection (medication regimen may have to be changed).

♦ Advise drinking 2–3 L of fluids daily to maintain adequate hydration (especially important if fever exists).

♦ Stress the importance of taking antibiotics for the entire time prescribed, even if signs and symptoms abate.

♦ *See Anti-infectives overview for more information.*

dienestrol

dye-en-ess'trol

dienoestrol: **DV, Ortho Dienestrol**
Class: Hormone, Estrogen

PEDS	PREG	GERI
👋	X	👋

D

Action Increases the volume and acidity of vaginal and cervical secretions and improves sexual functioning by replacing depleted estrogen levels and increasing DNA, RNA, and protein synthesis in responsive tissue. Also reduces FSH and LH from the pituitary.

Use/Therapeutic goal/Outcome

Atrophic vaginitis or kraurosis vulvae in postmenopausal women: Prevention of atrophic vaginitis and kraurosis vulvae; promotion of normal sexual functioning. **Outcome criteria:** Absence of vaginal and vulval symptoms (itching, burning, drainage); report of improved comfort and sexual functioning.

Dose range/Administration

Interaction alert: May alter hypoglycemic-agent requirements.

Adult: *Vaginal:* 1–2 applicators/day (6–12 g 0.01%-cream) for 1–2 wks; then 1/2 dose for 1–2 wks. *Maintenance dose:* 1 applicator 1–3 times/wk, 3 wks/mo, for 3–6 mos.

Clinical alert: Patient should remain recumbent for at least 30 min after dose is given to prevent leakage of drug (bedtime administration may be preferred).

Contraindications/Precautions

Contraindicated in hypersensitivity to estrogen, and in estrogen-dependent neoplasia, undiagnosed vaginal bleeding, cancer of the breast, thrombophlebitis, thromboembolic disease, and for prolonged therapy (>6 months). **Use with caution** in medical conditions that could be aggravated by fluid retention (asthma or cardiac, renal, or hepatic insufficiency), cerebrovascular disease, coronary artery disease, diabetes, gallbladder disease, uterine fibroids, and history of menstrual irregularities, or endometriosis.

👋 Contraindicated for children and pregnant or nursing mothers. Use with caution for the elderly (monitor for correct application).

Side effects/Adverse reactions

Hypersensitivity: vaginal burning and irritation. **GI:** nausea, vomiting, abdominal bloating, cramps. **CNS:** dizziness, migraine headache, depression. **CV:** edema, hypertension, thromboembolism. **Hem:** decreased glucose tolerance, hypercalcemia. **GU:** dysmenorrhea, vaginal candidiasis, uterine bleeding with excessive use, cystitis. **Skin:** urticaria, pigmentation. **Misc:** libido changes; breast tenderness, enlargement, and secretion.

Nursing implications/Documentation

Possible nursing diagnoses: Potential impaired skin integrity.

♦ Keep a record of blood pressure and weight; report hypertension and weight gain (systemic reactions can occur with intravaginal use).

♦ Cleanse vulva with non-deodorant or non-perfumed soap before application.

♦ Inspect condition of vaginal area before application; report increase in signs of vaginitis or inflammation of the vulva.

♦ Monitor diabetics for changes in hypoglycemic requirements.

Patient & family teaching/Home care

Possible nursing diagnoses: Sexual dysfunction; Impaired home maintenance management.

♦ Explain benefits and risks of estrogen therapy (estrogens are believed to improve female sexual functioning and reduce risk of osteoporosis and MI, but they are also associated with increased risk of cancer); provide a package insert and discuss specific information for this drug verbally.

♦ Demonstrate correct procedure for administration and observe return demonstration; caution not to wear tampons (sanitary napkin should be used).

♦ Caution to avoid use of perfumed or deodorant soaps.

♦ Advise that if a dose is missed, it should be given at the next dose time (the dose should never be doubled or exceeded).

♦ Point out that persistent vaginal symptoms and other systemic symptoms (e.g., blurred vision, edema, chest pain, depression) should be reported since they may be related to the medication.

♦ Warn that smoking can increase incidence of side effects.

♦ Inform women that withdrawal bleeding may occur if doses are suddenly stopped.

♦ Advise that sexual intercourse during therapy may cause skin irritation in partner (abstinence or use of a condom is recommended).

♦ Stress the importance of regular gynecologic exams (every 6–12 months), mammography (annually), and breast self-exam (monthly).

♦ Explore sexual concerns; encourage verbalizing feelings and concerns and seeking counseling as needed.

♦ Stress the need for diabetics to monitor blood sugars and report hyperglycemic trends (estrogen may alter antidiabetic-agent requirements).

diethylstilbestrol
dye-eth-il-stil-bess'trol

stilboestrol: **DES**

diethylstilbestrol diphosphate: ♣**Honvol, Stilphostrol**

Class: Hormone, Estrogen, Antineoplastic hormonal agent

PEDS	PREG	GERI
🖐	X	🖐

Action Promotes normal development and functioning of the female reproductive system by replacing depleted estrogens and increasing DNA, RNA, and protein synthesis in responsive tissue. Interferes with implantation of fertilized ova and reduces FSH and LH release from pituitary. Suppresses malignant cell growth of androgen-dependent prostatic and breast cancer by altering hormonal balance.

Use/Therapeutic goal/Outcome

Moderate to severe vasomotor symptoms of menopause: Relief of symptoms of menopause; replacement of natural estrogen levels. **Outcome criteria:** Report of improved sexual functioning and absence of hot flashes, excitability, insomnia, palpitations, vertigo, and myalgia; normalization of estrogen levels.

Advanced, inoperable, metastatic carcinoma of the breast in men and postmenopausal women; and advanced, inoperable, metastatic carcinoma of the prostate: Suppression of malignant-cell proliferation. **Outcome criteria:** Tumor, disease process regression or stabilization on radiologic and physical examination.

Dose range/Administration

Interaction alert: Effectiveness may be decreased by barbiturates. May alter requirements of antidiabetic agents and anticoagulants.

🖐 Give with or after food to decrease nausea.

Menopausal symptoms, hypogonadism, female castration, and primary ovarian failure: **Adult:** PO: 0.1–2 mg/day for 3 wks, then 1 wk off; continue monthly cycle.

Breast carcinoma: **Adult:** PO: 15 mg/day for at least 3 mos.

Prostatic cancer: **Adult:** PO: 1–3 mg/day diethylstilbestrol, then may reduce to 1 mg/day; or 50–200 mg diethylstilbestrol diphosphate tid. IM: *Initial dose:* 5 mg diethylstilbestrol diphosphate 2x/wk. *Maintenance dose:* Up to 4 mg 2x/wk. IV: *Initial dose:* 0.25 mg to 1 g/day diethylstilbestrol diphosphate for 5 days. *Maintenance dose:* 0.25 mg to 1g each week or 2 times/week.

Clinical alert: Do not allow enteric-coated tablets to be crushed or chewed. Lowest effective dose should be given (dose may be periodically reduced). Be sure that pregnancy is neither planned nor suspected before giving first dose; this drug has been associated with a high incidence of nonmalignant genital changes in offspring of mothers who have taken it during pregnancy (male and female offspring have an increased risk of reproductive-tract cancer).

Contraindications/Precautions

PREG X

Contraindicated in hypersensitivity to diethylstilbestrol, and in estrogen-dependent neoplasia, undiagnosed vaginal bleeding, thrombophlebitis, and thromboembolic disease. *Use with caution* in conditions that can be aggravated by fluid retention (asthma or cardiac, renal, or hepatic insufficiency), cerebrovascular or coronary artery disease, diabetes, gallbladder disease; history of seizures, migraines, or mental depression, or family history of genital or breast cancer or fibrocystic breast disease.

🖐 Contraindicated for children and pregnant or nursing mothers. Use with caution for the elderly.

Side effects/Adverse reactions

Hypersensitivity: abnormal/excessive genital bleeding, mastodynia, urticaria, leg cramps. *CNS:* dizziness, migraine headaches, depression (which may be severe). *CV:* thromboembolism, myocardial infarction, hypertension, pulmonary embolism, edema, increased risk of stroke. *Eye:* photosensitivity, increased myopia and astigmatism, steepening of the corneal curvature, (decreased visual acuity, intolerance to contact lenses). *Hem:* hyperglycemia, hypercalcemia, increased serum triglycerides. *GI:* anorexia, nausea, vomiting, diarrhea, constipation, abdominal cramps, weight loss or gain, increased appetite, excessive thirst, cholestatic jaundice, gallbladder disease. *GU:* breakthrough bleeding, dysmenorrhea/amenorrhea, cervical erosion, increase in size of uterine fibromas, endometrial carcinoma, Candida vaginitis, cystitis-like syndrome, testicular atrophy, impotence. *MS:* chorea, lethargy. *Skin:* acne, seborrhea, oily skin, erythema multiforme, hirsutism, alopecia. *Misc:* rapid weight gain, gynecomastia; breast tenderness, enlargement, or secretion; loss of libido, decreased glucose tolerance, folic acid deficiency.

Nursing implications/Documentation

Possible nursing diagnoses: Fluid volume excess; Body image disturbance.

◆ Keep a record of blood pressure and weight during therapy; report hypertension and weight gain.

◆ Document blood sugars to monitor diabetics for changes in hypoglycemic requirements.

Patient & family teaching/Home care

Possible nursing diagnoses: Altered sexuality patterns; Body image disturbance; Knowledge deficit; Impaired home maintenance management.

◆ Explain benefits and risks of estrogen therapy for women (estrogens are believed to improve female sexual functioning and reduce risk of osteoporosis, hypertension, and MI, but they may also be associated with increased risk of endometrial cancer); provide a package insert and discuss specific information for this drug verbally.

◆ Stress that this drug should be taken with, or immediately after, food to reduce nausea; point out that nausea usually diminishes after 1–2 weeks.

◆ Provide a calendar that clearly indicates drug-free days.

◆ Advise that missed doses should be taken as soon as possible, but not immediately before next dose.

◆ Point out that persistent vaginal symptoms or other systemic symptoms should be reported, as they may be related to the medication.

◆ Warn that smoking can increase incidence of side effects.

◆ Inform women that withdrawal bleeding may occur if doses are suddenly stopped.

◆ Stress the importance to women of regular gynecologic exams (every 6 months to 1 year), mammography (yearly), and breast self-exam (monthly).

◆ Reassure male patients that estrogen side effects will disappear after drug therapy ceases.

◆ Explore concerns about body image and sexual function; encourage the individual to seek counseling as needed.

◆ Stress the need for diabetics to monitor blood sugars and report hyperglycemic trends (estrogen may alter antidiabetic-agent requirements).

◆ *See Antineoplastic agents overview for more information.*

diflunisal

die-flu'ni-sal

Dolobid

Class: Non-narcotic analgesic, Nonsteroidal anti-inflammatory drug (NSAID)

PEDS	PREG	GERI
🖐	C	🖐

Action Produces analgesia and anti-inflammatory response through an unclear mechanism (action may be related to the drug's inhibition of prostaglandin synthesis).

Use/Therapeutic goal/Outcome

Anti-inflammatory: Reduction of pain and inflammation. *Outcome criteria:* After 2 weeks, report of reduced stiffness and swelling of joints; increased mobility.

Dose range/Administration

Interaction alert: Aspirin and antacid therapy may reduce effects. May enhance effects of anticoagulants.

🖐 **Give with a full glass of water or milk, or with meals.**

Adult/Child > 12 yrs: PO: 1000 mg, then 500 mg q8-12h. *Maximum dose:* 1500 mg/day. *For the elderly:* Start with 500 mg.

Clinical alert: Tablets should be swallowed whole, not chewed or crushed. Do not give to children with flu symptoms or chicken pox because of risk of Reye's syndrome.

Contraindications/Precautions

PREG
C

Contraindicated in hypersensitivity to diflunisal or aspirin. **Use with caution** in impaired renal function, active GI bleeding, history of peptic-ulcer disease, compromised cardiac function, and with anticoagulants.

🖐 **Contraindicated for children under 12 years, for children under 18 years with chickenpox or influenza-like symptoms, and for pregnant or nursing mothers. Use with caution for the elderly.**

Side effects/Adverse reactions

Hypersensitivity: itching, rashes, bronchospasm, anaphylaxis. *GI:* nausea, vomiting, dyspepsia, constipation, GI pain, diarrhea, dry mucus membranes, flatulence. *CNS:* somnolence, insomnia, dizziness, headache. *Ear:* tinnitus. *Skin:* sweating.

Nursing implications/Documentation

Possible nursing diagnoses: Pain; Impaired physical mobility.

◆ Be aware that this drug is a derivative of salicylic acid, but has a lesser effect on platelet function.

◆ Schedule doses so that drug is given *at least 1 hr* before maximum effect is needed; document and report inadequate pain control.

◆ Monitor for and report GI symptoms that may indicate peptic ulcer (nausea, pain, black stools).

◆ Observe the elderly for toxicity.

Patient & family teaching/Home care

Possible nursing diagnoses: Knowledge deficit; Impaired home maintenance management.

◆ Stress the need to take diflunisal with a full glass of water or milk, or with food to reduce GI symptoms; explain the importance of watching for symptoms of GI bleeding (black stools, persistent GI distress).

◆ Explain that full effects may not be noted for up to 2 weeks.

◆ Warn that use with antacids may reduce effectiveness.

◆ Advise reporting ringing of the ears, rashes, or visual changes.

◆ *See Narcotic and non-narcotic analgesics and Nonsteroidal anti-inflammatory drugs overviews for more information.*

digoxin/digitoxin

di-jox'in

digoxin: **Lanoxicaps, Lanoxin, ♥Novodigoxin**

digitoxin: **Crystodigin**

Class: ★**Cardiac glycoside prototype,** Positive inotrope, Antiarrhythmic

Antidote: digoxin immune FAB

PEDS	PREG	GERI
🖐	C	🖐

Action Increases force of contraction (positive inotropic effect) by inhibiting adenosine triphosphatase (ATPase), thus inhibiting the "sodium pump" and increasing intracellular calcium (calcium increases myocardial contractility). Controls supraventricular tachyarrhythmias by decreasing electrical impulse conduction in the SA and AV nodes. Reduces heart rate by decreasing sympathetic stimulation, increasing myocardial sensitivity to acetylcholine, and increasing vagal tone. A secondary effect is that of increased sodium and water excretion because of improved kidney perfusion.

Use/Therapeutic goal/Outcome

CHF: Improved cardiac output. **Outcome criteria:** Heart and respiratory rate within normal limits; absence of rales and signs and symptoms of CHF; improved activity tolerance; decreased cardiomegaly on chest X ray.

Atrial tachycardia, fibrillation and flutter: Restoration of normal sinus rhythm/control of tachycardia. **Outcome criteria:** Normal sinus rhythm on EKG.

Dose range/Administration

Interaction alert: Quinidine, verapamil, corticosteriods, diuretics and some antibiotics may increase digoxin level. Phenobarbital, phenytoin, antacids, kaolin-pectin, sulfasalazine, neomycin, cholestyramine, colestipol, and certain anti-cancer drugs may interfere with absorption. Beta-blockers and calcium channel blockers may cause additive depressant effect on AV-node conduction. Administration with calcium salts may cause arrhythmias.

Digoxin: Adult/Child > 10 yrs: PO, IV: *Loading dose:* 0.5–1.5 mg divided over 24-hr period. *Maintenance dose:* 0.125–0.5 mg daily or on alternate days. Larger doses may be necessary for treatment of arrhythmias. *The elderly:* 0.0625–0.25 mg/day. **Child 5–10 yrs:** PO: *Loading dose:* 15–35 mcg/kg/day. Half at once, the

remainder divided and given q4-8h. *Maintenance dose:* 25–35% of loading dose qd or divided bid. IV: *Loading dose:* 15–30 mcg/kg/day. Half the dose at once, then divide the remainder q4-8h. *Maintenance dose: 25–35% of loading dose give daily or bid.* **Child 2–5 yrs:** PO: *Loading dose:* 25–40 mcg/kg/day. Half the dose at once, then divide the remainder and give q4-8h. *Maintenance dose:* 25–35% of loading dose divided bid or tid. IV: *Loading dose:* 25–35 mcg/kg/day. Half the dose at once, then divide the remainder and give q4-8h. **Infants:** PO: *Loading dose:* 30–60 mcg/kg/day. Half the dose at once, then divide the remainder and give q4-8h. *Maintenance dose:* 25–35% of loading dose divided bid or tid. IV: *Loading dose:* 30–50 mcg/kg/day. Half the dose at once, then divide the remainder and give q4-8h. **Premature infants:** PO: *Loading dose:* 15–35 mcg/kg/day. Half the dose at once, then divide the remainder and give q4-8h. *Maintenance dose:* 20–30% of loading dose q24h. IV: *Loading dose:* 15–25 mcg/kg/day. Half the dose at once, then divide the remainder and give q4-8h. *Maintenance dose:* 20–30% of loading dose.

Digitoxin: Adult: PO: *Loading dose (rapid):* 0.6 mg; followed in 4–6 hr by 0.4 mg, then 0.2 mg in another 4–6 hrs. *Loading dose (gradual):* 0.2 mg bid for 4 days. *Maintenance dose:* 0.05 mg to 0.3 mg daily.

Clinical alert: Document apical pulse before administration; if < 60, or > 120, withhold drug and notify physician. Hold dose and report if PR interval > 0.24 seconds or if serum digoxin level > 2 ng/ml, or if digitoxin level > 35 ng/ml. Give IV doses slowly, over at least 5 min. Doses are highly individualized and adjusted according to clinical response, serum digoxin or digitoxin level, and serum potassium, magnesium, and calcium levels. Absorption of PO and IM digoxin is usually incomplete, and PO and IM doses are usually 20% higher than IV dose, depending on brand and formulation. **IM route is not recommended** because of injury to muscle and severe pain at injection site.

Contraindications/Precautions
PREG
C

Contraindicated in hypersensitivity to digoxin or digitalis, in ventricular fibrillation, with calcium administration, signs of digitalis toxicity, or serum digoxin level > 2 ng/ml, or serum digitoxin level > 35 ng/ml. **Use with caution** with digitalized patient undergoing elective cardioversion (Drug is often withheld 1–2 days prior to cardioversion to avoid development of ventricular arrhythmia. *Do not cardiovert if digitalis toxicity is suspected.*) **Use with caution** in the presence of acute myocardial infarction, heart block, constrictive pericarditis, cardiomyopathy, renal impairment, hypothyroidism, hypokalemia, and severe lung disease.

Use with caution for children, pregnant and nursing mothers, and the elderly.

Side effects/Adverse reactions

Hypersensitivity: rash. **CV:** premature ventricular contractions, junctional tachycardia, supraventricular arrhythmias, AV block, hypotension, bradycardia. **CNS:** weakness, fatigue, hallucinations, agitation, headaches, confusion, depression, malaise, dizziness, stupor, paresthesias. **Eye:** blurred vision, snowflakes, yellow-green halos around visual images (may be toxicity). **GI:** anorexia and nausea (these may be a sign of impending toxicity), vomiting, diarrhea, pain. **Hem:** blood dyscrasias. **Misc:** gynecomastia.

Nursing implications/Documentation

Possible nursing diagnoses: Activity intolerance; Fluid volume excess.

♦ Be sure to check baseline chest X ray, EKG, and laboratory studies (CBC, sodium, potassium, chloride, carbon dioxide, magnesium, BUN, creatinine, SGPT, and LDH) before giving first dose; monitor closely thereafter as indicated by clinical condition.

♦ Be aware that electrolyte imbalances (especially potassium), serum pH imbalances, and decreased oxygen saturation should be corrected to promote optimal effects.

♦ Document baseline respiration, lung sounds, heart rate, rhythm, and blood pressure before starting digoxin (post monitor strip on chart if available); monitor closely as indicated by condition.

♦ Assess apical-radial pulse for a full minute and document changes in rate, development of a pulse deficit, irregular rhythm, or regularization of previously irregular rhythm.

♦ Observe for and report signs of toxicity (heart rate < 60, nausea, vomiting, anorexia, or visual green halos); also monitor for abnormal serum level (0.9 to 2 ng/ml digoxin is therapeutic, 26–43 ng/ml digitoxin is therapeutic).

♦ Recognize that hypokalemia increases risk of digitalis toxicity.

♦ Coordinate care to provide frequent rest periods.

♦ Be aware that digoxin and digitoxin may produce false positive EKG changes during exercise testing.

Patient & family teaching/Home care

Possible nursing diagnoses: Knowledge deficit; Impaired home maintenance management.

♦ Explain that the purpose of this drug is to regulate and improve the pumping action of the heart.

♦ Stress that sudden weight gain, ankle edema, increasing cough or shortness of breath, or signs of toxicity (nausea, vomiting, seeing green halos) should be reported immediately.

♦ Teach how to assess pulse for decreased pulse rate, increased pulse rate, or pulse irregularities; stress that pulse < 60, or > 100, or increase in pulse irregularities should be reported.

♦ If taking diuretics, explain the need to maintain adequate potassium intake; obtain a list of foods that are high in potassium from dietician.

♦ Warn against substituting one brand of drug for another.

♦ *See Antiarrhythmics overview for more information.*

digoxin immune FAB *di-jox'in*

Digibind
Class: Antidote for digitalis toxicity

PEDS	PREG	GERI
♨	C	♨

Action Binds with molecules of digitalis, either digoxin or digitoxin, thus preventing them from binding at their site of action.

Use/Therapeutic goal/Outcome

Resolution of digitalis toxicity. **Outcome criteria:** Serum digoxin level within normal limits (0.9 to 2 ng/ml); or serum digitoxin level within normal limits (26–43 ng/ml).

Dose range/Administration

Adult: IV: 400–800 mg over 30 min. Bolus may be necessary if cardiac arrest is imminent. **Infants:** IV: 0.5 mg to 160 mg, depending upon weight in kg and serum drug levels. (Check package insert.)

Clinical alert: Use 0.22-micron filter. Place patient on continuous cardiac monitoring and have resuscitative equipment and drugs nearby before giving first dose.

Contraindications/Precautions

PREG
C

Contraindicated in hypersensitivity to sheep protein.

☙ **Use with caution for children and the elderly, and for those previously treated with this drug. Safe use for pregnant or nursing mothers has not been established (if toxicity is severe, use would be appropriate because the lives of both mother and infant are jeopardized).**

Side effects/Adverse reactions

Hypersensitivity: febrile reaction. *CV:* decreased cardiac output, atrial tachyarrhythmias. *Hem:* hypokalemia.

Nursing implications/Documentation

Possible nursing diagnoses: Potential for injury; Activity intolerance.

◆ Be aware that hypokalemia may aggravate effects of digitalis toxicity.

◆ Check serum digoxin or digitoxin level before giving digoxin immune fab (therapeutic levels are 0.9–2 ng/ml) for digoxin; 26–43 ng/ml for digitoxin).

◆ Document cardiac monitor strip at least every 8 hr and as significant changes are noted; record PR- and QRS-interval measurements at least every 8 hr (more frequently if necessary).

◆ Monitor for and report early signs of CHF (rales, fluid retention, difficulty breathing).

◆ Coordinate care to provide frequent rest periods.

Patient & family teaching/Home care

Possible nursing diagnoses: Knowledge deficit; Impaired home maintenance management.

◆ Explain that the purpose of this drug is to treat the adverse effects of having too much digitalis in the blood.

◆ Explore factors that may have contributed to overdosage; identify ways of preventing this in the future.

---

dye-hye-droe-er-got'a-meen
dihydroergotamine

dihydroergotamine mesylate: **D.H.E. 45, ☙Dihyder-got**

Class: Alpha-adrenergic blocker (sympathomimetic)

PEDS	PREG	GERI
☙	X	☙

Action Believed to relieve vascular headache by constricting blood vessels through inhibition of the effect of sympathomimetic amines (epinephrine, norepinephrine) at alpha-adrenergic receptor sites. Also has antiserotonin effects (serotonin is a potent vasodilator, which is implicated in the etiology of vascular headaches).

Use/Therapeutic goal/Outcome

Vascular headaches (short-term treatment): Relief of migraine headaches. *Outcome criteria:* Report of headache relief.

Dose range/Administration

Interaction alert: Use with oral contraceptives may cause increased breakthrough bleeding and increased risk of pregnancy.

Adult: IM, IV: 1 mg; may repeat q1h. *Maximum dose:* 3 mg/day or 6 mg/wk.

Clinical alert: Give dose at first sign of onset of migraine for optimum effect. Doses should be individualized to give minimum effective dose.

Contraindications/Precautions

PREG
X

Contraindicated in hypersensitivity to ergot preparations, and in peripheral vascular disease, coronary artery disease, hypertension, renal and hepatic dysfunction, and sepsis.

☙ **Contraindicated for pregnant or nursing mothers. Use with caution for the elderly. Safe use for children under 10 years has not been established.**

Side effects/Adverse reactions

Hypersensitivity: itching. *CV:* vasoconstriction, numbness and tingling in fingers and toes, chest pain, tachycardia or bradycardia. *GI:* nausea, vomiting. *MS:* muscle pain and weakness in extremities.

Nursing implications/Documentation

Possible nursing diagnoses: Pain; Ineffective individual coping.

◆ Have patient rate pain of headaches on a scale of 1–10.

◆ Identify dietary, emotional, physical, and environmental factors that precipitate or aggravate headaches.

◆ Provide a dark, quiet environment and holistic measures that promote comfort (e.g., cool washcloth for forehead).

Patient & family teaching/Home care

Possible nursing diagnoses: Ineffective individual coping; Impaired home maintenance management.

◆ Stress the need to treat headache as soon after onset as possible.

◆ Explore ways of avoiding stress, coping with stress, and eliminating environmental factors that trigger headaches.

◆ Teach holistic measures for relieving pain (e.g., relaxation techniques).

◆ Advise reporting numbness or tingling of fingers and toes (may be due to excessive vasoconstriction, which can be harmful).

◆ Point out that tobacco and alcohol should be avoided.

diltiazem   *dil-ti'a-zem*

Cardizem, Cardizem SR

Class: Antianginal, Calcium channel blocking agent, Antihypertensive, Antimigraine, Antiarrhythmic

PEDS	PREG	GERI
🖐	C	🖐

Action Inhibits calcium ion influx across the cell membrane, which results in increased availability of oxygen to the myocardium (by dilating coronary arteries) and decreased workload and oxygen demand of the heart (by reducing heart rate and force of contraction). Vasodilation causes a drop in blood pressure and systemic vascular resistance (afterload). Action in migraine is unclear.

Use/Therapeutic goal/Outcome

Angina pectoris: Promotion of myocardial oxygenation, reduction in myocardial oxygen demand, prevention of anginal (ischemic) attacks, improved activity tolerance. **Outcome criteria:** Patient reports decreased frequency and severity of anginal attacks, and increased activity tolerance.

Hypertension: Reduction in blood pressure. **Outcome criteria:** Blood pressure within normal limits.

Dose range/Administration

Interaction alert: Concomitant use with beta-blockers and digitalis glycosides may prolong cardiac conduction. May increase serum levels of digoxin (monitor closely). Use with antihypertensives and beta-blockers may cause hypotension. Cimetidine may decrease diltiazem metabolism (monitor for toxicity).

◩ **Give doses before meals and at bedtime.**

Adult: PO: 30–90 mg tid and at bedtime. Dose may be increased at 1–2 day intervals until optimum relief of pain is achieved. Should not exceed 360 mg/day. *Sustained release form:* Begin with 60–120 mg bid; adjust to 240–360 mg bid. The elderly may require lower dosages.

Clinical alert: Check pulse, blood pressure, and respiration before giving dose. Do not give in the presence of hypotension or bradycardia.

Contraindications/Precautions
PREG
C

Contraindicated in hypersensitivity to the drug, and in sick sinus syndrome, second- or third-degree heart block (unless a ventricular pacemaker is in place), when systolic blood pressure less than 90 mm Hg, heart rate less than 60, and in renal or hepatic failure. **Use with caution** in congestive heart failure (CHF), especially when a beta- blocker is also being used.

🖐 **Use with caution for the elderly. Safe use for pregnant or nursing mothers or for children has not been established.**

Side effects/Adverse reactions

Hypersensitivity: urticaria, pruritis. **CV:** CHF, arrhythmias, hypotension, palpitations, bradycardia, conduction abnormalities, flushing, edema. **CNS:** headache, syncope, drowsiness, fatigue, dizziness, nervousness, depression, insomnia, confusion, paresthesia, tremor. **GI:** nausea, dyspepsia, vomiting, diarrhea, constipation, transient elevation of liver enzymes. **GU:** polyuria, nocturia. **Skin:** petechiae; rash (may disappear even with continued use, but may progress to erythema multiforme or exfoliative dermatitis). **Eye:** photosensitivity.

Nursing implications/Documentation

Possible nursing diagnoses: Potential for injury; Activity intolerance.

◆ Keep a record of pulse and blood pressure before and after drug administration.

- Observe for postural hypotension; take blood pressure in both arms, and with patient sitting and standing, if possible.
- Supervise ambulation until response to drug has been determined.
- Coordinate care to provide frequent rest periods.

Patient & family teaching/Home care

Possible nursing diagnoses: Fear; Knowledge deficit; Impaired home maintenance management.

- Advise taking with meals to reduce GI upset.
- Explain that this drug controls blood pressure and reduces the workload of the heart.
- Stress the need to follow dose regimen closely—take the dose at the same times every day—and the need to return for medical follow-up.
- Advise changing positions slowly to avoid dizziness.
- Warn against taking any other drugs without checking with primary physician.
- If possible, teach the patient to self-monitor blood pressure and pulse; stress that persistent hypotension, hypertension, pulse irregularities, or dizziness should be reported.
- *See Antianginals, Calcium Channel Blockers, and Antihypertensives overviews for more information.*

dimenhydrinate
dye-men-hye'dri-nate

♠Andrumin, ♣Apo-Dimenhydrinate, Calm-X, Dimentabs, Dinate, Dommanate, Dramamine, Dramamine Chewable, Dramamine Liquid, Dramanate, Dramilin, Dramocen, Dramoject, Dymenate, ♣Gravol, Hydrate, Marmine, Motion-Aid, ♣Nauseatol, ♣Novodimenate, PMS-Dymenhydrinate, Reidamine, Tega-Vert, ♣Travamine, ♠Travs, Triptone Caplets, Wehamine

Class: Antiemetic, Antihistamine, Antivertigo agent, Sedative-hypnotic

PEDS	PREG	GERI
♨	B	♨

Action Relieves and prevents dizziness, nausea, and vomiting caused by motion, possibly by affecting neural pathways originating in the labyrinth (exact action unknown).

Use/Therapeutic goal/Outcome

Dizziness or motion sickness: Prevention or resolution of dizziness, nausea, and vomiting.

Outcome criteria: Report of absence of, or reduction in, feelings of dizziness and nausea with motion; absence of vomiting.

Dose range/Administration

Interaction alert: Because of CNS depressant effects, may increase effects of CNS depressants and alcohol. May mask ototoxicity caused by antibiotics. Do not mix parenteral preparation with other drugs.

🍎 **Give with food, milk, or full glass of water to minimize GI upset.**

Adult: PO: 50–100 mg q4h. RECT: 100 mg/day or bid. IM: 50 mg prn, not to exceed 300 mg/day. IV: 50 mg diluted in 10 ml NaCl injected over 2 min. **Child > 2 yrs:** PO, IM: 5 mg/kg/day, not to exceed 150 mg/day, in four equally divided doses.

Clinical alert: Give doses 30–60 min before travel, before meals, and at bedtime. Use parenteral solution only if absolutely clear; dilute solution for IV administration because it is very irritating to venous walls and may cause sclerosis.

Contraindications/Precautions
PREG
B

Contraindicated in hypersensitivity to dimenhydrinate. **Use with caution** in the presence of narrow-angle glaucoma, prostatic hypertrophy, seizure disorders.

🖐 **Contraindicated for infants under two years. Use with caution for the elderly. Safe use for pregnant or nursing mothers has not been established.**

Side effects/Adverse reactions

Hypersensitivity: extreme drowsiness, hypotension. **CNS:** dizziness, headache, drowsiness, poor coordination, nervousness, restlessness, insomnia (especially in children). **GI:** dry mucus membranes, anorexia, constipation, diarrhea. **CV:** hypotension, palpitations. **Eye:** blurred vision. **Ear:** ringing of the ears. **GU:** urinary frequency, dysuria, urinary retention.

Nursing implications/Documentation

Possible nursing diagnoses: Potential for injury; Altered nutrition: less than body requirements; Fluid volume deficit; Altered oral mucous membranes.

- Assess for presence of bowel sounds, pain, nausea, or vomiting before and after administering dimenhydrinate; hold drug and report if bowel sounds are absent.

♦ Determine cause of symptoms before giving antiemetics; ascertain that nausea and vomiting symptoms are not due to intestinal obstruction, increased intracranial pressure, or drug overdosage before giving first dose.

♦ Offer frequent mouth care.

♦ Supervise ambulation until response is determined.

♦ Document and monitor intake and output to detect dehydration.

♦ When able to tolerate liquids, begin with small amount of ice chips, then water, then clear liquids, then full liquids, then food.

Patient & family teaching/Home care

Possible nursing diagnoses: Knowledge deficit; Impaired home maintenance management.

♦ For treatment of motion sickness, teach that the drug should be taken 1 hr before travel.

♦ Stress that persistent nausea, vomiting, or abdominal discomfort should be reported.

♦ Explain that avoiding fatty foods and eating smaller and more frequent meals may reduce nausea.

♦ Advise against using alcohol or other CNS depressants.

♦ Point out that symptoms of drowsiness are likely to diminish after several days use; warn against driving or activities that require mental alertness until response is established.

♦ Emphasize the need to maintain good mouth care, especially when not taking liquids by mouth.

♦ Suggest that chewing sugarless gum may relieve symptoms of dry mouth.

♦ *See Antiemetics overview for more information.*

dinoprostone

dye-noe-prost'one

Prostin E₂

Class: Oxytocic, Prostaglandin, Abortifacient

PEDS	PREG	GERI
♨	C	♨

Action Produces strong uterine contractions, promoting elimination of uterine contents, by acting directly on the myometrium. Exact mechanism of action has not been determined. More effective in the second trimester of pregnancy than oxytocin.

Use/Therapeutic goal/Outcome

Second trimester abortion, missed abortion, intrauterine fetal death (up to 28 weeks gestation), benign hydatidaform mole: Stimulation of uterine contractions; expulsion of uterine contents. **Outcome criteria:** Within 30 hours, delivery of fetus and placenta; delivery of hydatidaform mole tissue.

Dose range/Administration

Interaction alert: Alcohol (IV or PO) may inhibit uterine activity. Other oxytocics may increase contractions and risk of uterine rupture or cervical laceration.

Adult: *Vaginal:* One 20 mg vaginal suppository inserted high in vagina (bring suppository to room temperature); may repeat q3-4h until abortion complete or labor initiated. *Maximum dose:* 240 mg; do not use for more than 2 days.

Clinical alert: This drug should be administered only in hospitals with intensive care and operating room facilities. A physician should be readily available. Keep the woman supine for 10–15 min after insertion of suppository. Sometimes an antiemetic and antidiarrheal may be ordered before dose is given.

Contraindications/Precautions

PREG
C

Contraindicated in hypersensitivity to dinoprostone or other oxytocics, and in acute pelvic inflammatory disease, infected endocervical lesions, uterine fibroids, cervical stenosis, and cardiac, pulmonary, liver, or kidney disease. **Use with caution** in history of asthma, hypotension, hypertension, anemia, diabetes, epilepsy; cervicitis, acute vaginitis, scarred uterus, or adrenal, kidney, liver, or cardiovascular disease.

♨ **Contraindicated for children and the elderly.**

Side effects/Adverse reactions

Hypersensitivity: rash, pruritus, bronchospasm, wheezing, dyspnea. **CNS:** headache, paresthesias, anxiety, weakness, syncope, dizziness, transient pyrexia (occurs in 50% of all patients), chills. **GI:** nausea, vomiting, diarrhea. **CV:** hypotension (with large doses), bradycardia, tachycardia. **MS:** joint inflammation, nocturnal leg cramps. **GU:** vaginal pain, vaginitis, uterine hypertonus.

Nursing implications/Documentation

Possible nursing diagnoses: Potential for infection; Pain; Impaired skin integrity.

- Follow hospital protocols and physician's orders for frequency of documentation of vital signs, contractions, and character of vaginal drainage; record more frequently if condition is unstable. (Keep in mind that 50% of patients experience a transient, self-limiting fever, sometimes as high as 102° F. This should be treated with sponging, rather than medication.)

- Assist with perineal skin care, especially if diarrhea is present; monitor closely for signs of infection or skin breakdown.

- Have the woman rate comfort level on a scale of 1–10; encourage using relaxation techniques; provide ordered analgesics, and report persistent, severe, unrelieved pain.

Patient & family teaching/Home care

Possible nursing diagnoses: Fear; Knowledge deficit.

- Explain that this drug stimulates labor-like uterine contractions; inform that expulsion of uterine contents usually is complete within 30 hr.

- Instruct the woman to stay in bed for 10–15 min after administration.

- Stress that vital signs, uterine contractions, and vaginal drainage will be monitored closely to ensure patient safety.

- Encourage both the woman and the labor coach to ask questions and verbalize fears or concerns.

- Teach the woman to report any sudden increase in discomfort or vaginal drainage.

diphenhydramine
dye-fen-hye'dra-meen

♣Allerdryl, AllerMax, Beldin, Belix, Bena-D, Bena-D 50, Benadryl, Benadryl Complete Allergy, Benahist 10, Benahist 50, Ben-Allergen 50, Benaphen, Benoject-10, Benoject-50, Benylin Cough, ♣Benylin Dietetic, ♣Benylin Expectorant, ♣Benylin Pediatric, Bydramine Cough, Compoz Diahist, Dihydrex, Diphenacen-50, Diphenadryl, Diphen Cough, Diphenhist, Dormarex 2, Fenylhist, Fynex, Hydramine, Hydramyn, Hydril, ♣Insomnal, Nervine Nighttime Sleep-Aid, Noradryl, Nordryl, Nytol with DPH, Sleep-Eze 3, Sominex, Sominex Liquid, Tusstat, Twilite, Valdrene, Wehdryl

Class: ★Antihistamine (H₁ receptor antagonist) prototype, Antivertigo, Antiemetic, Antitussive, Antiparkinson agent, Sedative-hypnotic

PEDS	PREG	GERI
🤚	C	🤚

Action Prevents but does not reverse histamine-mediated allergic responses by competing with histamine at the H₁ receptors especially those on smooth muscles of the bronchial tubes, GI tract, uterus, and blood vessels. Effects against parkinsonism and drug-induced extrapyramidal symptoms are apparently due to antagonism of cholinergic activity in the CNS. Suppresses the cough reflex by acting directly on the medulla. Acts as a sedative by depressing the CNS, and as a local anesthetic by preventing initiation and transmission of nerve impulses.

Use/Therapeutic goal/Outcome

Allergic conditions: Decrease in allergic response. **Outcome criteria:** Report and demonstration of relief of allergic symptoms (nasal secretions, sneezing, itching).

Sedation: Promotion of sleep, relaxation. **Outcome criteria:** Report of feeling relaxed or having slept well; observable relaxation or sleep.

Mild parkinsonism: Relief of mild symptoms. **Outcome criteria:** Demonstration of a decrease in excessive salivation, reduction in frequency and severity of rigidity and akinesia.

Motion sickness: Prevention or relief of nausea. **Outcome criteria:** Report of decreased frequency and severity of nausea episodes.

Nonproductive cough: Suppression of cough reflex. **Outcome criteria:** Report and demonstration of a decrease in coughing.

Dose range/Administration

Interaction alert: Use with CNS depressants or alcohol may cause excessive drowsiness. Do not give with MAOIs or anticholinergics.

🍴 Give with food or milk to reduce GI distress, unless given for motion sickness or as an antiemetic.

Allergies, motion sickness, parkinsonian symptoms: Adult/Child > 12 yrs: PO: 25–50 mg tid to qid, not to exceed 400 mg/day. IM, IV: 10–50 mg, to a maximum of 400 mg/day. **Child < 12 yrs:** PO, IM, IV: 5 mg/kg/day, in divided doses qid; maximum dose for children over 20 lb is 300 mg/day.

Sedation: Adult: PO, IM: 50 mg at bedtime, or 25–50 mg q4h prn, to a maximum of 400 mg/day.

Nonproductive Cough: Adult/Child > 12 yrs: PO: 25 mg q4h, to a maximum of 100 mg/day.

Child 6–12 yrs: PO: 12.5 mg q4h, to a maximum of 50 mg/day. **Child 2–6 yrs:** PO: 6.25 mg q4h, to a maximum of 25 mg/day.

Clinical alert: Expect reduced dosage for the elderly, and monitor closely for drowsiness and dizziness. This drug is the strongest sedative antihistamine. Children under 12 years should be given this drug only under direction of a physician. May give undiluted IV doses slowly. If given for motion sickness, give 30 min before travel.

Contraindications/Precautions
PREG C

Contraindicated in hypersensitivity to diphenhydramine or to chemically related antihistamines, and in acute asthma, and MAOI therapy. **Use with extreme caution** in narrow-angle glaucoma, prostatic hypertrophy, bladder-neck obstruction, stenosing peptic ulcer or GI obstruction. **Use with caution** in history of asthma, convulsive disorders, CNS depression, increased intraocular pressure, hyperthyroidism, hypertension, cardiovascular disease, and diabetes mellitus.

✋ **Contraindicated for premature infants, newborns, and nursing mothers. Use with caution for the elderly. Safe use in pregnancy and in children under 2 years has not been established.**

Side effects/Adverse reactions

Hypersensitivity: skin rash, urticaria, photosensitivity, anaphylaxis. **CNS:** drowsiness (high incidence), dizziness, headache, disturbed coordination, tingling, heaviness and weakness of hands, tremors, euphoria, nervousness, restlessness, insomnia, confusion, and (especially in children) hallucinations, excitement, fever, convulsions, coma. **CV:** palpitation, tachycardia, mild hypotension or hypertension. **Ear:** tinnitus, acute labyrinthitis, vertigo. **Resp:** dry nose and throat, nasal stuffiness, thickened bronchial secretions, wheezing, sensation of chest tightness. **GI:** dry mouth, epigastric distress, anorexia, nausea, vomiting, constipation, diarrhea. **GU:** urinary frequency or retention, dysuria.

Nursing implications/Documentation

Possible nursing diagnoses: Potential for injury; Fluid volume deficit.

♦ Determine and record known allergies; provide an environment that is free from allergens (especially sleeping areas).

♦ Provide favorite fluids and ensure adequate hydration (2 liters/day).

♦ With IV route, document blood pressure before and after dose.

♦ Recognize that this drug is a common component of OTC medications taken for insomnia, colds, and allergic responses.

Patient & family teaching/Home care

Possible nursing diagnoses: Knowledge deficit; Impaired home maintenance management.

♦ Advise taking this drug with food or milk if GI symptoms are experienced; if for motion sickness, advise taking on an empty stomach 30 min before travel, and before meals.

♦ Emphasize that dose should not be increased without physician's approval; explain that tolerance may occur, requiring a change in medication.

♦ Explain that the side effect of drowsiness should diminish after a few days of treatment.

♦ Warn that alcohol and other CNS depressants may cause excessive drowsiness; advise against driving until response is determined.

♦ Point out that avoiding pollens and staying in an air-conditioned environment may help reduce seasonal rhinitis.

♦ Suggest that coffee or tea may reduce drowsiness, and that sugarless gum or hard candy may relieve dry mouth.

♦ If used for sedation, explore reasons for insomnia and teach holistic ways of promoting sleep (see Antianxiety Agents, Sedatives, and Hypnotics classification overview).

♦ Explain that antihistamines should be stopped for 4 days before allergy testing to ensure accurate results.

♦ *See Antihistamines, Antianxiety agents, Sedatives, and Hypnotics, and Antiemetics overviews for more information.*

diphenoxylate

dye-fen-ox'i-late

diphenoxylate and atropine: **Diphenatol, Lofene, Logen, Lomanate, Lomotil, Lonox, Lo-Trol, Low-Quel, Nor-Mil**

Class: Antidiarrheal

Antidote: Naloxone for respiratory depression

PEDS	PREG	GERI	CONTROLLED SUBSTANCE
🖐	C	🖐	V

Action Diphenoxylate reduces intestinal motility by local and central action; atropine is present in subtherapeutic levels to discourage deliberate abuse.

Use/Therapeutic goal/Outcome

Diarrhea: Symptomatic control of acute and chronic diarrhea. **Outcome criteria:** Decreased frequency and liquid volume of bowel evacuations.

Dose range/Administration

Interaction alert: Increased CNS depression with sedatives, tranquilizers, narcotics, or alcohol. MAOIs may cause hypertensive crisis. Other anticholinergics increase effects. Naltrexone may block antidiarrheal effect and/or cause withdrawal symptoms.

Adult: PO: 2.5–5 mg bid to qid. **Child > 2 yrs:** PO: 0.3–0.4 mg/kg/day in 4 divided doses.

Clinical alert: Available in both tablet and liquid forms; use special dropper provided with liquid form to measure dose. Monitor young children for increased effects of atropine.

Contraindications/Precautions
PREG C

Contraindicated in hypersensitivity to any narcotic or anticholinergic, in jaundice, or for diarrhea caused by antibiotic-associated pseudomembranous colitis, infectious organisms, or poisoning. **Use with caution** in renal or hepatic impairment, dehydration, prostatic hypertrophy, urinary retention, glaucoma; respiratory, cardiovascular, or gallbladder disease; hypertension, hypothyroidism, hyperthyroidism, acute ulcerative colitis, intestinal atony, myasthenia gravis, and history of drug abuse.

🖐 **Contraindicated for infants under 2 years. Use with caution for pregnant or nursing mothers and the elderly.**

Side effects/Adverse reactions

Hypersensitivity: rash, itching, swelling of gums. **GI:** bloating, constipation, loss of appetite, nausea, vomiting, stomach pain, paralytic ileus, toxic megacolon, dry mouth. **CNS:** drowsiness, dizziness, mental depression, excitement, irritability. **Eye:** blurred vision. **Resp:** severe shortness of breath, respiratory depression. **CV:** rapid heart rate. **GI:** severe dryness of mouth, nose, and throat. **GU:** difficulty urinating. **Skin:** warmth, dryness, flushing. **Misc:** physical dependence after chronic use.

Nursing implications/Documentation

Possible nursing diagnoses: Constipation; Potential for injury.

♦ Monitor and record bowel sounds and frequency and consistency of stools.

♦ Expect acute diarrhea to improve within 48 hr; chronic diarrhea should improve within 10 days.

♦ Identify, report, and document signs of dehydration, especially in young children; dehydration may predispose to delayed diphenoxylate intoxication.

♦ Observe for respiratory depression, especially in children and the elderly.

♦ Monitor for anticholinergic effects, especially in children (urinary retention, blurred vision, fever, dryness of skin and mouth).

♦ Assess for symptoms of paralytic ileus or toxic megacolon (abdominal distention, constipation, loss of appetite, nausea and vomiting, stomach pain), especially in history of ulcerative colitis.

♦ Provide increased fluid intake and/or frequent mouth care to relieve dry mouth.

Patient & family teaching/Home care

Possible nursing diagnoses: Knowledge deficit; Potential for injury; Impaired home maintenance management.

♦ Caution against taking more than the prescribed amount or making up missed doses.

♦ Stress the importance of avoiding use of alcohol and other CNS depressants while taking diphenoxylate and atropine.

♦ Advise reporting if acute diarrhea does not diminish after 2 days, or if fever develops.

- ◆ Explain the need to avoid driving and operating dangerous machinery until response to drug has been determined.
- ◆ Point out the need for immediate medical attention if overdose is suspected.
- ◆ Warn that prolonged use may lead to physical dependence and tolerance to antidiarrheal effects.

dipyridamole
dye-peer-id'a-mole

♣*Apo-Dypyridamole, ♣Persantin, Persantine*
Class: Antiplatelet agent, Vasodilator

PEDS	PREG	GERI
♨	C	♨

Action Selectively dilates small resistance vessels of coronary vascular bed, possibly by causing accumulation of adenosine diphosphate (ADP), which produces vasodilation and reduces platelet adherence.

Use/Therapeutic goal/Outcome

Platelet adhesion in prosthetic heart valves, transient ischemic attacks: Prevention of thrombus formation or transient ischemic attacks. *Outcome criteria:* Absence of signs of thrombosis or transient ischemic attacks.

Dose range/Administration

Interaction alert: Enhances the effects of oral anticoagulants and heparin.

▯ **Give on an empty stomach unless GI symptoms are noted (then give with food).**
Inhibition of platelet adhesion: Adult: PO: 75–100 mg qid.
Transient ischemic attacks: Adult: PO: 400–800 mg daily in divided doses.

Contraindications/Precautions

PREG
C

Contraindicated in hypersensitivity to dipyridamole, acute myocardial infarction, and unstable angina. *Use with caution* in hypotension and concomitant anticoagulant therapy.
♨ **Use with caution for the elderly. Safe use for children and pregnant women has not been established.**

Side effects/Adverse reactions

Hypersensitivity: skin rash. *GI:* nausea, vomiting, and diarrhea. *CNS:* headache, dizziness, weakness. *CV:* peripheral vasodilation, flushing; excessive dosages may produce hypotension.

Nursing implications/Documentation

Possible nursing diagnoses: Activity intolerance; Pain.

- ◆ Document baseline circulatory status (presence and quality of peripheral pulses, skin color and temperature), and activity tolerance; monitor periodically thereafter.
- ◆ Monitor for dizziness and hypotension, especially when using high doses; supervise ambulation until response is determined.
- ◆ Observe for and report unusual bleeding (bruising, blood in urine or stools).

Patient & family teaching/Home care

Possible nursing diagnoses: Knowledge deficit; Impaired home maintenance management.

- ◆ Advise taking this drug on an empty stomach unless GI symptoms are noted (then may take with food).
- ◆ Stress that improvement in symptoms is usually gradual with dipyridamole, and that long-term therapy is necessary for optimal effects.
- ◆ Explain the need to change positions slowly to reduce dizziness; point out that side effects usually subside after a few weeks of therapy.
- ◆ *See Antianginals overview for more information.*

disopyramide
dye-soe-peer'a-mide

disopyramide: *Rhythmodan*
disopyramide phosphate: *Napamide, Norpace, Norpace CR, ♣Rythmodan LA*
Class: Antiarrhythmic (Class IA)

PEDS	PREG	GERI
♨	C	♨

Action Suppresses ventricular ectopy by prolonging the action potential and effective refractory period of atria, Purkinje fibers, and ventricles, and by increasing the threshold of excitability while reducing conduction velocity of the myocardium. Has anticholinergic, vagolytic, and negative inotropic effects.

Use/Therapeutic goal/Outcome

Premature ventricular contractions and nonsustained ventricular tachycardia: Suppression of ventricular ectopy, promotion of effective heartbeat. *Outcome criteria:* Absence of or decrease in ventricular ectopy on EKG; regular palpable pulses.

Dose range/Administration

Interaction alert: Use caution when given with antihypertensives, beta-blockers, calcium channel blockers, anticoagulants, and anticholinergics because of potential increased effects. Use with other antiarrhythmics may cause conduction disturbances.

Adult: PO: *Loading dose:* 300 mg, then 150–200 mg q6h; total 400–800 mg/day, < 400 mg/day for patients < 50 kg or who have impaired kidney, liver, or cardiac function. *Maintenance dose:* 100–200 mg q6h (available in capsules and suspension, and sustained-release capsules given q12h). In the presence of renal disease, dosage depends upon creatinine clearance: for 30–40 cc/min, give 100 mg q8h, for 15–30 cc/min, give 100 mg q12h, for 15 cc/min, give 100 mg q24h. ***Child:*** PO: Divide dose and give q6h. *< 1 yr:* 10–30 mg/kg/day. *1–4 yrs:* 10–20 mg/kg/day. *4–12 yrs:* 10–15 mg/kg/day. *12–18 yrs:* 6–15 mg/kg/day.

Clinical alert: Hold drug and report if heart rate is < 60/min or > 120/min. Place patient on continuous cardiac monitoring before initiating therapy. Hold drug and report if patient shows signs of CHF, if heart block develops, or if the QRS complex widens by more than 25 percent above baseline.

Contraindications/Precautions

PREG
C

Contraindicated in hypersensitivity to disopyramide, and in cardiogenic shock, conduction defects, or advanced heart block without the presence of a pacemaker. Avoid use in the presence of CHF. *Use with caution* in the presence of history of CHF, cardiomyopathy, urinary tract disease (especially prostatic hypertrophy), myasthenia gravis, glaucoma, or hepatic or renal impairment.

✋ **Use with caution for the elderly. Safe use for children and pregnant or nursing mothers has not been established.**

Side effects/Adverse reactions

Hypersensitivity: Allergic reactions are not listed. *CV:* hypotension, chest pain, dyspnea, CHF, heart block, conduction defects. *CNS:* dizziness, fatigue, syncope, insomnia, nervousness, depression. *GU:* urinary retention (especially with benign prostatic hypertrophy), impotence. *GI:* dry mouth, diarrhea, vomiting, abdominal pain, constipation. *Hem:* hypoglycemia, agranulocytosis. *Skin:* edema. *Eye:* blurry vision. *MS:* muscle weakness.

Nursing implications/Documentation

Possible nursing diagnoses: Potential for injury; Activity intolerance; Constipation; Altered patterns of urinary elimination.

◆ Be sure to check baseline chest X-ray, EKG, and laboratory studies (CBC, sodium, potassium, chloride, carbon dioxide, magnesium, BUN, creatinine, SGPT, and LDH) before giving first dose; monitor closely thereafter as indicated by clinical condition.

◆ Remember that oxygen requirements must be met, and that electrolyte imbalances (especially potassium and magnesium) and abnormal blood pH must be corrected, before expected antiarrhythmic effect can be seen; report abnormalities immediately.

◆ Document baseline vital signs, lung sounds, and cardiac monitor strip (measure and record PR, QRS, and QT segments) before giving first dose and at least every 8 hr; monitor closely until response is determined; report if prolongation in PR, QRS, or QT segment is noted.

◆ Monitor bowel elimination closely and provide adequate hydration and fiber intake; give laxative before problem becomes severe.

◆ Observe for urinary retention (anticholinergic effect).

◆ Supervise ambulation until response is determined.

◆ If dry mouth is experienced, provide special mouth care.

◆ Coordinate care to provide frequent rest periods.

Patient & family teaching/Home care

Possible nursing diagnoses: Fear; Knowledge deficit; Impaired home maintenance management.

◆ Explain that the purpose of this drug is to prevent arrhythmias and promote an effective heartbeat.

◆ Stress the need to follow dose regimen closely (the drug should be taken at the same time each day), and the need to return for medical follow-up for early detection of adverse reactions.

◆ Teach how to assess pulse for irregularities in rhythm and rate; stress that irregularities be reported.

◆ Stress that urinary retention, sudden weight gain, or shortness of breath should be reported immediately.

- Emphasize the need to pace activities, avoid stress, and plan for rest periods.

- Encourage learning CPR; reinforce that survival rate of cardiac arrest is greatly increased when CPR is initiated immediately.

- *See Antiarrhythmics overview for more information.*

disulfiram

dye-sul'fi-ram

Antabuse, Cronetal, Ro-Sulfiram

Class: Enzyme inhibitor, Alcohol deterrent

PEDS	PREG	GERI
🖐	X	🖐

Action Inhibits oxidation of alcohol, causing increased acetaldehyde blood levels, which results in the highly unpleasant *disulfiram reaction* (flushing, pounding headache, violent nausea and vomiting, thirst, sweating, fainting, weakness, anxiety, blurred vision, confusion, chest pain, palpitations, difficulty breathing, hypotension). *In severe reactions,* the patient may experience respiratory depression, arrhythmias, CHF, myocardial infarction, cardiovascular collapse, respiratory depression, seizures, unconsciousness, and even death. The reaction normally lasts 30 minutes to several hours, until alcohol is metabolized.

Use/Therapeutic goal/Outcome

Chronic alcoholism: Deterrence of desire for alcohol. *Outcome criteria:* Absence of disulfiram reaction; abstinence from alcohol.

Dose range/Administration

Interaction alert: May cause violent reaction if the person has ingested alcohol (even in small amounts) within the previous 12 hr. May cause psychosis if taken with metronidazole or isoniazid. Increases effects of anticoagulants, TCAs, diazepam, phenytoin (may lead to toxicity). Vitamin C may decrease disulfiram's effectiveness as an alcohol deterrent. Concurrent use with paraldehyde not recommended.

Adult: PO: For the first 1–2 weeks, give 250–500 mg in the morning or at bedtime (if drowsiness occurs). *Maintenance dose:* 125–500 mg (average is 250 mg) until person demonstrates self-control.

Clinical alert: Obtain *written* patient permission before beginning disulfiram.

Contraindications/Precautions

Contraindicated in hypersensitivity to disulfiram or rubber, and in alcohol intoxication, psychosis, cardiovascular disease. *Use with caution* in the presence of liver or kidney disease, diabetes, epilepsy, hypothyroidism, cerebral damage, elevated serum cholesterol.

🖐 **Contraindicated for pregnant women. Use with caution for the elderly.**

Side effects/Adverse reactions

Hypersensitivity: rashes, dermatitis, acne. *CNS:* fatigue, drowsiness, headache, confusion, depression, peripheral neuritis, polyneuritis. *Eye:* optic neuritis. *Resp:* dyspnea, respiratory depression. *Hem:* elevated serum cholesterol. *GI:* garlic-like or metallic taste in mouth. *GU:* impotence. *Misc:* mild to severe disulfiram reaction (see action).

Nursing implications/Documentation

Possible nursing diagnoses: Ineffective coping; Altered health maintenance.

- Be sure that the patient has not had any alcohol for 12 hr prior to giving dose.

- Monitor mental status and ability to abstain from alcohol.

- Expect that Vitamin B6 will be ordered to decrease cholesterol levels.

- Be aware that the side effects that are not related to alcohol ingestion should disappear within 2 weeks of therapy.

Patient & family teaching/Home care

Possible nursing diagnoses: Knowledge deficit; Impaired home maintenance management.

- Teach the effects of drinking alcohol while on disulfiram: Warn that a severe reaction (even death) may occur within 15 min, that reactions may occur up to 2 weeks after a single dose of disulfiram, and that with prolonged therapy, disulfiram tolerance does not occur, but the patient's sensitivity to alcohol actually *increases.*

- Reinforce the importance of *avoiding alcohol in all forms:* sauces, foods, salad dressing, cough syrups, mouthwashes, liniments, backrub and shaving lotions, and other external preparations.

- Warn against driving or hazardous activities until response is determined (may cause drowsiness).

- Advise wearing a medical alert bracelet to alert physicians that disulfiram is being taken.

dobutamine
doe-byoo'ta-meen

dobutamine hydrochloride: *Dobutrex*

Class: Direct-acting sympathomimetic amine, Beta-adrenergic agonist

PEDS	PREG	GERI
✋	C	✋

Action Increases myocardial contractility, stroke volume, and cardiac output by direct stimulation of cardiac beta$_1$ receptors (results in a positive inotropic effect and comparatively mild chronotropic, hypertensive, arrhythmogenic effects). At low doses, may activate dopamine receptors in vascular beds to produce vasodilating effects.

Use/Therapeutic goal/Outcome

Cardiac decompensation (cardiogenic shock): Increased myocardial contractility, cardiac output, and coronary blood flow. **Outcome criteria:** Clearing of lung fields, urinary output > 25 ml/hr, vital signs within normal limits, improved hemodynamic monitor measurements (cardiac output, pulmonary wedge pressures).

Dose range/Administration

Interaction alert: Do not mix with sodium bicarbonate or alkaline solutions. Dobutamine may be ineffective in increasing cardiac output when combined with beta-adrenergic blockers. MAOIs and tricyclic antidepressants increase presser effects. Often used with nitroprusside to increase cardiac output and lower pulmonary wedge pressure. May alter insulin requirements. Oxytocic drugs may cause persistent severe hypertension.

Adult: IV: 2.5 to 15 mcg/kg/min.

Clinical alert: Doses up to 40 mcg/kg/min have occasionally been used. Rate of administration and duration of therapy are individualized according to fluid requirements, cardiac response (changes in rate, ectopic activity), blood pressure, and urine output. Be sure hypovolemia has been corrected before starting dobutamine. Prepare dobutamine by adding 10 ml of D5W or sterile water diluent to 250 mg vial. Further dilution in at least 50 ml of D5W, 0.9% NaCl, or sodium lactate injection is required prior to administration. Dobutamine is also available in solution.

Contraindications/Precautions

PREG C

Contraindicated in hypersensitivity to sympathomimetic amines, and in idiopathic hypertrophic subaortic stenosis, and ventricular tachycardia. **Use with caution** in preexisting hypertension. Safe use after myocardial infarction has not been established.

✋ **Use with caution for pregnant women (if potential benefits outweigh unknown hazards to the fetus) and the elderly. Safe use for children has not been established.**

Side effects/Adverse reactions

Hypersensitivity: exaggeration of side effects. **CV:** increased heart rate and BP, ventricular ectopic activity, headache, nonspecific and anginal chest pain, palpitations. **Resp:** shortness of breath. **MS:** leg cramps (mild). **CNS:** nervousness, paresthesia, fatigue. **GI:** nausea.

Nursing implications/Documentation

Possible nursing diagnoses: Potential for injury; Activity intolerance.

• Ascertain accurate height and weight to assure accurate dose calculation.

• Document lung sounds, vital signs, and hemodynamic parameters before starting dobutamine; then at least hourly thereafter (record blood pressure and pulse every 5–15 min until response is determined, then hourly).

• Record and monitor intake and output hourly; report urine output less than 25–30 ml/hr.

• Keep patient in bed with side rails up; provide frequent rest periods.

Patient & family teaching/Home care

Possible nursing diagnoses: Knowledge deficit; Fear; Ineffective family coping.

• Explain that this drug will improve heart's ability to work as a pump.

• Stress that frequent monitoring of vital signs is needed to "fine tune" medication rate for optimum results.

• Emphasize that the nurses need to be told of new symptoms or uncomfortable feelings in case they indicate a need for medication adjustment.

• Stress the importance of remaining in bed.

◆ *See Adrenergics (sympathomimetics) overview for more information.*

docusate

dok'yoo-sate

docusate calcium: **Pro-Cal-Sof, Surfak**
docusate potassium: **Dialose, Diocto-K, Kasof**
docusate sodium: **Afko-Lube, Colace, ♣Coloxyl, ♣Coloxyl Enema Concentrate, Diocto, Dioeze, Diosuccin, Dio-Sul, Disonate, Di-Sosul, DOK-250, DOK Liquid, Doss 300, Doxinate, D-S-S, Duosol, Genasoft, Laxinate 100, Modane Soft, Pro-Sof, Pro-Sof 250, Pro-Sof Liquid Concentrate, Regulax SS, Regutol, Stulex**

Class: Emollient laxative, Stool softener

PEDS	PREG	GERI
✋	C	OK

Action Produces a soft stool mass by promoting permeation of liquid and fat into feces by means of reduced surface tension.

Use/Therapeutic goal/Outcome

Constipation: Promotion of regular evacuation of soft stool. *Outcome criteria:* Passage of soft, formed stool without straining (within 12–72 hr after first dose).

Dose range/Administration

Interaction alert: May interfere with the effectiveness of potassium-sparing diuretics or potassium supplements by promoting potassium loss through intestinal tract. May increase absorption of danthron, phenolphthalein, and mineral oil; products that combine these laxatives should be used with caution.

docusate calcium: **Adult:** PO: 50–240 mg/day. **Child:** PO: 50–150 mg/day.

docusate sodium: **Adult:** PO: 50–500 mg/day. Rectal: 4 ml unit. **Child:** PO: 40–120 mg/day. Rectal: 4 ml unit.

docusate potassium: **Adult:** PO: 100–300 mg/day. **Child:** PO: 100 mg/day.

Contraindications/Precautions

PREG C

Contraindicated in hypersensitivity to any emollient laxative, and in symptoms of appendicitis, undiagnosed rectal bleeding, fecal impaction or intestinal obstruction.

✋ **Use with caution for children under 6 years.**

Side effects/Adverse reactions

Hypersensitivity: rash. *GI:* abdominal cramping, throat irritation with liquid form only.

Nursing implications/Documentation

Possible nursing diagnoses: Pain.

♦ Give with 8 ounces of liquid; encourage increased fluid intake, especially in the elderly.

♦ Administer liquid forms in milk or fruit juice to improve palatability.

♦ Assess abdomen for bowel sounds and distention.

♦ Monitor and record character, frequency and amount of bowel evacuation.

♦ Monitor electrolyte studies for elevated levels of sodium, calcium, or potassium, depending on preparation used.

Patient & family teaching/Home care

Possible nursing diagnoses: Knowledge deficit; Impaired home maintenance management.

♦ Advise that results will usually occur within 1 to 3 days of continual use.

♦ Emphasize the need to drink 6 to 8 glasses of fluid daily to enhance effectiveness of docusate.

♦ Caution to avoid using docusate longer than 1 week unless instructed by physician.

♦ Warn against using mineral oil in combination with docusate.

♦ Stress the importance of dietary bulk, fluids, and exercise to prevent constipation.

♦ Point out that daily bowel movements are not necessary for each individual; regular evacuation of soft stool which does not require straining is an appropriate goal.

♦ *See Laxatives overview for more information.*

dopamine

doe'pa-meen

dopamine hydrochloride: **Intropin, ♦ ♣Revimine**

Class: Adrenergic agonist (sympathomimetic), Catecholamine, Vasopressor, Cardiac stimulant

PEDS	PREG	GERI
✋	C	✋

Action Dopamine increases myocardial contraction, cardiac output, stroke volume, glomerular filtration rate, sodium and water excretion, and (in low doses) renal blood flow by direct stimulation of beta$_1$ receptors, by variable stimulation of alpha receptors, and by releasing norepinephrine from its storage sites (causes a positive inotropic effect on the myocardium). Dopamine is an immediate precursor to norepinephrine.

Use/Therapeutic goal/Outcome

Shock syndrome due to trauma, MI, septicemia, open-heart surgery, renal failure, and CHF: Improvement of perfusion to vital organs and correction of hemodynamic imbalances. *Outcome criteria:* Blood pressure within normal range; urine output greater than 25 ml/hr; absence of clinical signs and symptoms of shock (confusion, restlessness, chest pain); hemodynamic monitor measurements (central venous pressure, cardiac output, pulmonary wedge pressure) within normal range.

Dose range/Administration

Interaction alert: Do not mix IV with any other drug. May be used with diuretics to provide an additive effect. Beta-blockers may reduce dopamine effects. Do not use with ergot alkaloids or MAOIs (may cause extreme elevation in blood pressure).

Adult: IV: 2–5 mcg/kg/min using controller; may increase by 5–10 mcg/kg/min. *Maximum dose:* 20–50 mcg/kg/min.

Clinical alert: Ascertain that reduced blood pressure is not a result of hypovolemia before starting dopamine (volume deficit should be corrected before starting vasopressors). Be aware that dopamine's effect is directly related to dose: 2–5 mcg/kg/min produces increased renal blood flow; 5–15 mcg/kg/min produces increased cardiac output and blood pressure, and some effects on renal blood flow; 15–50 mcg/kg/min produces increased blood pressure and *decreased* renal blood flow. Titrate dose carefully according to physician-prescribed parameters while carefully monitoring blood pressure, urine output, and clinical status. Be sure that the needle is in the vein, and monitor closely for infiltration. If infiltration occurs, stop dopamine immediately, notify physician, and be prepared to treat with 5–10 mg phentolamine (Regitine) in 10–15 ml normal saline (this may be injected into affected areas to minimize extravasation ischemia).

Contraindications/Precautions

PREG
C

Contraindicated in hypersensitivity to sympathomimetics and sulfites, and in pheochromocytoma, tachyarrhythmias, or ventricular fibrillation. *Use with caution* within 14 days before or after MAOIs, in cold injury, occlusive vascular disease, arterial embolism, and diabetic endarteritis.

✥ **Contraindicated for pregnant women (unless expected benefits outweigh risk to fetus). Use with caution for the elderly. Safe use for children has not been established.**

Side effects/Adverse reactions

Hypersensitivity: flushing, redness, or bluish coloration of skin; dizziness; rash; hives; itching; swelling of face, lips or eyelids; wheezing or difficulty breathing; exaggeration of side effects. *GI:* nausea, vomiting. *CV:* ectopic beats, tachycardia, anginal pain, palpitations, headache, hypotension, vasoconstriction (indicated by a disproportionate rise in diastolic pressure), aberrant conduction, bradycardia, widening QRS complex, elevated BP. *Resp:* dyspnea. *Skin:* necrosis and tissue sloughing with extravasation. *Eye:* mydriasis. *Hem:* azotemia.

Nursing implications/Documentation

Possible nursing diagnoses: Potential for injury; Activity intolerance; Sleep pattern disturbance.

◆ Ascertain accurate height and weight to assure accurate dose calculation.

◆ Document lung sounds, vital signs, and hemodynamic parameters before starting dopamine; then at least hourly thereafter (record blood pressure and pulse every 5–15 min until response is determined, then hourly).

◆ Record and monitor intake and output hourly; report urine output less than 25–30 ml/hr or sudden rapid increase in urine output.

◆ Monitor for and report any of the following: increased tachycardia, arrhythmias, marked decrease in pulse pressure (disproportionate rise in diastolic pressure), absence of peripheral pulses, or signs of peripheral vasoconstriction (cold, pale fingers and toes).

◆ Keep patient in bed with side rails up; provide frequent rest periods.

Patient & family teaching/Home care

Possible nursing diagnoses: Knowledge deficit; Fear; Ineffective family coping.

◆ Explain that this drug helps improve the pumping action of the heart and increases blood flow to vital organs.

◆ Point out that frequent monitoring of vital signs is needed to "fine tune" medication rate for optimum results.

◆ Emphasize that the nurses need to be told of new symptoms or uncomfortable feelings in case they indicate a need for medication adjustment.

♦ Stress the importance of remaining in bed.

♦ *See Adrenergics (sympathomimetics) overview for more information.*

doxapram   *dox'a-pram*

D

doxapram hydrochloride: *Dopram*
Class: Respiratory stimulant

PEDS PREG GERI
✋   C   ✋

Action Produces rapid onset (within 20–40 seconds) respiratory stimulation through direct medullary action (peak is in 1–2 min; duration is 5–10 min). Antagonizes narcotic-induced respiratory depression, but not analgesia. Increases tidal volume, respiratory rate, cardiac output, and blood pressure. May also increase salivation, gastric acid, and catecholamine release.

Use/Therapeutic goal/Outcome

Postanesthesia and drug-induced respiratory depression: Reversal of respiratory depression. *Outcome criteria:* Respirations within normal limits compared to baseline; return of cough and gag reflexes.

COPD with acute hypercapnia: Prevention of CO_2 retention. *Outcome criteria:* Respiratory rate within normal limits compared to baseline; arterial CO_2 within normal limits compared to baseline.

Dose range/Administration

Interaction alert: MAO inhibitors, sympathomimetics increase serious cardiovascular effects. Incompatible when mixed with alkaline solutions (thiopental sodium).

Postanesthesia respiratory depression: **Adult:** IV: *Injection:* 0.5–1 mg/kg injected slowly every 5 min prn (maximum total dose of 2 mg/kg). *Infusion:* Add 250 mg doxapram to 250 ml D5W or NS, infuse at 5 ml/min until response; maintain at 1–3 mg/min (maximum total dose of 4 mg/kg).

Drug-induced respiratory depression: **Adult:** IV: *Injection:* 1–2 mg/kg (depending on degree of depression) injected slowly, repeat in 5 min, and then repeat q1-2h (maximum daily dose of 3g). *Intermittent infusion:* After initial injection (1–2 mg/kg, repeat in 5 min), add 250 mg dox-

apram to 250 cc DSW or NS, and infuse at 1–3 cc/min for 2 hr. May repeat every 30 min to 2 hr to a maximum of 3 g/day.

COPD with hypercapnia: **Adult:** IV: Mix 400 mg doxapram in 180 cc D5W or NS (2 mg/ml), and infuse at 0.5–1 ml/min (1–2 mg/min). May increase rate to a maximum of 1.5 ml/min (3 mg/min). Do not infuse longer than 2 hr; additional doses are not recommended.

Clinical alert: This drug should be given only in the presence of a qualified professional (physician or nurse anesthetist), and suction, oxygen, and resuscitative equipment should be readily at hand. An airway should be established. Allow at least a 10-min interval between discontinuation of (inhalant) anesthesia and doxapram administration. An IV controller device should be used for infusion, and the site should be monitored for infiltration (drug may cause local irritation). Do not use with mechanical ventilation.

Contraindications/Precautions   PREG
                                           C

Contraindicated in hypersensitivity to doxapram, for intra-arterial injection, and in seizure disorders, head injury, heart failure, severe hypertension, CVA, neuromuscular disorders, flail chest, mechanically obstructed airway, pulmonary embolism, pneumothorax, restrictive lung disease, acute asthma, extreme dyspnea, and hypoxia not associated with hypercapnia. *Use with caution* in profound metabolic disorders, hyperthyroidism, pheochromocytoma, cerebral edema, increased CSF pressure, asthma, tachycardia or arrhythmias.

✋ **Contraindicated for newborns (because of benzyl alcohol). Use with caution for the elderly. Safe use for children under 12 years and for pregnant women has not been established.**

Side effects/Adverse reactions

Hypersensitivity: itching, bronchospasm, laryngospasm. *CNS:* fever, headache, dizziness, apprehension, disorientation, seizures, paresthesias, spasticity, bilateral Babinski sign. *CV:* variations in heart rhythm and rate, lowered T waves, chest pain and tightness, hypertension, phlebitis. *Resp:* difficult or rapid breathing, cough, bronchospasm, laryngospasm. *Skin:* flushing, sweating. *Eye:* dilated pupils. *GI:* nausea, vomiting, diarrhea. *GU:* urinary retention or incontinence.

Nursing implications/Documentation

Possible nursing diagnoses: Potential for injury; Potential for aspiration.

◆ Protect airway, position patient on side if possible, and suction as needed.

◆ Record vital signs, level of consciousness, respiratory status, and presence of reflexes, before administration and at least every 30 min thereafter.

◆ Monitor for (and report) signs of overdosage (increased arterial CO_2 or O_2 tension).

◆ Keep side rails up and monitor for hyperexcitability.

◆ Hold drug and report if sudden hypotension, dyspnea, or deterioration in ABGs occurs.

◆ Keep IV anticonvulsant (e.g., diazepam) at hand in case mechanical ventilation is necessary or if seizures occur.

Patient & family teaching/Home care

Possible nursing diagnoses: Fear; Sensory perceptual alterations.

◆ Explain all procedures briefly and in simple terms, even if the patient appears unconscious; reinforce that measures are being taken to provide for safety.

doxepin

dox'e-pin

doxepin hydrochloride: *Adapin, ◣Deptran, Sinequan, ♣Triadapin*

Class: Tricyclic antidepressant (TCA)

PEDS	PREG	GERI
♨	C	♨

Action Improves mood by increasing levels of the neurotransmitters norepinephrine and serotonin in the CNS. Produces more sedation than other TCAs. Has also been effective against intractable hiccups and chronic severe pain (exact mechanism of action is unclear).

Use/Therapeutic goal/Outcome

Depression (especially that associated with anxiety): Promotion of sense of well-being, ability to cope with daily living. *Outcome criteria:* After 2–4 weeks, report of feeling less depressed, less anxious, and more energetic and able to cope; return of normal sleeping and eating habits; demonstration of improved ability to problem solve and perform activities of daily living.

Dose range/Administration

Interaction alert: Barbiturates may reduce antidepressant blood levels and effects. Cimetidine and methylphenidate may increase blood levels. If given with epinephrine and norepinephrine, monitor for increased risk of hypertension. Avoid use with MAOIs (high risk of excitation, hyperpyrexia, and seizures). Give cautiously with thyroid drugs because it may increase CNS stimulation.

Adult: PO: Begin with 50–75 mg/day in divided doses or at bedtime. *Elderly:* 25–50 mg/day. *Maximum dose:* 300 mg/day if hospitalized; 150 mg/day for outpatients.

Clinical alert: Whenever possible give entire dose at bedtime. Adapin may contain tartrazine (FD&C Yellow No. 5) which may cause allergic reactions in some people (check package insert).

Contraindications/Precautions

PREG
C

Contraindicated in hypersensitivity to TCAs, for concomitant use with electroconvulsive therapy, and in elective surgery, acute recovery period of myocardial infarction, renal or hepatic disease, hyperthyroidism, glaucoma, prostatic hypertrophy, urinary retention, hypomania, mania, and suicidal tendency.

♨ **Contraindicated for children under 12 years and for pregnant or nursing mothers. Use with caution for adolescents and the elderly or debilitated.**

Side effects/Adverse reactions

Hypersensitivity: rash, itching, sensitivity to sunlight. *CNS:* drowsiness, dizziness, anxiety, headache, fatigue, agitation, extrapyramidal symptoms, sedation (especially the elderly). *CV:* orthostatic hypotension, palpitations, tachycardia, EKG changes, hypertension. *GI:* anorexia, dry mouth, nausea, vomiting, constipation, paralytic ileus. *GU:* urinary retention, decreased libido. *Eye:* blurred vision, eye pain. *Ear:* tinnitus. *Hem:* agranulocytosis.

Nursing implications/Documentation

Possible nursing diagnoses: Potential for injury; Constipation; Altered oral mucous membrane.

◆ Document mental status and vital signs at least twice a day until response to therapy has been established.

◆ Be sure that doses are swallowed (not hoarded).

- Monitor for orthostatic hypotension, dizziness, and drowsiness; supervise ambulation until response is established.

- Record intake and output, and observe for dehydration and urinary retention; provide special mouth care.

- Monitor for and report suicidal tendencies, increased depression, or excessive drowsiness (may require change in medication).

- Prevent constipation by monitoring bowel movements and encouraging adequate fiber and fluid intake; offer laxatives or stool softeners before the problem becomes severe.

Patient & family teaching/Home care

Possible nursing diagnoses: Ineffective coping (family and individual); Sleep pattern disturbance; Impaired home maintenance management.

- Stress that this medication helps reduce the depression that inhibits ability to make decisions and cope effectively (once the individual feels less depressed, it will be easier to take steps toward making healthy changes).

- Explain that side effects are often noted immediately, but they usually diminish after a few weeks; on the other hand, it is likely to take 2–4 weeks before *beneficial* effects are noted.

- Warn to change positions slowly to prevent dizziness.

- Point out the role of adequate nutrition, exercise, and sleep in combating depression.

- Emphasize that the effects of alcohol, sedatives, and tranquilizers may be potentiated.

- Caution to consult with physician before using OTC drugs; stress the need for ongoing medical follow-up.

- Recommend reporting continued depression; stress that doses should not be increased or stopped without checking with physician, because this may cause severe problems.

- Advise avoidance of driving and other potentially hazardous activities until response is established.

- Suggest using ice chips, hard candy, or gum to relieve side effect of dry mouth; stress the need for good mouth care.

- Warn women to report immediately if pregnancy is planned or suspected.

- *See Antidepressants overview for more information.*

doxorubicin

dox'-o-ru-bee-cin

doxorubicin hydrochloride: ◆*Adriamycin, Adriamycin PFS, Adriamycin RDF*
Class: ★Antineoplastic (antibiotic) agent prototype

PEDS	PREG	GERI
🖐	D	🖐

Action Kills rapidly growing cells (cancer, hair follicles, bone marrow, GI lining, ova, and sperm) by interfering with the synthesis of DNA, RNA, and protein, causing disruption of nucleic acid function. Is cell-cycle–phase nonspecific.

Use/Therapeutic goal/Outcome

Cancer of the breast, ovaries, bladder, lungs, thyroid, and stomach; osteogenic sarcomas; neuroblastoma; Wilms' tumor; Hodgkin's and non-Hodgkin's lymphomas; and acute lymphoblastic and myeloblastic leukemias: Elimination or suppression of malignant cell proliferation. *Outcome criteria:* Tumor and disease regression or stabilization on radiologic and physical examination for leukemias, absence of blasts in peripheral blood specimen.

Dose range/Administration

Interaction alert: Do not mix IV with any other drug. Radiation and other antineoplastics may cause cumulative bone marrow depression. Cyclophosphamide increases risk of hemorrhagic cystitis. Mercaptopurine increases risk of hepatotoxicity. Streptozocin may require dose adjustment. Barbiturates decrease cytotoxic effects.

Adult: IV: 60–90 mg/m^2 as a single dose q 3 wk; or 20 mg/m^2/wk as a single dose, or 30 mg/m^2/day for 3 days q 4 wk. *Maximum lifetime dose:* 550 mg/m^2 (increased incidence of cardiac toxicity). *Child:* IV: 30 mg/m^2/day for 3 days; repeat q 4 wk.

Clinical alert: This drug should be given only by nurses who are knowledgeable in the comprehensive management of the administration of antineoplastic agents. Doses may vary at physician's discretion. Repeat doses are held until it is ascertained that the patient has recovered sufficiently from toxicities of previous doses. Established protocols/policies for drug preparation, administration, and accidental skin contamination *must be followed closely* (gloves or double gloves are worn when handling drug; if the drug touches the skin, the area is washed immediately with plenty of soap and water).

Doxorubicin is given via bolus *slowly* over 5 min or diluted in 50–100 ml fluid to minimize inflammation and pain along the vein. This drug is a *potent* vesicant (can cause severe damage to tissues). *Prevention* of extravasation is essential. The drug is given by administering only when it is clear that the needle is in the vein (good blood return) and the infusion site is monitored *closely* for early signs of extravasation (pain and swelling at infusion site). If extravasation is suspected, the infusion is stopped *immediately*, the physician is notified, and protocols and policies for treatment are followed. Doxorubicin may also be given by instillation into the bladder, by intracavitary injection into the peritoneum, and by intra-arterial injection.

Contraindications/Precautions

PREG
D

Contraindicated in hypersensitivity to doxorubicin, myelosuppression, impaired cardiac function, or past cumulative dose of 550 mg/m^2.
Use with caution in hepatic impairment, depressed bone marrow, and active infections.

☞ **Contraindicated for pregnant or nursing mothers. Use with caution for children and the elderly.**

Side effects/Adverse reactions

Hypersensitivity: rash, urticaria, fever, chills, tachycardia, hypotension, anaphylaxis. **Hem:** hyperuricemia, leukopenia, thrombocytopenia, and anemia. **Skin:** hyperpigmentation of skin (especially in previously irradiated areas) and nails; dermatitis; complete alopecia (usually within 1 month); pain and erythema at injection site; cellulitis; ulceration and sloughing if extravasation occurs. **GI:** stomatitis; esophagitis; nausea; vomiting and diarrhea; hepatotoxicity. **CV:** cardiotoxicity (dysrhythmias, fatal CHF, hypertension, and irreversible cardiomyopathy), thrombophlebitis at injection site. **GU:** transient red urine, impotence, sterility, and amenorrhea. **Eye:** lacrimation and conjunctivitis.

Nursing implications/Documentation

Possible nursing diagnoses: Potential for infection; Potential for injury; Fatigue; Altered oral mucous membrane; Fluid volume deficit; Diarrhea; Altered nutrition: less than body requirements.

◆ *See important Nursing implications in Antineoplastic agents overview on page 72, which apply to all neoplastics. The interventions that follow are additional and specific to this drug only.*

◆ Monitor for and report early signs of cardiac toxicity (resting pulse > 100, difficulty breathing); stop drug and report immediately.

◆ Record vital signs, lung sounds, and skin condition on an ongoing basis, observing for signs of CHF (cardiac toxicity has occurred in 30% of patients 1–6 months after drug stopped if cumulative dose exceeded 550 mg/mm^2 of body surface area).

◆ Expect WBC, platelet and erythrocyte counts to drop to the nadir (lowest point) at 2 weeks with recovery in about 3 weeks.

Patient & family teaching/Home care

Possible nursing diagnoses: Knowledge deficit; Ineffective coping (individual and family); Hopelessness; Impaired home maintenance management.

◆ *See important Patient & family teaching in Antineoplastic agents overview on page 72, which apply to all neoplastics. The teachings that follow are additional and specific to this drug only.*

◆ Stress that shortness of breath, rapid pulse, or swelling of the ankles and feet should be reported immediately; they may require treatment.

◆ Warn that urine may have a reddish color for several days after treatment (stress that this is not blood).

◆ Explain that although nausea and vomiting may be severe, it should subside within 24–48 hours.

◆ *See Antineoplastic agents overview for more information.*

doxycycline

dox-i-sye'kleen

doxycycline: ♠*Doxylin*

doxycycline hyclate: *Doxy-100, Doxy-200, Doxy-Caps, Doxychel, Doxy-Lemmon, Doxy-Tabs, Vibramycin, Vibra-Tabs*

doxycycline hydrochloride: ♠*Cyclidox,* ♠*Doryx,* ♠*Vibramycin,* ♠*Vibramycin IV,* ♠*Vibra-Tabs 50*

Class: Anti-infective, Broad-spectrum tetracycline antibiotic

PEDS   PREG   GERI
☞   D   ☞

Action Limits bacterial growth (bateriostatic) by binding to the 30S ribosomal subunit and inhibiting protein synthesis.

Use/Therapeutic goal/Outcome

Infections (acne, gonorrhea, syphilis, susceptible gram-negative and gram-positive pathogens, trachoma, rickettsia, mycoplasma, and chlamydia): Resolution of infection. *Outcome criteria:* Absence of pathogenic growth on cultures, absence of clinical manifestations of infection (fever, pain, swelling, redness, heat, odor, drainage, productive cough, dysuria, frequency), normal WBC count, normal X rays.

Travelers' diarrhea: Prevention of diarrhea. *Outcome criteria:* Absence of diarrhea.

Dose range/Administration

Interaction alert: Avoid use with phenobarbital, carbamazepine, and alcohol (decreases antibiotic effect). To prevent interference with antibiotic absorption, give 1 hour before or 2 hours after antacids (including sodium bicarbonate) or laxatives containing aluminum, magnesium, or calcium. *Decreases* effects of penicillin and *increases* effect of anticoagulants. Give 2 hours before or 3 hours after iron products or zinc. May decrease effectiveness of oral contraceptives and increase breakthrough bleeding.

🖤 **Give with milk or food to reduce GI symptoms.**

Infections (syphilis, infections caused by susceptible gram-negative and gram-positive pathogens, trachoma, rickettsia, mycoplasma, and chlamydia): Adult/Child > 45 kg: PO: 100 mg q12h for 2 doses, then 100 mg/day. IV: 200 mg on the first day in single or divided doses, then 100–200 mg/day. *Child < 45 kg, > 8 yrs:* PO, IV: 4.4 mg/kg/day in divided doses q12h for 24 hrs, then 2.2 to 4.4 mg/day in divided doses.

Uncomplicated endocervical, urethral, or rectal infections: Adult: PO: 100 mg bid for at least 7 days.

Gonorrhea: Adult: PO: 200 mg initial dose, then 100 mg at hs, then 100 mg bid for 3 days; *or* 300 mg initial dose, repeat dose 1 hr later; *or* 100 mg bid for 7 days in combination with amoxicillin.

Syphilis: Adult: PO: 300 mg/day in divided doses for 10 days.

Prevention of travelers' diarrhea: Adult: PO: 100 mg/day.

Clinical alert: Protect IV doxycycline from light and infuse over a minimum of 1 hour (maximum 6 hours). Never give IM or SC. Taking outdated tetracyclines has been associated with fatal nephrotoxicity.

Contraindications/Precautions

Contraindicated in allergy to doxycycline or other tetracyclines or immunosuppression. *Use with caution* in impaired renal or liver function.

✋ **Contraindicated for children under 8 years (causes tooth discoloration and retards bone growth) and pregnant or nursing mothers. Use with caution for the elderly.**

Side effects/Adverse reactions

Hypersensitivity: (rare) itching, rashes, fever, anaphylaxis. *GI:* sore throat, glossitis, stomatitis, epigastric discomfort, nausea, cramps, diarrhea, enterocolitis, anogenital inflammation, hepatotoxicity with large IV doses. *Skin:* photosensitivity. *CNS:* dizziness, lightheadedness, headache, intracranial hypertension. *CV:* pericarditis. *Hem:* blood dyscrasias; thrombophlebitis (with IV route).

Nursing implications/Documentation

Possible nursing diagnoses: Potential for infection; Potential fluid volume deficit.

♦ Determine history of allergies, and (regardless of history) monitor closely for allergic reactions.

♦ Weigh patient and obtain baseline CBC, BUN, creatinine, liver function studies, and necessary culture specimens before administering first dose; monitor closely thereafter if therapy is prolonged.

♦ Encourage fluids, and record and monitor intake and output, to ensure adequate hydration and urine output.

♦ Monitor for and report symptoms of superinfection (mouth lesions, thrush, vaginal irritation, diarrhea, respiratory symptoms).

♦ If there is no improvement within 3–5 days, consult with physician to determine if antibiotic regimen should be re-evaluated (and new cultures drawn).

Patient & family teaching/Home care

Possible nursing diagnoses: Knowledge deficit, Impaired home maintenance management.

♦ Advise taking doxycycline with milk or food if GI symptoms are experienced.

♦ Advise avoiding exposure to sunlight; warn that photosensitivity may continue for weeks after drug has been discontinued.

♦ Teach the need to report persistent or new symptoms of illness (e.g., fever, mouth lesions, vaginal irritation, respiratory symptoms, diarrhea); medication may have to be changed.

♦ Explain the importance of taking antibiotics for the entire time prescribed, even if symptoms abate.

♦ Caution women that this drug may decrease effectiveness of oral contraceptives.

♦ *See Anti-infectives overview for more information.*

dronabinol
droe-na'bin-all

tetrahydrocannabinol: **Marinol**

Class: Antiemetic

PEDS	PREG	GERI	CONTROLLED SUBSTANCE
♨	**B**	♨	**II**

Action The exact mechanism of action has not been determined. Believed to relieve nausea and vomiting caused by cancer chemotherapy by effecting the CNS much in the same manner as marijuana and barbiturates. Often causes CNS depressions and other various psychoactive effects.

Use/Therapeutic goal/Outcome

Nausea or vomiting associated with chemotherapy, not manageable by conventional antiemetics: Prevention or resolution. **Outcome criteria:** Report of absence of, or reduction in, feelings of nausea; absence of vomiting.

Dose range/Administration

Interaction alert: Alcohol, barbiturates, or other CNS depressants may increase CNS depression. May alter effects of psychoactive drugs.

Adult: PO: Initial dose of 5 mg/M^2, 1–3 hr before chemotherapy, then q3-4h after chemotherapy, for a total of 4–6 doses/day. Dose may be increased by 2.5 mg/M^2 to a maximum of 15 mg/M^2 per dose.

Clinical alert: Be aware that dronabinol is available in 2.5-mg capsules, 5-mg capsules, and 10-mg capsules; the incidence of psychiatric symptoms increases with higher doses. Monitor closely for psychiatric side effects (e.g., hallucinations, muddled thinking, paranoia).

Contraindications/Precautions
PREG
B

Contraindicated in hypersensitivity to dronabinol or sesame oil, and for nausea and vomiting not related to chemotherapy. **Use with caution** in hypertension, heart disease, manic or depressive illness, schizophrenia, or use of other psychoactive drugs.

♨ **Use with caution for the elderly. Safe use for children and pregnant or nursing mothers has not been determined.**

Side effects/Adverse reactions

Hypersensitivity: severe psychiatric reactions. **CNS:** drowsiness, dizziness, anxiety, muddled thinking, perceptual difficulties, coordination problems, irritability, weird feeling, headache, fatigue, hallucinations, memory lapse, unsteadiness, ataxia, paranoia, depersonalization, disorientation, confusion, paresthesia. **CV:** tachycardia, hypotension, hypertension. **Eye:** visual distortions. **GI:** dry mouth.

Nursing implications/Documentation

Possible nursing diagnoses: Potential for injury; Altered thought processes; Sensory/perceptual alterations (visual and auditory); Fluid volume deficit; Altered oral mucous membrane.

♦ Assess for presence of bowel sounds, pain, nausea, or vomiting before and after administering antiemetics; hold drug and report if bowel sounds are absent.

♦ Record and monitor vital signs at least q4h (tachycardia, and both *hyper-* and *hypo*tension are common side effects).

♦ Observe for and report psychiatric side effects; provide reassurance and quiet environment.

♦ Offer frequent mouth care.

♦ Supervise ambulation until response is determined.

♦ Document and monitor intake and output to detect dehydration.

♦ When able to tolerate liquids, begin with small amount of ice chips, then water, then clear liquids, then full liquids, then food.

Patient & family teaching/Home care

Possible nursing diagnoses: Knowledge deficit; Impaired home maintenance management.

♦ Reinforce the need to follow dose administration times exactly as prescribed.

♦ Explain that even though this drug is much like marijuana (it is likely to be habit-forming and may cause psychoactive side effects), its beneficial effects in these types of situations has been demonstrated to be worth the risks involved.

- Teach the importance of having a responsible person stay with the person while he/she is under the effects of the drug; stress that the effects of this drug may persist for several days.

- Stress that persistent nausea, vomiting, or abdominal discomfort should be reported.

- Explain that avoiding fatty foods and eating smaller and more frequent meals may reduce nausea.

- Advise against using alcohol or other CNS depressants; warn against driving or activities that require mental alertness.

- Emphasize the need to maintain good mouth care, especially when not taking liquids by mouth; suggest that chewing sugarless gum may relieve symptoms of dry mouth.

- *See Antiemetics overview for more information.*

droperidol

droe-per'i-dole

♠Droleptan, Inapsine

Class: Antipsychotic, Antiemetic, Butyrophenone

PEDS	PREG	GERI
🖐	C	🖐

Action Reduces nausea and vomiting during surgical and diagnostic procedures by antagonizing emetic effects of narcotics and other drugs that act on the chemoreceptor trigger zone. Produces sedation and reduces anxiety and motor activity (without necessarily inducing sleep) by acting at subcortical level. Does not produce analgesia, but enhances analgesic effects of other drugs. Structurally and pharmacologically related to haloperidol.

Use/Therapeutic goal/Outcome

Premedication, adjunct to anesthesia, prevention of nausea and vomiting: Promotion of relaxation, and enhancement of analgesia. *Outcome criteria:* Absence of vomiting or retching; patient report of not feeling nauseated, feeling relaxed and comfortable.

Dose range/Administration

Interaction alert: Other CNS depressants potentiate sedation.

Premedication: Adult: IM, IV: 2.5–10 mg administered 30–60 min before procedure. *Child 2–12 yrs:* IM, IV: 1–1.5 mg/20–25 lbs. Dose should be titrated carefully.

Adjunct to general anesthesia: Adult: Induction dose: IV (preferable), IM: 0.22–0.275 mg/kg;

smaller doses may be adequate in some cases. *Maintenance dose:* IV: 1.25–2.5 mg.

Diagnostic procedures: Adult: IM: 2.5–10 mg administered 30–60 min before procedure. Additional doses of 1.25–2.5 mg may be administered, usually by IV injection.

Adjunct to regional anesthesia for additional sedation: Adult: IM, IV (slowly): 2.5–5 mg.

Clinical alert: Dosage is extremely individualized depending on age, height, weight, and health status. Administer IV only where there are emergency equipment and professionals qualified in endotracheal intubation. Emergency drugs should be nearby: hypotension and tachycardia commonly occur. Expect reduced dosage for children, the elderly, and debilitated.

Contraindications/Precautions

PREG C

Contraindicated in hypersensitivity to droperidol. *Use with caution* for the debilitated and other high-risk patients and in parkinsonism, hypotension, liver, kidney, or cardiac disease.

🖐 **Use with caution for the elderly. Safe use for children under 2 years and for pregnant women has not been established.**

Side effects/Adverse reactions

Hypersensitivity: laryngospasm, bronchospasm. *CV:* hypotension, tachycardia, peripheral dilatation. *CNS:* extrapyramidal symptoms (dystonia, akathisia, oculogyric crisis), drowsiness, dizziness, restlessness, hyperactivity, anxiety, seizures, hallucinations, depression. *Resp:* hypoventilation, bronchospasm, apnea. *Hem:* agranulocytosis. *Misc:* chills, shivering.

Nursing implications/Documentation

Possible nursing diagnoses: Potential for injury; Sensory/perceptual alterations (visual and auditory).

- Record vital signs before administration, and monitor closely for hypotension after administration.

- Employ measures to ensure safety (i.e., side rails up, call bell within reach, and no unsupervised smoking).

- Change the patient's position slowly to reduce occurrence of orthostatic hypotension.

- Monitor for and immediately report extrapyramidal signs—which may occur as late as 24–48 hr after administration.

- Recognize that droperidol is usually given with an analgesic. It may be used alone as an antiemetic during antineoplastic chemotherapy (this use is not FDA approved).

Patient & family teaching/Home care

Possible nursing diagnoses: Anxiety; Fear.

◆ Stress the need to remain in bed and to change positions slowly until blood pressure is stable.

◆ Explain procedures briefly and in simple terms, even if the patient appears asleep.

◆ *See Antipsychotics overview for more information.*

edrophonium
ed-roe-foe'nee-um

edrophonium chloride: *Enlon, Reversol, Tensilon*

Class: Cholinergic (parasympathomimetic), Anticholinesterase

Antidote: Atropine

PEDS	PREG	GERI
🖐	C	🖐

Action When given in appropriate doses, promotes impulse transmission from nerve cells to muscle cells by inhibiting the destruction of acetylcholine. Acetylcholine is responsible for facilitating impulse transmission from nerve cells to muscle cells. *Excessive or deficient* acetylcholine may cause *neuromuscular blockade.* Onset of action for IV route is almost immediate, but duration is only 6–24 min (repeated doses may be required).

Use/Therapeutic goal/Outcome

Diagnostic aid in myasthenia gravis (Tensilon test): Determination of presence of myasthenia gravis. **Outcome criteria:** Short-term (5–30 min) improvement of respiration, muscle strength, ptosis, and ability to speak and swallow indicates myasthenia gravis (positive test). Increased secretions and further weakness of muscles and respirations may indicate overdosage and cholinergic crisis.

Anesthesia recovery: Reversal of effects of nondepolarizing neuromuscular blocking agents (tubocurarine, gallamine, pancuronium) and promotion of neuromuscular impulse transmission. **Outcome criteria:** Ability to move arms and legs, breathe spontaneously, and demonstrate return of muscle strength.

Paroxysmal supraventricular tachycardia: Resolution of tachycardia. **Outcome criteria:** Pulse within normal range; absence of supraventricular tachycardia on EKG.

Dose range/Administration

Interaction alert: Procainamide and quinidine may inhibit action. Digitalis preparations may cause bradycardia. Other cholinergic drugs should be stopped before giving edrophonium chloride.

Diagnostic aid in myasthenia gravis (Tensilon test): Adult: IV: 1–2 mg over 15–30 sec; if no increase in muscle strength in 45 sec, then 8 mg more. **Child > 35 kg:** IV: 2 mg; if no response in 45 sec, then 1 mg q 45 sec. *Maximum dose:* 10 mg. **Child < 35 kg:** IV: 1 mg; if no response in 45 sec, then 1 mg q 45 sec. *Maximum dose:* 5 mg. **Infants:** IV: 0.5 mg.

To differentiate myasthenic from cholinergic crisis: Adult: IV: 1 mg; if no response in 1 min, then an additional 1 mg.

Reversal of neuromuscular blocking agents: Adult: IV: 10 mg over 30–45 sec; may repeat q 5–10 min. *Maximum dose:* 40 mg.

Paroxysmal supraventricular tachycardia: Adult: IV: 5–7 mg over 1 min. **Child:** IV: 2 mg in 1–2 min.

Clinical alert: For accurate dosage, use a TB syringe to draw up dose. This drug should be given only by physicians or nurse anesthetists who are qualified in its use. The patient should be attached to a cardiac monitor; atropine and resuscitative equipment should be readily available.

Contraindications/Precautions

PREG
C

Contraindicated in hypersensitivity to cholinergic agents and in bronchial asthma, intestinal or urinary obstruction and hypotension. **Use with caution** in cardiac disorders, asthma, peptic ulcer, and hyperthyroidism.

🖐 **Use with caution for children and the elderly (those > 50 years are particularly sensitive to drug). Safe use for pregnant or nursing mothers has not been established.**

Side effects/Adverse reactions

Hypersensitivity: exaggeration of side effects (severe side effects uncommon in safe dose range). **GI:** nausea, vomiting, abdominal cramps, diarrhea, excessive salivation. **CNS:** weakness. **Resp:** respiratory weakness and paralysis. **CV:** hypotension, bradycardia. **Skin:** flushing, sweating. **Eye:** miosis.

Nursing implications/Documentation

Possible nursing diagnoses: Potential for aspiration; Impaired swallowing.

- Monitor closely muscle strength and ability to chew, swallow and talk, for 1 hr after administration; document variations in strength, and pulse, respirations, and blood pressure every 3–5 min for the first half hour.
- For anesthetic reversal, protect airway by positioning the patient on his or her side and clearing oral secretions.
- Keep the patient in bed with side rails up until response is determined.

Patient & family teaching/Home care

Possible nursing diagnoses: Fear.

- Point out that the patient will be closely monitored to ensure safety.
- Reassure that measures are being taken to reverse weakness.
- Explain that this drug is not given in the home.
- *See Cholinergics overview for more information.*

enalapril
e-nal'a-pril

enalapril maleate: **♠Amprace, ♠Renitec, Vasotec**
enalaprilat: **Vasotec IV**

Class: Antihypertensive, Angiotensin converting enzyme inhibitor (ACE inhibitor)

PEDS	PREG	GERI
♒	C	♒

Action Reduces blood pressure by acting on the renin-angiotensin system. Inhibits angiotensin converting enzyme (ACE), thereby blocking the conversion of angiotensin I and angiotensin II, which is a very potent vasoconstrictor that also stimulates aldosterone secretion (causes kidney reabsorption of sodium and water). Enalapril thus prevents vasoconstriction and retention of sodium and water; and reduces peripheral vascular resistance (afterload), and pulmonary capillary wedge pressure (preload).

Use/Therapeutic goal/Outcome

Hypertension: Reduction of blood pressure. **Outcome criteria:** Blood pressure within normal limits.

Congestive Heart Failure: Resolution of CHF. **Outcome criteria:** Clear lungs, absence of edema; improved exercise tolerance; reduction of PVR, PCWP; urine output > 30 cc/hr.

Dose range/Administration

Interaction alert: Use with diuretics may increase hypotensive effect.

Adult: PO: 2.5–5 mg/day. Range 10–40 mg/day as a single dose or in divided doses. IV: 1.25 mg q6h (over at least 5 min).

Contraindications/Precautions
PREG C

Contraindicated in hypersensitivity to any ACE inhibitor. **Use with caution** in renal insufficiency, collagen vascular diseases, and patients receiving drugs that cause leukopenia or agranulocytosis.

✋ **May use safely for the elderly, but management at home should be carefully monitored. Safe use for children and pregnant women has not been established.**

Side effects/Adverse reactions

Hypersensitivity: rash; urticaria; angioedema; difficulty breathing; stridor; swelling of face, eyes, tongue and lips. **CV:** hypotension. **Hem:** agranulocytosis, neutropenia. **CNS:** headache, dizziness, fainting, insomnia, fatigue. **GI:** nausea, diarrhea.

Nursing implications/Documentation

Possible nursing diagnoses: Activity intolerance; Fatigue; Potential for injury.

- Assess mental status, and record pulse and blood pressure (lying, sitting, and standing, in both arms) before administration, and frequently thereafter until response is determined.
- Consult with physician to determine desired therapeutic range for blood pressure (be aware that some patients may require a slightly elevated blood pressure to perfuse vital organs).
- Ascertain that baseline CBC, electrolytes, BUN, creatinine, and liver function studies have been obtained before giving first dose; report abnormalities and monitor closely thereafter (WBC count should be performed every 2–3 weeks for the first 3 months, and periodically thereafter).
- Monitor for confusion, dizziness, bradycardia, and hypotension; hold drug and report immediately if these occur.
- Supervise ambulation until response is determined.
- Document and monitor daily weight, and intake and output; report significant negative or positive balance.

Patient & family teaching/Home care

Possible nursing diagnoses: Knowledge deficit; Impaired home maintenance management.

◆ Explain the importance of taking medication exactly as prescribed, even when feeling well.

◆ Stress the importance of good medical follow-up, explain that this drug reduces "wear and tear" on blood vessels and improves longevity and health.

◆ Teach how to monitor pulse and blood pressure; emphasize that syncope, hypertension or hypotension, or persistent dizziness should be reported.

◆ Advise changing positions slowly to avoid dizziness.

◆ Encourage daily monitoring of weight and reporting sudden weight gain (frequently is fluid retention).

◆ Point out the need to report symptoms of sore throat, fever, or malaise because they may indicate an abnormal WBC count.

◆ Warn against taking *any* OTC drugs without physician approval (some interactions can cause severe reactions).

◆ *See Antihypertensives overview for more information.*

encainide

en kay' nide

encainide hydrocholoride: *Enkaid*

Class: Antiarrhythmic (Class IC)

PEDS	PREG	GERI
👋	C	👋

Action Mechanism of action is unknown. Probably suppresses ventricular ectopy by slowing conduction, reducing membrane responsiveness, inhibiting automaticity, and increasing the ratio of the effective refractory period to the action potential duration.

Use/Therapeutic goal/Outcome

Life-threatening ventricular arrhythmias, premature ventricular contractions, and nonsustained ventricular tachycardia: Suppression of ventricular ectopy/promotion of effective heartbeat. *Outcome criteria:* Absence of or decrease in ventricular ectopy on EKG; regular palpable pulses.

Dose range/Administration

Interaction alert: Use with cimetidine may result in increased encainide levels.

Adult: PO: 25 mg q8h; after 3–5 days, may increase dose to 25–50 mg tid, if necessary. Allow at least 3 days before increasing dosage.

Clinical alert: This drug should be reserved for use with life-threatening arrhythmias only. An increased incidence of mortality has been found with the use of this agent for less serious arrhythmias. Place the patient on continuous cardiac monitoring prior to initiation of therapy. Patients receiving more than 200 mg/day should be hospitalized.

Contraindications/Precautions

PREG C

Contraindicated in hypersensitivity to encainide, cardiogenic shock, second- or third-degree heart block or bifasicular block (unless permanent pacemaker is in place to sustain cardiac rhythm if complete block should occur).

👋 **Use with caution for the elderly. Safe use for children and pregnant or nursing mothers has not been established.**

Side effects/Adverse reactions

Hypersensitivity: rash. *CNS:* dizziness, insomnia, headache, weakness, seizures. *CV:* development or aggravation of ventricular arrhythmias, produces dose-related changes in PR and QRS intervals, chest pain, palpitations. *GI:* nausea. *Eye:* visual disturbances.

Nursing implications/Documentation

Possible nursing diagnoses: Potential for injury; Activity intolerance.

◆ Be sure to check baseline chest X-ray, EKG, and laboratory studies (CBC, sodium, potassium, chloride, carbon dioxide, magnesium, BUN, creatinine, SGPT, and LDH) before giving first dose; monitor closely thereafter as indicated by clinical condition.

◆ Remember that oxygen requirements must be met, and that electrolyte imbalances (especially potassium and magnesium) and abnormal blood pH must be corrected, before expected antiarrhythmic effect can be seen; report abnormalities immediately.

◆ Document baseline vital signs, lung sounds, and cardiac monitor strip (measure and record PR and QRS segments) before giving first dose and at least every 8 hr; monitor closely until response is determined; report if prolongation in PR or QRS segment is noted.

◆ Supervise ambulation until response is determined.

- Coordinate care to provide for frequent rest periods.

Patient & family teaching/Home care

Possible nursing diagnoses: Fear; Knowledge deficit; Impaired home maintenance management.

- Explain that the purpose of this drug is to prevent arrhythmias and promote an effective heartbeat.
- Stress the need to follow dose regimen closely (the drug should be taken at the same time each day) and the need to return for medical follow-up for early detection of adverse reactions.
- Teach how to assess pulse for irregularities in rhythm and rate; stress that irregularities be reported.
- Emphasize the need to pace activities, avoid stress, and plan for rest periods.
- Encourage learning CPR; reinforce that survival rate of cardiac arrest is greatly increased when CPR is initiated immediately.

- *See Antiarrhythmics overview for more information.*

ephedrine

e-fed'rin

ephedrine hydrochloride: ♣*Fedrine*

ephedrine sulfate: *Ephed II, Efedron Nasal Jelly, Vatronol Nose Drops*

Class: ★**Adrenergic agonist (sympathomimetic) prototype,** Bronchodilator, Decongestant

PEDS	PREG	GERI
🖐	C	🖐

Action A potent sympathomimetic, ephedrine stimulates alpha and beta adrenergic receptors resulting in increased blood pressure, stimulation of the heart muscle (causing moderate tachycardia; increased cardiac output; and increase in coronary, cerebral, and muscle blood flow). Also causes constriction of arterioles, bronchodilation, relaxation of GI tract smooth muscle, dilation of pupils, and improvement in tone of the trigone and vesicle sphincter.

Use/Therapeutic goal/Outcome

Hypotension and shock: Elevation of blood pressure, improvement of perfusion of vital organs. **Outcome criteria:** Blood pressure within normal range; urine output over 25 ml/hr; absence of clinical signs and symptoms of shock (confu-

sion, restlessness, chest pain); hemodynamic monitor measurements (central venous pressure, cardiac output, pulmonary wedge pressure) within normal range.

Bronchospasm, nasal congestion: Reduction of airway resistance and improvement of air movement. **Outcome criteria:** Report of easier breathing, fewer episodes of wheezing; increased forced expiratory volume (FEV).

Dose range/Administration

Interaction alert: Monitor for additive effects if used with other sympathomimetics. Alpha-adrenergic blockers may reduce the vascular response, causing vasodilation. Beta-adrenergic blockers may block the cardiac and bronchodilating effects of ephedrine. Methyldopa and reserpine may reduce the vasopressor response of ephedrine. Do not use with MAOIs, tricyclic antidepressants, digitalis preparations, CNS stimulants or oxytocics.

Hypotension and shock: *Adult:* SC, IM: 25–50 mg; repeat if necessary. IV: 10–25 mg prn. *Maximum dose:* 150 mg/24 hr. *Child:* SC, IM, IV: 3 mg/kg/day in divided doses q4-6h.

Bronchodilator, nasal decongestant: *Adult:* PO: 12.5–50 mg bid to qid. *Maximum dose:* 400 mg/day in 6–8 equally divided doses. *Child:* PO: 2–3 mg/kg/day in divided doses q4-6h.

Nasal congestion: *Adult and Child:* Nasal: 3–4 drops 0.5% solution or a small amount of jelly on nasal mucosa prn, not more often than q4h. Do not use for longer than 3–4 days.

Clinical alert: For use in hypotension and shock, ascertain that reduced blood pressure is not a result of hypovolemia before giving ephedrine for hypotension (volume deficit should be corrected before starting vasopressors). If possible, avoid giving doses within 2 hr of bedtime to prevent insomnia.

Contraindications/Precautions
PREG
C

Contraindicated in hypersensitivity to sympathomimetics or sulfites and in narrow-angle glaucoma; within 14 days of MAOI therapy, and when vasopressors are contraindicated. *Use with caution* in diabetes or cardiovascular disease.

🖐 **Contraindicated for nursing mothers. Use with caution for children and the elderly. Safe use for pregnant women has not been established (has been used with spinal anesthesia in labor and delivery).**

Side effects/Adverse reactions

Hypersensitivity: flushing, redness, or bluish coloration of skin; dizziness; rash; hives; itching; swelling of face, lips, or eyelids; wheezing or difficulty in breathing; exaggeration of side effects. *CV:* palpitations, tachycardia, precordial pain, arrhythmias. *GU:* vesicle sphincter spasm, urinary retention, painful urination. *CNS:* headache, insomnia, sweating, nervousness, anxiety, tremor, weakness, hallucinations.

Nursing implications/Documentation

Possible nursing diagnoses: Potential for injury; Activity intolerance; Sleep pattern disturbance; Urinary retention.

◆ For IV route, document lung sounds, vital signs, and hemodynamic parameters before giving ephedrine; then at least hourly thereafter (record blood pressure and pulse every 5–15 min until response is determined, then hourly).

◆ When given for hypotension, record and monitor intake and output hourly; report urinary retention or output less than 25–30 ml/hr.

◆ Be aware that hypoxemia, and electrolyte and pH imbalances may reduce beneficial effects and increase adverse effects of ephedrine (these should be corrected as soon as possible).

◆ Monitor for and report angina or increased tachycardia or dysrhythmias.

◆ For IV route, keep patient in bed with side rails up; for IM and SC route, keep in bed until response is determined.

◆ Provide frequent rest periods.

Patient & family teaching/Home care

Possible nursing diagnoses: Knowledge deficit; Fear; Ineffective family coping.

◆ For hypotensive states, stress that frequent monitoring of vital signs is needed to "fine tune" medication dose for optimum results; stress the need to remain in bed.

◆ Point out that the nurses need to be told of new symptoms or uncomfortable feelings in case they indicate a need for medication adjustment.

◆ Warn against taking OTC drugs without physician's approval.

◆ For nasal route, have the patient demonstrate how to instill drops or jelly, and how to cleanse dropper with warm water between uses.

◆ See Adrenergics (sympathomimetics) overview for more information.

epinephrine
ep-i-nef'rin

epinephrine: *Adrenalin, Bronkaid Mist, ♣Bronkaid Mistometer, ♣Dysne Inhal, Primatine Mist Solution*

epinephrine bitartrate: *AsthmaHaler, Broniten Mist, Bronkaid Mist Suspension, Medihaler-Epi, Primatine Mist Suspension*

epinephrine hydrochloride: *Adrenalin Chloride, Epi-Pen, Epi-Pen JR, Sus-Phrine*

Class: ★Direct-acting adrenergic agonist (sympathomimetic) prototype, Bronchodilator

PEDS	PREG	GERI
✋	C	✋

Action Epinephrine acts directly on both beta and alpha receptors to produce sympathomimetic stimulation, causing increased myocardial contraction, bronchodilation, increased blood pressure, increased cardiac output and rate, constriction of bronchial arterioles, increased blood sugar, and decreased uterine contractions. Ophthalmic preparations lower intraocular pressure, by decreasing production and increasing outflow of aqueous humor. Topical applications stop bleeding through vasoconstriction.

Use/Therapeutic goal/Outcome

Cardiac arrest: Restoration of cardiac pumping action. *Outcome criteria:* Return of palpable pulses and improvement of cardiac rhythm on EKG.

Bronchospasm (asthma, bronchitis): Reduction of airway resistance, improved movement of air. *Outcome criteria:* Decreased wheezing, increased forced expiratory volume (FEV), increased ability to bring forth sputum; report of easier breathing, fewer episodes of wheezing.

Open-angle glaucoma: Reduction of aqueous humor formation. *Outcome criteria:* Upon measurement with tonometer, intraocular pressure within normal limits.

Anaphylactic shock: Correction of hemodynamic imbalances. *Outcome criteria:* Blood pressure, pulse, and respirations within normal limits.

Spinal anesthesia: Promotion of vasoconstriction. *Outcome criteria:* Prolonged effect of spinal anesthesia.

Uncontrolled bleeding: Promotion of hemostasis. *Outcome criteria:* Absence of bleeding.

Dose range/Administration

Interaction alert: Digoxin or general anesthetics may cause additive arrhythmic effects. High doses of digoxin may sensitize the heart to effects of epinephrine. Alpha-adrenergic blockers may cause hypotension. Beta-blockers may cause vasoconstriction and reflex bradycardia. Avoid guanethidine (may result in severe hypertension, arrhythmias, and prolonged mydriasis). Tricyclic antidepressants and certain antihistamines may increase effects.

Anaphylaxis and bronchospasm: Adult: SC, IM: 0.1–0.5 ml 1:1000 solution; may repeat q 10–15 min. IV: 0.1–0.25 ml 1:1000 solution. *Inhalation:* 1–2 breaths q 1–5 min. *Child:* SC: 0.01 ml (10 mcg)/kg 1:1000 solution q 20 min to 4 hr.

Cardiac arrest: Adult: IV: 0.5–1 mg 1:10,000 solution q 5 min prn during resuscitation. *Intracardiac:* 0.3–0.5 mg of 1:10,000 solution. May follow with 1–4 mcg/min epinephrine infusion. *Child:* IV: 10 mcg/kg 1:1000 solution q 5 min prn. *Intracardiac:* 5–10 mcg/kg 1:10,000 solution.

Anesthesia: Adult and Child: Intraspinal: 0.2–0.4 ml 1:1000 solution added to spinal anesthetic. *Local infiltration:* 1:500,000 to 1:50,000 solution mixed with anesthetic.

Acute asthma attacks: Adult and Child: Inhalation: 1 puff of 0.2 mg 1:100 solution; wait 1–2 minutes and give a second puff if needed. If no relief after 20 minutes, notify physician.

Hemostasis: Adult: Topical: A small amount of 1:50,000 to 1:1000 solution to stop bleeding.

Open-angle glaucoma: Adult: Ophthalmic: 1–2 drops 1–2% epinephrine bitartrate solution, frequency determined by tonometric readings; or 1 drop 0.5–2% epinephrine hydrochloride solution; or 0.5–1% epinephrine borate solution.

Clinical alert: Double check doses and concentration because these vary greatly with uses and intended goal. For IV route, document blood pressure every 3–5 min. Do not give IM doses into buttocks.

Contraindications/Precautions

PREG C

Contraindicated in hypersensitivity to sympathomimetics and sulfites, and in narrow-angle glaucoma, non-anaphylactic shock (hemorrhagic, traumatic, or cardiogenic), cardiac dilatation, coronary insufficiency, organic brain damage, arrhythmias, childbirth, and when vasopressor drugs might be contraindicated.

☙ **Contraindicated for pregnant or nursing mothers except in an emergency (excreted in breast milk). Use with caution for children and the elderly.**

Side effects/Adverse reactions

Hypersensitivity: bluish coloration of skin; dizziness; flushing or redness of skin; rash; hives; itching; swelling of face, lips or eyelids; wheezing or difficulty in breathing; exaggeration of side effects. *CNS:* nervousness, restlessness, insomnia, fear, tremors, headache. *CV:* cerebral hemorrhage, cardiac arrhythmias, myocardial infarction, anginal pain, palpitations, hypertension. *Resp:* bronchial and pulmonary edema. *GU:* urinary retention. *GI:* nausea, vomiting.

Nursing implications/Documentation

Possible nursing diagnoses: Potential for injury; Activity intolerance; Sleep pattern disturbance.

♦ Be aware that hypoxemia and electrolyte and pH imbalances may reduce beneficial effects and increase adverse effects of epinephrine (these should be corrected as soon as possible).

♦ For IV route, keep resuscitative equipment and drugs close at hand; monitor vital signs and EKG closely.

♦ Report sudden sharp increase in blood pressure, because this may require treatment (e.g., with nitrates).

♦ For IV route, keep patient in bed with side rails up; for IM and SC route, keep in bed until response is determined.

Patient & family teaching/Home care

Possible nursing diagnoses: Knowledge deficit; Fear; Ineffective family coping.

♦ For hypotensive states, stress that frequent monitoring of vital signs is needed to "fine tune" medication dose for optimum results; stress the need to remain in bed.

♦ Stress that the nurses need to be told of new symptoms or uncomfortable feelings in case they indicate a need for medication adjustment.

♦ Warn against taking OTC drugs without physician's approval.

♦ For ophthalmic route, teach the need to apply pressure over lacrimal duct to prevent systemic absorption and to report persistent irritation (slight stinging upon application is normal); warn that drops may stain soft contact lenses.

♦ For inhalation route, teach to begin administration immediately upon symptoms of wheezing, to take a second inhalation only if needed; stress the need to rinse mouth immediately after dose and to avoid swallowing any excess of drug.

♦ For bronchospasm, advise reporting immediately if symptoms are not relieved within 20 min.

♦ See Adrenergics (sympathomimetics) overview for more information.

ergoloid mesylates   *er'goe-loid mess'i-lates*

Hydergine, Circanol, Diapril

Class: Peripheral vasodilator, Cognitive adjuvant, Ergot alkaloid

PEDS	PREG	GERI
♨	C	♨

Action Exact mechanism of action is unknown. Produces peripheral vasodilation and decreases blood pressure and heart rate, primarily by central action. It is speculated that symptoms of cerebral arteriosclerosis are alleviated by increased cerebral metabolism, which improves cerebral vascular flow.

Use/Therapeutic goal/Outcome
Minimal brain dysfunction in the elderly (investigational use for Alzheimer's disease): Improved cerebral circulation. **Outcome criteria:** (per manufacturer): Client demonstrates decreased anxiety, fearfulness, depression, and fatigue; and improved appetite, mental alertness, energy, sociability, cooperation, and ability to perform self-care.

Dose range/Administration
♥ **Give with milk or food.**
Adult: PO, SL: 1 mg tid.
Clinical alert: Stress that SL tablet should not be crushed, but dissolved under tongue; advise not to eat, drink, or smoke until tablet is dissolved. This drug is available in PO tablet, SL tablet, and capsule form.

Contraindications/Precautions
PREG C
Contraindicated in hypersensitivity to ergoloid mesylates, and in acute or chronic psychosis. **Use with caution** in acute intermittent porphyria.

♨ **Monitor the elderly closely for accurate dose management. Safe use for children and pregnant women has not been established.**

Side effects/Adverse reactions
Hypersensitivity: skin rash. **CV:** orthostatic hypotension, lightheadedness, bradycardia. **Eye:** blurred vision. **Resp:** nasal stuffiness. **GI:** anorexia, nausea, vomiting, and cramps.

Nursing implications/Documentation
Possible nursing diagnoses: Activity intolerance; Potential for injury.

♦ Document baseline mental status and monitor closely thereafter.

♦ Monitor for dizziness and hypotension; supervise ambulation until response is determined.

♦ Report bradycardia or hypotension (may need to stop drug).

Patient & family teaching/Home care
Possible nursing diagnoses: Knowledge deficit; Impaired home maintenance management.

♦ Advise taking the oral preparation with food or milk.

♦ Stress the need to change positions slowly to reduce dizziness; point out that alcohol may increase vasodilation and dizziness.

♦ Warn that response to therapy is gradual (may take 3 to 4 weeks to see results) and that long-term therapy is usually required.

♦ See Antianginals overview for more information.

ergotamine   *er-got'a-meen*

ergotamine tartrate: **Ergomar, Ergostat, ♦Gynergen, Medihaler-Ergotamine**

Class: Alpha-adrenergic blocker (sympatholytic)

PEDS	PREG	GERI
♨	X	♨

Action Believed to relieve vascular headaches by constricting cerebral blood vessels through inhibition of the effect of sympathomimetic amines (epinephrine and norepinephrine) at alpha-adrenergic receptor sites and by antagonizing serotonin (implicated in the etiology of vascular headaches).

Use/Therapeutic goal/Outcome
Vascular headache: Relief of headaches. **Outcome criteria:** Patient report of headache relief.

Dose range/Administration

Interaction alert: Caffeine increases the rate of absorption. May interact with various OTC preparations, causing serious problems (check labels).

Adult: SL: 2 mg at start of migraine, then 1–2 mg q 30–60 min until attack abates. *Maximum dose:* 6 mg/day or 10 mg/wk. *Rectal:* 2 mg; may repeat in 1 hr. *Maximum dose:* 4 mg per attack or 10 mg/wk. *Inhalation:* 1 metered dose; may repeat in 5 min. *Maximum dose:* 6 doses in 24 hr or 15 doses/wk.

Clinical alert: Sublingual tablet and inhalation are the preferred routes because of rapid absorption.

Contraindications/Precautions

PREG
X

Contraindicated in hypersensitivity to ergot preparations, and in peripheral vascular disease, coronary artery disease, hypertension, renal and hepatic disease, anemia, infectious states, and malnutrition.

♨ **Contraindicated for children and pregnant women. Use with caution for nursing mothers and the elderly.**

Side effects/Adverse reactions

Hypersensitivity: itching. *CV:* numbness and tingling in extremities, chest pain, bradycardia or tachycardia. *GI:* nausea, vomiting, diarrhea. *CNS:* dizziness. *MS:* muscle weakness. *Misc:* acute ergotism (rare; vomiting, diarrhea, thirst, spasm of muscles, delirium, parethesias, seizures, cold skin), chronic ergotism (claudication, muscle weakness, pain, numbness, coldness, cyanosis of digits).

Nursing implications/Documentation

Possible nursing diagnoses: Pain; Ineffective individual coping.

◆ Have patient rate pain of headache on a scale of 1–10 before and after administration; report unrelieved pain.

◆ Identify dietary, emotional, physical, and environmental factors that precipitate or aggravate headaches.

◆ Provide a dark, quiet environment and holistic measures that promote comfort (e.g., cool washcloth for forehead).

◆ Monitor circulation to extremities to detect excessive vasoconstriction.

Patient & family teaching/Home care

Possible nursing diagnoses: Ineffective individual coping; Impaired home maintenance management.

◆ Stress the need to treat headache as soon after onset as possible.

◆ Explore ways of avoiding stress, coping with stress, and eliminating environmental factors that trigger headaches.

◆ Teach holistic measures for relieving pain (e.g., relaxation techniques).

◆ Advise reporting muscle weakness, numbness, or tingling of fingers and toes (may be due to excessive vasoconstriction, which can be harmful).

◆ Caution not to use OTC medications without physician's approval because of possible serious interactions.

◆ Warn that stopping this drug suddenly may cause a rebound effect that increases frequency and duration of headaches.

◆ Inform that exposure to cold may aggravate side effects.

◆ Point out that tobacco and alcohol should be avoided.

er-win'ee-ah a-spare'a-jun-ase

erwinia asparaginase

porton asparaginase

Class: Antineoplastic agent

PEDS   PREG   GERI
♨   D   ♨

Action Kills rapidly growing cells (cancer, hair follicles, bone marrow, GI lining, ova, and sperm) by depriving malignant cells of exogenous asparagine, which they require for protein synthesis. Is cell-cycle specific in the postmitotic G_2-phase.

Use/Therapeutic goal/Outcome

Acute lymphocytic leukemia (combination therapy only): Suppression of malignant cell proliferation. *Outcome criteria:* Absence of blasts in peripheral blood specimen.

Dose range/Administration

Interaction alert: Monitor for increased toxicity when administered with vincristine and prednisone. Decreases therapeutic effect of methotrexate. Other cytotoxic agents may cause severe myelosuppression.

Adult: IV, IM: 5000–10,000 IU/m^2/day for 7 days q 3 wk or 10,000–40,000 IU/m^2 every 2–3 weeks. Limit IM injections to 2 ml at one site. *Child:* IV, IM: 6000–10,000 IU/m^2/day for 14 days; or 1000 IU/kg for 10 days; or 60,000 IU/m^2 every other day for 12 doses. Limit IM injections to 2 ml at one site.

Clinical alert: Recognize that hypersensitivity reactions, including anaphylaxis, are common. This drug should be given to hospitalized patients only by nurses who are knowledgeable in the comprehensive management of the administration of antineoplastic agents. Doses may vary at physician's discretion. Repeat doses are held until it is ascertained that the patient has recovered sufficiently from toxicities of previous doses. Established protocols/policies for drug preparation, administration, and accidental skin contamination *must be followed closely* (gloves or double gloves are worn when handling drug; if the drug touches the skin, the area is washed immediately with plenty of soap and water). Erwinia asparaginase is diluted in 50–100 ml fluid and infused over a minimum of 30 min to minimize pain and inflammation. The solution should not be used if it is cloudy.

Contraindications/Precautions

PREG
C

Contraindicated in hypersensitivity to erwinia asparaginase and in pancreatitis. *Use with caution* in hepatic dysfunction.

🖐 **Contraindicated for pregnant or nursing mothers. Use with caution for children and the elderly.**

Side effects/Adverse reactions

Hypersensitivity: (common) respiratory distress, acute anaphylaxis, rashes, urticaria, arthralgia. *GI:* hepatotoxicity; pancreatitis; anorexia, nausea, vomiting. *GU:* acute renal failure, renal insufficiency, uric acid nephropathy. *CNS:* depression; drowsiness; confusion; agitation; hallucinations, Parkinson-like syndrome, headache, irritability. *Hem:* azotemia, hypofibrinogenemia, depression of clotting factors, thrombocytopenia, transient bone marrow depression, anemia, leukopenia. *Skin:* pain and erythema along injection site. *Misc:* fever, chills, and fatal hyperthermia.

Nursing implications/Documentation

Possible nursing diagnoses: Potential for infection; Potential for injury; Fatigue; Altered oral mucous membrane; Fluid volume deficit; Diarrhea; Altered nutrition: less than body requirements.

♦ *See important Nursing implications in Antineoplastic agents overview on page 72, which apply to all antineoplastics. The interventions that follow are additional and specific to this drug only.*

♦ Before administration, check that a hypersensitivity test has been documented at least 1 hr before dose (the patient may require desensitization); monitor closely for anaphylaxis and have emergency drugs and equipment on hand. (This drug may be useful for patients who are allergic to E. coli derived asparaginase, as cross-sensitivity does not occur.)

♦ Maintain a fluid intake of 2–3 L a day to prevent renal tubular damage from hyperuricemia secondary to cell lysis; record intake and output and report significant positive or negative balance.

♦ Observe for and report signs of pancreatic toxicity (abdominal pain, increased amylase levels).

♦ Monitor for drug-induced hyperglycemia and for CNS side effects.

Patient & family teaching/Home care

Possible nursing diagnoses: Knowledge deficit; Ineffective coping (individual and family); Hopelessness; Impaired home maintenance management.

♦ *See important Patient & family teaching in Antineoplastic agents overview on page 72, which apply to all antineoplastics. The teachings that follow are additional and specific to this drug only.*

♦ Stress the need to prevent kidney complications by drinking 2–3 L of fluid per day (if the patient can't keep fluids down, IV fluids may be necessary).

♦ *See Antineoplastic agents overview for more information.*

erythrityl tetranitrate

e-ri'thri-till

Cardilate

Class: Antianginal, Organic nitrate

PEDS	PREG	GERI
🖐	C	🖐

Action Decreases cardiac workload and myocardial oxygen demand by reducing left ventricular end-diastolic pressure (preload) and, to a lesser extent, by reducing systemic vascular resistance (afterload). Relaxes smooth muscle, particularly peripheral vascular smooth muscle, and has a vasodilating effect on large systemic arteries and veins, which decreases blood pressure. Also improves myocardial oxygen perfusion by promoting collateral circulation.

Use/Therapeutic goal/Outcome

Angina pectoris: Promotion of myocardial oxygenation, prevention of anginal (ischemic) attacks, improved activity tolerance. *Outcome criteria:* Patient reports decreased frequency and severity of angina attacks, and increased activity tolerance.

Dose range/Administration

Interaction alert: Antihypertensives and other antianginals may potentiate hypertensive effect.

▣ **Give oral doses 30 minutes before or 2–3 hours after meals for faster absorption.**

Adult: SL: 5–10 mg three to four times per day PRN, and as tolerated (before anticipated stress and, for nocturnal angina, at bedtime). PO: 10 mg tid. May be repeated as necessary up to 100 mg/day.

Clinical alert: Take blood pressure, pulse, and respirations prior to giving dose; hold dose and report if hypotension or bradycardia is present. If patient complains of tingling after taking sublingual dose, suggest holding in buccal pouch (cheek).

Contraindications/Precautions

PREG C

Contraindicated in hypersensitivity to nitrates, and in myocardial infarction accompanied by hypotension, severe anemia, head trauma, cerebral hemorrhage, and increased intracranial pressure.

🖐 **Use with caution in the elderly. Safe use for pregnant and nursing mothers and for children has not been established.**

Side effects/Adverse reactions

Hypersensitivity: rash. *CNS:* headache, dizziness. *CV:* palpitations, orthostatic hypotension, tachycardia, circulatory collapse, weakness, flushing. *GI:* nausea, vomiting, abdominal pain; sublingual use may cause local burning in the oral cavity while dissolving.

Nursing implications/Documentation

Possible nursing diagnoses: Potential for injury; Activity intolerance.

♦ Give sublingual doses at the first sign of angina; have the patient use a scale of 1 to 10 to rate pain before administration and 5 minutes after administration; report unrelieved pain immediately.

♦ Record pulse and blood pressure, before and after drug administration.

♦ Monitor for and report headache (usually can be treated with mild analgesics but may require dose adjustment); tolerance and decrease of headaches usually occur with long-term use.

♦ Observe for postural hypotension; take blood pressure in both arms, with patient sitting and standing, if possible.

♦ Supervise ambulation until response is determined.

♦ Coordinate care to provide frequent rest periods.

♦ Be aware that this drug is inactivated when exposed to heat, moisture, or air. Bottle and contents should be discarded 6 months after opening.

Patient & family teaching/Home care

Possible nursing diagnoses: Fear, Knowledge deficit; Impaired home maintenance management.

♦ Explain that antianginals help reduce the workload of the heart and improve coronary blood supply.

♦ Stress the need to follow the *scheduled* dose regimen closely (the drug should be taken at the same time each day) and the need to return for medical follow-up.

♦ Advise taking PO doses 30 minutes before meals and 2–3 hours after meals.

♦ Teach to take sublingual doses at the first sign of angina by wetting tablet with saliva and placing it under the tongue until completely dissolved.

♦ Emphasize the need to pace activities, avoid stress (emotional and physical), and plan for rest periods.

♦ Advise that tolerance to headache will develop with long-term use.

♦ Explain that an extra sublingual dose may be necessary during stress, or at bedtime if angina is nocturnal; teach that dose may be repeated every 10–15 minutes for 3 doses. If angina remains unrelieved, the patient should call paramedics.

- Advise changing positions slowly to avoid dizziness.
- Encourage keeping a record of angina attacks to show patterns; stress that an increase in frequency or severity should be reported.
- Stress that discontinuing this drug abruptly could precipitate coronary vasospasm and angina.
- Warn that drinking alcohol may cause fainting and hypotension.
- Emphasize that this drug can lose its effectiveness if exposed to moisture, heat, or air (keep in a cool place).
- *See Antianginals overview for more information.*

erythromycin

er-ith-roe-mye'sin

---

erythromycin base: ♣*Apo-Erythro base, A/T/S,* ♣*EMU-V, E-Mycin, Eryc, Erycette, Eryc Sprinkle, Eryderm, Erygel, Ery-Tab,* ♣*Erythromid, Ilotycin,* ♣*Novorythro, PCE Dispersatabs, Robimycin, Staticin*

erythromycin estolate: *Ilosone,* ♣*Novorythro*

erythromycin ethylsuccinate: ♣*Apo-Erythro-ES, E.E.S., E-Mycin E, EryPed, Erythrocin, Pediamycin, Wyamycin E.*

erythromycin gluceptate: *Ilotycin*

erythromycin lactobionate: *Erythrocin*

erythromycin stearate: ♣*Apo-Erythro-S, Erypar, Erythrocin,* ♣*Norvorythro, Wyamycin S*

Class: Anti-infective, Broad-spectrum antibiotic, Macrolide

PEDS	PREG	GERI
🖐	B	OK

Action Kills bacteria (bactericidal) or limits bacterial growth (bacteriostatic), depending upon concentration and susceptibility of the organism, by binding to the 50S ribosomal subunit, thus inhibiting protein synthesis.

Use/Therapeutic goal/Outcome

Infections (respiratory, pelvic inflammatory disease, endocarditis, skin and soft tissue, syphilis, Legionnaires' disease, endocervical or rectal infections, urogenital *Chlamydia trachomatis* during pregnancy, chlamydial conjunctivitis, Lyme disease): Prevention or resolution of infection. **Outcome criteria:** Absence of pathogenic growth on culture; absence of clinical manifestations of infection (redness, pain, swelling, fever, drainage, increased WBC count, productive cough); improvement of X rays.

Dose range/Administration

Interaction alert: Do not mix IV with any other drug. Clindamycin and lincomycin may block action of erythromycin. Use cautiously with theophylline and aminophylline (increase blood levels and risk of theophylline toxicity).

💊 **Give oral doses 1 hr before meals or 2 hr after meals, unless tablets are enteric coated or GI symptoms persist. Do not give with juice. However, give with food if GI symptoms persist.**

Respiratory, skin, and soft tissue infections (caused by Group A beta-hemolytic streptococci, Diplococcus pneumoniae, Mycoplasma pneumoniae, Corynebacterium diphtheriae, Bordetella pertussis, Listeria monocytogenes):
Adult: PO: 250–500 mg q6h (erythromycin base, esolate, stearate), or 400–800 mg q6h (erythromycin ethylsuccinate). IV: 15–20 mg/kg/day in divided doses, or as continuous infusion. **Child:** PO: 30–50 mg/kg/day (oral erythromycin salts) in divided doses q6h. IV: 15–20 mg/kg/day in divided doses q4-6h.

Endocarditis prophylaxis for dental surgery:
Adult: PO: 1 g (erythromycin base, estolate, stearate) 1 hr before procedure, then 500 mg 6 hr after. **Child:** PO: 20 mg/kg (erythromycin base, estolate, stearate) 1 hr before procedure, and 10 mg/kg 6 hr after.

Acute pelvic inflammatory disease (caused by Neisseria gonorrhoeae): **Adult:** IV: 500 mg (erythromycin gluceptate, lactobionate) q6h for 72 hours; then PO: 250 mg (erythromycin base, estolate, stearate) or 400 mg (erythromycin ethylsuccinate) q6h for 7 days.

Primary syphilis and other sexually transmitted diseases: **Adult:** PO: 500 mg qid for 7–30 days, depending on infection (CDC-recommended dosage). Usual duration of therapy for syphilis is 10 days.

Intestinal amebiasis: **Adult:** PO: 250 mg (erythromycin base, estolate, stearate) q6h for 10–14 days. **Child:** PO: 30–50 mg/kg/day (erythromycin base, estolate, stearate) in divided doses q6h for 10–14 days.

Chlamydia trachomatis infections:Newborn/Infant: PO: 50 mg/kg/day in 4 divided doses for 14 days (newborns) or 21 days (infants).
Ophthalmic: Apply a 1/2-inch ribbon of ointment to conjunctival sac of affected eye 2–6 times a day, depending on severity of infection.

Clinical alert: Give IV doses slowly over 60 minutes (dilute each 250 mg in a minimum of 100 cc IV solution) to reduce incidence of hypotension. Be aware that GI side effects associated with oral doses (nausea, vomiting, abdominal pain) may be severe, but abate with discontinuation of drug. Do not allow tablets to be chewed or crushed; do not give with juice.

Contraindications/Precautions

PREG B

Contraindicated in allergy to erythromycins, and in impaired liver function.

🖐 **Benzyl alcohol in lactobionate form can be fatal to neonates. Use with caution for pregnant or nursing mothers (has been used successfully during pregnancy to treat chlamydial infection); safety of other uses has not been established.**

Side effects/Adverse reactions

Hypersensitivity: itching, rashes, serum sickness, wheezing, fever, eosinophilia, dyspnea, generalized edema, anaphylaxis. **GI:** abdominal cramping, pain, nausea, vomiting, anorexia, pseudomembranous colitis, diarrhea; with erythromycin estolate, cholestatic jaundice. **CV:** (with IV route) pain, redness, swelling, thrombophlebitis at injection site. **Ear:** (with IV route) hearing loss with high doses. **Hem:** positive direct Coombs' test, slight elevation in SGOT, SGPT, BUN, and creatinine. **GU:** vaginitis. **CNS:** headache, dizziness, fatigue. **Misc:** superinfection.

Nursing implications/Documentation

Possible nursing diagnoses: Potential for infection; Diarrhea; Fluid volume deficit.

◆ Determine history of allergies, and (regardless of history) monitor closely for allergic reactions.

◆ Obtain baseline CBC, creatinine, liver function studies, and necessary cultures before administering first dose; monitor closely thereafter if therapy is prolonged.

◆ Encourage fluids, and record and monitor intake and output, to ensure adequate hydration; report significant negative or positive balance.

◆ Monitor for and report signs of superinfection (sore throat, fever, fatigue, thrush, vaginal discharge, diarrhea), and severe GI symptoms.

Patient & family teaching/Home care

Possible nursing diagnoses: Knowledge deficit; Impaired home maintenance management.

◆ Instruct to take doses with a full glass of water 1 hour before or 2 hours after meals (not juice, which inhibits absorption); may take with food only if GI symptoms persist.

◆ Teach the importance of reporting allergic symptoms, severe GI symptoms, signs and symptoms that do not abate, or *any* new signs and symptoms of discomfort that might indicate superinfection (medication regimen may have to be changed).

◆ Advise drinking 2–3 L of fluid daily to maintain adequate hydration (especially important if fever exists).

◆ Stress the importance of taking antibiotics for the entire time prescribed, even if signs and symptoms abate.

◆ *See Anti-infectives overview for more information.*

erythropoietin
ee-rith-row-poy'eh-tin

recombinant human erythropoietin (r-HuEPO): **Epogen, 🍁Eprex**

Class: Antianemic, Hormone, Human response modifier

PEDS	PREG	GERI
🖐	C	🖐

Action Stimulates red blood cell production by causing the erythroid tissues of the bone marrow to increase progenitor cell division and to produce precursor cells. (Erythropoietin is a naturally occurring hormone produced in the kidney. This preparation is produced by recombinant DNA techniques).

Use/Therapeutic goal/Outcome

Anemia due to decreased production of erythropoietin in end-stage renal disease: Stimulation of RBC production. **Outcome criteria:** After 2–6 weeks, increased hemoglobin, reticulocyte count, and hematocrit (target range 30–33%).

Clinical trials are being conducted for anemia in AIDS patients taking zidovudine, for patients receiving chemotherapy, and for patients with rheumatoid arthritis.

Dose range/Administration

Interaction alert: During hemodialysis, patients may require higher doses of heparin to prevent clotting in the artificial kidney and angioaccess.

Adult: IV, SC: *Initial dose:* 50 units/kg 3 times/wk. Monitor hematocrit closely, reduce dosage if hematocrit reaches 30–33, or increases > 4 points in < 2 wk; Individualize dose depending upon patient response. *Maintenance dose:* Usually ⅓ to ½ initial dose.

Clinical alert: Do not shake vial; shaking may inactivate the glycoprotein. Discard unused contents of vial; product contains no preservatives. This is a new drug, and information about dosage, administration, and adverse affects may change with additional clinical use. Erythropoietin is ineffective if iron levels are insufficient.

Contraindications/Precautions

PREG
C

Contraindicated in hypersensitivity to human albumin or to mammalian cell-derived products, and in uncontrolled hypertension.

〰 **Use with caution for the elderly (increased risk of thrombosis). Safe use for children and pregnant women has not been established.**

Side effects/Adverse reactions

Hypersensitivity: itching, rashes (rare and usually transient). **CV:** hypertension, chest pain, tachycardia. **Hem:** iron deficiency anemia, increased clotting of arteriovenous grafts, polycythemia. **CNS:** headache. **MS:** pelvic and limb pain (lasts only up to 12 hours, then disappears), seizures. **GI:** increased appetite. **Skin:** coldness, sweating (also transient).

Nursing implications/Documentation

Possible nursing diagnoses: Activity intolerance; Fatigue.

◆ Pace activities to allow for adequate rest.

◆ Monitor hematocrit weekly, report levels over 30–33% or increases more than 4 points in less than 2 weeks. (If there is a delayed response, the patient should be evaluated for iron or vitamin deficiency, occult blood loss, hemolysis, and for underlying infection, inflammatory or malignant process, hematologic disease.

◆ Be aware that as this drug improves anemic condition, the individual's sense of well-being and appetite will improve (may require dietary and dialysis prescription adjustment; monitor protein and potassium intake).

Patient & family teaching/Home care

Possible nursing diagnoses: Knowledge deficit; Impaired home maintenance management.

◆ Stress the importance of taking drug exactly as prescribed, and of returning for weekly hematocrits.

◆ Teach SC injection technique and observe return demonstration.

◆ Explain that if pelvic and long bone pain are experienced, the discomfort should abate after 12 hours.

◆ Stress the need for adequate intake of iron to achieve desired effects.

◆ Advise women to use contraceptives (fertility and sense of well-being improves when hematocrit reaches normal levels).

◆ Warn that as sense of well-being improves, it may be harder to stick to dietary restrictions (protein and potassium), but this is still very important.

◆ *See Antianemics overview for more information.*

esmolol hydrochloride

es'mo-lol

Brevibloc

Class: Selective beta-1 adrenergic blocking agent, Antiarrhythmic

PEDS	PREG	GERI
〰	C	〰

Action Reduces heart rate and blood pressure by inhibiting beta-1 receptors in the myocardium, thereby reducing its response to catecholamines (ultra-short-acting). Controls arrhythmias by blocking stimulation of cardiac pacemaker potentials.

Use/Therapeutic goal/Outcome

Hyperadrenergic response (associated with intubation and certain surgical procedures): Counteraction of hypertensive response. **Outcome criteria:** Blood pressure and heart rate within normal limits.

Supraventricular tachycardia: Suppression of supraventricular tachyarrhythmias. **Outcome criteria:** Absence of supraventricular tachycardia.

Dose range/Administration

Interaction alert: With morphine (which increases esmolol blood levels) or with reserpine or other catecholamine-depleting drugs, monitor for excessive hypotension and brady-cardia.

Adult: *IV:* *Loading dose:* 500 mcg/kg/min over 1 min. *Must be diluted before infusion to 10 mg/cc.* *Maintenance dose:* 50 mcg/kg/min over 4 min. *Titration procedure:* If desired response is not achieved within 5 min, repeat the 1-min loading dose, and increase the 4-min mainte-nance infusion to 100 mcg/kg/min. After 5 min, may repeat the 500 mcg/kg/min loading dose and increase maintenance infusion by incre-ments of 50 mcg/kg/min until desired heart rate (or excessive hypotension) is achieved. (Omit loading dose and use maintenance dose increments of 25 mcg/kg/min as desired end point is approached.) Do not exceed 200 mcg/kg/min.

Clinical alert: Monitor EKG and blood pressure closely during administration (excessive hypotension is common). Should not be used longer than 48 hours; when changing to a drug for long-term administration, do not abruptly discontinue esmolol infusion (wean according to package insert and patient response).

Contraindications/Precautions
PREG C

Contraindicated in hypersensitivity to esmolol, and in sinus bradycardia, second- or third-degree heart block (PR interval > 0.24 sec-onds), cardiogenic shock, CHF.

🖐 Use with caution for the elderly. Safe use for children and pregnant or nursing mothers has not been established.

Side effects/Adverse reactions

Hypersensitivity: hypotension with diaphoresis. *CV:* thrombophlebitis at injection site. *CNS:* dizziness, drowsiness, headache, agitation, fatigue. *GI:* nausea, vomiting.

Nursing implications/Documentation

Possible nursing diagnoses: Activity intolerance; Fatigue; Potential for injury.

◆ Assess mental status, and record pulse and blood pressure (if possible, lying, sitting, and standing, in both arms) before administration, and frequently thereafter until response is determined.

◆ Consult with physician to determine desired therapeutic range for blood pressure and heart rate (parameters for withholding the medica-tion should be written by physician).

◆ Ascertain that baseline CBC, electrolytes, BUN, creatinine, and liver function studies have been obtained before giving first dose;

report abnormalities and monitor closely there-after.

◆ Monitor for allergic reactions and for signs of confusion, dizziness, bradycardia, CHF, and hypotension; hold drug and report immediately if these occur.

◆ Keep patient in bed with side rails up during administration.

Patient & family teaching/Home care

Possible nursing diagnoses: Knowledge deficit; Anxiety.

◆ Explain that vital signs will be taken fre-quently to monitor blood pressure and cardiac response.

◆ Encourage the individual to verbalize unusual sensations and concerns.

◆ *See Beta Adrenergic Blockers and Antiarrhythmics overviews for more information.*

estrogen
es'troe-jen

conjugated estrogens (conjugated estrogenic sub-stances, conjugated oestrogens): 🌢 *C.E.S., Conju-gated Estrogens,* 🍁*C.S.D., Premarin, Premarin Intravenous, Progens*
Class: Hormone, Estrogen

PEDS PREG GERI
🖐   X   🖐

Action Enhances the functioning of the female reproductive system and increases the volume and acidity of vaginal and cervical secretions by replacing depleted estrogen levels and increasing DNA, RNA, and protein synthesis in responsive tissue. Also reduces FSH and LH from the pituitary. Maintains bone density by increasing calcitonin levels, which prevents bone reabsorption. Suppresses androgen-dependent malignant-cell growth by altering hormonal balance.

Use/Therapeutic goal/Outcome

Moderate to severe vasomotor symptoms associ-ated with menopause, female hypogonadism, and primary ovarian failure: Replacement of estro-gen; prevention or relief of menopausal symp-toms. *Outcome criteria:* Report of absence of menopausal symptoms (hot flashes, palpita-tions, vertigo); in developing females, presence of sexual development (breasts, pubic hair).

Atrophic vaginitis and kraurosis vulvae: Preven-tion or resolution of atrophic vaginitis and kraurosis vulvae. *Outcome criteria:* Absence of vaginal and vulval symptoms (itching, burning, drainage); report of improved comfort and sexual functioning.

Advanced, inoperable carcinoma of the breast in postmenopausal women and advanced, inoperable, metastatic carcinoma of the prostate: Suppression of malignant-cell growth. *Outcome criteria:* Tumor and disease process regression or stabilization on radiologic and physical exam.

Abnormal uterine bleeding due to hormonal imbalance: Restoration of estrogen levels. *Outcome criteria:* Absence of abnormal bleeding.

Postmenopausal osteoporosis: Prevention of bone loss and osteoporosis: *Outcome criteria:* Stabilization of bone density on radiologic examination; normal serum calcium levels.

Dose range/Administration

Interaction alert: May alter hypoglycemic and anticoagulant requirements. If given with tricyclic antidepressants, monitor for increased risk of toxicity.

🖐 **Give with food to decrease nausea.**

Menopausal symptoms: Adult: PO: 0.3 to 1.25 mg/day for 21 days, then 7 days off; repeat cycle. Regimen varies depending upon physician's orders; should be given in conjunction with progestins, except after hysterectomy.

Female hypogonadism: Adult: PO: 2.5 to 7.5 mg/day, bid or tid, for 20 days, then 10 days off; repeat cycle if menses does not occur. If menstruation begins, usually physician will prescribe a 20-day estrogen-progestin regimen.

Female castration and primary ovarian failure: Adult: PO: 1.25 mg/day for 21 days, then 7 days off. Repeat cycle if necessary.

Atrophic vaginitis and kraurosis vulvae: Adult: Vaginally: 2–4 g cream/wk for 3 wks, then 1 wk off. Repeat cycle as prescribed.

Breast cancer (postmenopausal): Adult: PO: 10 mg bid or tid.

Prostatic cancer: Adult: PO: 1.25 to 2.5 mg tid.

Abnormal uterine bleeding not related to cancer: Adult: IV, IM: 25 mg. Repeat in 6–12 hr if necessary.

Osteoporosis: Adult: PO: 0.625 mg/day for 21 days, then 7 days off. Repeat cycle as necessary.

Postpartum breast engorgement: Adult: PO: 3.75 mg q4h, for 5 doses, or 1.25 mg q4h for 5 days.

Clinical alert: Unless a woman has no uterus, estrogens should be given *in conjunction with progestins* to reduce risk of endometrial cancer. For IM and IV route, refrigerate before adding diluent; to mix, agitate gently. IM or IV is the preferred route for rapid treatment of uterine bleeding. For intravaginal application, give doses at bedtime or have patient lie down for 30 min after administration. Use the lowest effective dose for the shortest time to decrease incidence of side effects.

Contraindications/Precautions

PREG
X

Contraindicated in hypersensitivity to estrogens, and in thrombophlebitis, thromboembolic disease, and undiagnosed vaginal bleeding. *Use with caution* in medical conditions that could be aggravated by fluid retention (asthma, cardiac disease, epilepsy, hypertension, renal, and hepatic insufficiency); cerebrovascular or coronary artery disease; diabetes; gallbladder disease; history of seizures, migraines, or depression; ovarian, endometrial, breast, or estrogen-dependent cancer; and fibrocystic breast disease or endometriosis.

🖐 **Contraindicated for children and pregnant or nursing mothers. Use with caution for the elderly.**

Side effects/Adverse reactions

Hypersensitivity: abnormal or excessive genital bleeding, mastodynia, urticaria, leg cramps. *GI:* nausea, vomiting, diarrhea, constipation, anorexia, increased appetite, gallbladder disease. *CNS:* headache, migraine, dizziness. *Eye:* photosensitivity, increased myopia and astigmatism, steepening of the corneal curvature (visual acuity changes and intolerance to contact lenses). *CV:* increased risk of myocardial infarction, stroke, hypertension, thromboembolism, pulmonary embolism. *Hem:* hypercalcemia, folic acid deficiency. *GU:* breakthrough bleeding, change in menstrual flow, dysmenorrhea, candida vaginitis, cystitis-like syndrome, amenorrhea during and after treatment, increase in size of uterine fibromas, change in cervical erosion and amount of cervical secretions, endometrial carcinoma, feminization of genitalia, testicular atrophy, impotence. *MS:* weight gain or loss. *Skin:* acne, seborrhea, oily skin, pigmentation, hirsutism. *Misc:* breast tenderness and enlargement, loss of libido.

Nursing implications/Documentation

Possible nursing diagnoses: Altered sexuality patterns; Fluid volume excess.

• Keep a record of blood pressure and weight during therapy; report hypertension and weight gain.

• Document blood sugars to monitor diabetics for changes in hypoglycemic requirements.

Patient & family teaching/Home care

Possible nursing diagnoses: Altered sexuality patterns; Knowledge deficit; Impaired home maintenance management.

• Explain benefits and risks of estrogen therapy (estrogens in women are believed to improve female sexual functioning and reduce the incidence of osteoporosis, hypertension, and MI, but they may also be associated with increased risk of endometrial cancer); provide a package insert and discuss specific information for this drug verbally.

• Stress that this drug should be taken with, or immediately after, food to reduce nausea.

• Advise that missed doses should be taken as soon as possible, but not immediately before next dose.

• Warn that smoking can increase incidence of side effects.

• Inform women that withdrawal bleeding may occur if doses are suddenly stopped.

• Stress the importance to women of regular gynecologic exams (every 6 months to a year), mammography (yearly after age 40), and breast self-exam (monthly).

• If drug is taken on an on-off schedule, provide a calendar with drug-free days clearly marked.

• Point out the need for diabetics to monitor blood sugars and report hyperglycemic trends (estrogen may alter antidiabetic-agent requirements).

• Explore sexual concerns; encourage verbalizing feelings and concerns and seeking counseling as needed.

• For vaginal use, demonstrate technique for administration; advise wearing a sanitary napkin to protect underwear (tampons should not be used); point out that persistent vaginal symptoms and other systemic symptoms should be reported since they may be related to the medication; caution that sexual intercourse while drug is still present may cause irritation in partner (intercourse should be avoided until drug is absorbed).

estrogen with progestin   *proh-jess'tin*

ethinyl estradiol and ethynodiol diacetate, monophasic: *Demulen 1/35, Demulen 1/50*

ethinyl estradiol and levonorgestrel, monophasic: *Levlen, Nordette* triphasic: *Tri-Levlen, Triphasil*

ethinyl estradiol and norethindrone, monophasic: *Brevicon, Genora 0.5/35, Genora 1/35, Modicon, N.E.E. 1/35, Nelova 0.5/35 E, Nelova 1/35 E, Norcept-E 1/35, Norethin 1/35 E, Norinyl 1+35, Ortho-Novum 1/35, Ovcon-35, Ovcon-50* biphasic: *Nelova 10/11, Ortho Novum 10/11* triphasic: *Ortho Novum 7/7/7, Tri-Norinyl*

ethinyl estradiol and norethindrone acetate, monophasic: *Loestrin 21 1/20, Loestrin 21 1.5/30, Norlestrin 21 1/50, Norlestrin 21 2.5/50*

ethinyl estradiol and norgestrel, monophasic: *Lo/Ovral, Ovral*

ethinyl estradiol, norethindrone acetate, and ferrous fumarate, monophasic: *Loestrin Fe 1/20, Loestrin Fe 1.5/30, Norlestrin Fe 1/50, Norlestrin Fe 2.5/50*

mestranol and norethindrone, monophasic: *Genora 1/50, Nelova 1/50 M, Norethin 1/50 M, Norinyl 1+50, Ortho-Novum 1/50*

Class: Estrogen-progestin hormone, Contraceptive

PEDS	PREG	GERI
🤚	X	🤚

Action *Estrogen* blocks ovulation by preventing the release of the luteinizing hormone (known as LH, and responsible for development of the corpus luteum) and by suppressing secretion of the follicle-stimulating hormone (known as FSH, and responsible for follicle development). *Progestin* prevents ovulation, even if follicle development occurs, by inhibiting the preovulatory rise of LH; it inhibits sperm penetration by causing a thickening of the cervical mucus and prevents implantation of the fertilized ovum by altering the endometrium. Estrogen with progestin promotes regular menses by maintaining cyclic hormonal levels. *Estrogen-progestin combinations* come in varying concentrations, which significantly affect action.

Use/Therapeutic goal/Outcome

Contraception, polycystic ovarian disease, hypermenorrhea, endometriosis: Suppression of ovulation, prevention of pregnancy, resolution and prevention of ovarian cysts, suppression of endometrial proliferation. **Outcome criteria:**

Absence of pregnancy; absence or reduction in size of ovarian cyst on ultrasound; report of decreased pain associated with menstrual cycle and decreased menstrual flow.

Dose range/Administration

Interaction alert: Rifampin, barbiturates, phenylbutazone, phenytoin, anti-infective agents, and anticonvulsants may decrease contraceptive efficacy. May alter insulin and oral hypoglycemic dose requirements.

🖐 **Give with or after the evening meal or at bedtime to minimize nausea.**

Contraception: Adult: PO: 1 tablet/day; begin on day 5 of menstrual cycle for 20 or 21 days, then off 7 days. *28-tablet packs:* Extras are placebos or iron doses. *If 3 or more doses are missed:* Discard remaining tablets; another contraceptive method must be used. *Biphasic:* Color-1 tablet daily for 10 days, then color-2 tablet for 11 days. *Triphasic:* 1 tablet/day in manufacturer's specified sequence. *If 2 consecutive menstrual cycles are missed:* Rule out pregnancy before restarting dose.

Clinical alert: Make certain patient is not pregnant before beginning therapy (oral contraceptive use during pregnancy can cause fetal toxicity). Day 1 of menstrual cycle is first day of menstrual flow. Clarify dosage schedules with manufacturer's package inserts.

Contraindications/Precautions

PREG X

Contraindicated in hypersensitivity to estrogen–progestin combinations, and in undiagnosed abnormal vaginal bleeding, estrogen-dependent neoplasia, thrombophlebitis, thromboembolic disease, and cerebrovascular or coronary artery disease. *Use with caution* in asthma, renal and hepatic insufficiency, diabetes, gallbladder disease, seizure disorders, migraines, mental depression, family history of lupus erythematosus, rheumatic disease, or fibrocystic breast disease.

🖐 **Contraindicated for children and pregnant or nursing mothers. Use with caution for adolescents with incomplete bone growth, women over 40 years, and smokers over 35 years.**

Side effects/Adverse reactions

Hypersensitivity: abnormal/excessive vaginal bleeding, mastodynia, urticaria, paresthesia, acute porphyria. *CNS:* dizziness, migraine headaches, chorea, lethargy, mental depression (can be severe). *Eye:* optic neuritis, diplopia, retinal thrombosis, papilledema, increased degenerative changes in myopia and astigmatism, steepening of the corneal curvature (visual acuity changes and intolerance to contact lenses). *CV:* malignant hypertension, edema, thromboembolism, pulmonary embolism, myocardial infarction, increased risk of stroke. *Hem:* hypercalcemia, increased serum triglycerides, folic-acid deficiency. *GI:* anorexia, nausea, vomiting, diarrhea, constipation, abdominal cramps, increased appetite, excessive thirst, decreased glucose tolerance, jaundice, gallbladder disease, benign hepatic adenomas. *GU:* urinary tract infections, renal failure, breakthrough bleeding, dysmenorrhea, amenorrhea, cervical mucorrhea, cervical erosion, increase in uterine fibroma size, endometrial carcinoma, candida vaginitis, cystitis-like syndrome. *Skin:* acne, seborrhea, oily skin, erythema multiforme, hirsutism, alopecia. *Misc:* breast tenderness, enlargement, and secretion, changes in weight, loss of libido.

Nursing implications/Documentation

Possible nursing diagnoses: Pain; Fluid volume deficit.

◆ Document last menstrual period and absence of pregnancy before beginning oral contraceptive therapy.

◆ Record baseline weight and vital signs and periodically thereafter; report weight gain or hypertension.

◆ Report persistent diarrhea (drug should be discontinued if granulomous colitis develops).

Patient & family teaching/Home care

Possible nursing diagnoses: Knowledge deficit; Impaired home maintenance management.

◆ Stress the need to take this drug at the same time every day (preferably after the evening meal or at bedtime).

◆ Provide a package insert or list of risks and side effects that should be reported (dizziness, persistent headache, chest pain, abdominal pain, swelling of the feet or ankles).

◆ Reinforce that an alternate method of birth control should be used with the drug for the first month.

◆ Provide a calendar that clearly indicates drug days, rest days, and drug-free periods.

◆ Stress that 1 missed dose can be taken as soon as possible; 2 missed doses usually requires doubling the normal dose for 2 days

▶

and using additional birth control measures for 1 cycle. Missed doses in the middle of a cycle greatly increase the chances of pregnancy; an additional form of birth control should be used for remainder of cycle.

• Emphasize that 2 consecutively missed periods require stopping the drug and having a pregnancy test. (Progestin can cause serious problems when taken early in pregnancy.)

• Warn that breakthrough bleeding is not uncommon initially and should stop in 3–6 months; however, high-dose therapy may cause bleeding that requires dosage adjustment, so it should be reported (triphasic oral contraceptives may have less incidence of breakthrough bleeding).

• Stress that gynecologic examinations and PAP smears should be performed every 6 months.

• Teach breast self-examination (BSE) and observe return demonstration; emphasize that this should be performed monthly, and that women over 40 years should have annual mammograms.

• Advise avoiding tasks that require mental alertness or physical coordination if visual disturbances, dizziness, mental depression, or lightheadedness occurs.

• Explain that headache and nausea are not uncommon, but usually disappears by the fourth month; advise reporting severe nausea or vomiting (dose may be altered).

• Caution that cigarette smoking significantly increases the risk of fatal MI and CVA, and that the risk increases with age (over 35 years) and with the amount of smoking (more than 15–20 cigarettes a day).

• Caution against using the same drug for longer than 18 months; many physicians advise against using birth-control pills for longer than 5 years without periodically stopping the drug to assess normal cycle.

• Teach the importance of advising physicians and dentists that a birth control pill is being taken (birth control pills should be held for 1 month before major surgery to reduce risk of thromboembolism); stress the need to read the labels of OTC drugs to check for drug interactions.

• Provide a list of side effects that should be reported immediately (chest pain, shortness of breath, severe headache, visual disturbances such as flashing lights or blind spots, abdomi-

nal pain, swelling of hands or feet, stiffness or numbness in legs or buttocks).

• When this medication is discontinued, advise to use an alternative method of birth control for 3 months to avoid possible harm to fetus.

ethacrynic
eth-a-krin-ik

ethacrynic acid: *Edecrin,* ♠*Edecril*
ethacrynic sodium: *Edecrin sodium*
Class: Loop (high-ceiling) diuretic

PEDS	PREG	GERI
🖐	B	🖐

Action Promotes diuresis by inhibiting sodium and chloride reabsorption in the ascending loop of Henle, and in the proximal and distal tubules.

Use/Therapeutic goal/Outcome

Edema or ascites associated with renal disease, cirrhosis, lymphedema, CHF, malignancy, or heart disease: Promotion of diuresis, resolution of edema. *Outcome criteria:* Increased urine output; absence of rales and peripheral and sacral edema; in ascites, decreased abdominal girth. *Pulmonary edema:* Promotion of diuresis, resolution of pulmonary edema. *Outcome criteria:* Absence of rales; increased urine output; PWP and CVP within normal limits.

Dose range/Administration

Interaction alert: Aminoglycosides and other ototoxic drugs can potentiate ototoxicity. Corticosteroids may increase risk of GI bleeding. Potentiates effect of warfarin.

🍴 **Give with food to reduce GI upset.**

Edema: Adult: PO: 50 mg; increase to 50 mg bid the next day, and thereafter by 50–100 mg/day (divided bid). *Maximum dose:* 400 mg/day. Dose and frequency may be decreased once diuresis has occurred. *Child:* PO: 25 mg; may increase by 25 mg/day.

Pulmonary edema: Adult: IV: 50 mg (0.5–1 mg/kg) ethacrynic sodium over several min; dosage may be repeated once. (A single 100 mg dose has been used in critical situations.)

Clinical alert: Use the lowest effective dose. Give in morning (when possible) to avoid nocturnal diuresis.

Contraindications/Precautions
PREG B

Contraindicated in hypersensitivity to ethacrynic acid, and in anuria. *Use with caution* in cardiac disease, gout, diabetes, and pulmonary edema secondary to myocardial infarction.

🖐 **Contraindicated for infants and pregnant or nursing mothers. Use with caution for the elderly.**

Side effects/Adverse reactions

Hypersensitivity: rash, urticaria, dermatitis. *CV:* orthostatic hypotension, volume depletion, dehydration. *Hem:* agranulocytosis, leukopenia, thrombocytopenia, hypokalemia, asymptomatic hyperuricemia, fluid and electrolyte imbalances, hypocalcemia, hypomagnesemia, hyperglycemia, impaired glucose tolerance. *GI:* abdominal discomfort, diarrhea. *Ear:* transient (with rapid IV administration) and permanent deafness. *Misc:* hypochloremic alkalosis.

Nursing implications/Documentation

Possible nursing diagnoses: Fluid volume deficit; Altered patterns of urinary elimination; Potential for injury.

♦ Ascertain that baseline CBC, sodium, potassium, chloride, carbon dioxide, calcium, magnesium, BUN, creatinine, uric acid, and liver function studies have been obtained before giving first dose; report abnormalities and monitor closely thereafter.

♦ Give doses in early morning and early afternoon (if possible) to avoid nocturnal diuresis.

♦ Document and monitor blood pressure, daily weight, and intake and output; report significant discrepancies.

♦ Monitor for and report signs of fluid overload (auscultate lungs for rales; check feet, ankles, and sacrum for edema).

♦ Report diarrhea or impaired hearing (may need to discontinue drug).

♦ Be aware the diuretics often induce hypokalemia, which predisposes individuals to cardiac arrhythmias, cramping, and digoxin toxicity.

♦ Check with physician to determine dietary restrictions; if a low-salt, high-potassium diet is recommended, consult with dietician to plan a low-salt diet that includes foods and juices high in potassium (orange juice; banana; green leafy vegetables).

♦ Observe the elderly for extreme diuresis; monitor for orthostatic hypotension; supervise ambulation until response is determined.

Patient & family teaching/Home care

Possible nursing diagnoses: Knowledge deficit; Impaired home maintenance management.

♦ Advise taking this drug with meals to avoid GI symptoms.

♦ Before giving first dose, explain that the drug will increase the amount and frequency of urination.

♦ Emphasize the importance of taking this drug exactly as prescribed, and the importance of returning for medical follow-up.

♦ Explain that diuretics enhance the work of the kidney and reduce the workload of the heart.

♦ Recommend taking doses in early morning and early afternoon to prevent the need to disturb sleep to void.

♦ Explain that changing positions slowly helps prevent dizziness.

♦ Advise reporting dizziness, shortness of breath, swelling of hands and feet, diarrhea, ringing in the ears, hearing problems, or persistent sore throat; encourage daily monitoring of weight and reporting sudden weight gain.

♦ Provide a list of allowed foods and fluids; stress the need to stick to prescribed diet (explain the hazards of too much salt, or too little potassium).

♦ Warn against driving or activities that require alertness until response has been determined.

♦ *See Diuretics overview for more information.*

ethambutol

e-tham'byoo-tole

ethambutol hydrochloride: ✤*Etibi, Myambutol*
Class: Anti-infective, Antitubercular

PEDS	PREG	GERI
🖐	B	🖐

Action Limits tubercular bacterial growth (bacteriostatic action). Exact mechanism is unknown; may inhibit synthesis of a metabolite, which then impairs cellular metabolism.

Use/Therapeutic goal/Outcome

Tuberculosis (together with other antitubercular drugs) and other mycobacterial diseases: Resolution of infection. *Outcome criteria:* Absence of acid-fast bacilli on sputum cultures, decreased productive cough, normal temperature, improvement of X rays.

Dose range/Administration

🖐 **Give with meals.**

Adult/Child > 13 yrs: PO: *Initial treatment:* 15 mg/kg/day. *Retreatment:* 25 mg/kg/day for 60 days, then 15 mg/kg/day.

Clinical alert: In the presence of kidney impairment, expect decreased dosage.

Contraindications/Precautions
<small>PREG
B</small>

Contraindicated in hypersensitivity to ethambutol, and in optic neuritis. **Use with caution** in kidney disease, gout, diabetic retinopathy, cataracts, or occular defects.

🖐 **Contraindicated for children under 13 and nursing mothers. Use with caution for the elderly. Safe use during pregnancy has not been established (use with caution).**

Side effects/Adverse reactions

Hypersensitivity: itching, rashes, fever, anaphylaxis. **GI:** anorexia, nausea, vomiting, abdominal pain. **CNS:** dizziness, headache, confusion, peripheral neuritis, hallucinations. **Eye:** optic neuritis (vision loss and loss of color discrimination, especially red and green). **Hem:** elevated uric acid. **Misc:** malaise.

Nursing implications/Documentation

Possible nursing diagnoses: Potential for infection; Fatigue; Activity intolerance; Fluid volume deficit.

◆ Ascertain that baseline CBC, BUN, creatinine, and liver function studies are obtained, and that necessary culture specimens are collected, before starting ethambutol; monitor periodically thereafter, depending on clinical symptoms.

◆ If the patient is receiving more than 15 mg/kg/day, monitor for and report changes in visual acuity and color discrimination.

◆ Monitor and record intake and output and provide favorite fluids to ensure adequate hydration.

◆ Allow for a balance between rest and activity.

Patient & family teaching/Home care

Possible nursing diagnoses: Knowledge deficit; Impaired home maintenance management.

◆ Stress the importance of taking this drug as prescribed without missing doses, and the importance of long-term medical follow-up to avoid relapses or complications.

◆ Explain the need to report eye problems (these should stop within weeks or months after drug is stopped).

◆ Encourage the drinking of at least 2 L of fluid a day to maintain adequate hydration.

◆ *See Anti-infectives overview for more information.*

ethaverine
<small>*e-tha'ver-een*</small>

ethaverine hydrochloride: *Ethaquin, Ethatab, Ethavex-100, Isovex*

Class: Vasodilator, peripheral; Antispasmotic

PEDS	PREG	GERI
🖐	C	🖐

Action Dilates peripheral blood vessels by producing a direct relaxant effect on smooth muscle (inhibits phosphodiesterase). Closely resembles papaverine, but is reported to be 2 to 4 times more effective with fewer side effects.

Use/Therapeutic goal/Outcome

Vascular insufficiency (peripheral and cerebral): Prevention of spasm/dilation of vessels/ improved tissue perfusion. **Outcome criteria:** Signs of improved circulation or perfusion (report of absence of pain; improved pulse quality, and skin color and temperature); improved mental status.

Spastic conditions of the GI and GU tract: Prevention of spasm. **Outcome criteria:** Report of absence of abdominal pain; continence.

Dose range/Administration

🖐 **Give with meals.**

Adult: PO: 100–200 mg tid. *Sustained release form:* 150 mg q12h, up to 300 mg q12h.

Contraindications/Precautions
<small>PREG
C</small>

Contraindicated in hypersensitivity to ethaverine, and in complete AV block, serious arrhythmias, severe liver disease, glaucoma, coronary insufficiency, and pulmonary emboli.

🖐 **Use with caution for the elderly. Safe use for children and pregnant women has not been established.**

Side effects/Adverse reactions

Hypersensitivity: rash. **CNS:** headache. **CV:** flushing, vertigo, hypotension. **GI:** nausea, vomiting, dry throat, altered liver function. **Resp:** respiratory depression.

Nursing implications/Documentation

Possible nursing diagnoses: Activity intolerance; Potential for injury.

◆ Document baseline mental status, pain level, and circulatory status (presence and quality of peripheral pulses, skin color and temperature); monitor periodically thereafter.

◆ Monitor for dizziness and hypotension; supervise ambulation until response is determined.

Patient & family teaching/Home care

Possible nursing diagnoses: Knowledge deficit; Impaired home maintenance management.

◆ Advise taking with meals or immediately after meals.

◆ Stress the need to change positions slowly to reduce dizziness; point out that alcohol may increase vasodilation and dizziness.

◆ Warn that response to therapy is gradual, and that long-term therapy is usually required.

◆ Warn against driving or hazardous activities until response is determined.

ethosuximide

eth-oh-sux'i-mide

Zarontin

Class: ★**Anticonvulsant prototype,** Succinimide

PEDS ✋ | PREG C | GERI ✋

Action Limits seizure activity by elevating CNS threshold to convulsive stimuli (probably depresses the motor cortex).

Use/Therapeutic goal/Outcome

Petit mal (simple absence) and partial seizures with complex symptomatology: Limitation of seizure activity. ***Outcome criteria:*** Marked decrease or absence of seizures.

Dose range/Administration

Give with meals if GI distress is noted.

Adult/Child > 6 yrs: PO: 250 mg bid, may increase daily dosage every 4–7 days by 250 mg increments to a maximum of 1.5 g/day. ***Child 3–6 yrs:*** PO: 250 mg daily, or in divided doses bid. May increase daily dosage every 4–7 days by 250 mg increments to a maximum dose of 1.5 gm/day.

Monitor serum ethosuximide levels closely (therapeutic range is 40–80 mcg/ml) until stabilized. Monitor CBC every 3 months.

Contraindications/Precautions

PREG C

Contraindicated in hypersensitivity to succinimides, and in liver or renal disease.

✋ **Use with caution for the elderly. Safe use for children under 3 years and pregnant women has not been established.**

Side effects/Adverse reactions

Hypersensitivity: rash. ***Skin:*** Stevens-Johnson syndrome, skin eruptions, hirsutism, systemic lupus erythematosus. ***Hem:*** leukopenia, eosinophilia, aplastic anemia. ***CNS:*** dizziness, drowsiness, headache, hiccups, hyperactivity, inability to concentrate, confusion, psychological or psychiatric aberrations. May increase tendency for grand mal seizures. ***GI:*** nausea, vomiting, gum hypertrophy, anorexia. ***GU:*** urinary frequency, hematuria, vaginal bleeding, renal damage. ***Eye:*** blurred vision, photophobia, periorbital edema. ***Misc:*** increased libido.

Nursing implications/Documentation

Possible nursing diagnoses: Potential for injury; Potential for aspiration.

◆ Document history of seizures (type, frequency, duration, usual time they occur, precipitating factors, presence of an aura); initiate seizure precautions as indicated.

◆ Be aware that if this drug is used alone to treat mixed seizures, it may increase the frequency of generalized tonic-clonic (grand mal) seizures.

◆ Monitor for and report signs of hematological side effects (persistent fatigue, weakness, frequent infections).

Patient & family teaching/Home care

Possible nursing diagnoses: Fear; Self-esteem disturbance; Knowledge deficit; Impaired home maintenance management.

◆ Advise to take with meals if GI symptoms are noted.

◆ Stress the need for close medical follow-up; emphasize that persistent fatigue, weakness, fever, sore throat or infections may be signs of side effects that should be reported.

◆ Warn that stopping anticonvulsants suddenly can cause an increase in severity and frequency of seizures.

◆ Caution against driving until response is determined (may cause drowsiness at first).

• *See Anticonvulsants overview for more information.*

ethotoin

eth'oh-toyn

Preganone

Class: Anticonvulsant, Hydantoin

PEDS	PREG	GERI
🖐	D	🖐

Action Limits the spread of seizure activity, and reduces abnormal excitability in the motor cortex. Nerve impulses in the motor cortex are probably inhibited by an effect on sodium ion flux across neuronal cell membranes, but exact mechanism of anticonvulsant action is unknown. Less effective and toxic than phenytoin.

Use/Therapeutic goal/Outcome

Grand mal and partial seizures with complex symptomatology: Limitation of seizure activity. *Outcome criteria:* Marked decrease or absence of seizure activity.

Dose range/Administration

Interaction alert: Chronic alcohol use and folic acid may decrease effectiveness. Oral anticoagulants, antihistamines, chloramphenicol, cimetidine, some benzodiazepines, diazoxide, disulfiram, estrogens, isoniazid, phenothiazines, phenylbutazone, salicylates, and sulfonamides may increase risk of toxicity. The result of concurrent therapy with valproic acid, and with phenobarbital, is unpredictable. If given with phenacemide, monitor for paranoia.

🖤 **Give after food.**

Adult: PO: 250 mg qid. May increase gradually over several days up to 3 g/day in divided doses. *Child:* PO: 250 mg bid. May increase dosage gradually to a maximum 1.5 g/day (usual maintenance dose is 250 mg qid).

Clinical alert: Schedule doses as evenly as possible over a 24-hr period.

Contraindications/Precautions

PREG
D

Contraindicated in hypersensitivity to hydantoins and in liver or hematological disorders.

🖐 **High risk potential in pregnancy. Use with caution for children and the elderly.**

Side effects/Adverse reactions

Hypersensitivity: skin rash. *GI:* anorexia, nausea, vomiting, and (rarely) gingival hyperpla-

sia. *CNS:* drowsiness, and (rarely) ataxia. *Hem:* thrombocytopenia, leukopenia, agranulocytosis, megoblastic anemia. *Misc:* lymphadenopathy.

Nursing implications/Documentation

Possible nursing diagnoses: Potential for injury; Potential for aspiration.

• Document history of seizures (type, frequency, duration, usual time they occur, precipitating factors, presence of an aura); initiate seizure precautions as indicated.

• Monitor CBC monthly, and liver function studies periodically.

• Report signs of hematological side effects (persistent fatigue, sore throat, fever, infections).

• Be aware that this drug is usually used for those who are prone to gingival hyperplasia caused by phenytoin.

Patient & family teaching/Home care

Possible nursing diagnoses: Fear; Self-esteem disturbance; Knowledge deficit; Impaired home maintenance management.

• Advise to take this drug after meals if GI symptoms are noted.

• Stress the need for close medical follow-up; emphasize that persistent fatigue, weakness, fever, sore throat or infections may be signs of side effects that should be reported.

• Warn that stopping anticonvulsants suddenly can cause an increase in severity and frequency of seizures.

• Warn that drinking alcohol may reduce drug effectiveness.

• Caution against driving until response is determined (may cause drowsiness at first).

• *See Anticonvulsants overview for more information.*

ethylestrenol

eth-ill-ess'tre-nole

Maxibolin, ♠Orabolin

Class: Anabolic steroid

PEDS	PREG	GERI
🖐	X	🖐

Action Promotes body tissue-building processes and reverses catabolic processes by promoting protein anabolism and stimulating appetite.

Use/Therapeutic goal/Outcome

Catabolic state: Reversal of negative nitrogen balance and increased protein synthesis. **Outcome criteria:** Increased appetite, increased energy level, and weight gain.

Dose range/Administration

Interaction alert: Increases effect of insulin, oral hypoglycemics, and anticoagulants. Corticosteroids increase possibility of edema and severe acne. Avoid other hepatotoxic medications.

🖐 **Give with food or milk to minimize GI symptoms.**

Adult: PO: 4–8 mg/day. **Child:** PO: 1–3 mg/day, for maximum of 6 wks.

Clinical alert: Ethylestrenol therapy may be given intermittently (6 weeks of medication, then a 4-week drug-free period, then 6 weeks of medication) if indicated.

Contraindications/Precautions

PREG
X

Contraindicated in hypersensitivity to anabolic steroids, and in men with cancer of breast or prostate, women with hypercalcemia associated with breast cancer, hypercalcemia, and severe hepatic or renal impairment. **Use with caution** in cardiac, hepatic, or renal impairment; coronary artery disease; history of MI; diabetes mellitus; prostatic hypertrophy.

🖐 **Contraindicated for pregnant or nursing mothers. Use with caution for children and elderly men.**

Side effects/Adverse reactions

Hypersensitivity: rashes, anaphylaxis. **GU:** virilism of females (enlarged clitoris, deepening of voice, menstrual irregularities, unnatural hair growth or loss); virilism of prepubertal males (acne, enlarging penis, increased frequency of erections, unnatural hair growth); in older men, bladder irritability, breast soreness, gynecomastia, priapism, prostatic hypertrophy, prostatic carcinoma, testicular atrophy, suppression of spermatogenesis; decreased libido in both men and women. **Hem:** iron deficiency anemia, leukemia, suppression of clotting factors, hypercalcemia, decreased high-density lipoproteins (HDL), and increased low-density lipoproteins (LDL). **GI:** nausea, vomiting, diarrhea; hepatic dysfunction, carcinoma, or necrosis. **MS:** muscle cramps, premature epiphyseal closure in children. **Skin:** unexplained darkening, acne, edema.

Nursing implications/Documentation

Possible nursing diagnoses: Body image disturbance; Fluid volume excess.

◆ Record baseline blood pressure and weight.

◆ Assess for and report increased blood pressure, weight gain or evidence of edema or congestive failure.

◆ Monitor serum calcium levels; assess and document symptoms of hypercalcemia (nausea, vomiting, constipation, lethargy, muscle weakness).

◆ Monitor for changes in liver function tests and cholesterol levels.

◆ For diabetics, monitor glucose levels closely and observe for symptoms of hypoglycemia.

Patient & family teaching/Home care

Possible nursing diagnoses: Knowledge deficit; Impaired home maintenance management; Sexual dysfunction.

◆ Advise taking with food or milk to reduce gastric irritation.

◆ Suggest restriction of sodium intake to decrease fluid retention.

◆ Encourage a diet high in protein and calories to obtain maximum anabolic benefit.

◆ Caution women of child-bearing age to use reliable birth control methods and to stop drug immediately and report if they suspect pregnancy.

◆ For females, stress the importance of reporting the occurrence of masculinizing effects (abnormal growth of facial hair, deepening of voice, menstrual irregularities, enlarged clitoris).

◆ For males, advise reporting development of priapism, gynecomastia, or bladder irritability.

◆ For diabetics, caution about possible lowering of blood sugar; point out the need for adjustment of doses of insulin or oral antidiabetic agents.

◆ Inform parents of prepubertal children that X rays will be taken periodically to determine effect on bone growth.

◆ Caution to maintain close medical supervision for early detection of adverse reactions.

◆ Stress that using anabolic steroids for improvement of athletic performance may result in serious side effects that outweigh any advantages.

etidocaine

e-tid'oh-kane

etidocaine hydrochloride: *Duranest*

Class: Local anesthetic (amide-type)

PEDS	PREG	GERI
☙	B	☙

Action Produces local anesthesia by inhibiting sodium flux across the nerve cell membrane, thus preventing depolarization and generation and conduction of nerve impulses. Etidocaine has rapid onset (2–8 min), long duration (3–6 hr), and high potency and toxicity. When combined with epinephrine, action is prolonged.

Use/Therapeutic goal/Outcome

Central nerve blocks, epidural, peripheral and caudal anesthesia: Prevention of pain before, during, and after surgical and obstetric procedures. *Outcome criteria:* Patient report of numbness and absence of pain in anesthetized area. Patients receiving epidural anesthesia will demonstrate loss of motor function in anesthetized area.

Dose range/Administration

Interaction alert: Eflurane, halothane, and related drugs may produce arrhythmias if the etidocaine/epinephrine combination has been used. Dosages are for use *without* epinephrine.

Adult: Peripheral nerve block: 25–400 mg (5–80 cc) 0.5% solution, *or* 50–400 mg (5–40 cc) 1% solution. *Central nerve block:* 100–300 mg (10–30 cc) 1% solution, *or* 150–300 mg (10–20 cc) 1.5% solution. *Vaginal:* 50–200 mg (5–20 cc) 1% solution. *Caudal:* 100–300 mg (10–30 cc) 1% solution.

Clinical alert: These drugs should be administered only by clinicians thoroughly familiar with their use. Dose is highly individualized and depends upon the procedure, method of administration, area to be anesthetized, vascularity of tissue, patient condition and age, and individual tolerance. Maximum single dose is 4 mg/kg or 300 mg without epinephrine. With epinephrine, maximum dose is 5.5 mg/kg or 400 mg. This drug is not used for spinal anesthesia. Inadvertent intravascular injection may result in cardiovascular collapse, often refractory to therapy. Epinephrine in local anesthetic preparations may result in anginal pain, tachycardia, tremors, headache, restlessness, palpitations, dizziness, and hypertension. If doses are given without epinephrine, doses and intervals between injections are decreased. Have resuscitative drugs and equipment readily available.

Contraindications/Precautions

PREG B

Contraindicated in hypersensitivity to etidocaine or to other amide-type anesthetics, parabens, and bisulfites, and in acidosis, heart block, severe hemorrhage, severe hypotension, hypertension, cerebrospinal deformities or disease; for spinal block, epidural anesthesia in vaginal delivery, and for injection into inflamed or infected area. *Use with caution* in history of drug sensitivities, impaired cardiac function, renal or hepatic disease, severe shock, debilitated or severely ill patients.

☙ **Use with caution for the elderly. Safe use during pregnancy (except during labor), for nursing mothers, or for children under 14 years has not been established.**

Side effects/Adverse reactions

Hypersensitivity: skin rash, anaphylaxis. *CNS:* nervousness, headache, anxiety, excitement, convulsions followed by drowsiness, unconsciousness, respiratory arrest. *CV:* myocardial depression, arrhythmias, cardiac arrest, fetal bradycardia during delivery, maternal hypotension. *Eye:* blurred vision, pupillary constriction. *Ear:* tinnitus. *GI:* nausea, vomiting. *Misc:* inflammation, pain, and edema at injection site, backache.

Nursing implications/Documentation

Possible nursing diagnoses: Pain; Potential for injury.

♦ Be sure that history of allergies and accurate height and weight are recorded before procedure.

♦ Record vital signs ording to protocol, and monitor for and report immediately signs of systemic or hypersensitivity reactions.

♦ Determine from anesthesiologist or anesthetist whether there are any restrictions on patient positioning; post these at bedside.

♦ Administer oxygen and report first signs of CNS toxicity (restlessness, anxiety, tinnitus, dizziness, blurred vision, tremors, drowsiness).

♦ Monitor anesthetized area for level of sensation and motor function; watch for poor positioning and protect area from injury.

♦ Give prescribed pain medication as sensation begins to return, **before pain is severe**.

Patient & family teaching/Home care

Possible nursing diagnoses: Anxiety; Fear.

♦ Stress the need to protect areas of the body that have lost sensation.

♦ Explain rationale for taking prescribed pain medication before pain becomes too uncomfortable.

◆ *See Local anesthetics overview for more information.*

etoposide

e-toe-po'side

etoposide VP–16: *VePesid*

Class: Antineoplastic agent (plant alkaloid)

PEDS	PREG	GERI
✋	**D**	✋

Action Kills rapidly growing cells (cancer, hair follicles, bone marrow, GI lining, ova, and sperm) by arresting cell mitosis and inhibiting DNA synthesis. Is cell-cycle specific in G_2- and S-phases.

Use/Therapeutic goal/Outcome

Refractory testicular neoplasms, small-cell lung carcinoma, malignant lymphomas, leukemias, neuroblastomas, Kaposi's sarcoma and Hodgkin's disease: Elimination or suppression of malignant cell proliferation. *Outcome criteria:* Tumor and disease regression or stabilization on radiologic and physical examination; for leukemias, absence of blasts in peripheral blood specimen.

Dose range/Administration

Interaction alert: Use with etoposide, vindesine and warfarin may increase prothrombin time. Other cytotoxic agents can cause severe myelosuppression. BCNU (carmustine) may cause severe hepatotoxicity.

Testicular neoplasms: Adult: IV: 50–100 mg/m²/day for 5 days q 3–4 wk; or 100 mg/m² on days 1, 3, and 5, q 3–4 wk for 3–4 regimens.

Oat cell lung carcinoma: Adult: IV: 75–100 mg/m²/day for 3–5 days, q 3–4 wk. PO: Twice the IV dose rounded to the nearest 50 mg.

Malignant neoplasms: Adult: IV: 400–800 mg/m² for 3 days for 1–2 courses of therapy. High-dose 24-hr infusions are often used for brain tumors.

Kaposi's sarcoma: Adult: IV: 150 mg/m²/day for 3 days q 4 wk.

Clinical alert: This drug should be given only by nurses who are knowledgeable in the compre-hensive management of the administration of antineoplastic agents. Doses may vary at physician's discretion. Repeat doses are held until it is ascertained that the patient has recovered sufficiently from toxicities of previous doses. Established protocols/policies for drug preparation, administration, and accidental skin contamination *must be followed closely* (gloves or double gloves are worn when handling drug; if the drug touches the skin, the area is washed immediately with plenty of soap and water). Etoposide is diluted with D5W or normal saline solution to give a concentration of 0.2–0.4 mg/ml and infused over a minimum of 30 minutes (rapid infusion may cause transient hypotension).

Contraindications/Precautions

PREG D

Contraindicated in hypersensitivity to etoposide, and in bone marrow depression, severe hepatic or renal disease, and bacterial infections. Avoid giving intrathecally or intrapleurally (increased toxicity) and if platelet count $<100,000/mm^3$ or absolute neutrophil count $<1000/mm^3$ (may cause myelosuppression with infection and bleeding).

✋ **Contraindicated for pregnant or nursing mothers. Use with caution for the elderly (hypotension side effect may be severe). Safe use for children has not been established.**

Side effects/Adverse reactions

Hypersensitivity: chills, fever, bronchospasm, dyspnea, hypotension, anaphylaxis. *Hem:* myelosuppression (dose-related, and bone marrow recovers 20 days after therapy), leukopenia, thrombocytopenia, anemia. *Skin:* alopecia; rash; pain and erythema at injection site; cellulitis, ulceration, and sloughing if extravasation occurs. *GI:* anorexia, nausea, vomiting, diarrhea, stomatitis, hepatotoxicity. *CV:* hypotension (following rapid IV infusion), hypertension. *CNS:* headache, fatigue, and peripheral neuropathy. *GU:* nephrotoxicity.

Nursing implications/Documentation

Possible nursing diagnoses: Potential for infection; Potential for injury; Fatigue; Altered oral mucous membrane; Fluid volume deficit; Diarrhea; Altered nutrition: less than body requirements.

◆ *See important Nursing implications in Antineoplastic agents overview on page 72, which apply to all antineoplastics. The*

▶

etoposide 339

interventions that follow are additional and specific to this drug only.

♦ Document baseline blood pressure and every 30 minutes thereafter during infusion; hold drug and report if blood pressure less than 90 systolic is noted.

♦ Monitor for and report early signs of anaphylaxis (restlessness, tachycardia, dyspnea).

♦ Be aware that WBC, platelet, and erythrocyte counts usually drop to the nadir (lowest point) 1–2 weeks after administration.

♦ Keep patient in bed during infusion and supervise ambulation once allowed up because of risk of orthostatic hypotension.

♦ Increase fluid intake to 2–3 L a day to prevent renal tubular damage from hyperuricemia secondary to cell lysis; record intake and output and report significant negative or positive balance.

Patient & family teaching/Home care

Possible nursing diagnoses: Knowledge deficit; Ineffective family coping; Hopelessness; Impaired home maintenance management.

♦ *See important Patient & family teaching in Antineoplastic agents overview on page 72, which apply to all antineoplastics. The teachings that follow are additional and specific to this drug only.*

♦ Stress the need to prevent kidney complications by drinking 2–3 L of fluid per day (if the patient can't keep fluids down, IV fluids may be necessary).

♦ *See Antineoplastic agents overview for more information.*

Factor IX complex
fack'tor nine

Factor IX complex (human): **Konyne-HT, Profilnine Heat-Treated, Proplex T**

Class: Systemic hemostatic

PEDS	PREG	GERI
♨	C	♨

Action Directly replaces deficient factors that are essential to clotting.

Use/Therapeutic goal/Outcome

Factor II, VII, IX or X coagulation deficiencies (hemophilia B); anticoagulant overdosage: Promotion of normal clotting mechanism and control of bleeding episodes. **Outcome criteria:** Stable hemoglobin and hematocrit (within normal limits), coagulation studies within normal limits.

Dose range/Administration

Interaction alert: Do not mix with other IV solutions or medications.

Adult and Child: IV: Dose is individualized based upon weight, degree of deficiency, and bleeding severity, using the following formula:

Units required $= 0.8$ to $1 \times$ weight in kg $\times$ % desired increase in Factor IX.

A level of 60% of normal for clotting factors VII and IX is recommended for persons undergoing extensive surgery or dental procedures. This level should be maintained for 8 days.

Clinical alert: Warm to room temperature, then reconstitute lyophilized drug in each vial with 20 ml Sterile Water for Injection. Roll, *don't shake*, vial to mix. Keep refrigerated until ready to use, and use within 3 hours of reconstitution (solution is unstable). Store away from heat. Give slow IV push or slow infusion; do not exceed 10 ml/min.

Contraindications/Precautions
PREG C

Contraindicated in liver disease, suspected intravascular coagulation, or fibrinolysis.

✋ **Use with caution for neonates and infants (because of susceptability to hepatitis, which may be transmitted with Factor IX complex), pregnant or nursing mothers, and the elderly.**

Side effects/Adverse reactions

Hypersensitivity: persistent itching, rashes, chills, fever, headache. **GI:** viral hepatitis. **CV:** thromboembolic reactions; possible intravascular hemolysis in patients with blood types A, B, AB (due to trace amounts of blood groups A and B and isohemaglutinins). **Misc:** (with excessive infusion rate): transient fever, chills, headaches, flushing, and tingling.

Nursing implications/Documentation

Possible nursing diagnosis: Potential for injury.

♦ Document vital signs before beginning infusion and every 30 minutes thereafter.

♦ If tingling sensations, chills, fever, or headache occur, slow infusion rate and report immediately to physician.

♦ Determine whether hepatitis B vaccine has been administered; consult with physician to ascertain immunity prior to starting infusion (vaccine may have to be given).

• Protect the patient from bumping.

Patient & family teaching/Home care

Possible nursing diagnoses: Anxiety; Fear; Knowledge deficit.

• Explain that this drug helps to prevent bleeding.

• Encourage expressing fears or concerns so that these issues can be addressed.

famotidine
fam-ot′ih-deen

Pepcid, ◆*Pepcidine*

Class: Histamine (H₂) receptor antagonist, Antiulcer agent, Gastric acid secretion inhibitor

PEDS	PREG	GERI
🖐	B	🖐

Action Decreases basal and nocturnal secretion of gastric acid by inhibiting the action of histamine at the H_2 receptors in the gastric parietal cells; decreases gastric acid secretion in response to food or chemical stimulus.

Use/Therapeutic goal/Outcome

Duodenal ulcer: Promotion of healing and relief of pain. *Outcome criteria:* Report of absence of pain; hemoglobin and hematocrit within normal range; vital signs stable; stools negative for occult blood; endoscopic evidence of healing.

Prophylaxis of ulcer recurrence: Prevention. *Outcome criteria:* Report of absence of gastric pain; stable hemoglobin and hematocrit; stool and gastric secretions free of blood.

Hypersecretory conditions (e.g., Zollinger-Ellison syndrome): Control of hypersecretion of acid. *Outcome criteria:* Report of relief of epigastric pain; decreased diarrhea/steatorrhea; decreased acidity of gastric secretions.

Dose range/Administration

Interaction alert: Give antacids 1 hr before or after famotidine to avoid interference with cimetidine absorption. Famotidine does not inhibit hepatic metabolism of drugs, as do cimetidine and ranitidine.

🖐 **Give with food.**

Adult: PO: 40 mg at bedtime, or 20 to 40 mg bid with breakfast and at bedtime. IV: 20 mg q12h. *Maintenance dose:* 20 mg at bedtime. *Maximum dose:* 640 mg/day.

Clinical alert: Pediatric dosage has not been established. In moderate to severe renal fail-

ure, reduced doses should be used. Avoid rapid IV administration to prevent cardiac arrhythmias and hypertension.

Contraindications/Precautions
PREG
B

Contraindicated in hypersensitivity to histamine (H₂) receptor antagonists. *Use with caution* in severe renal impairment.

🖐 **Use with caution for children, pregnant or nursing mothers, and the elderly.**

Side effects/Adverse reactions

Hypersensitivity: rash, bronchospasm. *CNS:* headache, dizziness, confusion (especially in elderly patient with decreased renal function). *GI:* constipation, diarrhea.

Nursing implications/Documentation

Possible nursing diagnoses: Constipation; Potential for injury.

• Use oral suspension for those who are unable to swallow pills and for NG administration.

• Document bowel elimination and provide appropriate interventions for constipation.

• Give single dose or last dose of day at bedtime.

• Assess for and record changes in mental state, especially in the elderly.

Patient & family teaching/Home care

Possible nursing diagnoses: Knowledge deficit; Constipation; Impaired home maintenance management.

• Teach that single daily doses should be taken at bedtime.

• Advise smokers not to smoke after the bedtime dose to provide optimal suppression of nocturnal gastric acid secretion.

• Teach the need to avoid taking antacids within 1 hr of famotidine.

• Counsel smokers with active ulcer disease to stop smoking and to avoid the use of caffeine.

• Stress need to advise primary physician if dizziness, rash, or hallucinations develop or if "coffee grounds" vomitus or tarry stools occur.

◆ *See Histamine₂ Antagonists overview for more information.*

F

fat emulsions

Intralipid 10%, 20%, Liposyn 10%, 20%, Liposyn II 10%, 20%, Soyacal 10%, 20%, Travamulsion 10%, 20%

Class: Caloric, Lipid, Long chain fatty acid

PEDS	PREG	GERI
✋	C	✋

Action Promotes balanced nutritional state by supplying calories and essential fatty acids (10% solutions provide 1.1 kcal/ml and 20% solutions provide 2.2 kcal/ml.)

Use/Therapeutic goal/Outcome

Component of total parenteral nutrition: Prevention of fatty acid deficiency and provision of calories. **Outcome criteria:** Adequate calorie intake; maintenance or restoration of optimal weight.

Fatty acid deficiency: Prevention or correction of deficiency. **Outcome criteria:** Absence or improvement in symptoms of essential fatty acid deficiency (scaly dermatitis, alopecia, growth retardation, poor wound healing).

Dose range/Administration

Adult: IV: 500 cc infused over 4–6 hr, daily or twice weekly. *Maximum dose:* 2.5 g/kg/day.
Child: IV: 1 g/kg infused over 4 hr, rate of infusion should not exceed 100 ml/hr for 10% solution, or 50 ml/hr for 20% solution. *Maximum dose:* 4 g/kg/day.

Clinical alert: Fat emulsions are isotonic and may be infused either centrally or peripherally. Administer first dose slowly to assess for adverse reactions; for adults run 10% solution at 1 ml/min, or run 20% solution at 0.5 ml/min, for 15–30 minutes; for children run 10% solution at 0.1 ml/min, or run 20% solution at 0.05 ml/min, for 10–15 minutes. Rate may then be increased.

Contraindications/Precautions

PREG
C

Contraindicated in hypersensitivity to fat emulsions or eggs, and in hyperlipemia, or newborn hyperbilirubinemia. **Use with caution** in liver damage, diabetes mellitus, pulmonary disease, anemia or thrombocytopenia, or high risk of fat emboli.

✋ **Use with caution for newborns (especially low-birth-weight and premature infants), pregnant women, and the elderly.**

Side effects/Adverse reactions

Hypersensitivity: urticaria and pruritus. **CNS:** headache, dizziness, focal seizures. **Resp:** fat accumulation in lungs, dyspnea, pain in chest and back. **Hem:** hyperlipemia, hypercoagulability, thrombocytopenia, leukopenia. **GI:** nausea, vomiting, hepatomegaly. **Misc:** fever, chills, flushing, diaphoresis.

Nursing implications/Documentation

Possible nursing diagnoses: Potential for infection; Activity intolerance; Potential for injury; Pain.

♦ Inspect emulsion prior to infusion; discard if oil separation (oiliness) is observed; administer at room temperature and avoid shaking bottle before administration.

♦ Use tubing supplied with infusion to prevent interaction with polyvinyl chloride (PVC) tubing.

♦ Administer through separate site or by "piggy-backing" into line of amino acid solution below the filter; hang lipid infusion higher than TPN solution to prevent backflow. May also be added to some TPN solutions.

♦ Monitor closely (especially with initial infusion) for signs of adverse reactions.

♦ Do not use a filter because fat globules are too large.

♦ To prevent bacterial contamination, use a new tubing set for each infusion, and do not allow container to hang longer than 8 hours.

♦ Monitor lipid levels to detect failure to eliminate fat from the circulation; monitor liver function and hematology studies to detect adverse reactions.

♦ Assess infants closely for adverse reactions (fat clearance is lower in infants).

Patient & family teaching/Home care

Possible nursing diagnoses: Knowledge deficit; Impaired gas exchange; Potential for infection.

♦ Stress that the emulsion be inspected before administration to detect oil separation or oiliness.

♦ Teach aseptic technique for preparing and administering parenteral solutions.

♦ Point out the importance of using the provided tubing; teach caregiver to hang fat emulsion higher than amino acid solution (if "piggy-backing" method is used).

- Stress that fat emulsion be infused slowly over 4–6 hours.
- Teach proper method of discarding container, tubing, and needle.
- Emphasize the importance of regularly scheduled laboratory tests to monitor results of therapy.

fenoprofen

fen-oh-proe'fen

fenoprofen calcium: **Nalfon**

Class: Nonsteroidal anti-inflammatory drug (NSAID), Analgesic, Antipyretic, Antirheumatic agent

PEDS   PREG   GERI

Action Although the mechanism of action is unclear, fenoprofen calcium is believed to reduce inflammation by decreasing prostaglandin synthesis. Prostaglandin is a naturally occurring mediator of the inflammatory process found throughout body tissues.

Use/Therapeutic goal/Outcome

Pain and inflammation: Promotion of comfort and mobility; suppression of inflammation. *Outcome criteria:* Report of increased comfort with increased range of motion and ability to perform activities of daily life; reduction in or absence of joint stiffness, swelling, redness, and warmth.

Dose range/Administration

Interaction alert: Observe those receiving hydantoins, sulfonamides, or sulfonylureas for toxic effects of those drugs. Aspirin may decrease therapeutic effect of NSAID and increase risk of bleeding. Phenobarbital may enhance the metabolism of fenoprofen.

Give drug 30 min before or 2 hr after meals to enhance absorption unless GI symptoms occur (then give with food).
Rheumatoid arthritis: **Adult:** PO: 300–600 mg tid or qid, individualized.
Analgesia: **Adult:** PO: 200 mg q4-6h prn.
Clinical alert: Be aware that maximum dosage is 3200 mg/day. Improvement may be seen in a few days, but additional 2–3 weeks may be required to determine full benefits of therapy and therapeutic dose range.

Contraindications/Precautions

Contraindicated in hypersensitivity to fenoprofen, other NSAIDs, or aspirin, and in renal or hepatic impairment. *Use with caution* in peptic ulcer, history of bleeding, dysuria, cystitis, blood dyscrasias, cardiac decompensation, and impaired hearing.

Use with caution for the elderly. Safe use for children and pregnant women has not been determined (first two trimesters, preg B; third trimester, preg D).

Side effects/Adverse reactions

Hypersensitivity: asthma, rhinitis, urticaria, angioedema, and bronchospasm. *GI:* stomatitis, GI irritation and bleeding, nausea, constipation. *CV:* arrhythmias, peripheral edema. *Hem:* prolonged coagulation time, elevated serum transaminase, hyper- or hypoglycemia, elevated LDH, and alkaline phosphatase. *GU:* dysuria, cystitis, hematuria, nephrotic syndrome. *CNS:* headache, fatigue, somnolence, drowsiness, dizziness. *Ear:* difficulty hearing, tinnitus. *Eye:* blurred vision.

Nursing implications/Documentation

Possible nursing diagnoses: Pain; Impaired physical mobility.

- Establish a baseline for CBC, electrolytes, prothrombin time, BUN, creatinine, and liver function studies; monitor periodically thereafter if therapy is prolonged.
- Monitor for and report GI symptoms that may indicate peptic ulcer (nausea, pain, black stools).
- Record weight every other day; report edema or sudden weight gain.
- Observe for and report visual and auditory changes (periodic auditory tests are recommended if therapy is prolonged).
- For diabetics, monitor blood sugar closely since insulin requirements may change.

Patient & family teaching/Home care

Possible nursing diagnoses: Anxiety; Knowledge deficit.

- Point out that taking doses on an empty stomach enhances absorption, but if GI symptoms are experienced, it should be taken with milk or food.
- Explain the importance of watching for symptoms of GI bleeding (black stools, persistent GI distress).

- Stress the need to avoid aspirin, alcohol, and other OTC drugs (unless approved by physician) because of increased risk of GI bleeding.
- Instruct individuals to hold dose and report if any of the following side effects are experienced: vertigo, rashes, blood in urine, hearing or visual changes, sudden weight gain, edema.
- Warn against driving or operating machinery until response is established (may experience drowsiness, dizziness).
- Explain that full effects of therapy may not be realized up to 4 weeks.
- Reinforce the need for medical follow-up; advise telling dentist that fenoprofen is being taken.
- For diabetics, explain the importance of monitoring blood sugars with a blood glucose meter.
- *See Nonsteroidal anti-inflammatory drugs overview for more information.*

fentanyl

fen'ta-nil

fentanyl citrate: **Sublimaze**

fentamyul citrate with droperidol: **Innovar (see droperidol)**

Class: Narcotic analgesic, Opiate antagonist

Antidote: naloxone hydrochloride (Narcan)

PEDS	PREG	GERI	CONTROLLED SUBSTANCE
✋	C	✋	II

Action Alters both perception of and response to pain through an unclear mechanism. Believed to act by binding with opiate receptor sites in the CNS. Acts similarly to morphine and meperidine except that effects are seen more promptly and profoundly, duration is shorter, and there is less emetic activity.

Use/Therapeutic goal/Outcome

Adjunct to anesthesia (preoperatively, intraoperatively, and immediately postoperative): Promotion of comfort and relaxation. **Outcome criteria:** Report of comfort; absence of signs of pain (grimacing, frowning, restlessness, reluctance to move or cough) with increase in signs of comfort (relaxed facial expression); blood pressure and pulse within normal limits when compared to baseline.

Dose range/Administration

Interaction alert: Nitrous oxide and diazepam increase risk of cardiovascular depression. For up to 4 hours after giving fentanyl, give CNS depressants in reduced doses only (fentanyl increases CNS depressant effect). Do not mix IV with barbiturates. Anticholinergics and antiparkinsons may increase intraocular pressure. Do not give within 14 days of MAOIs therapy.

Preoperative medication: Adult: IM: 50-100 mcg 30–60 min before procedure.

Adjunct to general anesthesia: Adult: IV: 50–100 mcg q 2–3 min prn. *Child 2–12 yr:* IV: 1.7–2.6 mcg/kg.

Adjunct to regional anesthesia: Adult: IV: 50–100 mcg slowly over 1–2 min.

Postoperative analgesia, recovery room use: Adult: IM: 50–100 mcg q1-2h. IV: 12–30 mcg slowly over 1–2 min. *Child 2–12 yr:* IV: 2–3 mcg/kg.

Clinical alert: Dosage is highly individualized. IV doses should be given only by nurses who are qualified to administer IV narcotics and in the presence of a physician or nurse anesthetist qualified to perform intubation. Keep resuscitative equipment nearby.

Contraindications/Precautions

PREG
C

Contraindicated in hypersensitivity or intolerance to fentanyl, and in myasthenia gravis. *Use with caution* in increased intracranial pressure, respiratory problems, liver and kidney failure, and bradyarrhythmias.

✋ **Use with caution for children and the elderly. Safe use for pregnant and nursing mothers has not been established.**

Side effects/Adverse reactions

Hypersensitivity: itching, rash. *Resp:* respiratory depression, apnea (with large doses), bronchoconstriction. *CNS:* euphoria, profound sedation, coma. *CV:* bradycardia, hypotension. *GI:* vomiting. *MS:* muscle rigidity (Lead pipe syndrome) with rapid infusion. *Eye:* miosis.

Nursing implications/Documentation

Possible nursing diagnoses: Potential for aspiration; Potential for injury; Pain.

- Monitor closely for airway obstruction and keep suction at bedside until patient is recovered; be aware that respiratory depression lasts longer than analgesic effects.

- Record vital signs every 15 min if given via IV route and every 30 min if given IM (if given during childbirth, monitor neonate for respiratory depression).
- Watch closely for potential for injury; position extremities and head carefully; keep side rails up.
- Give before pain is severe.

Patient & family teaching/Home care

Possible nursing diagnoses: Fear; Sensory/perceptual alterations.

- Explain procedures briefly and in simple terms (even if the patient is not awake, he or she may be able to hear).
- Explain the rationale for reporting pain before it is severe.
- Reassure that things are going well and measures are being taken to ensure safety (even if the patient is not awake).
- *See Narcotic and non-narcotic analgesics overview for more information.*

ferrous (gluconate and sulfate)

ferrous gluconate: *Fergon, Ferralet, ♣Fertinic, ♣Novoferrogluc*

ferrous sulfate: *Feosol, Fer-in-Sol, ♠Feritard, ♣Fero-Grad, Fero-Gradumet, Ferolix, Ferospace, Ferralyn, ♠Fespan, Fesofor, Irospan, Mol-Iron, ♣Novoferrosulfa, Slow-Fe, Telefon*

Class: Antianemic

Antidote: deferoxamine

PEDS	PREG	GERI
✋	A	✋

Action Directly replaces iron, an essential component of hemoglobin.

Use/Therapeutic goal/Outcome

Iron deficiency and iron deficiency anemia: Replenishment of deficient iron blood levels, promotion of hemoglobin formation. *Outcome criteria:* Hemoglobin, hematocrit, and reticulocyte count, total serum iron–binding capacity, and serum iron within normal limits.

Dose range/Administration

Interaction alert: Antacids, Vitamin E, and pancreatic extracts reduce iron absorption; give at different times. Vitamin C increases iron absorption (may be beneficial). Chloramphenicol may delay response to iron replacement therapy.

▣ **Give between meals unless GI distress is experienced. Never give with milk (decreases absorption).**

Ferrous sulfate: *Adult:* PO: *Tablets, elixir:* 300–1500 mg/day divided doses tid. *Sustained-release preparations:* 225–525 mg q12-24h. *Child 6–12 yrs:* PO: 300 mg bid. *Infants:* PO: 3–6 mg/kg/day in divided doses.

Ferrous gluconate: *Adult:* PO: 200–600 mg tid. *Child 6–12 yrs:* PO: 300 mg/day, bid or tid. *Child < 6 yrs:* PO: 100–300 mg/day.

Clinical alert: Overdose may cause death.

Contraindications/Precautions

PREG A

Contraindicated in hypersensitivity to iron, and in hemolytic anemias (in absence of iron deficiency), hemochromatosis, hemosiderosis, cirrhosis of liver. *Use with caution* for long-term therapy and in peptic ulcer, regional enteritis, ulcerative colitis, alcoholism, repeated blood transfusions, and kidney or liver impairment.

🖑 **Use with caution for children (because of risk of overdosage) and the elderly.**

Side effects/Adverse reactions

Hypersensitivity: rare. *GI:* nausea, vomiting, stomach pain, constipation, black stools, staining of teeth (from elixir). *Misc:* acute iron toxicity (severe nausea and vomiting, abdominal cramping, diarrhea, and fever).

Nursing implications/Documentation

Possible nursing diagnoses: Altered nutrition: less than body requirements; Constipation; Fatigue.

- If using elixir, give with orange juice to enhance absorption, (use a straw to prevent staining of teeth, and provide mouth rinse immediately after).
- If GI distress occurs, obtain order for enteric-coated tablets, or ask if lower doses could be given more frequently.
- To prevent constipation, provide fiber, fruits, and at least 2–4 liters of water or juice per day, unless contraindicated.
- Pace activities to allow for adequate rest.
- Monitor hemoglobin and reticulocyte count.

Patient & family teaching/Home care

Possible nursing diagnosis: Impaired home maintenance management.

- Emphasize that GI symptoms may be reduced by taking with food (not milk); teach the need to mix elixir with juice, to use a straw, and to rinse mouth.

- Explain that stools may be dark black or green, which is harmless; advise reporting persistent GI distress.

- With extended-release form, advise reporting if stools are not black; iron may not be properly released.

- Teach the importance of preventing constipation through diet, adequate fluid intake, and exercise.

- Warn about the dangers of iron overdose; stress the importance of keeping it out of reach of children, and of calling the emergency room or poison control center *immediately* if overdose is suspected. Ipecac syrup should be kept readily available.

- Recommend that if doses are missed, the regular dose schedule should be followed, rather than doubling dose to make up for missed dose.

- Teach dietary sources high in iron (fish, liver, chicken, and green, leafy vegetables), and explain that increased dietary iron intake may decrease the need for iron replacement.

- *See Antianemics overview for more information.*

flavoxate

fla-vox'ate

flavoxate hydrochloride: *Urispas*
Class: urinary antispasmodic (spasmolytic)

PEDS	PREG	GERI
✋	C	✋

Action Inhibits bladder spasms by relaxing smooth muscles of the urinary tract (also causes some local anesthesia and analgesia).

Use/Therapeutic goal/Outcome

Symptomatic relief of dysuria, urinary frequency and urgency, nocturia, incontinence, and suprapubic pain: Promotion of normal patterns of urinary elimination, and relief of associated discomfort. **Outcome criteria:** Demonstration of normal patterns of urinary elimination; report of relief of symptoms.

Dose range/Administration

Adult: PO: 100–200 mg tid or qid.

Contraindications/Precautions

PREG
C

Contraindicated in hypersensitivity to flavoxate hydrochloride, and in GI or urinary tract obstruction. **Use with caution** in glaucoma.

✋ **Contraindicated for nursing mothers. Use with caution for the elderly (may cause confusion). Safe use in pregnancy and children under 12 years has not been established.**

Side effects/Adverse reactions

Hypersensitivity: itching, rash. **CNS:** headache, dizziness, drowsiness, nervousness, poor concentration, confusion (especially in the elderly). **GI:** nausea, vomiting, dry mouth and throat, abdominal pain, constipation with high doses. **Eye:** visual disturbances. **CV:** palpitations, tachycardia. **Hem:** eosinophilia. **Misc:** fever.

Nursing implications/Documentation

Possible nursing diagnoses: Altered patterns of urinary elimination; Pain.

- Monitor and record time and amount of urination.

- Provide favorite fluids to maintain adequate hydration.

- Monitor the elderly for confusion.

Patient & family teaching/Home care

Possible nursing diagnoses: Knowledge deficit; Impaired home maintenance management.

- Explain the importance of drinking at least 2 quarts of fluid a day, even if it causes more frequent urination.

- Explain that dry mouth is a common side effect.

- Point out that suppressed sweating may predispose the individual to heat stroke on hot days.

- Warn that drowsiness, dizziness, and blurred vision may be experienced at the beginning of therapy; caution to avoid driving or activities that require mental alertness until effects are known.

- Reinforce the importance of reporting persistent or new symptoms.

- Offer number and address of local support groups available for help with dealing with incontinence (e.g., Simon Foundation; PO Box 835; Wilmette, IL 60091).

flecainide acetate

fle-kay'nide

Tambocor

Class: Antiarrhythmic (Class 1C)

PEDS	PREG	GERI
✋	C	✋

Action Suppresses ventricular ectopy by prolonging conduction in all parts of the heart, particularly the AV node and His-Purkinje system. Has membrane-stabilizing effect. Increases ventricular refractory period.

Use/Therapeutic goal/Outcome

Life-threatening ventricular arrhythmias, including sustained and nonsustained ventricular tachycardia, and premature ventricular contractions: Suppression of ventricular ectopy, promotion of effective heartbeat. **Outcome criteria:** Absence of or decrease in ventricular ectopy on EKG; regular palpable pulses.

Dose range/Administration

Interaction alert: Monitor for increased toxicity when given with amiodarone, cimetidine, digoxin, and propranolol.

Adult: PO: 100 mg q8h or q12h. May be increased by 50 mg increments up to a maximum of 400 mg/day; do not increase dosage more frequently than once every 4 days. Full effect may not be seen for 3 to 5 days. (Patient may be on lidocaine until then.)

Clinical alert: This drug should be reserved for life-threatening arrhythmias only, because it can induce potentially fatal arrhythmias, and increase mortality rate when used in less serious arrhythmias. Place patient on cardiac monitor before therapy and monitor continuously until response is determined.

Contraindications/Precautions

PREG C

Contraindicated in hypersensitivity to flecainide and amide-type anesthetics, and in cardiogenic shock and heart block (unless a pacemaker is present). **Use with caution** in presence of congestive heart failure or cardiomyopathy.

✋ **Use with caution for the elderly. Safe use for children and pregnant or nursing mothers has not been established.**

Side effects/Adverse reactions

Hypersensitivity: rash. **CV:** arrhythmias, sinus arrest, chest pain, dose-related prolongation of PR, QRS, and QT intervals. **CNS:** dizziness, headache, fatigue, insomnia, depression, nervousness, tremor, weakness, syncope. **GI:** flatulence, dry mouth, nausea, vomiting, constipation. **Resp:** dyspnea. **Eye:** blurred vision. **Ear:** tinnitus. **Misc:** fever.

Nursing implications/Documentation

Possible nursing diagnoses: Potential for injury; Activity intolerance.

◆ Be sure to check baseline chest X-ray, EKG, and laboratory studies (CBC, sodium, potassium, chloride, carbon dioxide, magnesium, BUN, creatinine, SGPT, and LDH) before giving first dose; then monitor closely as indicated by clinical condition.

◆ Remember that oxygen requirements must be met, and electrolyte imbalances (especially potassium and magnesium) and abnormal blood pH must be corrected, before expected antiarrhythmic effect can be seen; report abnormalities immediately.

◆ Document baseline vital signs, lung sounds, and cardiac monitor strip (measure and record PR and QRS segments) before giving first dose and at least every 8 hr; monitor closely until response is determined; report prolongation in PR or QRS segment.

◆ If a pacemaker is in place, determine pacing threshold 1 week before and 1 week after initiating therapy (timing of pacemaker may need adjustment).

◆ Supervise ambulation until response is determined.

◆ Coordinate care to provide frequent rest periods.

Patient & family teaching/Home care

Possible nursing diagnoses: Fear; Knowledge deficit; Impaired home maintenance management.

◆ Explain that the purpose of this drug is to prevent arrhythmias and promote an effective heartbeat.

◆ Stress the need to follow dose regimen closely (the drug should be taken at the same time each day), and the need to return for medical follow-up to detect adverse reactions early.

◆ Teach how to assess pulse for irregularities in rhythm and rate; stress that irregularities be reported.

F

- Emphasize the need to pace activities, avoid stress, and plan for rest periods.

- Encourage learning CPR; reinforce that survival rate of cardiac arrest is greatly increased when CPR is initiated immediately.

◆ *See Antiarrhythmics overview for more information.*

floxuridine

flox-yoor'i-deen

FUDR

Class: Antineoplastic (antimetabolite) agent

PEDS	PREG	GERI
✍	D	✋

Action Kills rapidly growing cells (cancer, hair follicles, bone marrow, GI lining, ova, and sperm) by inhibiting DNA, RNA, and protein synthesis (thymidylate antagonist). Drug is cell-cycle specific in the S-phase.

Use/Therapeutic goal/Outcome

Cancer of the bile duct, brain, breast, gallbladder, head, and neck; palliative treatment of advanced GI adenocarcinoma that has metastasized to the liver, pancreas, and biliary tract: Elimination or suppression of malignant cell proliferation. *Outcome criteria:* Tumor and disease regression or stabilization on radiologic and physical examination.

Dose range/Administration

Interaction alert: Cimetidine, radiation therapy, and other cytotoxic agents may cause increased toxicity.

Adult: *Intra-arterial:* 0.1 to 0.6 mg/kg/day for 1–6 weeks. *Hepatic artery injection:* 0.4–0.6 mg/kg/day for 1–6 weeks.

Clinical alert: This drug should be given only by nurses who are knowledgeable in the comprehensive management of the administration of antineoplastic agents. Doses may vary at physician's discretion and are held until the patient has sufficiently recovered from toxicities of previous doses. Protocols for drug preparation, administration, and accidental skin contamination must be followed. Gloves or double gloves must be worn when handling floxuridine (skin contamination may cause a local reaction). Contaminated areas should be washed with large amounts of soap and water. Floxuridine should be diluted in 50–100 ml D5W or saline and given via pump into the chosen artery continuously over 1–6 weeks.

Contraindications/Precautions

Contraindicated in hypersensitivity to floxuridine and in compromised nutritional status, depressed bone marrow function, and serious infections. ***Use with caution*** in impaired liver or kidney function, and in previous exposure to high-dose pelvic irradiation or the use of alkylating agents.

✍ **Contraindicated for pregnant or nursing mothers. Use with caution for the elderly. Safe use for children has not been established.**

Side effects/Adverse reactions

Hypersensitivity: rash, urticaria, itching, flushing. ***Hem:*** cumulative myelosuppression, anemia, leukopenia, and thrombocytopenia; elevated serum transaminase, bilirubin, and alkaline phosphatase; decreased plasma albumin. ***GI:*** esophagopharyngitis; anorexia, nausea, and vomiting; GI hemorrhage; stomatitis; enteritis; abdominal cramping and diarrhea; cholangitis, jaundice, and chemical hepatitis (indication to stop drug). ***GU:*** renal failure. ***CNS:*** hiccups; lethargy, depression, malaise, and weakness; nystagmus; vertigo; cerebellar ataxia; convulsions. ***Eye:*** blurred vision, photophobia, lacrimation. ***CV:*** myocardial ischemia, angina; complications of intra-arterial administration (arterial aneurysm, ischemia, and thrombosis; thrombophlebitis). ***Skin:*** dermatitis, erythema, pruritus; bleeding and infection at catheter site; pain and inflammation at infusion site.

Nursing implications/Documentation

Possible nursing diagnoses: Potential for infection; Potential for injury; Fatigue; Altered oral mucous membrane; Fluid volume deficit; Diarrhea; Altered nutrition: less than body requirements.

◆ *See important Nursing implications in Antineoplastic agents overview on page 72, which apply to all antineoplastics. The interventions that follow are additional and specific to this drug only.*

- Hold dose and report if severe GI distress or skin reactions are noted; examine mouth for ulcers before each dose.

- Monitor for and report early signs of CNS toxicity (changes in mental status, numbness or tingling of extremities, muscle weakness, balance problems).

- Increase fluid intake to 2–3 L a day to prevent renal tubular damage from hyperuricemia secondary to cell lysis.
- Expect WBC nadir (lowest point) at 1 week and platelet nadir at 10 days.

Patient & family teaching/Home care

Possible nursing diagnoses: Knowledge deficit; Ineffective coping (individual and family); Hopelessness; Impaired home maintenance management.

- *See important Patient & family teaching in Antineoplastic agents overview on page 72, which apply to all antineoplastics. The teachings that follow are additional and specific to this drug only.*
  - Point out that drinking 2–3 L a day helps prevent kidney complications.
  - Stress that it can take 1–6 weeks for therapeutic effects to be seen.
  - Explain the need to report balance problems, muscle weakness, numbness, or tingling of extremities.
- *See Antineoplastic agents overview for more information.*

fluconazole

flew-kon'a-zol

Diflucan

Class: Anti-infective, Antifungal, Antibiotic

PEDS	PREG	GERI
॥	C	॥

Action
Has broad-spectrum fungistatic action (limits fungal growth). Believed to act by inhibiting fungal cytochrome P-450 sterol and C-14 alpha-demethylation, causing a loss of normal sterols in the cell and altering the cell membrane.

Use/Therapeutic goal/Outcome
Cryptococcal meningitis, candidal infections (oropharyngeal, esophageal, and serious systemic infections including urinary tract infections, peritonitis, and pneumonia): Elimination of pathogenic fungi. **Outcome criteria:** Absence of pathogenic fungal growth on culture; absence of clinical manifestations of infection (redness, pain, swelling, fever, drainage, productive cough, increased WBC count).

Dose range/Administration
Interaction alert: Do not mix IV with any other drug. May increase effect of oral anticoagu-

lants (monitor prothrombin time carefully) and oral hypoglycemics (monitor for hypoglycemia). May significantly increase levels of phenytoin and cyclosporine, requiring careful monitoring of serum levels of these drugs. Diuretics may increase fluconazole levels. Rifampin may enhance metabolism of fluconazole, which may require an increase in dosage. Because this is a new drug, interaction studies have not been completed (check with pharmacist for most up-to-date information).

Oropharyngeal candidiasis: Adult: PO, IV: 200 mg the first day, then 100 mg/day for at least 2 wk after symptoms resolve.

Esophageal candidiasis: Adult: PO, IV: 200 mg the first day, then 100 mg/day (doses as high as 400 mg/day have been used) for at least 3 wk total and at least 2 weeks after symptoms resolve.

Systemic candidiasis: Adult: PO, IV: 400 mg the first day, then 200 mg/day for at least 4 wk total and at least 2 wk after symptoms resolve.

Cryptococcal meningitis: Adult: PO, IV: 400 mg/day until clinical response, then 200 mg/day (doses as high as 400 mg/day have been used) for 10–12 wk after cerebrospinal fluid culture becomes negative. *For suppression of relapse (in AIDS):* 200 mg/day.

Clinical alert: Give IV doses as an infusion at a rate not to exceed 200 mg/hr; do not use cloudy solutions. This drug is absorbed almost equally as well when administered by mouth as when administered intravenously.

Contraindications/Precautions

PREG C

Contraindicated in hypersensitivity to fluconazole. **Use with caution** in renal failure.

॥ **Use with caution for the elderly. Safe use for children (has been used effectively in a small number of children 3–13 yr) and pregnant or nursing mothers has not been established.**

Side effects/Adverse reactions

Hypersensitivity: itching, rashes (in patients with AIDS, may require discontinuation of drug if lesions progress). **GI:** nausea, vomiting, diarrhea, abdominal pain, hepatotoxicity. **CNS:** headache.

Nursing implications/Documentation

Possible nursing diagnoses: Potential for infection; Altered oral mucous membrane; Fluid volume deficit.

- Be sure that cultures are drawn before giving first dose; record status of signs and symptoms of infection before administration, and daily thereafter.

- Provide preferred fluids, monitor intake, and encourage drinking at least 2 L a day.

- Provide special mouth care.

- In impaired kidney function, expect reduced dosage because fluconazole is cleared primarily by the kidneys.

- Recognize that patients with AIDS and cryptococcal meningitis or recurrent esophageal candidiasis usually require maintenance therapy to avoid relapse.

Patient & family teaching/Home care

Possible nursing diagnoses: Knowledge deficit; Impaired home maintenance management.

- Explain that this is a relatively new antifungal that has a low incidence of side effects and is almost equally effective when taken by mouth or intravenously.

- Point out the importance of taking fluconazole for the entire time prescribed, even if symptoms subside.

- Stress the need for performing daily oral hygiene and reporting oral inflammation or ulceration early.

- *See Anti-infectives overview for more information.*

flucytosine (5-FC)

floo-sye'toe-seen

Ancobon

Class: Anti-infective, Antifungal

PEDS	PREG	GERI
OK	C	✋

Action Believed to act by selectively penetrating fungal cells (where it is converted to fluorouracil, a known metabolic antagonist) and inhibiting protein synthesis. Can be fungicidal (kills fungi) or fungistatic (limits fungal growth), depending upon drug concentration and susceptibility of the organisms.

Use/Therapeutic goal/Outcome

Severe fungal infections caused by susceptible *Candida* and *Cryptococcus* (given with amphotericin B): Resolution of infection. **Outcome criteria:** Absence of pathogenic growth on culture; absence of clinical manifestations of infection (redness, pain, swelling, fever, drainage, increased WBC count).

Dose range/Administration

Adult/Child > 50 kg: PO: 50–150 mg/kg/day divided q6h. **Adult/Child < 50 kg:** PO: 1.5–4.5 g/m²/day divided q6h.

Clinical alert: Reduce risk of GI symptoms (nausea, vomiting) by giving capsules over a 15 minute period, rather than all at once.

Contraindications/Precautions

PREG C

Contraindicated in hypersensitivity to flucytosine. **Use with caution** in bone marrow depression, and impaired kidney or liver function.

✋ **Contraindicted for pregnant women or those in childbearing years. Use with caution for the elderly.**

Side effects/Adverse reactions

Hypersensitivity: (rare) itching, rashes. **GI:** nausea, vomiting, bloating, diarrhea. **CNS:** headache, dizziness, drowsiness, confusion. **Hem:** bone marrow depression, anemia, leukopenia, thrombocytopenia. **Misc:** elevated SGOT, SGPT, alkaline phosphatase, creatinine, BUN.

Nursing implications/Documentation

Possible nursing diagnoses: Potential for infection; Altered nutrition: less than body requirements.

- Obtain necessary cultures before starting flucytosine; monitor periodically throughout treatment to detect resistance.

- Monitor CBC to determine clinical response or presence of hematological side effects.

- Record and monitor intake and output, and ensure adequate hydration (report excessive negative or positive balance).

- Document and report diarrhea.

- Monitor serum drug level (therapeutic range is 25–120 mcg/ml) and report abnormalities.

Patient & family teaching/Home care

Possible nursing diagnoses: Knowledge deficit; Impaired home maintenance management.

- Assure that dose is correct, even though 8–10 capsules must be taken at once.

- Stress the importance of taking the drug for the entire time prescribed, even if symptoms abate (long-term treatment, from 2 weeks to 3 months, may be required).

- ♦ Explain that unusual feelings or discomfort should be reported in case they are side effects that should be treated.
- ♦ *See Anti-infectives overview for more information.*

fluorouracil

flur-rah-yoor'a-sil

5-FU: *Adrucil, Efudex, Fluoroplex*

Class: Antineoplastic (antimetabolite) agent

PEDS	PREG	GERI
🖐	**D**	🖐

Action Kills rapidly growing cells (cancer, hair follicles, bone marrow, GI lining, ova, and sperm) by inhibiting DNA and RNA synthesis and enzyme reactions (pyrimidine antagonist). Drug is cell cycle specific in the S-phase.

Use/Therapeutic goal/Outcome

Cancer of the colon, rectum, breast, stomach and pancreas (used palliatively for carcinomas not amenable to surgery or irradiation): Reduction or suppression of malignant cell proliferation. *Outcome criteria:* Tumor and disease regression or stabilization on radiologic and physical examination.

Actinic keratosis and superficial basal cell carcinoma: Elimination of abnormal and malignant cell growth. *Outcome criteria:* After 1–2 months, normal reepithelialization; absence of abnormal tissue.

Dose range/Administration

Interaction alert: Radiation therapy and other cytotoxic agents may cause severe myelosuppression.

Adult: IV: 12 mg/kg/day for 4 days. If no toxicity, give 6 mg/kg on days 6, 8, 10, and 12. Discontinue therapy after 12th day. Repeat dosage at 30-day intervals, or give maintenance dose of 10–15 mg/kg/wk. *Maximum dose:* 1 g/wk. *Hepatic arterial infusion:* 22.5 mg/kg in 150 ml of D/5W over 8 hr for 5–21 days.

Actinic or solar keratoses: Adult and Child: Topical: 1–5% cream or solution, bid to lesion, for 2–6 weeks.

Superficial basal cell carcinoma: Adult and Child: Topical: 5% cream or solution bid for 3–6 weeks.

Clinical alert: This drug should be given IV only by nurses who are knowledgeable in the comprehensive management of the administration of antineoplastic agents. Doses may vary at physician's discretion and are held until the patient sufficiently recovers from toxicities of previous doses. Protocols for drug preparation, administration, and accidental skin contamination must be followed. Gloves or double gloves must be worn when handling fluorouracil (skin contamination may cause a local reaction). Contaminated areas should be washed with large amounts of soap and water. Daily doses of fluorouracil should not exceed 800 mg (600 for the elderly or debilitated). It should be given by slow IV push over 2–5 minutes (more effective) or diluted in 50–100 ml fluid over 2–8 hr to minimize toxic effects. If the drug crystalizes during administration, it should be taken down and warmed, then shaken vigorously and cooled to room temperature before using.

Contraindications/Precautions

PREG
D

Contraindicated in hypersensitivity to fluorouracil, poor nutritional status, potentially serious infections, depressed bone marrow function, or in those who have had surgery within 30 days. *Use with extreme caution* with pelvic irradiation or alkylating agents. *Use with caution* in impaired hepatic/renal function, chronic debilitating illness, and depressed bone marrow reserve.

🖐 **Contraindicated for pregnant or nursing mothers. Use with caution for children and the elderly.**

Side effects/Adverse reactions

Hypersensitivity: urticaria, fever, tachycardia, hypotension. *Hem:* anemia, leukopenia (WBC nadirs in 9–14 days after first dose), thrombocytopenia (platelet nadirs in 14 days). *GI:* anorexia, nausea, and vomiting (30–50% of patients); stomatitis; esophagopharyngitis; diarrhea. *CNS:* malaise, lethargy, acute cerebellar syndrome. *Eye:* photophobia, lacrimation, decreased vision. *CV:* angina, myocardial ischemia; arterial ischemia, aneurysm, or thrombosis; thrombophlebitis. *GU:* renal failure. *Skin:* maculopapular rash, reversible alopecia, nail changes, diffuse erythema, and increased pigmentation; pain and erythema at injection site; cellulitis.

Nursing implications/Documentation

Possible nursing diagnoses: Potential for infection; Potential for injury; Fatigue; Altered oral mucous membrane; Fluid volume deficit; Diarrhea; Altered nutrition: less than body requirements.

- *See important Nursing implications in Antineoplastic agents overview on page 72, which apply to all antineoplastics. The interventions that follow are additional and specific to this drug only.*
  - Hold drug and report immediately if changes in mental status, diarrhea, stomatitis, or GI bleeding occur (monitor stools for occult blood) and check mouth for ulcers before each dose.
  - Observe for dizziness, balance problems, or weakness (signs of cerebellar dysfunction) which may occur after the drug has been stopped; supervise ambulation to prevent injury.
  - Report cardiac symptoms (angina, tachycardia, dysrhythmias) immediately.
  - For topical preparation, avoid contact with eyes, nose, mouth, or skin; avoid occlusive dressings at administration site.
  - Be aware that toxicity may be delayed (1–3 weeks).
  - Expect blood counts to drop to the lowest point in 1–3 weeks.

Patient & family teaching/Home care

Possible nursing diagnoses: Knowledge deficit; Ineffective coping (individual and family); Hopelessness; Impaired home maintenance management.
- *See important Patient & family teaching in Antineoplastic agents overview on page 72, which apply to all antineoplastics. The teachings that follow are additional and specific to this drug only.*
  - Stress the importance of avoiding exposure to direct sunlight.
  - Explain the need to report changes in vision, chest pain, pulse irregularities, balance problems, or muscle weakness.
  - **With topical use**
    - Teach how to apply ointment; observe return demonstration.
    - Warn that area of skin being treated may look worse during the course of treatment until healing is complete (about 1–2 months).
    - Stress that the skin must be protected from injury (avoid abrasive soaps, tight-fitting clothes, chemical irritants, exposure to sunlight).
- *See Antineoplastic agents overview for more information.*

fluoxetine

floo-ox'e-teen

Prozac

Class: Bicyclic antidepressant

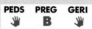

PEDS   PREG   GERI

    B

Action Improves mood by increasing levels of the neurotransmitter serotonin in the CNS (selectively inhibits the uptake of serotonin). Has little or no effect on other neurotransmitters or receptor sites.

Use/Therapeutic goal/Outcome

Short term treatment of non-hospitalized individuals with major depression disorders: Promotion of sense of well-being, ability to cope with daily living. ***Outcome criteria:*** After 2–4 weeks, report of feeling less depressed, less anxious, and more energetic and able to cope; return of normal sleeping and eating habits; demonstration of improved ability to problem solve and perform activities of daily living.

Dose range/Administration

Interaction alert: Alcohol or other CNS depressants may cause excessive sedation. May prolong the action and half-life of diazepam. If given with warfarin or digoxin, monitor for increased risk of digoxin or warfarin toxicity. Avoid use with MAOIs because of limited knowledge of safety of using these two drugs together.

Adult: PO: Begin with 20 mg every morning. If no response after 4 weeks, may increase to 20 mg bid upon rising and at noon. *Maximum dose:* 80 mg/day; for the elderly, 60 mg/day.

Clinical alert: Do not give this drug in the afternoon or evening because of common side effect of nervousness and insomnia. Because this drug is relatively new, expect additional information resulting from increased use.

Contraindications/Precautions

PREG
B

Contraindicated in hypersensitivity to fluoxetine. ***Use with caution*** for those with suicidal tendencies.

Use with caution during the first trimester of pregnancy, and for the elderly or debilitated. Safe use for children and nursing mothers has not been established.

Side effects/Adverse reactions

Hypersensitivity: itching, rashes, chills, trouble breathing. ***CNS:*** drowsiness, dizziness, anxiety, headache, fatigue, agitation, sedation, insomnia, weird dreams. **CV:** palpitations, angina pectoris, tachycardia, bradycardia, dysrhythmias, hypertension. **GI:** changes in taste, appetite changes, dry mouth, indigestion, diarrhea, nausea, vomiting, constipation. **Resp:** nasal congestion, upper respiratory infection, pharyngitis, cough, sinusitis. **GU:** dysmenorrhea, urinary frequency or retention, decreased libido, impotence. **Eye:** visual changes. **Ear:** tinnitus. **MS:** muscle pain, weight loss.

Nursing implications/Documentation

Possible nursing diagnoses: Potential for injury; Diarrhea; Constipation; Altered oral mucous membrane.

◆ Document mental status and vital signs at each visit.

◆ Be sure that doses are swallowed (not hoarded).

◆ Monitor for dizziness and drowsiness; supervise ambulation until response is established.

◆ Monitor for and report suicidal tendencies, increased depression, excessive nervousness or agitation (may require change in medication).

Patient & family teaching/Home care

Possible nursing diagnoses: Ineffective coping (family and individual); Sleep pattern disturbance; Impaired home maintenance management.

◆ Stress that this medication helps reduce the depression that inhibits ability to make decisions and cope effectively (once the individual feels less depressed, it will be easier to take steps toward making healthy changes).

◆ Point out that doses should not be taken in the afternoon or evening because of side effect of insomnia.

◆ Explain that it is likely to take 2–4 weeks before beneficial effects are noted.

◆ Discuss the role of adequate nutrition, exercise, and sleep in combating depression.

◆ Stress that the effects of alcohol, sedatives, and tranquilizers may be potentiated.

◆ Caution to consult with physician before using OTC drugs; stress the need for ongoing medical follow-up.

◆ Warn about side effect of constipation or diarrhea. Teach the role of fluids, fiber, and exercise in preventing constipation; advise reporting persistent diarrhea.

◆ Advise avoidance of driving and other potentially hazardous activities until response is established.

◆ Suggest using ice chips, hard candy, or gum to relieve side effect of dry mouth; stress the need for good mouth care.

◆ *See Antidepressants overview for more information.*

fluoxymesterone
floo-ox-i-mess'te-rone

Android-F, Halotestin, Ora-Testryl

Class: Androgen, Antineoplastic agent

PEDS	PREG	GERI
🖐	X	🖐

Action Stimulates development and maintenance of male sex organs; induces development of male secondary sex characteristics; stimulates sperm production; increases body size by stimulating growth of skeletal muscles.

Use/Therapeutic goal/Outcome

Androgen deficiency/hypogonadism: Correction of deficiency. **Outcome criteria:** Absence or improvement of deficiency symptoms (delayed development of male secondary sex characteristics, impotence, or male climacteric).

Breast cancer: Palliation of inoperable metastatic disease for women 1–5 years postmenopause; suppression of hormone-responsive tumors. **Outcome criteria:** Evidence of decreased tumor and metastatic activity; decreased bone pain.

Dose range/Administration

Interaction alert: Increases effect of insulin, oral hypoglycemics, and anticoagulants. Corticosteroids increase possibility of edema and severe acne. Avoid other hepatotoxic medications.

🍴 **Give with food to minimize GI distress.**

Deficiency: Adult: PO: 5 mg 1–4 times a day. **Child:** PO: 2.5–10 mg/day for 4–6 mos.

Breast cancer: Adult: PO: 10–40 mg/day.

Contraindications/Precautions
PREG X

Contraindicated in hypersensitivity to androgens, lactose or tartrazine, and in severe renal, hepatic, or cardiac disease, hypercalcemia, breast or prostatic cancer in men, and genital bleeding. **Use with caution** in diabetes mellitus, prostatic hypertrophy, gynecomastia, history of MI, and cardiac failure.

✋ **Contraindicated for pregnant or nursing mothers. Use with caution for children and elderly men.**

Side effects/Adverse reactions

Hypersensitivity: rashes, anaphylaxis. *GU:* virilism of females (enlarged clitoris, deepening of voice, menstrual irregularities, unnatural hair growth or loss); virilism of prepubertal males (acne, enlarging penis, increased frequency of erections, unnatural hair growth); in older men, bladder irritability, breast soreness, gynecomastia, priapism, prostatic hypertrophy, prostatic carcinoma, epididymitis, increased libido. *Hem:* polycythemia, hypercalcemia, decreased high-density lipoproteins (HDL), and increased low-density lipoproteins (LDL). *GI:* nausea, vomiting, obstructive jaundice; hepatic dysfunction, carcinoma, or necrosis. *MS:* premature epiphyseal closure in children. *Skin:* unexplained darkening, acne, edema.

Nursing implications/Documentation

Possible nursing diagnoses: Body image disturbance; Fluid volume excess.

♦ Monitor serum calcium levels; assess, report and document symptoms of hypercalcemia (vomiting, constipation, polyuria, lethargy and muscle weakness).

♦ For elderly men, monitor for difficult or frequent urination.

♦ Record baseline blood pressure and weight.

♦ Assess for and report decreased urine output, edema, increased blood pressure, weight gain, and congestive failure.

♦ Monitor electrolyte and cholesterol levels and liver function tests.

♦ For diabetics, monitor glucose levels and observe for symptoms of hypoglycemia.

Patient & family teaching/Home care

Possible nursing diagnoses: Knowledge deficit; Impaired home maintenance management; Sexual dysfunction.

♦ Advise taking oral tablets with meals to minimize gastric distress.

♦ Suggest restricting sodium intake to decrease fluid retention.

♦ Caution women of child-bearing age to use reliable birth control and to stop drug and report any suspicion of pregnancy.

♦ For women, stress the importance of reporting the occurrence of masculinizing effects (abnormal growth of facial hair, deepening of voice, menstrual irregularities, enlarged clitoris).

♦ For men, advise reporting priapism, gynecomastia, or bladder irritability.

♦ For diabetics, caution about possible lowering of blood sugar and need for adjustment of doses of insulin or oral antidiabetic agents.

♦ Inform parents of prepubertal children that X rays will be taken periodically to determine effect on bone growth.

♦ Caution to maintain close medical supervision for early detection of adverse reactions.

♦ Warn that using high doses of androgens for improvement of athletic performance may result in serious side effects that outweigh any advantages.

fluphenazine

floo-fen'azeen

fluphenazine decanoate: ♦ ♠*Modecate Decanoate, Prolixin Decanoate*

fluphenazine enanthate: ♣*Moditen Enanthate, Prolixin Enanthate*

fluphenazine hydrochloride: ♠*Anatensol,* ♣*Apo-Fluphenazine,* ♣*Moditen HCL,* ♣*Moditen HCL-HP, Permitil, Prolixin.*

Class: Phenothiazine antipsychotic

PEDS	PREG	GERI
✋	C	✋

Action Exact mechanism of action has not been determined. Believed to produce calmness and alleviate psychiatric symptoms (disorders of perception, thought, consciousness, mood, affect, and social interaction) by blocking dopamine receptors in the limbic system. Blocks peripheral muscarinic, adrenergic, and histamine receptors. Also has some effect on the hypothalamus and pituitary gland, causing changes in regulation of body temperature and endocrine function. A dose of 2 mg of fluphenazine is therapeutically equivalent to 100 mg of chlorpromazine. Preparations with enanthate and decanoate esters are mixed in oil; these have a delayed onset of action (24–96 hr) and a long duration of action (may last up to 3–4 weeks).

Use/Therapeutic goal/Outcome

Chronic schizophrenia and psychotic disorders: Promotion of reality orientation, elimination of agitation and hyperactivity. ***Outcome criteria:*** Demonstration of reality orientation, and ability to problem solve and interact with others; absence of hyperactive and agitated behavior.

Dose range/Administration

Interaction alert: Antacids reduce absorption; separate doses of antacid and phenothiazines by at least 2 hr. Alcohol and other CNS depressants may cause excessive sedation. Lithium may decrease phenothiazine effects. May decrease the effect of centrally acting antihypertensives.

Psychotic disorders: fluphenazine hydrochloride. *Adult:* PO: 0.5–10 mg q4h. *For severely disturbed patients:* Up to 20 mg/day. *For the elderly:* Begin with 1–2.5 mg/day, use lowest effective dose. IM: Use 1/2 to 1/3 oral dose. *Child > 12 yrs:* PO: 0.25–0.75 one to four times a day. *Maximum dose:* 10 mg/day. IM: Use 1/2 to 1/3 oral dose.

Chronic schizophrenia: fluphenazine enanthate or decanoate. *Adult/Child > 12 yrs:* IM: *Enanthate: Initial dose:* 25 mg. *Maintenance dose:* 25 mg every 2 wk. *Decanoate: Initial dose:* 12.5–25 mg. *Maintenance dose:* 25–100 mg prn (usually every 2–4 wks).

Clinical alert: Be aware that Prolixin *Concentrate* and Permital *Concentrate* (which both contain 5 mg/cc) are 10 times more concentrated than Prolixin *Elixir* (which contains 0.5 mg/ml). Dilute concentrate in milk, fruit juice, or soft food just before giving dose. Avoid skin contact with liquid and parenteral forms (may cause contact dermatitis). Keep IV diphenhydramine available in case of side effect of acute dystonic reaction.

Contraindications/Precautions
PREG
C

Contraindicated in hypersensitivity to fluphenazine or phenothiazines, and in coma or CNS depression. *Use with caution* in seizure disorders, hypertension, Parkinsonism, poorly controlled diabetes mellitus, asthma, emphysema, narrow-angle glaucoma, cardiac disease, hypotension, paralytic ileus, liver disease, prostatic hypertrophy, and bone marrow depression.

✴ **Contraindicated for children under 12 years and nursing mothers. Use with caution for adolescents and the elderly or debilitated. Safe use for pregnant women has not been established.**

Side effects/Adverse reactions

Hypersensitivity: rash, contact dermatitis. *CNS:* extrapyramidal reactions (pseudoparkinsonism, akathisia [restless need to keep moving], dystonia, tardive dykinesia), neuroleptic malignant syndrome (fever, tachycardia, tachypnea, profuse diaphoresis), EEG changes, dizziness. *CV:* orthostatic hypotension, palpitations, dysrhythmias, EKG changes. *GI:* appetite changes, dry mouth, constipation, abnormal liver function. *GU:* urinary retention or hesitancy, dark urine, impaired ejaculation, priapism, amenorrhea. *Eye:* blurred vision. *Skin:* photosensitivity, jaundice. *MS:* weight gain. *Hem:* agranulocytosis. *Misc:* gynecomastia, galactorrhea. *After abrupt withdrawal of long-term therapy:* gastritis, nausea, vomiting, lightheadedness, tremors, feeling of warmth or cold, diaphoresis, tachycardia, headache, insomnia.

Nursing implications/Documentation

Possible nursing diagnoses: Potential for injury; Constipation; Altered oral mucous membrane.

♦ Record mental status and vital signs before and one hr after administration during initial phase of treatment, then bid until response to therapy has been established, then periodically thereafter.

♦ Check CBC, liver function, BUN, and creatinine before giving first dose and periodically thereafter.

♦ Be sure that PO doses are swallowed (not hoarded).

♦ Monitor for orthostatic hypotension, dizziness, and drowsiness; supervise ambulation until response is established.

♦ Record weight every 2 weeks; report significant weight gain.

♦ Provide special mouth care; observe for and report oral ulcers.

♦ Prevent constipation by monitoring bowel movements and encouraging adequate fiber and fluid intake; offer laxatives or stool softeners before problem becomes severe.

♦ Report persistent sore throat, fever, and malaise, because these may indicate agranulocytosis (drug may have to be discontinued).

♦ Monitor for (and report immediately) signs of neuroleptic malignant syndrome (muscle rigidity, tremors, high fever, tachycardia); this is a rare, but potentially fatal, side effect.

Patient & family teaching/Home care

Possible nursing diagnoses: Sleep pattern disturbance; Impaired home maintenance management.

* Emphasize the need to continue medication, even when feeling well (for compliance problems, explain that the enanthate and decanoate forms can make administration more simple because injections are as infrequent as weekly or every 6 weeks).

* Warn to change positions slowly to prevent dizziness.

* Stress that the effects of alcohol, sedatives, and CNS depressants may be potentiated.

* Caution to consult with physician before using OTC drugs; stress the need for ongoing medical follow-up.

* Provide a list of side effects that should be reported: involuntary movements, muscular rigidity, tremors, fever, respiratory distress, tachycardia, persistent sore throat.

* Point out that doses should not be increased or stopped without checking with physician.

* Caution to wear a sunscreen (number 15), protective clothing, and sunglasses when out in the sun.

* Advise avoidance of driving and other potentially hazardous activities until response has been established.

* Suggest using ice chips, hard candy, or gum to relieve side effect of dry mouth; stress the need for good mouth care.

* Warn women to report if pregnancy is planned or suspected.

* See Antipsychotics overview for more information.

Flurazepam

flure-az'e-pam

flurazepam hydrochloride: ✸*Apo-flurazepam, Dalmane, Durapam,* ✸*Novoflupam,* ✸*Sam-Pam*

Class: Hypnotic, anxiolytic (antianxiety), benzodiazepine, psychotropic

PEDS	PREG	GERI		CONTROLLED SUBSTANCE
🖐	NR	🖐		IV

Action Produces sleep, probably by acting upon the limbic system, thalamus, and hypothalamus of the central nervous system (exact mode and site of action unknown).

Use/Therapeutic goal/Outcome

Short-term insomnia (less than 4 weeks): Promotion of sleep. ***Outcome criteria:*** Report of having slept well.

Dose range/Administration

Interaction alert: Cimetidine, alcohol, narcotics, analgesics, antihistamines, and other CNS depressants intensify CNS depression. ***Adult: Under 65 yrs:*** PO: 15–30 mg at bedtime (may repeat once). ***Adult: Over 65 yrs:*** 15 mg at bedtime. Capsules may be opened and mixed with fluid or food for easier swallowing.

Clinical alert: If desired effect is not achieved, wait 2–4 days before considering increase in dosage or change in medication. This drug accumulates within the body, and therefore full effects are not always observed until 2–4 days after medication is started.

Contraindications/Precautions

PREG
NR

Contraindicated in hypersensitivity or intolerance to flurazepam hydrochloride. ***Use with caution*** for history of benzodiazepine hypersensitivity, depression, suicidal tendencies, and impaired liver or kidney function.

🖐 Use with caution for the elderly. Safe use for children and for pregnant or nursing mothers has not been established.

Side effects/Adverse reactions

Hypersensitivity: rashes. ***CNS:*** lethargy, drowsiness, dizziness, hangover; rarely, paradoxical excitement, confusion, and blurred vision. ***GI:*** nausea, vomiting, diarrhea. ***Misc:*** drug tolerance and dependence.

Nursing implications/Documentation

Possible nursing diagnoses: Potential for injury; Sensory/perceptual alterations (visual and auditory).

* Document mental status before administration, monitor patient activity closely following administration, and employ appropriate measures to ensure safety (i.e., side rails up, call bell within reach, and no unsupervised smoking).

* Hold dose and report if respiratory depression, severe pain, or signs of overdosage (constricted pupils, somnolence, hypotension, clammy skin, cyanosis) are present.

* Be sure that doses are swallowed (not hoarded).

* Be aware that sedatives and hypnotics *do not provide pain relief* (patient may need an analgesic as well).

* Monitor for and report signs of overdosage (slurred speech, continued somnolence, respira-

tory depression, confusion) and tolerance (increased anxiety and/or increased wakefulness).

Patient & family teaching/Home care

Possible nursing diagnoses: Sleep pattern disturbance; Ineffective coping (family and individual); Impaired home maintenance management.

♦ Explore problems that may contribute to insomnia or anxiety, and ways of coping effectively with these problems (stress that effective coping can promote restful sleep).

♦ Explain the importance of daily exercise in promoting rest and encourage the person to establish a method for getting enough exercise (e.g., daily walks).

♦ Stress that drug tolerance and dependence can occur, and that the drug should be used only when holistic measures (e.g., quiet music, relaxation techniques) don't work.

♦ Emphasize that the effects of alcohol, other sedatives, and tranquilizers may be potentiated and should be avoided.

♦ Reinforce the importance of consulting with physician before using OTC drugs, and of returning for medical follow-up.

♦ Advise avoidance of driving and other potentially hazardous activities while under the effects of the medication.

♦ Advise that morning "hangover" is common and that this should be reported if it continues.

♦ *See Antianxiety Agents, Sedatives, and Hypnotics overview for more information.*

flurbiprofen (ophthalmic) *flure-by-pro'fen*

flurbiprofen sodium: **Ocufen**

Class: Nonsteroidal Anti-inflammatory drug (NSAID), Opthalmic

PEDS	PREG	GERI
♦	C	♦

Action Reduces inflammation of the eye by inhibiting prostaglandin synthesis; reverses prostaglandin-induced vasodilation, leukocytosis, and increased permeability. Prostaglandin is a naturally occurring mediator of the inflammatory process which is found throughout body tissues.

Use/Therapeutic goal/Outcome

Intraoperative procedures: Prevention of miosis (abnormal contraction of the pupils). **Outcome criteria:** Report of improved vision in diminished light; normal dilation of pupil.

(Investigational uses) Reduction of inflammation following cataract surgery, uveitis syndromes, and cystoid macular edema.

Dose range/Administration

Adult: *Ophthalmic: Operative procedures:* 1 drop 0.03% solution q 30 min beginning 2 hr before surgery; up to total of 4 drops. *Anti-inflammatory:* 1 drop 0.03% solution q4h for 1–3 wk.

Contraindications/Precautions

PREG
C

Contraindicated in hypersensitivity to flurbiprofen, other NSAIDs, and aspirin, and in dendritic keratitis.

✋ **Use with caution for the elderly. Safe use for children under 14 years and pregnant women has not been established.**

Side effects/Adverse reactions

Hypersensitivity: itching, irritation. **Eye:** occular irritation, transient stinging or burning, delay in wound healing.

Nursing implications/Documentation

Possible nursing diagnoses: Pain; Sensory/perceptual alterations (visual).

♦ Follow administration protocol carefully prior to surgery.

♦ Monitor for and report delayed wound healing.

Patient & family teaching/Home care

Possible nursing diagnoses: Fear; Knowledge deficit.

♦ Demonstrate how to instill eye drops and have patient or caretaker return demonstration.

♦ Warn not to rub eyes, even after administration.

♦ Advise reporting stinging, burning, or irritation to physician.

♦ *See Nonsteroidal anti-inflammatory drugs overview for more information.*

F

flurbiprofen (systemic)
flure-by-pro'fen

Ansaid, ♣Froben

Class: Nonsteroidal anti-inflammatory drug (NSAID), Analgesic, Antipyretic

PEDS	PREG	GERI
🖐	B	🖐

Action Reduces inflammation probably by inhibiting synthesis and/or release of prostaglandin. Prostaglandin is a naturally occurring mediator of the inflammatory process which is found throughout body tissue. Acts on hypothalamus to produce vasodilation. Inhibits platelet aggregation.

Use/Therapeutic goal/Outcome

Mild to moderate pain and inflammation: Promotion of comfort and mobility; suppression of inflammation. **Outcome criteria:** Report of increased comfort with increased range of motion and ability to perform activities of daily life; reduction in or absence of joint stiffness, swelling, redness, and warmth.

Dose range/Administration

Interaction alert: Since this drug is protein-bound, observe those receiving hydantoins, sulfonamides, and sulfonylureas for toxicity. Aspirin may decrease the therapeutic effect of NSAIDs and increase risk of bleeding. Antihypertensive effects of beta-blocking agents may be decreased.

🍴 **Give with food or milk to reduce GI distress.**

Adult: PO: Up to 100 mg bid, tid, or qid.

Clinical alert: Dosage is individualized, but should not exceed 100 mg per dose and 200–300 mg/day. May give with antacid to those with GI irritation or history of peptic ulcer.

Contraindications/Precautions
PREG B

Contraindicated in hypersensitivity to flurbiprofen, other NSAIDs, or aspirin. **Use with caution** in history of GI bleeding, renal or hepatic impairment, and coagulation defects.

🖐 **Use with caution for the elderly. Safe use for children under 14 years and pregnant women has not been established.**

Side effects/Adverse reactions

Hypersensitivity: chills, fever, anaphylactic reaction (bronchospasm, angiospasm, asthmatic symptoms). **GI:** dyspepsia, diarrhea, bleeding, abdominal pain, nausea, vomiting. **Hem:** elevated liver enzymes (SGPT, SGOT), hyperuricemia, elevated BUN and creatinine, platelet aggregation inhibition. **CNS:** headache, nervousness, dizziness. **CV:** hypertension, fluid weight gain. **Eye:** visual disturbance, blurring. **Ear:** tinnitus. **CU:** urinary tract infection.

Nursing implications/Documentation

Possible nursing diagnoses: Pain; Impaired physical mobility.

♦ Establish a baseline for CBC, electrolytes, prothrombin time, BUN, creatinine, and liver function studies; if therapy is prolonged, monitor periodically thereafter.

♦ Monitor for and report GI symptoms that may indicate peptic ulcer (nausea, pain, black stools).

♦ Record weight every other day; report edema or sudden weight gain.

♦ Observe for and report visual and auditory changes (periodic auditory tests are recommended if therapy is prolonged).

♦ For diabetics, monitor blood sugar closely since insulin requirements may change.

Patient & family teaching/Home care

Possible nursing diagnoses: Altered health maintenance; Knowledge deficit.

♦ Advise taking doses with food to reduce GI symptoms. Explain the importance of watching for symptoms of GI bleeding (black stools, persistent GI distress).

♦ Stress the need to avoid aspirin, alcohol, and other OTC drugs (unless approved by physician) because of increased risk of GI bleeding.

♦ Instruct individuals to hold dose and report if any of the following side effects are experienced: vertigo, rashes, blood in urine, hearing or visual changes, sudden weight gain, edema.

♦ Warn against driving or activities that require alertness until response is determined (may cause drowsiness and dizziness at first; this should be transient).

♦ Reinforce the need for medical follow-up; advise telling dentist that flurbiprofen is being taken.

♦ For diabetics, explain the importance of monitoring blood sugars with a blood glucose meter.

- *See Nonsteroidal anti-inflammatory drugs overview for more information.*

flutamide

floot'-a-mide

Eulexin, Euflex

Class: Antineoplastic agent, Antihormone

PEDS ✋ PREG D GERI ✋

Action Inhibits malignant cellular growth of androgen-responsive tumors by blocking androgen uptake needed for tumor growth.

Use/Therapeutic goal/Outcome

Metastatic prostatic carcinoma (stage 2): Suppression of malignant cell proliferation. **Outcome criteria:** Tumor and disease regression or stabilization on radiologic and physical examination.

Dose range/Administration

Adult: PO: 250 mg q8h for total of 750 mg/day.

Clinical alert: Must be used in conjunction with luteinizing hormone-releasing hormone agonist (e.g., leupromide).

Contraindications/Precautions

PREG D

Contraindicated in hypersensitivity to flutamide. **Use with caution** in liver disorders.

✋ **Contraindicated for pregnant or nursing mothers. Safe use for children is not established. Use with caution for the elderly.**

Side effects/Adverse reactions

Hypersensitivity: urticaria, hypotension. **GU:** loss of libido, impotence. **GI:** nausea, vomiting, diarrhea; elevated AST, ALT, bilirubin; hepatitis. **CV:** edema, hypertension. **Skin:** rash, photosensitivity. **Misc:** gynecomastia.

Nursing implications/Documentation

Possible nursing diagnoses: Fluid volume deficit; Self-esteem disturbance; Altered nutrition: less than body requirements.

- *See important Nursing implications in Antineoplastic agents overview.*
  - Recognize that combination therapy is necessary to achieve maximum results.

Patient & family teaching/Home care

Possible nursing diagnoses: Knowledge deficit; Impaired home maintenance management; Ineffective coping (individual and family).

- *See important Patient & family teaching in Antineoplastic agents overview.*
  - Explain that this treatment is a form of medical castration that is equally as effective as removal of the testicles; encourage voicing concerns about sexuality.
- *See Antineoplastic agents overview for more information.*

folic acid

fo'lik

Folvite, ✦Novofolacid

Class: Vitamin B9; Water-soluble vitamin, Antianemic

PEDS ✋ PREG A GERI OK

Action Required for production of RBCs, WBCs, and platelets, and for nucleoprotein synthesis.

Use/Therapeutic goal/Outcome

Folic acid deficiency, and megaloblastic or macrocytic anemia: Maintenance of adequate blood levels of folic acid for patients with inadequate intake or increased requirements. **Outcome criteria:** Increase in RBC, WBC, and platelet counts; reversal of symptoms of folic acid deficiency (glossitis, diarrhea, constipation, weight loss, irritability, diffuse muscular pain, insomnia, depression and pallor).

Dose range/Administration

Interaction alert: Large doses of folic acid may be needed with long-term adrenocorticosteroids or analgesic therapy, and with estrogen, phenytoin anticonvulsants or sulfonamides. May increase metabolism of phenytoin, resulting in decreased seizure control. Inhibits antimicrobial effect of pyrimethamine. Folate antagonists (methotrexate, pyrimethamine, trimethoprim) inhibit action of folic acid.

Adult and Child: PO: 100 mcg to 1 mg/day. IM, IV, SC: 250 mcg to 1 mg/day.

Clinical alert: Diagnosis of pernicious anemia must be ruled out before folic acid therapy is initiated to avoid undetected neurologic deterioration.

Contraindications/Precautions

PREG A

Contraindicated in hypersensitivity to folic acid; in undiagnosed anemia, or as sole agent in treatment of pernicious anemia.

✋ **Parenteral preparations containing benzyl alcohol are contraindicated for infants (may result in fatal toxicity).**

▶

Side effects/Adverse reactions

Hypersensitivity: fever or skin rash. *GU:* (with large doses) yellow discoloration of urine.

Nursing implications/Documentation

Possible nursing diagnosis: Impaired skin integrity.

♦ Be aware that oral administration is preferred.

♦ Do not mix other medications in same syringe for IM injections.

♦ Assess skin for possible allergic response.

Patient & family teaching/Home care

Possible nursing diagnosis: Knowledge deficit.

♦ Teach dietary sources of folic acid; i.e., vegetables, fruits, organ meats; explain that heat destroys folic acid.

♦ Discourage self-medication with large doses of vitamins.

♦ Advise of possibility of yellow discoloration of urine with large doses.

♦ Point out that excessive use of alcohol increases requirement for folic acid.

furosemide
fur-os'e-myd

♣Apo-Furosemide, ♣Furoside, Lasix, Myrosimide, ♣Novosemide, ♣Uritol, ♠Urex, ♠Urex-M

Class: ★**Loop (high-ceiling) diuretic prototype,** Antihypertensive

PEDS	PREG	GERI
✋	C	✋

Action Promotes diuresis by preventing sodium and chloride reabsorption in the ascending loop of Henle, and in the proximal and distal tubules. Promotes potassium and hydrogen ion excretion and decreases urinary ammonium ion concentration and pH. Lowers blood pressure by reducing plasma and extra-cellular volume.

Use/Therapeutic goal/Outcome

Hypertension: Promotion of diuresis, reduction of blood pressure. *Outcome criteria:* Increased urinary output, blood pressure within normal limits.

Pulmonary edema: Adjunctive therapy, promotion of diuresis, resolution of pulmonary edema. *Outcome criteria:* Significant diuresis; absence of rales; CVP and PAP within normal limits.

Edema associated with CHF, liver cirrhosis, renal pathology: Promotion of diuresis, resolution of edema. *Outcome criteria:* Increased urine output; absence of rales, and peripheral and sacral edema.

Dose range/Administration

Interaction alert: Aminoglycosides and other ototoxic drugs can increase risk of ototoxicity. Clofibrate can potentiate effect. Nonsteroidal anti-inflammatory drugs, indomethacin, and probenicid can decrease effect. IV furosemide with chloral hydrate can cause flushing and sweating.

Hypertension: Adult: PO: 40 mg bid; individualize dose, depending on response. May repeat q6-8h, may increase each dose by 20–40 mg.

Acute pulmonary edema: Adult: IV: 40 mg over 1–2 min; may repeat in 1 hr prn; if response is inadequate, increase dose by 40 mg. *Maximum dose:* 200 mg. *Child:* IM or IV: 1mg/kg; may increase by 1 mg/kg q2h. *Maximum dose:* 6 mg/kg.

Edema: Adult: PO: 20–80 mg. *Maximum dose:* 600 mg/day. IM (least desirable route): 20–40 mg; may repeat q2h, and may increase each dose by 20 mg. IV: 20–40 mg over 2 min; may repeat q2h; may increase each dose by 20 mg. *Child:* PO/IV: 2 mg/kg/day. Increase by 1–2 mg/kg q6-8h prn. *Maximum dose:* 6 mg/kg/day.

Acute renal failure: Adult: IV: 100–200 mg over 1–2 min.

Chronic renal failure: Adult: PO: 80 mg/day. Increase by 80–120 mg/day prn.

Clinical alert: Give in morning and early afternoon to avoid nocturnal diuresis. Use IV route for children only when PO route is not feasible.

Contraindications/Precautions
PREG C

Contraindicated in hypersensitivity to furosemide or sulfonamides, and in anuria. *Use with caution* in the presence of cardiogenic shock, advanced hepatic cirrhosis, or history of systemic lupus erythematosus or gout.

✋ **Use with caution for children, pregnant or nursing mothers, and the elderly.**

Side effects/Adverse reactions

Hypersensitivity: rash, urticaria, dermatitis. *CV:* orthostatic hypotension, volume depletion, dehydration. *Hem:* hypokalemia, asymptomatic hyperuricemia, fluid and electrolyte imbalance, hyperglycemia, impaired glucose tolerance, hypocalcemia, hypomagnesemia, leukopenia, agranulocytosis, thrombocytopenia. *Ear:* transient (with rapid IV administration)

F

and permanent deafness. *GI:* abdominal discomfort, diarrhea. *Skin:* increased sensitivity to sunlight, yellow pigmentation. *Misc:* hypochloremic alkalosis

Nursing implications/Documentation

Possible nursing diagnoses: Fluid volume deficit; Altered patterns of urinary elimination; Potential for injury.

♦ Ascertain that baseline CBC, sodium, potassium, chloride, carbon dioxide, calcium, magnesium, BUN, creatinine, uric acid, and liver function studies have been obtained before giving first dose; report abnormalities and monitor closely thereafter.

♦ Give doses in early morning and early afternoon (if possible) to avoid nocturnal diuresis.

♦ For bedridden patients, keep bedpan close at hand.

♦ Document and monitor blood pressure, daily weight, and intake and output; report significant discrepancies.

♦ Monitor for and report signs of fluid overload (auscultate lungs for rales; check feet, ankles, and sacrum for edema) and of toxicity (fever, ringing in the ears, sore throat).

♦ Be aware that diuretics often induce hypokalemia, which predisposes individuals to cardiac arrhythmias, cramping, and digoxin toxicity.

♦ Check with physician to determine dietary restrictions; if a low-salt, high-potassium diet is recommended, consult with dietician to plan a low-salt diet that includes foods and juices high in potassium (orange juice; banana; green leafy vegetables).

♦ Observe the elderly for extreme diuresis; monitor for orthostatic hypotension; supervise ambulation until response is determined.

Patient & family teaching/Home care

Possible nursing diagnoses: Knowledge deficit; Impaired home maintenance management.

♦ Before giving first dose, explain that the drug will increase the amount and frequency of urination.

♦ Emphasize the importance of taking this drug exactly as prescribed, and the importance of ongoing medical follow-up.

♦ Explain that diuretics enhance the work of the kidney and reduce the workload of the heart.

♦ Recommend taking doses in early morning and early afternoon to prevent the need to disturb sleep to void.

♦ Explain that changing positions slowly helps prevent dizziness.

♦ Advise reporting dizziness, shortness of breath, swelling of hands and feet, and symptoms of fever, sore throat, hearing problems, and ringing in the ears; encourage daily monitoring of weight and reporting sudden weight gain.

♦ Provide a list of allowed foods and fluids; stress the need to stick to prescribed diet (explain the hazards of too much salt, or too little potassium).

♦ Warn against driving or activities that require alertness until response has been determined.

♦ *See Diuretics and Antihypertensives overviews for more information.*

gallamine

gal'a-meen

gallamine triethiodide: *Flaxedil*

Class: Nondepolarizing neuromuscular blocker, Skeletal-muscle relaxant

Antidote: Neostigmine methylsulfate

PEDS	PREG	GERI
✋	C	✋

Action Relaxes or paralyzes skeletal muscles (depending on dose) by competing with acetylcholine for cholinergic receptor sites, thereby inhibiting neuromuscular transmission. Does not alter consciousness or thought processes.

Use/Therapeutic goal/Outcome

Endotracheal intubation, adjunct to general anesthesia, mechanical ventilation, reduction of fractures and dislocations, and during pharmacologically or electrically induced seizures: Facilitation of endotracheal tube tolerance; relaxation of skeletal muscle. *Outcome criteria:* Tolerance of endotracheal intubation and mechanical ventilation; diminished or absent voluntary and reflexive movement.

Dose range/Administration

Interaction alert: Ether, methoxyflurane, fluoroxene, certain antibiotics (aminoglycosides and polymyxins) barbiturates, and narcotic analgesics may increase the effect of gallamine.

Adult/Child > 1 mo: IV: 1 mg/kg. Single dose < 100 mg. May repeat half dose after 30 min.

Child < 1 mo, > 5 kg: IV: 0.25–0.75 mg/kg. May repeat 0.01–0.05 mg/kg q 30–40 min.

Clinical alert: Gallamine should be given only by physicians and nurses who are familiar with its use, and in the presence of a physician, nurse anesthetist, or respiratory therapist who is qualified to manage endotracheal intubation.

Contraindications/Precautions

PREG
C

Contraindicated in hypersensitivity to gallamine or iodides, and in myasthenia gravis, shock, cardiac disease, hypertension, hypoalbuminemia, hyperthyroidism, impaired renal function, and respiratory depression.

🖐 **Use with caution for children, pregnant women, and the elderly.**

Side effects/Adverse reactions

Hypersensitivity: anaphylaxis. *Resp:* respiratory paralysis, increased bronchial secretions. *CV:* tachycardia. *MS:* residual muscle weakness.

Nursing implications/Documentation

Possible nursing diagnoses: Impaired communication; Pain; Potential for aspiration; Potential for injury.

♦ Ascertain that baseline CBC, electrolytes, BUN, creatinine, liver function, chest X ray, and EKG studies are posted on chart before drug administration (report abnormalities).

♦ Protect airway, position for drainage of oropharyngeal secretions (if possible), and keep suction at bedside until the patient is fully alert; have emergency equipment and drugs available.

♦ Monitor and record vital signs every 15 min until stable; report abnormalities that might indicate potential complications.

♦ Recognize that this drug may *paralyze*, but does not relieve pain (provide analgesics if pain is suspected, anticipate human needs).

♦ Monitor for potential for injury: protect eyes if there is no blink reflex (tape shut); watch positioning of all extremities (provide range of motion exercises if therapy is prolonged).

Patient & family teaching/Home care

Possible nursing diagnoses: Anxiety; Fear.

♦ Explain all procedures, even if the person seems unconscious (the ability to hear may be present).

♦ Reassure individual that muscle paralysis, weakness, or stiffness will subside.

ganciclovir

gan-sye'klow-veer

Cytovene
Class: Antiviral

PEDS	PREG	GERI
🖐	C	🖐

Action Inhibits replication of the cytomegalovirus (CMV) by blocking viral DNA synthesis.

Use/Therapeutic goal/Outcome

CMV retinitis in immunocompromised individuals: Resolution of CMV infection. **Outcome criteria:** Normal retina upon ophthalmic exam.

Dose range/Administration

Interaction alert: Probenecid increases ganciclovir levels. Avoid use with zidovudine (increases risk of granulocytopenia). Cytotoxic agents increase toxic effects, especially stomatitis and hematologic effects. Use with imipenem-cilastatin has been associated with reports of seizure activity.

Adult: IV: *Induction:* 5 mg/kg q12h for 2–3 wk. *Maintenance dose:* 5 mg/kg/day, or 6 mg/kg/day 5 days a week.

Clinical alert: During preparation, avoid contacting skin with ganciclovir, which is alkaline. Do not give via bolus; give over 1 hr via infusion. In decreased renal function, expect reduced dosage.

Contraindications/Precautions

PREG
C

Contraindicated in hypersensitivity to ganciclovir or acyclovir. **Use with caution** in decreased renal function, neutropenia, and thrombocytopenia.

🖐 **Contraindicated for nursing mothers. Avoid use for pregnant women. Use with caution for children under 12 years and the elderly.**

Side effects/Adverse reactions

Hypersensitivity: itching, rashes, fever, chills. *Hem:* granulocytopenia, thrombocytopenia, neutropenia, anemia, eosinophilia. *GI:* nausea, vomiting, anorexia, diarrhea, abdominal pain, hemorrhage. *CNS:* drowsiness, confusion, dizziness, headache, bizarre thoughts and dreams, psychoses, tremors, paresthesias. *CV:* dysrhythmias, hypertension, hypotension, phlebitis at injection site. *GU:* hematuria, impaired kidney function. *Eye:* retinal detachment in patients with CMV retinitis.

Nursing implications/Documentation

Possible nursing diagnoses: Fluid volume deficit; Altered thought processes; Potential for injury.

♦ Ensure adequate hydration by providing adequate fluids and keeping a record of fluid intake.

♦ Check neutrophil and platelet counts every 2 days during twice-daily doses and at least weekly thereafter. Hold dose and report if neutrophil count < 500/mm^3 or platelet count < 25,000/mm^3.

♦ Monitor mental status; report confusion or bizarre thought processes and employ safety precautions as needed.

Patient & family teaching/Home care

Possible nursing diagnoses: Knowledge deficit; Impaired home maintenance management.

♦ Stress that regular eye exams are essential because this drug does not cure the condition and retinitis may continue during and after treatment.

♦ Explain the need for close monitoring of blood work for early detection of adverse side effects.

♦ Advise that the patient may be at risk for retinal detachment; advise reporting deterioration in vision immediately.

♦ Advise significant others to report bizarre thoughts or behavior.

♦ *See Ant-infectives overview for more information.*

gemfibrozil
gem-fi'broe-zil

Lopid

Class: Antilipemic

PEDS	PREG	GERI
🖐	B	🖐

Action Reduces serum lipid levels by inhibiting peripheral lipolysis and decreasing hepatic extraction of free fatty acids. Thought to increase high-density lipoprotein (HDL) fractions, which may inhibit the progression of atherosclerosis. Increases very-low-density lipoprotein (VLDL) and low-density lipoprotein (LDL) clearance.

Use/Therapeutic goal/Outcome

Hypertriglyceridemia and hypercholesterolemia (type IIB): Reduction of serum lipid levels. *Outcome criteria:* Serum lipid levels within normal range.

Dose range/Administration

Interaction alert: Potentiates the effects of anticoagulants.

▯ **Give 30 minutes before morning and evening meal.**

Adult: PO: 1.2 g/day in two divided doses. *Range:* 900 mg – 1.5 g.

Contraindications/Precautions
PREG B

Contraindicated in hypersensitivity to this drug, and in hepatic or renal dysfunction (including primary biliary cirrhosis), and pre-existing gallbladder disease.

🖐 **Use with caution for the elderly. Safe use for children and pregnant or nursing mothers has not been established.**

Side effects/Adverse reactions

Hypersensitivity: rash, dermatitis, pruritus, urticaria. *GI:* abdominal or epigastric pain, diarrhea, nausea, vomiting, flatulence. *CNS:* headache, dizziness. *Hem:* blood dyscrasias, elevated liver enzymes. *Eye:* blurred vision. *MS:* painful extremities.

Nursing implications/Documentation

Possible nursing diagnoses: Diarrhea; Altered nutrition: more than body requirements.

♦ Monitor for and report diarrhea or persistent GI symptoms.

♦ Assess history and physical exam to rule out liver, kidney, or gallbladder disease before giving first dose.

Patient & family teaching/Home care

Possible nursing diagnoses: Altered health maintenance; Knowledge deficit; Impaired home maintenance management.

♦ Explain that the purpose of this drug is to reduce serum cholesterol and decrease the risk of cardiovascular disease.

♦ Emphasize the need to reduce other cardiac risk factors (obesity, smoking, high cholesterol diet, sedentary lifestyle), and help develop a plan to reduce these.

- ◆ Stress that persistent GI symptoms and bleeding or bruising tendencies should be reported.

- ◆ Reinforce that this drug will have to be taken for a long time and that ongoing medical follow-up of cholesterol level studies is essential.

- ◆ *See Antilipemics overview for more information.*

gentamicin

jen-ta-mye'sin

gentamicin: *Gentacidin*

gentamicin sulfate: ◆ ✿*Cidomycin, Garamycin, Garamycin Ophthalmic, Gentafain, Genoptic, Jenamicin*

Class: ★*Anti-infective (aminoglycoside) prototype,* Antibiotic

PEDS	PREG	GERI
🤚	C	🤚

Action Kills bacteria (bactericidal) by binding to the ribosomes, thereby disrupting bacterial protein synthesis.

Use/Therapeutic goal/Outcome

Serious infections (caused by *Pseudomonas aeruginosa, Escherichia coli, Proteus, Klebsiella, Serratia, Enterobacter, Citrobacter, Staphylococcus*): Resolution of infection. **Outcome criteria:** Absence of pathogenic growth on cultures, absence of clinical manifestations of infection (fever, pain, swelling, redness, heat, odor, drainage, productive cough, dysuria, urinary frequency, elevated WBC count, abnormal X rays).

Dose range/Administration

Interaction alert: Do not mix IV with any other drug. Loop diuretics (e.g., furosemide) increase risk of nephrotoxicity and ototoxicity. Dimenhydrinate may mask symptoms of ototoxicity. Use cautiously with other aminoglycosides, amphotericin B, methoxyflurane, and cisplatin, and cephalosporins (increased risk of toxicity).

Serious systemic infections caused by susceptible organisms: **Adult:** IM, IV: 3 mg/kg/day, in divided doses q8h. (For IV use, dilute in 50–200 ml NS or D5W; administer over 30–60 min. May give IV push if necessary). *For life-threatening infection,* may give up to 5 mg/kg/day in divided doses q6-8h. **Child:** IM, IV: 2–2.5 mg/kg q8h. **Infant/Neonate > 1 week:** IM, IV: 2.5 mg/kg q8h. **Neonate < 1 week:** IM, IV: 2.5 mg/kg q12h.

Meningitis: **Adult:** Intrathecal: May give 4–8 mg/day in addition to systemic therapy. **Child:** Intrathecal: May give 1–2 mg/day in addition to systemic therapy.

Endocarditis prophylaxis for GI or GU surgery or procedures: **Adult:** IM, IV: 1.5 mg/kg 30–60 min before procedure and q8h after, for 2 doses (given with aqueous penicillin G or ampicillin). **Child:** IM, IV: 2.5 mg/kg 30–60 min before procedure and q8h after, for 2 doses (given with aqueous penicillin G or ampicillin).

Post hemodialysis to maintain therapeutic blood levels: **Adult:** IM, IV: 1–1.7 mg/kg after each dialysis. **Child:** IM, IV: 2 mg/kg after each dialysis.

External ocular infections (conjunctivitis, keratoconjunctivitis, corneal ulcers, blepharitis, blepharoconjunctivitis, meibomianitis, and dacryocystitis) caused by susceptible organisms: **Adult and Child:** Ophthalmic: *Ophthalmic drops:* 1 or 2 drops (0.3% solution) in affected eye q4h (for severe infections, up to 2 drops qh). *Ophthalmic ointment:* Apply a thin strip (about 1 cm) to conjunctival sac bid or qid.

Primary and secondary bacterial infections, superficial burns, skin ulcers, infected insect bites and stings, infected abrasions and lacerations: **Adult/Child > 1 yr:** *Topical:* Gently rub in a small amount tid or qid.

Clinical alert: In impaired renal function, the initial dose should follow the regular dosing guidelines, but subsequent doses and frequency of doses should be determined by serum gentamicin levels and renal function studies. Schedule blood drawing for peak levels 1 hour after IM dose, or 30–60 minutes after IV dose. Schedule blood drawing for trough levels just before next dose. Therapeutic peak levels are 4–10 mcg/ml; therapeutic trough levels are 1–2 mcg/ml. Peak levels exceeding 12 mcg/ml and trough levels exceeding 2 mgc/ml are associated with toxicity; monitoring of peak and trough levels is especially important for ototoxicity if hearing ability is difficult to evaluate (e.g., in very young and elderly patients).

Contraindications/Precautions

PREG
C

Contraindicated in hypersensitivity to gentamicin or other aminoglycoside antibiotics. *Use with caution* in impaired renal function, hearing loss or tinnitus, vertigo or dizziness, fever, dehydration, parkinsonism, neuromuscular diseases. Safe use for more than 14 days has not been established.

🤚 **Use with caution for neonates, premature babies, infants, and the elderly. Safe use** for pregnant or nursing mothers has not been established (fetal deafness has occurred).

Side effects/Adverse reactions

Hypersensitivity: itching, burning, rashes, drug fever, arthralgia, laryngeal edema, anaphylaxis. *Ear:* ototoxicity (hearing loss, tinnitus). *CNS:* headache, dizziness, weakness, lethargy, tremors, neuromuscular blockade with respiratory depression. *GI:* anorexia, nausea, vomiting, stomatitis. *GU:* nephrotoxicity (oliguria, proteinuria, hematuria, decreased creatinine clearance, increased serum BUN and creatinine).

Nursing implications/Documentation

Possible nursing diagnoses: Potential for infection; Fluid volume deficit.

◆ Determine history of allergies, and (regardless of history) monitor closely for allergic reactions.

◆ Weigh patient, and obtain baseline renal function studies, hearing ability, and culture specimens before administering first dose.

◆ Monitor renal function (urine output, specific gravity, serum BUN and creatinine, creatinine clearance) and report signs of decreased function.

◆ Encourage fluid intake, and document and monitor intake and output, to ensure adequate hydration and prevent renal damage from chemical irritation of renal tubules.

◆ Monitor for and report symptoms of ototoxicity (hearing loss, tinnitus, vertigo) and superinfection (mouth lesions, thrush, vaginal irritation, diarrhea, respiratory symptoms).

◆ If there is no response within 3–5 days, consult with physician to determine whether drug regimen should be re-evaluated, and new cultures drawn.

Patient & family teaching/Home care

Possible nursing diagnoses: Knowledge deficit; Impaired home maintenance management.

◆ Advise reporting ear symptoms (e.g., full feeling, hearing loss, ringing of the ears) immediately.

◆ Teach the need to report new signs and symptoms of illness (e.g., fever, mouth lesions, vaginal irritation, diarrhea, respiratory symptoms) since medication may have to be changed.

◆ Explain the importance of taking antibiotics for the entire time prescribed, regardless of absence of signs and symptoms, and of maintaining hydration (drinking at least 2 L is recommended).

◆ *See Anti-infectives overview for more information.*

glipizide
glip'i-zide

Glucotrol, ✦*Minidiab*
Class: Antidiabetic (oral hypoglycemic), Second-generation sulfonylurea
Antidote: D$_{50}$W, glucagon

PEDS	PREG	GERI
🤚	C	🤚

Action Reduces serum glucose and promotes cellular nutrition by stimulating insulin release in beta cells of the pancreas (not effective if beta cells have ceased to function). Onset of action occurs within 15–30 min when taken on an empty stomach; peak action is in 1–2 hr, and duration of action is 12–24 hr.

Use/Therapeutic goal/Outcome

Mild to moderately severe, stable, Type II (noninsulin-dependent) diabetes mellitus; for those not controlled by meal plan and weight control: Normalization of blood glucose levels, glycemic control. *Outcome criteria:* Absence of clinical symptoms of hypoglycemia (confusion, shakiness, weakness, diaphoresis, apprehension) together with blood glucose studies that demonstrate glycemic control (fasting blood sugar: 100–140 mg/dl is good control; 140–200 mg/dl is fair control).

Dose range/Administration

Interaction alert: Food delays the absorption of glipizide. Anabolic steroids, insulin, chloramphenicol, oral anticoagulants, salicylates, NSAID's, MAOI's, phenylbutazone, sulfonamides, and clofibrate may *increase* hypoglycemic activity. Corticosteroids, rifampin, glucagon, calcium channel blockers, thyroid preparations, and thiazide diuretics may *decrease* hypoglycemic activity and exacerbate diabetic symptoms. Beta-blockers and clonidine may mask and prolong hypoglycemic reactions. Alcohol ingestion may significantly alter hypoglycemic activity and cause disulfiram-like reaction (flushing, vomiting, headache).

Adult: PO: 5 mg/day, 30 min before the first meal. May increase to maintenance dose of

▶

10–15 mg/day. Doses > 15 mg should be divided and given 30 min before morning and evening meals.

Clinical alert: Because glipizide is a sulfonylurea, assess for allergy to sulfa before giving first dose. Check blood glucose levels 3 times a day during transition from an insulin regimen to glipizide. Recognize that dose requirements vary with age, food intake, activity levels, and concurrent medical problems. Monitor the elderly closely for hypoglycemic reactions.

Contraindications/Precautions

PREG
C

Contraindicated in hypersensitivity to glipizide and in Type I diabetes mellitus, uncontrolled diabetes mellitus, and severe renal, hepatic, or endocrine impairment. ***Use with caution*** in allergy to sulfa, and in Type II diabetics who require surgery, experience trauma, or are compromised by an infection (may require insulin).

Contraindicated for children and pregnant women (usually require insulin). Use with caution for the elderly.

Side effects/Adverse reactions

Hypersensitivity: itching, rashes, erythema, eczema, urticaria, maculopapular eruptions, photosensitivity. ***GI:*** anorexia, nausea, vomiting, constipation, diarrhea, and cholestatic jaundice. ***CNS:*** headache, dizziness, and drowsiness. ***Hem:*** hypoglycemia, leukopenia, thrombocytopenia, agranulocytosis, aplastic and hemolytic anemia.

Nursing implications/Documentation

Possible nursing diagnoses: Potential for injury; Impaired skin integrity; Impaired tissue integrity; Altered nutrition: more than body requirements; Altered nutrition: less than body requirements.

◆ Keep a record of blood sugars taken before each meal and before bedtime snack; report persistent trends or significant episodes of hyperglycemia or hypoglycemia.

◆ Monitor food intake; notify physician when the patient is not eating.

◆ Monitor daily weights, especially during periods of illness.

◆ If signs of hypoglycemia (tremors, sweating, sudden weakness, pale skin, anxiety, confusion, agitation) are noted, confirm by a capillary blood glucose test first, then give 15 g of a fast-acting carbohydrate (4 oz of fruit juice, 4–6

pieces of hard candy, a tablespoon of sugar or honey). If blood glucose monitoring equipment is not immediately available, then give carbohydrate and check glucose level later.

◆ If signs of hyperglycemia (extreme thirst, frequent urination, fatigue, blurred vision) are noted, confirm by blood glucose meter and report immediately.

Patient & family teaching/Home care

Possible nursing diagnoses: Knowledge deficit; Impaired home maintenance management.

◆ Explain that oral hypoglycemics control blood sugars but do not cure diabetes; stress that regular exercise, careful regulation of diet and medication, close monitoring of blood sugars, and medical supervision help promote health and prevent the long-term complications of diabetes (heart, kidney, eyes).

◆ Explain that taking doses 30 minutes before meals enhances absorption.

◆ Point out that diet, activity, weight fluctuation, illness and emotional stress can affect hypoglycemic medication requirements.

◆ Stress that everything on meal plan should be eaten, especially carbohydrates, but that concentrated sweets should be avoided.

◆ Teach the signs and symptoms of hypoglycemia and hyperglycemia; advise that a fast-acting carbohydrate (4 oz of fruit juice, 4–6 pieces of hard candy, 1 tablespoon of honey or sugar) should be given for suspected *hypo*glycemia (suspected *hyper*glycemia should be reported immediately).

◆ Advise reporting persistent symptoms of nausea, vomiting, fatigue, thirst, frequent urination.

◆ Suggest carrying some form of fast-acting carbohydrate (e.g., small box of raisins) for treatment of hypoglycemia.

◆ Warn against use of alcohol and OTC drugs without physician's approval.

◆ Recommend wearing a medical alert bracelet to alert others to hypoglycemics use.

◆ Point out the need for wearing a sunscreen (SPF #15) because of side effect of photosensitivity.

◆ *See Antidiabetics overview for more information.*

glucagon

gloo'kah-gon

Class: ★**Antihypoglycemic prototype,** Antidote

PEDS	PREG	GERI
OK	**B**	**OK**

Action Raises blood glucose by promoting conversion of hepatic glycogen to glucose. Acts as an antidote for beta-adrenergic blocker overdosage by exerting a positive inotropic and chronotropic action on the heart.

Use/Therapeutic goal/Outcome

Severe insulin-induced hypoglycemia: Reversal of hypoglycemia. ***Outcome criteria:*** Blood sugar over 60–80 mg/dl.

Dose range/Administration

Interaction alert: Do not mix IV with any other drug or in chloride solutions because this causes a precipitate to form. Phenytoin may increase hyperglycemic effect.

Adult and Child: SC, IM, IV: 0.5–1 mg stat; may repeat in 5–25 min if needed.

Clinical alert: Be prepared to start an IV to give 10–50% dextrose and water (especially if the patient is unstable or in a deep coma because glucagon may not be effective). Attach unconscious patients to a cardiac monitor and have resuscitative drugs and equipment readily available. Recognize the elderly may require slightly higher than normal blood sugar to reverse clinical symptoms of hypoglycemia. Upon wakening, the patient should replenish glycogen stores by eating a meal.

Contraindications/Precautions

PREG
B

Contraindicated in hypersensitivity to glucagon or protein compounds, and in pheochromocytoma. ***Use with caution*** in insulinoma.

Side effects/Adverse reactions

Hypersensitivity: itching, rashes, shortness of breath. ***GI:*** nausea and vomiting. ***Hem:*** hyperglycemia.

Nursing implications/Documentation

Possible nursing diagnoses: Potential for aspiration; Potential for injury.

♦ Ascertain baseline blood sugar before giving first dose and monitor closely thereafter.

♦ Monitor closely for airway obstruction; position on side if possible (patients often vomit upon awakening).

Patient & family teaching/Home care

Possible nursing diagnoses: Knowledge deficit; Impaired home maintenance management.

♦ Explore factors that contributed to hypoglycemic episode and identify ways of avoiding episodes in the future.

♦ Teach how to recognize hypoglycemic episodes and how to administer glucagon; stress the need for getting immediate emergency aid (prolonged severe hypoglycemia can result in brain damage).

♦ Point out the need to eat a meal after glucagon is taken and hypoglycemia resolved.

♦ Stress that all severe hypoglycemic events should be reported.

glyburide

gly'boor-ide

DiaBeta, ♥**Euglucon, Micronase**

Class: Antidiabetic (oral hypoglycemic), Second-generation sulfonylurea

Antidote: $D_{50}W$, glucagon

PEDS	PREG	GERI
🤚	**B**	🤚

Action Reduces serum glucose and promotes cellular nutrition by stimulating insulin release in beta cells of the pancreas (not effective if beta cells have ceased to function). Onset of action occurs within 15–60 minutes; peak action is in 2–8 hours, and duration of action is 10–24 hours.

Use/Therapeutic goal/Outcome

Mild to moderately severe, stable, Type II (noninsulin-dependent) diabetes mellitus; for those not controlled by meal plan and weight control alone: Normalization of blood glucose levels, glycemic control. ***Outcome criteria:*** Absence of clinical symptoms of hypoglycemia (confusion, shakiness, weakness, diaphoresis, apprehension) together with blood glucose studies that demonstrate glycemic control (fasting blood sugar: 100–140 mg/dl is good control; 140–200 mg/dl is fair control).

Dose range/Administration

Interaction alert: Alcohol, anabolic steroids, insulin, chloramphenicol, oral anticoagulants, salicylates, MAOI's, phenylbutazone, sulfonamides, and clofibrate may *increase* hypoglycemic activity. Glucocorticoids, rifampin, glucagon, calcium channel blockers, thyroid preparations, oral contraceptives, and thiazide

►

diuretics may *decrease* hypoglycemic activity and exacerbate diabetic symptoms. Alcohol ingestion may cause a disulfiram-like reaction (facial reddening, headache, nausea, and vomiting. Beta-blockers and clonidine may mask and prolong hypoglycemic reactions.

Adult: PO: 2.5–5 mg/day, with the first meal, may increase by 2.5 mg q wk up to a maximum dose of 20 mg. Larger doses may be taken as a single dose or in divided doses with morning and evening meals. *For the elderly:* 1.25 mg, increase gradually prn.

Clinical alert: Because glyburide is a potent second-generation sulfonylurea, assess for allergy to sulfa before giving first dose. Check blood glucose levels 3 times a day during transition from an insulin regimen to glyburide. Recognize that dose requirements vary with age, food intake, activity levels, and concurrent medical problems. Monitor the elderly closely for hypoglycemic reactions; they are likely to require slightly higher fasting blood sugars to prevent clinical symptoms of hypoglycemia.

Contraindications/Precautions

PREG
B

Contraindicated in hypersensitivity to glyburide and in Type I diabetes mellitus, uncontrolled diabetes mellitus, and severe renal, hepatic, or endocrine impairment. *Use with caution* in allergy to sulfa, cardiac disease, and Type II diabetics who require surgery, experience trauma, or are compromised by an infection (may require insulin).

➹ **Contraindicated for children and pregnant women (insulin required). Use with caution for the elderly.**

Side effects/Adverse reactions

Hypersensitivity: itching, erythema, urticaria, rash. *GI:* nausea, heartburn, epigastric fullness, hepatotoxicity. *Hem:* hypoglycemia, leukopenia, thrombocytopenia, aplastic and hemolytic anemia, agranulocytosis. *CNS:* headache, dizziness, weakness, paresthesia. *Skin:* photosensitivity. *MS:* joint pain.

Nursing implications/Documentation

Possible nursing diagnoses: Potential for injury; Impaired skin integrity; Impaired tissue integrity; Altered nutrition: more than body requirements; Altered nutrition: less than body requirements.

♦ Keep a record of blood sugars taken upon rising in the morning and 30 minutes before each meal and before bedtime snack; report persis-

tent trends or significant episodes of hyperglycemia or hypoglycemia.

♦ Monitor food intake; notify physician when the patient is not eating.

♦ Monitor daily weights, especially during periods of illness.

♦ If signs of hypoglycemia (tremors, sweating, sudden weakness, pale skin, anxiety, confusion, agitation) are noted, confirm by a capillary blood glucose test first, then give 15 g of a fast-acting carbohydrate (4 oz of fruit juice, 4–6 pieces of hard candy, 1 tablespoon of sugar or honey). If blood glucose monitoring equipment is not immediately available, then give carbohydrate and check glucose level later.

♦ If signs of hyperglycemia (extreme thirst, frequent urination, fatigue, blurred vision) are noted, confirm by blood glucose meter and report immediately.

Patient & family teaching/Home care

Possible nursing diagnoses: Knowledge deficit; Impaired home maintenance management.

♦ Explain that hypoglycemics control blood sugar but do not cure diabetes; stress that regular exercise, careful regulation of diet and medication, close monitoring of blood sugars, and medical supervision help promote health and prevent the long-term complications of diabetes (heart, kidney, eyes).

♦ Point out that diet, activity, weight fluctuation, illness, and emotional stress can affect hypoglycemic medication requirements.

♦ Stress that everything on meal plan should be eaten, especially carbohydrates, but that concentrated sweets should be avoided.

♦ Teach the signs and symptoms of hypoglycemia and hyperglycemia; advise that a fast-acting carbohydrate (4 oz of fruit juice, 4–6 pieces of hard candy, 1 tablespoon of honey or sugar) should be given for suspected *hypo*glycemia (suspected *hyper*glycemia should be reported immediately).

♦ Advise reporting persistent symptoms of nausea, vomiting, fatigue, thirst, frequent urination.

♦ Suggest carrying some form of fast-acting carbohydrate (e.g., small box of raisins) for treatment of hypoglycemia.

♦ Warn against use of alcohol and OTC drugs without physician's approval.

♦ Recommend wearing a medical alert bracelet to alert others to hypoglycemics use.

- Point out the need for wearing a SPF #15 sunscreen because of side effect of photosensitivity.
- *See Antidiabetics overview for more information.*

glycopyrrolate

glye-koe-pyr'roe-late

Robinul, Robinul Forte

Class: Anticholinergic, Cholinergic blocker (parasympatholytic)

Antidote: Physostigmine

PEDS	PREG	GERI
✋	B	✋

Action Reduces respiratory, salivary, and gastric secretions and reverses neuromuscular blockade caused by nondepolarizing neuromuscular blockers by inhibiting the cholinergic (muscarinic) actions of acetylcholine at parasympathetic postganglionic sites.

Use/Therapeutic goal/Outcome

Adjunctive therapy in peptic ulcer disease: Reduction in gastric acidity. *Outcome criteria:* Report of decrease in GI symptoms.

Preoperative medication: Suppression of respiratory secretions and cholinergic effects of surgery (i.e., dysrhythmias, hypotension). *Outcome criteria:* Report of feeling dry and thirsty; absence of dysrhythmias; blood pressure within normal range.

Anesthesia recovery: Reversal of effects of nondepolarizing neuromuscular blockers. *Outcome criteria:* Spontaneous respirations; demonstration of return of muscle strength, ability to move limbs; pulse within normal range.

Dose range/Administration

Interaction alert: Do not mix with IV solutions containing sodium bicarbonate. Alcohol, antihistamines, and amantadine may increase anticholinergic effects.

- Give PO doses 30 min to 1 hr before meals.
GI disorders: Adult: PO: 1–2 mg tid ac.
Preoperative: Adult: IM: 0.1–0.2 mg 30–60 min before anesthesia.
Reversal of neuromuscular blockers: Adult: IV: 0.2 mg for each 1 mg of neostigmine, or 5 mg of pyridostigmine. May be given by direct IV injection or diluted in dextrose solution.

Clinical alert: Be aware that there is a small margin for toxicity with this drug; monitor clinical response closely and keep physostigmine readily available for use as an antidote.

Contraindications/Precautions

PREG B

Contraindicated in hypersensitivity to glycopyrrolate and in narrow-angle glaucoma, asthma, obstructive diseases of GI or urinary tract, and myasthenia gravis. *Use with caution* in hot environments (drug-induced heatstroke is possible), and cardiac disease, hypertension, and renal and hepatic disease.

- Use with caution for the elderly. Safe use for pregnant or nursing mothers has not been established.

Side effects/Adverse reactions

Hypersensitivity: rash, hives. *GI:* dry mouth, constipation. *GU:* urinary hesitancy and retention. *Eye:* blurred vision, dilated pupils, increased intraocular pressure. *CV:* palpitations, tachycardia. *CNS:* disorientation, drowsiness, dizziness, weakness. *Skin:* decreased sweating.

Nursing implications/Documentation

Possible nursing diagnoses: Potential for injury; Urinary retention; Constipation.

- Have patient void before doses; monitor intake and output because this drug can cause voiding difficulties.

- Monitor the elderly and debilitated for increased incidence of side effects; document and report changes in mental status.

- Relieve dry mouth by providing frequent mouth care and keeping ice chips at the bedside.

- Monitor for constipation; provide adequate fluids and fiber (laxatives and/or stool softeners should be given before problem is severe).

Patient & family teaching/Home care

Possible nursing diagnoses: Knowledge deficit; Impaired home maintenance management.

- Point out the need to take this drug 30–60 min before meals.

- Explain that dry mouth is a transient side effect.

- Warn that this drug may cause drowsiness and dizziness; caution to change position slowly.

- Advise against driving until response is determined.

• Stress the need to avoid OTC cold medications.

• Emphasize that this drug should not be discontinued abruptly, because this may precipitate adverse reactions.

◆ *See Anticholinergics overview for more information.*

gold sodium thiomalate *thye-oh-mah'late*

Myochrysine

Class: Antirheumatic, Gold compound, Disease modifying agent

PEDS	PREG	GERI
☜	C	☚

Action Suppresses joint inflammation by inhibiting the release of lysosomal enzymes, decreasing phagocytosis, and modifying the immune response.

Use/Therapeutic goal/Outcome

Rheumatoid arthritis: Modification or suppression of disease; prevention of damage to affected joints. *Outcome criteria:* (After 8–12 weeks) Reduction in swelling of affected joints; decreased sedimentation rate; improved grip strength; decreased use of analgesics; report of decreased morning stiffness, increased ability to ambulate, and decreased fatigue.

Dose range/Administration

Interaction alert: Immunosuppressants and cytotoxic drugs may increase the risk of blood dyscrasias.

Adult: IM: *Loading dose:* 10 mg wk 1, then 25 mg wk 2 and 3, then 25–50 mg/wk to total of 1000 mg. *Maintenance dose:* 25–50 mg q 2–4 wk. **Child:** IM: 10 mg wk 1, then 1 mg/kg/wk. *Maximum single dose:* 25 mg.

Clinical alert: Administer *only* deep IM into the upper outer quadrant of the gluteal region, using a 21–gauge, 1 1/2–inch needle. Observe immediately after injection for possibility of nitritoid reaction (flushing, dizziness, sweating, and hypotension) or anaphylaxis. Have epinephrine readily available to treat life-threatening reactions.

Contraindications/Precautions
PREG
C

Contraindicated in hypersensitivity to gold or other heavy metals, and in thrombocytopenia with previous gold therapy and systemic lupus erythematosus. **Use with caution** in blood dyscrasias, diabetes mellitus, hepatic or renal disease, eczema, and with medications known to cause blood dyscrasias.

☜ **Contraindicated for nursing mothers. Use with caution for children, pregnant women, and the elderly.**

Side effects/Adverse reactions

Hypersensitivity: itching; difficulty breathing or swallowing; swelling of face, lips, or eyelids; bradycardia; syncope; and anaphylactic shock. **Skin:** painful, pruritic skin rashes. **CV:** nitritoid reaction (flushing, dizziness, sweating, and hypotension) immediately after injection. **Hem:** thrombocytopenia, aplastic anemia. **GI:** soreness of tongue, gums, or throat; metallic taste; mouth ulcers. **GU:** albumin, protein, or RBCs in urine; nephrotic syndrome.

Nursing implications/Documentation

Possible nursing diagnoses: Impaired skin integrity; Altered oral mucous membrane.

◆ Assess for mouth ulcers, easy bruising or bleeding, and rashes prior to each subsequent dose to detect early signs of toxicity.

◆ Recognize that gold injections will not reverse *existing* joint damage.

◆ Monitor results of blood and platelet counts and hepatic and renal function tests.

◆ For mild reactions, expect that therapy will be temporarily discontinued and restarted at lower dose; for severe reactions or with evidence of hypersensitivity or thrombocytopenia, therapy will be discontinued permanently.

Patient & family teaching/Home care

Possible nursing diagnoses: Knowledge deficit; Impaired home maintenance management; Potential for injury.

◆ Explain that response to therapy does not usually occur for at least 8–12 weeks.

◆ Inform that joint pain may occur for 1 or 2 days after an injection with the first few injections.

◆ Stress the need to remain under close medical supervision and have blood and urine testing done as frequently as recommended, usually after every other dose.

◆ Teach that dermatitis is the most common adverse reaction to gold therapy and is frequently preceded by itching and hives; mouth ulcers are the second most common reaction and may be preceded by a metallic taste.

These early symptoms must be reported promptly.

◆ Point out that dermatitis and mouth ulcers may occur up to many months after discontinuing the medication; their development is usually accompanied by marked improvement in the arthritis.

◆ Warn to avoid exposure to sunlight to prevent photosensitivity reaction or rash.

griseofulvin
gri-see-oh-ful'vin

griseofulvin microsize: ♠*Fulcin, Fulvicin-U/F, Grifulvin V, Grisactin,* ♠*Grisovin,* ♠*Grisovin 500, Grisovin-FP*

griseofulvin ultramicrosize: *Fulvicin P/G, Grisactin-Ultra,* ♠*Grisostatin, Gris-PEG*

Class: Anti-infective, Antifungal

PEDS	PREG	GERI
🖐	C	OK

Action Arrests fungal cell division (fungistatic) by disrupting mitotic spindle structure. Also binds to keratin–producing cells, making keratin resistant to disease.

Use/Therapeutic goal/Outcome
Tinea (ringworm) infections not responsive to topical treatment and caused by *Trichophyton, Microsporum,* or *Epidermophyton*: Resolution of infection. *Outcome criteria:* Absence of pathogenic growth on 3 successive cultures.

Dose range/Administration
Interaction alert: Avoid alcohol (may cause tachycardia, flushing, diaphoresis). Decreases effectiveness of oral contraceptives and anticoagulants. Barbiturates decrease griseofulvin absorption (give griseofulvin in 3 divided doses per day).

🖐 **Give with or after meals.**

Tinea corpus, tinea pedis, tinea capitis (when caused by trychophyton, microsporum, or Epidermophyton): **Adult:** PO: *Microsize:* 500 mg/day in single or divided doses (up to 1 g/day for severe infections). *Ultramicrosize:* 330–375 mg/day in single or divided doses.

Tinea pedis and tinea unguium (onychomycosis): **Adult:** PO: *Microsize:* 750 mg to 1 g/day. *Ultramicrosize:* 660–750 mg/day. **Child:** PO: *Microsize:* 11 mg/kg/day in single or divided doses. *Ultramicrosize:* 7.3 mg/kg/day in single or divided doses.

Clinical alert: Increase drug absorption by administering dose with a high-fat meal; verify whether preparation is microsize or ultramicrosize.

Contraindications/Precautions
PREG C

Contraindicated in hypersensitivity to griseofulvin, and in porphyria or liver failure. *Use with caution* in penicillin sensitivity, lupus erythematosus.

🖐 **Avoid use for pregnant women or children less than 2 years.**

Side effects/Adverse reactions
Hypersensitivity: itching, rashes, urticaria, angioneurotic edema. *GI:* oral thrush, nausea, excessive thirst, vomiting, flatulence, diarrhea. *CNS:* headache (usually abates after regimen is established), fatigue, difficulty performing routine activities, confusion, psychosis. *GU:* proteinuria. *Hem:* leukopenia, granulocytopenia (drug should be discontinued). *Skin:* photosensitivity. *Misc:* porphyria; estrogenlike effect on children.

Nursing implications/Documentation
Possible nursing diagnoses: Potential for infection; Impaired skin integrity.

◆ Obtain necessary cultures before starting griseofulvin; and monitor cultures periodically during treatment to detect organism resistance.

◆ Monitor closely for allergic response if patient is allergic to penicillin (cross-sensitivity is possible).

◆ Monitor CBC weekly for at least a month.

◆ Report and document confusion or changes in effect.

Patient & family teaching/Home care
Possible nursing diagnoses: Knowledge deficit; Impaired home maintenance management.

◆ Stress the importance of taking this drug for the entire time prescribed, even if symptoms abate (long-term treatment may be required).

◆ Point out that taking doses with food reduces GI symptoms, and that fatty foods increase absorption.

◆ Caution women that this drug reduces effect of oral contraceptives.

◆ Advise avoidance of alcohol and direct sunlight, advise using a strong sunscreen when outside.

◆ *See Anti-infectives overview for more information.*

guanabenz

gwan'a-benz

Wytensin

Class: Antihypertensive, Alpha-2 adrenergic agonist

PEDS	PREG	GERI
🖐	C	🖐

Action Reduces blood pressure and heart rate by activating alpha receptors in the CNS, which decreases sympathetic outflow to the heart, kidneys, and peripheral vasculature.

Use/Therapeutic goal/Outcome

Hypertension: Reduction of blood pressure. *Outcome criteria:* Blood pressure within normal limits.

Dose range/Administration

Interaction alert: Use with alcohol, narcotics, and other CNS depressants may increase sedative effect.

Adult: PO: 4 mg bid; may increase every 1–2 weeks by 4–8 mg/day. *Maximum dose:* 32 mg bid.

Clinical alert: Give last dose at bedtime to maintain blood pressure control overnight.

Contraindications/Precautions

PREG C

Contraindicated in hypersensitivity to guanabenz. *Use with caution* in vascular or coronary insufficiency, recent myocardial infarction, severe renal or hepatic failure, cerebrovascular disease.

🖐 **Use with caution for the elderly. Safe use for children and pregnant or nursing mothers has not been established.**

Side effects/Adverse reactions

Hypersensitivity: rash, pruritis. *CV:* orthostatic hypertension, bradycardia, severe rebound hypotension. *CNS:* headache, dizziness, sedation, drowsiness, ataxia, weakness, depression. *GI:* dry mouth. *GU:* sexual dysfunction.

Nursing implications/Documentation

Possible nursing diagnoses: Activity intolerance; Fatigue; Potential for injury.

◆ Assess mental status, and record pulse and blood pressure (lying, sitting, and standing, in both arms) before administration, and frequently thereafter until response is determined.

◆ Consult with physician to determine desired therapeutic range for blood pressure (be aware that some patients may require a slightly elevated blood pressure to perfuse vital organs).

◆ Ascertain that baseline CBC, electrolytes, BUN, creatinine, and liver function studies have been obtained before giving first dose; report abnormalities and monitor closely thereafter.

◆ Monitor for allergic reactions, and for confusion, dizziness, bradycardia, arrhythmias, hypotension; hold drug and report immediately if these occur.

◆ Supervise ambulation until response is determined.

◆ Be aware that this drug should be discontinued slowly to avoid rebound hypertension.

◆ Document and monitor daily weight, and intake and output; report significant negative or positive balance.

Patient & family teaching/Home care

Possible nursing diagnoses: Altered sexuality patterns; Knowledge deficit; Impaired home maintenance management.

◆ Explain the importance of taking medication exactly as prescribed, even when feeling well; stress the importance of not withdrawing medication abruptly and of taking last dose at bedtime.

◆ Stress the importance of good medical follow-up, explain that this drug reduces "wear and tear" on blood vessels, and improves longevity and health.

◆ Teach how to monitor pulse and blood pressure; emphasize that syncope, hypertension or hypotension, palpitations, tachycardia, or persistent dizziness should be reported.

◆ Advise changing positions slowly to avoid dizziness.

◆ Encourage daily monitoring of weight and reporting sudden weight gain (frequently is fluid retention).

◆ Explain that driving should be avoided until response is determined (may cause drowsiness); use with alcohol may increase drowsiness.

◆ Warn against discontinuing drug abruptly or taking *any* OTC drugs without physician approval (some interactions can cause severe reactions).

◆ Explain that this drug may affect sexual activity; counsel individuals with concerns.

◆ *See Antihypertensives overview for more information.*

guanadrel

gwahn'a-drel

Hylorel

Class: Antihypertensive, Adrenergic blocking agent

PEDS	PREG	GERI
🖐	B	🖐

Action Lowers blood pressure by inhibiting norepinephrine release and storage in peripheral adrenergic nerve endings.

Use/Therapeutic goal/Outcome

Hypertension: Reduction of blood pressure. **Outcome criteria:** Blood pressure within normal limits.

Dose range/Administration

Interaction alert: Use with diuretics increases hypotensive effects. If given with potassium-sparing diuretics, monitor for hyperkalemia. Use within one week of (or concurrently with) MAO inhibitors may cause severe hypertension; withdrawal of MAO inhibitors at least 1 week prior to initiation of guanadrel therapy is recommended. Phenothiazines, tricyclic antidepressants, and indirect-acting sympathomimetics may also inhibit hypotensive effect.

Adult: PO: 5 mg bid; may increase to 20–75 mg/day (or higher) in divided doses. Dose is highly individualized.

Clinical alert: This drug should be discontinued prior to surgery to reduce the risk of cardiac complications.

Contraindications/Precautions

PREG B

Contraindicated in hypersensitivity to guanadrel, and in CHF, pheochromocytoma. **Use with caution** in cerebrovascular or peripheral vascular disease, febrile states, renal and hepatic impairment, and asthma.

🖐 **Use with caution for the elderly. Safe use for children and pregnant women has not been established.**

Side effects/Adverse reactions

Hypersensitivity: rash, urticaria. **CV:** orthostatic hypotension, edema. **CNS:** dizziness, faintness, drowsiness, fatigue. **GU:** impotence, ejaculation disturbances. **GI:** diarrhea.

Nursing implications/Documentation

Possible nursing diagnoses: Activity intolerance; Fatigue; Potential for injury.

♦ Assess mental status, and record pulse and blood pressure (lying, sitting, and standing, in both arms) prior to administration, and frequently thereafter until response is determined.

♦ Consult with physician to determine desired therapeutic range for blood pressure (be aware that some patients may require a slightly elevated blood pressure to perfuse vital organs).

♦ Ascertain that baseline CBC, electrolytes, BUN, creatinine, and liver function studies have been obtained before giving first dose; report abnormalities and monitor closely thereafter.

♦ Monitor for allergic reactions and for confusion, dizziness, bradycardia, hypotension and diarrhea; hold drug and report immediately if these occur.

♦ Supervise ambulation until response is determined.

♦ Document and monitor daily weight, and intake and output; report significant negative or positive balance.

Patient & family teaching/Home care

Possible nursing diagnoses: Altered sexuality patterns; Knowledge deficit; Impaired home maintenance management.

♦ Explain the importance of taking medication exactly as prescribed, even when feeling well.

♦ Stress the importance of good medical follow-up, explain that this drug reduces "wear and tear" on blood vessels and improves longevity and health.

♦ Teach how to monitor pulse and blood pressure; emphasize that syncope, hypertension or hypotension, chest pain, or persistent dizziness should be reported.

♦ Advise changing positions slowly to avoid dizziness.

♦ Encourage daily monitoring of weight and reporting sudden weight gain (frequently is fluid retention).

♦ Warn against drinking alcohol or taking *any* OTC drugs without physician approval (some interactions can cause severe reactions).

♦ Explain that this drug may alter sexual ability; explore concerns and seek consultation as needed.

♦ *See Antihypertensives overview for more information.*

guanethidine

gwahn-eth'i-deen

Class: Antihypertensive, Adrenergic blocking agent

PEDS	PREG	GERI
☙	C	☙

Action Reduces blood pressure by inhibiting norepinephrine release and storage in peripheral adrenergic nerve endings.

Use/Therapeutic goal/Outcome

Hypertension: Reduction of blood pressure. *Outcome criteria:* Blood pressure within normal limits (after 1–3 weeks of therapy).

Dose range/Administration

Interaction alert: Amphetamines, antidepressants, ephedrine, and phenothiazines may decrease hypotensive effect. Levodopa may increase effect. Do not use within 1 week of MAO inhibitors.

Adult: PO: 10mg/day; may increase weekly or monthly by 10 mg/day as tolerated. *Maintenance dose:* 25–50 mg/day. *Maximum dose:* 300 mg/day. **Child:** PO: 0.2 mg/kg/day. *Maintenance dose:* 0.3 mg/kg/day.

Clinical alert: Monitor the elderly for increased hypotensive effects. A warm environment may increase hypotensive effect. Report if fever is present (may require decrease in dosage).

Contraindications/Precautions

PREG C

Contraindicated in hypersensitivity to guanethidine, and in CHF, pheochromocytoma, and tartrazine allergy. **Use with caution** in patients with diabetes, cardiac disease, ulcer disease, cerebrovascular insufficiency, asthma, febrile state, and hepatic or renal impairment.

☙ **Use with caution for children and the elderly. Safe use in pregnant and nursing mothers has not been established.**

Side effects/Adverse reactions

Hypersensitivity: rash, urticaria. **CV:** orthostatic hypotension, bradycardia, edema, CHF, arrhythmias, angina. **CNS:** dizziness, weakness, syncope. **GI:** diarrhea, dry mouth, weight gain. **Resp:** nasal stuffiness. **GU:** impotence, inhibition of ejaculation.

Nursing implications/Documentation

Possible nursing diagnoses: Activity intolerance; Fatigue; Potential for injury; Diarrhea.

◆ Assess mental status, and record pulse and blood pressure (lying, sitting, and standing, in both arms) prior to administration, and frequently thereafter until response is determined.

◆ Consult with physician to determine desired therapeutic range for blood pressure (be aware that some patients may require a slightly elevated blood pressure to perfuse vital organs).

◆ Ascertain that baseline blood sugar, CBC, electrolytes, BUN, creatinine, and liver function studies have been obtained before giving first dose; report abnormalities and monitor closely thereafter.

◆ Monitor for allergic reactions and for confusion, dizziness, arrhythmias or hypotension; hold drug and report immediately if these occur.

◆ Supervise ambulation until response is determined.

◆ Document and monitor daily weight, and intake and output; report significant negative or positive balance.

◆ Be aware that this drug should be withheld before surgery.

Patient & family teaching/Home care

Possible nursing diagnoses: Knowledge deficit; Impaired home maintenance management; Altered sexuality patterns.

◆ Explain the importance of taking medication exactly as prescribed, even when feeling well.

◆ Stress the importance of good medical follow-up, explain that this drug reduces "wear and tear" on blood vessels and improves longevity and health.

◆ Teach how to monitor pulse and blood pressure; emphasize that syncope, hypertension or hypotension, chest pain, or persistent dizziness should be reported.

◆ Advise changing positions slowly to avoid dizziness.

◆ Encourage daily monitoring of weight and reporting sudden weight gain (frequently is fluid retention).

◆ Warn against drinking alcohol or taking *any* OTC drugs without physician approval (some interactions can cause severe reactions).

- Advise avoiding driving or hazardous activities until response is determined (may cause drowsiness).
- Teach that this drug may cause dry mouth; suggest using ice chips, sugarless gum, or hard candy.
- Explain that this drug may alter sexual activity; explore concerns.
- *See Antihypertensives overview for more information.*

guaifenesin

gweye-fen'e-sin

Anti-Tuss, ♣Balminil Expectorant, Baytussin, Breonesin, Colrex, Cremacoat–2, Dilyn, Gee-Gee, GG-CEN, Glycotuss, Glytuss, Guiatus, Halotussin, Humbid L.A., Malotuss, Naldecon Senior-EX, ♣Neo-Spec, Nortussin, ♣Resyl, Robafen, Robitussin

Class: Expectorant, Antitussive

PEDS	PREG	GERI
OK	C	OK

Action Reduces viscosity, adhesiveness, and surface tension of respiratory secretions by increasing production of respiratory fluids.

Use/Therapeutic goal/Outcome

Dry non-productive cough: Relief of cough.
Outcome criteria: Report and demonstration of decreased cough and increased ability to expectorate mucous.

Dose range/Administration

Adult/Child > 12 yrs: PO: 100–400 mg q4-6h to a maximum of 2.4 gm/day. **Child 6–11 yrs:** PO: 50–100 mg q4-6h to a maximum of 600 mg/day. **Child 2–6 yrs:** PO: 50 mg q4h to a maximum of 300 mg/day.

Contraindications/Precautions

PREG **C**

Contraindicated in hypersensitivity to guiafenesin, and chronic cough or cough with excess secretions.

Side effects/Adverse reactions

Hypersensitivity: none listed. **GI:** low incidence of nausea, vomiting. **CNS:** drowsiness.

Nursing implications/Documentation

Possible nursing diagnoses: Fluid volume deficit; Potential for infection.

- Assure adequate hydration by providing at least 2000 cc fluids per day.

- Monitor for and report increased cough and/or sputum production.
- Consult with physician regarding use of humidity.

Patient & family teaching/Home care

Possible nursing diagnoses: Knowledge deficit; Impaired home maintenance management.

- Teach the importance of maintaining adequate hydration; advise asking physician about use of humidity.
- Caution that onset of shortness of breath (or increasing shortness of breath) with activity should be reported immediately.
- For smokers, reinforce that smoking should be avoided, at least until well again.
- *See Antitussives, Expectorants, and Mucolytics overview for more information.*

guanfacine

gwahn'fa-seen

Tenex

Class: Antihypertensive, Alpha-adrenergic agonist

PEDS	PREG	GERI
✋	B	✋

Action Reduces blood pressure and heart rate by activating alpha-2 receptors in the CNS, which decreases sympathetic outflow to the heart, kidneys, and peripheral vasculature.

Use/Therapeutic goal/Outcome

Hypertension: Reduction of blood pressure.
Outcome criteria: Blood pressure within normal limits.

Dose range/Administration

Interaction alert: Use with alcohol, narcotics and central nervous system depressants may increase sedative effect.

Adult: PO: 1 mg/day at bedtime. May increase every 3–4 weeks by 1 mg/day. *Maximum dose:* 3 mg/day.

Contraindications/Precautions

PREG **B**

Contraindicated in hypersensitivity to guanfacine, and in depression, suicidal tendencies, electroconvulsive therapy, ulcer disease. **Use with caution** in coronary insufficiency, cerebrovascular disease, recent myocardial infarction, and hepatic or renal failure.

Use with caution for nursing mothers and the elderly. Safe use for children and pregnant women has not been established.

Side effects/Adverse reactions

Hypersensitivity: rash, pruritis. *CNS:* headache, dizziness, sedation, weakness, fatigue. *GI:* dry mouth, constipation. *GU:* impotence.

Nursing implications/Documentation

Possible nursing diagnoses: Activity intolerance; Fatigue; Potential for injury; Altered oral mucus membrane.

◆ Assess mental status, and record pulse and blood pressure (lying, sitting, and standing, in both arms) before administration, and frequently thereafter until response is determined.

◆ Consult with physician to determine desired therapeutic range for blood pressure (be aware that some patients may require a slightly elevated blood pressure to perfuse vital organs).

◆ Ascertain that baseline CBC, electrolytes, BUN, creatinine, and liver function studies have been obtained before giving first dose; report abnormalities and monitor closely thereafter.

◆ Monitor for allergic reactions and for confusion, dizziness, bradycardia, arrhythmias, hypotension; hold drug and report immediately if these occur.

◆ Supervise ambulation until response is determined.

◆ Document and monitor daily weight, and intake and output report significant negative or positive balance.

◆ Provide frequent mouth care.

Patient & family teaching/Home care

Possible nursing diagnoses: Altered sexuality patterns; Knowledge deficit; Impaired home maintenance management.

◆ Explain the importance of taking medication exactly as prescribed, even when feeling well; stress the importance of not withdrawing medication abruptly and of taking doses at bedtime.

◆ Stress the importance of good medical follow-up, explain that this drug reduces "wear and tear" on blood vessels and improves longevity and health.

◆ Teach how to monitor pulse and blood pressure; emphasize that syncope, hypertension or hypotension, palpitations, tachycardia, or persistent dizziness should be reported.

◆ Advise changing positions slowly to avoid dizziness.

◆ Encourage daily monitoring of weight and reporting sudden weight gain (may be fluid retention).

◆ Explain that driving should be avoided until response is determined (may cause drowsiness); use with alcohol may increase drowsiness.

◆ Warn against discontinuing drug abruptly or taking *any* OTC drugs without physician approval (some interactions can cause severe reactions).

◆ If dry mouth is experienced, encourage frequent mouth care and suggest using sugarless gum, ice chips, or hard candy.

◆ Explain that this drug may affect sexual activity; counsel individuals with concerns.

◆ *See Antihypertensives overview for more information.*

halazepam

hal-az'e-pam

Paxipam

Class: Antianxiety agent, Benzodiazepine

PEDS	PREG	GERI	CONTROLLED SUBSTANCE
🖐	D	🖐	IV

Action Produces CNS depression and relaxation, and increases seizure threshold by potentiating the action of gamma-aminobuteric acid (GABA), which reduces neuronal activity in all regions of the CNS. Promotes muscle relaxation by inhibiting spinal motor reflex pathways. Decreases anxiety by inhibiting cortical and limbic arousal.

Use/Therapeutic goal/Outcome

Short-term treatment of anxiety (less than 4 months): Alleviation of symptoms of apprehension, muscle tension, and insomnia. *Outcome criteria:* Report of feeling more calm, sleeping better, and coping better; observable signs of decreased anxiety (decreased motor activity, reduced muscle tension, decrease in pulse and blood pressure).

Dose range/Administration

Interaction alert: Alcohol and other CNS depressants may cause excessive sedation. Cimetidine increases blood levels.

🖐 **Give with food or milk if GI upset is noted.**

Adult: PO: 20–40 mg tid or qid. *Usual dose range:* 80–160 mg/day (as much as 600 mg/day has been given). *For the elderly:* 20 mg/day or bid.

Clinical alert: When discontinuing drug, taper dose gradually, rather than withdrawing abruptly, to avoid withdrawal symptoms. Halazepam accumulates in the body, and elimination after discontinuation may take weeks.

Contraindications/Precautions

PREG D

Contraindicated in hypersensitivity or intolerance to halazepam or other benzodiazepines, and in narrow-angle glaucoma, and psychiatric disorders without anxiety. ***Use with caution*** in psychosis, depression, suicidal tendencies, or impaired liver or kidney function.

🖐 **Contraindicated for pregnant or nursing mothers. Use with caution for the elderly or debilitated. Safe use for children has not been established.**

Side effects/Adverse reactions

Hypersensitivity: itching, rash, exaggeration of side effects. ***CNS:*** lethargy, drowsiness, headache, dizziness, confusion, tremors, insomnia, ataxia, depression. ***CV:*** hypotension, transient tachycardia and bradycardia. ***Resp:*** respiratory depression. ***GI:*** dry mouth, anorexia, nausea, vomiting, constipation, diarrhea. ***GU:*** urinary retention. ***Eye:*** blurred vision, mydriasis. ***Misc:*** drug tolerance and dependence.

Nursing implications/Documentation

Possible nursing diagnoses: Potential for injury; Constipation.

◆ Record baseline blood pressure; monitor closely if dizziness is experienced. Supervise ambulation until response is determined.

◆ Be sure that doses are swallowed (not hoarded).

◆ Provide a quiet environment that is conducive to rest.

◆ Monitor bowel elimination and provide adequate fluids and fiber to prevent constipation; offer laxatives before the problem is severe.

Patient & family teaching/Home care

Possible nursing diagnoses: Anxiety; Fear; Ineffective individual coping; Impaired home maintenance management.

◆ Advise taking this drug with milk or food if GI symptoms are noted.

◆ Help the individual identify stressors that contribute to anxiety and ways of coping effectively; stress that effective coping strategies can reduce the need for medication.

◆ Explain the importance of daily exercise in relieving stress, and encourage establishing a plan for getting enough exercise (e.g., daily walks).

◆ Point out that drug tolerance and dependence can occur, and that the drug should be used only when holistic measures (e.g., quiet music, relaxation techniques) are not effective.

◆ Emphasize that the effects of alcohol, other sedatives and CNS depressants, and tranquilizers may be potentiated (these should be avoided).

◆ Advise avoidance of driving and other potentially hazardous activities until response is established.

◆ *See Antianxiety agents/Sedatives/Hypnotics overview for more information.*

haloperidol

ha-loe-per'i-dole

🍁**Apo-Haloperidol, Haldol, Halperon,** 🍁**Novoperidol,** 🍁**Peridol,** 🐾**Serenace**

haloperidol decanoate: ***Haldol Decanoate,*** 🍁**Haldol LA**

Class: Antipsychotic butyrophenone, Antidyskinetic

PEDS	PREG	GERI
🖐	C	🖐

Action Exact mechanism of action has not been determined. Believed to produce calmness and alleviate psychiatric symptoms (disorders of perception, thought, consciousness, mood, affect, and social interaction) by blocking dopamine receptors in the limbic system. Blocks peripheral muscarinic, adrenergic, and histamine receptors. Also has some effect on the hypothalamus and pituitary gland, causing changes in regulation of body temperature and endocrine function. A dose of 2 mg of haloperidol is therapeutically equivalent to 100 mg of chlorpromazine. Although haloperidol does produce sedation in some patients, it is the least sedating of all the antipsychotics.

H

Use/Therapeutic goal/Outcome

Chronic schizophrenia, psychotic disorders, and agitation associated with senile dementia: Promotion of reality orientation, elimination of agitation and hyperactivity. *Outcome criteria:* Demonstration of reality orientation, and ability to problem solve and interact with others; absence of hyperactive and agitated behavior.

Tourette's syndrome: Control of tics and involuntary verbal utterances associated with Tourette's syndrome. *Outcome criteria:* Absence of tics and verbal utterances.

Hyperactivity in children: Elimination of excessive motor activity in children. *Outcome criteria:* Demonstration (by child) and report (by parent) of normalization of motor activity.

Dose range/Administration

Interaction alert: Alcohol and other CNS depressants may cause excessive sedation. Use with lithium may cause lethargy and confusion and possible brain damage. If given with methyldopa, monitor for symptoms of dementia.

◆ **Give with food or milk to avoid GI upset.**

Psychotic disorders: **Adult:** PO: *Initial dose:* 0.5–5 mg bid or tid. *Maximum dose:* 100 mg/day in divided doses. *For the elderly:* Initial dose of 0.5–2 mg bid or tid. IM: 2–5 mg q1-8h prn. **Child 3–12 yrs:** PO: 0.05–0.15 mg/day in divided doses.

Chronic schizophrenia: **Adult:** IM: Using decanoate preparation, 10–15 times the established oral dose every 4 wks. *Maximum dose:* 100 mg.

Tourette's syndrome: **Adult:** PO: 0.5–5 mg bid or tid; increase prn. *Maximum dose:* 100 mg/day in divided doses.

Hyperactivity: **Child > 3 yrs:** PO: 0.05–0.075 mg/kg/day. *Maximum dose:* 6 mg/day.

Clinical alert: Dosage varies depending upon severity of symptoms and patient response. Keep IV diphenhydramine available in case of acute dystonic reaction.

Contraindications/Precautions

PREG C

Contraindicated in hypersensitivity to haloperidol, and in CNS depression and comatose states. *Use with caution* in seizure disorders, hypertension, parkinsonism, asthma, emphysema, narrow-angle glaucoma, cardiac disease, hypotension, and liver disease.

🖐 **Contraindicated for children under 3 years and nursing mothers. Use with caution for older children and the elderly or debili-** tated. **Safe use for pregnant women has not been established.**

Side effects/Adverse reactions

Hypersensitivity: rash. **CNS:** high incidence of extrapyramidal reactions (pseudoparkinsonism, akathisia [restless need to keep moving], dystonia, tardive dykinesia), neuroleptic malignant syndrome (fever, tachycardia, tachypnea, profuse diaphoresis), EEG changes, dizziness. **CV:** orthostatic hypotension, palpitations, dysrhythmias, EKG changes. **GI:** appetite changes, dry mouth, constipation, abnormal liver function. **GU:** urinary retention or hesitancy, impaired ejaculation, amenorrhea. **Eye:** blurred vision. **Hem:** leukopenia, agranulocytosis, hyperglycemia. **Skin:** photosensitivity, jaundice. **MS:** weight gain. **Misc:** gynecomastia, galactorrhea. *After abrupt withdrawal of long-term therapy:* gastritis, nausea, vomiting, lightheadedness, tremors, feeling of warmth or cold, diaphoresis, tachycardia, headache, insomnia.

Nursing implications/Documentation

Possible nursing diagnoses: Potential for injury; Constipation; Altered oral mucous membrane.

◆ Document mental status and vital signs before and 1–2 hr after administration during initial phase of treatment, then bid until response to therapy has been established, then periodically thereafter.

◆ Check CBC, liver function, BUN, and creatinine before giving first dose and periodically thereafter.

◆ Be sure that PO doses are swallowed (not hoarded).

◆ Monitor for orthostatic hypotension, dizziness, and drowsiness; supervise ambulation until response is established.

◆ Record weight every 2 weeks; report significant weight gain.

◆ Provide special mouth care; observe for and report oral ulcers.

◆ Prevent constipation by monitoring bowel movements and providing adequate fiber and fluid intake; offer laxatives or stool softeners before problem becomes severe.

◆ Report persistent sore throat, fever, and malaise, because these may indicate agranulocytosis (drug may have to be discontinued).

◆ Monitor for (and report immediately) signs of neuroleptic malignant syndrome (muscle rigidity, tremors, high fever, tachycardia); this is a rare, but potentially fatal, side effect.

Patient & family teaching/Home care

Possible nursing diagnoses: Sleep pattern disturbance; Impaired home maintenance management.

♦ Emphasize the need to continue medication, even when feeling well.

♦ Warn to change positions slowly to prevent dizziness.

♦ Stress that the effects of alcohol, sedatives and CNS depressants, and tranquilizers may be potentiated.

♦ Caution to consult with physician before using OTC drugs; stress the need for ongoing medical follow-up.

♦ Provide a list of side effects that should be reported: involuntary movements, muscular rigidity, tremors, fever, respiratory distress, tachycardia, persistent sore throat.

♦ Point out that doses should not be increased or stopped without checking with physician.

♦ Caution to wear a sunscreen (number 15), protective clothing, and sunglasses when out in the sun.

♦ Advise avoidance of driving and other potentially hazardous activities until response has been established.

♦ Suggest using ice chips, hard candy, or gum to relieve side effect of dry mouth; stress the need for good mouth care.

♦ Warn women to report if pregnancy is planned or suspected.

♦ *See Antipsychotics overview for more information.*

heparin

(hep'a-rin)

heparin calcium: ♥*Calcilean, Calciparine, ♠Caprin, ♠Unicaprin-Ca*

heparin sodium: ♥*Hepalean, Heparin Lock Flush Solution (Tubex), Hep Lock, Liquaemin Sodium, ♠Uniparin*

Class: ★**Parenteral anticoagulant prototype**

Antidote: Protamine sulfate

PEDS	PREG	GERI
🖐	C	🖐

Action Inhibits blood coagulation. Low (prophylactic) doses prevent the conversion of prothrombin to thrombin; high (therapeutic) doses prevent the conversion of fibrinogen to fibrin. Heparin prevents *extension* of clots, but does not dissolve *existing* clots.

Use/Therapeutic goal/Outcome

Anticoagulant: Prevention of thrombus formation or thrombus extension (common high-risk situations include phlebitis, peripheral vascular disease, pulmonary embolus, myocardial infarction, atrial fibrillation, prolonged immobility, cardiac and vascular surgery, cerebral thrombosis, dialysis, arterial and Swan-Ganz pressure monitoring, and the presence of a capped intravenous catheter). **Outcome criteria:** Prolonged PTT, usually 1.5 to 2 times the normal (normal mean is 26.5 seconds).

Dose range/Administration

Interaction alert: Risk of bleeding increases with concurrent oral anticoagulants, thrombolytic enzymes, or drugs that affect platelet function (salicylates, dipyridamole, nonsteroidal anti-inflammatory agents). Do not mix in the same solution with antibiotics.

Myocardial infarction, pulmonary embolus, and deep vein thrombosis: Adult: IV: *Intermittent:* bolus dose of 5,000–10,000 units; followed by maintenance dosage of 5,000–10,000 units q4-6h, depending on current PTT. *Continuous infusion:* 20,000–40,000 units/day, depending on current PTT. **Child:** IV: *Intermittent:* bolus dose of 50 units/kg; followed by maintenance dosage of 50–100 units/kg q4h, depending on current PTT. *Continuous infusion:* 20,000 units/m^2/day, depending on current PTT.

Prophylaxis of thrombus formation: Adult: SC: *Loading dose:* 10,000–20,000 units (usually given after an IV bolus of 5,000 units); followed by maintenance dosage of 5,000–10,000 units q8-12h, or 15,000–20,000 units q12h (use concentrated solution; do not aspirate syringe on injection; do not rub site after injection; do not give in arms or legs).

Flushings: Heparin lock flush: IV: 10–100 units q8-12h (use concentration of 10 units/cc). **Arterial line flush:** Intra-arterial: 1 unit heparin per cc normal saline, maintained in a flush bag with pump. **Pulmonary artery catheter flush:** Intra-arterial: 1 unit heparin per cc normal saline, *or* 2 units heparin per cc normal saline maintained in a flush bag with pump (concentration depends upon hospital policy).

Clinical alert: Read vial labels carefully to be sure of the concentration of heparin in solution; heparin is available in many different concentrations. Be aware that heparin dosage is *highly* individualized, depending on age, indication, and individual response. A test dose of 1,000 units SC should be given to people with a history of asthma or multiple allergies.

Contraindications/Precautions
PREG
C

Contraindicated in hypersensitivity to heparin; and in active bleeding, conditions that cause a bleeding tendency (e.g., hemophilia, severe thrombocytopenia); blood dyscrasias; anticipated impending surgery; threatened abortion; recent surgery of the eye, brain, or spinal cord; GI ulcers; open wounds; subacute bacterial endocarditis; advanced renal or liver disease. **Never** administer intramuscularly.

👐 **Use with caution for children and the elderly, and for menstruating and pregnant women (especially during the last trimester of pregnancy and in the immediate postpartum period).**

Side effects/Adverse reactions

Hypersensitivity: (rare): anaphylaxis; fever; pruritis; rhinitis; conjunctivitis; tearing; rashes; itching, tingling, numbing, and burning sensations of the hands and feet; headache. **Hem:** predominant side effect is hemorrhage, either local or systemic. **CV:** white clot syndrome; (IV route) pain, redness, swelling, and phlebitis at injection site. **Skin:** (SC route) pain, itching, swelling, bruising at injection site.

Nursing implications/Documentation

Possible nursing diagnoses: Potential for injury; Impaired skin integrity.

♦ Ascertain that baseline CBC, BUN, creatinine, liver function studies, and PTT are established before giving first dose; report abnormalities.

♦ Assess for history of bleeding conditions before giving first dose.

♦ Monitor PTT (at least daily) until therapeutic range has been achieved and is stable.

♦ Schedule PTT to be drawn 30 minutes before the next *intermittent* IV dose; draw blood from arm opposite the continuous IV infusion.

♦ Report PTT *below* therapeutic range because of potential for thrombus formation; report PTT *above* therapeutic range because of potential for bleeding.

♦ Chart anticoagulant therapy on the same record that all medications are charted to avoid an oversight that the patient is being anticoagulated; use a flow sheet to monitor PTT levels to ascertain safe dosage.

♦ Monitor closely for occult or overt bleeding: check gums for bleeding; assess skin for bruising; and observe for tarry stools, GI bleeding, or hematuria (may signify onset of hemorrhage). Elderly females are at higher risk of hemorrhage.

♦ Keep protamine sulfate (heparin antidote) on hand for ready use.

♦ *For continuous IV infusion,* regulate flow with a controller or pump.

♦ *For SC administration,* change needle after withdrawing heparin from vial so that no medication is left on needle tip; rotate injection sites and avoid scars, muscles, and a 2-inch diameter around the umbilicus; use a 25- or 27-gauge needle, bunch skin to ensure **intrafat** injection, and inject at a 90-degree angle (inject without aspirating; do not rub site after injection).

♦ Apply pressure to venipuncture sites for at least 5 minutes after blood is drawn, and observe closely for hematomas.

♦ Avoid unnecessary IM injections of other medications, especially into the buttocks (because of risk of retroperitoneal bleeding).

♦ Ensure that anticoagulant therapy is discontinued prior to surgical or invasive procedures.

Patient & family teaching/Home care

Possible nursing diagnoses: Knowledge deficit; Impaired home maintenance management.

♦ *For SC administration,* emphasize the importance of using proper deep intrafat SC injection technique; have the patient/caregiver demonstrate injection technique several times before discharge.

♦ Explain the rationale for avoiding activities that may cause bumping or injury, and for reporting signs of bleeding (bruising, blood in urine/stool).

♦ Explain that aspirin, other salicylates, and ibuprofen also have anticoagulant effects and should be avoided; warn against the use of *any* OTC drugs without physician's approval.

♦ Stress the importance of taking doses at the same time every day without missing doses, and encourage the person to record doses as soon as they are taken. (A forgotten dose should be taken as soon as possible.)

♦ Emphasize that abdominal or flank pain, heavy menstrual flow, or signs and symptoms of bleeding (e.g., bruising, blood in urine or stools) should be reported; dose adjustment may be indicated.

♦ Explain the importance of informing dentists and other physicians of anticoagulant therapy.

♦ Recommend using a soft toothbrush to avoid gum injury, and an *electric* razor to prevent cuts.

♦ Encourage wearing a bracelet or carrying an ID card that states that the person is taking an anticoagulant.

♦ *See Anticoagulants and Thrombolytic Enzymes overview for more information.*

hepatitis B vaccine

hepatitis B vaccine (plasma derived): *Heptavax-B*

hepatitis B vaccine (recombinant): *Engerix-B, Recombivax HB, Recombivax HB Dialysis Formulation*

Class: Vaccine, Immunizing agent

PEDS	PREG	GERI
🤚	C	🤚

Action Promotes active immunity to hepatitis B virus by inducing protective antibody (anti-HBs) formation. The recombinant form of this vaccine is the first vaccine to be made by gene splicing.

Use/Therapeutic goal/Outcome

Hepatitis B prophylaxis for individuals at risk for contracting hepatitis B infection: Prevention of hepatitis B infection. *Outcome criteria:* After 2 weeks, presence of protective anti-HBs antibody titer; absence of clinical symptoms of hepatitis B.

Dose range/Administration

Interaction alert: Effectiveness may be reduced by immunosuppressive agents (may require higher vaccine dosage).

Hepatitis B vaccine (plasma-derived): Adult/Child > 10 yrs: IM: 20 mcg adult formulation initially, repeat dose 30 days and 6 mos later. *Child < 10 yrs/Neonate:* IM: Give 10 mcg pediatric formulation initially, repeat dose 30 days and 6 mos later.

Recombinant hepatitis B vaccine (Energix B): Same dose and schedule, except for *Adults on immunosuppressive therapy or dialysis:* 40 mcg adult formulation, divided in two equal doses injected in two different sites, repeat dose 30 days and 6 mos later.

Recombinant hepatitis B vaccine (Recombivax HB): Adult: IM: 10 mcg adult formulation initially, repeat dose 30 days and 6 mos later. *Adults on immunosuppressive therapy or dialysis:* Use dialysis formulation, which contains 40 mcg/ml; 40 mcg initially, repeat 30 days and 6 mos later. *Child 11–19 yrs:* IM: 5 mcg pediatric formulation initially, repeat 30 days and 6 mos later. *Child < 11 yrs:* IM: 2.5 mcg pediatric formulation initially, repeat 30 days and 6 mos later. *Neonate:* IM: *If mother is HBsAg-negative:* 2.5 mcg pediatric formulation initially, repeat 30 days and 6 mos later. *If mother is HBsAg-positive:* 5 mcg pediatric formulation initially, repeat 30 days and 6 mos later.

Clinical alert: Double check labels and physician's orders *carefully* to be sure you have the right type and brand of vaccine (concentrations vary). Shake vial before withdrawing dose. According to the CDC, this vaccine is significantly more effective when injected into the deltoid muscle, rather than the buttocks (it is absorbed better). For infants and young children, use the thigh. May be given SC to patients at risk for bleeding (e.g., hemophiliacs).

Contraindications/Precautions

PREG
C

Contraindicated in hypersensitivity to vaccine or any of its ingredients (alum or thimerosal). *Use with caution* in compromised cardiopulmonary status, active infections, or fever.

🤚 **Use with caution for children and the elderly. Safe use for pregnant or nursing mothers has not been established.**

Side effects/Adverse reactions

Hypersensitivity: itching, urticaria, rash, angioedema. *GI:* anorexia, nausea, vomiting, diarrhea, and abdominal pain. *CNS:* headache, dizziness. *Skin:* erythema, swelling, induration, pain at the injection site. *Misc:* fever, chills, fatigue, and myalgia (may be delayed).

Nursing implications/Documentation

Possible nursing diagnosis: Potential for infection.

♦ Document and specify presence of immune deficiency or history of exposure to infectious disease.

• Recognize that it is highly recommended by the Advisory Committee on Immunization Practices that persons that are at high risk of coming in contact with hepatitis B virus be immunized for hepatitis B.

• People at high risk include nurses, student nurses, physicians, dentists, morticians, embalmers, those who come in contact with blood or feces, international travelers, and populations with high infection rates (Alaskan Eskimos, Haitian and Indochinese refugees).

Patient & family teaching/Home care

Possible nursing diagnoses: Fear; Knowledge deficit.

• Encourage verbalizing fears and concerns; stress that there is no risk of contracting AIDS or hepatitis B through this vaccine: point out that side effects are minimal, compared to those of hepatitis B infection.

• Advise that pain, redness, and tenderness at injection site may persist for several hours.

• Explain that immunity lasts for 5 years; after which a booster will maintain immunity.

• For dialysis or immunosuppressed patients, reinforce that they return to confirm immunity.

hydralazine
hye-dral'a-zeen

hydralazine hydrochloride: **Alazine, Apresoline,** ✦**Novo-Hylazin,** ♠**Supres**

Class: ★**Antihypertensive prototype,** Peripheral vasodilator

PEDS	PREG	GERI
🖐	C	🖐

Action Reduces blood pressure by directly relaxing vascular smooth muscle, dilating peripheral blood vessels, thereby decreasing peripheral and systemic vascular resistance. Increases cardiac output (CO), stroke volume, and renal and cerebral blood flow.

Use/Therapeutic goal/Outcome

Hypertension: Reduction of blood pressure. **Outcome criteria:** Blood pressure within normal limits.

Congestive heart failure: Resolution of heart failure. **Outcome criteria:** Absence of rales; improved activity tolerance, pulmonary artery pressure, central venous pressure; cardiac output within normal limits, urine output > 30 cc/hr.

Dose range/Administration

Interaction alert: Use with diuretics and MAO inhibitors potentiates effect of hydralazine.

🖐**Give with food to increase plasma levels.**

Adult: PO: 10 mg qid; may increase after 2–4 days to 25 mg qid, after 2 weeks to 50 mg qid. *Maximum dose:* 300 mg/day. IV/IM : 10–40 mg q4-6h. **Child:** PO: 0.75 mg/kg/day divided into 4 doses. Maximum dose is 7.5 mg/kg/day (increase slowly). IV/IM : 1.75–3.5 mg/kg/day in 4 divided doses.

Clinical alert: Administer IV by direct bolus (not diluted); do not exceed 10 mg/minute. Monitor patients sensitive to aspirin for allergic reactions because some forms of this drug contains tartrazine.

Contraindications/Precautions
PREG
C

Contraindicated in hypersensitivity to hydralazine or to tartrazine or parabens (which are present in some preparations); in coronary artery disease, rheumatic mitral valvular disease, myocardial infarction, tachycardia, lupus erythematosus. **Use with caution** in cerebrovascular accident and advanced renal disease.

🖐 **Use with caution for the elderly. Safe use for children and pregnant women has not been established.**

Side effects/Adverse reactions

Hypersensitivity: rash, urticaria, pruritus. **CV:** tachycardia, palpitations, orthostatic hypotension, arrhythmias. **CNS:** headache, peripheral neuritis. **GI:** nausea, vomiting, diarrhea, anorexia, obstructive jaundice. **MS:** arthralgia. **Misc:** lupus-like syndrome, weight gain, sodium retention, fever, chills.

Nursing implications/Documentation

Possible nursing diagnoses: Activity intolerance; Fatigue; Potential for injury.

• Assess mental status, and record pulse and blood pressure (lying, sitting, and standing in both arms) prior to administration, and frequently thereafter until response is determined.

• For IV route, document blood pressure every 5 minutes until stable, then every 15 minutes during hypertensive crisis.

• Consult with physician to determine desired therapeutic range for blood pressure (be aware that some patients may require a slightly elevated blood pressure to perfuse vital organs).

• Ascertain that baseline, CBC, electrolytes, BUN, creatinine, and liver function studies have been obtained before giving first dose; report abnormalities and monitor closely thereafter.

• Monitor for allergic reactions and for confusion, dizziness, rales, arrhythmias, angina, hypotension, lupus-like syndrome (sore throat, fever, muscle and joint pain, skin rash); hold drug (or decrease IV rate) and report immediately if these occur.

• Supervise ambulation until response is determined (patients on IV route should remain in bed).

• Document and monitor daily weight, and intake and output; report significant negative or positive balance.

Patient & family teaching/Home care

Possible nursing diagnoses: Knowledge deficit; Impaired home maintenance management.

• Explain the importance of taking antihypertensive medications exactly as prescribed, even when feeling well.

• Advise taking this drug with food to reduce GI symptoms.

• Stress the importance of good medical follow-up, explain that this drug reduces "wear and tear" on blood vessels and improves longevity and health.

• Teach how to monitor pulse and blood pressure; emphasize that syncope, hypertension or hypotension, or persistent dizziness should be reported.

• Advise changing positions slowly, to avoid dizziness.

• Encourage daily monitoring of weight and reporting sudden weight gain (frequently fluid retention).

• Point out that symptoms of sore throat, fever, muscle and joint pain, skin rash should be reported.

• Warn against taking **any** OTC drugs without physician approval (some interactions can cause severe reactions).

• *See Antihypertensives overview for more information.*

hydrochlorothiazide *hydro-klor-o-thy'a-zyde*

✤*Apo-Hydro, Dichlotride,* ✤*Diuchlor H, Esidrix, HydroDIURIL, Mictrin,* ✤*Natrimax,* ✤*Novohydrazide Oretic, Thiuretic,* ✤*Urozide*

Class: ★**Thiazide diuretic prototype**, Antihypertensive

PEDS	PREG	GERI
✋	B	✋

Action Promotes sodium chloride, potassium, and water excretion by inhibiting the reabsorption of sodium in the early portion of the distal tubule. Lowers blood pressure by reducing plasma and extra-cellular volume.

Use/Therapeutic goal/Outcome

Hypertension: Promotion of diuresis, reduction of blood pressure. **Outcome criteria:** After 3–4 days, blood pressure within normal limits.
Edema: Promotion of diuresis, resolution of edema. **Outcome criteria:** Increased urine output; weight loss; absence of rales and peripheral and sacral edema.

Dose range/Administration

Interaction alert: Cholestyramine and colestipol decrease intestinal absorption. Diazoxide potentiates the hyperuricemic, hyperglycemic, and hypotensive effects. Nonsteroidal anti-inflammatory drugs may decrease effects. Do not give concomitantly with lithium. Give cautiously with corticosteroids, antidiabetics, lanoxin, and skeletal muscle relaxants.

🥄**Give with food to enhance absorption.**

Hypertension: Adult: PO: 25–100 mg/day in 1–2 doses.

Edema: Adult: PO: 25–100 mg once or twice daily. **Child > 6 mos:** PO: 1–2 mg/kg/day in divided doses. **Child < 6 mos:** PO: 3 mg/kg/day.

Clinical alert: Give in morning to prevent nocturnal diuresis.

Contraindications/Precautions
PREG B

Contraindicated in hypersensitivity to sulfonamides or thiazides, and in anuria. **Use with caution** in patients with renal or hepatic dysfunction, systemic lupus erythematosus, gout, asthma, allergic bronchitis, diabetes, pancreatitis, arteriosclerosis, and debilitated states.

✋ **Contraindicated for pregnant or nursing mothers. Use with caution for children and the elderly.**

Side effects/Adverse reactions

Hypersensitivity: rash, urticaria, dermatitis with photosensitivity, purpura, pneumonitis, vasculitis, fever. **Hem:** hypokalemia, hyperglycemia, azotemia, impaired glucose tolerance, asymptomatic hyperuricemia, electrolyte imbalances, metabolic alkalosis, hypercalcemia, lipid abnormalities, aplastic anemia, agranulocytosis, leukopenia, thrombocytopenia. **CV:** volume depletion, dehydration, orthostatic hypotension. **GI:** anorexia, nausea, pancreatitis, hepatic encephalopathy. **Misc:** gout.

Nursing implications/Documentation

Possible nursing diagnoses: Fluid volume deficit; Altered patterns of urinary elimination; Potential for injury.

♦ Ascertain that baseline CBC, sodium, potassium, chloride, carbon dioxide, calcium, magnesium, BUN, creatinine, uric acid, and liver function studies have been obtained before giving first dose; report abnormalities and monitor closely thereafter.

♦ Document and monitor blood pressure, pulse, daily weight, and intake and output; report significant discrepancies.

♦ Monitor for hyperglycemia because of risk of thiazide diabetes.

♦ Observe for and report signs of fluid overload (auscultate lungs for rales; check feet, ankles, and sacrum for edema).

♦ Be aware the diuretics often induce hypokalemia, which predisposes individuals to cardiac arrhythmias, cramping, and digoxin toxicity.

♦ Check with physician to determine dietary restrictions; if a low-salt, high-potassium diet is recommended, consult with dietician to plan a low-salt diet that includes foods and juices high in potassium (orange juice; banana; green leafy vegetables).

♦ Observe the elderly for extreme diuresis (may require lower doses); monitor for orthostatic hypotension; supervise ambulation until response is determined.

Patient & family teaching/Home care

Possible nursing diagnoses: Knowledge deficit; Impaired home maintenance management.

♦ Before giving first dose, explain that the drug will increase the amount and frequency of urination.

♦ Advise taking this drug with food to enhance absorption.

♦ Emphasize the importance of taking this drug exactly as prescribed, and the importance of returning for medical follow-up.

♦ Explain that diuretics enhance the work of the kidney and reduce the workload of the heart.

♦ Recommend taking doses in early morning and early afternoon to prevent the need to disturb sleep to void.

♦ Explain that changing positions slowly helps prevent dizziness.

♦ Advise reporting dizziness, shortness of breath, swelling of hands and feet, or persistent sore throat; encourage daily monitoring of weight and reporting sudden weight gain.

♦ Warn that hyperglycemia is common; advise reporting thirst, fatigue, or weight loss.

♦ Provide a list of allowed foods and fluids; stress the need to stick to prescribed diet (explain the hazards of too much salt, or too little potassium).

♦ Warn against driving or activities that require alertness until response has been determined.

♦ Advise avoidance of OTC drugs unless approved by physician. Suggest using a (Number 15) sunscreen when outside because of photosensitivity (avoid products containing PABA).

♦ *See Diuretics and Antihypertensives overviews for more information.*

hydrocortisone
hye-droe-kor'ti-sone

hydrocortisone: *Acticort, Aeroseb-HC, Carmol HC, Cetacort, Cort-Dome, Cortef, Cortenema, Cortinal, Cortizone 5, Cortril, Cremesone, Delacort, DermiCort, Dermolate, Durel-Cort, Ecosone, HC Cream, H1-Cor-2.5, ♣Hycort, Hycortole, Hydrocortex, Hydrocortone, Hytone, Ivocort, Maso-Cort, Microcort, Orabase HCA, Penecort, Proctocort, Rhus Tox HC, Rocort, ♠Squibb-HC, Unicort*

hydrocortisone acetate: *Biosone, Cortaid, ♣Cortamed, Cortef, ♣Corticreme, Cortifoam, ♠Dermacort, ♠Dermacort Ointment, Epifoam, Hydrocortisone Acetate, Hydrocortone Acetate, Mycort Lotion, Proctofoam-HC*

hydrocortisone cypionate: *Cortef*

hydrocortisone sodium phosphate: *Hydrocortone phosphate* hydrocortisone sodium succinate: *A-HydroCort, Solu-Cortef*

hydrocortisone valerate: *Westcort Cream*

Class: ★**Adrenocorticosteroid (naturally occurring glucocorticoid) prototype**, Steroidal anti-inflammatory, Immunosuppressant

PEDS	PREG	GERI
♆	C	♆

Action Suppresses inflammation by inhibiting accumulation of inflammatory cells, reducing dilatation and permeability of capillaries, and inhibiting release of chemical mediators of inflammation. Modifies immune response by suppressing cell-mediated immune reactions. Provides physiologic glucocorticoid and mineralocorticoid activity when endogenous hormones are diminished.

Use/Therapeutic goal/Outcome

Adrenocortical insufficiency: Replacement of deficient endogenous hormones. *Outcome criteria:* Improved appetite, decreased fatigue, normal blood pressure, normal skin color and turgor, report of improved sense of well-being.

Inflammatory or allergic conditions: Symptomatic relief. *Outcome criteria:* Decreased symptoms associated with condition being treated.

Dose range/Administration

Interaction alert: May decrease effectiveness of anticoagulants and antidiabetics. Vaccines may lead to diminished antibody response and serious infection. Potassium-depleting diuretics may cause severe hypokalemia. Alcohol or medications known to cause gastric irritation may cause gastric bleeding. Drugs that increase metabolism of corticosteroids (e.g., phenytoin, barbiturates, ephedrine, and rifampin) and those that decrease its absorption (e.g., cholestyramine, colestipol, and antacids) may decrease hydrocortisone levels, requiring an increase in hydrocortisone dosage.

🍎 **Give oral doses with food or milk to reduce gastric distress.**

Adult: PO: 20–240 mg/day. IM: 15–240 mg/day. IV: 100–500 mg/day. *Rectal: Retention enema:* 100 mg hs for 21 days. *Foam applicator:* 90 mg qd to bid for 2–3 wk. *Child:* PO: 2–8 mg/kg/day. IM: 0.6–4 mg/kg q12-24h. *Adult and Child: Topical:* Apply sparingly to affected area bid to qid. *Ophthalmic:* Thin strip bid to qid.

Clinical alert: Give single daily doses in the morning to reduce adrenal suppression. For replacement therapy, give 2/3 of daily dose in the morning and 1/3 in evening to simulate endogenous secretion. Give IM doses deep into gluteal muscle to lessen muscle atrophy. May also be injected directly into joints, soft tissues, or lesions.

Contraindications/Precautions

PREG
C

Contraindicated in hypersensitivity to corticosteroids or paraben preservatives present in some preparations, and in active peptic-ulcer disease, active tuberculosis or fungus infections, and herpes of eyes, lips, or genitals. *Use with caution* in acquired immunodeficiency syndrome (AIDS), hypertension, thrombophlebitis, congestive heart failure, diabetes mellitus, hypothyroidism, glaucoma, osteoporosis, myasthenia gravis, and history of bleeding ulcers, seizure disorder, or mental illness.

♆ **Use with caution for children, pregnant or nursing mothers, and the elderly.**

Side effects/Adverse reactions

Hypersensitivity: rash, hives, hypotension, respiratory distress, anaphylaxis. *CNS:* euphoria, restlessness, insomnia, hallucinations, depression, psychosis. *Eye:* glaucoma, cataracts. *MS:* impaired growth in children. *CV:* thrombophlebitis, embolism, irregular heartbeat. *GI:* increased appetite, oral candidiasis. *Misc:* hyperglycemia, withdrawal syndrome.

With prolonged use: Skin: acne; increased hair growth; thin, shiny skin; ecchymosis or petechiae; delayed wound healing. *GI:* nausea, vomiting, GI bleeding, pancreatitis. *MS:* osteoporosis; pain in hip, back, ribs, arms, or legs; muscle wasting. *CV:* hypertension, edema, hypokalemia. *GU:* menstrual irregularity. *Misc:* increased susceptibility to infection; Cushingoid appearance (moon-face and buffalo hump); withdrawal syndrome or acute adrenal insufficiency.

Nursing implications/Documentation

Possible nursing diagnoses: Potential for infection; Body image disturbance; Fluid volume excess; Altered oral mucous membrane.

◆ Assess for hypersensitivity reactions, especially with parenteral administration.

◆ Record baseline weight, blood pressure, and electrolyte levels.

• Apply topical cream sparingly to clean, moist skin; occlusive dressing will increase absorption.

• Assess and record improvement in condition being treated so dosage can be decreased as early as possible.

• Monitor electrolyte levels to detect sodium retention and potassium loss; assess for development of edema and/or muscle weakness, and document and report abnormal findings.

• Monitor for signs of infection and slowed wound healing.

• During dose reduction, monitor for symptoms of adrenal insufficiency (hypotension, hypoglycemia, weight loss, vomiting, and diarrhea).

• Recognize that use of hydrocortisone for inflammatory and allergic conditions is limited because it causes sodium retention and potassium loss.

Patient & family teaching/Home care

Possible nursing diagnoses: Knowledge deficit; Impaired home maintenance management; Body image disturbance; Impaired skin integrity.

• Explain the need to take oral doses with food or milk.

• Advise reporting unusual weight gain; swelling of lower extremities; muscle weakness; black tarry stools; vomiting of blood; epigastric burning; puffing of face; menstrual irregularities; prolonged sore throat, fever, cold, or infections; also stress the need to report symptoms of adrenal insufficiency (fatigue, anorexia, nausea, vomiting, diarrhea, weight loss, weakness, dizziness, depression, and mood swings).

• Caution not to take OTC or prescription drugs without consulting primary physician.

• For long-term therapy, advise carrying card indicating need for additional systemic steroids in case of trauma or surgery.

• Counsel to adhere to prescribed dose schedule and not to discontinue medication against medical advice.

• Emphasize importance of medical follow-up for evaluation of therapy.

• Advise against drinking alcohol while taking hydrocortisone to decrease risk of ulcers.

• Teach rectal administration technique; caution to report signs of rectal irritation or infection.

• See Adrenocorticosteroids overview for more information.

hydromorphone
hye-droe-mor'fone

hydromorphone hydrochloride: **Dilaudid, Dilaudid-HP**

Class: Narcotic analgesic

Antidote: naloxone hydrochloride (Narcan)

PEDS PREG GERI

CONTROLLED SUBSTANCE
II

Action Alters both the perception of and response to pain through an unclear mechanism. Believed to act by binding with opiate receptors at many CNS sites. Suppresses cough reflex by direct action on the cough center in the medulla. This drug is structurally similar to morphine but has an analgesic effect 8–10 times more potent, more rapid onset, shorter duration of action, less hypnotic effect, and less tendency to cause nausea and vomiting.

Use/Therapeutic goal/Outcome

Moderate to severe pain: Relief of pain. **Outcome criteria:** Report of comfort; absence of signs of pain (grimacing, frowning, restlessness, reluctance to move or cough) with increase in signs of comfort (relaxed facial expression); blood pressure and pulse within normal limits when compared to baseline.

Dose range/Administration

Interaction alert: Alcohol and CNS depressants increase effects. Reduce dose if used with general anesthetics, narcotic analgesics, tranquilizers, sedatives, hypnotics, tricyclic antidepressants, or MAO inhibitors.

Adult: PO: 1–6 mg q4-6h (available in 1, 2, 3, and 4 mg tablets). IM, SC, IV: 2–4 mg q4-6h prn or around the clock. *Rectal:* 3 mg hs, prn, or q6-8h around the clock.

Clinical alert: Be aware that Dilaudid HP, a highly concentrated form (10 mg/ml), is available to administer smaller volumes. Give IV doses slowly over 3–5 min while monitoring for respiratory depression and hypotension. Expect decreased dosage for the elderly or debilitated. Check respirations and blood pressure before giving hydromorphone. Hold drug and report if respirations < 12, or if there is hypotension. Keep naloxone readily available in case of respiratory depression.

Contraindications/Precautions

Contraindicated in hypersensitivity to hydromorphone, and in increased intracranial pressure or status asthmaticus. **Use with caution** in respiratory depression, increased cerebrospinal fluid pressure, hepatic or renal disease, hypothyroidism, shock, Addison's disease, alcoholism, seizures, head injury, severe CNS depression, brain tumor, bronchial asthma, and COPD.

👋 **Safe dose for children must be individualized by physician. Use with caution for the elderly or debilitated. Safe use for pregnant or nursing mothers has not been established (preg D for high dosage at term; otherwise, preg C).**

Side effects/Adverse reactions

Hypersensitivity: (rare) rashes, hives, itching, facial swelling. **CNS:** euphoria, mood changes, convulsions with large doses, extreme somnolence, coma, physical dependence. **Resp:** respiratory depression. **CV:** hypotension, bradycardia. **GI:** nausea, vomiting, constipation, ileus. **GU:** urinary retention. **Skin:** induration from repeated subcutaneous injections. **MS:** skeletal-muscle flaccidity.

Nursing implications/Documentation

Possible nursing diagnoses: Pain; Anxiety; Potential for injury; Constipation.

♦ Have patient rate pain on a scale of 1–10 before and after medication is given; report and record inadequate pain control.

♦ Ascertain that there is not an acute abdominal problem before giving hydromorphone (may mask or worsen pain of cholecystitis, obstruction, or appendicitis).

♦ Document pulse, respirations, and blood pressure immediately before and 1 hr after administration.

♦ Monitor closely for risk factors for injury; keep side rails up and supervise ambulation if allowed out of bed.

♦ Give before pain is severe for best effects.

♦ Document and monitor bowel function to detect constipation; provide adequate fluid and fiber; give laxatives before problem is severe.

♦ Be aware of potential for psychic and physical dependence after prolonged use (withdrawal symptoms are similar to those of morphine, but occur sooner).

Patient & family teaching/Home care

Possible nursing diagnoses: Sensory/perceptual alterations; Knowledge deficit.

♦ Explain the rationale for reporting pain/discomfort before it is severe.

♦ Advise ambulatory patients to refrain from activities that require alertness and to seek assistance if there is any question about ability to get out of bed (e.g., if there is weakness or light headedness).

♦ Explain procedures briefly and in simple terms.

♦ Warn not to exceed prescribed dose because of overdose, dependence, and abuse potential (instead of increasing dose regimen, unsatisfactory pain relief should be reported).

♦ Stress that alcohol and other CNS depressants may cause excessive sedation.

♦ *See Narcotic and non-narcotic analgesics overview for more information.*

hydroxocobalamin *hy-drox-oh-koe-bal'a-min*

Alpha-Ruvite, Codroxomin, Droxomin, Rubesol-LA
Class: Vitamin B_{12}, Antianemic, Water-soluble vitamin

PEDS	PREG	GERI
OK	A	OK

Action Promotes fat and carbohydrate metabolism and protein synthesis by acting as a coenzyme; promotes normal growth, cell reproduction, maturation of RBCs and synthesis of nucleoprotein and myelin by metabolism of methionine, folic acid, and malonic acid.

Use/Therapeutic goal/Outcome

Vitamin B_{12} deficiency or malabsorption, pernicious anemia: Adequate blood levels of Vitamin B_{12}. **Outcome criteria:** Increased reticulocyte and RBC count; absence or improvement in symptoms of deficiency (paresthesias, anorexia, fatigue, and red, sore tongue).

Dose range/Administration

Interaction alert: Chloramphenicol may inhibit the hematopoietic activity of hydroxocobalamin.

Adult: IM: *Loading dose:* 30–50 mcg/day for 5–10 days. *Maintenance dose:* 100–200 mcg/month. **Child:** IM: *Loading dose:* 30–50 mcg/day for 2 wk. *Maintenance dose:* 30–100 mcg/month.

Contraindications/Precautions

Contraindicated in hypersensitivity to hydroxo-cobalamin or to cobalt, and in optic nerve atrophy. *Use with caution* in history of gout.

Side effects/Adverse reactions

Hypersensitivity: Rash, hives, wheezing, anaphylaxis. *CV:* peripheral vascular thrombosis, CHF, pulmonary edema. *Hem:* hypokalemia. *Misc:* pain at injection site.

Nursing implications/Documentation

Possible nursing diagnoses: Activity intolerance; Altered peripheral tissue perfusion.

♦ For those with history of sensitivities, administer intradermal test dose before beginning therapy.

♦ Do not mix in syringe with other medications or solutions.

♦ Do not administer IV, except for small amounts in parenteral nutrition solutions.

♦ Monitor potassium level, reticulocyte and RBC count, hemoglobin, and Vitamin B_{12} levels.

♦ Assess for CHF and pulmonary edema in cardiac patients.

Patient & family teaching/Home care

Possible nursing diagnoses: Knowledge deficit; Impaired home maintenance management.

♦ For dietary deficiency, identify foods high in Vitamin B_{12} (meats, fish, egg yolk, aged cheeses).

♦ For pernicious anemia or noncorrectable malabsorption, advise that Vitamin B_{12} injections must be continued throughout life to prevent irreversible neurologic damage.

♦ Explain that the stinging, burning sensation that may occur after injection is transient.

hydroxyurea

hye-drox'ee-yo-rhe-ah

Hydrea
Class: Antineoplastic (antimetabolite) agent

PEDS	PREG	GERI
☙	D	☙

Action Kills rapidly growing cells (cancer, hair follicles, bone marrow, GI lining, ova, and sperm) by inhibiting DNA synthesis and damaging DNA strands (incorporates thymidine into DNA); does not interfere with RNA or protein synthesis. Drug is cell-cycle specific in the S-phase.

Use/Therapeutic goal/Outcome

Melanoma; chronic myelocytic leukemia; cancer of the head and neck; recurrent, inoperable ovarian cancer: Elimination or suppression of malignant cell proliferation. *Outcome criteria:* After 6 weeks, tumor and disease regression or stabilization on radiologic and physical examination; for leukemia, absence of blasts in peripheral blood specimen.

Dose range/Administration

Interaction alert: Radiation therapy and other cytotoxic agents may cause severe myelosuppression.

Adult: PO: *Single dose:* 80 mg/kg every 3 days. *Continuous therapy:* 20–30 mg/kg/day.

Clinical alert: If the patient cannot chew, empty capsule contents into water and give immediately. Calculate drug dosage on basis of actual or ideal body weight (whichever is lower). When hydroxyurea is used in combination with radiation therapy, it should be started at least 7 days before radiation therapy begins. Hold drug and report if platelets <100,000/mm³ or WBC <4000/mm³. Leukopenia can occur in 10 days.

Contraindications/Precautions

Contraindicated in hypersensitivity to hydroxyurea, and severe myelosuppression. *Use with caution* in preexisting renal disorders, infection, or previous radiation (increased toxicity; dose reduction is usually required).

☙ **Contraindicated for pregnant or nursing mothers. Use with caution for the elderly. Safe use for children has not been established.**

Side effects/Adverse reactions

Hypersensitivity: rash, urticaria, pruritus. *Hem:* cumulative and dose-limiting bone marrow suppression, anemia, thrombocytopenia, leukopenia; increased BUN and serum creatinine levels, hyperuricemia. *GI:* anorexia, nausea, and vomiting; stomatitis; diarrhea; and constipation; elevated hepatic enzymes. *Skin:* maculopapular rash. *GU:* nephrotoxicity. *CNS:* fever, dizziness, confusion, hallucinations, convulsions. *Misc:* chills, malaise.

Nursing implications/Documentation

Possible nursing diagnoses: Potential for infection; Potential for injury; Fatigue; Altered oral mucous membrane; Fluid volume deficit; Diarrhea; Altered nutrition: less than body requirements.

◆ *See important Nursing implications in Antineoplastic agents overview on page 72, which apply to all antineoplastics. The interventions that follow are additional and specific to this drug only.*

♦ Increase fluid intake to 2–3 L a day to prevent renal tubular damage from hyperuricemia secondary to cell lysis.

Patient & family teaching/Home care

Possible nursing diagnoses: Knowledge deficit; Ineffective coping (individual and family); Hopelessness; Impaired home maintenance management.

◆ *See important Patient & family teaching in Antineoplastic agents overview on page 72, which apply to all antineoplastics. The teachings that follow are additional and specific to this drug only.*

♦ Point out that it may take 6 weeks for a response to therapy to occur.

♦ Advise immediately reporting visual or auditory hallucinations or difficulty breathing.

♦ Stress that drinking 2–3 L a day helps prevent kidney complications.

◆ *See Antineoplastic agents overview for more information.*

ibuprofen

eye-byoo'proe-fen

Advil, ♦*Amersol,* ♦*Apo-Ibuprofen,* ♠*Brufen, CapProfen, Haltran, Ibuprin,* ♠*Inflam, Medipren, Midol-200, Motrin,* ♦*Novoprofen, Nuprin, Pamparin-IB,* ♠*Rafen, Rufen, Trendar*

Class: Nonsteroidal anti-inflammatory drug (NSAID), Analgesic, Antipyretic, Antirheumatic

PEDS   PREG   GERI
🖑   🖑   🖑

Action Reduces inflammation and pain by inhibiting synthesis and/or release of prostaglandin. Decreases uterine contractility by inhibiting intrauterine prostaglandins. Prostaglandin is a naturally occurring mediator of the inflammatory process which is found throughout body tissue. Acts on hypothalamus to produce vasodilation. Inhibits platelet aggregation.

Use/Therapeutic goal/Outcome

Pain and inflammation: Promotion of comfort and mobility; suppression of inflammation. **Outcome criteria:** Report of increased comfort with increased range of motion and ability to perform activities of daily life; reduction in or absence of joint stiffness, swelling, redness, and warmth.

Primary dysmenorrhea: Reduction of uterine hyperactivity (cramping). **Outcome criteria:** Report of increased comfort and increased activity level.

Dose range/Administration

Interaction alert: Since this drug becomes protein-bound, patients receiving hydantoins, sulfonamides, and sulfonylureas should be observed for toxicity. In those receiving coumarin-type anticoagulants, prothrombin time may be prolonged. Aspirin may decrease therapeutic effect of NSAID and increase risk of bleeding.

🖱 **Give 1 hr before or 2 hr after meals, unless GI distress is noted (then give with meals).**
Arthritis: **Adult:** PO: 300–800 mg tid or qid.
Mild to moderate pain: **Adult:** PO: 200–400 mg q4-6h prn.
Primary dysmenorrhea: **Adult:** PO: 400 mg q4h prn.

Clinical alert: Dosage individualized, not to exceed 3200 mg/day. Renal failure has been reported with high doses. Be aware that ibuprofen is available in lower doses OTC, but that some people increase dosage by taking more than the recommended dose (question carefully). Expect decreased dosage for the elderly and those with renal impairment.

Contraindications/Precautions

PREG
🖑

Contraindicated in hypersensitivity to ibuprofen, other NSAIDs, or aspirin, or in acute asthma, nasal polyps, or active GI disease.
Use with caution in history of renal or hepatic impairment, GI bleeding, and intrinsic coagulation defects.

🖑 **Use with caution for the elderly. Safe use for children under 14 years and pregnant women has not been established (first two trimesters, preg B; in third trimester, preg D).**

Side effects/Adverse reactions

Hypersensitivity: rash, pruritus, urticaria, asthmatic symptoms, bronchospasm, and angioedema. **GI:** GI irritation. **CNS:** dizziness, headache, drowsiness. **Ear:** tinnitus. **Eye:** visual disturbances. **Hem:** prolonged bleeding time, elevated liver enzymes. **GU:** nephrotic syndrome. **Skin:** edema. **GU:** cystitis, dysuria, hematuria. **Hem:** hypo- or hyperglycemia.

Nursing implications/Documentation

Possible nursing diagnoses: Pain; Impaired physical mobility.

♦ Establish a baseline for CBC, electrolytes, prothrombin time, BUN, creatinine, and liver function studies; if therapy is prolonged, monitor periodically thereafter.

♦ Schedule doses so that they are given at least 1 hr before maximum mobility is needed.

♦ Monitor for and report GI symptoms that may indicate peptic ulcer (nausea, pain, black stools).

♦ Record weight every other day; report edema or sudden weight gain.

♦ Observe for and report visual and auditory changes (periodic auditory tests are recommended if therapy is prolonged).

♦ For diabetics, monitor blood sugar closely since insulin requirements may change.

Patient & family teaching/Home care

Possible nursing diagnoses: Altered health maintenance; Knowledge deficit.

♦ Advise taking this drug with food to reduce GI symptoms.

♦ Explain the importance of watching for symptoms of GI bleeding (black stools, persistent GI distress).

♦ Explain that full effect of drug may not be realized for up to 3 weeks.

♦ Stress the need to avoid aspirin, alcohol, and other OTC drugs (unless approved by physician) because of increased risk of GI bleeding.

♦ Instruct individuals to hold dose and report if any of the following side effects are experienced: vertigo, rashes, blood in urine, hearing or visual changes, sudden weight gain, edema.

♦ Warn against driving or activities that require alertness until response is determined (may cause drowsiness and dizziness at first; this should be transient).

♦ Reinforce the need for medical follow-up; advise telling dentist that they are taking ibuprofen.

♦ For diabetics, explain the importance of monitoring blood sugars with a blood glucose meter.

♦ *See Nonsteroidal anti-inflammatory drugs overview for more information.*

ifosfamide
eye-fos'fa-mide

Ifex

Class: Antineoplastic (alkylating) agent

PEDS	PREG	GERI
🖐	D	🖐

Action Kills rapidly growing cells (cancer, hair follicles, bone marrow, GI lining, ova, and sperm) by interfering with DNA replication and RNA transcription through alkylation (cross-linking of DNA occurs). Is cell-cycle–phase nonspecific, affecting both actively dividing cells and dormant (resting) cells.

Use/Therapeutic goal/Outcome

Refractory germ cell testicular cancer, sarcomas, carcinoma of the lung, and non-Hodgkin's lymphomas: Reduction, elimination of malignant cell proliferation. **Outcome criteria:** Tumor and disease regression or stabilization on radiologic and physical examination.

Dose range/Administration

Interaction alert: Allopurinol and barbiturates may increase hepatotoxicity. Radiation therapy or other cytotoxic agents can cause severe myelosuppression.

Adult: IV: 1.2 g/m^2 per day for 5 days. Repeat q 3–4 wk.

Clinical alert: This drug should be given only by nurses who are knowledgeable in the comprehensive management of administration of antineoplastic agents. Dose may vary at physician's discretion, and should be given slowly over 30–60 minutes. Repeat doses are held until it is ascertained that the patient has recovered sufficiently from toxicities of previous doses. Established protocols and policies for drug preparation, administration, and accidental skin contamination must be followed closely (gloves or double gloves are worn when handling drug; if the drug touches the skin, the area is washed immediately with plenty of soap and water). Check urine before each dose; hold dose and report if microscopic or gross hematuria is present. Often given with Mesna or another protective agent to prevent hemorrhagic cystitis.

Contraindications/Precautions

PREG
D

Contraindicated in hypersensitivity to ifosfamide, and severe myelosuppression. **Use with caution** in impaired renal (increased risk of CNS toxicity) and liver function.

🖐 **Contraindicated for pregnant or nursing mothers. Use with caution for the elderly. Safe use for children has not been established.**

Side effects/Adverse reactions

Hypersensitivity: rash, urticaria, erythema. *GU:* hematuria, hemorrhagic cystitis (occurs in 50% of patients), renal toxicity, dysuria, urinary frequency. *GI:* nausea and vomiting; elevated liver enzymes, hepatotoxicity. *Hem:* leukopenia, thrombocytopenia, myelosuppression. *CNS:* somnolence, confusion, depressive psychoses, hallucinations, coma. *Skin:* alopecia; pain, burning, and inflammation at injection site.

Nursing implications/Documentation

Possible nursing diagnoses: Potential for infection; Potential for injury; Fatigue; Altered oral mucous membrane; Fluid volume deficit; Diarrhea; Altered nutrition: less than body requirements.

♦ *See important Nursing implications in Antineoplastic agents overview on page 72, which apply to all antineoplastics. The interventions that follow are additional and specific to this drug only.*

♦ Check urine before each dose; hold dose and report if microscopic or gross hematuria is present.

♦ Monitor closely for toxicity, which may occur with a low therapeutic range.

♦ Maintain a fluid intake of at least 2–3 L per day (this is essential to prevent cystitis and may require IV fluids if intake is low).

♦ Expect that a continuous bladder irrigation of normal saline may be ordered to prevent cystitis.

♦ Monitor for and report signs of CNS toxicity (changes in mental status, balance problems).

♦ Expect WBC to drop to the nadir (lowest point) in 7–14 days, with recovery by day 21.

Patient & family teaching/Home care

Possible nursing diagnoses: Knowledge deficit; Ineffective coping (individual and family); Hopelessness; Impaired home maintenance management.

♦ *See important Patient & family teaching in Antineoplastic agents overview on page 72, which apply to all antineoplastics. The teachings that follow are additional and specific to this drug only.*

♦ Stress that changes in mental status or problems with balance should be reported; such problems may require reduction in dosage.

♦ Explain that drinking 2–3 L is essential to prevent cystitis; point out the need to void frequently, at least once during the night, to prevent prolonged contact of metabolites with bladder mucosa.

♦ *See Antineoplastic agents overview for more information.*

imipenem

i-mi-pen'em

imipenem with cilastatin sodium: *Primaxin*
Class: Anti-infective, Beta-lactam antibiotic

PEDS   PREG   GERI
🖐   C   🖐

Action Imipenem kills bacteria (bactericidal) by disrupting cell wall synthesis, which makes the bacteria more susceptible to osmotic pressure and lysis. *Cilastatin* prevents imipenem degradation by enzymes in the kidney, making it also effective for urinary tract infections. This drug is effective against most known microorganisms (*very* broad spectrum).

Use/Therapeutic goal/Outcome

Severe infections (lower respiratory tract, urinary tract, intraabdominal and gynecological, bacterial septicemia, bone and joint, skin and soft tissue, endocarditis) caused by *Staphylococcus, Streptococcus, Escherichia coli, Klebsiella, Proteus, Enterobacter, Pseudomonas aeruginosa* and *Bacteroides:* Resolution or prevention of infection. *Outcome criteria:* Absence of pathogenic growth on cultures, absence of clinical manifestations of infection (fever, pain, swelling, redness, heat, odor, drainage, productive cough, dysuria), normal WBC count, normal X rays.

Dose range/Administration

Adult: IV: 250 mg to 1 g q6-8h. *Maximum dose:* 4 g/day or 50 mg/kg/day, whichever is less.

Clinical alert: Never give IV bolus. Give 250–500 mg doses over 20–30 minutes; give 1 g doses over 40–60 minutes. If nausea occurs, reduce IV rate.

Contraindications/Precautions

PREG
C

Contraindicated in hypersensitivity to imipenem or cilastatin. **Use with caution** in history of allergy to penicillins or cephalosporins (these drugs are chemically similar), in history of seizure disorders, and in reduced kidney function.

Use with caution for the elderly. Safe use for children and pregnant or nursing mothers has not been established.

Side effects/Adverse reactions

Hypersensitivity: itching, rashes, fever, difficulty breathing, anaphylaxis. **GI:** nausea, vomiting, diarrhea, pseudomembranous colitis. **CV:** hypotension; pain, redness, swelling, thrombophlebitis at injection site. **CNS:** seizures (especially in decreased kidney function), confusion, dizziness, tremors. **Misc:** superinfection.

Nursing implications/Documentation

Possible nursing diagnoses: Potential for infection; Fluid volume deficit.

◆ Obtain culture specimens and baseline lab studies (CBC, BUN, creatinine, electrolytes, liver function) before administering first dose; monitor closely thereafter if therapy is prolonged.

◆ Monitor those allergic to penicillin or cephalosporins closely for allergic response (symptoms of hypotension and hyperventilation are associated with onset of allergic reaction).

◆ Provide preferred fluids, and record and monitor intake and output, to ensure adequate hydration and urine output; report decreased urinary output.

◆ Monitor for and report symptoms of superinfection (mouth lesions, thrush, vaginal irritation, diarrhea).

◆ Schedule peak serum lab studies to be drawn 1 hour after completion of IV dose; schedule trough levels 30 minutes before IV dose.

Patient & family teaching/Home care

Possible nursing diagnoses: Knowledge deficit; Impaired home maintenance management.

◆ Teach the need to report new symptoms of illness (e.g., fever, mouth lesions, vaginal irritation, diarrhea); medication change may be necessary.

◆ Explain the importance of drinking plenty of fluids and taking antibiotics for the entire time prescribed, even if symptoms abate.

◆ *See Anti-infectives overview for more information.*

imipramine

im-ip'ra-meen

imipramine hydrochloride: ✦*Apo-Imipramine,* ✦*Impril,* ✦*Imiprin, Janimine,* ✦*Novo-Pramine, Presamine Tripramine, Tofranil*

imipramine pamoate: *Tofranil-PM*

Class: ★Tricyclic antidepressant (TCA) prototype

PEDS PREG GERI
         D

Action Improves mood by increasing levels of the neurotransmitters norepinephrine and serotonin in the CNS. (Blocks neurotransmitter reuptake into presynaptic neurons by inhibiting the "amine pump." Reuptake normally terminates the action of neurotransmitters.) Believed to prevent enuresis by its anticholinergic activity and by CNS stimulation, causing earlier arousal when full bladder is sensed. Has been effective for relieving chronic severe neurogenic pain (exact mechanism of action is unclear). Has moderate anticholinergic and sedating effects.

Use/Therapeutic goal/Outcome

Major depressive disorders: Promotion of sense of well-being, ability to cope with daily living. **Outcome criteria:** After 2–4 weeks, report of feeling less depressed, more energetic and able to cope; return of normal sleeping and eating habits; demonstration of improved ability to problem solve and perform activities of daily living.

Phobias: Particularly agorophobia: Prevention of panic attacks. **Outcome criteria:** Report of absence of panic attacks.

Childhood enuresis: Prevention of bed-wetting. **Outcome criteria:** Absence of bed-wetting.

Dose range/Administration

Interaction alert: Barbiturates may reduce antidepressant blood levels and effects. Cimetidine and mathylphenidate may increase blood levels. If given with epinephrine and norepinephrine, monitor for increased risk of hypertension. Avoid use with MAOIs (risk of excitation, hyperpyrexia, and seizures). Give cautiously with thyroid drugs because it may increase CNS stimulation and cardiac arrhythmias.

🐾 **Give with (or immediately after) food to reduce GI symptoms.**

Depression/Phobias: Adult/Child > 12 yrs: PO: 75–100 mg/day in divided doses or at hs for the first 14 days. May increase by increments of 25–50 mg to a maximum of 300 mg/day. IM: Use only if absolutely necessary.

Childhood enuresis: Child: PO: 25–50 mg at bedtime.

Clinical alert: Whenever possible give entire dose at bedtime. This drug may contain tartrazine (FD&C Yellow No. 5), which has caused allergic responses in some patients (check package insert).

Contraindications/Precautions

PREG D

Contraindicated in hypersensitivity to TCAs, for concomitant use with electroconvulsive therapy, in elective surgery, and acute recovery period of myocardial infarction. *Use with caution* in renal or hepatic disease, hyperthyroidism, glaucoma, prostatic hypertrophy, urinary retention, hypomania, mania, and suicidal tendency.

✋ **Contraindicated for pregnant or nursing mothers and for treating depression in children under 6 years. Use with caution for adolescents and the elderly or debilitated.**

Side effects/Adverse reactions

Hypersensitivity: rash, sensitivity to sunlight. *CNS:* drowsiness, dizziness, anxiety, headache, fatigue, agitation, extrapyramidal symptoms, sedation (especially the elderly). *CV:* orthostatic hypotension, palpitations, tachycardia, EKG changes, hypertension. *GI:* anorexia, dry mouth, nausea, vomiting, constipation, paralytic ileus. *GU:* urinary retention, decreased libido. *Eye:* blurred vision. *Ear:* tinnitus. *Hem:* agranulocytosis.

Nursing implications/Documentation

Possible nursing diagnoses: Potential for injury; Constipation; Altered oral mucous membrane.

◆ Document mental status and vital signs at least twice a day until response to therapy has been established.

◆ Be sure that doses are swallowed (not hoarded).

◆ Monitor for orthostatic hypotension, dizziness, and drowsiness; supervise ambulation until response is established.

◆ Record intake and output, and observe for dehydration or urinary retention; provide special mouth care.

◆ Monitor for and report suicidal tendencies, increased depression, or excessive drowsiness (may require change in medication).

◆ Prevent constipation by monitoring bowel movements and encouraging adequate fiber and fluid intake; offer laxatives or stool softeners before the problem becomes severe.

Patient & family teaching/Home care

Possible nursing diagnoses: Ineffective coping (family and individual); Sleep pattern disturbance; Impaired home maintenance management.

◆ Stress that this medication helps reduce the depression that inhibits ability to make decisions and cope effectively (once the individual feels less depressed, it will be easier to take steps toward making healthy changes).

◆ Explain that side effects are often noted immediately, but they usually diminish after a few weeks; on the other hand, it is likely to take 2–4 weeks before *beneficial* effects are noted (the patient may feel worse before feeling better).

◆ Warn to change positions slowly to prevent dizziness.

◆ Point out the role of adequate nutrition, exercise, and sleep in combating depression.

◆ Emphasize that the effects of alcohol, sedatives, and tranquilizers may be potentiated.

◆ Caution to consult physician before using OTC drugs; stress the need for ongoing medical follow-up.

◆ Recommend reporting continued depression; stress that doses should not be increased or stopped without checking with physician because this may cause severe problems.

- ◆ Advise avoidance of driving and other potentially hazardous activities until response is established.

- ◆ Suggest using ice chips, hard candy, or gum to relieve side effect of dry mouth; stress the need for good mouth care.

- ◆ Warn women to report immediately if pregnancy is planned or suspected.

- ◆ Refer mothers of children with enuresis to incontinence specialists to employ holistic method of preventing bet-wetting.

- ◆ *See Antidepressants overview for more information.*

immune globulin
glob'u-lin

immune globulin intramuscular (IGIM, IG, gamma globulin): *Gamastan, Gammar*

immune globulin intravenous (IGIV): *Gamimune N, Gammagard, Sandoglobulin, Venoglobulin-I*

Class: Immunizing agent

PEDS	PREG	GERI
🖐	C	🖐

Action Provides passive immunity to a variety of infections by increasing antibody titer.

Use/Therapeutic goal/Outcome

Combined immunodeficiency and primary immunoglobulin deficiency syndromes, agammaglobulinemia, hypogammaglobulinemia, modification of measles, measles vaccine complications, and exposure to hepatitis A, hepatitis B, measles, poliomyelitis, chickenpox, and exposure to rubella during the first trimester of pregnancy: Enhancement of immune response, prevention or suppression of infectious disease process. *Outcome criteria:* Increased antibody titer (in immunodeficiency, IgG serum concentrations greater than 200mg/dl); absent or diminished signs and symptoms of infectious disease.

Idiopathic Thrombocytopenic Purpura (ITP): Reversal of thrombocytopenia. *Outcome criteria:* Increased platelet count.

Dose range/Administration

Interaction alert: Immune globulin antibodies may suppress response to live virus vaccines (measles, mumps, rubella) if given within 3 months, resulting in failure to develop active immunity. Do not mix IV with any other drug.

Prophylaxis in immunodeficiency diseases: Adult and Child: IM: Initially, 1.2 ml/kg, then 0.6 ml/kg q 2-4 wks (maximum single dose of

30–50 ml for adults and 20–30 ml for children). IV: (*Gamimune N*) 100–200 mg/kg (2–4 ml/kg) monthly; may be increased to 400 mg/kg (8 ml/kg) or given more frequently. (*Gammagard*) 200–400 mg/kg monthly. (*Sandoglobulin*) 200 mg/kg monthly, may be increased to 300 mg/kg monthly or given more frequently. (*Venoglobulin-I*) 200 mg/kg monthly, may be increased to 300–400 mg/kg monthly or given more frequently.

Hepatitis A exposure (within 2–6 weeks): Adult and Child: IM: 0.02–0.04 ml/kg immediately after (or before) exposure. *Do not give after onset of clinical symptoms.*

Measles exposure and complications of measle vaccine: Adult and Child: IM: 0.25 ml/kg, within 6 days after exposure. *Maximum dose: 15 ml. For complications of vaccine,* give immediately. Children over 15 months who have not been vaccinated should be vaccinated 3 months later.

Chicken pox exposure: Adult and Child: IM: 0.6–1.2 ml/kg as a single dose.

Poliomyelitis exposure: Adult and Child: IM: 0.3–0.4 ml/kg within 7 days of exposure.

Rubella exposure (in the first trimester of pregnancy): Adult: IM: 0.2–0.4 ml/kg immediately after exposure.

Idiopathic thrombocytopenic purpura: Adult: IV: (*Gamimune N or Sandoglobulin*) 400 mcg/kg for 2–5 days. (*Gammagard*) 1 g/kg as a single dose; up to 3 doses may be given on alternate days.

Clinical alert: IGIM (for intramuscular use) and IGIV (for intravenous use) are NOT interchangeable. Read labels carefully to assure that correct type is used. Give IM doses > 5 ml in divided doses deeply into large muscles (preferably anterior thigh or ventrogluteal site). Use a controller for IV administration; consult with physician for infusion rate, which varies with product. Monitor vital signs closely during IV infusion: stop IV and report if hypotension is noted. Have resuscitative equipment and emergency drugs (epinepherine, diphenhydramine, corticosteroids) readily available in case of anaphylaxis.

Contraindications/Precautions
PREG
C

Contraindicated in hypersensitivity to immune globulin or drug preservatives (thimerosal, maltose), and for hepatitis A if more than 6 weeks have passed since exposure or after onset of clinical symptoms, in IgA deficiency (anaphylaxis could occur due to IgA antibody production). **Use with caution** IM for thrombocytopenia or bleeding disorders.

🖐 **Use with caution for children and the elderly. Safe use for pregnant or nursing mothers has not been established.**

Side effects/Adverse reactions

Hypersensitivity: itching, rashes, wheezing, dyspnea, angioedema, fever, chills, sweating, (with IV use) hypotension, chest tightness, anaphylaxis. *CNS:* headache, dizziness. *Skin:* pain and inflammation at injection site. *MS:* muscle stiffness at injection site. *GI:* nausea, abdominal pain. *GU:* nephrotic syndrome. *Misc:* flu-like syndrome (joint pain, fatigue).

Nursing implications/Documentation

Possible nursing diagnoses: Potential for infection; Potential for injury.

♦ Document and specify presence of immune deficiency or history of exposure to infectious disease.

♦ If patient is immunosuppressed, keep people with respiratory symptoms out of the room.

♦ During IV administration, keep patient in bed with side rails up and call bell within reach. If hypotension occurs, reduce IV rate.

♦ Observe closely for hypersensitivity reactions (more likely with IV and large IM doses).

♦ Monitor CBC closely for signs of infection (especially for those with thrombocytopenic purpura).

Patient & family teaching/Home care

Possible nursing diagnoses: Fear; Knowledge deficit; Impaired home maintenance management.

♦ Explain that this drug helps prevent or reduce the severity of various infectious diseases; for those with thrombocytopenia, explain that it will help increase platelets and ability to clot.

♦ Encourage verbalizing fears and concerns; stress that the patient will be monitored closely for optimal results and early detection of side effects.

♦ Advise that pain, redness, and tenderness at injection site may persist for several hours.

♦ Stress that allergic symptoms (itching, rashes, difficulty breathing, chest tightness) should be reported immediately.

indapamide
in-dap'a-mide

✦*Lozide, Lozol,* ♠*Natrilix*
Class: Thiazide-like diuretic, Vasodilator, Antihypertensive

PEDS	PREG	GERI
🖐	B	🖐

Action Enhances the excretion of sodium and water by inhibiting sodium reabsorption in the nephron. Lowers blood pressure by reducing plasma and extra-cellular volume. Decreases peripheral resistance by a direct vasodilating action that may result from a calcium channel blocking action.

Use/Therapeutic goal/Outcome

Hypertension: Reduction in blood pressure. *Outcome criteria:* Blood pressure within acceptable range.

Edema: Resolution of edema. *Outcome criteria:* Increased urine output; absence of peripheral and sacral edema.

Dose range/Administration

Interaction alert: If given with diazoxide, monitor for increased effects and hyperuricemic effects. Concurrent use with lithium is not recommended.

🖐 **Administer with or after meals to increase bioavailability.**

Adult: PO: 2.5 mg/day. May be increased to 5 mg/day.

Clinical alert: Give in the morning to prevent nocturnal diuresis.

Contraindications/Precautions
PREG
B

Contraindicated in hypersensitivity to sulfonamide-derived agents, and in anuria. *Use with caution* in severe renal or hepatic impairment, diabetes, history of gout.

🖐 **Use with caution for the elderly. Safe use for children and pregnant or nursing mothers has not been established.**

Side effects/Adverse reactions

Hypersensitivity: purpura, rash, dermatitis with photosensitivity, respiratory distress, anaphylaxis, blood dyscrasias. *CV:* orthostatic hypotension, muscle cramps. *CNS:* headache, irritability, nervousness. *Hem:* electrolyte imbalances, volume depletion, dehydration, hyperuricemia, metabolic acidosis. *GI:* anorexia, nausea, pancreatitis.

►

Nursing implications/Documentation

Possible nursing diagnoses: Fluid volume deficit; Altered patterns of urinary elimination; Potential for injury.

• Ascertain that baseline CBC, sodium, potassium, chloride, carbon dioxide, calcium, magnesium, BUN, creatinine, uric acid, and liver function studies have been obtained before giving first dose; report abnormalities and monitor closely thereafter.

• Document and monitor blood pressure, pulse, daily weight, and intake and output; report significant discrepancies.

• Observe for and report signs of fluid overload (auscultate lungs for rales; check feet, ankles, and sacrum for edema).

• Check with physician to determine dietary restrictions; consult with dietician to plan diet.

• Observe the elderly for extreme diuresis (may require lower doses); monitor for orthostatic hypotension; supervise ambulation until response is determined.

Patient & family teaching/Home care

Possible nursing diagnoses: Knowledge deficit; Impaired home maintenance management.

• Before giving first dose, explain that the drug will increase the amount and frequency of urination.

• Emphasize the importance of taking this drug exactly as prescribed, and the importance of returning for medical follow-up.

• Explain that diuretics enhance the work of the kidney and reduce the workload of the heart.

• Recommend taking dose in early morning to prevent the need to disturb sleep to void.

• Explain that changing positions slowly helps prevent dizziness.

• Advise reporting dizziness, shortness of breath, muscle weakness or spasms, swelling of hands and feet, or persistent sore throat; encourage daily monitoring of weight and reporting sudden weight gain.

• Provide a list of allowed foods and fluids; stress the need to stick to prescribed diet (explain the hazards of too much salt, or too little potassium).

• Warn against driving or activities that require alertness until response has been determined.

• Advise avoidance of OTC drugs unless approved by physician.

♦ *See Diuretics and Antihypertensives overviews for more information.*

indomethacin

in-doe-meth'a-sin

♣**Apo-Indomethacin,** ♠**Arthrexin, Indometh,** ♣♠**Indocid,** ♣**Indocid SR, Indocin, Indocin SR, Indomed,** ♣**Novomethacin,** ♠**Rheumacin, Zendole**

indomethacin sodium trihydrate: ♣**Apo-Indomethacin,** ♣**Indocid, Indocin IV, Indometh, Novomethacin**

Class: Nonsteroidal anti-inflammatory drug (NSAID), Analgesic, Antipyretic

PEDS	PREG	GERI
🤚	🤚	🤚

Action Reduces inflammation and pain by inhibiting synthesis and/or release of prostaglandin. Decreases uterine contractility by inhibiting intrauterine prostaglandins. Prostaglandin is a naturally occurring mediator of the inflammatory process which is found throughout body tissue. Decreases mobility of leukocytes and vascular permeability of inflamed tissue.

Use/Therapeutic goal/Outcome

Pain and inflammation: Promotion of comfort and mobility; suppression of inflammation. **Outcome criteria:** Report of increased comfort with increased range of motion and ability to perform activities of daily life; reduction in or absence of joint stiffness, swelling, redness, and warmth.

Patent ductus arteriosis: Closure of patent ductus arteriosis. **Outcome criteria:** Diminished width of pulse pressure and elimination of or reduction in "machinery" or systolic murmur.

(Investigational use) Premature labor: Inhibition of uterine contractions. **Outcome criteria:** Absence of premature uterine contractions.

Dose range/Administration

Interaction alert: Since this drug becomes protein-bound, observe patients receiving hydantoins, sulfonamides, or sulfonylureas for toxicity. Aspirin may decrease therapeutic effect of NSAIDs and increase risk of bleeding. Probenecid may enhance the effect of indomethacin. Indomethacin may antagonize furosemide and thiazide diuretics, beta-adrenergic blocking agents, and captopril. Salicylates and corticosteroids may increase the possibility of GI ulceration.

🖐 **Give this drug with food or antacid.**

Moderate to severe pain: Adult: PO: 25–50 mg bid to tid. May increase doses weekly by 25 mg if tolerated. *Maximum dosage:* 150–200 mg/day.

Bursitis or tendonitis: Adult: PO: 75–150 mg/day in divided doses for 1–2 wk.

Gouty arthritis: Adult: PO: 50 mg tid until pain is tolerable; then rapidly reduce dose to termination (in 3–5 days).

Patent ductus arteriosis: Infant < 2 days: IV: *Initial dose:* 0.2 mg/kg. Then 2 doses of 0.1 mg/kg each. **Infant 2–7 days:** Same initial dose, then 3 doses of 0.2 mg/kg each. **Infant > 7 days:** Same initial dose, then 2 doses of 0.25 mg/kg each. A second course of therapy may be required.

Premature labor: Adult: PO or RECT: *Loading dose:* 100 mg. *Maintenance dose:* Maximum of 50 mg q4-6h tapered to lowest possible dose (300 mg/day should be sustained).

Contraindications/Precautions

PREG
🖐

Contraindicated in hypersensitivity to indomethacin, other nonsteroidal anti-inflammatory drugs, or aspirin, or in history of or currently active GI disease, and nasal polyps associated with angioedema. **Use with caution** in history of psychiatric illness, epilepsy, Parkinson's disease, renal or hepatic impairment, coagulation defects, and comprised cardiac function.

🖐 **Contraindicated for nursing mothers. Use with caution for the elderly. Safe use for children under 14 years (except for patent ductus arteriosis in neonates) and pregnant women has not been established (first two trimesters, preg B; in third trimester, preg D).**

Side effects/Adverse reactions

Hypersensitivity: asthma symptoms, urticaria, nasal polyps, angioedema, and bronchospasm. **GI:** epigastric distress, nausea, peptic ulcers. **CNS:** headache, dizziness, fatigue, muscle weakness, ataxia, aggravation of depression or other psychiatric disturbances, epilepsy, and parkinsonism. **CV:** peripheral edema. **Eye:** visual disturbances such as blurring. **Hem:** elevated LDH, serum transaminase, and alkaline phosphatase; increased AST, ALT, bilirubin, BUN; positive direct Coombs' test; hyperkalemia; hyperglycemia in diabetics; prolonged bleeding time; and decreased platelet count, hemoglobin, and hematocrit. **Misc:** reactivation of latent infections.

Nursing implications/Documentation

Possible nursing diagnoses: Pain; Impaired physical mobility.

♦ Establish a baseline for CBC, electrolytes, prothrombin time, BUN, creatinine, and liver function studies; if therapy is prolonged, monitor periodically thereafter.

♦ Schedule doses so that drug is given at least 1 hr before maximum mobility is needed.

♦ Monitor for and report GI symptoms that may indicate peptic ulcer (nausea, pain, black stools); also watch for signs of bleeding tendencies (check urine and gums).

♦ Record weight every other day; report edema or sudden weight gain.

♦ For diabetics, monitor blood sugar closely since insulin requirements may change.

Patient & family teaching/Home care

Possible nursing diagnoses: Altered health maintenance; Knowledge deficit.

♦ Advise taking doses with food to reduce GI symptoms; explain the importance of watching for symptoms of GI bleeding (black stools, persistent GI distress).

♦ Explain that it will take 3–5 days to produce desired effects.

♦ Stress the need to avoid aspirin, alcohol, and other OTC drugs (unless approved by physician) because of increased risk of GI bleeding.

♦ Instruct to hold drug and report if any of the following side effects are experienced: vertigo, rashes, blood in urine, hearing or visual changes, sudden weight gain, edema.

♦ Warn against driving or activities that require alertness until response is determined (may cause drowsiness and dizziness at first; this should be transient).

♦ Reinforce the need for medical follow-up; advise telling dentist that indomethacin is being taken.

♦ For diabetics, explain the importance of monitoring blood sugars with a blood glucose meter.

♦ *See Nonsteroidal anti-inflammatory drugs overview for more information.*

insulin

in'su-lin

Rapid—acting insulin: insulin injection (regular insulin, crystalline zinc insulin): **▲Actrapid HM, ▲Actrapid HM Penfill, ▲Actrapid MC, ▲Actrapid MC Penfill, Beef Regular Iletin II, Humulin R, ▲Hypurin Neutral, ▲Insulin 2, Novolin R, Novolin R Penfill, Pork Regular Iletin II, Regular (Concentrated) Iletin II, Regular Iletin I, Regular Purified Pork Insulin, Velosulin, ▲Velosulin Human, Velosulin Insuject.**

insulin zinc suspension, prompt (semilente): **Semilente Iletin I, Semilente Insulin, ▲Semilente MC Pork, Semilente Purified Pork**

Intermediate-acting insulin: isophane insulin suspension (neutral protamine Hagedorn Insulin, NPH): **Beef NPH Iletin II, Humulin N, ▲Humulin NPH, ▲Hypurin Isophane, ▲Insulatard, Insulatard Human, Insulatard NPH, ▲Isotard MC, Novolin N, NPH Iletin I, NPH Insulin, NPH Purified Pork, Pork NPH Iletin II, ▲Protaphane HM, ▲Protaphane HM Penfill, ▲Protaphane MC**

insulin zinc suspension (lente): **Humulin L, Lente Iletin I, Lente Iletine II, Lente Insulin, ▲Lente MC, Lente Purified Pork Insulin, ▲Monotard HM, ▲Monotard MC, Novolin L**

Long—acting insulin: protamine zinc suspension (PZI): **Protamine, Zinc & Iletin I, Protamine, Zinc & Iletin II (Beef), Protamine, Zinc & Iletin II (Pork), ▲Protamine Zinc Insulin MC**

insulin zinc suspension, extended (ultralente): **Ultralente Iletin I, Ultralente Insulin, Ultralente Purified Beef, ▲Ultratard HM, ▲Ultratard MC**

Insulin mixture: isophane insulin suspension with insulin injection: **▲Actraphane HM, ▲Actraphane HM Penfill, ▲Actraphane MC, Mixtard, ▲Mixtard Human, Novolin 70/30**

Class: ★**Antidiabetic prototype (insulin)**, hormone

Antidote: $D_{50}W$, glucagon

PEDS	PREG	GERI
OK	B	OK

Action Reduces serum glucose and enhances cellular nutrition by allowing glucose to pass from the bloodstream into liver and muscle cells; promotes protein synthesis by moving amino acids into cells; prevents the breakdown of fats as a source of energy by promoting the metabolism of carbohydrates. Also reduces serum potassium, phosphate, and lactate. Pharmacokinetics are listed as follows:

Insulin	Onset	Peak	Duration
Regular IV	10–30 min	15–30 min	30–60 min
Regular SC	30–60 min	2–5 hr	5–7 hr
Semilente	1–2 hr	5–10 hr	12–16 hr
NPH	1–2 hr	4–12 hr	24–28 hr
Lente	1–3 hr	6–15 hr	24–28 hr
PZI	4–8 hr	14–24 hr	36 hr
Ultralente	4–8 hr	10–30 hr	36 hr
Mixture	15–60 min	2–8 hr	24 hr

Use/Therapeutic goal/Outcome

Type I (insulin-dependent, or IDDM) diabetes mellitus, and Type II (noninsulin-dependent, or NIDDM) diabetes mellitus, hyperglycemia, ketoacidosis, and diabetic coma: Normalization of blood glucose levels. *Outcome criteria:* Absence of clinical symptoms of hypoglycemia (confusion, shakiness, weakness, diaphoresis, apprehension) together with blood glucose studies that demonstrate glycemic control (fasting blood sugar: 100–140 mg/dl is good control, 140–200 mg/dl is fair control; for gestational diabetics, a fasting blood sugar less than 100 mg/dl, preferably 60–80 mg/dl, is good control.)

Dose range/Administration

Interaction alert: Never mix NPH insulin with semilente, ultra, or ultralente insulin. Use mixtures of short and intermediate insulins within 5 minutes of mixing to avoid conversion of short-acting insulin to longer-acting insulin. Corticosteroids and thiazide diuretics diminish insulin response (monitor for hyperglycemia). Beta-adrenergic blockers potentiate hypoglycemic effects of insulin and may mask clinical signs of hypoglycemia. Thyroid preparations, estrogens, and smoking may increase risk of hyperglycemia. Alcohol, MAOIs, salicylates, and tetracycline may prolong hypoglycemia.

Maintenance therapy for Type I diabetes mellitus and Type II diabetes inadequately controlled by diet and oral agents: **Adult and Child:** SC: Dose individualized by physician and adjusted according to serum glucose levels, activity, diet and tolerance. Give doses before meals, immediately after checking blood sugar.

Diabetic ketoacidosis (regular insulin only): **Adult:** IV, SC: 25–150 units IV immediately, followed by additional doses q1h, based on hourly blood sugars until stable, then change to SC q6h; or 50–100 units IV with 50–100 units SC immediately, then additional SC doses q2-6h based on blood sugars; or IV bolus of 0.33 units/kg or smaller boluses of 5–10 units, followed by 7–10 units/hr continuous infusion. **Child:** IV, SC: 0.5 to 1 unit/kg, half

IV and half SC, then 0.5 to 1 unit/kg IV q1-2h based on blood sugars; or 0.1 unit/kg IV bolus, then continuous infusion of 0.1 unit/kg/hr until blood sugar drops to 250 mg/dl, then begin SC dosing.

Clinical alert: **Read all labels carefully because insulin comes in different forms and concentrations.** For IV route use regular insulin only because other insulin preparations are suspensions that can cause harm if given IV. Human insulin is used during pregnancy, for those who are hypersensitive to pork and beef, and when glycemic control is difficult. Dose requirements vary with age, food intake, activity levels, and concurrent medical problems.

Contraindications/Precautions

PREG
B

Contraindicated in coma unless blood sugars done immediately before dose, and (for pork and beef insulins) in hypersensitivity to pork or beef.

🖐 **Use with caution for pregnant women (insulin requirements may increase drastically).**

Side effects/Adverse reactions

Hypersensitivity: rashes; lymphadenopathy, development of antiinsulin antibodies, swelling, itching, and redness at injection site. *Skin:* lipoatrophy and lipohypertrophy at injection site (except for human insulin). *Hem:* hypoglycemia, hyperinsulinism resulting in rebound hyperglycemia (Somogyi effect) and insulin resistance. *Misc:* clinical signs and symptoms of mild hypoglycemia (hunger, shakiness, weakness, apprehension, sweating), moderate hypoglycemia (gait disturbances, confusion, agitation, visual disturbances), and severe hypoglycemia (seizures, coma).

Nursing implications/Documentation

Possible nursing diagnoses: Potential for injury; Impaired skin integrity; Impaired tissue integrity; Altered nutrition: more than body requirements; Altered nutrition: less than body requirements.

♦ Ascertain baseline blood sugar before giving first dose and monitor closely thereafter; check blood glucose ½ hr before each meal and before hs snack. Keep a record of blood sugars, and report persistent trends in hyperglycemia or hypoglycemia or isolated episodes of significant hypoglycemia or hyperglycemia.

♦ Monitor food intake; notify physician when patient is not eating.

♦ Recognize that diabetics are at special risk for electrolyte imbalance, kidney failure, cardiac disease, vascular pathology, GI symptoms (nausea, vomiting, constipation, diarrhea), and neuropathy; monitor electrolytes (especially potassium), BUN, and creatinine carefully, and report abnormalities.

♦ Record and monitor daily weights, especially during periods of illness; notify physician of significant weight gain or loss.

♦ Establish a plan for rotation of injection sites; document injection sites and allow about 1 inch between injection sites (try not to reuse a site for 6–8 weeks).

♦ Observe injection sites for manifestations of lipoatrophy and lipohypertrophy (less common for individuals using human insulin).

♦ If signs of hypoglycemia (shakiness, sweating, sudden weakness, pale skin, anxiety, confusion, agitation) are noted, confirm by a capillary blood glucose test first, then give 15 g of a fast-acting carbohydrate (4 oz of fruit juice, 4–6 pieces of hard candy, 1 tablespoon of sugar or honey). If blood glucose meter is not immediately available, then give carbohydrate and check glucose level later.

♦ If signs of hyperglycemia (extreme thirst, frequent urination, fruity breath, lethargy, coma) are noted, confirm by blood glucose meter and report immediately to physician; expect administration of IV regular insulin and rehydration with normal saline solution (before infusing an insulin drip, prime the tubing with 50–100 ml of solution).

♦ Monitor neonates of mothers who have received insulin for hyperglycemia or hypoglycemia.

Patient & family teaching/Home care

Possible nursing diagnoses: Knowledge deficit; Impaired home maintenance management.

♦ Explain that insulin controls blood sugars but does not cure diabetes. Stress that medical supervision and careful regulation of insulin and diet, based upon frequent blood sugar monitoring, help promote health and prevent the long-term complications of diabetes (heart, kidney, eyes).

♦ Emphasize that diet, activity, illness, and emotional stress greatly affect insulin requirements (especially in children); stress that hypoglycemia may be caused by excess exercise, profuse sweating, skipped or delayed meals, or decreased carbohydrate intake.

• Stress that everything on meal plan should be eaten, especially carbohydrates, but that concentrated sweets should be avoided.

• Point out that insulin should be continued during illness despite inability to tolerate food (insulin requirements may even increase), and that physician should be contacted.

• Teach the signs and symptoms of hypoglycemia and hyperglycemia; explain the importance of checking blood sugar when symptomatic. If a glucose monitoring device is not available, advise that a fast-acting carbohydrate (4 oz of fruit juice, 4–6 pieces of hard candy, 1 tablespoon of honey or sugar) should be given if these symptoms of *hypo*glycemia should appear. Symptoms of *hyper*glycemia should be reported immediately to the physician.

• Emphasize that those with Type I diabetes, particularly children, are more prone to ketoacidosis than those with Type II diabetes. During stress or illness, advise checking urine for ketones when blood sugar is greater than 240 mg/dl.

• Advise reporting persistent symptoms of nausea, vomiting, fatigue, thirst, and frequent urination.

• Suggest carrying some form of fast-acting carbohydrate (e.g., hard candy or raisins) for treatment of hypoglycemia.

• Warn against drinking alcohol and taking OTC drugs without physician's approval.

• Demonstrate how to manage technique of insulin self-injection, including all the teaching points listed below.

• Review species (whether pork, beef, or human), brand, and type of insulin; stress that insulin brands should not be switched or mixed.

• Explain importance of storing insulin in a refrigerator, unless it is used within 1 month (then it may be stored at room temperature). Prefilled syringes are stable for 3 weeks with refrigeration.

• Suggest keeping an extra vial of insulin on hand.

• Teach the need to roll cloudy insulin before preparing doses (avoid shaking), and to inspect vials of cloudy insulin for clumping or frosting (vials that are granular, discolored, or expired should be discarded). Explain that the only insulin that should be clear is regular insulin (if it is not, it should be discarded).

• Inform that most insulin syringes come in U-100 and that syringes are sold in sizes of 0.3 ml, 0.5 ml and 1 ml (0.3 ml and 0.5 ml are marked in increments of 1 unit, 1-ml size is marked in increments of 2 units). Stress that syringes should never be shared; used syringes should be disposed of in a closed, puncture-proof container.

• Demonstrate technique for mixing two insulins in one syringe and observe return demonstration.

• Provide an insulin injection chart that depicts injection sites; stress that rotation reduces risk of lipodystrophy. Advise that insulin is usually given SC (not IM) 15–60 min before meals so that peak effectiveness will coincide with increased blood sugar levels.

• For adults, explain that injection angle should be 90 degrees, for children, 45 degrees. Stress that aspiration is not recommended.

• Advise those planning to engage in active sports to inject insulin into the abdomen or buttocks to prevent rapid insulin absorption from actively used limbs (helps prevent hypoglycemia).

• Stress need to report allergic reactions immediately.

• Recommend wearing a medical alert bracelet to alert others to insulin use and risk of hypoglycemia.

• Assist those with visual impairment to select appropriate equipment, and suggest contacting local community resources such as the local chapter of the American Diabetes Association for support.

• *See Antidiabetics overview for more information.*

interferon

in-ter-fere'-on

alfa-2a, recombinant (rIFN–A): *Roferon-A*
interferon alfa-2b, recombinant (IFN–alpha 2): *Intron-A*

Class: Antineoplastic agent, Biological response modifier

PEDS	PREG	GERI
✋	C	✋

Action Suppresses malignant tumor cell proliferation by destroying viral RNA, and activates the body's immune mechanism by the attachment of interferons to specific membrane receptors on the cell's surface.

Use/Therapeutic goal/Outcome

Hairy cell leukemia, condylomata acuminata, Kaposi's sarcoma, malignant melanoma: Elimination or suppression of malignant cell proliferation. ***Outcome criteria:*** Tumor and disease regression or stabilization on radiologic and physical examination; for leukemias, absence of blasts in peripheral blood specimen.

Dose range/Administration

Interaction alert: Reduced clearance of aminophylline when given concurrently. CNS depressants increase risk of adverse CNS effects. Use with other cytotoxic agents may cause severe myelosuppression.

Hairy cell leukemia: Adult (alfa-2a): IM, SC: *Induction dose:* 3 million IU/day for 16–24 weeks. *Maintenance dose:* 3–6 million IU, 3 times a week. ***Adult (alfa-2b):*** IM, SC: *Induction and maintenance dose:* 2 million IU/m^2, 3 times a week.

Condylomata acuminata: Adult (alfa-2b): *Intralesion:* (by physician) 1 million IU, 3 times a week for 3 weeks; may be used for 5 lesions at a time.

Kaposi's sarcoma: Adult (alfa-2a): IM, SC: *Induction dose:* 36 million IU/day for 10–12 weeks. *Maintenance dose:* 36 million IU, 3 times a week. ***Adult (alfa-2b):*** IM, SC: 30 million IU/m^2, 3 times a week.

Clinical alert: Obtain baseline laboratory results prior to therapy. If platelet count is <50,000/mm^3, hold drug and report (dosage may be reduced by 50% or therapy stopped). Administer SC rather than IM for those with a platelet count <100,000/mm^3. For alpha-2a, leukocyte count drops to nadir (lowest point) at 22–38 days and platelet count drops at 17–19 days; recovery occurs within a few weeks after therapy is stopped. With alpha-2b, platelet and WBC counts drop to the nadir (lowest point) within 3–5 days, and recovers 3–5 days after therapy is stopped.

Contraindications/Precautions

PREG C

Contraindicated in hypersensitivity to interferon, and in unstable angina, and CHF. ***Use with caution*** in severe cardiac, renal or hepatic disease, seizure disorders, CNS dysfunction, pulmonary disease, chickenpox, herpes zoster, myelosuppression, bleeding tendencies, and diabetes.

Contraindicated for children and pregnant or nursing mothers. Use with caution for the elderly.

Side effects/Adverse reactions

Hypersensitivity: urticaria, angioedema, bronchoconstriction, anaphylaxis. ***GI:*** anorexia, nausea, vomiting, diarrhea, change in taste sensation, stomatitis, abnormal liver function. ***MS:*** weight loss. ***Hem:*** neutropenia, leukopenia, thrombocytopenia, anemia. ***CNS:*** dizziness, confusion, paresthesias, depression, sleep disturbances, amnesia. ***Resp:*** cough, dyspnea. ***CV:*** hypotension, hypertension, chest pain, edema, dysrhythmias, CHF. ***Eye:*** visual disturbances. ***Skin:*** partial alopecia, rash, dry skin, itching, flushing, diaphoresis. ***GU:*** transient impotence, dysmenorrhea. ***Misc:*** flu-like syndrome with fatigue, myalgia, headache, chills, and arthralgia (occurs in the majority of patients; symptoms subside as therapy continues).

I

Nursing implications/Documentation

Possible nursing diagnoses: Potential for infection; Potential for injury; Fatigue; Altered oral mucous membrane; Fluid volume deficit; Diarrhea, Altered nutrition: less than body requirements.

◆ *See important Nursing implications in Antineoplastic agents overview on page 72, which apply to all antineoplastics. The interventions that follow are additional and specific to this drug only.*

◆ Monitor for and report CNS side effects (confusion, dizziness, tingling or numbness of the extremities) and CV side effects (chest pain, changes in cardiac rhythm, hyper- or hypotension); be aware that prolonged cough or difficulty breathing may be signs of pulmonary toxicity.

◆ Consult with physician about use of mild antipyretics and analgesics to relieve the common side effect of flu-like syndrome; plan doses at bedtime to minimize these symptoms.

◆ Increase fluid intake to 2–3 L a day prior to starting interferon; document and monitor intake and output (report significant negative or positive balance).

◆ If the platelet count is less than 50,000 mm^3, use SC route.

◆ Be aware that if there is no response after 6 weeks of therapy, interferon should be discontinued.

Patient & family teaching/Home care

Possible nursing diagnoses: Knowledge deficit; Ineffective family coping; Hopelessness; Impaired home maintenance management.

- *See important Patient & family teaching in Antineoplastic agents overview on page 72, which apply to all antineoplastics. The teachings that follow are additional and specific to this drug only.*

  - Stress the need to drink 2–3 L of fluid per day (if the patient can't keep fluids down, IV fluids may be necessary).
  - Reassure that flu-like side effects are likely to diminish as the body becomes accustomed to dosage; advise that taking doses at bedtime and using acetominophen can help reduce symptoms.
  - Ascertain that the patient or caretaker is able to manage SC administration; point out that different brands of interferon are not interchangeable (the 2a and the 2b have different dosages).
  - Advise reporting changes in mental status, muscle weakness, numbness or tingling of extremities, persistent cough, or difficulty breathing, palpitations, or chest pain immediately.
  - Point out that CNS depressants and alcohol should be avoided.

- *See Antineoplastic agents overview for more information.*

eye'oh-di-nay-ted gli'ser-all

iodinated glycerol

Iophen Elixir, Myodine, Organidin, R-Ger Elixir

Class: Expectorant

PEDS	PREG	GERI
✋	X	✋

Action Enhances ability to expectorate by stimulating respiratory tract secretory glands, which reduces viscosity and adhesiveness of the secretions. The efficacy of this drug has not been established.

Use/Therapeutic goal/Outcome

Bronchial asthma, bronchitis, emphysema, chronic sinusitis: Promotion of expectoration, removal of secretions. ***Outcome criteria:*** Report and demonstration of increased ability to bring forth mucous; clearing of lung fields.

Dose range/Administration

When possible, give doses with a full glass of water to promote hydration.

Adult: PO: *Tablets:* 60 mg qid. *Solution:* dilute 20 drops in liquid qid. *Elixir:* 5 cc qid. ***Child:*** PO: Up to half the adult dose, based on weight.

Contraindications/Precautions

PREG X

Contraindicated in hypersensitivity to iodides. ***Use with caution*** in thyroid disease.

✋ **Contraindicated in pregnancy and lactation. Monitor children and the elderly for adequate dose management.**

Side effects/Adverse reactions

Hypersensitivity: rash. ***GI:*** gastric and intestinal irritation, parotitis, mouth and throat ulcers, increased salivation, metallic taste. ***Hem:*** reversible iodism. ***Resp:*** rhinitis. ***CNS:*** headache. ***With prolonged use:*** iodism, hypothyroidism.

Nursing implications/Documentation

Possible nursing diagnoses: Ineffective airway clearance; Fluid volume deficit.

- Record lung sounds and sputum production to monitor effectiveness; report cough that lasts longer than a week.
- Provide preferred fluids to promote hydration.

Patient & family teaching/Home care

Possible nursing diagnoses: Knowledge deficit; Impaired home maintenance management.

- Advise reporting a rash or an increase in breathing problems, because it may indicate a need to stop this drug.
- Stress the importance of adequate hydration; advise taking doses with a full glass of water.
- Point out that increased environmental humidity with decreased environmental irritants (e.g., smoke) can minimize aggravating factors.
- Advise reporting a cough that persists longer than a week.

- *See Antitussives, Expectorants, and Mucolytics overview for more information.*

iodoquinol
eye-oh-do-kwin'ole

♣ Diodoquin, Moebiquin, Yodoxin

Class: Anti-infective, Amebicide, Antiprotozoal

PEDS	PREG	GERI
🖐	C	🖐

Action Kills amoebas (amebical action) in the intestinal lumen. Exact mechanism of action has not been established.

Use/Therapeutic goal/Outcome

Intestinal amoebas: Elimination of intestinal amoebas. *Outcome criteria:* Absence of amoebas in stools for 1 year (then person is considered cured).

Dose range/Administration

🖐 **Give after meals to reduce GI symptoms (may crush and give with syrup or something sweet).**

Adult: PO: 630–650 mg tid for 20 days. *Maximum dose:* 2 g/day. **Child:** PO: 30–40 mg/kg/day divided bid or tid for 20 days. Wait 2–3 weeks if repeat course is necessary.

Clinical alert: Report diarrhea that lasts longer than 3 days.

Contraindications/Precautions

PREG C

Contraindicated in hypersensitivity to iodoquinol, iodine, or 8–hydroxyquinoline, and in renal or liver disease, severe thyroid disease, optic neuropathy.

🖐 **Use with caution in children (more likely to have side effects) and the elderly. Safe use for pregnant or nursing mothers has not been established.**

Side effects/Adverse reactions

Hypersensitivity: itching, rashes, hives. **GI:** anorexia, cramping, nausea, vomiting, diarrhea, constipation, epigastric discomfort, gastritis, anal itching or irritation. **Skin:** boils. **Eye:** optic neuritis, optic atrophy, permanent loss of vision. **CNS:** neurotoxicity (higher doses), weakness, vertigo, malaise, headache, nervousness, retrograde amnesia, ataxia, peripheral neuropathy. **Misc:** thyroid enlargement, fever, chills.

Nursing implications/Documentation

Possible nursing diagnoses: Potential for infection; Fluid volume deficit.

◆ Obtain necessary cultures before first dose (stool specimens should go to the lab while still warm).

◆ Provide preferred fluids; monitor and document intake and output to ensure adequate hydration.

◆ Determine other family members or close contacts who should be evaluated for intestinal amoebas.

Patient & family teaching/Home care

Possible nursing diagnoses: Knowledge deficit, Impaired home maintenance management.

◆ Advise holding medication and reporting symptoms of allergy (see hypersensitivity side effects) or blurred vision.

◆ Teach the importance of good handwashing after bowel movements and of daily cleansing of toilets.

◆ Point out the need to take iodoquinol for the entire time prescribed, even if symptoms abate.

◆ Stress that a cure is not certain until stools have been negative for 1 year; therefore, the person should return for follow-up lab studies.

◆ *See Anti-infectives overview for more information.*

ipecac syrup
ip'i-kak

Class: Emetic

PEDS	PREG	GERI
OK	C	🖐

Action Induces vomiting by acting centrally on the chemoreceptor trigger zone and locally on the gastric mucosa.

Use/Therapeutic goal/Outcome

Emergency treatment of noncaustic poison or drug ingestion: Prevention of absorption of poisons or drugs. *Outcome criteria:* Vomiting within 30 min of administration.

Dose range/Administration

Interaction alert: Since ipecac syrup neutralizes the effect of activated charcoal, hold activated charcoal doses until *after* vomiting has occurred.

Adult: PO: 15 ml, followed by 1–2 glasses of water. May repeat in 20–30 min if vomiting hasn't occurred. **Child < 1 yr:** PO: 5–10 ml followed by 1/2–1 glass of water. May repeat in 20–30 min if vomiting hasn't occurred. **Child > 1 yr:** PO: 15 ml, followed by 1/2–1 glass of water. May repeat in 20–30 min if vomiting hasn't occurred.

Clinical alert: Do not confuse with *ipecac fluidextract*, which is 14 times stronger. Look specifically for both words, *ipecac syrup* (not just ipecac) on the label. No more than 2 doses should be given because of cardiotoxicity.

Contraindications/Precautions

Contraindicated in hypersensitivity to ipecac and in those who have a history of esophageal stricture or other esophageal disease, those who are semicomatose, inebriated, unconscious, seizing, in shock, or with depressed gag reflex (because of risk of aspiration); in ingestion of strong acids, alkalis, other corrosive substance, strychnine, petroleum, or volatile oils.

Ⓦ **Contraindicated for pregnant or nursing mothers. Use with caution for the elderly.**

Side effects/Adverse reactions

Hypersensitivity: prolonged "dry heaves."

If the drug is not vomited, but absorbed: **CNS:** CNS depression. **CV:** cardiac arrhythmias. **GI:** diarrhea, (with violent vomiting) hematemesis, esophageal rupture.

Nursing implications/Documentation

Possible nursing diagnoses: Potential for aspiration; Fear.

◆ Determine exact type of ingested substance, and be sure substance is not caustic before administration of ipecac.

◆ To speed desired effects, be sure full amount of water is taken, and encourage activity (e.g., gently bounce small children on lap).

◆ If child refuses fluids, may add small amount of sugar, food coloring, and/or flavoring to water to make it more desirable.

◆ Have a large emesis basin readily available, and supply parents with a gown/apron for protection.

◆ Notify physician if vomiting doesn't occur within 20–30 min (second dose or lavage may be necessary).

◆ Offer frequent mouth care.

Patient & family teaching/Home care

Possible nursing diagnoses: Impaired home maintenance management.

◆ Advise keeping ipecac syrup available at home, but stress the need for calling poison control *before* giving ipecac; suggest keeping poison control phone number with ipecac with a note stating "call poison control first."

◆ Teach that ipecac syrup can be purchased OTC in small doses and that doses should be replaced yearly.

◆ Explore whether the home is "child proof" and reinforce the importance of prevention.

◆ Caution that ipecac has been known to be chronically abused by bulimics.

ipratropium

i-pra-troe'pee-um

Atrovent

Class: Anticholinergic bronchodilator

PEDS   PREG   GERI
 Ⓦ   B   Ⓦ

Action Produces bronchodilation by inhibiting cholinergic receptors of bronchial smooth muscle.

Use/Therapeutic goal/Outcome

Bronchospasm associated with COPD: Reduction in airway resistance; improvement of air movement. *Outcome criteria:* Report of decrease in or absence of respiratory distress; improved forced expiratory volume (FEV).

Dose range/Administration

Adult: *Inhal:* 2 inhalations (26 mcg) qid, and prn, to a maximum of 12 inhalations in 24 hr.

Clinical alert: Monitor for and report deterioration in symptoms. Not for rapid relief of acute bronchospasm, because its effect is not noted for 15 min.

Contraindications/Precautions

Contraindicated in hypersensitivity to ipratropium, atropine, or related anticholinergics. *Use with caution* in narrow-angle glaucoma, prostatic hypertrophy, or bladder-neck obstruction.

Ⓦ **Use with caution for the elderly. Safe use for children and pregnant women has not been established.**

Side effects/Adverse reactions

Hypersensitivity: skin rash, hives. **CNS:** nervousness, headache, dizziness. **Resp:** cough, worsening of symptoms. **CV:** palpitations. **GI:** nausea, upset stomach, dry mouth. **Eye:** blurred vision.

Nursing implications/Documentation

Possible nursing diagnoses: Activity intolerance; Ineffective breathing pattern.

♦ Determine and record known allergies; provide an environment that is free from allergens (e.g., use air conditioning).

♦ Document lung sounds, respirations, pulse, and blood pressure, before and after dose administration, until response is determined.

♦ Provide favorite fluids, and monitor intake and output to ensure adequate hydration (at least 2 L a day is recommended).

Patient & family teaching/Home care

Possible nursing diagnoses: Knowledge deficit; Impaired home maintenance management; Fear.

♦ Explain that this drug will enlarge air passages and make breathing easier.

♦ Point out that stress and exercise can aggravate wheezing and bronchospasm, and that relaxation, controlled breathing techniques, and controlled exercise programs can help reduce severity and frequency of wheezing episodes.

♦ Give written and verbal instructions on how to use inhalers (shake container, exhale completely, hold mouthpiece to mouth with canister upside down, inhale deeply through mouth while pressing the canister base once, hold breath a few seconds, remove mouthpiece and exhale, then wait 1 minute and repeat).

♦ Instruct to report deterioration in symptoms, instead of increasing dose.

♦ Warn that accidental spraying in the eyes may cause blurred vision.

♦ Teach that inhaling ipratropium 5 minutes before cromolyn or steroid inhalers produces bronchodilation and allows better medication deposits deep in the airways.

♦ *See Bronchodilators and Cholinergics overviews for more information.*

iron dextran

Hydextran, Imferon, K-FeRON
Class: Antianemic

PEDS	PREG	GERI
♌	C	♌

Action Directly replaces iron, an essential component of hemoglobin.

Use/Therapeutic goal/Outcome

For iron deficiency anemia: Replenishment of deficient iron blood levels, promotion of hemoglobin formation. **Outcome criteria:** Hemoglobin, hematocrit, reticulocyte count, serum iron-binding capacity, and serum iron within normal limits.

Dose range/Administration

Interaction alert: Do not mix IV doses with any other drug. Mix only with NS.

Adult: IM: Z-Track, after test dose of 0.5 cc. **Adults > 50 kg:** 50 mg the first day, then up to 250 mg qod until the total calculated dose is given (calculated from tables by physician). **Adults < 50 kg:** use pediatric dose. IV: (Check hospital policy to ensure that iron dextran may be given IV. IV route is not recommended unless IM route is unfeasible [safety of IV administration is controversial].) 15–30 mg on the first day; may increase by 10 mg/day until hemoglobin level returns to normal. *Maximum dose:* 100 mg/day. Have physician determine IV rate; monitor vital signs closely (some reactions are severe). **Child:** IM: Z-track, after a test dose of 0.5 cc. **Children 9–50 kg:** maximum of 100 mg/day. **Infants 3.5–9 kg:** maximum of 25 mg/day.

Clinical alert: Use only if oral administration of iron is impossible or ineffective. Discontinue oral doses before starting parenteral administration. Give a 0.5 cc test dose before the first therapeutic dose, because allergic reactions can be severe. Wait at least 1 hour before administering therapeutic dose. Dosage is determined by physician from tables or by calculating according to weight with an appropriate formula (there are several).

Contraindications/Precautions
PREG
C

Contraindicated in hypersensitivity to iron dextran in hemochromatosis, hemosiderosis, and for all anemias except iron deficiency anemias. **Use with caution** in asthma, allergies, alcoholism, repeated blood transfusions, rheumatoid arthritis, ankylosing spondylitis, impaired liver or kidney function.

♘ **Safe use for pregnant women, and of IV route for children, has not been established. Use with caution for children and the elderly.**

Side effects/Adverse reactions

Hypersensitivity: itching, rash, fever, chills, muscle and joint pain, dyspnea, severe anaphylaxis. **GI:** abdominal pain, nausea, vomiting, metallic taste. **CV:** rapid IV rate may cause hypotension, precordial pain or pressure, tachycardia, fatal arrhythmias, shock; IV administration may also cause phlebitis. **Hem:** (with IV route) hemosiderosis. **Skin:** pain, sterile abscess, and brown discoloration of skin at IM site. **Misc:** lymphadenopathy.

Nursing implications/Documentation

Possible nursing diagnoses: Activity intolerance; Altered nutrition: less than body requirements; Fatigue; Impaired skin integrity.

♦ For IM route, use Z-track technique to avoid leakage into subcutaneous tissue. Use 2–3 inch 19G or 20G needle; change needle after withdrawing solution and before injecting (never inject into deltoid; preferred site is ventrogluteal muscle of the buttocks).

♦ Report allergic reaction immediately; if route is IV, stop infusion immediately and report. After IV administration, keep patient in bed for 15–30 minutes.

♦ Monitor hemoglobin, hematocrit, and reticulocyte count to determine therapeutic effect.

♦ Provide a balance between rest and activity.

Patient & family teaching/Home care

Possible nursing diagnoses: Knowledge deficit; Impaired home maintenance management.

♦ Teach the dietary sources high in iron (fish, liver, chicken, and leafy, green vegetables); emphasize that increased dietary iron intake may reduce the need for iron replacement.

♦ Instruct the patient to report shortness of breath and unusual symptoms immediately.

♦ Stress the need to balance daily activities to allow for adequate rest.

♦ *See Antianemics overview for more information.*

isocarboxazid

eye-soe-kar-box'a-zid

Marplan

Class: Monoamine oxidase inhibitor (MAOI), Antidepressant

PEDS	PREG	GERI
🖐	C	🖐

Action Improves mood by promoting accumulation of the neurotransmitters norepinephrine, serotonin, and dopamine in the CNS (inhibits monoamine oxidase, the major enzyme responsible for the breakdown of neurotransmitters).

Use/Therapeutic goal/Outcome

Major depressive disorders that have not responded to other treatment, including TCAs: Promotion of sense of well-being, ability to cope with daily living. **Outcome criteria:** After 2–4 weeks, report of feeling less depressed, less anxious, and more energetic and able to cope; return of normal sleeping and eating habits; demonstration of improved ability to problem solve and perform activities of daily living.

Dose range/Administration

Interaction alert: MAOIs such as this drug have a strong potential for severe and unpredictable side effects when taken with other medications: check with pharmacist to ascertain most recent information on interactions. It is known that use with alcohol, barbiturates, sedatives, narcotics, dextromethorphan, and TCAs have produced a variety of problems; use with amphetamines, ephedrine, levodopa, meperidine, metaraminol, phenylephrine, and phenylpropanolamine can cause severe hypertension. Monitor diabetics for altered hypoglycemic requirements. There is a potential for fatal hypertensive crisis if taken with tryptophan or food or beverages containing tyramine (aged cheese or wine, beer, avocados, chicken livers, chocolate, bananas, soy sauce, meat tenderizers, salami, or bologna).

Adult: PO: Begin with 30 mg/day in divided dose. When improvement is noted, decrease to lowest dose that relieves symptoms (usually 10–20 mg).

Clinical alert: Because of the many unpredictable food and drug interactions (see Interaction alert), monitor diet and medication regimen closely. Hold drug and report if hypertension is noted. Keep phentolamine (Regitine) available to treat hypertension.

Contraindications/Precautions

PREG
C

Contraindicated in hypersensitivity to MAOIs, and in cardiac, renal, or hepatic disease, alcoholism, hypertension, and pheochromocytoma. **Use with caution** in suicidal tendency, seizure disorders, psychosis, diabetes mellitus, and hyperactive behavior.

🖐 **Contraindicated for children under 16 years, pregnant or nursing mothers, and the elderly.**

Side effects/Adverse reactions

Hypersensitivity: rash. **CNS:** insomnia, dizziness, anxiety, headache, restlessness, hyperreflexia, tremors, muscle twitching, mania, confusion, memory impairment, fatigue, sedation. **CV:** orthostatic hypotension, palpitations, dysrhythmias, hypertensive crisis. **GI:** anorexia, dry mouth, nausea, diarrhea, constipation. **GU:** urinary frequency, decreased libido. **Eye:** blurred vision. **MS:** weight gain.

Nursing implications/Documentation

Possible nursing diagnoses: Potential for injury; Diarrhea; Constipation; Altered oral mucous membrane.

♦ Document mental status and vital signs daily until response to therapy has been established; then periodically thereafter.

♦ Check CBC, liver function, BUN, and creatinine before giving first dose and periodically thereafter.

♦ Be sure that doses are swallowed (not hoarded).

♦ Monitor for orthostatic hypotension, dizziness, and drowsiness; supervise ambulation until response is established.

♦ Record weights every 2 weeks; report significant weight gain.

♦ Monitor for and report suicidal tendencies, increased depression, or excessive hyperactivity.

♦ Prevent constipation by monitoring bowel movements and encouraging adequate fiber and fluid intake; offer laxatives or stool softeners before the problem becomes severe. Report diarrhea.

♦ Check with pharmacy and dietary department to determine dietary restrictions for MAOIs; continue restrictions for 10 days after stopping drug because effects last a long time.

Patient & family teaching/Home care

Possible nursing diagnoses: Ineffective coping (family and individual); Sleep pattern disturbance; Impaired home maintenance management.

♦ Stress that this medication helps reduce the depression that inhibits ability to make decisions and cope effectively (once the individual feels less depressed, it will be easier to take steps toward making healthy changes).

♦ Provide a list of foods that must be avoided; emphasize the need to stick to restrictions.

♦ Explain that side effects are often noted immediately, but they usually diminish after a few weeks; on the other hand, it is likely to take 2–4 weeks before *beneficial* effects are noted (the patient may feel worse before feeling better).

♦ Warn to change positions slowly to prevent dizziness.

♦ Point out the role of adequate nutrition, exercise, and sleep in combating depression.

♦ Emphasize that the effects of alcohol, sedatives, and tranquilizers may be potentiated.

♦ Caution to consult physician before using OTC drugs; stress the need for ongoing medical follow-up.

♦ Recommend reporting continued depression; stress that doses should not be increased or stopped without checking with physician (may cause severe problems).

♦ Advise avoidance of driving and other potentially hazardous activities until response is established.

♦ Suggest using ice chips, hard candy, or gum to relieve side effect of dry mouth; stress the need for good mouth care.

♦ Warn women to report if pregnancy is planned or suspected.

♦ *See Antidepressants overview for more information.*

isoetharine

eye-soe-eth'a-reen

isoetharine hydrochloride: **Arm-a-Med Isoetharine, Beta-2, Bisorine, Bronkosol, Dey-Dose Isoetharine, Dey-Dose Isoetharine S/F, Dey-Lute Isoetharine, Disposa-a-Med Isoetharine**
isoetharine mesylate: **Bronkometer**

Class: Respiratory smooth muscle relaxant, Beta-adrenergic agonist, Bronchodilator

PEDS	PREG	GERI
🖐	C	🖐

Action Produces bronchodilation by stimulating beta-2 receptors of the bronchi. It has a rapid onset (immediate, with peak in 5–15 min) and long duration of action (1–4 hr) while producing few cardiac side effects.

Use/Therapeutic goal/Outcome

Bronchospasm and asthma: Reduction of airway resistance, improved movement of air. **Outcome criteria:** Decreased wheezing; increased forced expiratory volume (FEV); increased ability to bring forth sputum; report of easier breathing, fewer episodes of wheezing.

Dose range/Administration

Interaction alert: Propranolol and other beta-blockers may antagonize the bronchodilation effect of isoetharine.

Adult: *Inhalation: Hand nebulizer: 3–7 puffs, undiluted. Metered dose nebulizer (mesylate): 1–2 breaths q4h prn (1 min between puffs to assess effect). IPPB/oxygen aerosolization: 0.25–1 ml diluted 1:3 with NS or other diluent.*

Clinical alert: Give doses upon rising, before meals, and 2 hr before bedtime for optimum results.

Contraindications/Precautions

PREG C

Contraindicated in hypersensitivity to sympathomimetics or to sulfites, in use with other sympathomimetics such as epinephrine, and in cardiac disease. **Use with caution** in hypertension, congestive heart failure, hyperthyroidism, coronary artery disease, diabetes mellitus, tuberculosis, and history of seizures.

🖐 **Use with caution for the elderly. Safe use for pregnant women requires evaluation of risks and benefits. Safe use for children has not been established.**

Side effects/Adverse reactions

Hypersensitivity: bluish coloration of skin; dizziness; flushing or redness of skin; rash; hives; itching; swelling of face, lips or eyelids; wheezing or difficulty in breathing; exaggeration of side effects. **CV:** dysrhythmias, palpitations, cardiac arrest, hypertension. **GI:** nausea. **CNS:** headache, anxiety, tension, restlessness, tremor, weakness, excitement.

Nursing implications/Documentation

Possible nursing diagnoses: Potential for injury; Activity intolerance; Ineffective breathing pattern.

◆ Record lung sounds, respirations, pulse, and blood pressure before and after dose administration until response is determined.

◆ Provide favorite fluids and monitor intake and output to ensure adequate hydration (at least 2 L a day is recommended).

◆ Hold drug and report if paradoxical bronchospasm occurs (usually occurs after excessive use).

◆ When diluted with water, be aware that sputum may be pink after inhalations (drug oxidation causes the pink color).

Patient & family teaching/Home care

Possible nursing diagnoses: Knowledge deficit; Fear; Ineffective family coping.

◆ Explain that this drug will enlarge air passages and make breathing easier, and that effects should be noted immediately (peak effect in 5–15 min, duration 1–4 hr).

◆ Warn against excessive use (may cause increased constriction of air passages); advise reporting unrelieved symptoms.

◆ Point out that stress and exercise can aggravate wheezing and bronchospasm, and that learning relaxation and controlled breathing techniques can help reduce severity and frequency of episodes of wheezing.

◆ Explain that this drug may turn sputum pink and that this is not blood.

◆ Give verbal and written instructions for proper use and cleansing of inhaler; have individual or caregiver demonstrate technique before going home.

◆ Warn against taking OTC drugs without physician's approval.

◆ For bronchospasm, advise reporting immediately if symptoms are not relieved within 20 min.

◆ *See Adrenergics (sympathomimetics) overview for more information.*

isoniazid (INH)

eye-soe-nye'a-zid

DOW-Isoniazid, ✦Isotamine, Laniazid, Nydrazid, ✦PMS-Isoniazid

Class: ★Anti-infective prototype, Antitubercular

PEDS	PREG	GERI
🖐	C	🖐

Action Kills tubercle bacilli (bactericidal action) or limits their growth (bacteriostatic action) by inhibiting synthesis and disrupting the cell wall.

Use/Therapeutic goal/Outcome

Treatment and prevention of tuberculosis: Prevention or resolution of tubercular infection. **Outcome criteria:** Absence of acid-fast bacilli on sputum cultures, decreased productive cough, normal temperature, improvement of X rays.

Dose range/Administration

Interaction alert: Give isoniazid at least 1 hr before aluminum-containing antacids and laxatives (they may decrease drug absorption). Increases blood levels and toxicity of phenytoin. Monitor for decreased therapeutic effectiveness if given with corticosteroids. Carbamazepine, rifampin, and alcohol increase risk of liver toxicity. Avoid disulfiram (may cause changes in behavior and coordination).

🖤 **Give with meals if GI symptoms occur.**

Primary treatment of active tuberculosis: Concomitant administration of at least one other antitubercular drug is recommended. **Adult:** PO, IM: 5 mg/kg/day in a single dose (up to 300 mg/day) for 6 mos to 2 yrs. **Child:** PO, IM: 10–20 mg/kg/day in a single dose (up to 300–500 mg/day) for 18 mos to 2 yrs.

Preventive therapy: **Adult:** PO: 300 mg daily for 1 yr. **Child:** PO: 10 mg/kg/day in a single dose (up to 300 mg/day) for 1 yr.

Clinical alert: Monitor for side effect of psychosis; report symptoms of liver toxicity (malaise, decreased appetite, dark urine, jaundice), especially in the elderly.

Contraindications/Precautions
PREG C

Contraindicated in hypersensitivity to isoniazid, and in history of INH-related problems. *Use with caution* in chronic kidney or liver disease, diabetes, cataracts and other eye defects.

✋ **Use with caution for children under 13 yrs and the elderly (increased risk of severe hepatic side effects). Safe use during pregnancy has not been established (although it has been used).**

Side effects/Adverse reactions

Hypersensitivity: itching, rashes, fever, lymphadenopathy, vasculitis. *GI:* Nausea, vomiting, dry mouth, epigastric discomfort, constipation, hepatitis. *CNS:* peripheral neuropathy, headache, drowsiness, seizures, memory impairment, lethargy, depression, confusion, psychosis. *Hem:* agranulocytosis, aplastic anemia, hemolytic anemia, eosinophilia, thrombocytopenia, methemoglobinemia, pyridoxine-responsive hypochromic anemia, hyperglycemia. *Eye:* optic neuritis and atrophy. *Misc:* lupus-like syndrome, pyridoxine deficiency.

Nursing implications/Documentation

Possible nursing diagnoses: Potential for infection; Fatigue; Activity intolerance; Fluid volume deficit; Constipation.

♦ Ascertain that baseline CBC, BUN, creatinine, and liver function studies are obtained, and that necessary culture specimens are col-

lected before starting isoniazid; monitor periodically thereafter, depending on clinical symptoms.

♦ Monitor and record intake and output and provide favorite fluids to ensure adequate hydration.

♦ Allow for a balance between rest and activity.

♦ Monitor for and report symptoms of peripheral neuropathy; pyridoxine may be given to prevent this problem.

Patient & family teaching/Home care

Possible nursing diagnoses: Knowledge deficit; Impaired home maintenance management.

♦ Teach the need to take with meals. Stress the importance of taking this drug as prescribed without missing doses, and the importance of long-term medical follow-up to avoid relapses or complications.

♦ Advise avoiding alcohol to reduce risk of liver toxicity.

♦ Encourage drinking at least 2 L of fluid a day to maintain adequate hydration.

♦ *See Anti-infectives overview for more information.*

isoproterenol
eye-soe-proe-ter'a-nole

isoproterenol: *Aerolone, Dey Dose Isoproterenol, Dispos-a-Med Isoproterenol, Isuprel, Vapo-Iso*

isoproterenol hydrochloride: *Isuprel, Isuprel Mistometer, Norisodrine Aerotrol*

isoproterenol sulfate: *Medihaler-Iso*

Class: Beta-adrenergic agonist, Sympathomimetic, Bronchodilator

PEDS	PREG	GERI
✋	C	✋

Action Produces sympathomimetic effects by acting on both beta-1 and beta-2 receptors of the heart, bronchi, skeletal muscle vasculature, and GI tract: Cardiac stimulation produces positive inotropic and chronotropic actions, increasing cardiac output and venous return; relaxation of the bronchial tree produces bronchodilation; peripheral vasodilation produces a drop in blood pressure.

Use/Therapeutic goal/Outcome

Asthma or bronchospasm: Reduction of airway resistance; improved movement of air. *Out-*

come criteria: Decreased wheezing, increased forced expiratory volume (FEV), increased ability to bring forth sputum; report of easier breathing, fewer episodes of wheezing.

Heartblock and ventricular dysrhythmias: Cardiac stimulation, promotion of effective heartbeat and blood pressure. **Outcome criteria:** Palpable pulses, stabilization of vital signs, improvement of cardiac rhythm on EKG.

Shock: Promotion of effective blood pressure, profusion of vital organs. **Outcome criteria:** Systolic blood pressure > 100; absence of clinical signs of shock (restlessness, confusion, pallor, urine output < 25 ml/hr).

Dose range/Administration

Interaction alert: Propranolol and other beta-blockers reduce effects. Tricyclic antidepressants may increase risk for arrhythmias. MAOIs increase vasopressor effects. Other sympathomimetics increase effects.

Asthma, bronchospasm: Adult and Child: *Metered-dose inhaler:* 1 breath; repeat in 2–5 min if no relief. *Maintenance dose:* 1–2 breaths 4–6 times daily, not more than q3-4h, not more than 2 breaths at one time. *Hand-bulb nebulizer:* 5–15 deep breaths 1:200 solution, or 3–7 breaths 1:100 solution; repeat in 5–10 min if no relief. *IPPB/oxygen aerosolization:* 0.5 ml 1:200 solution diluted to 2–2.5 ml with water or isotonic saline, delivered over 5–10 min up to 5 times a day.

Heart block and ventricular dysrhythmias (i. hydrochloride): Adult: IV: 0.2–0.06 mg, then 0.01–0.2 mg/min prn. IM: 0.2 mg, then 0.02–1 mg prn. **Child:** IM, IV: Half the adult dose.

Shock (i. hydrochloride): Adult and Child: IV: 0.5 mcg/min; increase prn. *Maximum dose:* 5 mcg. Mix 1 mg (5 ml) in 500 ml D5W.

Clinical alert: When using isoproterenol for asthma or bronchospasm, give dose at earliest onset of symptoms and 2 hr before bedtime (to avoid insomnia). When given for shock, ascertain that hypotension is not due to hypovolemia before starting dose (volume deficit should be corrected before starting vasopressors). Use IV controller and titrate according to blood pressure, heart rate, urine output, and, if available, central venous pressure and pulmonary wedge pressure device. Be aware that sublingual doses are poorly and erratically absorbed.

Contraindications/Precautions

Contraindicated in hypersensitivity to sympathomimetics and sulfites, with epinephrine, in cardiac dysrhythmias associated with tachycardia, and in central hyperexcitability. **Use with caution** in hypertension, cardiac disease, renal disease, diabetes, prostatic hypertrophy, glaucoma, and tuberculosis.

✋ **Use with caution for children, pregnant women, and the elderly.**

Side effects/Adverse reactions

Hypersensitivity: bluish coloration of skin; dizziness; flushing or redness of skin; rash; hives; itching; swelling of face, lips or eyelids; wheezing or difficulty in breathing; exaggeration of side effects. **CV:** tachycardia, precordial distress, pain. **CNS:** flushing of face, sweating, mild tremors, headache, nervousness. **GI:** nausea, vomiting, buccal ulcerations. **Resp:** severe, prolonged asthma attack.

Nursing implications/Documentation

Possible nursing diagnoses: Potential for injury; Activity intolerance; Ineffective breathing pattern.

◆ **Use by inhalation**

◆ Record lung sounds, respirations, pulse, and blood pressure before and after dose administration until response is determined.

◆ Provide favorite fluids and monitor intake and output to ensure adequate hydration (at least 2 L a day is recommended).

◆ When isoproterenol is diluted with water, be aware that sputum may be pink after inhalations (from drug oxidation).

◆ **Parenteral use**

◆ Place patient on cardiac monitor and keep emergency equipment and drugs readily available (external or temporary pacemaker may be necessary).

◆ Obtain written parameters from physician for titration of IV drips (rate is usually adjusted according to heart rate, blood pressure, and urine output and usually decreased or stopped for angina or heart rate > 110–130).

◆ Document pulse, blood pressure, and respirations every 5 min until stable, then every 15 min, then every 1/2–1 hr; document urine output every 1 hr.

◆ Report immediately if precordial distress, angina, or a heart rate > 130 is noted (increased risk of cardiac problems).

Patient & family teaching/Home care

Possible nursing diagnoses: Knowledge deficit; Fear; Ineffective family coping.

- **Use by inhalation**
  - Explain that this drug will enlarge air passages and make breathing easier.
  - Warn that excessive use may cause tolerance (reduced effectiveness); advise reporting unrelieved symptoms.
  - Point out that stress and exercise can aggravate wheezing and bronchospasm, and that learning relaxation and controlled breathing techniques can help reduce severity and frequency of episodes of wheezing.
  - Explain that this drug may turn sputum pink and that this is not blood.
  - Warn against taking OTC drugs without physician's approval.
  - Give verbal and written instructions for proper use and cleansing of inhaler (clear nasal passages and throat, breathe out slowly and completely, place mouthpiece well into mouth, inhale deeply as dose is released from nebulizer, hold breath for several seconds, remove mouthpiece and exhale; for powdered inhaler, the patient should not inhale deeply because of risk of systemic absorption). Have the individual or caregiver demonstrate technique before going home.
- **Parenteral use**
  - Explain that this drug improves heart rate and blood pressure; reassure that vital signs will be taken frequently to ensure optimum drug effect.
  - Stress that symptoms of discomfort should be reported immediately in case they are related to the medication.
- *See Adrenergics (sympathomimetics) overview for more information.*

isosorbide dinitrate
eye-soe-sor'bide

♣Apo-ISDN, ♣Cedocard-SR, ♣Coronex, Dilatrate-SR, Iso-Bid, Isonate, Isorbid, Isordil, Isotrate, ♣Novosorbide, Sorbitrate, Sorbitrate Sustained Action

Class: Antianginal, Organic nitrate

PEDS	PREG	GERI
🖐	C	🖐

Action Decreases cardiac workload and myocardial oxygen demand by reducing left ventricular end-diastolic pressure (preload), and to a lesser extent, by reducing systemic vascular resistance (afterload). Relaxes smooth muscle, particularly peripheral vascular smooth muscle, and has a vasodilating effect on large systemic arteries and veins, which decreases blood pressure. Also improves myocardial oxygen perfusion by promoting collateral circulation.

Use/Therapeutic goal/Outcome

Angina pectoris: Promotion of myocardial oxygenation, resolution or prevention of anginal (ischemic) attacks, improvement in activity tolerance. *Outcome criteria:* Patient reports decreased frequency and severity of angina, and demonstrates activity tolerance.

Dose range/Administration

Interaction alert: Antihypertensives and other vasodilators may potentiate hypotensive effects.

🥄 **Give oral doses 30 minutes before or 2–3 hours after meals for faster absorption.**

Adult: SL: 2.5–10 mg q2-3h during acute attacks; q4-6h prophylactically. PO: (chewable): 5–10 mg prn q2-3h for prophylaxis. PO: (tablet): 5–30 mg q6h. PO: (sustained release): 40 mg q6-12h.

Clinical alert: Check blood pressure and heart rate prior to giving dose; hold drug and report if hypotension or tachycardia is present.

Contraindications/Precautions
PREG C

Contraindicated in hypersensitivity to nitrates, and in myocardial infarction accompanied by hypotension, severe anemia, head trauma, cerebral hemorrhage, and increased intracranial pressure.

🖐 **Use with caution in the elderly. Safe use for pregnant and nursing mothers and for children is not established.**

Side effects/Adverse reactions

Hypersensitivity: rash. **CNS:** headache, dizziness, weakness, fainting. **CV:** orthostatic hypotension, tachycardia, palpitations, flushing. **GI:** nausea, vomiting, sublingual burning. **Skin:** cutaneous vasodilation, flushing.

Nursing implications/Documentation

Possible nursing diagnoses: Potential for injury; Activity intolerance.

- Give sublingual doses at the first sign of angina; have the patient use a scale of 1 to 10 to rate pain immediately before and 5 minutes

▶

after administration; report unrelieved pain immediately.

- Keep a record of pulse and blood pressure, before and after drug administration.

- Monitor for and report headache (a side effect usually treated with mild analgesics; tolerance of headache usually occurs with long-term use).

- Observe for postural hypotension; take blood pressure in both arms, with patient sitting and standing if possible.

- Supervise ambulation until response to drug is determined.

- Coordinate care to allow frequent rest periods.

Patient & family teaching/Home care

Possible nursing diagnoses: Fear; Knowledge deficit; Impaired home maintenance management.

- Explain that antianginals help reduce the workload of the heart and improve coronary blood supply.

- Advise taking oral doses 30 minutes before meals or 2–3 hours after meals.

- Teach to take sublingual doses at the first sign of angina: tablet should be wet with saliva and placed under the tongue until completely dissolved.

- Emphasize the need to pace activities, avoid stress (emotional and physical), and plan for rest periods.

- Explain that an extra sublingual dose may be necessary during stress, or at bedtime if angina is nocturnal; teach that dose may be repeated every 10–15 minutes for 3 doses. If angina is unrelieved, the patient should call paramedics.

- Advise changing positions slowly to avoid dizziness.

- Explain that tolerance to headache will develop with long-term use.

- Encourage keeping a record of angina attacks to observe pattern; stress that an increase in frequency or severity should be reported.

- Stress that discontinuing this drug abruptly could precipitate coronary vasospasm.

- Warn that drinking alcohol may cause fainting and hypotension.

- Emphasize that this drug could be ineffective if exposed to moisture, heat, or air (keep in a cool dark place).

- *See Antianginals overview for additional information.*

isotretinoin

eye-soe-tret'i-noyn

Accutane, ♦Roaccutane

Class: Antiacne agent, Keratinization stabilizer, Synthetic retinoid

PEDS	PREG	GERI
🖐	X	🖐

Action Decreases secretion of sebum by reducing size and activity of sebaceous glands. Inhibits keratinization and inflammation.

Use/Therapeutic goal/Outcome

Severe recalcitrant cystic acne unresponsive to conventional therapy: Improvement or clearing of skin condition. *Outcome criteria:* After 2–6 months, decreased erythema, tenderness; oiliness of skin; decreased number of comedones; reduction of cystic and acneiform lesions.

Dose range/Administration

Interaction alert: Tetracycline or minocycline may cause papilledema, headache and visual disturbances (benign intracranial hypertension). Vitamin A supplements increase potential for toxic effects. Alcohol may potentiate elevation of serum triglycerides. Topical antiacne agents may potentiate drying effect of isotretinoin.

🖐 **Give with meals.**

Adult: PO: 0.5–1 mg/kg/day in 2 divided doses for 15–20 wk.

Clinical alert: Expect that dose may be adjusted after 2 or more weeks based on toxicity and clinical response. If second course of treatment is necessary, it should not be initiated until at least 8 weeks after completion of first course. Recognize that initial response may be an apparent aggravation of acne; this should subside after 4–6 weeks.

Contraindications/Precautions

PREG
X

Contraindicated in hypersensitivity to Vitamin A or its derivatives or to parabens preservatives. **Use with caution** in coronary artery disease, diabetes mellitus, obesity, liver disease, or high alcohol intake.

⚓ **Contraindicated for children, pregnant or nursing mothers, and the elderly (no information available for use in the elderly).**

Side effects/Adverse reactions

Hypersensitivity: rash. *Skin:* chapped lips, thinning hair, photosensitivity, dry skin, peeling palms and soles. *Eye:* burning, redness, itching, dryness, corneal opacities. *MS:* pain, tenderness or stiffness of muscles or joints. *GI:* dry mouth, bleeding gums, abdominal pain, severe diarrhea, rectal bleeding, elevated liver function studies. *Resp:* epistaxis, dry nostrils. *Misc:* elevated triglycerides, altered blood glucose control in diabetics.

Nursing implications/Documentation

Possible nursing diagnoses: Impaired skin integrity; Pain.

◆ Record negative results of pregnancy test 2 weeks prior to starting treatment; initiate therapy on second or third day of next normal menstrual period.

◆ Monitor results of triglycerides and liver function studies closely; report elevated levels immediately (especially liver function).

◆ For diabetics, monitor blood glucose levels and watch for signs of hyper- or hypoglycemia.

◆ Provide mild analgesics (e.g., acetaminophen) to alleviate side effect of muscle stiffness and tenderness.

◆ Monitor for eye irritation or visual changes; report and record abnormal findings.

Patient & family teaching/Home care

Possible nursing diagnoses: Knowledge deficit; Impaired home maintenance management; Body image disturbance.

◆ Point out the need to take isotretinoin with meals; caution not to crush capsule.

◆ Explain that the acne may get worse at the beginning of treatment but will decrease in 4–6 weeks; improvement may continue for 6–8 weeks after treatment is completed.

◆ For those with excessive bleeding and scabbing, advise checking with physician to establish a plan of cleansing and treating lesions; point out that expert advise on how to deal with this problem will help reduce scarring.

◆ Warn women that fetal abnormalities occur with use of drug and that reliable contraception is necessary during therapy and for 1 month after drug is discontinued; provide written warnings of hazards of pregnancy.

◆ For sexually active women, recommend monthly pregnancy test; advise to discontinue isotretinoin and to notify physician immediately if pregnancy is suspected.

◆ Caution not to take Vitamin A supplements or multivitamin preparations containing Vitamin A to avoid additive toxic effects.

◆ Advise avoiding skin cleansers, medicated soaps, cosmetics with drying effects, or alcohol-containing preparations (e.g., shaving lotions, shaving creams, perfumed toiletries).

◆ Stress the need to avoid drinking alcohol because alcohol also increases triglyceride levels, and may increase risk of liver toxicity.

◆ Caution contact lense wearers that they may experience discomfort because of increased eye dryness.

◆ Suggest the use of sugarless gum or ice to relieve dry mouth.

◆ Advise against donating blood during therapy or for 30 days after completion to eliminate danger of transfusion to a pregnant woman.

◆ Warn to use sunscreen (SFP #15) or protective clothing during exposure of skin to sunlight or ultraviolet light.

◆ Stress the importance of medical follow-up for monitoring clinical response and/or development of toxic reactions (liver problems can be serious).

◆ Point out that improvement may continue for 6–8 weeks after course is completed.

◆ Advise reporting visual changes or episodes of severe abdominal pain with diarrhea or rectal bleeding.

◆ Explain that acne is difficult for all young people; recognize the impact on body image, and encourage verbalizing feelings, frustrations, and concerns.

isoxsuprine
eye-sox'syoo-preen

isoxsuprine hydrochloride: **Vasodilan, Vasoprine**
Class: Vasodilator, Beta-adrenergic agonist

PEDS	PREG	GERI
🖐	C	🖐

Action Decreases vascular resistance and increases blood flow in skeletal muscles by activating beta-adrenergic receptor sites in vascular smooth muscles. Produces cardiac stimulation, uterine relaxation, and possibly bronchodilation. High doses may inhibit platelet aggregation and decrease blood viscosity.

Use/Therapeutic goal/Outcome

Adjunctive treatment of peripheral and cerebral vascular insufficiency spasm: Improvement of tissue perfusion. *Outcome criteria:* Presence of satisfactory pulse quality, skin color and temperature; absence of episodes of altered mental and motor capabilities.

Dose range/Administration

Adult: PO: 10–20 mg tid or qid. IM: 5–10 mg bid or tid.

Contraindications/Precautions

**PREG
C**

Contraindicated in hypersensitivity to isoxsuprine; hypotension, tachycardia, postpartum. *Use with caution* in bleeding disorders, severe cerebrovascular and coronary artery disease, and recent myocardial infarction.

⚕ **Use with caution for the elderly. Safe use in children and pregnancy has not been established (has been used to prevent premature labor).**

Side effects/Adverse reactions

Hypersensitivity: Severe rash. *CV:* hypotension, palpitations. When used to delay premature labor, hypotension and irregular and rapid heartbeat may occur in mother and fetus. *CNS:* dizziness. *GI:* nausea, vomiting, and abdominal distension.

Nursing implications/Documentation

Possible nursing diagnoses: Activity intolerance; Potential for injury.

♦ Document baseline mental status and circulatory status (presence and quality of peripheral pulses, skin color and temperature); monitor periodically thereafter.

♦ Monitor for dizziness and hypotension; supervise ambulation until response is determined.

Patient & family teaching/Home care

Possible nursing diagnoses: Knowledge deficit; Impaired home maintenance management.

♦ Stress the need to change positions slowly to reduce dizziness.

kanamycin

kan-a-mye'sin

kanamycin sulfate: ♠*Kanasig, Kantrex, Klebcil*
Class: Anti-infective, Aminoglycoside antibiotic

PEDS	PREG	GERI
⚕	**D**	⚕

Action Kills bacteria (bactericidal) by binding to the ribosomes, thereby disrupting bacterial protein synthesis.

Use/Therapeutic goal/Outcome

Serious infections (caused by Escherichia coli, Proteus, Klebsiella pneumoniae, Enterobacter aerogenes, Serratia marcescens, Acinetobacter) and preoperative bowel sterilization: Resolution of infection. *Outcome criteria:* Absence of pathogenic growth on cultures, absence of clinical manifestations of infection (fever, pain, swelling, redness, heat, odor, drainage, productive cough, dysuria, frequency, increased WBC count, abnormal X rays).

Adjunctive treatment of liver failure: Elimination of ammonia-producing bacteria. *Outcome criteria:* Decreased blood ammonia.

Dose range/Administration

Interaction alert: Do not mix IV with any other drug. Loop diuretics (e.g., furosemide) increase risk of nephrotoxicity and ototoxicity. Dimenhydrinate may mask symptoms of ototoxicity. Use cautiously with other aminoglycosides, amphotericin B, methoxyflurane, cisplatin, and cephalosporins (increased risk of toxicity).

Serious infections caused by susceptible organisms: Adult and Child: IM: 15 mg/kg/day, in divided doses q8-12h deep into large muscle mass. IV: 15 mg/kg/day, in divided doses q8-12h (dilute 500 mg in 200 cc NS or D5W, infuse over 2–3 hr). *Maximum dose:* 1.5 g/day. *Neonate:* IM, IV: 15 mg/kg/day, in divided doses q12h.

Preoperative bowel sterilization: Adult: PO: 1 g qh for 4 doses, then 4 doses q4h; or 1g qh for 4 doses then q6h for 36–72 hrs.

Liver failure: Adult: PO: 8–12 g/day in divided doses.

Clinical alert: Schedule blood drawing for peak levels 1 hour after IM dose or 30–60 minutes after IV dose. Schedule blood drawing for trough levels just before next dose. Peak levels should not exceed 30 mcg/ml; trough levels should not exceed 5–10 mcg/ml.

Contraindications/Precautions

Contraindicated in hypersensitivity to kanamycin or other aminoglycoside antibiotics, in history of drug-induced hearing loss, vertigo, tinnitus, for long-term use, and (PO route) in systemic infection, or intestinal obstruction. *Use with caution* in impaired renal function, and dehydration.

✋ **Contraindicated for pregnant or nursing mothers. Use with caution for infants and the elderly.**

Side effects/Adverse reactions

Hypersensitivity: itching, burning, rashes, exfoliative dermatitis, drug fever, blood dyscrasias, arthralgia, anaphylaxis. *Ear:* ototoxicity (hearing loss, tinnitus). *CNS:* headache, dizziness, weakness, lethargy, tremors; neuromuscular blockade leading to respiratory arrest. *GU:* nephrotoxicity (oliguria, proteinuria, cells in urine, hematuria, decreased creatinine clearance, increased serum BUN and creatinine).

Nursing implications/Documentation

Possible nursing diagnoses: Potential for infection; Fluid volume deficit.

◆ Determine history of allergies and (regardless of history) monitor closely for allergic reactions.

◆ Weigh patient and obtain baseline renal function studies, hearing ability, and culture specimens before administering first dose.

◆ Monitor renal function (urine output, specific gravity, serum BUN and creatinine, creatinine clearance) and report signs of decreased function.

◆ Encourage fluid intake, and document and monitor intake and output, to ensure adequate hydration and prevent renal damage from chemical irritation of renal tubules.

◆ Monitor for and report symptoms of ototoxicity (hearing loss, tinnitus, vertigo) and superinfection (mouth lesions, thrush, vaginal irritation, diarrhea, respiratory symptoms).

◆ If there is no response within 3–5 days, consult with physician to determine whether drug regimen should be re-evaluated and new cultures drawn.

Patient & family teaching/Home care

Possible nursing diagnoses: Knowledge deficit; Impaired home maintenance management.

◆ Teach the need to report ear symptoms (e.g., full feeling, ringing of the ears, difficulty hearing) and symptoms of superinfection (mouth sores, diarrhea, persistent infections).

◆ Explain the importance of taking antibiotics for the entire time prescribed, even if symptoms abate, and of maintaining adequate hydration (drinking at least 2 L is recommended).

◆ *See Anti-infectives overview for more information.*

kaolin and pectin *kay'oh-lin and pek'tin*

♣*Donnagel-MB,* ♣*Kao-Con, Kaopectate, Kaopectate Concentrate, Kao-tin, Kapectolin, K-P, K-Pek*

Class: Antidiarrheal

PEDS	PREG	GERI
✋	C	✋

Action Provides symptomatic relief of diarrhea by absorbing bacteria, toxins, and irritants from GI tract and soothing irritated mucosa.

Use/Therapeutic goal/Outcome

Diarrhea: Symptomatic control of mild to moderate diarrhea. *Outcome criteria:* Reduction of fluid content and frequency of bowel movements.

Dose range/Administration

Interaction alert: Give doses at least 2–3 hours before other oral medication to avoid interference with absorption.

Adult: PO: 45–90 ml concentrate or 60–120 ml regular strength after each loose bowel movement. *Child:* PO: 15–45 ml concentrate or 30–60 ml regular strength after each loose bowel movement.

Clinical alert: Shake suspension *well* before administering.

Contraindications/Precautions

Use with caution in dehydration, asthma, peptic ulcer, and heart disease.

✋ **Contraindicated in children under 3 years. Use with caution for pregnant or nursing mothers and the elderly.**

Side effects/Adverse reactions

Hypersensitivity: none listed. *GI:* constipation, fecal impaction (especially in infants or elderly, debilitated patients).

Nursing implications/Documentation

Possible nursing diagnoses: Constipation.

♦ Identify, report, and record signs of dehydration, especially in children and the elderly.

♦ Assess and document quality of bowel sounds and frequency and consistency of stools.

Patient & family teaching/Home care

Possible nursing diagnoses: Knowledge deficit; Impaired home maintenance management.

♦ Explain the need to take this drug after each loose bowel movement until diarrhea is controlled.

♦ Stress the need to report if diarrhea is not controlled within 48 hr and/or if fever develops.

♦ Explain that kaolin and pectin should be taken 2–3 hr before taking other medications.

♦ Suggest dietary treatment of diarrhea, especially for young children.

ketamine

keet'a-meen

ketamine hydrochloride: *Ketalar*

Class: Dissociative anesthetic

PEDS	PREG	GERI
👋	C	👋

Action Produces profound *dissociative anesthesia* (a feeling of dissociation from the environment) by an unknown mechanism (possibly acts on cortical and limbic receptors in the brain). May increase muscle tone and salivation.

Use/Therapeutic goal/Outcome

Induction of anesthesia and as an adjunct to mild anesthetics during short procedures: Promotion of comfort. *Outcome criteria:* Absence of observable signs of pain (grimacing, frowning, restlessness, withdrawal from painful stimulus); blood pressure and pulse within normal limits compared to baseline.

Dose range/Administration

Interaction alert: Atropine, morphine, or meperidine may increase depth and duration of ketamine-induced anesthesia. May potentiate neuromuscular blocking action of tubocurarine. If the patient is taking thyroid hormones, monitor for elevated blood pressure and tachycardia. Do not mix in the same syringe with diazepam or with barbiturates because they are incompatible.

Adult and Child: IV: 1–2 mg/kg, given slowly over 1 min. May be repeated in titrated doses depending on patient response. IM: 5–10 mg/kg. May be repeated in increments of half the full initial dose.

Clinical alert: This drug should be given IV only by those specifically qualified to manage the use of IV anesthetics. Expect reduced dosage for children and the elderly. Give adults IM doses in deltoid for more rapid effects. Keep emergency drugs and resuscitation equipment readily available.

Contraindications/Precautions

PREG
C

Contraindicated in hypersensitivity to ketamine, and in increased intracranial pressure, psychiatric disorders, increased intraocular pressure, congestive heart failure, and in patients for whom an increase in blood pressure or heart rate would be hazardous. *Use with caution* in chronic alcoholism, convulsive disorders, or concurrent use of thyroid hormone replacements.

👋 **Use with caution for children and the elderly. Safe use for pregnant or nursing mothers has not been established.**

Side effects/Adverse reactions

Hypersensitivity: rare. **CNS:** emergence reactions (tremors, tonic-clonic movements, dissociative or floating sensations, hallucinations, vivid illusions, delirium). **CV:** increase or decrease in blood pressure and pulse rate, arrhythmias. **Resp:** respiratory stimulation, depression, or apnea, laryngospasm. **Eye:** diplopia, nystagmus, increase in intraocular pressure. **MS:** enhanced skeletal muscle tone and clonic movements. **GI:** hypersalivation, anorexia, nausea, vomiting. **Misc:** local pain and skin eruption at injection site; transient erythema, rash.

Nursing implications/Documentation

Possible nursing diagnoses: Potential for injury; Potential for aspiration; Sensory/perceptual alterations (visual and auditory).

♦ Record vital signs before administration, and every 5–15 min after administration (check protocol).

♦ Monitor for increased salivation and potential for vomiting; protect airway, and keep suction equipment at the bedside.

♦ During recovery, keep environment quiet (low lighting if possible), minimize tactile, verbal, and visual stimuli; monitor closely for potential for injury (this drug may cause confusion and excitement).

♦ Recognize that ketamine may produce hallucinations as the patient emerges from anesthesia (may be relieved by diazepam).

♦ Be aware that because this drug is a hallucinogen, it is a popular "street" drug.

Patient & family teaching/Home care

Possible nursing diagnoses: Anxiety; Fear.

♦ Caution to avoid driving, hazardous activities, and alcohol for at least 24 hr after procedure.

ketoconazole

kee-to-con'a-zol

Nizoral

Class: Anti-infective, Antifungal

PEDS	PREG	GERI
♨	C	♨

Action Kills fungi (fungicidal) by inhibiting ergosterol synthesis, which increases cell membrane permeability and allows leakage of intracellular components.

Use/Therapeutic goal/Outcome

Systemic candidiasis, chronic mucocutaneous candidiasis, oral thrush, candiduria, coccidioidomycosis, histoplasmosis, nonmeningeal blastomycosis, chromomycosis, and paracoccidoidomycosis; severe cutaneous dermatophyte infections resistant to topical therapy and griseofulvin: Resolution of infection. *Outcome criteria:* After 1–6 weeks of therapy, absence of pathogenic growth on culture; absence of clinical manifestations of infection (redness, pain, swelling, fever, drainage, increased WBC count).

Dose range/Administration

Interaction alert: Acidic conditions are necessary for drug to dissolve; allow 2 hours after doses of antacids, anticholinergics, or H_2 blockers, before giving ketoconazole to ensure adequate absorption. Do not use with rifampin or isoniazid (decreases antifungal effect).

☞ **Give oral doses with meals to reduce GI symptoms.**

Adult/Child > 40 kg: PO: *Initial dose:* 200 mg qd. If no response, increase to 400 mg qd. *Topical:* Apply cream to affected areas and surrounding skin once or twice daily. *Child 20–40*

kg: PO: 100 mg (1/2 tablet) qd. *Child < 40 kg:* PO: 50 mg (1/4 tablet) qd.

Clinical alert: Monitor closely for first–dose anaphylaxis. Have emergency drugs readily available.

Contraindications/Precautions

PREG C

Contraindicated in hypersensitivity to ketoconazole, and for less serious conditions, such as mild fungus infections of the skin or nails (potential liver toxicity). *Use with caution* in impaired kidney or liver function.

☞ **Contraindicated for nursing mothers. Safe use for children under 2 years and pregnant women has not been established.**

Side effects/Adverse reactions

Hypersensitivity: itching, rashes, urticaria, anaphylaxis. *GI:* nausea, vomiting, diarrhea, constipation, abdominal pain, hepatoxicity, elevated liver enzymes. *CNS:* headache, dizziness. *Hem:* hemolytic anemia. *GU:* impotence, decreased sperm count, menstrual irregularities. *Misc:* breast tenderness, gynecomastia in males.

Nursing implications/Documentation

Possible nursing diagnoses: Potential for infection; Altered nutrition: less than body requirements; Altered oral mucous membrane.

♦ Obtain necessary cultures before starting ketoconazole.

♦ If nausea persists, even if given with meals, check with physician whether daily dose can be given in two divided doses.

♦ Record and monitor intake and output, and ensure adequate hydration (report excessive negative or positive balance).

♦ Monitor for symptoms of hepatotoxicity (jaundice, fatigue, persistent nausea, anorexia, dark urine, pale stools); if on prolonged therapy, monitor liver function studies.

♦ If the individual has achlorhydria, give with dilute hydrochloride acid (consult with physician for order); use a straw to avoid contact with teeth.

♦ For topical route, report worsening in condition or failure to improve after 3 days (may require change in medication).

Patient & family teaching/Home care

Possible nursing diagnoses: Knowledge deficit; Impaired home maintenance management.

K

• Explain that taking doses with meals helps reduce GI symptoms.

• Stress the importance of taking the drug for the entire time prescribed, even if symptoms abate (long-term treatment may be required).

• Teach the need to report persistent nausea, vomiting, fatigue, yellowish color of skin, dark urine, pale stools, as they may indicate liver problems.

• Advise avoidance of antacids to ensure drug absorption; stress that no OTC drugs should be taken without checking with the physician, and that alcohol may cause excessive vomiting..

• For topical route, stress the need to continue treatment for at least 2 weeks after skin is clear; advise reporting worsening in condition or failure to improve after 3 days.

• *See Anti-infectives overview for more information.*

K ketoprofen

kee-toe'proe-fen

Orudis, ❦OrudisE, ❦OrudisSR, Rhodis

Class: Nonsteroidal anti-inflammatory drug (NSAID), Analgesic, Antipyretic, Antirheumatic

PEDS	PREG	GERI
👋	👋	👋

Action Reduces inflammation by inhibiting prostaglandin and leukotriene synthesis. Prostaglandin is a naturally occurring mediator of the inflammatory process found throughout body tissue. Inhibits bradykinin activity, thus decreasing constriction of smooth muscle and pain receptor stimulation. Also has lysosomal membrane stabilizing action.

Use/Therapeutic goal/Outcome

Pain and inflammation: Promotion of comfort and mobility; suppression of inflammation. *Outcome criteria:* Report of increased comfort with increased range of motion and ability to perform activities of daily life; reduction in or absence of joint stiffness, swelling, redness, and warmth.

Dose range/Administration

Interaction alert: Aspirin and probenecid increase plasma level of this drug; aspirin also increases risk of bleeding. Coumarin-type anticoagulants increase risk of GI bleeding. Thiazide diuretics decrease potassium and chloride levels.

💊 **Give with milk or antacid to prevent gastric irritation.**

Adult: PO: 50–300 mg in 3–4 divided doses. *Initial dose:* 75 mg tid or 50 mg qid. *Maximum dose:* 300 mg/day. *Rect:* 100 mg bid.

Contraindications/Precautions

PREG
👋

Contraindicated in hypersensitivity to ketoprofen, aspirin, other NSAIDs, and in active GI disease or severe kidney impairment. *Use with caution* in mild to moderate kidney or hepatic impairment, myasthenia gravis, cardiovascular disease, coagulation defects.

👋 Use with caution for the elderly. Safe use for children and pregnant women has not been determined (first two trimesters, preg B; in third trimester, preg D).

Side effects/Adverse reactions

Hypersensitivity: asthma, urticaria, rash, and pruritus. *GI:* dry mouth, dyspepsia, nausea, abdominal pain, diarrhea, constipation, flatulence, (with suppository) rectal irritation. *CNS:* nervousness, dizziness, headache, insomnia. *Hem:* prolonged coagulation time. *Ear:* tinnitus. *Eye:* visual disturbance. *CV:* tachycardia, hypertension, edema. *GU:* kidney and hepatic toxicity.

Nursing implications/Documentation

Possible nursing diagnoses: Pain; Impaired physical mobility.

• Establish a baseline for CBC, electrolytes, prothrombin time, BUN, creatinine, and liver function studies; if therapy is prolonged, monitor periodically thereafter.

• Monitor for and report GI symptoms that may indicate peptic ulcer (nausea, pain, black stools).

• Record weight every other day; report edema or sudden weight gain.

• For diabetics, monitor blood sugar closely since insulin requirements may change.

Patient & family teaching/Home care

Possible nursing diagnoses: Altered health maintenance; Knowledge deficit.

• Advise taking doses with food to reduce GI symptoms.

• Explain the importance of watching for symptoms of GI bleeding (black stools, persistent GI distress).

- Stress the need to avoid aspirin, alcohol, and other OTC drugs (unless approved by physician) because of increased risk of GI bleeding.
- Instruct individuals to hold dose and report if any of the following side effects are experienced: vertigo, rashes, blood in urine, hearing or visual changes, sudden weight gain, edema.
- Warn against driving or activities that require alertness until response is determined.
- Reinforce the need for medical follow-up; advise telling dentist that ketoprofen is being taken.
- For diabetics, explain the importance of monitoring blood sugars with a blood glucose meter.
- *See Nonsteroidal anti-inflammatory drugs overview for more information.*

ketorolac

ket'or-oe-lak

ketorolac tromethamine: *Toradol*

Class: Non-narcotic analgesic, Nonsteroidal anti-inflammatory drug (NSAID)

PEDS	PREG	GERI
✋	B	✋

Action Relieves pain by blocking generation of pain impulses (peripheral action). Reduces inflammation and fever by inhibiting prostaglandin synthesis. Inhibits platelet aggregation and may prolong bleeding time.

Use/Therapeutic goal/Outcome

Mild to moderate pain: Relief of pain. *Outcome criteria:* Report of greater comfort; absence of signs of discomfort (frowning, restlessness, crying).

Dose range/Administration

Interaction alert: May increase action of anticoagulants, methotrexate, and lithium. Aspirin and other salicylates may enhance action of ketorolac.

Adult: IM: *Loading dose:* 30–60 mg *Maintenance dose:* 15–30 mg q6h. *Maximum daily dose:* 150 mg the first day and 120 mg/day thereafter.

Clinical alert: If pain returns within 3–5 hours, the next dose may be increased by 50%. Patients under 50 kg, > 65 years old, or with decreased renal function should receive reduced dosage.

Contraindications/Precautions

Contraindicated in hypersensitivity to ketorolac, aspirin, or other salicylates, and in those with syndrome of nasal polyps, and for long-term use. *Use with caution* in Vitamin-K deficiency, hypoprothrombinemia, bleeding disorders, decreased kidney or liver function, and in history of GI ulcers.

✋ **Contraindicated for children. Use in pregnant women only if clearly needed, when no safer alternative is available. Use with caution for nursing mothers and the elderly.**

Side effects/Adverse reactions

Hypersensitivity: rashes, anaphylaxis, asthma. *GI:* nausea, vomiting, GI distress, diarrhea. *CNS:* drowsiness, dizziness, headache. *CV:* vasodilation.

Nursing implications/Documentation

Possible nursing diagnoses: Pain; Impaired physical mobility.

- Recognize that this drug has a low incidence of side effects and has been very effective in the short-term management of postoperative bone pain.
- Assess comfort level (have patient rate pain on a scale of 1–10 before and after administration); report and record unrelieved pain.
- If fever is present, take temperatures immediately before doses to obtain a true reading.

Patient & family teaching/Home care

Possible nursing diagnoses: Knowledge deficit; Impaired home maintenance management.

- Stress the need to report pain before it is too uncomfortable; explain that dosage may need to be increased, especially during the first two days.
- Point out that this drug is not a narcotic and is not addicting.
- *See Narcotic and non-narcotic analgesics and Nonsteroidal anti-inflammatory drugs overviews for more information.*

labetalol

la-bet'a-lole

labetalol hydrochloride: ***Normodyne, ♠Presolol, Trandate***

Class: Adrenergic blocking agent (alpha & beta), Antihypertensive

PEDS	PREG	GERI
🖐	C	🖐

Action Reduces blood pressure by blocking alpha-adrenergic receptors (causing vasodilation and decreased peripheral vascular resistance) and beta-adrenergic receptors (slowing atrial and AV-node conduction). Depresses renin secretion.

Use/Therapeutic goal/Outcome

Hypertension, prompt reduction of blood pressure during hypertensive crisis; control of hypertension. ***Outcome criteria:*** Blood pressure within normal range.

Dose range/Administration

Interaction alert: Labetalol reduces the reflex tachycardia caused by nitroglycerin and may increase antihypertensive effects. With cimetidine, monitor for excessive hypotension and bradycardia. Other antihypertensives increase hypotensive effects. May alter antidiabetic agent requirements.

🖐 **Administer with or after meals to increase bioavailability.**

Adult: PO: 100 mg bid; may increase by 100 mg every 2–3 days. *Maintenance dose:* 200–400 mg bid. IV: *Repeated injection:* 20 mg (0.25 mg/kg) over 2 min; then 40–80 mg every 10 min prn until desired response or a maximum of 300 mg has been given. *Continuous infusion:* Mix 200 mg labetalol in 200 cc D5W (concentration 1 mg/cc). Infuse at a rate of 2 mg/min with an infusion pump, and stop when desired response is achieved. May repeat infusion q6-8h prn; when possible, start oral administration when supine diastolic blood pressure begins to rise (200 mg PO, then 200–400 mg in 6–12 hr, then titrate to patient response).

Clinical alert: With IV route, keep patient supine for 3 hours after infusion. Document vital signs every 5 minutes until stable; monitor closely for excessive hypotension.

Contraindications/Precautions

PREG
C

Contraindicated in hypersensitivity to labetalol, and in bronchial asthma, uncontrolled CHF, second- or third-degree heart block (PR interval > 0.24 seconds), severe bradycardia, and cardiogenic shock. ***Use with caution*** in pheochromocytoma, impaired hepatic function or jaundice, diabetes mellitus, and peripheral vascular disease.

🖐 **Use with caution for the elderly. Safe use for children and pregnant or nursing mothers has not been established.**

Side effects/Adverse reactions

Hypersensitivity: rash. ***CV:*** orthostatic hypotension, arrhythmias, CHF, peripheral vascular disease. ***CNS:*** dizziness, fatigue, vivid dreams, insomnia, headache. ***Resp:*** increased airway resistance, nasal stuffiness. ***GI:*** nausea, vomiting, diarrhea. ***GU:*** urinary retention, sexual dysfunction. ***Skin:*** numbness and tingling of scalp.

Nursing implications/Documentation

Possible nursing diagnoses: Activity intolerance; Fatigue; Potential for injury.

♦ Assess mental status, and record pulse and blood pressure (if possible, lying, sitting, and standing, in both arms) before administration, and frequently thereafter until response is determined.

♦ Consult with physician to determine desired therapeutic range for blood pressure and heart rate (parameters for withholding the medication should be written by physician).

♦ Ascertain that baseline CBC, electrolytes, BUN, creatinine, and liver function studies have been obtained before giving first dose; report abnormalities and monitor closely thereafter.

♦ Monitor for allergic reactions and signs of confusion, dizziness, bradycardia, CHF, and hypotension; hold drug and report immediately if these occur.

♦ Supervise ambulation until response is determined.

♦ Document and monitor daily weight, and intake and output; report significant negative or positive balance.

Patient & family teaching/Home care

Possible nursing diagnoses: Knowledge deficit; Impaired home maintenance management; Altered sexuality patterns.

♦ Explain the importance of taking this drug exactly as prescribed, even when feeling well;

warn not to discontinue drug abruptly (may precipitate angina).

◆ Stress the importance of good medical follow-up, explain that this drug reduces "wear and tear" on blood vessels, reduces the workload of heart, and improves longevity and health.

◆ Teach how to monitor pulse and blood pressure; emphasize that syncope, hypertension or hypotension, or persistent dizziness should be reported; provide pulse and blood pressure parameters for withholding medication.

◆ With IV route, explain that vital signs are taken frequently to monitor blood pressure and cardiac response; stress the need to stay in bed.

◆ With oral route, advise changing positions slowly, to avoid dizziness.

◆ Encourage daily monitoring of weight, and reporting sudden weight gain (frequently fluid retention).

◆ Warn against drinking alcohol or taking *any* OTC drugs without physician approval (some interactions can cause severe reactions).

◆ Explain that this drug may alter sexual activity; counsel about concerns.

◆ *See Beta Adrenergic Blockers and Anti-hypertensives overviews for more information.*

lactulose

lak'tyoo-lose

Cephulac, Cholac, Chronulac, Constilac, Duphalac, ✦*Lactulax*

Class: Stimulant laxative, Ammonia detoxicant

PEDS	PREG	GERI
∜	C	∜

Action Increases peristalsis and promotes bowel evacuation by acidifying the colon and causing fermentative osmosis; promotes trapping of ammonia in colon by acidification of colon contents.

Use/Therapeutic goal/Outcome

Constipation: Promotion of short-term relief. *Outcome criteria:* Evacuation of soft stool mass (within 24–48 hrs).

Hyperammonemia: Prevention and treatment of portal system encephalopathy and hepatic coma. *Outcome criteria:* Reduction of blood ammonia concentrations and improved mental state.

Dose range/Administration

Interaction alert: Effectiveness will be decreased when taken with oral anti-infectives because of reduction in bacteria levels in colon.

Laxative: **Adult:** PO: 15–30 ml.

Hyperammonemia: **Adult:** PO: 30–45 ml/day. RECT: 30–45 ml in 100 ml of water as retention enema.

Clinical alert: In the initial treatment of dangerously high ammonia levels, dose may be repeated every hour to induce rapid effect; subsequent doses may be adjusted to produce 2–3 soft stools daily.

Contraindications/Precautions

PREG
C

Contraindicated in hypersensitivity to lactulose. Use with caution in diabetics.

∜ **Use with caution for pregnant or nursing mothers and the elderly. Safe use for children has not been established.**

Side effects/Adverse reactions

Hypersensitivity: none listed. *GI:* Cramping, diarrhea, intestinal bloating, increased thirst. *Misc:* hypokalemia, dehydration.

Nursing implications/Documentation

Possible nursing diagnoses: Diarrhea; Pain.

◆ Give single daily dose before breakfast for best results.

◆ Administer mixed with fruit juice, citrus-flavored carbonated beverage, or milk to enhance palatability.

◆ Encourage fluid intake of at least 6–8 full glasses daily to improve response to medication and to avoid dehydration.

◆ In hepatic coma, lactulose enema may be given and should be retained for 30–60 min; do not administer alkaline agents such as soap suds as cleansing enema.

◆ Assess and record mental status during therapy for hepatic encephalopathy.

◆ Monitor and document bowel sounds and frequency and character of bowel evacuation.

◆ Do not give any other laxatives to patient being treated with lactulose for hyperammonemia.

Patient & family teaching/Home care

Possible nursing diagnoses: Knowledge deficit; Impaired home maintenance management.

- ◆ Suggest mixing lactulose with milk, juice, or carbonated beverages to increase palatability.
- ◆ Stress the importance of dietary bulk, fluids, and exercise to prevent constipation.
- ◆ Caution not to take other laxatives while using lactulose for ammonia-reducing effects.
- ◆ For reduction of ammonia levels, advise that 2–3 bowel movements per day is desired effect.
- ◆ *See Laxatives overview for more information.*

leucovorin
loo-koe-vor'in

leucovorin calcium (folinic acid): *Wellcovorin*

Class: Antianemic, Antidote to folic acid antagonists

PEDS	PREG	GERI
✋	C	✋

Action (Similar to folic acid.) Required for production of RBCs, WBCs, and platelets, and for nucleoprotein synthesis; competes with folic acid antagonists for transport into cells, especially bone marrow and GI tract cells.

Use/Therapeutic goal/Outcome

Megaloblastic anemia: Provides adequate levels of folate when oral folic acid therapy is not feasible. **Outcome criteria:** Normal CBC, weight gain; report of absence of fatigue.

Antidote to folic acid antagonists: Protection from hematopoietic and reticuloendothelial effects of unintentional or therapeutic high doses of methotrexate, pyrimethamine, and trimethoprim. **Outcome criteria:** RBC, WBC, and platelet counts within acceptable range; nontoxic blood level of folic acid antagonist.

Dose range/Administration

Interaction alert: Large doses decrease anticonvulsant effects of phenobarbital, phenytoin, and primidone. Concurrent use with fluorouracil may increase therapeutic and toxic effects of fluorouracil.

Megaloblastic anemia: Adult and Child: PO, IM: 1 mg/day.

Antidote to folic acid antagonists: Adult and Child: PO, IV, IM: 5–15 mg/day.

Methotrexate "rescue": Adult and Child: PO, IV, IM: 10 mg/m^2 q6h for 72 hr; individualize dose based on serum creatinine, tumor type, methotrexate dose and route of administration.

Clinical alert: Administer by parenteral route if nausea and vomiting preclude oral administration or when dose is greater than 25 mg.

Contraindications/Precautions

Contraindicated in hypersensitivity to leucovorin (or to lactose contained in oral tablets), and in undiagnosed anemia or pernicious anemia. **Use with caution** in renal disease, aciduria (pH < 7), ascites, pleural or peritoneal effusions, GI obstruction, and dehydration.

✋ **Use with caution for children taking anticonvulsants (may cause increase in seizures), pregnant or nursing mothers, and the elderly.**

Side effects/Adverse reactions

Hypersensitivity: rash, pruritis, urticaria, bronchospasm. **Skin:** local pain and irritation at injection site. **CNS:** seizures in susceptible children.

Nursing implications/Documentation

Possible nursing diagnoses: Pain; Potential for injury.

- ◆ For treatment of folic acid antagonist overdose, administer first dose of leucovorin within 1 hour; increase fluid intake to enhance renal excretion.
- ◆ In history of seizure disorders, monitor for reoccurrence.

Patient & family teaching/Home care

Possible nursing diagnosis: Knowledge deficit.

- ◆ For treatment of deficiency, teach patient the important food sources of folic acid (fruits, nuts, vegetables, bran, and yeast).
- ◆ For methotrexate rescue, emphasize importance of spacing doses evenly around the clock, and the importance of not missing any doses; advise to report any problems with prescribed schedule.
- ◆ Stress the need to maintain close medical supervision and to have blood tests done as ordered.

leuprolide
loo-proe'lide

leuprolide acetate: ◆*Lucrin, Lupron, Lupron Depot*

Class: Antineoplastic agent, Antihormone

PEDS	PREG	GERI
✋	B	✋

Action Inhibits malignant cellular growth of gonadotropin-responsive tumors by desensitizing pituitary receptors and suppressing luteinizing hormone and testosterone levels.

Use/Therapeutic goal/Outcome

Advanced prostatic cancer (palliative treatment): Suppression of malignant cell proliferation. *Outcome criteria:* Tumor and disease regression or stabilization on radiologic and physical examination.

Dose range/Administration

Adult: SC: 1 mg/day. IM: (Lupron Depot) 7.5 mg/mon.

Clinical alert: Initial response to leuprolide acetate causes an increase in follicle-stimulating and luteinizing hormone, which leads to a transient increase in testosterone. These levels decrease in 2–4 weeks.

Contraindications/Precautions

PREG
B

Contraindicated in hypersensitivity to leuprolide acetate or benzyl alcohol (used in leuprolide injection).

🖐 **Contraindicated for children and pregnant or nursing mothers. Use with caution for the elderly.**

Side effects/Adverse reactions

Hypersensitivity: itching, rash. *CNS:* anxiety, dizziness, headache, paresthesia, lethargy, insomnia. *Eye:* blurred vision. *Resp:* difficulty breathing, pleural rub, pulmonary fibrosis. *CV:* CHF, peripheral edema, thrombophlebitis, pulmonary emboli, dysrhythmias, MI. *Hem:* decreased hematocrit, hemoglobin. *GI:* anorexia, nausea, vomiting, sour taste in mouth, constipation, bleeding. *GU:* impotence, decrease in testes size, hematuria, difficulty urinating. *Skin:* alopecia, local reactions at injection site. *Misc:* transient bone pain during the first week of treatment, decreased libido, hot flashes.

Nursing implications/Documentation

Possible nursing diagnoses: Fluid volume deficit; Altered patterns of urinary elimination; Self-esteem disturbance; Altered nutrition: less than body requirements.

◆ *See important Nursing implications in Antineoplastic agents overview.*

◆ Document and monitor urinary elimination; report hematuria or difficulty voiding.

◆ Record daily weights; report weight gain more than 2 lb in a day.

◆ Monitor serum testosterone and acid phosphatase levels, (should increase the first two

weeks and then drop to levels consistent with medical castration).

Patient & family teaching/Home care

Possible nursing diagnoses: Knowledge deficit; Impaired home maintenance management; Altered sexuality patterns.

◆ *See important Patient & family teaching in Antineoplastic agents overview.*

◆ If bone pain or hot flashes are experienced, reassure that these are transient and usually subside with continued therapy.

◆ Ascertain that the patient or caretaker can demonstrate management of SC injections.

◆ Encourage monitoring daily weights and reporting edema or weight gain greater than 2 lb in a day.

◆ Explore sexual concerns; refer to a specialist for counseling if necessary.

◆ *See Antineoplastic agents overview for more information.*

levamisole

lee-vam'i-sole

L

levamisole hydrochloride: *Ergamisol*
Class: Immunomodulator, Biologic response modifier

PEDS PREG GERI
🖐   C   🖐

Action Exact mechanism of action is unclear. Appears to restore depressed immune function rather than stimulate response to above-normal levels: stimulates formation of antibodies to various antigens; enhances T-cell responses by stimulating T-cell activation and proliferation; potentiates monocyte and macrophage functions, including phagocytosis and chemotaxis; increases neutrophil mobility, adherence, and chemotaxis. Has cholinergic activity.

Use/Therapeutic goal/Outcome

Duke's stage C colon cancer (used only after surgical resection and in combination with fluorouracil): Enhancement of immunity and prevention of cancer cell proliferation. *Outcome criteria:* Absence of recurrence of tumor growth on X ray or biopsy.

Dose range/Administration

Interaction alert: Alcohol may cause disulfiram-like reaction (nausea, vomiting, flushing, headache, chest pain).

Adult: PO: 50 mg q8h for 3 days starting 7–30 days after surgery, with 450 mg/m^2/day IV flurorouracil for 5 days starting 21–34 days after surgery. *Maintenance dose:* 50 mg q8h for 3 days every 2 weeks for 1 yr, with 450 mg/m^2 of IV fluorouracil weekly starting 28 days after the initial 5-day course.

Clinical alert: Since this drug is indicated only for concomitant use with IV fluorouracil, nurses who are giving this drug should become familiar with the comprehensive management of the patient receiving IV fluorouracil (see fluorouracil).

Contraindications/Precautions

PREG
C

Contraindicated in hypersensitivity to levamisole. **Use with caution** in bone-marrow depression, renal impairment, infection, and seizure disorders.

♨ Contraindicated for nursing mothers. Use with caution in the elderly. Safe use for children and pregnant women has not been established.

Side effects/Adverse reactions

Hypersensitivity: rashes, dermatitis, flu-like symptoms. **GI:** nausea, vomiting, diarrhea, stomatitis, altered taste, anorexia, abdominal pain. **Hem:** agranulocytosis (may be asymptomatic, but often accompanied by onset of fever and chills, sometimes fatal), leukopenia, thrombocytopenia. **Skin:** hair loss. **CNS:** dizziness, headache, paresthesia, ataxia. **Ear:** abnormal hearing. **Eye:** blurred vision, conjunctivitis.

Nursing implications/Documentation

Possible nursing diagnoses: Potential for infection; Altered oral mucous membrane; Diarrhea.

♦ Check baseline CBC with differential platelets, electrolytes, and liver function tests before first dose; thereafter, monitor CBC with differential and platelets weekly before fluorouracil doses, and check electrolytes and liver function studies every 3 months for 1 yr.

♦ Report onset of fever and chills immediately (may indicate agranulocytosis).

Patient & family teaching/Home care

Possible nursing diagnoses: Knowledge deficit; Fear; Body image disturbance; Ineffective individual coping.

♦ Point out that studies have shown that the use of this drug with fluorouracil has demon-

strated a significant reduction in tumor recurrence.

♦ Stress the importance of reporting onset of fever, chills, and flu-like symptoms immediately.

levodopa (L-dopa)

lee-voe-doe'pa

Dopar, Larodopa, Levopa, Parda, Rio-Dopa
Class: Antiparkinsons, Dopaminergic agent

PEDS	PREG	GERI
♨	C	♨

Action Converts to dopamine (a neurotransmitter) in extrapyramidal centers of the brain, restoring depleted dopamine levels (thought to cause parkinsonian symptoms). It is the precursor of dopamine, and it crosses the blood-brain barrier.

Use/Therapeutic goal/Outcome

Parkinsonism: Control of parkinsonian symptoms, promotion of mobility. **Outcome criteria:** Absence of or decrease in tremors, rigidity, akinesia, and drooling; improvement in gait, balance, posture, speech, and handwriting.

Dose range/Administration

Interaction alert: Effects of levodopa may be decreased by antipsychotics, phenytoin, Vitamin B6 (pyridoxine), multivitamins containing B6 (pyridoxine), reserpine, and benzodiazepines. Levodopa may enhance the effect of antihypertensive drugs, and the cardiovascular effects of sympathomimetic drugs such as amphetamine, ephedrine, and epinephrine (monitor for dysrythmias). The therapeutic effects of levodopa may be potentiated by propranolol, methyldopa, and anticholinergics. Avoid concomitant use of levodopa and tricyclic antidepressants or MAO inhibitors (may result in tachycardia and hypertension). May alter dose requirement of antidiabetics.

♥ Give with meals.

Adult: PO: 0.5 to 1 g daily in divided doses (bid to qid); increase by increments of not more than 0.75 g every 3–7 days, until maximum of 8 g/day is reached.

Clinical alert: Dosage is highly individualized, depending on clinical response and incidence of side effects (dose should be carefully titrated to lowest effective dose). Report muscle twitching and eyelid twitching immediately (may indicate toxicity).

Contraindications/Precautions

Contraindicated in hypersensitivity to levodopa or tartrazine, and in narrow-angle glaucoma, melanoma, skin lesions, psychosis, recent use of MAO inhibitors. **Use with caution** in patients with cardiovascular disease; renal, hepatic, or respiratory disorders; seizures; diabetes; asthma; peptic ulcer; and endocrine disorders.

🖐 **Use with caution for the elderly. Safe use for pregnant or nursing mothers and for children has not been established.**

Side effects/Adverse reactions

Hypersensitivity: rash, flushing. **CV:** orthostatic hypotension, tachycardia, hypertension. **GI:** anorexia, nausea, vomiting, abdominal pain, dry mouth, bitter taste, constipation, diarrhea, hepatotoxicity. **CNS:** involuntary movements, ataxia, muscle twitching, weakness, confusion, agitation, behavioral changes, insomnia, nightmares, depression. **Eye:** blurred vision, spasm or closing of eyelids. **GU:** urinary retention, incontinence, brown urine. **Skin:** dark-colored sweat. **Misc:** increased sexual drive.

Nursing implications/Documentation

Possible nursing diagnoses: Potential for injury; Impaired physical mobility; Fluid volume deficit.

◆ Establish a baseline profile of patient's abilities and disabilities to differentiate between desired responses and drug-induced side effects.

◆ Recognize that levodopa is available in combination with carbidopa (carbidopa-levodopa), which is likely to decrease the required dose of levodopa by 75 percent, which reduces the incidence of side effects.

◆ Monitor vital signs closely during periods of dose adjustment; record at least bid.

◆ For those on long-term therapy, periodically check blood sugar, and liver and kidney function studies.

◆ Have patient dangle legs before ambulating (because of risk of postural hypotension); supervise ambulation until response is determined.

◆ Be aware that a medically supervised drug holiday may reduce dose requirement.

Patient & family teaching/Home care

Possible nursing diagnoses: Self-care deficit; Impaired home maintenance management.

◆ Point out the need to take this drug with food to reduce GI symptoms.

◆ Caution not to increase or decrease dosage without the physician's approval; stress the need for ongoing medical follow-up.

◆ Advise that multivitamin labels should be checked to be sure they do not contain Vitamin B6 (pyridoxine), which reverses the effects of levodopa.

◆ Explain that the patient may need increased help with self-care until stabilized on dose regimen.

◆ Advise reporting muscle twitching or eyelid twitching, because this may indicate drug toxicity.

◆ Inform that after long-term therapy, sometimes patients experience a worsening of symptoms and unexpected rigidity, tremor, and/or inability to move; this should be reported immediately because it may require a temporary drug holiday or change in dosing schedule.

◆ *See Antiparkinsons overview for more information.*

levorphanol tartrate

lee-vor'fa-nole

Levo-Dromoran

Class: Narcotic analgesic

Antidote: naloxone hydrochloride (Narcan)

PEDS	PREG	GERI	CONTROLLED SUBSTANCE
🖐	B	🖐	II

Action Alters both perception of and response to pain by binding with opiate receptors at many CNS sites; has properties and actions similar to morphine (it is a synthetic morphine derivative).

Use/Therapeutic goal/Outcome

Moderate to severe pain: Relief of pain. **Outcome criteria:** Report of comfort; absence of observable signs of pain (grimacing, frowning, restlessness, reluctance to move or cough), with increase in signs of comfort (relaxed facial expression, decreased restlessness); blood pressure and pulse within normal limits when compared to baseline.

Dose range/Administration

Interaction alert: General anesthetics, other narcotic analgesics, tranquilizers, sedatives, hypnotics, alcohol, tricyclic antidepressants, and MAOI therapy increases CNS depression (reduce levorphanol doses).

Adult: PO, SC: 2–3 mg q6-8h prn or around the clock.

Clinical alert: Expect decreased dosage for the elderly or debilitated. Check respirations and blood pressure before giving levorphanol. Hold drug and report if respirations < 12, or if there is hypotension. Keep naloxone readily available in case of respiratory depression.

Contraindications/Precautions

PREG
B

Contraindicated in hypersensitivity to levorphanol tartrate and in acute alcoholism, bronchial asthma, increased intracranial pressure, respiratory depression, and anoxia. *Use with caution* in hepatic or renal disease, hypothyroidism, Addison's disease, seizures, head injury, severe CNS depression, brain tumor, COPD, or shock.

☙ **Contraindicated for children and pregnant or nursing mothers. Use with caution for the elderly or debilitated.**

Side effects/Adverse reactions

Hypersensitivity: rash. *CNS:* dizziness, sedation, euphoria, convulsions (large doses), physical dependence. *Resp:* respiratory depression. *GI:* nausea, vomiting, constipation. *CV:* hypotension, bradycardia. *GU:* urinary retention.

Nursing implications/Documentation

Possible nursing diagnoses: Pain; Anxiety; Potential for injury.

◆ Have patient rate pain on a scale of 1–10 before and after medication is given; report and record inadequate pain control.

◆ Document pulse, respirations, and blood pressure immediately before and 1 hr after administration until response is determined (then check qid if hospitalized).

◆ Monitor closely for risk factors for injury; keep side rails up and supervise ambulation if allowed out of bed.

◆ Give before pain is severe for best effects.

◆ Be aware of potential for psychic and physical dependence after prolonged use (withdrawal symptoms are similar to those of morphine).

Patient & family teaching/Home care

Possible nursing diagnoses: Sensory/perceptual alterations; Knowledge deficit.

◆ Warn that this drug has a bitter taste.

◆ Explain the rationale for reporting pain/discomfort before it is severe.

◆ Advise those who are ambulatory to refrain from activities that require alertness and to seek assistance if there is any question about ability to get out of bed (e.g., if there is weakness or light headedness).

◆ Explain procedures briefly and in simple terms.

◆ Warn not to exceed prescribed dose because of overdose, dependence, and abuse potential (instead of increasing dose regimen, unsatisfactory pain relief should be reported).

◆ Stress that alcohol and other CNS depressants may cause excessive sedation.

◆ *See Narcotic and non-narcotic analgesics overview for more information.*

levothyroxine

lee-voe-thye-rox'een

levothyroxine sodium (T_4 or L-thyroxine sodium): ✦*Eltroxin, Levoid, Levothroid, Levoxine,* ➥*Oroxine, Synthroid, Synthrox*

Class: Thyroid hormone

PEDS	PREG	GERI
☙	A	☙

Action Accelerates rate of cellular metabolism by increasing blood levels of thyroid hormone (resulting in increased metabolic rate, cardiac output, oxygen consumption, body temperature, and blood volume, and promotion of growth and development).

Use/Therapeutic goal/Outcome

Hypothyroidism, cretinism, myxedema coma, nontoxic goiter: Replacement of deficient circulating thyroid hormones, promotion of normal metabolism. *Outcome criteria:* Increased T_3 and T_4 levels, weight loss, increased appetite, decreased fatigue, normal skin and hair texture, normal heart rate, normal growth and development.

Dose range/Administration

Interaction alert: Give at least 1 hr before or 4 hours after giving cholestyramine and colestipol (they impair levothyroxine absorption). Increases effects of anticoagulants, and tricyclic antidepressants. Monitor those receiving digoxin for digitalis toxicity. Catecholamines increase risk of coronary insufficiency (report chest pain). May alter insulin requirements.

🖐 **Give 1 hour before meals or 2 hours after meals for best absorption.**

Thyroid hormone replacement: Adult: PO, IM, IV: (PO unless contraindicated.) 25–50 mcg/day qAM, then increase by 25–50 mcg q1-4 wks prn. *Maintenance dose:* 25–75 mcg/day. *Maximum dose:* 100–200 mcg. *For the elderly:* 25 mcg/day qAM, increase by 25 mcg q3-4 wks prn. *Child:* PO: A single dose, then change dose q1-4 wks prn. *< 6 mos:* 25–50 mcg/day. *6–12 mos:* 50–75 mcg/day. *1–5 yr:* 75–100 mcg/day. *6–12 yr:* 100–150 mcg/day.

Myxedema coma: Adult: IV: 0.2–0.5 mg; if no response, give a second dose of 0.1–0.3 mg. *Maintenance dose:* PO: 50–200 mcg/day starting on day 2, when condition stabilizes.

Cretinism: Child: PO: Use thyroid hormone dose above.

Clinical alert: Do not substitute different brands or generic brands for this drug unless approved by physician (they may not be bio-equivalent). Prepare IV doses immediately before administration. Individual response and dose requirement for thyroid hormones *vary greatly.*

Contraindications/Precautions

Contraindicated in hypersensitivity to levothyroxine, and in adrenal insufficiency, myocardial infarction, thyrotoxicosis. *Use with caution* in angina, ischemia, or hypertension.

🖐 **Use with caution for children, pregnant or nursing mothers, and the elderly.**

Side effects/Adverse reactions

Hypersensitivity: itching, rashes. Other side effects are usually dose related. *CNS:* headache, nervousness, insomnia, tremors. *CV:* palpitations, tachycardia, arrhythmias, angina, hypertension. *GI:* increased appetite, nausea, abdominal cramps, diarrhea. *GU:* change in menstrual flow or cycle. *MS:* weight loss, leg cramps. *Misc:* sweating, heat intolerance. *In children:* partial hair loss, pseudotumor cerebri.

Nursing implications/Documentation

Possible nursing diagnoses: Altered nutrition: less than body requirements; Altered nutrition: more than body requirements.

♦ Record and monitor pulse and blood pressure at least once a day during initial treatment; also document daily weights.

♦ Check T_4 and TSH levels after 6 weeks of therapy for therapeutic range (level below normal indicates need for increase in dose).

♦ For patients over 40 or with a history of cardiovascular disease, monitor for and report symptoms of cardiovascular disease (chest pain, tachycardia, dyspnea).

♦ If radioactive iodine uptake tests are necessary, discontinue drug 4 weeks before test.

♦ For children, monitor growth and development every 3–6 months.

♦ If giving Synthroid tablets, monitor for and report allergic symptoms such as bronchial asthma. (Synthroid has a yellow dye that may produce allergic symptoms.)

Patient & family teaching/Home care

Possible nursing diagnoses: Knowledge deficit; Impaired home maintenance management.

♦ Emphasize the importance of taking this drug daily as prescribed (avoid generic or different brands; take doses at the same time every day, preferably in the morning to prevent insomnia; do not skip or double up on doses).

♦ Explain that this medication is likely to be needed for life, and that medical follow-up is necessary to ensure health.

♦ Advise reporting signs and symptoms of increased fatigue or nervousness, palpitations or tachycardia, chest pain.

♦ Explain that symptoms of hypothyroidism may persist for several months.

♦ Stress that this drug is potentially dangerous and should not be used for simple weight loss or fatigue.

♦ Explain that foods with iodine (iodized salt, some seafood, soybeans, tofu) should be avoided.

♦ Warn that temporary hair loss may occur with children.

♦ Point out the need to tell other physicians a thyroid medication is being taken.

♦ Stress that pregnant women need to return for medical follow-up (dosage may need adjusting during pregnancy and after birth).

♦ *See Thyroid Hormones overview for more information.*

lidocaine (anesthetic)   *lye'doe-kane*

Lidocaine hydrochloride (local): *Ardecaine, Caine–2, Dalcaine, Dilocaine, Lidoject–2, Nervocaine, Rocaine, Stanacaine, Xylocaine*

Class: ★**Local anesthetic (amide-type) prototype**

PEDS	PREG	GERI
☜	B	☜

Action Produces local anesthesia by inhibiting sodium flux across the nerve cell membrane, thus preventing depolarization and generation and conduction of nerve impulses. Lidocaine has a rapid onset, moderate duration, moderate potency and duration. When combined with epinephrine, action is prolonged.

Use/Therapeutic goal/Outcome

Local anesthesia, peripheral nerve block, caudal and spinal block: Prevention of pain during surgical, obstetrical, and dental procedures. *Outcome criteria:* Patient report of numbness, and absence of pain in anesthetized area. Patients undergoing regional anesthesia (caudal, spinal block) will demonstrate loss of motor function in anesthetized area.

Dose range/Administration

Interaction alert: Lidocaine increases the neuromuscular blocking action of succinylcholine, decamethonium, and tubocurarine. For epidural and spinal anesthesia, use only solutions without preservatives. Dosages listed are for use *without* epinephrine except as noted.

Adult: Caudal (during delivery) and epidural (thoracic): Use 200–300 mg (20–30 cc) of a 1% solution. Caudal (during surgery): Use 225–300 mg (15–20 cc) of a 1.5% solution. Epidural (lumbar): Use 225–300 mg (15–20 cc) of a 1.5% solution *or* 200–300 mg (10–15 cc) of a 2% solution. Maximum dose is 200–300 mg/h. Spinal block: Use 75–100 mg (1.5–2 cc) of a 5% solution with 7.5% dextrose. If combined with epinephrine, dosage and interval should be increased. Anesthesia other than spinal: Use no more than 4.5 mg/kg or 300 mg in a single dose. With epinephrine use no more than 7 mg/kg or 500 mg. Do not repeat dose more frequently than q2h. Topical anesthesia: Apply a small amount (jelly, ointment, cream, solution) of 2.5–5% anesthetic to desired area.

Clinical alert: These drugs should be administered only by clinicians thoroughly familiar with their use. Dose is highly individualized and depends upon the procedure, method of administration, area to be anesthetized, vascularity of tissues, condition of patient, and individual tolerance. Epinephrine in local anesthetic preparations may result in angina, tachycardia, tremors, headache, restlessness, palpitations, dizziness, and hypertension. With epidural use, a 2–5 cc test dose should be given at least 5 minutes before giving rest of dose to verify position of catheter or needle. Have resuscitative drugs and equipment readily available.

Contraindications/Precautions   PREG B

Contraindicated in hypersensitivity to lidocaine or other amide-type local anesthetics. Do not use lidocaine anesthetic in the presence of severe trauma or sepsis, blood dyscrasias, supraventricular arrhythmias, Stokes-Adams syndrome, untreated sinus bradycardia, severe degree of sinoatrial, atrioventricular, and intraventricular heart block. *Use with caution* in liver or kidney disease, CHF, marked hypoxia, respiratory depression, hypovolemia, shock, myasthenia gravis, debilitated patients, family history of malignant hyperthermia; topical opthalmic use, topical applications over large body areas; use over prolonged periods, use in severe or extensive trauma or skin disorders.

☜ **Use with caution for the elderly. Safe use for pregnant or nursing mothers and for children has not been established; use with caution.**

Side effects/Adverse reactions

Hypersensitivity: urticaria, rash, edema, anaphylaxis. *CNS:* drowsiness, dizziness, light-headedness, restlessness, confusion, irritability, apprehension, euphoria, wild excitement, numbness of lips or tongue and other paresthesias including sensations of heat and cold, chest heaviness, difficulty speaking, difficulty breathing or swallowing, muscular twitching, tremors, psychosis. **In high doses:** convulsions. *Resp:* respiratory depression and arrest. *CV:* hypotension, bradycardia, conduction disorders (heart block, cardiovascular collapse, cardiac arrest). *Ear:* tinnitus, decreased hearing. *Eye:* blurred or double vision, impaired color perception. *GI:* anorexia, nausea, vomiting. *Skin:* excessive perspiration.

Nursing implications/Documentation

Possible nursing diagnoses: Pain; Potential for injury.

◆ Be sure that history of allergies and accurate height and weight are recorded before procedure.

- Record vital signs according to protocol, and monitor for and report immediately signs of systemic or hypersensitivity reactions.
- Determine from anesthesiologist or anesthetist whether there are any restrictions on patient positioning; post these at bedside.
- Monitor anesthetized area for level of sensation and motor function; watch for poor positioning and protect area from injury.
- Prevent contacting eyes with topical preparation.
- Give prescribed pain medication as sensation begins to return, **before pain is severe**.

Patient & family teaching/Home care

Possible nursing diagnoses: Anxiety; Fear.
- Stress the need to protect areas of the body that have lost sensation.
- Explain rationale for taking prescribed pain medication before pain becomes too uncomfortable.
- Warn that oral topical anesthetics may interfere with swallowing reflex; explain the importance of not eating or drinking for one hour after use (especially for children and the elderly or debilitated).
- *See Local Anesthetics overview for more information.*

lidocaine (systemic) *lye'doe-kane*

lidocaine hydrochloride: *Lido-Pen Auto-Injector, Xylocaine, ✦✦Xylocard*

Class: ★Antiarrhythmic prototype (Class IB)

PEDS	PREG	GERI
ॶ	B	ॶ

Action Suppresses ventricular ectopy by increasing excitability threshold of the ventricles, by depressing automaticity of the His-Purkinje system, and by decreasing the duration of the action potential in Purkinje fibers and ventricles. At usual serum concentrations, does not cause atrioventricular or ventricular conduction disturbances, or affect myocardial contractility.

Use/Therapeutic goal/Outcome

Premature ventricular contractions, ventricular tachycardia, and ventricular fibrillation: Suppression of ventricular ectopy, promotion of effective heartbeat. *Outcome criteria:* Absence of or decrease in ventricular ectopy on EKG; palpable regular pulses.

Dose range/Administration

Interaction alert: Monitor for lidocaine toxicity when given with beta-blockers, cimetidine. Monitor for cardiodepressant effects when using phenytoin concomitantly.

Adult: IV: Initial injection: Give bolus of 50–100 mg (1–1.5 mg/kg) at a rate of 25–50 mg/min. Give one reduced dose to the elderly and to patients weighing less than 50 kg, with CHF, or with hepatic impairment. If initial bolus does not control arrhythmia, repeat injection in 5 min. *Do not give more than 300 mg in a 1-hr period.* Continuous infusion: Continuous IV infusion (via pump) is recommended to maintain effective blood levels and prevent recurrent arrhythmias. Infusions may be administered at the rate of 1–4 mg/min, by diluting 1 g in 500 cc (or 2g in 1L) of D5W. Do not exceed flow rate of 4 mg/min. IM: (Use IM route only if no IV is available.) 300 mg in the deltoid muscle only or thigh (for self-injection). *Child:* IV: 1 mg/kg bolus followed by an infusion of 30 mcg/kg/minute.

Clinical alert: Observe cardiac monitor closely for widened QRS and PR segments or aggravated arrhythmia. Keep resuscitative equipment and drugs nearby. Slow IV rate and immediately report dizziness, confusion, restlessness, or tremors (may indicate toxicity, and can precede seizures).

Contraindications/Precautions

PREG
B

Contraindicated in hypersensitivity to lidocaine and amide-type anesthetics, and in Adams-Stokes syndrome, Wolff-Parkinson-White syndrome, and in the absence of a pacemaker for patients with severe heart block, intraventricular conduction delays, and complete heart block with ventricular "escape" beats (lidocaine may abolish the action of the ventricular focus that maintains heartbeat). *Use with caution* for patients weighing less than 50 kg, and for patients with CHF, or hepatic or renal dysfunction.

ॶ **Use with caution for the elderly. Safe use for pregnant or nursing mothers and for children has not been determined; use with caution.**

Side effects/Adverse reactions

Hypersensitivity: itching, rashes, swelling, difficulty breathing. *CNS:* confusion, anxiety, slurred speech, restlessness, lightheadedness, drowsiness, numbness, twitching, tremors, lethargy, unconsciousness, convulsions. **CV:** hypotension, bradycardia, cardiac arrest, thrombophlebitis at IV site. **Eye:** visual disturbances. **Ear:** tinnitus, transient deafness. **Resp:** respiratory depression. **GI:** anorexia, nausea, vomiting. **Misc:** sensations of heat and cold.

Nursing implications/Documentation

Possible nursing diagnoses: Potential for injury; Activity intolerance.

♦ Check for allergies to local anesthetics of the amide type prior to giving; hold drug and report immediately if these are noted.

♦ Be sure to check baseline chest X-ray, EKG, and laboratory studies (CBC, sodium, potassium, chloride, carbon dioxide, magnesium, BUN, creatinine, SGPT, and LDH) before giving first dose (or as soon as possible after giving first dose); monitor closely thereafter as indicated by clinical condition.

♦ Remember that oxygen requirements must be met, and that electrolyte imbalances (especially potassium and magnesium) and abnormal blood pH must be corrected, before expected antiarrhythmic effect can be seen; report abnormalities immediately.

♦ Document baseline vital signs, lung sounds, and cardiac monitor strip (measure and record PR and QRS segments) before giving first dose and at least every 8 hr; monitor closely until response is determined; report if prolongation in PR or QRS segment is noted.

♦ Keep patient in bed with side rails up until response is determined.

♦ Coordinate care to provide frequent rest periods.

Patient & family teaching/Home care

Possible nursing diagnoses: Fear; Knowledge deficit; Impaired home maintenance management.

♦ Explain that the purpose of this drug is to prevent arrhythmias and promote an effective heartbeat.

♦ Stress that the patient notify nurses if dizziness, visual disturbances, or "strange feeling" is experienced; these may be related to the medication.

♦ Emphasize the need to pace activities, avoid stress, and plan for rest periods.

♦ *See Antiarrhythmics overview for more information.*

liothyronine

lye-oh-thy'roe-neen

liothyronine sodium (T_3): **Cyronine, Cytomel, ♠Tertroxin**

Class: Thyroid hormone

PEDS	PREG	GERI
🖐	A	🖐

Action Accelerates rate of cellular metabolism by increasing blood levels of thyroid hormone (resulting in increased metabolic rate, cardiac output, oxygen consumption, body temperature, blood volume, and promotion of growth and development in children). Has a rapid onset of action and a short duration, which makes it useful when a rapid effect is needed.

Use/Therapeutic goal/Outcome

Hypothyroidism, myxedema coma, nontoxic goiter, thyroid hormone replacement: Replacement of deficient circulating thyroid hormones, promotion of normal metabolism. **Outcome criteria:** Increased T_3 and T_4 levels, weight loss, normal heart rate, increased appetite, decreased fatigue, normal skin and hair texture, normal growth and development.

T_3 suppression test in patients with borderline high iodine thyroid uptake test: Differentiation of hyperthyroidism from euthyroidism. **Outcome criteria:** I-131 scan demonstrating level of thyroid iodine uptake.

Dose range/Administration

Interaction alert: Give at least 1 hour before or 4 hours after giving cholestyramine and colestipol (they impair liothyronine absorption). Increases effects of anticoagulants, and tricyclic antidepressants. Monitor those taking digoxin for digitalis toxicity. Catecholamines, increase risk of coronary insufficiency (report chest pain). May alter insulin requirements.

🥄 **Give 1 hour before meals or 2 hours after meals for best absorption.**

Thyroid hormone replacement: Adult: PO: 25 mcg/day qAM, then increase by 12.5–25 mcg q1-2 wks prn. *Maintenance dose:* 25–75 mcg/day. *For the elderly:* 5 mcg/day, then increase q1-2 wks prn.

Nontoxic goiter: Adult: PO: 5 mcg/day qAM, then increase by 12.5–25 mcg q1-2 wks prn. (for the elderly, 5 mcg/wk). *Maintenance dose:* 75 mcg/day. **Child:** PO: 5 mcg/day qAM, then increase by 5 mcg q3-4 days prn.

Myxedema: *Adult:* PO: 5 mcg/day qAM, increase by 5–10 mcg q1-2 wks prn. *Maintenance dose:* 50–100 mcg/day.

T₃ suppression test: **Adult:** PO: 75–100 mcg/day qAM for 7 days, then do I-131 scan.

Clinical alert: Do not substitute different brands or generic brands for this drug unless approved by physician (they may not be bio-equivalent). Individual response and dose requirement for thyroid hormones *vary greatly.*

Contraindications/Precautions

PREG
A

Contraindicated in hypersensitivity to liothyronine and in adrenal insufficiency, myocardial infarction, thyrotoxicosis. **Use with caution** in angina, myocardial ischemia, or hypertension.

✋ **Use with caution for children, pregnant or nursing mothers, and the elderly.**

Side effects/Adverse reactions

Hypersensitivity: itching, rashes. Other side effects are usually dose related. **CNS:** headache, nervousness, insomnia, tremors. **CV:** palpitations, tachycardia, dysrhythmias, angina, hypertension. **GI:** increased appetite, nausea, abdominal cramps, diarrhea. **GU:** change in menstrual flow or cycle. **MS:** weight loss, leg cramps. **Misc:** sweating, heat intolerance.

Nursing implications/Documentation

Possible nursing diagnoses: Altered nutrition: less than body requirements; Altered nutrition: more than body requirements.

♦ Record and monitor pulse and blood pressure at least once a day during initial treatment; also document daily weights.

♦ Monitor T₄ and TSH levels for therapeutic range (level below normal indicates need for increase in dose).

♦ For patients over 40 or with a history of cardiovascular disease, monitor for and report symptoms of cardiovascular disease (chest pain, tachycardia, dyspnea).

♦ If radioactive iodine uptake tests are necessary, discontinue drug 4 weeks before test.

♦ For children, monitor growth and development every 3–6 months.

Patient & family teaching/Home care

Possible nursing diagnoses: Knowledge deficit; Impaired home maintenance management.

♦ Emphasize the importance of taking this drug daily as prescribed (avoid generic or different brands; take doses at the same time every day, preferably in the morning to prevent insomnia; do not skip or double up on doses).

♦ Explain that this medication is likely to be needed for life, and that medical follow-up is necessary to ensure health.

♦ Advise reporting signs and symptoms of increased fatigue or nervousness, palpitations or tachycardia, chest pain.

♦ Explain that symptoms of hypothyroidism may persist for several months.

♦ Stress that this drug is potentially dangerous and should not be used for simple weight loss or fatigue.

♦ Point out the need to tell other physicians that thyroid medication is being taken.

♦ *See Thyroid Hormones overview for more information.*

liotrix

lye'oh-trix

L

Euthroid, Thyrolar
Class: Thyroid hormone

PEDS	PREG	GERI
✋	A	✋

Action Accelerates rate of cellular metabolism by increasing blood levels of thyroid hormone (resulting in increased metabolic rate, cardiac output, oxygen consumption, body temperature, and blood volume, and promotion of growth and development). Liotrix is a synthetic combination of T₃ and T₄.

Use/Therapeutic goal/Outcome

Hypothyroidism: Replacement of deficient circulating thyroid hormones, promotion of normal metabolism. **Outcome criteria:** Increased T₃ and T₄ levels, normal heart rate, weight loss, increased appetite, decreased fatigue, normal skin and hair texture, normal growth and development.

Dose range/Administration

Interaction alert: Give at least 1 hour before or 4 hours after giving cholestyramine and colestipol (they impair liotrix absorption). Increases effects of anticoagulants, and tricyclic antidepressants. Monitor those taking digoxin for digitalis toxicity. Catecholamines increase risk of coronary insufficiency (report chest pain). May alter insulin requirements.

☐ **Give 1 hour before meals or 2 hours after meals for best absorption.**

Adult and Child: PO: 15–30 mg/day qAM, then increase by 15–30 mg q1-2 wks prn (for children, q 2 wks; for the elderly, q6-8 wks).

Clinical alert: Do not substitute different brands or generic brands for this drug unless approved by physician (they may not be bio-equivalent). Individual response and dose requirements for thyroid hormones *vary greatly.*

Contraindications/Precautions

PREG A

Contraindicated in hypersensitivity to liotrix, and in adrenal insufficiency, myocardial infarction, thyrotoxicosis. **Use with caution** in angina, ischemia, or hypertension.

🖑 **Use with caution for children, pregnant or nursing mothers, and the elderly.**

Side effects/Adverse reactions

Hypersensitivity: itching, rashes. Other side effects are usually dose related. **CNS:** headache, nervousness, insomnia, tremors. **CV:** palpitations, tachycardia, arrhythmias, angina, hypertension. **GI:** increased appetite, nausea, abdominal cramps, diarrhea. **GU:** change in menstrual flow or cycle. **MS:** weight loss, leg cramps. **Misc:** sweating, heat intolerance.

Nursing implications/Documentation

Possible nursing diagnoses: Altered nutrition: less than body requirements; Altered nutrition: more than body requirements.

♦ Record and monitor pulse and blood pressure at least once a day during initial treatment; also document daily weights.

♦ Monitor T_4 and TSH levels for therapeutic range (level below normal indicates need for increase in dose).

♦ For patients over 40 or with a history of cardiovascular disease, monitor for and report symptoms of cardiovascular disease (chest pain, tachycardia, dyspnea).

♦ If radioactive iodine uptake tests are necessary, discontinue drug 4 weeks before test.

♦ For children, monitor growth and development every 3–6 months.

♦ For Euthroid, monitor for allergic reaction (bronchial asthma) because it contains a yellow dye to which some are allergic.

Patient & family teaching/Home care

Possible nursing diagnoses: Knowledge deficit; Impaired home maintenance management.

♦ Emphasize the importance of taking this drug daily as prescribed (avoid generic or different brands; take doses at the same time every day, preferably in the morning to prevent insomnia; do not skip or double up on doses).

♦ Explain that this medication is likely to be needed for life, and that medical follow-up is necessary to ensure health.

♦ Advise reporting signs and symptoms of increased fatigue or nervousness, palpitations or tachycardia, chest pain.

♦ Explain that symptoms of hypothyroidism may persist for several months.

♦ Stress that this drug is potentially dangerous and should not be used for simple weight loss or fatigue.

♦ *See Thyroid Hormone overview for more information.*

lisinopril

li-sin'o-pril

Prinivil, Zestril

Class: Antihypertensive, Angiotensin converting enzyme (ACE) inhibitor

PEDS 🖑 **PREG** C **GERI** 🖑

Action Reduces blood pressure by acting on the renin-angiotensin system: Inhibits angiotensin converting enzyme (ACE), thereby blocking the conversion of angiotensin I to angiotensin II, which is a very potent vasoconstrictor that also stimulates aldosterone secretion (causes kidney reabsorption of sodium and water). Lisinopril thus prevents vasoconstriction and retention of sodium and water.

Use/Therapeutic goal/Outcome

Hypertension: Blood pressure within normal limits. **Outcome criteria:** Blood pressure readings within normal limits.

Dose range/Administration

Interaction alert: Potassium supplements or potassium-sparing diuretics may increase risk of hyperkalemia. Diuretics increase hypotensive effects (may require dose adjustment).

Adult: PO: 10 mg/day; may increase gradually to 20–40 mg/day.

Clinical alert: For those with kidney impairment, expect lower dosage.

Contraindications/Precautions

Contraindicated in hypersensitivity to any ACE inhibitor. **Use with caution** in impaired renal function.

☟ Use with caution for the elderly. Safe use for children and pregnant or nursing mothers has not been established.

Side effects/Adverse reactions

Hypersensitivity: angioedema of face, extremities, lips, tongue, glottis and larynx; rash. **CNS:** dizziness, headache, fatigue, decreased libido. **CV:** hypotension, chest pain. **Resp:** upper respiratory symptoms, including cough. **GI:** diarrhea, vomiting. **GU:** acute renal impairment, proteinuria. **Hem:** hyperkalemia, neutropenia, agranulocytosis.

Nursing implications/Documentation

Possible nursing diagnoses: Activity intolerance; Fatigue; Potential for injury.

♦ Assess mental status, and record pulse and blood pressure before administration, and frequently thereafter until response is determined.

♦ Consult with physician to determine desired therapeutic range for blood pressure (be aware that some patients may require a slightly elevated blood pressure to perfuse vital organs).

♦ Ascertain that baseline CBC, electrolytes, BUN, creatinine, and liver function studies have been obtained before giving first dose; report abnormalities and monitor closely thereafter (WBC counts should be performed every 2–3 weeks for the first 3 months, and periodically thereafter).

♦ Monitor for allergic reactions and for confusion, dizziness, bradycardia, or hypotension; hold drug and report immediately if these occur.

♦ Supervise ambulation until response is determined.

♦ Document and monitor daily weight, and intake and output; report significant negative or positive balance.

Patient & family teaching/Home care

Possible nursing diagnoses: Knowledge deficit; Impaired home maintenance management.

♦ Explain the importance of taking medication exactly as prescribed, even when feeling well.

♦ Stress the importance of good medical follow-up, explain that this drug reduces "wear and tear" on blood vessels, thus improving longevity and health.

♦ Teach how to monitor pulse and blood pressure; emphasize that syncope, hypertension or hypotension, or persistent dizziness should be reported.

♦ Advise changing positions slowly to avoid dizziness.

♦ Encourage daily monitoring of weight and reporting sudden weight gain (frequently is fluid retention).

♦ Instruct people to report symptoms of sore throat, fever, or malaise, because they may indicate an abnormal WBC count.

♦ Warn against taking *any* OTC drugs without physician approval (some interactions can cause severe reactions).

♦ *See Antihypertensives overview for more information.*

lithium

li'thee-um

L

lithium carbonate: ♠*Camcolit,* ♣*Carbolith,* ♥*Duralith, Eskalith, Eskalith CR, Lithane,* ♠*Lithicarb,* ♣*Lithizine, Lithobid, Lithonate, Lithotabs,* ♠*Priadel*

lithium citrate: *Cibalith-S*

Class: Antimania agent

PEDS ☟ PREG D GERI ☟

Action Exact mechanism of action is unknown. Believed to normalize mood and alleviate and prevent symptoms associated with bipolar disorder by decreasing the release of neurotransmitters in the brain. A naturally occurring salt, lithium also effects nerve function by substituting for sodium ions, which are essential regulators of nerve function. Serum lithium levels peak within hours of administration, but clinical effects do not appear for 1–2 weeks.

Use/Therapeutic goal/Outcome

Manic and depressive bipolar affective disorders, recurring depressive episodes in unipolar illness: Elimination or prevention of mood swings, promotion of reality orientation and ability to interact with others. **Outcome criteria:** After 1–3 weeks, absence of episodes of mania (rapid speech, increased psychomotor

►

lithium 433

activity, sleeplessness, inability to concentrate); report of absence of episodes of severe depression (extreme feelings of sadness, that nothing is worthwhile); demonstration of reality orientation, and ability to problem solve and interact with others.

Dose range/Administration

Interaction alert: Use extreme caution if given with diuretics, which increase reabsorption of lithium; monitor for lithium toxicity. Monitor for toxicity if given with carbamazepine, probenecid, indomethacin, methyldopa, and piroxicam. Aminophylline, sodium bicarbonate, and sodium chloride may increase lithium excretion. Use with haloperidol and thioridazine may cause encephalopathic syndrome (tremors, weakness, extrapyramidal symptoms). May alter hypoglycemic requirements of diabetics (monitor blood sugar closely).

🖢 **Give with meals to reduce nausea.**

Acute mania: Adult: PO: 300–600 tid. *Depressive states: Maintenance dose:* 300 mg tid. Lithium citrate (liquid form) contains 8 mEq per 5 ml of lithium, which is equal to 300 mg lithium carbonate.

Clinical alert: Dilute liquid form in a flavored drink. Recognize that the elderly tend to retain lithium and are more susceptible to toxicity. Lithium should only be used when the person can return for monitoring of serum lithium levels (there is a narrow margin of safety and toxicity can be fatal). Therapeutic levels of lithium for initial therapy are 1–1.5 mEq/L; for maintenance therapy, 0.7–1.2 mEq/L. Levels should never exceed 2 mEq/liter. Blood samples should be drawn 8–12 hr after the previous dose.

Contraindications/Precautions

PREG **D**

Contraindicated in hypersensitivity to lithium, and in cardiac disease, angina pectoris, severe dehydration and sodium depletion, hyperthyroidism, situations in which serum lithium level cannot be monitored closely. *Use with caution* in diabetes or hyperexcitable states.

✋ **Contraindicated for children under 12 years, nursing mothers, and during the first trimester of pregnancy. Risks versus benefits must be weighed before use in second and third trimesters. Use with caution for adolescents and the elderly or debilitated.**

Side effects/Adverse reactions

Hypersensitivity: itching, rashes, allergic vasculitis with ankle and wrist edema. *Hem:* reversible leukocytosis, hyponatremia. *GU:* polyurea, glycosuria, incontinence, renal toxicity (with long-term use). *GI:* dry mouth, thirst, anorexia, nausea, vomiting, diarrhea, metallic taste. *CV:* EKG changes (reversible), dysrhythmias, peripheral circulatory collapse. *CNS:* drowsiness, headache, confusion, tremors, restlessness, dizziness, stupor, lethargy, blackouts, coma, seizures, EEG changes, deterioration in organic brain syndrome, ataxia, weakness, impaired speech, hyperexcitability. *Skin:* drying and thinning of hair. *Misc:* goiter, hypothyroidism, transient hyperglycemia.

Nursing implications/Documentation

Possible nursing diagnoses: Potential for injury; Fluid volume deficit; Altered oral mucous membrane.

◆ Document and report history of heart disease, kidney disease, decreased thyroid function, or diabetes.

◆ Check EKG, BUN, creatinine, creatinine clearance, T_3, T_4, and FBS before giving first dose.

◆ Check serum lithium levels and electrolytes weekly (daily for high-risk patients) at first, then monthly once response is established.

◆ Monitor sodium intake to ensure steady daily intake (because of the close relationship between sodium and lithium levels, change in sodium intake is likely to cause changes in lithium levels).

◆ Document and report excessive sweating or fluid loss (may alter serum sodium and lithium levels).

◆ Provide favorite fluids to ensure adequate hydration and relieve dry mouth; until response is established, record and monitor intake and output to ensure 2.5–3 liters of fluid per day.

◆ Expect early side effects of nausea, dry mouth, thirst, frequent urination, drowsiness, and hand tremors to diminish after 6 weeks.

◆ Hold dose and report if side effects of vomiting, diarrhea, vertigo, extreme tremors, or muscle weakness are noted.

Patient & family teaching/Home care

Possible nursing diagnoses: Sleep pattern disturbance; Impaired home maintenance management.

♦ Stress that although it takes 2–3 weeks before beneficial effects are noted, lithium has helped many people with manic-depressive illnesses to live normal lives.

♦ Explain that side effects are often noted at the beginning of treatment, but they should diminish after 6 weeks; point out that tolerating the early side effects is worth the beneficial effects that are noted after 1–3 weeks.

♦ Point out the need to report early symptoms of toxicity (diarrhea, loss of appetite, nausea, vomiting, drowsiness, slurred speech, muscle weakness, and trembling).

♦ Explain that the patient must return for periodic laboratory studies to ensure safe dosage.

♦ Teach the need to take lithium with food, to increase fluid intake to 10–12 glasses per day, to avoid excessive sweating, and to maintain a steady salt intake.

♦ Emphasize the need to continue medication, even when feeling well.

♦ Caution that drinking alcohol may cause severe reactions and problems with lithium toxicity.

♦ Advise avoidance of driving and other potentially hazardous activities until response has been established.

♦ Suggest using ice chips, hard candy, or gum to relieve side effect of dry mouth; stress the need for good mouth care.

♦ Warn women to report if pregnancy is planned or suspected.

lomustine

low'mus-teen

CeeNu

Class: Antineoplastic (nitrosourea alkylating) agent

PEDS	PREG	GERI
🤚	D	🤚

Action Kills rapidly growing cells (cancer, hair follicles, bone marrow, GI lining, ova, and sperm) by interfering with DNA replication and RNA transcription through alkylation (cross-linking of DNA occurs). Is cell-cycle–phase nonspecific, affecting both actively dividing cells and dormant (resting) cells.

Use/Therapeutic goal/Outcome

Brain tumors, Hodgkin's lymphoma, melanoma, renal cell and lung cancer, gastric and colorectal adenocarcinoma, multiple myeloma: Elimination or suppression of malignant cell proliferation. **Outcome criteria:** Tumor and disease regression or stabilization on radiologic and physical examination.

Dose range/Administration

Interaction alert: Barbiturates, other cytotoxic agents, and radiation therapy can cause severe myelosuppression. Succinylcholine potentiates effects of lomustine. Allopurinol may cause increased bone marrow depression.

🔲 **Give 2-4 hours after meals to reduce nausea and enhance drug absorption**

Adult and Child: PO: 130 mg/m² as a single dose q 6 wk while platelets are >100,000/mm³ or WBC >4,000/mm³.

Clinical alert: Monitor for toxicity, which is expected to occur with a low therapeutic index. WBC, platelet, and erythrocyte count should drop to the nadir (lowest point) in 3–7 weeks. Dosage adjustments will be required for those with severe myelosuppression.

Contraindications/Precautions

PREG D

Contraindicated in hypersensitivity to lomustine, severe leukopenia, and thrombocytopenia (cumulative hematologic toxicity).

🤚 **Contraindicated for pregnant or nursing mothers. Use with caution for children and the elderly.**

Side effects/Adverse reactions

Hypersensitivity: rash, fever, hypotension, anaphylaxis. **Hem:** leukopenia (lasting 1–2 weeks) beginning 6 weeks after therapy; thrombocytopenia (occurring at 4–5 weeks and lasting 1–2 weeks) beginning about 1 month after therapy; anemia; and lowered hematocrit (nadir occurs in 4–7 weeks). **GI:** nausea and vomiting (lasting 1–3 days) beginning 3–5 hr after drug ingestion; stomatitis; hepatotoxicity. **GU:** azotemia and renal failure. **Resp:** pulmonary infiltrate, fibrosis. **CNS:** lethargy, ataxia, and dysarthria. **Skin:** alopecia.

Nursing implications/Documentation

Possible nursing diagnoses: Potential for infection; Potential for injury; Fatigue; Altered oral mucous membrane; Fluid volume deficit; Diarrhea; Altered nutrition: less than body requirements.

- See important Nursing implications in Antineoplastic agents overview on page 72, which apply to all antineoplastics. The interventions that follow are additional and specific to this drug only.

  - Report if the person vomits within 60 minutes of taking dose (dose may be lost).

  - Monitor for and report early signs of CNS toxicity (numbness or tingling of the extremities, balance problem) or pulmonary toxicity (persistent cough, dyspnea, chest pain).

  - Be aware that therapeutic response is often accompanied by toxicity.

Patient & family teaching/Home care

Possible nursing diagnoses: Knowledge deficit; Ineffective coping (individual and family); Hopelessness; Impaired home maintenance management.

- See important Patient & family teaching in Antineoplastic agents overview on page 72, which apply to all antineoplastics. The teachings that follow are additional and specific to this drug only.

  - Explain that taking lomustine 2–3 hr after a meal enhances its absorption; teach that lomustine comes in capsules of three different strengths and that a combination of capsules equals a single dose.

  - Point out that drinking 2–3 L a day helps prevent kidney complications.

  - Stress the need to report chest pain, dyspnea, persistent cough, problems with balance, or numbness or tingling of extremities.

- See Antineoplastic agents overview for more information.

loperamide

loe-per'a-mide

Imodium, Imodium A-D
Class: Antidiarrheal

PEDS	PREG	GERI
🖐	B	✋

Action Reduces intestinal motility and slows intestinal transit time by direct effect on the nerves of the intestinal wall.

Use/Therapeutic goal/Outcome

Diarrhea: Symptomatic control of acute and chronic diarrhea; reduction of volume of ileostomy drainage. **Outcome criteria:** Decreased frequency and liquid volume of bowel evacuations.

Dose range/Administration

Interaction alert: Narcotic analgesics increase risk of severe constipation.

Acute diarrhea: Adult: PO: *Initial dose:* 4 mg, then 2 mg after each loose stool. *Maximum dose:* 16 mg/day. **Child 2–5 yrs:** 1 mg tid first day, then 1 mg/10 kg only after loose stool. **Child 5–8 yrs:** 2 mg bid first day, then 1 mg/10 kg only after loose stool. **Child 8–12 yrs:** 2 mg tid first day, then 1 mg/10 kg only after loose stool. *Maximum dose:* same as first day dose.

Chronic diarrhea: Adult: PO: 4–8 mg/day, in 1 or 2 doses.

Clinical alert: For children under 5 years, administer oral solution. Use special dropper provided to measure dose.

Contraindications/Precautions

PREG **B**

Contraindicated in hypersensitivity to loperamide, and in diarrhea caused by antibiotic-associated pseudomembranous colitis or infectious organisms. **Use with caution** in ulcerative colitis, dehydration, and liver dysfunction.

🖐 **Contraindicated for infants under 2 years. Use with caution for pregnant or nursing mothers and the elderly.**

Side effects/Adverse reactions

Hypersensitivity: rash. **GI:** abdominal distention, constipation, dry mouth, nausea, vomiting. **CNS:** drowsiness, dizziness.

Nursing implications/Documentation

Possible nursing diagnoses: Constipation; Potential for injury; Pain.

- Assess and record bowel sounds and frequency and consistency of stools.

- Monitor for symptoms of toxic megacolon (abdominal distention, constipation, drowsiness, anorexia, nausea and vomiting, and fever), especially for patients with ulcerative colitis.

- Identify, report, and document signs of dehydration, especially in young children and the elderly.

- Provide increased fluid intake and/or frequent mouth care to relieve dry mouth.

- Discontinue loperamide after 48 hr if diarrhea is not improved, fever persists, or stools become bloody or mucoid.

Patient & family teaching/Home care

Possible nursing diagnoses: Knowledge deficit; Impaired home maintenance management.

♦ Caution against taking more than the prescribed amount or making up missed doses.

♦ Advise reporting if diarrhea does not improve within 48 hr.

♦ Explain the need to avoid driving and operating dangerous machinery until response to drug has been determined.

lorazepam

lor-a'ze-pam

Alzapam, ✦Apo-Lorazepam, Ativan, Loraz, ✦Novolorazem

Class: Antianxiety agent, Sedative-hypnotic, Benzodiazepine

PEDS	PREG	GERI	CONTROLLED SUBSTANCE
♨	**D**	♨	**IV**

Action Produces CNS depression and relaxation, and increases seizure threshold by potentiating the action of gamma-aminobuteric acid (GABA), which reduces neuronal activity in all regions of the CNS. Promotes muscle relaxation by inhibiting spinal motor reflex pathways. Decreases anxiety by inhibiting cortical and limbic arousal. Because lorazepam has a short half-life, it has fewer cumulative effects than other benzodiazepines.

Use/Therapeutic goal/Outcome

Short-term treatment of anxiety or agitation: Alleviation of symptoms of apprehension, agitation, muscle tension, and insomnia. **Outcome criteria:** Report of feeling calmer, sleeping better, and coping better; observable signs of decreased anxiety or agitation (decreased motor activity, reduced muscle tension, decrease in pulse and blood pressure).

Sedation (pre-procedure and during procedure): Promotion of relaxation, amnesia of discomforts of procedure. **Outcome criteria:** Report of feeling relaxed; not remembering discomfort.

Insomnia: Promotion of sleep. **Outcome criteria:** Report of having slept well; observed sleep.

Dose range/Administration

Interaction alert: Alcohol and other CNS depressants may cause excessive sedation.

Anxiety/agitation: Adult: PO: 2–6 mg daily in divided doses. *Maximum dose:* 10 mg/day. *For the elderly:* 1–2 mg/day in divided doses.

Sedation: Adult: PO: 1–4 mg 30 min before procedure. IV: 0.05 mg/kg (maximum 2 mg for patients > 50 yrs, maximum 4 mg for patients < 50 yrs.) immediately before procedure. IM: same as IV dose, 1–2 hr before procedure.

Insomnia: Adult: PO: 2–4 mg hs. *For the elderly:* 1 mg.

Clinical alert: For IV route, dilute dose with an equal amount of NS; administer slowly at a rate not to exceed 2 mg/min. Give IM doses deep into large muscle mass. When discontinuing drug, taper doses, rather than withdrawing abruptly.

Contraindications/Precautions

PREG D

Contraindicated in hypersensitivity or intolerance to lorazepam or other benzodiazepines, and in narrow-angle glaucoma, and shock.

Use with caution in psychosis, depression, suicidal tendencies, or impaired liver or kidney function.

♨ **Contraindicated for pregnant or nursing mothers. Use with caution for adolescents and the elderly or debilitated. Safe use for children under 12 years has not been established.**

Side effects/Adverse reactions

Hypersensitivity: itching, rash, exaggeration of side effects. **CNS:** lethargy, drowsiness, headache, dizziness, confusion, ataxia, tremors, depression. **CV:** hypotension, transient tachycardia and bradycardia. **Resp:** respiratory depression. **GI:** dry mouth, anorexia, nausea, vomiting, constipation, diarrhea. **Eye:** blurred vision, mydriasis. **Hem:** leukopenia. **Misc:** drug tolerance and dependence.

Nursing implications/Documentation

Possible nursing diagnoses: Potential for injury; Constipation.

♦ Record baseline blood pressure; monitor closely if dizziness is experienced.

♦ Supervise ambulation until response is determined; monitor the elderly for prolonged effects.

♦ Keep those who have received parenteral doses in bed with side rails up.

♦ Be sure that doses are swallowed (not hoarded).

♦ Provide a quiet environment that is conducive to rest.

+ Monitor bowel elimination and provide adequate fluids and fiber to prevent constipation; offer laxatives before the problem is severe.

Patient & family teaching/Home care

Possible nursing diagnoses: Anxiety; Fear; Ineffective individual coping; Impaired home maintenance management.

+ Help the individual identify stressors that contribute to anxiety and ways of coping effectively; stress that effective coping strategies can reduce the need for medication.

+ Explain the importance of daily exercise in relieving stress, and encourage establishing a plan for getting enough exercise (e.g., daily walks).

+ Point out that drug tolerance and dependence can occur, and that the drug should be used on a short-term basis.

+ Emphasize that the effects of alcohol, other sedatives and CNS depressants, and tranquilizers may be potentiated (these should be avoided).

+ Advise avoidance of driving and other potentially hazardous activities until response is established.

+ *See Antianxiety agents/Sedatives/Hypnotics overview for more information.*

lovastatin

low-va-stat'in

Mevacor

Class: Antilipemic

PEDS	PREG	GERI
♥	X	♥

Action Reduces serum levels of both total cholesterol and low-density-lipoprotein (LDL) cholesterol by inhibiting the action of HMG CoA reductase (enzyme necessary for cholesterol production); produces moderate increase in levels of high-density lipoproteins (HDL).

Use/Therapeutic goal/Outcome

Primary hypercholesterolemia (types IIA and IIB): Reduction of serum cholesterol levels, increase in HDL-cholesterol level, decrease in LDL-cholesterol level. *Outcome criteria:* Decreased level of serum cholesterol within 4 to 6 weeks of the initiation of therapy.

Dose range/Administration

Interaction alert: Cholestyramine and clofibrate potentiate lovastatin action.

Give with evening meal (absorption is enhanced, and inhibition of cholesterol synthesis is enhanced because cholesterol synthesis is naturally greater in the evening).

Adult: PO: 20 mg/day. May increase monthly. *Maximum dose:* 80 mg in single or divided doses.

Clinical alert: Establish that normal liver function exists prior to giving first dose, and periodically thereafter.

Contraindications/Precautions

PREG
X

Contraindicated in hypersensitivity to the drug, and in active liver disease, unexplained elevated transaminase levels, myositis, marked elevation of CPK, and renal failure. *Use with caution* in alcoholics, and in the presence of opacities of ocular lens.

Contraindicated for pregnant or nursing mothers. Use with caution for the elderly. Safe use for children has not been established.

Side effects/Adverse reactions

Hypersensitivity: skin rashes. *GI:* nausea, gas, diarrhea, constipation, abdominal pain, indigestion, CPK elevation, liver dysfunction. *CNS:* headache, fatigue, insomnia. *MS:* myalgia, myositis. *Eye:* opacities of ocular lens.

Nursing implications/Documentation

Possible nursing diagnoses: Constipation; Diarrhea; Altered nutrition: more than body requirements.

+ Watch for and report muscle pain or tenderness associated with fever and malaise.

+ Monitor for constipation or diarrhea; establish a plan to prevent constipation; report diarrhea to physician.

Patient & family teaching/Home care

Possible nursing diagnoses: Altered health maintenance; Knowledge deficit; Impaired home maintenance management.

+ Explain that the purpose of this drug is to reduce serum cholesterol and to decrease the risk of cardiovascular disease.

+ Stress the need to take this drug with evening meal for best effect.

+ Warn against drinking alcohol while on lovastatin.

- ◆ Emphasize the need to reduce other cardiac risk factors (obesity, smoking, high cholesterol diet, sedentary lifestyle), and help develop a plan to reduce these.

- ◆ Reinforce that this drug will have to be taken for a long time, and that ongoing medical follow-up of cholesterol and liver-function studies is essential.

- ◆ Stress that unexplained muscle pain accompanied by fever or malaise should be reported immediately.

- ◆ *See Antilipemics overview for more information.*

loxapine

lox'a-peen

loxapine hydrochloride: ◆*Loxapac, Loxitane C, Loxitane I.M.*

loxapine succinate: ◆*Loxapac, Loxitane*

Class: Dibenzoxazepine antipsychotic

PEDS	PREG	GERI
🖐	C	🖐

Action Exact mechanism of action has not been determined. Believed to produce calmness and alleviate psychiatric symptoms (disorders of perception, thought, consciousness, mood, affect, and social interaction) by blocking dopamine receptors in the limbic system. Blocks peripheral muscarinic, adrenergic, and histamine receptors. Also has some effect on the hypothalamus and pituitary gland, causing changes in regulation of body temperature and endocrine function. A dose of 10 mg of loxapine is therapeutically equivalent to 100 mg of chlorpromazine.

Use/Therapeutic goal/Outcome

Schizophrenia and psychotic disorders: Promotion of reality orientation, reduction in agitated hyperactivity. *Outcome criteria:* Demonstration of reality orientation and ability to problem solve and interact with others; absence of hyperactive and agitated behavior.

Dose range/Administration

Interaction alert: Alcohol and other CNS depressants may cause excessive sedation.

🖐 **Give with food or milk to avoid GI upset.**

Adult: PO: *Initial dose:* 10–25 mg bid, depending upon severity of symptoms. Increase rapidly to 30–50 mg bid to qid. *Maximum dose:* 250 mg/day. IM: 12.5–50 mg q4-6h prn. Change to oral route as soon as possible.

Clinical alert: Dilute liquid form with juice just before giving. Use IM route only if the individual is bedfast or able to be closely monitored; keep lying down for ½ hour after injection to avoid acute hypotensive effects. Keep IV diphenhydramine available in case of side effect of acute dystonic reaction.

Contraindications/Precautions

PREG
C

Contraindicated in hypersensitivity to loxapine, and in CNS depression, comatose states. *Use with caution* in seizure disorders, hypertension, parkinsonism, narrow-angle glaucoma, cardiac disease, hypotension, liver damage, and prostatic hypertrophy.

🖐 **Contraindicated for children under 16 years and nursing mothers. Use with caution for the elderly or debilitated. Safe use for pregnant women has not been established.**

Side effects/Adverse reactions

Hypersensitivity: rash. *CNS:* sedation, extrapyramidal reactions (pseudoparkinsonism, akathisia [restless need to keep moving], dystonia, tardive dykinesia), neuroleptic malignant syndrome (fever, tachycardia, tachypnea, profuse diaphoresis), EEG changes, dizziness. *CV:* orthostatic hypotension, palpitations, dysrhythmias, EKG changes. *GI:* appetite changes, dry mouth, constipation, abnormal liver function. *GU:* urinary retention or hesitancy, impaired ejaculation, amenorrhea. *Eye:* blurred vision. *Hem:* leukopenia, agranulocytosis, hyperglycemia. *Skin:* photosensitivity, jaundice. *MS:* weight gain. *Misc:* gynecomastia, galactorrhea.

Nursing implications/Documentation

Possible nursing diagnoses: Potential for injury; Constipation; Altered oral mucous membrane.

- ◆ Document mental status and vital signs before and 1–2 hr after administration during initial phase of treatment, then bid until response to therapy has been established, then periodically thereafter.

- ◆ Be sure that PO doses are swallowed (not hoarded).

- ◆ Monitor for orthostatic hypotension, dizziness, and drowsiness; supervise ambulation until response is established.

- ◆ Provide special mouth care; observe for and report oral ulcers.

• Prevent constipation by monitoring bowel movements and encouraging adequate fiber and fluid intake; offer laxatives or stool softeners before problem becomes severe.

• Report persistent sore throat, fever, and malaise, because these may indicate agranulocytosis (drug may have to be discontinued).

• Monitor for (and report immediately) signs of neuroleptic malignant syndrome (muscle rigidity, tremors, high fever, tachycardia); this is a rare, but potentially fatal, side effect.

Patient & family teaching/Home care

Possible nursing diagnoses: Sleep pattern disturbance; Impaired home maintenance management.

• Emphasize the need to continue medication, even when feeling well.

• Warn to change positions slowly to prevent dizziness.

• Stress that the effects of alcohol, sedatives and other CNS depressants, and tranquilizers may be potentiated.

• Caution to consult with physician before using OTC drugs; stress the need for ongoing medical follow-up.

• Provide a list of side effects that should be reported: involuntary movements, muscular rigidity, tremors, fever, respiratory distress, tachycardia, persistent sore throat.

• Caution to wear a sunscreen (number 15) and sunglasses when out in the sun.

• Advise avoidance of driving and other potentially hazardous activities until response has been established.

• Suggest using ice chips, hard candy, or gum to relieve side effect of dry mouth; stress the need for good mouth care.

• Warn women to report if pregnancy is planned or suspected.

• *See Antipsychotics overview for more information.*

magaldrate
mag'al-drate

♣*Antiflux, Lowsium, Riopan*
Class: Antacid

PEDS	PREG	GERI
♨	C	♨

Action Neutralizes existing stomach acid and reduces pepsin activity by elevating gastric pH.

Use/Therapeutic goal/Outcome

Hyperacidity and gastroesophageal reflux: Reduction of acid concentration within the esophagus and stomach. **Outcome criteria:** Report of decreased pain and upper GI irritation.

Dose range/Administration

Interaction alert: Do not give other oral medications for 2 hr after magaldrate to ensure their absorption. Separate doses of magaldrate from doses of enteric coated drugs by 1 hr (causes enteric coated drugs to be released while still in the stomach).

Adult: PO: *Liquid:* 5–10 ml between meals and hs. *Tablets:* 480–960 mg between meals and hs.
Child: PO: Individualize dose.

Clinical alert: Giving doses 1 and 3 hr after meals and at bedtime enhances therapeutic effects. Shake liquid form well before giving and follow with water or milk. After giving via nasogastric tube, flush with water. Using combination of aluminum and magnesium salts usually prevents constipation or diarrhea. Low sodium content makes magaldrate useful for patients on sodium restrictions.

Contraindications/Precautions
PREG
C

Contraindicated in hypersensitivity to aluminum or magnesium products. **Use with caution** in renal impairment, decreased GI motility or obstruction, colostomies or ileostomies, and dehydration or fluid restriction.

⚠ **Use with caution for children and the elderly.**

Side effects/Adverse reactions

Hypersensitivity: rare. **GI:** stomach cramps, constipation, or diarrhea. **CNS:** neurotoxicity. **Misc:** phosphate depletion, osteomalacia, osteoporosis, hypermagnesemia.

Nursing implications/Documentation

Possible nursing diagnoses: Potential for injury; Pain.

• Monitor bowel elimination; record character and color of stools.

Patient & family teaching/Home care

Possible nursing diagnoses: Knowledge deficit; Impaired home maintenance management.

• Advise that the liquid form of magaldrate is more effective than tablet form; palatability may be increased by refrigeration.

• Teach to shake liquid preparation vigorously to achieve uniform suspension, and to follow with water to assure passage into stomach.

• Point out the need to chew chewable tablets well before swallowing and to follow with water for maximum effectiveness.

• For ulcers, advise taking medication 1 and 3 hr after eating and at bedtime for best results.

• Caution to continue taking magaldrate under medical supervision for 4 to 6 weeks after ulcer symptoms have subsided.

• Advise those who self-medicate with antacids to seek medical advice if symptoms recur frequently or persist longer than 2 weeks.

magnesium salicylate

Doan's Pills, Durasal, Magan, Mobidin

Class: Analgesic, Nonsteroidal anti-inflammatory drug (NSAID), Salicylate

PEDS	PREG	GERI
🤚	C	🤚

Action Produces analgesia by an ill-defined effect on the hypothalamus (central action) and by blocking generation of pain impulses (peripheral action, which may involve inhibition of prostaglandin synthesis). Reduces inflammation by inhibiting prostaglandin synthesis and synthesis or action of other mediators of the inflammatory response. Reduces fever by acting on the hypothalamic heat-regulating center to cause peripheral vasodilation which increases peripheral blood supply, and promotes heat loss through sweating and cooling by evaporation. This drug is sodium-free and does not affect platelet aggregation.

Use/Therapeutic goal/Outcome

Inflammation: Reduction of pain and inflammation. *Outcome criteria:* After 2 weeks, report of reduced pain and stiffness; observable decrease in swelling and increase in mobility.

Pain: Relief of pain. *Outcome criteria:* Report of less discomfort.

Dose range/Administration

Interaction alert: Increases hypoglycemic activity of antidiabetic agents. Avoid use with oral anticoagulants and heparin because of increased risk of bleeding. Ammonium chloride and other urine acidifiers increase risk of toxicity. High doses of antacids, other urine alkalinizers, and corticosteroids reduce effects.

🍵 **Give with a large glass of water, food, milk, or low dose of antacid to minimize GI effects.**

Adult: PO: 600 mg tid to qid; may increase to 4 g/day in divided doses.

Clinical alert: Do not give to children with chicken pox or influenza-like infections because of association with Reye's syndrome. Monitor the elderly for increased risk of toxicity.

Contraindications/Precautions

PREG
C

Contraindicated in hypersensitivity to salicylates, and in peptic ulcer, chronic renal insufficiency, GI bleeding, liver damage, bleeding disorders, and before surgery. *Use with caution* in Vitamin K deficiency, and hypoprothrombinemia.

🤚 **Contraindicated for children under 12 years, children under 18 years with chickenpox or influenza-like symptoms, and for pregnant or nursing mothers. Use with caution for older children and the elderly.**

Side effects/Adverse reactions

Hypersensitivity: rash, hives, itching, anaphylaxis, and asthma. *GI:* GI distress, bleeding, abnormal liver-function studies, hepatitis. *Misc:* salicylism (dizziness, drowsiness, tinnitus, hearing loss, nausea, vomiting); hypermagnesemia with high doses in patients with renal insufficiency.

Nursing implications/Documentation

Possible nursing diagnoses: Pain; Impaired physical mobility.

• Monitor for and report GI symptoms that may indicate peptic ulcer (nausea, pain, black stools).

• Observe the elderly for toxicity.

Patient & family teaching/Home care

Possible nursing diagnoses: Knowledge deficit; Impaired home maintenance management.

• Explain the importance of watching for symptoms of GI bleeding (black stools, persistent GI distress).

• Point out that long-term use of salicylates (or use in high doses) is likely to increase risk of bleeding and that those taking this drug on a long-term basis should be followed by a physician.

• Advise telling physician and dentist if magnesium salicylate is taken on a regular basis.

- Warn not to use other drugs containing aspirin at the same time.

- Stress that those under 18 years with flu-like symptoms or chicken pox should not receive aspirin or this drug (because of risk of developing Reye's syndrome).

- *See Narcotic and non-narcotic analgesics and Nonsteroidal anti-inflammatory drugs overviews for more information.*

magnesium salts

magnesium citrate: *Citroma, Citro-Nesia, Magnesium Citrate*

magnesium hydroxide: *Magnesia, Milk of Magnesia*

magnesium sulfate: *Epson salts*

Class: Saline hyperosmotic laxative

PEDS	PREG	GERI
✋	B	✋

Action Promotes increased peristalsis and bowel evacuation by drawing water into lumen of small intestine.

Use/Therapeutic goal/Outcome

Constipation and preparation for surgery or diagnostic studies: Evacuation of fecal material from colon. *Outcome criteria:* Evacuation of soft stool mass (within 1/2–3 hr).

Edema and inflammation (epsom salts only): Reduction in inflammation/edema. *Outcome criteria:* Patient demonstrates and reports decreased pain, inflammation, and edema.

Dose range/Administration

Interaction alert: Effectiveness of oral anticoagulants, digitalis glycosides, tetracycline, and phenothiazines may be reduced in the presence of magnesium.

- **Give on an empty stomach with a full glass of water for faster effect.**

magnesium citrate: **Adult:** PO: 240 ml as one dose. **Child 2–5 yrs:** PO: 4–12 ml as one dose. **Child 6–12 yrs:** PO: 50–100 ml as one dose.

magnesium hydroxide: **Adult:** PO: *600-mg tabs:* 6–12 tablets; *300-mg tabs:* 12–24 tablets; *Liquid:* 30–60 ml. **Child:** PO: *600-mg tabs:* 3–6 tablets. *300-mg tabs:* 6–12 tabs. *Liquid:* 5–30 ml.

Magnesium sulfate: **Adult:** PO: 10–15 g in the morning or midafternoon (may be chilled and

flavored with lemon or orange juice). **Child:** PO: 5–10 g in the morning or midafternoon (may be chilled and flavored with lemon or orange juice).

Contraindications/Precautions

Contraindicated in hypersensitivity to saline laxatives, and in symptoms of appendicitis or intestinal obstruction, undiagnosed rectal bleeding, renal impairment, dehydration, congestive heart failure, hypertension, and in those with a colostomy or ileostomy.

✋ **Use with caution for children, pregnant or nursing mothers, and the elderly.**

Side effects/Adverse reactions

Hypersensitivity: rash, difficulty breathing. *GI:* cramping, diarrhea, gas formation, increased thirst. *CNS:* confusion, dizziness. *CV:* irregular heartbeat. *MS:* muscle weakness. *Skin:* irritation around rectal area. *Hem:* hypermagnesia, hypokalemia, fluid and electrolyte imbalance. *Misc:* edema, laxative dependence.

Nursing implications/Documentation

Possible nursing diagnoses: Impaired skin integrity; Diarrhea.

- Administer early in day to reduce sleep interruption.

- Encourage fluid intake of at least 6–8 full glasses daily to improve response and to avoid dehydration.

- Assess for abdominal distention and bowel sounds.

- Monitor and record frequency, appearance, and amount of stool evacuated.

- Assess perianal area and provide appropriate measures for good hygiene.

- Observe for signs of magnesium toxicity (thirst, drowsiness, dizziness) or electrolyte imbalance (confusion, irregular heartbeat, muscle cramps, unusual fatigue or weakness).

Patient & family teaching/Home care

Possible nursing diagnoses: Knowledge deficit.

- Stress the importance of drinking at least 6–8 full glasses of liquids each day and following directions for safe use of product.

- Point out that laxatives should not be used for longer than 1 week without consulting a physician.

- For the elderly, advise avoiding magnesium laxatives unless prescribed by physician.

- Teach the importance of dietary bulk, fluids, and exercise to prevent constipation.

- *See Laxatives overview for more information.*

magnesium sulfate

mag-neez'ee-um

Class: Anticonvulsant, Magnesium replacement agent

Antidote: Calcium gluconate

PEDS	PREG	GERI
🖐	C	🖐

Action When given parenterally, stops convulsions by decreasing acetylcholine release from motor nerve terminals (causes peripheral neuromuscular blockade); also depresses the CNS, and musculature (smooth, skeletal, and cardiac). Reduces the frequency and intensity of uterine contractions.

Use/Therapeutic goal/Outcome

Seizures associated with hypomagnesemia, toxemia of pregnancy, acute nephritis, and hyperthyroidism: Restoration of normal serum magnesium levels, prevention and limitation of seizures. *Outcome criteria:* Serum magnesium levels within normal range (1.3–2.1 mEq/L); absence of seizures.

Premature labor: Prevention of uterine contractions. *Outcome criteria:* Absence of uterine contractions.

Dose range/Administration

Interaction alert: Neuromuscular blocking agents increase neuromuscular blockade.

Pre-eclampsia and eclampsia: Adult: IM: Following an initial IV dose of 4 g (see below), give 4 g into alternate buttocks q4h. IV: Dilute 4 g in 250 cc of D5W and infuse at a rate not to exceed 150 mg/min. May give in conjunction with 4 g injected deep IM into each buttock; *or* may follow with an IV infusion at 1–4 g/hr.

Hypomagnesemic seizures: Adult: IM: 1 g q4-6h, depending upon response and magnesium blood levels. IV: 1–2 g of 10% solution, given over 15 min; follow with the IM dose schedule (1 g q4-6h), depending on blood magnesium levels. *Child:* IM: 100 mg/kg q4-6h, depending upon response and magnesium blood levels. IV: 100 mg/kg in a 1–3% solution given very slowly, depending upon response and magnesium blood levels.

Clinical alert: Hold parenteral doses and report if respirations are less than 16 per min, if urine output is less than 100 cc in the previous 4 hr, or if knee jerk reflex is absent. When giving IV, document vital signs at least every 15 min; do not infuse faster than 150 mg/min (complaint of "feeling hot" may be related to rapid IV rate). Monitor for and report heart block or slowing of heart rate.

Contraindications/Precautions

PREG B

Contraindicated in hypersensitivity to magnesium sulfate, and in myocardial damage, heart block. PO use is contraindicated in the presence of GI distress, impaired renal function, concomitant use of digitalis. *Use with caution* with other CNS depressants or neuromuscular blocking agents.

🖐 **Use with caution for the elderly and children and during labor.**

Side effects/Adverse reactions

Hypersensitivity: rash. *CNS:* confusion, muscle weakness, flaccid paralysis, depressed reflexes, hypothermia. *CV:* complete heart block, hypotension, depressed cardiac function, circulatory collapse, hypocalcemia. *Resp:* respiratory paralysis. *Skin:* sweating, flushing.

Nursing implications/Documentation

Possible nursing diagnoses: Potential for injury; Potential for aspiration; Sensory/perceptual alterations.

- Initiate seizure precautions upon admission and keep calcium gluconate readily available in case of hypermagnesemia.

- Check most recent serum electrolyte and magnesium level studies before giving dose; hold dose and report if magnesium level is within normal range (4 mEq/ml produces early signs of toxicity such as respiratory depression, cathartic effects, extreme thirst, sedation, confusion, feeling of warmth, or absence of knee jerk reflex).

- When given within 24 hr of birth, monitor neonates for signs of toxicity.

- Document intake and output and monitor for fluid retention.

M

Patient & family teaching/Home care

Possible nursing diagnoses: Fear; Knowledge deficit; Impaired home maintenance management.

♦ If used as a laxative, warn that magnesium sulfate tastes salty, and is likely to produce profound bowel evacuation.

♦ For parenteral use, stress the need for close medical supervision.

♦ *See Anticonvulsants and Laxatives overviews for more information.*

mannitol
man'i-tol

Osmitrol

Class: ★Osmotic diuretic prototype

PEDS	PREG	GERI
🖐	C	🖐

Action Increases flow of water into extracellular fluid by elevating blood plasma osmolality. Promotes diuresis by increasing osmolality of glomerular filtrate, which promotes water and electrolyte retention in the lumen of the nephron, increasing rate and volume of urine. Reduces intraocular pressure and intracranial pressure by creating an osmotic gradient between plasma and ocular fluids, and between plasma and CSF.

Use/Therapeutic goal/Outcome

Acute renal failure: Promotion of diuresis. *Outcome criteria:* Increased urine output; improvement in serum creatinine and BUN.

Increased intracranial pressure (ICP): Reduction in intracranial pressure. *Outcome criteria:* Upon measurement via ICP monitor, intracranial pressure within acceptable range.

Increased intraocular pressure (IOP): Reduction of intraocular pressure. *Outcome criteria:* Reduced intraocular pressure, when measured with tonometer.

Poisoning: Promotion of diuresis, which increases elimination of toxic substances. *Outcome criteria:* Negative toxicology studies and improved clinical studies.

Dose range/Administration

Interaction alert: Reduces therapeutic effect of most drugs eliminated by the kidneys.

Renal failure: Adult: IV: *Test dose:* 200 mg/kg over 3–5 min, may repeat once. *Therapeutic dose:* 50–100 g/day in divided portions, using 5–25% solution at a rate to maintain a urine flow of 30-50 cc/hr.

Increased ICP, IOP: Adult: IV: 1.5–2 g/kg of a 15–25% solution over 30–60 min.

Poisoning: Adult: IV: 5–25% solution, infused continuously to maintain urine flow of 100–500 cc/hr. *Maximum dose:* 200 g.

Measurement of GFR: Adult: IV: 100 ml of 20% solution mixed with 180 ml sodium chloride; administer at a rate of 20 ml/min.

Clinical alert: Do not use in the same IV tubing as other drugs or blood transfusion; use a filter on tubing; warm bottle and shake if crystals are noted, then cool to body temperature before giving.

Contraindications/Precautions
PREG C

Contraindicated in hypersensitivity to drug, severe CHF, pulmonary congestion or edema, intracranial bleeding, dehydration, anuria, progressive renal disease after initiation of mannitol therapy. **Use with caution** with hypokalemia or hyponatremia, hypovolemia, or significant renal or cardiopulmonary impairment.

🖐 **Contraindicated for children under 12 years. Use with caution for the elderly. Safe use for pregnant or nursing mothers has not been established.**

Side effects/Adverse reactions

Hypersensitivity: rash, hives. **CNS:** headache, confusion, dizziness, convulsions, rebound increase in intracranial pressure 8–12 hr after diuresis. **CV:** tachycardia, circulatory overload, pulmonary edema, angina, dehydration. **Hem:** fluid and electrolyte imbalances, water intoxication. **GI:** dry mouth, thirst, nausea, vomiting. **GU:** urinary retention. **Eye:** blurred vision. **Ear:** loss of hearing. **Skin:** necrosis if extravasation occurs.

Nursing implications/Documentation

Possible nursing diagnoses: Fluid volume deficit; Altered patterns of urinary elimination; Potential for injury.

♦ Ascertain that baseline CBC, sodium, potassium, chloride, carbon dioxide, calcium, magnesium, BUN, creatinine, uric acid, and liver function studies have been obtained before giving first dose; report abnormalities and monitor closely thereafter.

♦ Monitor closely for hypokalemia and hyponatremia.

♦ Document and monitor hourly vital signs and urine output; report abnormal vital signs, urine output less than 30 cc/hr, and significant negative or positive balance in cumulative summaries.

♦ Monitor for and report signs of fluid overload (auscultate lungs for rales; check feet, ankles, and sacrum for edema).

♦ Monitor for extravasation and phlebitis because this drug is very irritating to the tissues.

♦ Keep patients in bed with side rails up and call bell in reach until stable.

Patient & family teaching/Home care

Possible nursing diagnoses: Fear; Knowledge deficit.

♦ Before giving first dose, explain that the drug will enhance the work of the kidneys and reduce the work of the heart by reducing fluid overload.

♦ Explain that vital signs and urine output will be monitored frequently to ensure safe dosage and fluid replacement.

♦ Stress that fluid intake limitations may be necessary, even though the patient is thirsty.

♦ Explain that changing positions slowly helps prevent dizziness.

♦ Encourage voicing of questions and concerns.

♦ *See Diuretics overviews for more information.*

maprotiline
ma-proe'ti-leen

maprotiline hydrochloride: *Ludiomil*

Class: Tetracyclic antidepressant

PEDS	PREG	GERI
♨	B	♨

Action Improves mood by increasing levels of the neurotransmitter norepinephrine in the CNS. (Blocks neurotransmitter reuptake into presynaptic neurons by inhibiting the "amine pump." Reuptake normally terminates the action of neurotransmitters.)

Use/Therapeutic goal/Outcome

Major depressive disorders and depressive phase of manic-depression: Promotion of sense of well-being, ability to cope with daily living. *Outcome criteria:* After 2–4 weeks, report of feeling less depressed, less anxious, and more energetic and able to cope; return of normal sleeping and eating habits; demonstration of improved ability to problem solve and perform activities of daily living.

Dose range/Administration

Interaction alert: Barbiturates may reduce antidepressant blood levels and effects. Cimetidine and methylphenidate may increase blood levels. If given with epinephrine and norepinephrine, monitor for increased risk of hypertension. Avoid use with MAOIs (risk of excitation, hyperpyrexia, and seizures).

Adult: PO: 75 mg daily for 14 days, may increase up to 150 mg/day. *Maximum dose:* Hospitalized patients: 300 mg/day; outpatients 225 mg/day. *For the elderly:* Begin with 25 mg/day, increase gradually to 50–75 mg/day if needed.

Clinical alert: Whenever possible give entire dose at bedtime to reduce daytime sedation.

Contraindications/Precautions
PREG B

Contraindicated in hypersensitivity to maprotiline or TCAs, for concomitant use with electroconvulsive therapy, and in elective surgery, seizure disorders or acute recovery period of myocardial infarction. *Use with caution* in renal or hepatic disease, hyperthyroidism, glaucoma, prostatic hypertrophy, urinary retention, hypomania, mania, alcoholism, and suicidal tendency.

♨ **Contraindicated for children and nursing mothers. Use with caution for pregnant women and the elderly or debilitated.**

Side effects/Adverse reactions

Hypersensitivity: rash, swelling, itching. *CNS:* drowsiness, dizziness, anxiety, headache, fatigue, agitation, extrapyramidal symptoms, sedation (especially the elderly), seizures. *CV:* orthostatic hypotension, palpitations, tachycardia, EKG changes, hypertension. *GI:* anorexia, dry mouth, nausea, vomiting, constipation, paralytic ileus. *GU:* urinary retention, decreased libido. *Eye:* blurred vision. *Ear:* tinnitus. *Skin:* sensitivity to sunlight. *Hem:* agranulocytosis. *Misc:* (After abrupt withdrawal following long-term therapy) headache, malaise, nausea.

Nursing implications/Documentation

Possible nursing diagnoses: Potential for injury; Constipation; Altered oral mucous membrane.

♦ Document mental status and vital signs at least daily until response to therapy has been established.

♦ Be sure that doses are swallowed (not hoarded).

* Monitor for orthostatic hypotension, dizziness, and drowsiness; supervise ambulation until response is established.

* Record intake and output, and observe for dehydration or urinary retention; provide special mouth care.

* Monitor for and report suicidal tendencies, increased depression, or excessive drowsiness (may require change in medication).

* Prevent constipation by monitoring bowel movements and providing adequate fiber and fluid intake; offer laxatives or stool softeners before the problem becomes severe.

Patient & family teaching/Home care

Possible nursing diagnoses: Ineffective coping (family and individual); Sleep pattern disturbance; Impaired home maintenance management.

* Stress that this medication helps reduce the depression that inhibits ability to make decisions and cope effectively (once the individual feels less depressed, it will be easier to take steps toward making healthy changes).

* Explain that side effects are often noted immediately, but they usually diminish after a few weeks; on the other hand, it is likely to take 2–4 weeks before *beneficial* effects are noted (the patient may feel worse before feeling better).

* Warn to change positions slowly to prevent dizziness.

* Point out the role of adequate nutrition, exercise, and sleep in combating depression.

* Emphasize that the effects of alcohol, sedatives, and tranquilizers may be potentiated.

* Caution to consult physician before using OTC drugs; stress the need for ongoing medical follow-up.

* Recommend reporting continued depression; stress that doses should not be increased or stopped without checking with physician because this may cause severe problems.

* Advise avoidance of driving and other potentially hazardous activities until response is established.

* Suggest using ice chips, hard candy, or gum to relieve side effect of dry mouth; stress the need for good mouth care.

* *See Antidepressants overview for more information.*

mebendazole

me-ben'da-zole

Vermox

Class: Anti-infective, Anthelmintic, Antibiotic

PEDS	PREG	GERI
✋	C	OK

Action Vermicidal, kills helminths (intestinal worms) in an infected host by inhibiting their ability to absorb glucose and other nutrients.

Use/Therapeutic goal/Outcome

Pinworm, roundworm, whipworms, hookworms, tapeworms: Elimination of intestinal helminths. **Outcome criteria:** Expulsion of worms, followed by 3 negative stool samples after completion of treatment; for pinworms, perianal swabs negative for 7 days.

Dose range/Administration

🥄 **Give with food to reduce GI symptoms; with fatty foods to enhance absorption.**
Pinworm: Adult/Child > 2 yrs: PO: 100 mg in one dose.

Roundworm, whipworm, hookworm: Adult/Child > 2 yrs: PO: 100 mg bid for 3 days.

Clinical alert: Be aware that although worms may be eliminated, eggs may survive and cause reinfection; therefore a *second course of treatment*, 3 weeks later, is recommended. Tablets may be chewed or swallowed whole.

Contraindications/Precautions

PREG
C

Contraindicated in hypersensitivity to mebendazole. **Use with caution** in Crohn's disease, ulcerative colitis, or liver function impairment.

🖐 **Contraindicated for pregnant or nursing mothers. Safe use for children under 2 years has not been established.**

Side effects/Adverse reactions

Hypersensitivity: (rare) rash. **GI:** abdominal discomfort, transient diarrhea.

Nursing implications/Documentation

Possible nursing diagnoses: Potential for infection; Diarrhea; Situational low self-esteem.

* Practice meticulous handwashing before and after contact with the patient or changing of bed linens or clothing.

* Record character of all stools, and inspect them closely for worms, before and during therapy (stool specimens must go to the lab while still warm).

• Determine close contacts (family members, playmates, babysitters with long-term contact), who should be also treated.

Patient & family teaching/Home care

Possible nursing diagnoses: Knowledge deficit; Impaired home maintenance management.

• Explore feelings and concerns, and explain that this common childhood illness is not associated with "dirtiness" of the child or family.

• Point out that because this drug is poorly absorbed, eating fatty foods and taking high doses provides best drug levels.

• Teach how to recognize pinworms, roundworms, and ova.

• Stress the importance of preventing reinfection or spread of infection by treating all family members and close contacts, taking the medication exactly as prescribed, washing foods especially carefully, meticulously washing hands after bowel movements, cutting nails short, changing clothing every day, keeping fingers out of mouth, having infected individuals sleep alone, eliminating ova by washing all linens daily in hot water (without shaking them), vacuuming and damp-mopping the house daily, cleaning the toilet with disinfectant daily.

• Advise infected individuals to wear gloves when preparing food.

◆ *See Anti-infectives overview for more information.*

mechlorethamine   *me-klor-eth′a-meen*

mechlorethamine hydrochloride (nitrogen mustard): *Mustargen*

Class: Antineoplastic (alkylating) agent

PEDS 🖐   **PREG D**   **GERI** 🖐

Action Kills rapidly growing cells (cancer, hair follicles, bone marrow, GI lining, ova, and sperm) by interfering with DNA replication and RNA transcription through alkylation (cross-linking of DNA occurs). Is cell-cycle–phase nonspecific, affecting both actively dividing cells and dormant (resting) cells. With intracavitary use, produces adherance of serosal-surface by inflammation and sclerosis.

Use/Therapeutic goal/Outcome

Hodgkin's disease and non-Hodgkin's lymphomas, lymphosarcomas, mycosis fungoides, malignant effusions (pleural, peritoneal, pericardial), bronchogenic carcinoma, polycythemia vera, and cancer of the breast and ovaries: Elimination or suppression of malignant cell proliferation. **Outcome criteria:** Tumor and disease regression or stabilization on radiologic and physical examination; for effusions, X-ray evidence of resolution of effusion; for polycythemia, CBC within normal limits.

Dose range/Administration

Interaction alert: Increased incidence of blood dyscrasias when given with amphotericin B.

Adult: IV: 0.4 mg/kg or 6–10 mg/m^2 as a single or divided dose q 3–6 wk. *Intracavitarily:* 10–20 mg by physician.

Clinical alert: This drug should be given only by nurses who are knowledgeable in the comprehensive management of the administration of antineoplastic agents. Doses may vary at physician's discretion and are held until the patient has sufficiently recovered from toxicities of previous doses. Protocols for drug preparation, administration, and accidental skin contamination must be followed. Gloves or double gloves must be worn when handling mechlorethamine (skin contamination may cause a local reaction). Contaminated areas should be washed with large amounts of soap and water. Mechlorethamine is a potent vesicant and is given via bolus over 1–3 min into a running IV line. Giving doses at night with a sedative and an antiemetic helps reduce nausea, which occurs in 90% of patients. Extravasation should be prevented by monitoring the infusion site closely. If extravasation occurs, the infusion should be stopped immediately and protocols for treatment followed.

Contraindications/Precautions   **PREG D**

Contraindicated in hypersensitivity to mechlorethamine, infectious disease, herpes zoster, and preexisting myelosuppression. Intracavitary use is contraindicated with concurrent use of bone marrow suppressants.

🖐 **Contraindicated for pregnant or nursing mothers. Use with caution for the elderly. Safe use for children has not been established.**

Side effects/Adverse reactions

Hypersensitivity: urticaria, tachycardia, hypotension. **Hem:** thrombosis and thrombophlebitis with insufficient drug dilution; anemia, leukopenia, and thrombocytopenia (within

10–14 days); hemorrhagic diathesis; hyperuricemia, granulocytopenia, lymphocytopenia. *GI:* nausea, vomiting, and diarrhea; metallic taste in mouth immediately after dose; stomatitis. *CNS:* vertigo, paresthesias, and peripheral neuropathy. *Ear:* tinnitus and impaired hearing. *Skin:* alopecia, pruritus; herpes zoster, and pain and erythema at injection site; cellulitis, ulceration, and sloughing if extravasation occurs.

Nursing implications/Documentation

Possible nursing diagnoses: Potential for infection; Potential for injury; Fatigue; Altered oral mucous membrane; Fluid volume deficit; Diarrhea; Altered nutrition: less than body requirements.

◆ *See important Nursing implications in Antineoplastic agents overview on page 72, which apply to all antineoplastics. The interventions that follow are additional and specific to this drug only.*

• After intracavity injection, turn patient from side to side every 5–10 min for 1 hr to distribute drug; be prepared for a paracentesis 24–26 hr after administration to remove remaining fluid.

• After intraperitoneal injection, monitor for and report abdominal pain (pain is unusual).

• After intrapericardial injection, monitor for dysrhythmias and pericardial bleeding.

• Report rash as it may be hypersensitivity or herpes.

• Monitor for and report early signs of CNS toxicity (numbness or tingling of the extremities, balance problem).

• Increase fluid intake to 2–3 L a day to prevent renal tubular damage from hyperuricemia secondary to cell lysis.

• Be aware that therapeutic response is often accompanied by toxicity.

Patient & family teaching/Home care

Possible nursing diagnoses: Knowledge deficit; Ineffective coping (individual and family); Hopelessness; Impaired home maintenance management.

◆ *See important Patient & family teaching in Antineoplastic agents overview on page 72, which apply to all antineoplastics. The teachings that follow are additional and specific to this drug only.*

• Point out that drinking 2–3 L a day helps prevent kidney complications.

• For intra-abdominal cavity dose, explain that a paracentesis will be done a day later to remove excess fluid.

• Stress the need to report skin rash, increasing pain, hearing deficits, problems with balance, or numbness or tingling of extremities.

◆ *See Antineoplastic agents overview for more information.*

meclizine
mek'li-zeen

meclizine hydrochloride: ◣*Ancolan, Antivert, Antivert/25, Antivert/50,* ❧*Bonamine, Bonine, Dizmiss, Meni-D, Ru-Vert M*

Class: Antiemetic, Antivertigo, Antihistamine, H_1-receptor antagonist

PEDS	PREG	GERI
✋	B	✋

Action Relieves and prevents dizziness, nausea, and vomiting caused by motion, possibly by affecting neural pathways originating in the labyrinth. Exact mechanism of action has not been determined.

Use/Therapeutic goal/Outcome

Dizziness or motion sickness: Prevention or resolution of dizziness, nausea, and vomiting. *Outcome criteria:* Report of absence of, or reduction in, feelings of dizziness and nausea with motion; absence of vomiting.

Dose range/Administration

Interaction alert: May potentiate CNS depressants. May mask ototoxicity of other drugs.

🖐 **Give with food, milk, or full glass of water to reduce GI symptoms.**

Dizziness: Adult: PO: 25–100 mg/day in divided doses.

Motion sickness: Adult: PO: 25–50 mg 1 hr before travel, and daily for duration of journey.

Clinical alert: Be aware that this antihistamine has a slower onset and longer duration than other antihistamines.

Contraindications/Precautions
PREG
B

Contraindicated in hypersensitivity to meclizine. *Use with caution* in narrow-angle glaucoma, GI or GU disorders, and seizure disorders.

ᴟ Contraindicated for children and pregnant or nursing mothers. Use with caution for the elderly.

Side effects/Adverse reactions

Hypersensitivity: extreme drowsiness, hypotension. **CNS:** drowsiness, fatigue. **GI:** dry mouth.

Nursing implications/Documentation

Possible nursing diagnoses: Potential for injury; Fluid volume deficit; Altered oral mucous membrane.

• Determine cause of symptoms before giving meclizine hydrochloride.

• Offer frequent mouth care.

• Supervise ambulation until response is determined.

• When able to tolerate liquids, begin with small amount of ice chips, then water, then clear liquids, then full liquids, then food.

Patient & family teaching/Home care

Possible nursing diagnoses: Knowledge deficit; Impaired home maintenance management.

• Teach that the drug should be taken 1 hr before travel, with milk, food, or a full glass of water.

• Stress that persistent dizziness, nausea, vomiting, or abdominal discomfort should be reported.

• Explain that avoiding fatty foods and eating smaller and more frequent meals may reduce nausea.

• Advise against using alcohol or other CNS depressants.

• Point out that symptoms of drowsiness are likely to diminish after several days use; warn against driving or activities that require mental alertness until response is determined.

• Encourage frequent mouth care; suggest that chewing sugarless gum may relieve symptoms of dry mouth.

◆ See Antiemetics overview for more information.

meclofenamate   *me-kloe-fen-am'ate*

meclofenamate sodium: ***Meclomen***

Class: Nonsteroidal anti-inflammatory drug (NSAID), Analgesic, Antipyretic

PEDS	PREG	GERI
ᴟ	ᴟ	ᴟ

Action Exact mechanism to reduce inflammation unclear. Believed to inhibit prostaglandin synthesis and binding at receptor sites. Prostaglandin is a naturally occurring mediator of inflammatory response that is found in tissue throughout the body.

Use/Therapeutic goal/Outcome

Pain and inflammation: Promotion of comfort and mobility: suppression of inflammation. **Outcome criteria:** Report of increased comfort with increased range of motion and ability to perform activities of daily life; reduction in or absence of joint stiffness, swelling, redness, and warmth.

(Investigational use) Acute gouty arthritis: Reduction in inflammation. **Outcome criteria:** Same as above.

Dose range/Administration

Interaction alert: This drug increases the effect of coumarin-type anticoagulants. Use with aspirin increases risk of bleeding.

🖐 **Give with food, milk, or antacid to prevent gastric irritation.**

Adult: PO: 50–400 mg/day in divided doses tid or qid. Dosage individualized; begin at low dose, then increase gradually.

Clinical alert: Do not exceed 400 mg/day. Improvement may be seen in 2–4 days, but 2–3 weeks are usually required to obtain optimum therapeutic effect.

Contraindications/Precautions
PREG
ᴟ

Contraindicated in hypersensitivity to meclofenamate, aspirin, or other NSAIDs; in severe debilitating rheumatoid arthritis, active GI disease, coagulation defects, and severe renal or hepatic impairment. **Use with caution** in impaired cardiovascular or renal function.

ᴟ Contraindicated for nursing mothers. Use with caution for the elderly. Safe use for children under 14 years and pregnant women has not been established (first two trimesters, preg B; in third trimester, preg D).

Side effects/Adverse reactions

Hypersensitivity: rash, urticaria, asthma, dyspnea, bronchospasm, and anaphylaxis. **GI:** nausea, diarrhea, gastric irritation and bleeding. **Hem:** agranulocytosis and aplastic anemia. **CNS:** drowsiness, headache, dizziness. **Eye:** visual disturbances. **Ear:** tinnitus. **CV:** edema, palpitations.

▶

Nursing implications/Documentation

Possible nursing diagnoses: Pain; Impaired physical mobility.

♦ Establish a baseline for CBC, electrolytes, prothrombin time, BUN, creatinine, and liver function studies; if therapy is prolonged, monitor periodically thereafter (this drug will initially increase BUN, creatinine, alkaline phosphatase, bilirubin, and transaminase).

♦ Monitor for and report GI symptoms that may indicate peptic ulcer (nausea, pain, black stools).

♦ Record weight every other day; report edema or sudden weight gain.

♦ For diabetics, monitor blood sugar closely since insulin requirements may change.

Patient & family teaching/Home care

Possible nursing diagnoses: Altered health maintenance; Knowledge deficit.

♦ Explain that meclofenamate will take 2–3 weeks to achieve desired effects.

♦ Advise taking doses with food to reduce GI symptoms.

♦ Explain the importance of watching for symptoms of GI bleeding (black stools, persistent GI distress).

♦ Stress the need to avoid aspirin, alcohol, and other OTC drugs (unless approved by physician) because of increased risk of GI bleeding.

♦ Instruct individuals to hold dose and report if any of the following side effects are experienced: vertigo, rashes, blood in urine, hearing or visual changes, sudden weight gain, edema.

♦ Warn against driving or activities that require alertness until response is determined (may experience drowsiness at first).

♦ Reinforce the need for medical follow-up; advise telling dentist that meclofenamate is being taken.

♦ For diabetics, explain the importance of monitoring blood sugars with a blood glucose meter.

♦ *See Nonsteroidal anti-inflammatory drugs overview for more information.*

medroxyprogesterone

medroxyprogesterone acetate: *Amen, Curretab, Cycrin, Depo-provera, Provera*

Class: Progestational hormone, Antineoplastic agent

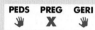

PEDS	PREG	GERI
✋	X	✋

Action Increases progestin levels by providing an exogenous source of progestin (progestin inhibits release of luteinizing hormone [LH], converts a proliferative endometerium to a secretory endometrium, thickens and reduces amount of cervical mucus, suppresses ovulation, and inhibits spontaneous uterine contractions). Suppresses progression of some cancers by altering hormonal balance.

Use/Therapeutic goal/Outcome

Secondary amenorrhea: Promotion of hormonal balance and regular menses. ***Outcome criteria:*** Regular menses.

Abnormal uterine bleeding due to hormonal imbalance: Cessation of bleeding; promotion of hormonal balance and regular menses. ***Outcome criteria:*** Cessation of bleeding; regular menses.

Renal and endometrial carcinoma: Promotion of hormonal environment that is unfavorable to cancer growth. ***Outcome criteria:*** Decrease in tumor growth on X rays.

Dose range/Administration

Interaction alert: Rifampin decreases progestin effectiveness.

🍂 **Give with food or milk to decrease GI effects.**

Secondary amenorrhea: Adult: PO: 5–10 mg/day for 5–10 days.

Abnormal uterine bleeding due to hormonal imbalance: Adult: PO: 5–10 mg/day for 5–10 days, usually beginning on day 16 or 21 of cycle. If bleeding is controlled, give 2 subsequent high-dose cycles.

Renal and endometrial carcinoma: Adult: IM: 400 mg to 1 g/wk. *Maintenance dose:* May be as low as 400 mg/mo.

Clinical alert: FDA guidelines require that patients read the package insert explaining possible progestin side effects before they receive their first dose. Give IM doses deep into large muscle (not deltoid) because they are painful.

Contraindications/Precautions

Contraindicated in hypersensitivity to medroxyprogesterone acetate or progestins, and in thromboembolic disease, cerebral pathology, liver disease, undiagnosed vaginal bleeding, missed abortion, known or suspected malignancy of the breast, and as a diagnostic test for pregnancy. *Use with caution* in history of epilepsy, migraine, asthma, cardiac or renal dysfunction, or diabetes.

🖐 **Contraindicated for children and pregnant or nursing mothers. Use with caution for the elderly.**

Side effects/Adverse reactions

Hypersensitivity: pruritus, rash, erythema, anaphylaxis. *CV:* edema, hypertension, thrombophlebitis, pulmonary embolism, cerebral thrombosis, embolism. *Hem:* hyperglycemia. *GI:* nausea, changes in appetite. *CNS:* headache, dizziness, nervousness, pyrexia, insomnia, somnolence, mental depression. *Eye:* retinal thrombosis, optic neuritis; proptosis; diplopia; sudden, partial, or complete loss of vision. *GU:* breakthrough bleeding, change in menstrual flow, amenorrhea, premenstrual-like syndrome, cystitis-like syndrome, cervical erosion, and changes in cervical secretions. *Skin:* urticaria, acne, alopecia, hirsutism. *Misc:* changes in libido, weight gain or loss.

Nursing implications/Documentation

Possible nursing diagnoses: Altered sexuality patterns; Pain.

♦ Check for pregnancy before giving first dose to women of childbearing years (this drug is associated with serious fetal abnormalities when taken during pregnancy).

♦ Report severe headache or visual disturbances immediately.

Patient & family teaching/Home care

Possible nursing diagnoses: Altered sexuality patterns; Knowledge deficit; Impaired home maintenance management.

♦ Stress that this drug should be taken with food to reduce nausea.

♦ Teach the need to hold dose and report if severe headaches, dizziness, visual disturbances, or numbness or tingling of the arms and legs is experienced.

♦ Advise women to report immediately if pregnancy is planned or suspected.

♦ Point out the importance of regular gynecologic exams (every 6 months to 1 year), mammography (yearly after age 40), and breast self-exam (monthly).

♦ If drug is taken on an on-off schedule, give the patient a calendar with drug-free days clearly marked.

♦ Explore sexual concerns; encourage verbalizing feelings and concerns and seeking counseling as needed.

♦ *See Antineoplastic agents overview for more information.*

mefenamic acid   *me-fe-nam'ik*

🍁*Ponstan, Ponstel*

Class: Nonsteroidal anti-inflammatory drug (NSAID), Analgesic, Antipyretic

PEDS	PREG	GERI
🖐	C	🖐

Action Reduces inflammation by inhibiting prostaglandin synthesis. Decreases uterine contractility by inhibiting intrauterine prostaglandins. Prostaglandin is a naturally occurring mediator of the inflammatory process which is found throughout body tissue.

Use/Therapeutic goal/Outcome

Pain and inflammation: Promotion of comfort and mobility; suppression of inflammation. *Outcome criteria:* Report of increased comfort with increased range of motion and ability to perform activities of daily life; reduction in or absence of joint stiffness, swelling, redness, and warmth.

Primary dysmenorrhea: Reduction of uterine hyperactivity (cramping). *Outcome criteria:* Report of pain relief and increased activity level.

Dose range/Administration

Interaction alert: Coumarin-type anticoagulants prolong prothrombin time. Hydantoins, sulfonamides, or sulfonylureas increase risk for drug toxicity. Corticosteroids, salicylates (including aspirin), and other NSAIDs increase risk of bleeding and GI ulcers.

🖐 **Give with food, milk, or antacid to prevent GI irritation.**

Arthritis: Adult: PO: *Initial dose:* 500 mg, then 250 mg q6h prn. *Child > 14 yr:* PO: *Initial dose:* 500 mg, then 250 mg q4h prn.

Primary dysmenorrhea: **Adult:** PO: *Initial dose:* 500 mg, then 250 mg q6h prn for 2–3 days. May begin before onset of menses.

Clinical alert: Do not give mefenamic acid for longer than 1 week. If rash develops, discontinue doses promptly.

Contraindications/Precautions
PREG
C

Contraindicated in hypersensitivity to mefenamic acid, and in history of upper or lower GI ulceration, bleeding or inflammation, or impaired renal function. *Use with caution* in impaired hepatic function, blood dyscrasias (especially coagulation defects), asthma, diabetes mellitus, and hypersensitivity to aspirin.

✋ **Use with caution for the elderly. Safe use for children under 14 years and pregnant women has not been determined.**

Side effects/Adverse reactions

Hypersensitivity: rash, urticaria, pruritus, asthma, and bronchospasm. *Hem:* agranulocytosis, hyperglycemia, aplastic anemia, hypoprothrombinemia, (prolonged use). *CNS:* dizziness, drowsiness, headache. *GI:* gastric irritation, diarrhea, nausea, vomiting, abdominal cramps. *GU:* dysuria, hematuria.

Nursing implications/Documentation

Possible nursing diagnoses: Pain; Impaired physical mobility.

♦ Establish a baseline for CBC, electrolytes, prothrombin time, BUN, creatinine, and liver function studies; if therapy is prolonged, monitor periodically thereafter.

♦ Monitor for and report GI symptoms that may indicate peptic ulcer (nausea, pain, black stools).

♦ Record weight every other day; report edema or sudden weight gain.

♦ If rash or diarrhea develop, hold dose and report immediately.

♦ For diabetics, monitor blood sugar closely since insulin requirements may change.

Patient & family teaching/Home care

Possible nursing diagnoses: Anxiety; Knowledge deficit; Impaired home maintenance management.

♦ Advise taking doses with food to reduce GI symptoms.

♦ Explain the importance of watching for symptoms of GI bleeding (black stools, persistent GI distress).

♦ Stress the need to avoid aspirin, alcohol, and other OTC drugs (unless approved by physician) because of increased risk of GI bleeding.

♦ Instruct individuals to hold dose and report if any of the following side effects are experienced: rashes, diarrhea, blood in urine, hearing or visual changes, sudden weight gain, edema.

♦ Warn against driving or activities that require alertness until response is determined.

♦ Reinforce the need for medical follow-up; advise telling dentist that mefenamic acid is being taken.

♦ For diabetics, explain the importance of monitoring blood sugars with a blood glucose meter.

♦ *See Nonsteroidal anti-inflammatory drugs overview for more information.*

megestrol
meh-jees'trole

megestrol acetate: *Megace,* ♦*Megostat*

Class: Antineoplastic agent, Antihormone

PEDS	PREG	GERI
✋	X	✋

Action Inhibits malignant cellular growth of gonadotropin-responsive tumors by desensitizing pituitary receptors and suppressing release of luteinizing hormone.

Use/Therapeutic goal/Outcome

Recurrent, inoperable, or metastatic endometrial or breast cancer (palliative treatment; not used as the sole agent): Suppression of malignant cell proliferation. *Outcome criteria:* Tumor and disease regression or stabilization on radiologic and physical examination.

Dose range/Administration

🥄 **Give with meals if GI distress occurs.**

Breast carcinoma: **Adult:** PO: 40 mg, qid for at least 2 months.

Endometrial carcinoma: **Adult:** PO: 40–320 mg/day in equally divided doses for at least 2 months.

Contraindications/Precautions
PREG
X

Contraindicated in hypersensitivity to megestrol acetate. *Use with caution* in history of thrombophlebitis.

♚ **Contraindicated for children and pregnant or nursing mothers. Use with caution for the elderly.**

Side effects/Adverse reactions

Hypersensitivity: urticaria, fever, chills. *GI:* anorexia. *GU:* breast tenderness, gynecomastia, dysfunctional uterine bleeding when drug is discontinued. *CNS:* carpal tunnel syndrome (soreness and tenderness of muscles of thumbs), mood swings. *CV:* deep-vein thrombosis. *Skin:* alopecia.

Nursing implications/Documentation

Possible nursing diagnoses: Fluid volume deficit; Self-esteem disturbance; Potential for injury; Altered nutrition: less than body requirements.

◆ *See important Nursing implications in Antineoplastic agents overview.*

♦ Monitor for and report vaginal bleeding.

♦ Observe for increased risk of thrombophlebitis.

♦ Check strength in hands every visit; report thumb weakness or soreness.

Patient & family teaching/Home care

Possible nursing diagnoses: Impaired home maintenance management; Knowledge deficit.

◆ *See important Patient & family teaching in Antineoplastic agents overview.*

♦ Stress that doses should be taken exactly on schedule (without missing or doubling up on doses) to maintain therapeutic levels.

♦ Advise reporting vaginal bleeding, edema, or pain and swelling of leg veins.

◆ *See Antineoplastic agents overview for more information.*

melphalan

mel'fa-lan

L-phenylalanine mustard: **Alkeran**

Class: Antineoplastic (nitrogen mustard alkylating) agent

PEDS	PREG	GERI
♚	**D**	♚

Action Kills rapidly growing cells (cancer, hair follicles, bone marrow, GI lining, ova, and sperm) by interfering with DNA replication and RNA transcription through alkylation (cross-linking of DNA occurs). Is cell-cycle–phase nonspecific, affecting both actively dividing cells and dormant (resting) cells.

Use/Therapeutic goal/Outcome

Multiple myeloma; and breast, ovarian, and testicular cancer: Elimination or suppression of malignant cell proliferation. *Outcome criteria:* Tumor and disease regression or stabilization on radiologic and physical examination.

Dose range/Administration

Interaction alert: Radiation therapy and other cytotoxic agents can cause severe myelosuppression.

▣ **Give on an empty stomach to increase drug absorption.**

Multiple myeloma: Adult: PO: 6 mg/day for 2–3 wk. Then stop drug for 4 wk or until leukocyte and platelet counts begin to increase. Then a maintenance dose of 2–4 mg/day while WBC > 4000/mm^3 and platelets >100,000/mm^3. *Alternate dose:* 0.15 mg/kg/day for 7 days or 0.25 mg/kg/day for 5 days q 4–6 wk. Wait for WBC and platelets to recover (4–6 weeks) then 0.05 mg/kg/day.

Ovarian carcinoma: Adult: PO: 0.2 mg/kg/day for 5 days q 4–5 wk, depending on myelosuppression.

Clinical alert: Monitor for toxicity, which is expected to occur with a low therapeutic index; drug therapy is designed to obtain significant myelosuppression to be effective (nadir, or lowest point, occurs at 14–21 days).

Contraindications/Precautions

PREG
D

Contraindicated in hypersensitivity to melphalan, severe leukopenia, thrombocytopenia, or anemia. *Use with caution* in impaired renal function (dose reduction may be necessary).

♚ **Contraindicated for pregnant and nursing mothers. Use with caution for the elderly. Safe use for children has not been established.**

Side effects/Adverse reactions

Hypersensitivity: urticaria, pruritus, exanthema, anaphylaxis. *Hem:* delayed and cumulative leukopenia, thrombocytopenia, and agranulocytosis (usually occurs within 4 weeks), hyperuricemia. *GI:* nausea and vomiting, stomatitis and oral ulceration, diarrhea. *Resp:* pulmonary fibrosis and pneumonitis. *GU:* amenorrhea.

Nursing implications/Documentation

Possible nursing diagnoses: Potential for infection; Potential for injury; Fatigue; Altered oral mucous membrane; Fluid volume deficit; Diar-

▶

M

rhea; Altered nutrition: less than body requirements.

- *See important Nursing implications in Antineoplastic agents overview on page 72, which apply to all antineoplastics. The interventions that follow are additional and specific to this drug only.*
  - Monitor for and report early signs of pulmonary toxicity (persistent cough, dyspnea, chest pain).
  - Increase fluid intake to 2–3 L a day to prevent renal tubular damage from hyperuricemia secondary to cell lysis.
  - Be aware that therapeutic response is often accompanied by toxicity.

Patient & family teaching/Home care

Possible nursing diagnoses: Knowledge deficit; Ineffective coping (individual and family); Hopelessness; Impaired home maintenance management.

- *See important Patient & family teaching in Antineoplastic agents overview on page 72, which apply to all antineoplastics. The teachings that follow are additional and specific to this drug only.*
  - Explain that taking melphalan on an empty stomach enhances its absorption.
  - Point out that drinking 2–3 L a day helps prevent kidney complications.
  - Stress that persistent cough, dyspnea, or chest pain should be reported.
- *See Antineoplastic agents overview for more information.*

menadiol

men-a-dye'ole

menadiol sodium diphosphate: ♣*Snykavite, Synkayvite*
Class: Vitamin K4; Prothrombogenic

PEDS	PREG	GERI
🖐	🖐	**OK**

Action Increases clotting ability by promoting hepatic formation of essential clotting factors (II, VII, IX, and X).

Use/Therapeutic goal/Outcome

Hypoprothrombinemia (secondary to obstructive jaundice, biliary fistula, antibacterials, salicylates): Prevention or control of bleeding.

Outcome criteria: Absence or control of bleeding; prothrombin time within 2 seconds of control.

Dose range/Administration

Interaction alert: Decreases effect of oral anticoagulants. Antacids, cholestyramine, colestipol, and mineral oil decrease oral absorption. Broad spectrum antibiotics, sufonamides, quinidine and salicylates may increase dose requirement.
Adult: PO: 5–10 mg/day. IM, SC: 5–15 mg/day or bid. *Child:* PO: 5–10 mg/day. IM, SC: 5–10 mg/day or bid.

Contraindications/Precautions

PREG
🖐

Contraindicated in hypersensitivity to menadiol. *Use with caution* in hepatic function impairment, and glucose-6-phosphate dehydrogenase (G6PD) deficiency.

🖐 **Contraindicated during last few weeks of pregnancy (preg X, near term), during labor, and for treatment of neonates. Use with caution for other children and pregnant women (preg C during first eight months).**

Side effects/Adverse reactions

Hypersensitivity: pruritus, urticaria, and rash. *Hem:* hyperbilirubinemia in neonates, hemolysis with G6PD deficiency. *GI:* unusual taste. *Skin:* redness, pain or swelling at injection site. *Misc:* facial flushing.

Nursing implications/Documentation

Possible nursing diagnosis: Impaired tissue integrity.

- With SC or IM injections, assess for irritation at injection site and provide comfort measures.
- Monitor prothrombin times and report significant changes to physican so that dosage can be regulated effectively.

Patient & family teaching/Home care

Possible nursing diagnosis: Knowledge deficit.

- Caution patient not to take other medications without consulting primary physician.
- Stress the importance of follow-up medical exams and blood studies.

meperidine

me-per'i-deen

meperidine hydrochloride (pethidine hydrochloride):
Demerol, Pethadol

Class: Narcotic analgesic

Antidote: naloxone hydrochloride (Narcan)

PEDS	PREG	GERI		CONTROLLED SUBSTANCE
✋	B	✋		II

Action Alters perception of and response to pain by an unclear mechanism. Believed to act by binding with opiate receptors at various CNS sites and altering the release of neurotransmitters from afferent nerves sensitive to painful stimuli.

Use/Therapeutic goal/Outcome

Moderate to severe pain and pre-procedure sedation: Relief of pain, promotion of relaxation. *Outcome criteria:* Report of increased comfort; absence of signs of pain (grimacing, frowning, restlessness, reluctance to move or cough), with increase in signs of comfort (relaxed facial expression, decreased restlessness); blood pressure and pulse within normal limits when compared to baseline.

Dose range/Administration

Interaction alert: Do not mix parenterally with barbiturates (they are incompatible). Other narcotic analgesics, general anesthetics, phenothiazines, sedative/hypnotics, tricyclic antidepressants, and alcohol increase risk of respiratory depression, hypotension, and profound sedation. Barbiturates, amphetamines, and cimetidine may increase CNS stimulation or depression. Do not use with isoniazid therapy or within 14 days of MAOI therapy.

▢ **Give meperidine syrup with a full glass of water because it has an anesthetic effect on mucous membranes.**

Moderate to severe pain: Adult: PO, IM, SC, IV: 50–150 mg q3-4h prn or around the clock. *Child:* PO, SC, IM: 1 mg/kg q4-6h prn or around the clock. *Maximum dose:* 100 mg.

Pre-procedure medication: Adult: SC, IM: 50–100 mg 30–90 min before procedure. *Child:* SC, IM: 1–2 mg/kg 30–90 min before procedure. *Maximum dose:* 100 mg.

Clinical alert: Expect decreased dosage for the elderly or debilitated. Avoid SC route because it is painful and irritating to tissues. Be aware that PO meperidine is less than half as effective as parenteral route, and that patient-controlled analgesia (PCA) via PCA pump may give best pain relief for terminally ill patients and for immediate postoperative period. Check respirations and pulse before giving meperidine; hold dose and report if respirations < 12, or if there is hypotension. Keep naloxone readily available in case of respiratory depression.

Contraindications/Precautions
PREG B

Contraindicated in hypersensitivity to meperidine hydrochloride. *Use with caution* in increased intracranial pressure, head injury, acute asthma attack, COPD, respiratory depression, compromised ability to maintain blood pressure, CNS depression, supraventricular tachycardias, convulsive disorders, acute abdominal conditions, impaired liver or kidney function, Addison's disease, hypothyroidism, urethral stricture, prostatic hypertrophy, and alcoholism.

✋ **Contraindicated for pregnant or nursing mothers (except during labor). Use with caution for children under 12 years and the elderly or debilitated.**

Side effects/Adverse reactions

Hypersensitivity: (rare) rash, hives, itching, swelling of face. *CNS:* lightheadedness, dizziness, sedation, physical dependence, convulsions with large doses. *Resp:* respiratory depression, respiratory arrest. *CV:* circulatory depression, shock, cardiac arrest, hypotension, phlebitis after IV injection. *GI:* nausea, vomiting. *Skin:* sweating, pain at injection site, local tissue irritation and induration after SC injection.

Nursing implications/Documentation

Possible nursing diagnoses: Pain; Anxiety; Potential for injury.

◆ Have patient rate pain on a scale of 1–10 before and after medication is given; report and record inadequate pain control.

◆ Determine whether a less potent analgesic might effectively relieve pain (narcotic analgesics should be used in the smallest effective dose compatible with the patient's needs).

◆ Consider alternating meperidine with a non-narcotic analgesic (ASA, ibuprofen, acetaminophen) to improve pain control while requiring lower narcotic doses.

◆ Give analgesics before pain is severe for best effects.

▶

- Document pulse, respirations, and blood pressure immediately before and 1 hr after administration until response is determined (then check 4 times a day if hospitalized).
- Monitor closely for risk factors for injury; keep side rails up and supervise ambulation if allowed out of bed; be aware that IV administration may abolish corneal reflex (protect eyes).
- Be aware of potential for psychic and physical dependence after prolonged use (withdrawal symptoms are similar to those of morphine).
- Encourage coughing and deep breathing; splint painful areas with a pillow.
- Monitor neonates of mothers who received this drug during labor for respiratory depression.

Patient & family teaching/Home care

Possible nursing diagnoses: Sensory/perceptual alterations; Impaired home maintenance management.

- Explain the rationale for taking analgesics before pain is too severe.
- Advise those who are ambulatory to refrain from activities that require alertness and to seek assistance if there is any question about ability to get out of bed (e.g., if there is weakness or light headedness).
- If nausea, vomiting, dizziness, or hypotension is noted, advise staying in bed with head down (helps relieve symptoms).
- Stress the need to adhere to prescribed dose regimen because of risk of overdose, dependence, and abuse potential (instead of increasing dosage regimen, unsatisfactory pain relief should be reported).
- Warn that alcohol and other CNS depressants may cause excessive sedation.
- *See Narcotic and non-narcotic analgesics overview for more information.*

mephenytoin

me-fen'i-toyn

Mesantoin

Class: Anticonvulsant, Hydantoin

PEDS	PREG	GERI
🖐	C	🖐

Action Limits the spread of seizure activity, and reduces abnormal excitability in the motor cortex. Nerve impulses in the motor cortex are probably inhibited by an effect on sodium ion flux across neuronal cell membranes, but exact mechanism of anticonvulsant action is unknown. Incidence of ataxia, gingival hyperplasia, GI distress, and hirsutism is lower than that of phenytoin, but incidence of sedation and serious toxic reactions (fatal blood dyscrasias) is higher; therefore mephenytoin usefulness is limited. Ineffective for petit mal seizures.

Use/Therapeutic goal/Outcome

Grand mal, focal, Jacksonian, and psychomotor seizures refractory to other anticonvulsants: Limitation of seizure activity. **Outcome criteria:** Marked decrease or absence of seizure activity.

Dose range/Administration

Interaction alert: Alcohol and folic acid may decrease effectiveness. Oral anticoagulants, antihistamines, chloramphenicol, cimetidine, some benzodiazepines, diazoxide, disulfiram, estrogens, isoniazid, phenothiazines, phenylbutazone, salicylates, and sulfonamides may increase risk of toxicity. The result of concomitant therapy with valproic acid, and with phenobarbital, is unpredictable.

Adult: PO: 50–100 mg daily. May increase daily dosage weekly by increments of 50–100 mg, to a maximum of 200 mg tid. **Child:** PO: Dose must be individualized. Begin with 25–50 mg daily. May increase daily dosage weekly by increments of 25–50 mg, to a maximum of 200 mg q8h.

Clinical alert: Schedule doses as evenly as possible over a 24-hr period to maintain constant blood levels (therapeutic drug level is 25–40 mcg/ml). Monitor lab studies for abnormalities that may indicate serious and life threatening side effects. Check CBC and platelet count every 2 weeks for up to 2 weeks after full maintenance dose has been attained; then every month for 1 year, and every 3 months thereafter; check liver function studies periodically.

Contraindications/Precautions

PREG C

Contraindicated in hypersensitivity to mephenytoin or hydantoins.

🖐 Use with caution for the elderly. Safe use for pregnant and nursing mothers has not been established.

Side effects/Adverse reactions

Hypersensitivity: rashes, exfoliative dermatitis. **Hem:** leukopenia, agranulocytosis, thrombocytopenia. **CNS:** drowsiness, dizziness, choreiform movements, insomnia. **Eye:** photophobia, conjunctivitis, diplopia, and nystagmus. **Misc:** fever, pain, lymphadenopathy.

Nursing implications/Documentation

Possible nursing diagnoses: Potential for injury; Potential for aspiration.

◆ Document history of seizures (type, frequency, duration, usual time they occur, precipitating factors, presence of an aura); initiate seizure precautions as indicated.

◆ Hold dose and report if signs of hematological side effects (persistent fatigue, sore throat, fever, infections) are noted.

Patient & family teaching/Home care

Possible nursing diagnoses: Fear; Self-esteem disturbance; Knowledge deficit; Impaired home maintenance management.

◆ Stress the need for close medical follow-up; emphasize that persistent fatigue, weakness, fever, sore throat or infections may be signs of side effects that should be reported.

◆ Warn that stopping anticonvulsants suddenly can cause an increase in severity and frequency of seizures.

◆ Warn that drinking alcohol may reduce drug effectiveness.

◆ Caution against driving until response is determined (may cause drowsiness at first).

◆ *See Anticonvulsants overview for more information.*

mephobarbital

me-foe-bar'bi-tal

Mebaral

Class: Anticonvulsant, Sedative, Barbiturate

PEDS	PREG	GERI	CONTROLLED SUBSTANCE
✋	**D**	✋	**IV**

Action Limits seizure activity by increasing nerve cell firing threshold (exact mechanism is unknown). Sedative action, properties, precautions and adverse reactions are similar to those of phenobarbital, but mephobarbital's lower potency means that larger doses are required for anticonvulsant effect.

Use/Therapeutic goal/Outcome

Grand mal and partial seizures: Limitation of seizure activity. **Outcome criteria:** Marked decrease or absence of seizure activity.

Sedation in management of delirium tremens, acute agitation, and anxiety: Promotion of relaxation. **Outcome criteria:** Reports of feeling less agitated and more relaxed; observable signs of relaxation (more quiet, less restless).

Dose range/Administration

Interaction alert: MAO inhibitors, alcohol, narcotics, and other CNS depressants may cause excessive sedation. May decrease the effects of oral anticoagulants, estrogens, oral contraceptors, doxycycline, and corticosteroids. Rifampin may decrease mephobarbital effects.

Adult: PO: 400–600 mg once daily, or in divided doses. **Child: > 5 yrs:** PO: 32–64 mg 3–4 times a day. **Child: < 5 yrs:** PO: 16–32 mg 3–4 times a day.

Clinical alert: For nocturnal seizures in adults, give total dose or largest dose at bedtime. Monitor the elderly and young for paradoxical excitement.

Contraindications/Precautions

PREG D **M**

Contraindicated in hypersensitivity to barbiturates, and in obstructive respiratory disease with dyspnea, or hepatic, renal, or cardiac dysfunction. **Use with caution** in alcoholism, hyperthyroidism, and fever.

✋ **Use with caution for the elderly and children. Safe use in pregnancy is not established.**

Side effects/Adverse reactions

Hypersensitivity: exfoliative dermatitis, and Stevens-Johnson syndrome. **CNS:** lethargy, dizziness, hangover, irritability, and paradoxical excitement. **GI:** nausea, vomiting. **Resp:** respiratory depression.

Nursing implications/Documentation

Possible nursing diagnoses: Potential for injury; Sensory/perceptual alterations.

◆ Document history of seizures (type, frequency, duration, usual time they occur, precipitating factors, presence of an aura); initiate seizure precautions as indicated.

◆ Hold drug and report if there is excessive sedation or respiratory depression.

◆ Keep side rails up and supervise ambulation until response is determined.

• Monitor CBC, BUN, creatinine, and drug level periodically (most of this drug is metabolized to phenobarbital; therapeutic phenobarbital levels are 15–40 mcg/ml).

Patient & family teaching/Home care

Possible nursing diagnoses: Fear; Self-esteem disturbance; Knowledge deficit; Impaired home maintenance management.

• Warn that stopping anticonvulsants suddenly can cause an increase in severity and frequency of seizures.

• Warn that drinking alcohol may reduce drug effectiveness.

• Caution against driving until response is determined (likely to cause drowsiness).

• Advise women that oral contraceptives may not be as effective when taking mephobarbital.

• *See Antianxiety Agents, Sedatives, and Hypnotics, and Anticonvulsants overviews for more information.*

mepivacaine
me-piv'a-kane

mepivacaine hydrochloride: **Carbocaine, Cavacaine, Isocaine**

Class: Local anesthetic (amide-type)

PEDS	PREG	GERI
✋	C	✋

Action Produces local anesthesia by inhibiting sodium flux across the nerve cell membrane, thus preventing depolarization and generation and conduction of nerve impulses. Mepivacaine has moderate potency and toxicity, begins to act within 15 min and lasts up to 3 hr. When combined with the vasoconstrictor levonordefrin, action may be prolonged.

Use/Therapeutic goal/Outcome

Local infiltration, nerve block, caudal, and epidural anesthesia: Prevention of pain during surgical and obstetrical procedures. **Outcome criteria:** Report of numbness and absence of pain in anesthetized area. Patients undergoing regional anesthesia will demonstrate loss of motor function in anesthetized area.

Dose range/Administration

Adult: *Therapeutic nerve block (for pain management)*: 50–200 mg 1% solution or 100–400 mg 2% solution. *Maximum dose*: 7 mg/kg, 500 mg per dose or 1 g/day. Do not repeat more frequently than every 90 min. *Transvagi-*

nal block or infiltration: Up to 400 mg (40 cc) 1% solution. *Paracervical block*: Up to 100 mg (10 cc) 1% solution on each side (200 mg total) per 90 min period. *Caudal and epidural block*: Up to 150–300 mg (15–30 cc) 1% solution *or* 150–375 mg (10–25 cc) 1.5% solution *or* 200–400 mg (10–20 cc) 2% solution. **Child:** *Therapeutic nerve block (for pain management)*: Maximum single dose 5–6 mg/kg. Dose and interval may be increased if given with levonordefrin (used only for dental procedures).

Clinical alert: These drugs should be administered only by clinicians thoroughly familiar with their use. Dose is highly individualized depending on the procedure, method of administration, area to be anesthetized, vascularity of tissue, and on patient condition, tolerance, and response. Keep resuscitative drugs and equipment immediately available.

Contraindications/Precautions
PREG C

Contraindicated in hypersensitivity to mepivacaine or to other amide-type anesthetics, or to methylparaben (multiple-dose vial only). **Use with caution** in severe arrhythmias, shock, or heart block, in liver or kidney disease, and for the debilitated or acutely ill.

🖐 **Use with caution for children and the elderly (reduce dosage). Safe use for pregnant women has not been established (may effect fetal development); used for obstetrical anesthesia and analgesia.**

Side effects/Adverse reactions

Hypersensitivity: rash, cutaneous lesions of delayed onset, urticaria, edema, anaphylaxis. **CNS:** excitation, depression, drowsiness, tremors, convulsions, chills. **CV:** arrhythmias, vasodilatation, hypotension, myocardial depression, bradycardia, hypertension, cardiac arrest. **Resp:** respiratory arrest. **GI:** nausea, vomiting. **Eye:** blurred vision. **Ear:** tinnitus.

Nursing implications/Documentation

Possible nursing diagnoses: Pain; Potential for injury.

• Be sure that history of allergies and accurate height and weight are recorded before procedure.

• Record vital signs according to protocol, and monitor for and report immediately signs of systemic or hypersensitivity reactions.

• Determine from anesthesiologist or anesthetist whether there are any restrictions on patient positioning; post these at bedside.

- Monitor anesthetized area for level of sensation and motor function; watch for poor positioning, and protect area from injury.

- Give prescribed pain medication as sensation begins to return, **before pain is severe.**

Patient & family teaching/Home care

Possible nursing diagnoses: Anxiety; Fear.

- Stress the need to protect areas of the body that have lost sensation.

- Explain rationale for taking prescribed pain medication before pain becomes too uncomfortable.

◆ *See Local anesthetics overview for more information.*

mercaptopurine   *mer-kap-toe-pyoor'een*

6-MP, 6-Mercaptopurine: *Purinethol*

Class: Antineoplastic (antimetabolite) agent

PEDS	PREG	GERI
🤚	D	🤚

Action Kills rapidly growing cells (cancer, hair follicles, bone marrow, GI lining, ova, and sperm) by inhibiting DNA and RNA synthesis. Drug is cell-cycle specific for the S-phase.

Use/Therapeutic goal/Outcome

Acute lymphocytic leukemias, acute and chronic myelogenous leukemia, and acute and chronic myeloblastic and myelocytic leukemia (mainly in combination chemotherapy): Elimination or suppression of malignant cell proliferation. *Outcome criteria:* Tumor and disease regression or stabilization on radiologic and physical examination; for leukemias, absence of blasts on examination of peripheral blood specimen.

Dose range/Administration

Interaction alert: Drug dosage should be reduced 35–75% if given with allopurinol (allopurinol inhibits oxidation of mercaptopurine and increases bone marrow depression). Radiation therapy and other cytotoxic agents can cause severe myelosuppression. If given with warfarin, monitor daily PT (may alter anticoagulant activity).

🖐 **Give with meals to decrease GI upset.**

Adult: PO: 1.5 to 2.5 mg/kg or 80–100 mg/m²/day; may increase to 5 mg/kg/day. *Child:* PO: 50–70 mg/m²/day; may increase to 5 mg/kg/day after 4 wk if dose is effective.

Clinical alert: Expect that dosage will be increased until symptoms of toxicity are evident. Discontinue at first sign of significant drop in WBC count (blood count will continue to drop for several days after drug is stopped). Expect decreased dosage for those with renal impairment (nephrotoxicity may occur with drug accumulation). WBC, platelets, and erythrocytes should drop to the lowest point (nadir) in 14 days. Hold dose and report if platelets <100,000/mm³ or WBC <4000/mm³.

Contraindications/Precautions   PREG D

Contraindicated in hypersensitivity to mercaptopurine. *Use with caution* in hepatic or renal dysfunction, and concomitant use of hepatotoxic drugs (increased risk of liver toxicity).

🖐 **Contraindicated for pregnant or nursing mothers. Use with caution for children and the elderly.**

Side effects/Adverse reactions

Hypersensitivity: urticaria, fever, tachycardia, and hypotension. *Hem:* hyperuricemia, leukopenia, anemia, and thrombocytopenia (all may last several days after drug is stopped). *GI:* hepatotoxicity (jaundice, cholestasis, ascites); nausea, vomiting, and anorexia (25–30% of patients); painful oral ulcers; abdominal pain; diarrhea. *GU:* oliguria, hematuria. *Skin:* hyperpigmentation.

Nursing implications/Documentation

Possible nursing diagnoses: Potential for infection; Potential for injury; Fatigue; Altered oral mucous membrane; Fluid volume deficit; Diarrhea; Altered nutrition: less than body requirements.

◆ *See important Nursing implications in Antineoplastic agents overview on page 72, which apply to all antineoplastics. The interventions that follow are additional and specific to this drug only.*

- Increase fluid intake to 2–3 L a day to prevent renal tubular damage from hyperuricemia secondary to cell lysis.

- Be aware that this drug may cause a falsely elevated value for serum glucose.

Patient & family teaching/Home care

Possible nursing diagnoses: Knowledge deficit; Ineffective coping (individual and family); Hopelessness; Impaired home maintenance management.

M

▶

- See important Patient & family teaching in Antineoplastic agents overview on page 72, which apply to all antineoplastics. The teachings that follow are additional and specific to this drug only.
  - Stress that it may take 2–4 weeks (or longer) for a response to therapy to occur.
  - Point out that drinking 2–3 L a day helps prevent kidney complications.
- See Antineoplastic agents overview for more information.

mesalamine

mez-al'a-meen

Rowasa, ♣*Salofalk*

Class: Rectal anti-inflammatory

PEDS	PREG	GERI
☜	B	☜

Action Reduces inflammation by inhibiting production of prostaglandin in the colon and inhibiting mucosal production of metabolites associated with inflammatory bowel disease.

Use/Therapeutic goal/Outcome

Ulcerative colitis, proctosigmoiditis, and Procititis: Reduction of inflammation and ulceration of bowel mucosa. *Outcome criteria:* Absence of abdominal pain and blood in stools; decreased frequency of bowel movements; sigmoidoscopic evidence of decreased inflammation.

Dose range/Administration

Interaction alert: Sulfasalazine increases risk of renal toxicity.

Adult: RECT: Suspension: 4 g at bedtime for 3–6 wk. Suppository: 500 mg bid to tid for 3–6 wk.

Clinical alert: Give at bedtime and encourage patient to retain suspension until morning.

Contraindications/Precautions

PREG B

Contraindicated in hypersensitivity to mesalamine, sulfasalazine, salicylates, or sulfites. *Use with caution* in renal impairment.

☜ Use with caution for children, pregnant or nursing mothers, and the elderly.

Side effects/Adverse reactions

Hypersensitivity: acute intolerance syndrome (cramping, acute abdominal pain, bloody diarrhea, fever, severe headache, rash). *GI:* cramps, abdominal pain, diarrhea, nausea, anal irritation. *CNS:* headache. *GU:* renal toxicity.

Nursing implications/Documentation

Possible nursing diagnoses: Pain; Diarrhea.
- Obtain history to rule out previous intolerance to sulfasalazine.
- Administer as retention enema, after a bowel movement, if possible.
- Monitor for and report development of acute intolerance symptoms (fever, rash, bloody diarrhea, acute abdominal pain, severe headache).
- Assess and record bowel sounds and character and frequency of stools.
- Observe for anal irritation; employ appropriate measures to protect area from breakdown.

Patient & family teaching/Home care

Possible nursing diagnoses: Knowledge deficit; Impaired home maintenance management.
- Teach that the enema should be administered at bedtime, after a bowel movement.
- Teach method for administration (shake container well; remove cover from applicator tip; lie on left side; insert applicator tip into rectum and squeeze container steadily to discharge suspension).
- Stress the importance of retaining suspension overnight.
- Advise to stop drug and report development of fever, rash, or severe gastrointestinal distress.
- Advise reporting development of rectal irritation.
- Point out the need to avoid foods that exacerbate diarrhea and to maintain a well-balanced, low-residue, high-protein diet.
- Caution to avoid cold foods and smoking, which increase bowel motility.
- Emphasize the need to maintain medical supervision during course of treatment.

mesoridazine

mez-oh-rid'a-zeen

mesoridazine besylate: *Serentil*

Class: Phenothiazine antipsychotic

PEDS	PREG	GERI
☜	C	☜

Action Exact mechanism of action has not been determined. Believed to produce calmness and alleviate psychiatric symptoms (disorders of

M

perception, thought, consciousness, mood, affect, and social interaction) by blocking dopamine receptors in the limbic system. Blocks peripheral muscarinic, adrenergic, and histamine receptors. Also has some effect on the hypothalamus and pituitary gland, causing changes in regulation of body temperature and endocrine function. A dose of 50 mg of mesoridazine is therapeutically equivalent to 100 mg of chlorpromazine.

Use/Therapeutic goal/Outcome

Schizophrenia, schizoaffective disorders, psychosis: Promotion of reality orientation. *Outcome criteria:* Demonstration of reality orientation, and ability to problem solve and interact with others.

Behavior disturbances associated with chronic mental problems: Elimination of uncooperative and hyperactive behavior. *Outcome criteria:* Demonstration of increased ability to cooperate with others; absence of hyperactivity (increased periods of calmness).

Nonpsychotic anxiety, and acute and chronic alcoholism: Promotion of calmness, improved ability to cope with activities of daily living (ADLs). *Outcome criteria:* Report of feeling more calm and able to cope with ADLs, and demonstration of decreased restlessness/agitation.

Dose range/Administration

Interaction alert: Antacids may reduce absorption; separate doses of antacid and phenothiazines by at least 2 hr. Alcohol and other CNS depressants may cause excessive sedation. Barbiturates may decrease phenothiazine effects.

Psychosis: Adult: PO: 50 mg tid, increasing to 100–400 mg/day in divided doses. IM: 25 mg; repeat in 30–60 min if needed and tolerated. *Maximum dose:* (for severe psychosis) 200 mg/day.

Nonpsychotic anxiety: Adult: PO: 10 mg tid, increasing to 30–150 mg/day.

Alcoholism: Adult: PO: 25 mg bid, increasing to 50–200 mg/day.

Behavioral disorders: Adult: PO: 25 mg tid, increasing to 75–300 mg/day.

Clinical alert: Avoid skin contact with liquid and parenteral forms (may cause contact dermatitis). Before IM doses, count respirations and check blood pressure; hold dose and report if respirations are less than 12/min or if the patient is hypotensive. Keep IV diphenhydramine available in case of side effect of acute

dystonic reaction. If compliance is a problem, consider using liquid form.

Contraindications/Precautions

PREG C

Contraindicated in hypersensitivity to mesoridazine or to phenothiazines, and in CNS depression, comatose states. *Use with caution* in seizure disorders, hypertension, parkinsonism, poorly controlled diabetes mellitus, asthma, emphysema, narrow-angle glaucoma, cardiac disease, hypotension, paralytic ileus, liver damage, prostatic hypertrophy, and bone marrow depression.

☙ **Contraindicated for nursing mothers. Use with caution for adolescents and the elderly or debilitated. Safe use for children under 12 years and pregnant women has not been established.**

Side effects/Adverse reactions

Hypersensitivity: rash, contact dermatitis. *CNS:* sedation, extrapyramidal reactions (pseudoparkinsonism, akathisia [restless need to keep moving], dystonia, tardive dykinesia), neuroleptic malignant syndrome (fever, tachycardia, tachypnea, profuse diaphoresis); EEG changes, dizziness. *CV:* orthostatic hypotension, palpitations, dysrhythmias, EKG changes. *GI:* appetite changes, dry mouth, constipation, abnormal liver function. *GU:* urinary retention or hesitancy, priapism, dark urine, impaired ejaculation, amenorrhea. *Eye:* blurred vision, photophobia. *Skin:* photosensitivity, jaundice. *MS:* weight gain. *Hem:* hyperglycemia, transient leukopenia, agranulocytosis. *Misc:* galactorrhea, gynecomastia. *After abrupt withdrawal of long-term therapy:* gastritis, nausea, vomiting, lightheadedness, tremors, feeling of warmth or cold, diaphoresis, tachycardia, headache, insomnia.

Nursing implications/Documentation

Possible nursing diagnoses: Potential for injury; Constipation; Altered oral mucous membrane.

♦ Record mental status and vital signs before and 1 hr after administration during initial phase of treatment, then bid until response to therapy has been established, then periodically thereafter.

♦ Check CBC, liver function, BUN, and creatinine before giving first dose and periodically thereafter.

♦ Be sure that doses are swallowed (not hoarded).

• Monitor for orthostatic hypotension, dizziness, and drowsiness; supervise ambulation until response is established.

• Record weight every 2 weeks; report significant weight gain. Provide special mouth care; observe for and report oral ulcers.

• Prevent constipation by monitoring bowel movements and encouraging adequate fiber and fluid intake; offer laxatives or stool softeners before problem becomes severe.

• Report persistent sore throat, fever, and malaise, because these may indicate agranulocytosis (drug may have to be discontinued).

• Monitor for (and report immediately) signs of neuroleptic malignant syndrome (muscle rigidity, tremors, high fever, tachycardia); this is a rare, but potentially fatal, side effect.

Patient & family teaching/Home care

Possible nursing diagnoses: Sleep pattern disturbance; Impaired home maintenance management.

• Emphasize the need to continue medication, even when feeling well.

• Warn to change positions slowly to prevent dizziness.

• Stress that the effects of alcohol, sedatives and other CNS depressants, and tranquilizers may be potentiated.

• Caution to consult with physician before using OTC drugs; stress the need for ongoing medical follow-up.

• Teach the need to report persistent sore throat, fever, and fatigue.

• Point out that doses should not be increased or stopped without checking with physician.

• Caution to wear a sunscreen (number 15), protective clothing, and sunglasses when out in the sun.

• Advise avoidance of driving and other potentially hazardous activities until response is determined.

• Suggest using ice chips, hard candy, or gum to relieve side effect of dry mouth; stress the need for good mouth care.

• Warn women to report if pregnancy is planned or suspected.

• *See Antipsychotics overview for more information.*

metaproterenol
met-a-pro-ter'e-nole

metaproterenol sulfate: *Alupent, Arm-a-Med Metaproterenol, Dey-Dose Metaproterenol, Dey-Med Metaproterenol, Metaprel*

Class: Sympathomimetic, Adrenergic agonist, Smooth muscle relaxant (respiratory), Bronchodilator, Tocolytic

PEDS	PREG	GERI
🤚	C	🤚

Action Produces sympathomimetic action by acting on beta-2 receptors, causing relaxation of the smooth muscle of the bronchi, uterus, and blood vessels supplying skeletal muscles.

Use/Therapeutic goal/Outcome

Bronchospasm (asthma, bronchitis, emphysema): Reduction of airway resistance, promotion of air movement. **Outcome criteria:** Decreased wheezing; increased forced expiratory volume (FEV); increased ability to bring forth sputum; report of easier breathing, fewer episodes of wheezing.

Dose range/Administration

Interaction alert: Beta adrenergic blockers such as propranolol may reduce bronchodilating effects.

Adult/Child > 9 yr or 27 kg: PO: 20 mg q6-8h. *Inhalation:* 2–3 breaths, not more than q3-4h. *Maximum daily dose:* 12 breaths. **Child 6–9 yr or < 27 kg:** PO: 10 mg q6-8h.

Clinical alert: If both PO route and inhalation route are being taken, monitor for increased risk of toxicity. For best effects, give metaproterenol doses 5 min before steroid inhalations.

Contraindications/Precautions
PREG
C

Contraindicated in hypersensitivity to metaproterenol and sympathomimetic amines, and in tachycardia, hypertension, and hyperthyroidism.

🤚 Use with caution for the elderly. Safe use for children (under 6 years for oral use and under 12 years for aerosol use), women of childbearing age, and pregnant or nursing mothers has not been established.

Side effects/Adverse reactions

Hypersensitivity: exaggeration of side effects. *CNS:* nervousness, weakness, drowsiness, tremor. *CV:* tachycardia, hypertension, palpi-

M

tation. *GI:* nausea, vomiting, bad taste. *GU:* difficulty in micturition. *MS:* muscle cramps.

Nursing implications/Documentation

Possible nursing diagnoses: Potential for injury; Activity intolerance; Ineffective breathing pattern.

♦ Record lung sounds, respirations, pulse, and blood pressure before and after dose administration until response is determined.

♦ Provide favorite fluids and monitor intake and output to ensure adequate hydration (at least 2 L a day is recommended).

♦ Hold drug and report immediately if paradoxical bronchospasm occurs.

Patient & family teaching/Home care

Possible nursing diagnoses: Knowledge deficit; Fear; Ineffective family coping.

♦ Explain that this drug will enlarge air passages and make breathing easier.

♦ Warn that paradoxical bronchospasm can occur (teach the need to hold dose and report immediately if this should happen, rather than increase dose).

♦ Point out that stress and exercise can aggravate wheezing and bronchospasm, and that learning relaxation and controlled breathing techniques can help reduce severity and frequency of episodes of wheezing.

♦ Give written and verbal instructions on how to use inhalers (shake container, exhale slowly and completely through nose, inhale deeply while administering aerosol, hold breath for a few seconds, then exhale slowly; allow 2 min between inhalations). Have individual or caregiver demonstrate technique before going home.

♦ Warn against taking OTC drugs without physician's approval.

♦ *See Adrenergics (sympathomimetics) overview for more information.*

metaraminol

met-a-ram'i-nole

metaraminol bitartrate: *Aramine*

Class: Adrenergic agonist, Sympathomimetic, Vasopressor

PEDS	PREG	GERI
🖐	D	🖐

Action Produces sympathomimetic action by acting on alpha-adrenergic receptors (causing vas-

oconstriction) and beta-1 receptors (causing positive inotropic effects on the heart). Its vasoconstricting action increases pulmonary arterial pressure and produces a sustained rise in blood pressure (systolic and diastolic), but reduces blood flow to the kidneys and other vital organs.

Use/Therapeutic goal/Outcome

Prevention and treatment of hypotension and shock: Improvement of blood pressure. **Outcome criteria:** Blood pressure greater than 90–100 systolic; absence of clinical signs of shock (confusion, restlessness, rapid weak pulse, urine output less than 25 ml/hr).

Dose range/Administration

Interaction alert: Do not mix IV with any other drugs. Ergot alkaloids, furazolidone, guanethidine, or tricyclic antidepressants may increase pressor effects. Do not give with cyclopropane, halothane, or within 14 days of MAOI therapy. Digitalis may sensitize the myocardium to metaraminol. May alter insulin requirement.

Prevention of hypotension: Adult: SC, IM: 2–10 mg. Wait 10 min before giving additional dose (to avoid additive effects). **Child:** SC, IM: 0.1 mg/kg. Wait 10 min before giving additional dose (to avoid additive effects).

Treatment of hypotension and shock: Adult: IV: 0.5–5 mg bolus, then an infusion of 15–100 mg in 500 ml of D5W or NS, titrated according to blood pressure. **Child:** IV: 0.01 mg/kg bolus, then an infusion of 1 mg in 25 ml of D5W or NS, titrated according to blood pressure.

Clinical alert: Ascertain that hypotension is not due to hypovolemia before giving first dose (volume deficit should be corrected before giving vasopressors). Use an IV controller device to regulate IV infusion; monitor closely for infiltration (stop infusion immediately and report, because this drug is extremely irritating to tissues). Obtain blood pressure parameters for increasing or decreasing IV rate from physician. Place patient on a continuous cardiac monitor and have emergency drugs and equipment readily available.

Contraindications/Precautions

PREG
D

Contraindicated in hypersensitivity to sympathomimetics and sulfites, in use within 14 days of MAOI therapy, and in pulmonary edema, cardiac arrest, untreated hypoxia, hypercapnia, acidosis, and peripheral or mesenteric thrombosis.

♨ Use with caution for children and the elderly. Safe use for pregnant women has not been established.

Side effects/Adverse reactions

Hypersensitivity: bluish coloration of skin; dizziness; flushing or redness of skin; rash; hives; itching; swelling of face, lips, or eyelids; wheezing or difficulty in breathing; exaggeration of side effects. *CV:* ventricular tachycardia, dysrhythmias, hypertension and hypotension upon stopping the drug, palpitations, bradycardia, precordial pain. *CNS:* headache, flushing, tremors, dizziness, apprehension, restlessness, pallor. *Skin:* tissue necrosis, sloughing at injection site. *GI:* nausea, vomiting.

Nursing implications/Documentation

Possible nursing diagnoses: Potential for injury; Activity intolerance; Sleep pattern disturbance.

♦ Record and monitor pulse, blood pressure, and respirations every 5 min until stable, then every 15 min, then every 1/2–1 hr.

♦ Record urine output hourly; report urine output less than 30 ml/hour.

♦ Keep patient in bed with side rails up.

♦ When weaning off metaraminol bitartrate, taper dose slowly, while closely monitoring blood pressure (be aware that this drug has a prolonged action and may have cumulative effects).

Patient & family teaching/Home care

Possible nursing diagnoses: Knowledge deficit; Fear; Ineffective family coping.

♦ For hypotensive states, stress that frequent monitoring of vital signs is needed to "fine tune" medication dose for optimum results; stress the need to remain in bed.

♦ Stress that the nurses need to be told of new symptoms or uncomfortable feelings in case they indicate a need for medication adjustment.

♦ *See Adrenergics (sympathomimetics) overview for more information.*

metaxalone   *met-ax'ah-lone*

Skelaxin

Class: Skeletal-muscle relaxant (centrally acting)

PEDS	PREG	GERI
♨	C	♨

Action Relaxes skeletal muscle by producing CNS depression. Mode of action may be related to its sedative properties.

Use/Therapeutic goal/Outcome

Sprains and other musculoskeletal trauma: Relief of muscle spasms without loss of voluntary muscle function; relief of pain. *Outcome criteria:* Increased range of motion and ability to perform activities of daily life; report of relief of pain, anxiety, and tension.

Dose range/Administration

Interaction alert: CNS effects may be additive to those of other CNS depressants and alcohol.

🍎 **Give with food to prevent gastric distress.**

Adult/Child > 12 yrs: PO: 800 mg tid or qid.

Contraindications/Precautions   PREG C

Contraindicated in hypersensitivity to metaxalone, and in tendency to drug-induced anemias. *Use with caution* in epilepsy, and impaired renal or hepatic function.

♨ Use with caution for pregnant women and the elderly. Safe use for children under 12 years and nursing mothers has not been established.

Side effects/Adverse reactions

Hypersensitivity: light rash with or without pruritus. *GI:* nausea, vomiting, GI distress, hepatotoxicity. *CNS:* dizziness, headache, drowsiness, nervousness, agitation, exacerbation in grand mal epilepsy. *Hem:* leukopenia, hemolytic anemia.

Nursing implications/Documentation

Possible nursing diagnoses: Impaired physical mobility; Potential for injury; Pain.

♦ Monitor comfort level and range of motion before and after dose is given.

♦ Monitor for and report abnormal liver function studies or signs of hepatotoxicity (jaundice, fever, abdominal discomfort).

♦ Supervise ambulation until risk of drowsiness, loss of balance, or dizziness is determined.

♦ Observe for and report hypersensitivity reaction to physician immediately.

♦ Be aware that false-positive Benedict's glucose tests may occur.

Patient & family teaching/Home care

Possible nursing diagnoses: Knowledge deficit; Impaired home maintenance management.

♦ Explain the importance of taking doses with food to avoid gastric distress.

♦ Stress the need to contact physician immediately if side effects occur.

♦ Warn against operating machinery, driving, or taking alcohol or other CNS depressants—especially if drowsiness or dizziness is present (early therapy response should be determined).

♦ Teach to avoid OTC drugs unless approved by physician.

♦ *See Skeletal-muscle relaxants overview for more information.*

methacholine

meth-a-koe'lin

methacholine chloride: *Provocholine*

Class: Cholinergic bronchoconstrictor, Diagnostic agent

PEDS	PREG	GERI
✋	C	✋

Action Produces bronchoconstriction in individuals with bronchial airway hyperreactivity by cholinergic stimulation. Methacholine-induced bronchoconstriction lasts longer than acetylcholine-induced bronchoconstriction, and asthmatics are more sensitive to both agents than nonasthmatics.

Use/Therapeutic goal/Outcome

Diagnosis of bronchial airway hyperreactivity in the absence of clinically apparent asthma: Determination of presence of bronchial airway hyperactivity. *Outcome criteria:* Within 5 min of administration, a 20% reduction in forced expiratory volume (FEV) from baseline is diagnostic for asthma.

Dose range/Administration

Interaction alert: Beta-adrenergic blockers prolong or exaggerate bronchoconstrictive effect. Do not give within 24 hr of administration of sustained-release aminophylline or theophylline; both are bronchodilators that will interfere with results. Antihistamines and decongestants and other bronchodilators should be held for 12 hours before the test (except for prednisone).

Adult: Inhal: Begin with a low concentration (0.025 mg/ml). Give 5 inhalations from dosimeter, and progressively increase concentration to

a maximum of 10 mg/ml (for use by physician only).

Clinical alert: Withhold respiratory medications (except prednisone) the morning of test (see Interaction alert). A beta-adrenergic agonist is usually administered after methacholine challenge to return FEV to normal. Atropine and equipment to support ventilation must be readily available.

Contraindications/Precautions

PREG
C

Contraindicated in hypersensitivity to methacholine or similar agents, and in clinically obvious asthma, history of wheezing, low baseline pulmonary function, and concomitant use of beta-adrenergic blockers. *Use with caution* in cardiovascular disease with bradycardia, epilepsy, irritability of the vagus nerve, peptic ulcers, thyroid disease, or urinary tract obstruction.

🖐 **Use with caution for the elderly. Safe use has not been established and drug should be avoided for children under 6 years and for pregnant or nursing mothers.**

Side effects/Adverse reactions

Hypersensitivity: itching. **CNS:** headache, lightheadedness. **Resp:** throat irritation, severe bronchospasm.

Nursing implications/Documentation

Possible nursing diagnoses: Potential for injury; Ineffective breathing pattern.

♦ Report if patient has had an influenza vaccine within 3 weeks (test may be held, although false positive results are common).

♦ Document lung sounds, pulse, respirations and blood pressure, before, during, and immediately after drug administration.

♦ Keep patient seated or in bed during test; supervise ambulation after test until dizziness and other adverse responses have been ruled out.

Patient & family teaching/Home care

Possible nursing diagnoses: Anxiety; Fear.

♦ Explain that wheezing, coughing, throat irritation, headache, itching, and dizziness may be caused by this drug, and that they will be relieved with a second drug immediately after the test.

♦ Caution the patient to stay seated or in bed until nurse is present to supervise ambulation.

M

methadone

meth'a-done

methadone hydrochloride: *Dolophine, Methadone,* ➤*Physeptone*

Class: Narcotic analgesic, Opiate agonist

Antidote: naloxone hydrochloride (Narcan)

PEDS	PREG	GERI	CONTROLLED SUBSTANCE
🖐	B	🖐	II

Action Prevents opiate withdrawal symptoms and alters both perception of and response to pain through an unclear mechanism. Believed to act by binding with opiate receptors at many CNS sites.

Use/Therapeutic goal/Outcome

Severe pain: Relief of pain. *Outcome criteria:* Report of reduced pain.

Heroin detoxification and temporary maintenance: Suppression of heroin withdrawal symptoms. *Outcome criteria:* Report and demonstration of relief of withdrawal symptoms (insomnia, anxiety, anorexia, abdominal pain, weakness, sweating, headache, hot and cold flashes).

Narcotic abstinence syndrome: Elimination of compulsive craving and euphoric effects of IV narcotics. *Outcome criteria:* Report of absence of craving for narcotics; demonstration of abstinence from use of other narcotics.

Dose range/Administration

Interaction alert: Alcohol, cimetidine, and CNS depressants increase methadone effects. Barbiturates, pentazocine, phenytoin, and rifampin reduce methadone effects. Ammonium chloride, other urine acidifiers, and phenytoin, reduce analgesic effect.

Severe Pain: Adult: PO, SC, IM: 2.5–10 mg q3-4h prn. Parenteral doses > 10 mg not recommended.

Detoxification: Adult: PO: 15–40 mg/day. Doses highly individualized, adjusted to maintain tolerable level of withdrawal symptoms.

Maintenance treatment: Adult: PO: 20–120 mg/day. Doses highly individualized. Doses > 120 mg/day require special state and federal approval.

Clinical alert: Oral dose is half as effective as parenteral dose. Give doses of tablets completely dissolved in 120 ml of orange juice or powdered citrus drink so that it cannot be injected (oral liquid form is legally required in maintenance programs). Be aware that special

state and federal approval is necessary before methadone can be given to children. Keep naloxone readily available in case of overdose.

Contraindications/Precautions

PREG B

Contraindicated in hypersensitivity to methadone hydrochloride and for obstetric analgesia (potential newborn respiratory depression). *Use with caution* in severe renal, cardiac, or hepatic impairment; Addison's disease; acute abdominal conditions; hypothyroidism; prostatic hypertrophy; urethral stricture; increased intracranial pressure; head injury; CNS or respiratory depression; asthma; and COPD.

🖐 Use with caution for the elderly or debilitated. Safe use for children and pregnant or nursing mothers has not been established.

Side effects/Adverse reactions

Hypersensitivity: (rare) rash, hives, itching, swelling of face. *CNS:* drowsiness, sedation, extreme somnolence, coma, physical dependence, convulsions with large doses. *CV:* transient hypotension, circulatory collapse. *GI:* nausea, vomiting, constipation. *GU:* urinary retention, impotence. *Resp:* respiratory depression. *Skin:* local tissue irritation, induration after repeated subcutaneous administration. *MS:* skeletal-muscle flaccidity.

Nursing implications/Documentation

Possible nursing diagnoses: Constipation; Pain; Sensory/perceptual alterations.

♦ For maintenance use, obtain physician order for stool softener or laxative because of potentially severe constipation.

♦ Record and monitor patient's circulatory, respiratory, and bowel-function status.

♦ Observe for marked sedation resulting from cumulative effect of frequent doses.

♦ Be aware that adequate maintenance is achieved with one daily dose. There is no advantage to divided doses, except in cases of severe, chronic pain.

♦ Use IM route when repeated parenteral doses are required.

♦ Recognize that a regimented scheduling (around the clock) is beneficial in severe, chronic pain; tolerance may develop with long-term use, requiring a higher dose to achieve the same degree of analgesia.

♦ Monitor for abstinence symptoms that may not appear for 36–72 hr after last dose and

M

may persist 10–14 days. Usually symptoms are mild (insomnia, anxiety, anorexia, abdominal pain, weakness, sweating, headache, hot and cold flashes).

• For detoxification treatment to suppress abstinence symptoms, be aware that drug is given orally in decreasing doses over a maximum of 21 days; if treatment exceeds 21 days, the patient is considered to be on maintenance.

• When used for drug addiction, give additional analgesic if pain control is necessary.

• For methadone-addicted mothers, refer to social worker for follow-up care of children (evaluation of methadone exposure).

Patient & family teaching/Home care

Possible nursing diagnoses: Ineffective individual coping; Fear.

• Advise those who are ambulatory to change positions slowly to alleviate adverse reactions such as dizziness or feeling faint.

• Warn against performing activities that require alertness.

• Encourage using psychiatric, social, and vocational rehabilitation services available through methadone maintenance program.

• Caution about the potential dangers of use with alcohol.

• Warn that severe constipation is common with maintenance regime; stress the need to increase fluid and fiber intake, to exercise daily, and to use laxatives before problem is severe.

• Point out that most side effects are gone after several weeks.

• Instruct family to report signs of overdose (principally respiratory depression) immediately.

• Explain prescribed treatment regimen to facilitate maximum compliance with therapy; reinforce that methadone maintenance programs provide coordinated psychiatric, social, and vocational rehabilitation that are vital to recovery from drug addiction.

• *See Narcotic and non-narcotic analgesics overview for more information.*

methamphetamine *meth-am-fet'a-meen*

methamphetamine hydrochloride: *Desoxyn, Desoxyn Gradumet*

Class: Cerebral stimulant, sympathomimetic, amphetamine, anorectic agent

PEDS	PREG	GERI	CONTROLLED SUBSTANCE
🤚	C	🤚	II

Action *In adults,* has a stimulant effect, *in hyperactive children,* a "paradoxical" calming effect. Probably stimulates the CNS by its action on the cerebral cortex and reticular activating system, where it promotes nerve impulse transmission by releasing stored norepinephrine from nerve terminals.

Use/Therapeutic goal/Outcome

Short-term appetite suppression: Reduction in desire for food. **Outcome criteria:** Report of lack of appetite.

Attention Deficit Disorders with Hyperactivity (ADDH): Promotion of ability to concentrate and pay attention. **Outcome criteria:** Demonstration of increased attention span; increased ability to sit quietly.

Dose range/Administration

Interaction alert: Use within 14 days of MAO inhibitors may cause severe hypertensive crisis. May alter insulin requirements. Antacids, sodium bicarbonate, and acetazolamide may potentiate effect; ammonium chloride, ascorbic acid, phenothiazines, and haloperidol may reduce effect.

Short-term appetite suppression: Adult: PO: 2.5–5 mg, 30 min before meals (up to tid); or one sustained-release 5–15 mg tablet daily before breakfast.

Attention Deficit Disorder with Hyperactivity (ADDH): Child 6 yrs and older: PO: 2.5–5 mg daily or bid, with weekly increments of 5 mg prn. Usual therapeutic dose is 20–25 mg/day.

Clinical alert: Give doses at least 6 hr before bedtime to prevent insomnia. For treatment of ADDH in children, monitor for need to *decrease* dose; that is, watch for lessening effectiveness (this drug is usually stopped after puberty). For people with epilepsy, be aware that amphetamines may decrease seizure threshhold.

M

Contraindications/Precautions

PREG C

Contraindicated in hypersensitivity or intolerance to methamphetamine, glaucoma, symptomatic cardiac disease, angina, moderate to severe hypertension, hyperthyroidism, arteriosclerosis, agitation, history of drug abuse, or use within 14 days of MAO inhibitors. Desoxyn 15 mg is contraindicated in allergy to tartrazine. *Use with caution* for diabetics.

🖐 **Contraindicated for children under 6 years. Use with caution for the elderly and for children with Tourette's disease. Safe use for pregnant or nursing mothers has not been established.**

Side effects/Adverse reactions

Hypersensitivity: itching, rashes. *CNS:* insomnia, restlessness, tremors, hyperactivity, talkativeness, irritability, headache, dizziness. *CV:* tachycardia, hypertension, hypotension. *GI:* anorexia, metallic taste, nausea, vomiting, dry mouth, cramps, diarrhea, constipation. *GU:* impotence, changes in libido. *Misc:* growth suppression in children.

Nursing implications/Documentation

Possible nursing diagnoses: Altered thought processes; Sleep pattern disturbance; Constipation; Altered nutrition: less than body requirements.

◆ Question about the use of beverages and OTC drugs that contain caffeine.

◆ Monitor attention span and ability to concentrate, and report and document changes in status (dosage may need to be adjusted).

◆ Provide decaffeinated beverages.

◆ Document blood pressure at least daily when beginning therapy, and periodically once stabilized.

◆ Document daily weights and keep a record of food intake to ensure adequate nutrition.

◆ Prevent side effect of constipation by monitoring bowel movements, ensuring adequate hydration, and providing fruits, juices, and vegetables (use laxatives only when necessary).

Patient & family teaching/Home care

Possible nursing diagnoses: Knowledge deficit; Impaired home maintenance management.

◆ Explain that this drug has a high potential for abuse, and should only be taken as prescribed, and under continuous medical supervision.

◆ If used as an appetite suppressant, reinforce the importance of enrolling in a behavior modification weight reduction program.

◆ Stress the importance of checking labels for caffeine content and recognizing that caffeine may increase drug effects.

◆ Emphasize that side effect of constipation can be avoided by drinking plenty of fluids, eating fruits and fiber, ensuring adequate exercise, and using mild laxatives when necessary.

◆ For use with children

Teach the need to monitor physical and mental growth, and to report growth failure and behavior extremes (dosage may have to be adjusted); explain that dosage will probably be reduced as child progresses to puberty, and that periodic "drug holidays" may be planned to determine if the drug is still necessary.

◆ *See Cerebral Stimulants overview for more information.*

methazolamide

meth-a-zoe'la-mide

Neptazane

Class: Carbonic anhydrase inhibitor

PEDS	PREG	GERI
🖐	C	🖐

Action Lowers intraocular pressure by inhibiting carbonic anhydrase, thus reducing the rate of aqueous humor formation.

Use/Therapeutic goal/Outcome

Adjunctive treatment of chronic simple (open-angle) and secondary glaucoma, and preoperatively for acute angle-closure glaucoma: Reduction of rate of intraocular pressure. *Outcome criteria:* Decreased intraocular pressure when measured with tonometer.

Dose range/Administration

🖐 **Give with food to minimize GI upset.**
Adult: PO: 50-100 mg bid or tid.

Contraindications/Precautions

PREG C

Contraindicated in hypersensitivity to sulfonamides and derivatives (thiazide diuretics), and in hyponatremia, hypokalemia or other electrolyte imbalances, renal or hepatic dysfunction, adrenal insufficiency, obstructive pulmonary disease, hyperchloremic acidosis, and chronic noncongestive angle-closure glaucoma.

🖐 **Contraindicated for pregnant women. Use with caution for the elderly. Safe use for** children and nursing mothers has not been established.

Side effects/Adverse reactions

Hypersensitivity: rash, fever, hives, itching.
CNS: drowsiness, paresthesias, convulsions, weakness, nervousness, dizziness, confusion, ataxia, headache. *GI:* nausea, vomiting, diarrhea, anorexia, weight loss. *Hem:* aplastic anemia, hemolytic anemia, leukopenia, hypokalemia, hyperuricemia. *Eye:* myopia. *GU:* renal calculi. *Misc:* hyperchloremic acidosis, photosensitivity.

Nursing implications/Documentation

Possible nursing diagnoses: Fluid volume deficit; Altered patterns of urinary elimination; Potential for injury.

♦ Ascertain that baseline CBC, sodium, potassium, chloride, carbon dioxide, calcium, magnesium, BUN, creatinine, uric acid, and liver function studies have been obtained before giving first dose; report abnormalities and monitor closely thereafter.

♦ Question about eye symptoms.

♦ Supervise ambulation until response is determined.

Patient & family teaching/Home care

Possible nursing diagnoses: Knowledge deficit; Impaired home maintenance management.

♦ Before giving first dose, explain that the drug will increase the amount and frequency of urination.

♦ Advise taking this drug with food to reduce GI symptoms.

♦ Emphasize that vision damage can occur unnoticed; stress that ongoing follow-up for measurement of intraocular pressure is essential.

♦ Stress that eye pain, muscle cramping, and edema should be reported, and that hypokalemia is a common side effect.

methenamine
meth-en′a-meen

methenamine hippurate: *Hiprex,* ♣*Hip-Rex, Urex*
methenamine mandelate: *Mandameth, Mandelamine,* ♣*Sterine*
Class: Urinary tract anti-infective

PEDS	PREG	GERI
♥	C	♥

Action In acidic urine, kills bacteria (bactericidal) by decomposing to generate formaldehyde, a nonspecific bactericidal chemical.

Use/Therapeutic goal/Outcome

Chronic urinary tract infection: Elimination or prevention of infection. *Outcome criteria:* Absence of growth on urine culture; report of absence of dysuria, frequency.

Dose range/Administration

Interaction alert: Do not mix with sulfonamides or alkalinizing agents, such as antacids (urine must be acidic for action). Acetazolamide diminishes effects of methenamine.

♥ **Give after meals and at bedtime to minimize GI distress (enteric-coated tablets are available to reduce continued distress).**
Adult/Child > 12 yrs: PO: *Hippurate:* 1 g bid. *Mandelate:* 1 g qid. *Child 6–12 yrs:* PO: *Hippurate:* 500 mg bid. *Mandelate:* 500 mg qid, or 50 mg/kg/day in 3 divided doses. *Child < 6 yrs:* PO: *Mandelate:* 50 mg/kg/day in 4 divided doses.

Clinical alert: Stress importance of fluid intake of 2 L a day (not more, or urine will be diluted and effect of formaldehyde will be reduced), and of promoting urine acidity by drinking acidic juices (cranberry, plum, prune) and by limiting intake of alkaline food (vegetables, citrus products, milk, peanuts). Monitor the elderly for septic shock.

Contraindications/Precautions
PREG
C

Contraindicated in allergy or intolerance to methenamine, and in renal insufficiency, liver disease, gout, severe dehydration. *Use oral suspension with caution* in susceptibility to lipid pneumonia.

♥ **Use oral suspension with caution for the elderly or debilitated. Safe use of all forms for pregnant or nursing mothers, and of hippurate for children under 6 years has not been established.**

Side effects/Adverse reactions

Hypersensitivity: itching, rashes, stomatitis.
GI: anorexia, nausea, vomiting, diarrhea, cramping, elevated liver enzymes. *GU:* (with high doses) dysuria, frequency, hematuria, albuminuria, crystalluria.

Nursing implications/Documentation

Possible nursing diagnoses: Altered patterns of urinary elimination; Fluid volume deficit.

M

♦ Obtain urine for culture and sensitivity, and ensure that necessary lab studies (e.g., CBC, BUN, creatinine, liver function) are done before administering first dose; monitor closely thereafter if therapy is prolonged.

♦ Provide acidic juices (*not* citrus), and document and monitor intake and output, to maintain adequate hydration (see clinical alert).

♦ Monitor urine pH (may use nitrazine paper) to maintain urine pH at 5.5 or less (patient may have to take up to 12 g of ascorbic acid daily to achieve desired acidity).

Patient & family teaching/Home care

Possible nursing diagnoses: Knowledge deficit; Impaired home maintenance management.

♦ Explain that taking this drug after meals and at bedtime may help reduce GI symptoms.

♦ Provide a list of fluids and foods that should be encouraged or avoided (see clinical alert).

♦ Advise reporting symptoms that do not abate after 3–5 days, new symptoms of illness (fever, sore throat), or symptoms of allergy (itching, rashes).

♦ Stress the importance of taking this drug without missing doses for the entire time prescribed, even if symptoms disappear (if a dose is missed, take it as soon as possible).

♦ *See Anti-infectives overview for more information.*

methicillin

meth-i-sill'in

methicillin sodium: **♦Metin, Staphcillin**

Class: ★Anti-infective (penicillinase–resistant penicillin) prototype, Antibiotic

PEDS	PREG	GERI
♛	B	♛

Action Broad-spectrum, usually bactericidal antibiotic; kills bacteria by inhibiting cell wall synthesis. Resistant to bacterial penicillinases (enzymes that degrade some penicillins).

Use/Therapeutic goal/Outcome

Systemic infections (caused by penicillinase-producing staphylococci): Resolution of infection. **Outcome criteria:** Absence of pathogenic growth on cultures, absence of clinical manifestations of infection (fever, pain, redness, heat, swelling, odor, dysuria, drainage), normal WBC count, improvement of X rays.

Dose range/Administration

Interaction alert: Probenecid inhibits excretion of methicillin and may be given to increase serum levels of the drug. Do not mix this drug IV with any other drug. Give at least 1 hour before bacteriostatic antibiotics for optimal effect.

Adult: IM, IV: 1–3 g q6h (IV use, mix in 50 cc of NS and infuse at 10 cc/h). **Child:** IM: 100 mg/kg/day, in divided doses q6h. IV: 200–300 mg/kg/day, in divided doses q6h.

Clinical alert: For those on sodium-restrictions, recognize that since this drug contains sodium, sodium intake may have to be further reduced.

Contraindications/Precautions

PREG B

Contraindicated in allergy to penicillin. **Use with caution** in cephalosporin sensitivity, history of allergic responses (e.g., other drugs, hay fever, asthma), and renal insufficiency.

♛ **Use with caution for children, the elderly, and pregnant or nursing mothers.**

Side effects/Adverse reactions

Hypersensitivity: itching, rashes, urticaria, fever, difficulty breathing, anaphylaxis. **GI:** nausea, vomiting, anorexia, glossitis, stomatitis, diarrhea, pseudomembranous colitis. **CV:** pain, redness, swelling, thrombophlebitis at injection site. **GU:** acute interstitial nephritis. **Hem:** slight elevation in SGOT and SGPT. **Misc:** bone marrow depression, superinfection.

Nursing implications/Documentation

Possible nursing diagnoses: Potential for infection; Diarrhea.

♦ Determine history of allergies, and (regardless of history) monitor closely for allergic reactions.

♦ Obtain baseline CBC, creatinine, eosinophil count, and necessary cultures before administering first dose; monitor closely thereafter if therapy is prolonged.

♦ Encourage fluids, and record and monitor intake and output, to ensure adequate hydration; report significant negative or positive balance.

♦ Monitor for and report signs of superinfection (sore throat, fever, fatigue, thrush, vaginal discharge, diarrhea).

Patient & family teaching/Home care

Possible nursing diagnoses: Knowledge deficit; Impaired home maintenance management.

- Teach the importance of reporting allergic symptoms, diarrhea, signs and symptoms that do not abate, or *any* new signs and symptoms of discomfort that might indicate superinfection (medication regimen may have to be changed).

- Advise drinking 2–3 L of fluids daily to maintain adequate hydration (especially important if fever exists).

- Stress the importance of taking antibiotics for the entire time prescribed, even if signs and symptoms abate.

- *See Anti-infectives overview for more information.*

methimazole

meth-im'a-zole

Tapazole

Class: Thyroid hormone antagonist

PEDS	PREG	GERI
☜	D	☜

Action Interferes with synthesis of thyroid hormones (T_3 and T_4) by blocking oxidation of idodine, thus inhibiting its ability to combine with tyrosine to form thyroxin. May also inhibit the coupling of diiodotyrosine and monoiodotyrosine, preventing formation of thyroxine and triiodothyronine.

Use/Therapeutic goal/Outcome

Hyperthyroidism and thyrotoxic crisis (especially in Graves' disease): Suppression of secretion of thyroid hormones, promotion of normal metabolism. *Outcome criteria:* After 3 weeks, decreased T_4 levels; weight gain; normal pulse rate; decreased sweating and diarrhea.

Preparation for thyroidectomy: Reduction of vascularity of the thyroid gland (reduced risk of bleeding) and promotion of normal metabolism. *Outcome criteria:* Decrease in thyroid size.

Dose range/Administration

Interaction alert: May increase effects of anticoagulants (monitor for hypoprothrombinemia manifested by increased bruising, bleeding).

☞ **Give with meals to reduce GI distress.**

Hyperthyroidism: Adult: PO: 5–20 mg tid, depending upon severity of hyperthyroidism; continue until euthyroid, then maintenance dose 5–30 mg daily to tid. *Maximum dose:* 150 mg/day. *Child:* PO: 0.4 mg/kg/day in divided doses q8h; continue until euthyroid, then maintenance dose 0.2 mg/kg/day in divided doses q8h.

Preparation for thyroidectomy: Adult and Child: PO: Give hyperthyroidism dose with iodine for 10 days.

Thyrotoxic crisis: Adult and Child: PO: Give hyperthyroidism dose with iodine and propranolol.

Clinical alert: Give drug at the same time every day to maintain therapeutic levels. Hold dose and report if the following appear: rashes, enlarged cervical lymph nodes, peripheral nonpitting edema, petechiae, ecchymosis, persistent fatigue, or signs of bone marrow depression (fever, chills, sore throat). Doses greater than 30 mg/day are more frequently associated with adverse effects such as agranulocytosis.

Contraindications/Precautions

**PREG
D**

Contraindicated in hypersensitivity to methimazole. *Use with caution* in infection, bone marrow depression, and liver disease.

☙ **Contraindicated for nursing mothers and in the first trimester of pregnancy. Use with caution later in pregnancy and for children and the elderly.**

Side effects/Adverse reactions

Hypersensitivity: itching, rashes, drug fever. Other side effects are usually dose related and usually subside after the first 3 weeks of therapy. *GI:* nausea, vomiting, decreased appetite, loss of taste, diarrhea, salivary gland enlargement, hepatitis. *CNS:* headache, drowsiness, dizziness. *Hem:* agranulocytosis, leukopenia, thrombocytopenia. *GU:* irregular menses, nephritis. *MS:* joint pain, muscle pain, paresthesia. *Skin:* jaundice, hyperpigmentation, hair loss. *Misc:* lymphadenopathy, lupus-like syndrome.

Nursing implications/Documentation

Possible nursing diagnoses: Altered nutrition: less than body requirements; Altered nutrition: more than body requirements.

- Observe for and report signs of hypothyroidism (fatigue, weight gain, drowsiness), overdose (hepatitis, jaundice, peripheral edema, heat intolerance, sweating, palpitations, tachycardia, CNS irritability), or blood dyscrasias (sore throat, fever, chills, mouth sores).

- Document vital signs at least daily during initial treatment.

- Monitor T_4 levels every month, then every 2–3 months once stable, for therapeutic range;

report abnormalities (level below or above normal range indicates need for dose adjustment).

♦ For prolonged treatment, monitor CBC and liver function studies.

♦ Record and monitor input and output and provide 3–4 L of fluids a day, unless contraindicated; also record and monitor daily weights (report significant discrepancies).

Patient & family teaching/Home care

Possible nursing diagnoses: Knowledge deficit; Impaired home maintenance management.

♦ Emphasize the importance of taking this drug at the same time with meals every day, exactly as prescribed. If a dose is missed, advise taking it as soon as possible or with next dose; if more than a single dose is missed, advise checking with physician.

♦ Teach to report signs and symptoms of overdosage and hypersensitivity (see Clinical alert).

♦ Advise checking with physician whether iodized salt and foods (seafood, some breads) should be avoided.

♦ Stress the importance of returning for medical follow-up (blood work).

♦ *See Thyroid Hormone Antagonists overview for more information.*

methocarbamol
meth-oh-kar'ba-mole

Delaxin, Marbaxin-750, Robomol, Robaxin

Class: Skeletal-muscle relaxant (centrally acting), Antispasmodic

PEDS	PREG	GERI
✋	C	✋

Action Relaxes skeletal muscle by inhibitng central synaptic reflexes in the descending reticular formation and spinal cord.

Use/Therapeutic goal/Outcome

Spasticity associated with acute, painful musculoskeletal conditions: Reduction of muscle spasm without loss of voluntary motor function; relief of pain. **Outcome criteria:** Increased range of motion and ability to perform activities of daily life; report of relief of pain, anxiety, and tension.

Adjunct therapy in tetanus management: Control of neuromuscular manifestations (especially convulsions) and head and neck rigidity. **Outcome criteria:** Decreased spasticity and tightness in jaw with increased ability to swallow.

Dose range/Administration

Interaction alert: The CNS effects may be additive to those of other CNS depressants and alcohol. Use cautiously with pyridostigmine bromide.

🍴 **Give PO dose with food to prevent gastric distress.**

Spasticity: Adult: PO: 1.5 g qid for 2–3 days, then 1 g qid. IM: 0.5–1 g q8h prn. IV: 1–3 g/day, for not more than 3 days. *IV infusion:* maximum 1 g methocarbamol in 250 ml NS or D5W.

Tetanus: Adult: IV: 1–2 g, may repeat q6h until nasogastric tube can be inserted for administration. **Child:** IV: 15 mg/kg, may repeat q6h prn.

Clinical alert: Do not give SC; for IM, use Z-tract technique in gluteal region only. For IV route, observe closely for extravasation and keep the patient lying down for at least 15 minutes to reduce episodes of postural hypotension; dangle before allowing to stand.

Contraindications/Precautions
PREG
C

Contraindicated in hypersensitivity to methocarbamol, and in renal impairment (IV route) and comatose states. **Use with caution** in epilepsy, CNS depression, acidosis, and in combination with anticholinesterase preparations.

✋ **Use with caution for children under 12 years and the elderly. Safe use for older children and pregnant women has not been determined.**

Side effects/Adverse reactions

Hypersensitivity: urticaria, pruritus, rash, conjunctivitis, nasal congestion, headache, blurred vision, fever, anaphylaxis. **CNS:** lightheadedness, dizziness, syncope, drowsiness, flushing, fever. **GI:** nausea, metallic taste, anorexia, GI distress. **CV:** phlebitis, hypotension, bradycardia. **GU:** urine discoloration. **With IV use:** fainting, seizures, bradycardia, weakness, nystagmus, thrombophlebitis at site of infusion.

Nursing implications/Documentation

Possible nursing diagnoses: Potential for injury; Pain.

♦ Supervise out-of-bed activities.

♦ If on prolonged therapy, monitor for and report abnormal laboratory studies, especially WBC and renal function.

Patient & family teaching/Home care

Possible nursing diagnoses: Knowledge deficit; Impaired home maintenance management.

◆ Advise taking this drug with food to reduce GI symptoms.

◆ Warn that urine may turn brown, black, or green while on this drug.

◆ Stress the importance of changing position slowly to avoid hypotensive episodes (sit up, flex arms and legs to promote vasoconstriction).

◆ Caution to lie down (on floor if necessary) if there is a feeling of faintness. Teach to monitor pulse and report if bradycardia or tachycardia are noted.

◆ Explain the need to contact physician if **hypersensitivity** (rash, headache, fever) reaction develops and avoid OTC drugs without physician approval.

◆ Stress the importance of continuing total treatment plan, including rest, physical therapy, and other measures (e.g., relaxation techniques).

◆ Caution against driving until response is determined; stress that alcohol and other CNS depressants should be avoided.

◆ *See Skeletal-muscle relaxants overview for more information.*

methotrexate

meth-oh-trex'ate

methotrexate sodium: *Folex, Mexate, Rheumatrex*

Class: ★Antineoplastic (antimetabolite) agent prototype

PEDS	PREG	GERI
✋	**D**	✋

Action Kills rapidly growing cells (cancer, hair follicles, bone marrow, GI lining, ova, and sperm) by inhibiting the enzyme that breaks down folic acid, thus impairing DNA synthesis and cell replication (purine and thymidine antagonist). Inhibits lymphocyte multiplication (has immunosuppressive activity).

Use/Therapeutic goal/Outcome

Trophoblastic neoplasms (choriocarcinoma, chorioadenoma destruens, hydatidiform mole); acute lymphocytic and lymphoblastic leukemia; advanced lymphosarcoma; epidermoid carcinoma of the head and neck; cancer of the breast, testes, lung, and colon; mycosis fungoides: Elimination or suppression of malignant cell prolif-

eration. *Outcome criteria:* Tumor and disease regression or stabilization on radiologic and physical examination; for leukemias, absence of blasts in peripheral blood specimen.

Psoriasis: Promotion of normal skin integrity. *Outcome criteria:* Absence of or decrease in skin lesions.

Rheumatoid arthritis: Reduction in inflammation. *Outcome criteria:* Decrease in pain and swelling.

Dose range/Administration

Interaction alert: Aspirin, sulfa drugs, alcohol, phenylbutazone, PABA, ibuprofen, chloramphenicol, phenytoin, probenecid, sulfonamides, tetracyclines, other antineoplastic agents, and radiation therapy increase toxicity. Hepatotoxicity is increased with alcohol use (may lead to a coma). May alter anticoagulant requirements. Folic acid and related vitamins may alter response to methotrexate (do not give together).

🥄 **Give oral doses 1–2 hours before meals.**

Trophoblastic neoplasms: **Adult:** PO, IM: 15–30 mg/day for 5 days; repeat after 1 week. Regimen may be repeated 5 times.

Leukemia: **Adult and Child:** PO, IM, IV: *Acute phase:* 3.3 mg/m^2/day for 4–6 weeks. (With predisone, 60 mg/m^2/day.) PO, IM: *Maintenance dose:* 20–30 mg/m^2 twice weekly. IV: 2.5 mg/kg q 2 wk.

Meningeal Leukemia: **Adult and Child:** *Intrathecal:* 12 mg/m^2, every 2–5 days until CSF is normal. Use powder vials without preservatives; dilute with 0.9% NaCl.

Lymphosarcomas: **Adult:** PO, IM, IV: 0.625 to 2.5 mg/kg/day.

Mycosis fungoides: **Adult:** PO: 2.5 to 10 mg/day. IM: 50 mg/wk or 25 mg twice weekly.

Psoriasis: **Adult:** PO, IM, IV: 10–25 mg/wk as a single dose (5–10 mg test dose recommended 1 wk before therapy).

Rheumatoid Arthritis: **Adult:** PO, IM, IV: 7.5 to 15 mg/wk; or 2.5 to 5.0 mg in 3 doses, 12 hr apart, each week. May increase to 20 mg/wk.

Clinical alert: The route of choice for methotrexate is PO (to reduce risk of infection). PO doses should be given in the evening with an antacid to reduce GI symptoms. IV doses should be given only by nurses who are knowledgeable in the comprehensive management of the administration of antineoplastic agents. Doses may vary at physician's discretion and are held until the patient has sufficiently recovered from toxicities of previous doses. Leucovorin rescue (a protocol for administration of leucovorin that reduces *systemic* toxicity, but does not interfere with tumor cell absorption of methotrexate) is necessary for doses greater than 100 mg. Protocols for drug preparation, administration, and accidental skin contamination must be followed. Gloves or double gloves must be worn when handling methotrexate. Contaminated areas should be washed with large amounts of soap and water.

Contraindications/Precautions

PREG
D

Contraindicated in hypersensitivity to methotrexate, and in blood dyscrasias (anemia, leukopenia), severe renal or hepatic disorders, poor nutritional status, decreased bone marrow reserve, and malignant effusions in pleural space or abdomen. **Use with caution** in infection, peptic ulcer disease, ulcerative colitis, or chronic debilitating disease.

✋ **Contraindicated for pregnant or nursing mothers. Use with caution for children and the elderly.**

Side effects/Adverse reactions

Hypersensitivity: urticaria, chills, fever, pruritus, tachycardia, hypotension. **Hem:** leukopenia, thrombocytopenia anemia, hyperuricemia. **GI:** gingivitis, pharyngitis, stomatitis, ulcerations and bleeding of portions of the GI tract, anorexia, nausea, vomiting, diarrhea and melana, hepatotoxicity, hepatic fibrosis. **GU:** tubular necrosis. **CNS:** drowsiness, tremors, ataxia, convulsions, and brain atrophy; headache, nuchal rigidity, somnolence, paresis, and paraplegia with intrathecal use. **Resp:** chronic interstitial obstructive pulmonary disease. **Skin:** photosensitivity, acne, dry skin, alopecia; pain and erythema at injection site.

Nursing implications/Documentation

Possible nursing diagnoses: Potential for infection; Potential for injury; Fatigue; Altered oral mucous membrane; Fluid volume deficit; Diarrhea; Altered nutrition: less than body requirements.

◆ *See important Nursing implications in Antineoplastic agents overview on page 72, which apply to all antineoplastics. The interventions that follow are additional and specific to this drug only.*

◆ Monitor for and report oral ulcerations (may be the first sign of toxicity) and persistent

cough, dyspnea, or chest pain (may be a sign of pulmonary toxicity).

◆ Observe for CNS toxicity (numbness or tingling of the extremities, footdrop, wristdrop, muscle weakness, balance problems, changes in mental status).

◆ Check stools for occult blood (hemorrhage may occur rapidly); report diarrhea, as it may indicate need to hold dose.

◆ Increase fluid intake to 2–3 L a day to prevent renal tubular damage from hyperuricemia secondary to cell lysis.

◆ Expect that sodium bicarbonate tablets will be given to alkalinize the urine and prevent drug crystallization; monitor urine pH and report pH less than 6.5 (may require dose change).

◆ Report changes in vision.

◆ Be aware that WBC and platelet counts will nadir (drop to the lowest point) in 1–2 weeks.

Patient & family teaching/Home care

Possible nursing diagnoses: Knowledge deficit; Ineffective coping (individual and family); Hopelessness; Impaired home maintenance management.

◆ *See important Patient & family teaching in Antineoplastic agents overview on page 72, which apply to all antineoplastics. The teachings that follow are additional and specific to this drug only.*

◆ Emphasize the need to take doses exactly on time.

◆ Point out that drinking 2–3 L a day helps prevent kidney complications.

◆ Stress the need to report oral ulcers, diarrhea, persistent cough, dyspnea, chest pain, numbness or tingling of extremities, balance problems, and changes in mental status or vision.

◆ Explain that alcohol should be avoided because of increased hepatotoxicity.

◆ Teach that OTC drugs should be avoided unless approved by physician.

◆ *See Antineoplastic agents overview for more information.*

methotrimeprazine *meth-oh-trye-mep'ra-zeen*

methotrimeprazine hydrochloride: *Levoprome,*
❦*Nozinan*

Class: Sedative-hypnotic, Non-narcotic analgesic,
Phenothiazine

PEDS	PREG	GERI
🖐	C	🖐

Action Produces sedation by acting on the limbic
system, thalamus, and hypothalamus of the
CNS. Other actions include antiemetic, antipruritic, local anesthetic, weak anticholinergic
properties, amnesia, and elevated pain threshold.

Use/Therapeutic goal/Outcome

*Pre-procedure sedation; moderate to severe pain
in the nonambulatory:* Relief of pain, promotion
of relaxation. *Outcome criteria:* Report of
increased comfort and feeling more relaxed;
absence of signs of discomfort (frowning, restlessness, crying).

Psychosis: Promotion of relaxation and reality
orientation. *Outcome criteria:* Report of feeling more calm; demonstration of reality orientation and ability to interact with others.

Dose range/Administration

Interaction alert: Do not give with MAO inhibitors or antihypertensives. CNS depressants,
alcohol, and narcotics increase sedation. Do not
mix in the same syringe as any other drug
(except for atropine or scopolomine).

🍂 **Give PO doses with meals.**

Sedation, analgesia: Adult/Child > 12 yrs: IM:
10–20 mg q4-6h prn. *For the elderly:* 5–10 mg
q4-6h prn.

Preoperative medication: Adult/Child > 12 yrs:
IM: 2–20 mg 45 min to 3 hr before procedure.

Postoperative analgesia: Adult/Child > 12 yrs:
IM: 2.5–7.5 mg q4-6h; adjust dose prn.

Psychosis: Adult: PO: 6–25 mg daily in three
divided doses. May increase to 50–75 mg daily
in divided doses.

Clinical alert: Check respirations and blood pressure before giving IM dose. Hold drug and
report if respirations are less than 12 or if
hypotension is noted. Give deep IM into large
muscle mass; rotate injection sites. IV injection
is not recommended. After IM injection, keep
patient in bed until response is determined
(hypotension is common).

Contraindications/Precautions

Contraindicated in hypersensitivity to phenothiazines or bisulfite and in severe cardiac,
renal or hepatic disease, history of convulsive
disorders, previous overdose of CNS depressant,
and coma. *Use with caution* in cardiac disease,
those who may incur serious consequences
from a sudden decrease in blood pressure, and
women of childbearing age.

🖐 **Contraindicated for children under 12
years and for pregnant or nursing mothers. Use with caution for the elderly or
debilitated.**

Side effects/Adverse reactions

Hypersensitivity: excessive sedation, severe
hypotensive effects. *CV:* orthostatic hypotension, palpitations. *CNS:* drowsiness, amnesia,
extrapyramidal symptoms, disorientation,
euphoria, headache, slurred speech. *GI:* dry
mouth, nausea, vomiting. *GU:* difficulty urinating. *Skin:* injection-site swelling, pain,
inflammation. *Resp:* nasal congestion. *Misc:*
(long-term) agranulocytosis and other blood
dyscrasias, weight gain.

Nursing implications/Documentation

Possible nursing diagnoses: Pain; Anxiety;
Potential for injury.

◆ For use as an analgesic

◆ Have patient rate pain on a scale of 1–10
before and after medication is given; report
and record inadequate pain control.

◆ Give analgesics before pain is severe for best
effects.

◆ If faintness is experienced, have patient lie
flat and check blood pressure immediately
(phenylephrine, methoxamine, or levarterenol
may be given to treat hypotension).

◆ Monitor closely for risk factors for injury;
keep patient in bed with side rails up.

◆ Recognize that this drug is effective as an
analgesic when there is concern about respiratory depression.

◆ For use in psychosis

◆ Monitor for orthostatic hypotension; record
blood pressure bid until response is established.

Patient & family teaching/Home care

Possible nursing diagnoses: Sensory/perceptual
alterations; Impaired home maintenance management.

M

▶

- **For use as an analgesic**
  - Explain the rationale for taking analgesics before pain is too severe.
  - Stress that the patient should remain in bed while taking this drug.
- **For use in psychosis**
  - Explain that this drug helps reduce anxiety.
  - Caution to change position slowly to prevent dizziness.
  - Warn that alcohol and other CNS depressants may cause excessive sedation.
- *See Antianxiety agents, sedatives and hypnotics and Narcotic and non-narcotic analgesics overviews for more information.*

methsuximide

meth-sux'i-mide

Celontin

Class: Anticonvulsant, Succinimide

PEDS	PREG	GERI
🖐	C	🖐

Action Limits seizure activity, probably by depressing the motor cortex and elevating the firing threshold of cortical neurons (exact mechanism is unknown).

Use/Therapeutic goal/Outcome

Absence (petit mal) seizures that are resistant to other drugs: Limitation of seizure activity. *Outcome criteria:* Marked decrease or absence of seizures.

Dose range/Administration

Adult and Child: PO: 300 mg daily for the first week. May increase weekly prn by 300 mg increments, to a maximum of 1.2 g/day in divided doses.

Clinical alert: Be aware that this drug is associated with a high incidence of adverse effects.

Contraindications/Precautions

Contraindicated in hypersensitivity to succinimides. **Use with caution** in liver or kidney disease.

🖐 **Use with caution for children and the elderly. Safe use in pregnancy and lactation has not been established.**

Side effects/Adverse reactions

Hypersensitivity: itching, rashes, fever, hiccups, periorbital edema. **Hem:** eosinophilia, leukopenia, monocytosis, systemic lupus erythemato-

sus. **CNS:** drowsiness, dizziness, ataxia, irritability, headache, depression, behavioral changes, insomnia. **GI:** nausea and vomiting. **Eye:** visual disturbances.

Nursing implications/Documentation

Possible nursing diagnoses: Potential for injury; Potential for aspiration.

- Document history of seizures (type, frequency, duration, usual time they occur, precipitating factors, presence of an aura); initiate seizure precautions as indicated.
- Monitor CBC every 3 months, and check urinalysis and liver function studies every 6 months.

Patient & family teaching/Home care

Possible nursing diagnoses: Fear; Self-esteem disturbance; Knowledge deficit; Impaired home maintenance management

- Stress the need for close medical follow-up; advise reporting new symptoms in case they are related to taking methsuximide.
- Warn that stopping anticonvulsants suddenly can cause an increase in severity and frequency of seizures.
- Explain that this drug may turn urine pink or brown.
- Caution against driving until response is determined (may cause drowsiness).
- *See Anticonvulsants overview for more information.*

methyclothiazide

meth-i-kloe-thye'a-zide

Aquatensen, ♣Duretic, Enduron, ♠Enduron M

Class: Thiazide diuretic, Antihypertensive

PEDS	PREG	GERI
🖐	D	🖐

Action Promotes sodium chloride, potassium, and water excretion by inhibiting sodium reabsorption in the early portion of the distal tubule. Lowers blood pressure by reducing plasma and extra-cellular volume.

Use/Therapeutic goal/Outcome

Hypertension: Promotion of diuresis, reduction of blood pressure. **Outcome criteria:** After 3–4 days, blood pressure within normal limits. **Edema:** Promotion of diuresis, resolution of edema. **Outcome criteria:** Increased urine output; weight loss; absence of rales and peripheral and sacral edema.

Dose range/Administration

Interaction alert: Cholestyramine and colestipol may inhibit intestinal absorption. Diazoxide may potentiate the antihypertensive, hyperuricemic, and hyperglycemic effect. Nonsteroidal anti-inflammatory drugs may decrease effects. Do not give concomitantly with lithium. Give cautiously with corticosteroids, antidiabetics, lanoxin, and skeletal muscle relaxants.

Adult: PO: 2.5–10 mg/day. *Child:* 0.05–0.2 mg/kg/day.

Clinical alert: Give in morning to prevent nocturnal diuresis. Antihypertensive effects may not occur for 3–4 days.

Contraindications/Precautions

PREG
D

Contraindicated in hypersensitivity to sulfonamides or thiazides, and in anuria. *Use with caution* in renal and hepatic disease, systemic lupus erythematosus, gout, asthma, multiple allergies, bronchitis, diabetes, pancreatitis, arteriosclerosis, and debilitated states.

✋ **Contraindicated for pregnant or nursing mothers. Use with caution for children and the elderly.**

Side effects/Adverse reactions

Hypersensitivity: rash, urticaria, dermatitis with photosensitivity. *Hem:* hypokalemia, hyperglycemia, impaired glucose tolerance, asymptomatic hyperuricemia, fluid and electrolyte imbalances, metabolic alkalosis, hypercalcemia, lipid abnormalities, aplastic anemia, agranulocytosis, leukopenia, thrombocytopenia. *CV:* volume depletion, orthostatic hypotension, dehydration. *GI:* anorexia, nausea, pancreatitis, hepatic encephalopathy. *Misc:* gout.

Nursing implications/Documentation

Possible nursing diagnoses: Fluid volume deficit; Altered patterns of urinary elimination; Potential for injury.

◆ Ascertain that baseline CBC, sodium, potassium, chloride, carbon dioxide, calcium, magnesium, BUN, creatinine, uric acid, and liver function studies have been obtained before giving first dose; report abnormalities and monitor closely thereafter.

◆ Document and monitor blood pressure, pulse, daily weight, and intake and output; report significant discrepancies.

◆ Observe for and report signs of fluid overload (auscultate lungs for rales; check feet, ankles, and sacrum for edema).

◆ Be aware that diuretics often induce hypokalemia, which predisposes individuals to cardiac arrhythmias, cramping, and digoxin toxicity.

◆ Check with physician to determine dietary restrictions; if a low-salt, high-potassium diet is recommended, consult with dietician to plan a low-salt diet that includes foods and juices high in potassium (orange juice; banana; green leafy vegetables).

◆ Observe the elderly for extreme diuresis (may require lower doses); monitor for orthostatic hypotension; supervise ambulation until response is determined.

Patient & family teaching/Home care

Possible nursing diagnoses: Knowledge deficit; Impaired home maintenance management.

◆ Before giving first dose, explain that the drug will increase the amount and frequency of urination.

◆ Emphasize the importance of taking this drug exactly as prescribed, and the importance of returning for medical follow-up.

◆ Explain that diuretics enhance the work of the kidney and reduce the workload of the heart.

◆ Recommend taking doses in early morning and early afternoon to prevent the need to disturb sleep to void.

◆ Explain that changing positions slowly helps prevent dizziness.

◆ Advise reporting dizziness, shortness of breath, swelling of hands and feet, or persistent sore throat; encourage daily monitoring of weight and reporting sudden weight gain.

◆ Provide a list of allowed foods and fluids; stress the need to stick to prescribed diet (explain the hazards of too much salt, or too little potassium).

◆ Warn against driving and activities that require alertness until response has been determined.

◆ Advise avoidance to OTC drugs unless approved by physician. Suggest using a (Number 15) sunscreen when outside because of photosensitivity (avoid products with PABA).

◆ *See Diuretics and Antihypertensives overviews for more information.*

M

methylcellulose

meth-ill-sell′yoo-lose

Citrucel, Cologel

Class: Bulk-forming laxative

PEDS	PREG	GERI
🖐	C	🖐

Action Promotes normal peristalsis and bowel motility by increasing bulk and moisture content of stool.

Use/Therapeutic goal/Outcome

Constipation: Promotion of regular evacuation of soft stool. **Outcome criteria:** Passage of soft, formed stool without straining (usually within 12–24 hr after initial dose, but may take up to 3 days).

Dose range/Administration

Interaction alert: Oral anticoagulants, digitalis glycosides, and salicylates should be separated from methylcellulose by a 2 hr interval to prevent decreased absorption of these medications due to physical binding.

Adult: PO: 5–20 ml or 1 packet/day to tid.
Child: PO: 5 ml or 1 tsp/day to tid.

Clinical alert: Mix in 8-oz glass of water or juice and give immediately, before congealing takes place.

Contraindications/Precautions

PREG
C

Contraindicated in hypersensitivity to any bulk-forming laxative, and in dysphagia, symptoms of appendicitis, undiagnosed rectal bleeding, and intestinal obstruction.

🖐 **Use with caution for children under 6 years and the elderly.**

Side effects/Adverse reactions

Hypersensitivity: rash, itching, difficulty breathing. **GI:** esophageal blocking, intestinal impaction.

Nursing implications/Documentation

Possible nursing diagnoses: Constipation.

◆ Give each dose with 8-oz glass of water and encourage increased fluid intake.

◆ Avoid administration before meals to prevent interference with appetite.

◆ Assess abdomen for bowel sounds and distention.

◆ Monitor and record character, frequency, and amount of stool evacuated.

Patient & family teaching/Home care

Possible nursing diagnoses: Knowledge deficit; Impaired home maintenance management.

◆ Caution not to swallow methylcellulose in dry form to prevent obstruction of the GI tract.

◆ Stress the importance of drinking 6–8 glasses of liquid daily, and taking each dose of methylcellulose with 8 ounces of water or juice to provide enough fluid for the desired action to take place.

◆ Caution not to take methylcellulose at bedtime, to reduce risk of intestinal obstruction.

◆ Advise against taking other oral medicines within 2 hours of methylcellulose to avoid decreased absorption due to binding.

◆ Stress the importance of dietary bulk, fluids, and exercise to prevent constipation; caution that high intake of bran, when combined with methylcellulose, increases the risk of impaction.

◆ Point out that daily bowel movements are not necessary for each individual; regular evacuation of soft stool which does not require straining is an appropriate goal.

◆ *See Laxatives overview for more information.*

methyldopa

meth-il-doe′pa

Aldomet, ♣Aldometm, ♣Apo-Methyldopa, ♣Dopamet, ♣Hydopa, ♣Novomedopa

Class: Antihypertensive, Adrenergic inhibiting agent

PEDS	PREG	GERI
🖐	B	🖐

Action Reduces blood pressure, possibly by stimulating central alpha-adrenergic receptors and blocking sympathetic outflow from the brain to the heart, kidneys, and peripheral vasculature, thereby resulting in vasodilation and bradycardia. May act as a "false neurotransmitter," and may inhibit plasma renin activity.

Use/Therapeutic goal/Outcome

Hypertension: Reduction of blood pressure. **Outcome criteria:** Blood pressure within normal limits.

Dose range/Administration

Interaction alert: Anesthetics, alcohol, diuretics, narcotics, levodopa, quinidine, vasodilators, and other antihypertensives can potentiate the hypotensive effects. Amphetamines, catecholamines, tricyclic antidepressants, MAO inhibitors, phenothiazines, sympathomimetics, and vasopressors can antagonize the hypotensive effects. Use with haloperidol can cause psychiatric disturbances.

Adult: PO: 250 mg bid or tid for 48 hr; may increase every 2 days as needed. *Maintenance dose:* 500–2000 mg/day in 2–4 divided doses. *Maximum dose:* 3000 mg/day. IV: 250–500 mg q6h prn, dilute in D5W and give over 30–60 min. *Maximum dose:* 1000 mg q6h. **Child:** PO: 10–65 mg/kg/day in 2–4 divided doses. IV: 20–40 mg/kg/day in 4 divided doses. *Maximum dose:* 65 mg/kg/day.

Clinical alert: During IV administration, document pulse, respirations, and blood pressure every 30 minutes until stable, then every 2 hours.

Contraindications/Precautions

PREG
B

Contraindicated in hypersensitivity to methyldopa, and in hepatic disease, blood dyscrasias, pheochromocytoma and labile hypertension. **Use with caution** in history of impaired renal or liver function, cerebrovascular disease, angina, or mental depression.

☙ Use with caution for children and the elderly. Safe use for pregnant women has not been established.

Side effects/Adverse reactions

Hypersensitivity: rash, urticaria, fever. **CV:** orthostatic hypotension, edema, bradycardia, angina, myocarditis. **CNS:** decreased mental acuity, headache, dizziness, weakness, sedation, depression, nightmares, psychotic disturbance. **GI:** dry mouth, diarrhea, pancreatitis, hepatic necrosis. **Hem:** eosinophilia, thrombocytopenia, granulocytopenia, hemolytic anemia. **Skin:** foot ulcerations, skin eruptions. **Resp:** nasal stuffiness. **GU:** impotence. **Misc:** SLE-like symptoms, lymphadenopathy, weight gain, sodium and fluid retention, lactation, gynecomastia.

Nursing implications/Documentation

Possible nursing diagnoses: Activity intolerance; Fatigue; Potential for injury.

◆ Assess mental status, and record pulse and blood pressure (lying, sitting, and standing, in both arms) prior to administration, and frequently thereafter until response is determined.

◆ Consult with physician to determine desired therapeutic range for blood pressure (be aware that some patients may require a slightly elevated blood pressure to perfuse vital organs).

◆ Ascertain that baseline CBC, electrolytes, BUN, creatinine, liver function studies, and direct Coombs test have been obtained before giving first dose; report abnormalities and monitor closely thereafter.

◆ Monitor for allergic reactions and confusion, dizziness, bradycardia, arrhythmias, hypotension; hold drug and report immediately if these occur.

◆ Supervise ambulation until response is determined.

◆ Document and monitor daily weight, and intake and output; report significant negative or positive balance.

Patient & family teaching/Home care

Possible nursing diagnoses: Altered sexuality patterns; Knowledge deficit; Impaired home maintenance management.

◆ Explain the importance of taking medication exactly as prescribed, even when feeling well; stress the importance of last doses at bedtime.

◆ Stress the importance of good medical follow-up, explain that this drug reduces "wear and tear" on blood vessels, and improves longevity and health.

◆ Teach how to monitor pulse and blood pressure; emphasize that syncope, hypertension or hypotension, palpitations, tachycardia, persistent dizziness, fatigue, chills, fever, or GI symptoms should be reported.

◆ Advise changing positions slowly to avoid dizziness.

◆ Encourage daily monitoring of weight and reporting sudden weight gain (frequently is fluid retention).

◆ Explain that driving should be avoided until response is determined (may cause drowsiness); use with alcohol may increase drowsiness.

◆ Warn against discontinuing drug abruptly or taking *any* OTC drugs without physician approval (some interactions can cause severe reactions).

◆ Inform that urine may appear dark in toilets cleaned with bleach.

◆ Explain that this drug may affect sexual activity; counsel individuals with concerns.

◆ *See Antihypertensives overview for more information.*

M

methylergonovine

meth-ill-er-go-noe'veen

methylergonovine maleate: **Methergine**

Class: Oxytocic; Hormone

PEDS	PREG	GERI
✋	C	✋

Action Improves uterine tone and reduces post-partum bleeding by directly stimulating uterine and vascular smooth-muscle contraction.

Use/Therapeutic goal/Outcome

Postpartum or postabortion uterine atony and bleeding: Improvement in uterine tone; reduction in bleeding. **Outcome criteria:** Sustained uterine tone; reduction in bleeding.

Dose range/Administration

Interaction alert: Dopamine, oxytocin, regional anesthetics, other vasoconstrictors and ergot alkaloids may cause excessive vasoconstriction.

Adult: IM, IV: 0.2 mg q2-4h, maximum 5 doses. *May follow with PO if needed:* 0.2 mg q6-12h for 2–7 days; not longer than 7 days.

Clinical alert: Dilute IV doses (used in emergencies only) in 5 ml normal saline and give slowly, over 1 min, while closely monitoring blood pressure and uterine response; hold dose and report if severe hypertension is noted. Never add doses to existing IVs. This drug should never be used for the induction or augmentation of labor; it may be used during the third stage of labor, but only after delivery of the anterior shoulder or placenta.

Contraindications/Precautions

PREG
C

Contraindicated in hypersensitivity to methyl-ergonovine, for prolonged use, and in venoatrial shunts, mitral-valve stenosis, threatened abortion, labor induction, hypertension, and eclampsia. **Use with caution** in obliterative vascular disease, cardiac disease, hypocalcemia, sepsis, and liver or kidney disease.

✋ **Contraindicated for pregnant women prior to delivery of fetus and placenta. Use with caution for adolescents and older mothers.**

Side effects/Adverse reactions

Hypersensitivity: rash, pruritus. **GI:** nausea, vomiting, diarrhea; foul taste. **GU:** uterine cramping. **CNS:** headache, seizures, dizziness, hallucinations. **Ear:** tinnitus. **Resp:** dyspnea, nasal congestion. **CV:** hypertension (may be severe if IV drug is given too rapidly), hypotension, transient chest pains, thrombophlebitis, palpitations. **MS:** leg cramps. **Skin:** diaphoresis. **Misc:** water intoxication.

Nursing implications/Documentation

Possible nursing diagnoses: Potential for injury; Pain.

◆ Monitor lochia and palpate fundus to determine uterine tone and amount of blood loss; report persistent atony of uterus or increase in vaginal bleeding.

◆ Expect contractions to begin immediately after IV route, 2–5 min after IM injection, and 5–15 min after PO administration; cramping may continue for 45 min after IV route and 3 hours after PO or IM administration.

◆ Record vital signs at least every 4 hours (more frequently if unstable).

◆ During IV administration, keep mother in bed with side rails up and call-bell within reach; supervise ambulation after IM route.

◆ Have patient rate comfort level on a scale of 1–10; encourage using relaxation techniques and provide ordered analgesics; report persistent severe unrelieved pain.

Patient & family teaching/Home care

Possible nursing diagnoses: Fear; Knowledge deficit; Impaired home maintenance management.

◆ Explain that this drug increases uterine cramping to reduce bleeding; stress that uterine tone, vaginal bleeding, and vital signs will be monitored frequently to assure optimum results.

◆ Point out that while uterine cramping may be uncomfortable, severe pain should be reported immediately.

◆ Encourage asking questions and verbalizing fears or concerns.

◆ If discharged before oral dose regimen is completed, emphasize the need to take doses on time (doses should not be doubled if a dose is missed).

◆ Stress the importance of reporting uterine bleeding that persists after dosing stops.

M

methylphenidate

meth-ill-fen'i-date

methylphenidate hydrochloride: *Ritalin, Ritalin SR*
Class: Cerebral stimulant, piperidine

PEDS	PREG	GERI	CONTROLLED SUBSTANCE
✋	C	✋	II

Action *In adults,* produces central nervous system stimulation, *in hyperactive children,* a "paradoxical" calming effect by releasing stored norepinephrine from nerve terminals in the brain.

Use/Therapeutic goal/Outcome

Narcolepsy: Promotion of alertness; reduction in episodes of narcolepsy. **Outcome criteria:** Reduction in episodes of narcolepsy; report of feeling more alert and less fatigued.
Attention Deficit Disorders with Hyperactivity (ADDH): Promotion of ability to concentrate or pay attention. **Outcome criteria:** Demonstration of increased attention span; increased ability to sit quietly.

Dose range/Administration

Interaction alert: Use within 14 days of MAO inhibitors may cause severe hypertensive crisis. May alter insulin requirements of diabetics, and anticonvulsant medication requirements of people with seizure disorders.

🖐 **Give on empty stomach to increase absorption.**
Narcolepsy: Adult: PO: 10 mg bid to tid *after meals* (may give up to 50 mg/day).

Attention Deficit Disorder with Hyperactivity (ADDH): Child > 6 years: PO: 5 mg *before breakfast and lunch,* with weekly increments of 5–10 mg prn (maximum of 50 mg/day).

Clinical alert: Give doses at least 6 hr before bedtime to prevent insomnia. If sustained-release tablets are used, warn the patient not to chew them. For treatment of ADDH in children, monitor for need to *decrease* dose; that is, watch for lessening effectiveness (this drug is usually stopped after puberty). May decrease seizure threshhold for people with epilepsy.

Contraindications/Precautions

PREG C

Contraindicated in hypersensitivity or intolerance to methylphenidate, cardiac disease, hypertension, severe anxiety, agitation, parkinsonism, history of drug abuse, or use within 14 days of MAO inhibitors. **Use with caution** for patients with seizure disorders, Tourette's syndrome, psychosis, hypertension, cardiovascular disease, or diabetes.

🖐 **Contraindicated for children under 6 years. Use with caution for the elderly. Safe use for pregnant and nursing mothers has not been established.**

Side effects/Adverse reactions

Hypersensitivity: itching, rashes, joint pain, bruising. **CNS:** insomnia, restlessness, tremors, hyperactivity, irritability, headache, dizziness, Tourette's disease. **CV:** palpitations, tachycardia, hypertension, hypotension. **GI:** anorexia, metallic taste, nausea, vomiting, dry mouth, cramps, diarrhea. **Misc:** growth suppression in children.

Nursing implications/Documentation

Possible nursing diagnoses: Altered thought processes; Sleep pattern disturbance; Altered nutrition: less than body requirements.

♦ Question carefully use of beverages and OTC drugs that contain caffeine.

♦ Monitor attention span or ability to concentrate, and report and document changes in status (drug dosage may need to be adjusted).

♦ Provide decaffeinated beverages, and give doses at least 6 hr before bedtime to prevent insomnia.

♦ Record blood pressure at least daily when beginning therapy, and periodically once stabilized.

♦ Document daily weights and keep a record of food intake to ensure adequate nutrition.

Patient & family teaching/Home care

Possible nursing diagnoses: Knowledge deficit; Impaired home maintenance management.

♦ Explain that this drug has a high potential for abuse, and should only be taken as prescribed, and under continuous medical supervision.

♦ Stress the importance of checking labels for caffeine content and avoiding caffeine (may increase drug effects).

♦ For use with children

Teach the need to monitor physical and mental growth, and to report growth failure and behavior extremes (dosage may have to be adjusted); explain that dosage will probably be reduced as child progresses to puberty, and that periodic "drug holidays" may be planned to determine if the drug is still necessary.

- *See Cerebral Stimulants overview for more information.*

meth-ill-pred-niss'oh-lone

methylprednisolone

methylprednisolone: *Medrol, Meprolone*

methylprednisolone acetate: *depMedalone, Depoject, Depo-Medrol, Depopred, Depo-Predate, D-Med, Duralone, Durameth, Medralone, Medrol, Medrol Enpak, Medrone, Methylone, M-Prednisol, Rep-Pred*

methylprednisolone sodium succinate: *A-MethaPred, ♣Medrol, Solu-Medrol*

Class: Synthetic adrenocorticosteroid, Intermediate-acting glucocorticoid, Steroidal anti-inflammatory, Immunosuppressant

PEDS	PREG	GERI
♨	C	♨

Action Suppresses inflammation by inhibiting accumulation of inflammatory cells, reducing dilatation and permeability of capillaries, and inhibiting release of chemical mediators of inflammation. Modifies immune response by suppressing cell-mediated immune reactions.

Use/Therapeutic goal/Outcome

Inflammatory, allergic, and immune conditions: Symptomatic relief. *Outcome criteria:* Decreased symptoms associated with condition being treated.

Spinal cord injury: Reduced destruction of nerve fibers in spinal cord. *Outcome criteria:* Decreased loss of sensory and motor function below level of injury.

Dose range/Administration

Interaction alert: May decrease effectiveness of anticoagulants and antidiabetics. Vaccines may lead to diminished antibody response and serious infection. Potassium-depleting diuretics may cause severe hypokalemia. Alcohol or medications known to cause gastric irritation may cause gastric bleeding. Drugs that increase metabolism of corticosteroids (e.g., phenytoin, barbiturates, ephedrine, and rifampin) and those that decrease its absorption (e.g., cholestyramine, colestipol, and antacids) may reduce methylprednisolone levels, requiring an increase in methylprednisolone dosage.

🖐 **Give oral doses with food or milk to decrease gastric irritation.**

Inflammatory, allergic, and immune conditions: *Adult:* PO: 4–48 mg/day. IV, IM: 10–120 mg qd to q 2 wk prn. *Rectal:* 40 mg 3–7 times/wk for 2 or more wk. *Child:* PO: 0.117–1.67 mg/kg/day in 3–4 divided doses. IV: 0.5 mg/kg/day. IM: 0.139–0.835 mg/kg q12-24h. *Rectal:* 0.5–1 mg/kg qd to qod for 2 or more wk. *Adult and Child:* *Topical:* Apply sparingly to affected area bid to qid.

Spinal cord injury: *Adult and Child:* IV: 30 mg/kg over 15 min, then in 45 min continuous infusion 5.4 mg/kg/hr for 23 hr.

Clinical alert: Give single daily or alternate-day doses in the morning to reduce adrenal suppression. Give IM doses deep into gluteal muscle to lessen muscle atrophy. Administer rectal doses as a retention enema or slow continuous drip; shake suspension well. May also be injected directly into joints, soft tissues, or lesions.

Contraindications/Precautions

PREG
C

Contraindicated in hypersensitivity to corticosteroids or to tartrazine (present in some preparations), and in active peptic ulcer disease, active tuberculosis or fungus infections, and herpes of eyes, lips, or genitals. *Use with caution* in acquired immunodeficiency syndrome (AIDS), hypertension, thrombophlebitis, congestive heart failure, diabetes mellitus, hypothyroidism, glaucoma, osteoporosis, myasthenia gravis, and history of bleeding ulcers, seizure disorder, or mental illness.

♨ **Use with caution for children, pregnant or nursing mothers, and the elderly.**

Side effects/Adverse reactions

Hypersensitivity: rash, hives, hypotension, respiratory distress, anaphylaxis. *CNS:* euphoria, restlessness, insomnia, hallucinations, depression, psychosis. *Eye:* glaucoma, cataracts. *MS:* impaired growth in children. *CV:* thrombophlebitis, embolism, irregular heartbeat. *GI:* increased appetite, oral candidiasis. *Misc:* hyperglycemia, withdrawal syndrome.

With prolonged use: *Skin:* acne; increased hair growth; thin, shiny skin; ecchymosis or petechiae; delayed wound healing. *GI:* nausea, vomiting, GI bleeding, pancreatitis. *MS:* osteoporosis; pain in hip, back, ribs, arms, or legs; muscle wasting. *CV:* hypertension, edema, hypokalemia. *GU:* menstrual irregularity. *Misc:* increased susceptibility to infection; Cushingoid appearance (moon-face and buffalo hump); withdrawal syndrome, or acute adrenal insufficiency.

Nursing implications/Documentation

Possible nursing diagnoses: Potential for infection; Body image disturbance; Fluid volume excess.

◆ Monitor for hypersensitivity reactions, especially with parenteral administration.

◆ Record baseline weight, blood pressure, and electrolyte levels.

◆ Apply topical cream sparingly to clean, moist skin; occlusive dressing will increase absorption.

◆ Assess and record improvement in condition being treated so dosage can be decreased as early as possible.

◆ Monitor electrolyte levels to detect sodium retention and potassium loss; monitor for edema and/or muscle weakness and document findings.

◆ Observe for signs of infection and slowed wound healing.

◆ During dose reduction, assess for signs and symptoms of adrenal insufficiency (hypotension, hypoglycemia, weight loss, vomiting, and diarrhea).

Patient & family teaching/Home care

Possible nursing diagnoses: Knowledge deficit; Impaired home maintenance management; Impaired physical mobility; Impaired skin integrity.

◆ Explain the need to take oral doses with food or milk.

◆ Advise against drinking alcohol while taking methylprednisolone to decrease ulcer potential.

◆ Teach rectal administration technique; caution to report signs of rectal irritation or infection.

◆ For long-term therapy, advise wearing a medical alert medal indicating the need for additional systemic steroids in case of trauma or surgery.

◆ Caution against taking OTC or prescription drugs without consulting primary physician.

◆ Advise reporting unusual weight gain; swelling of lower extremities; muscle weakness; black tarry stools; vomiting of blood; epigastric burning; puffing of face; menstrual irregularities; prolonged sore throat, fever, cold, or infections; also stress the need to report symptoms of adrenal insufficiency (fatigue, anorexia, nausea, vomiting, diarrhea, weight loss, weakness, dizziness, depression, and mood swings).

◆ Counsel to adhere to prescribed dose schedule and not to discontinue medication against medical advice.

◆ Reinforce the importance of medical follow-up for evaluation of therapy.

◆ *See Adrenocorticosteroids overview for more information.*

methyltestosterone *meth-ill-tess-toss'te-rone*

Android, Metandren, Metandren Linguets, Oreton Methyl, ♠Testomet, Testred, Virilon

Class: Androgen, Antineoplastic agent

PEDS	PREG	GERI
🖐	X	🖐

Action Stimulates development and maintenance of male sex organs; induces development of male secondary sex characteristics; stimulates sperm production; increases body size by stimulating growth of skeletal muscles.

Use/Therapeutic goal/Outcome

Androgen deficiency/hypogonadism: Correction of deficiency. **Outcome criteria:** Absence or improvement of deficiency symptoms (delayed development of male secondary sex characteristics, impotence, or male climacteric).

Breast cancer: Palliation of inoperable metastatic disease for women 1–5 years postmenopause; suppression of hormone-responsive tumors. **Outcome criteria:** Evidence of decreased tumor and metastatic activity; decreased bone pain.

Dose range/Administration

Interaction alert: Increases effect of insulin, oral hypoglycemics, and anticoagulants. Corticosteroids increase possibility of edema and severe acne. Avoid other hepatotoxic medications.

🍃 **Give oral doses with food to minimize GI distress.**

Deficiency: Adult: PO: 10–50 mg/day. Buccal: 5–25 mg/day. **Child:** PO: 5–25 mg/day for 4–6 mos. Buccal: 2.5–12.5 mg/day for 4–6 mos.

Breast cancer: Adult: PO: 50 mg 1–4 times a day. Buccal: 25 mg 1–4 times a day.

Clinical alert: For buccal administration, place tablet in mouth against cheek; allow 30–60 minutes for tablet to dissolve before eating or drinking.

Contraindications/Precautions

Contraindicated in hypersensitivity to androgens, lactose, or tartrazine dye, and in severe renal, hepatic, or cardiac disease; hypercalcemia; breast or prostatic cancer in men; and genital bleeding. **Use with caution** in diabetes mellitus, prostatic hypertrophy, gynecomastia, history of MI, and cardiac failure.

🖐 **Contraindicated for pregnant or nursing mothers. Use with caution for children and elderly men.**

Side effects/Adverse reactions

Hypersensitivity: rashes, bronchospasm, anaphylaxis. **GU:** virilism of females (enlarged clitoris, deepening of voice, menstrual irregularities, unnatural hair growth or loss); virilism of prepubertal males (acne, enlarging penis, increased frequency of erections, unnatural hair growth); in older men, bladder irritability, breast soreness, gynecomastia, priapism, prostatic hypertrophy, prostatic carcinoma, epididymitis, increased libido. **Hem:** polycythemia, hypercalcemia, decreased high-density lipoproteins (HDL), increased low-density lipoproteins (LDL). **GI:** nausea, vomiting, stomatitis with buccal administration; hepatic dysfunction, carcinoma, or necrosis. **MS:** premature epiphyseal closure in children. **Skin:** edema, unexplained darkening, acne, pain or swelling at injection site.

Nursing implications/Documentation

Possible nursing diagnoses: Body image disturbance; Fluid volume excess.

♦ Assess oral mucous membrane for signs of irritation.

♦ Monitor serum calcium levels; assess, report, and document symptoms of hypercalcemia (vomiting, constipation, polyuria, lethargy, and muscle weakness).

♦ For elderly men, monitor for difficult or frequent urination.

♦ Record baseline blood pressure and weight.

♦ Monitor for and report decreased urine output, edema, increased blood pressure, weight gain, and congestive failure.

♦ Monitor electrolyte and cholesterol levels and liver function tests.

♦ For diabetics, monitor glucose levels and assess for symptoms of hypoglycemia.

Patient & family teaching/Home care

Possible nursing diagnoses: Knowledge deficit; Impaired home maintenance management; Sexual dysfunction; Altered oral mucous membrane.

♦ Advise taking oral tablets with meals to minimize gastric distress.

♦ For buccal administration, teach to place tablet inside cheek and not to eat, drink, or smoke until tablet is dissolved; instruct to rinse mouth with water after tablet is dissolved and to alternate areas used.

♦ Caution to restrict sodium intake to decrease fluid retention.

♦ Caution women of child-bearing age to use reliable birth control and to stop drug and report any suspicion of pregnancy.

♦ For women, stress the importance of reporting the occurrence of masculinizing effects (abnormal growth of facial hair, deepening of voice, menstrual irregularities, enlarged clitoris).

♦ For men, advise reporting development of priapism, gynecomastia, or bladder irritability.

♦ For diabetics, caution about possible lowering of blood sugar and need for adjustment of doses of insulin or oral antidiabetic agents.

♦ Inform parents of prepubertal children that X rays will be taken periodically to determine effect on bone growth.

♦ Caution to maintain close medical supervision for early detection of adverse reactions.

♦ Warn that use of high doses of androgens for improvement of athletic performance may result in serious side effects that outweigh any advantages.

methysergide

meth-i-ser'jide

methysergide maleate: ◆**Deseril, Sansert**
Class: Adrenergic blocker (sympatholytic), Serotonin antagonist

PEDS	PREG	GERI
🖐	C	🖐

Action Believed to relieve vascular headaches by inhibiting the effects of serotonin, a neurotransmitter and potent vasodilator that is believed to play a role in vascular headaches; it also inhibits the release of serotonin from platelets and histamine from mast cells.

Use/Therapeutic goal/Outcome

Vascular headache: Prevention of migraine, cluster, or vascular headaches. **Outcome criteria:** After 3 weeks, report of absence or decrease in migraine, cluster, and vascular headaches.

Dose range/Administration

🖐 **Give with meals.**

Adult: PO: 4–8 mg/day in divided doses tid.

Clinical alert: Methysergide maleate should be stopped for 3–4 weeks every 6 months because of high incidence of side effects.

Contraindications/Precautions

Contraindicated in hypersensitivity to methysergide maleate. **Use with caution** in fibrotic processes, valvular heart disease, hypertension, peripheral vascular disease, hypertension, sepsis, pulmonary disease, rheumatoid arthritis, renal and hepatic disease, serious infections, and debilitated states. **Use with caution** in cardiac disease.

🖐 **Contraindicated for children and pregnant or nursing mothers. Use with caution for those over 40 years.**

Side effects/Adverse reactions

Hypersensitivity: rash, eosinophilia. **CNS:** insomnia, drowsiness, confusion, excitement, vertigo, hallucinations, euphoria, weakness. **CV:** peripheral edema; impaired circulation; chest pain; tachycardia; numb, cold, painful extremities (because of vasoconstriction). **GI:** nausea, vomiting, diarrhea, constipation, heartburn. **Skin:** facial flushing, hair loss. **Misc:** cardiac fibrosis (thickening of valves with murmurs), retroperitoneal fibrosis (abdominal pain, fatigue, fever, urinary obstruction, paresthesia), pleuropulmonary fibrosis (chest pain, dyspnea).

Nursing implications/Documentation

Possible nursing diagnoses: Pain; Ineffective individual coping.

♦ Check for baseline studies of cardiac status, renal function, CBC, and sedimentation rate prior to starting drug; these should be checked periodically thereafter.

♦ Have patient rate pain of headache on a scale of 1–10 before and after administration; report and record unrelieved pain.

♦ Identify dietary, emotional, physical, and environmental factors that precipitate or aggravate headaches.

♦ Provide a dark, quiet environment and holistic measures that promote comfort (e.g., cool washcloth for forehead) if headache is present.

♦ Report immediately if fibrotic complications are suspected (see miscellaneous side effects).

Patient & family teaching/Home care

Possible nursing diagnoses: Ineffective individual coping; Impaired home maintenance management.

♦ Teach that taking this drug with food helps reduce GI symptoms.

♦ Stress the need to treat headache as soon after onset as possible.

♦ Explore ways of avoiding stress, coping with stress, and eliminating environmental factors that trigger headaches.

♦ Teach holistic measures for relieving pain (e.g., relaxation techniques).

♦ Advise reporting new symptoms in case they are related to the medication.

♦ Emphasize the need for ongoing medical supervision.

♦ Caution not to use OTC medications without physician's approval because of possible serious interactions.

♦ Warn that stopping this drug suddenly may cause a rebound effect that increases frequency and duration of headaches.

♦ Inform that exposure to cold may aggravate side effects.

♦ Point out that tobacco and alcohol should be avoided.

metoclopramide

met-oh-kloe-pra'mide

metoclopramide hydrochloride: 🍁*Maxeran*, 🦘*Maxolon*, 🦘*Maxolon High Dose*, Reglan

Class: Cholinergic, Parasympathomimetic, Antiemetic

PEDS	PREG	GERI
🖐	B	🖐

Action Relieves and prevents nausea and vomiting associated with chemotherapy by elevating CTZ (chemoreceptor trigger zone) threshold and enhancing gastric emptying. Reduces gastroesophageal reflux and diabetic gastric stasis by increasing resting tone of the esophageal sphincter and increasing upper GI motility. Facilitates intubation of the small bowel by promoting gastric emptying.

Use/Therapeutic goal/Outcome

Nausea or vomiting: Prevention or resolution. **Outcome criteria:** Report of absence of, or reduction in, feelings of nausea; absence of vomiting.

Gastric stasis/Gastroesophageal reflux: Promotion of gastric emptying; reduction in gastroesophageal reflux, heartburn, esophagitis. **Outcome criteria:** Report of absence of heartburn, indigestion, pain, acid taste in mouth, nausea.

Small bowel intubation: Facilitation of procedure. **Outcome criteria:** X-ray evidence of small bowel intubation.

Dose range/Administration

Interaction alert: Because of CNS depressant effects, may increase effects of other CNS depressants and alcohol. Avoid giving with psychotropic drugs because it is likely to increase extrapyramidal side effects. May alter insulin requirements and dosage of other drugs affected by rate of GI absorption.

■ **Give 30 minutes before meals.**

Nausea and vomiting associated with chemotherapy: **Adult:** IV: 2 mg/kg q2h for 5 doses, beginning 30 min prior to chemotherapy.
Small bowel intubation: **Adult:** IV: 10 mg given over 1–2 min. **Child < 6 yrs:** IV: 0.1 mg/kg. **Child 6–14 yrs:** IV: 2.5–5 mg over 1–2 min.

Delayed gastric emptying associated with diabetic gastrointestinal stasis: **Adult:** PO: 10 mg, 30 min ac and hs.

Gastroesophageal reflux: **Adult:** PO: 10–15 mg, 30 min ac and hs prn.

Clinical alert: Give IV doses slowly because rapid administration may cause intense transient anxiety and restlessness, followed by drowsiness. For slower administration, may be diluted in 50 ml D5W, normal or half strength saline solution, or Ringers lactate solution, and administered over at least 15 min.

Contraindications/Precautions

**PREG
B**

Contraindicated in hypersensitivity to metoclopramide, procaine, or procainamide, and in coma, depression, suspected bowel obstruction, seizure disorders, Parkinsonism, or with drugs which cause extrapyramidal reactions. **Use with caution** in liver or kidney failure.

☟ **Use with caution for children and the elderly. Safe use for pregnant or nursing mothers has not been determined.**

Side effects/Adverse reactions

Hypersensitivity: rash, extreme drowsiness, tardive dyskinesia, and symptoms of parkinsonism (especially in the elderly). **CNS:** drowsiness, restlessness, fatigue. **GI:** constipation, diarrhea.

Nursing implications/Documentation

Possible nursing diagnoses: Potential for injury; Constipation; Fluid volume deficit; Altered oral mucous membranes.

◆ Assess for presence of bowel sounds, pain, nausea, or vomiting before and after administering antiemetics; hold drug and report if bowel sounds are absent.

◆ Determine cause of symptoms before giving antiemetics; ascertain that nausea and vomiting symptoms are not due to intestinal obstruction, increased intracranial pressure, or drug overdosage before giving first dose.

◆ Offer frequent mouth care.

◆ Supervise ambulation until response is determined.

◆ Monitor elderly patients for symptoms of parkinsonism, which may be treated with diphenhydramine.

◆ Document and monitor intake and output to detect dehydration; monitor bowel movements to detect constipation.

◆ Provide adequate fiber and fluids to prevent constipation.

◆ Monitor for and report immediately early signs of extrapyramidal side effects.

◆ When able to tolerate liquids, begin with small amount of ice chips, then water, then clear liquids, then full liquids, then food.

Patient & family teaching/Home care

Possible nursing diagnoses: Knowledge deficit; Impaired home maintenance management.

◆ Teach that the drug should be taken 30 min before meals and at bedtime.

◆ Stress that persistent nausea, vomiting, or abdominal discomfort should be reported.

◆ Discuss the role of fiber, fluids, and exercise in preventing constipation.

◆ Teach signs of extrapyramidal side effects and stress that these should be reported immediately.

◆ Explain that avoiding fatty foods and eating smaller and more frequent meals may reduce nausea.

M

- ◆ Advise against using alcohol or other CNS depressants; warn against driving or activities that require mental alertness until response is determined.

- ◆ Emphasize the need to maintain good mouth care, especially when not taking liquids by mouth; suggest that chewing sugarless gum may relieve symptoms of dry mouth.

- ◆ *See Antiemetics overview for more information.*

metocurine

met-oh-kyoo'reen

metocurine iodide: *Metubine*

Class: Skeletal-muscle relaxant, Nondepolarizing neuromuscular blocker

Antidote: Neostigmine methylsulfate

PEDS	PREG	GERI
🖐	C	🖐

Action Relaxes or paralyzes skeletal muscles (depending on dose) by competing with acetylcholine for cholinergic receptor sites thereby inhibiting neuromuscular transmission. Does not alter consciousness, pain threshold, or thought processes.

Use/Therapeutic goal/Outcome

Endotracheal intubation, adjunct to general anesthesia, reduction of fractures and dislocations, and during pharmacologically or electrically induced seizures: Facilitation of endotracheal tube tolerance; relaxation of skeletal muscle. **Outcome criteria:** Tolerance of endotracheal intubation and mechanical ventilation; diminished or absent voluntary and reflexive movement.

Dose range/Administration

Interaction alert: Do not mix with alkaline solutions, barbiturates, meperidine, or morphine (precipitate may form). Halothane, diethyl ether, methoxyflurane, aminoglycoside antibiotics, thiazide diuretics, succinylcholine, and quinidine may increase the effects of metocurine.

Surgery: Adult: IV: *With cyclopropane:* 2–4 mg (average of 2.68 mg). *With ether:* 1.5–3 mg (average of 2.1 mg). *With nitrous oxide:* 4–7 mg (average of 4.79 mg). Supplemental doses of 0.5 to 1 mg may be required.

Endotracheal intubation: Adult: IV: 0.2–0.4 mg.

Electroshock therapy: Adult: IV: 1.75–5.5 mg (average of 2–3 mg).

Clinical alert: Metocurine should be given over 30–60 seconds only by physicians and nurses who are familiar with its use, and in the presence of a physician, nurse anesthetist, or respiratory therapist who is qualified to manage endotracheal intubation.

Contraindications/Precautions

PREG C

Contraindicated in hypersensitivity to metocurine or iodides, and in asthma. **Use with caution** in renal, hepatic, or pulmonary impairment; myasthenia gravis; electrolyte imbalance; debilitated patients; dehydration, thyroid disorders; and collagen diseases.

🖐 **Use with caution for pregnant women and the elderly. Safe use for children has not been established.**

Side effects/Adverse reactions

Hypersensitivity: (rare) flushing, itching, wheezing. **Resp:** dose-related prolonged apnea and bronchospasm, respiratory depression. **CNS:** dizziness. **CV:** tachycardia, circulatory depression, hypotension.

Nursing implications/Documentation

Possible nursing diagnoses: Impaired communication; Pain; Potential for aspiration; Potential for injury.

- ◆ Ascertain that baseline CBC, electrolytes, BUN, creatinine, liver function, chest X ray, and EKG studies are posted on chart before drug administration (report abnormalities).

- ◆ Protect airway, position for drainage of oropharyngeal secretions (if possible), and keep suction at bedside until the patient is fully alert; have emergency equipment and drugs available.

- ◆ Monitor and record vital signs every 15 min until stable; report abnormalities that might indicate potential complications.

- ◆ Recognize that this drug may *paralyze*, but does not relieve pain (provide analgesics if pain is suspected, anticipate human needs).

- ◆ Monitor for potential for injury: protect eyes if there is no blink reflex (tape shut); watch positioning of all extremities (provide range of motion exercises if therapy is prolonged).

- ◆ Document and monitor intake and output every 2–4 hours for 24 hours postoperatively.

Patient & family teaching/Home care

Possible nursing diagnoses: Anxiety; Fear.

- Explain all procedures, even if the person seems unconscious (the ability to hear may be present).
- Reassure individual that muscle weakness, paralysis, or stiffness will subside.

metolazone
me-toe'la-zone

Diulo, Microx, Zaroxolyn
Class: Thiazide-like diuretic

PEDS	PREG	GERI
✋	D	✋

Action Promotes excretion of sodium and water by inhibiting the reabsorption of sodium and chloride in the early portion of the distal tubule. Lowers blood pressure by reducing plasma and extra-cellular volume.

Use/Therapeutic goal/Outcome

Hypertension: Promotion of diuresis, reduction of blood pressure. **Outcome criteria:** After 3–4 days, blood pressure within normal limits.

Edema: Promotion of diuresis, resolution of edema. **Outcome criteria:** Increase in urinary output; weight loss; absence of rales and peripheral and sacral edema.

CHF: Promotion of diuresis, resolution of CHF. **Outcome criteria:** Absence of rales; non-distended neck veins; CVP/PAP within normal limits.

Dose range/Administration

Interaction alert: Cholestyramine and colestipol decrease intestinal absorption. Diazoxide potentiates the antihypertensive, hyperglycemic, and hyperuricemic effects.

🖐 **Administer with food to decrease GI upset.**
Hypertension: Adult: PO: 2.5–5 mg/day.
Edema in kidney disease: Adult: PO: 5–20 mg/day.
Edema in CHF: Adult: PO: 5–20 mg/day.

Clinical alert: Give in morning to avoid nocturnal diuresis. Be aware that antihypertensive response may not occur for 3–4 days. Extended tablets and prompt tablets must not be substituted for one another.

Contraindications/Precautions

Contraindicated in hypersensitivity to metolazone or sulfonamides, and in anuria, hypokalemia and hepatic coma. **Use with caution** in gout, allergies, hepatic or renal dysfunction.

🖐 **Contraindicated for children and pregnant or nursing mothers. Use with caution for the elderly.**

Side effects/Adverse reactions

Hypersensitivity: rash, urticaria, dermatitis with photosensitivity, pneumonitis, vasculitis. **Hem:** hypokalemia, hyperglycemia, azotemia, impaired glucose tolerance, asymptomatic hyperuricemia, electrolyte imbalance, metabolic alkalosis, hypercalcemia, lipid abnormalities, aplastic anemia, agranulocytosis, leukopenia, thrombocytopenia. **CV:** volume depletion, dehydration, orthostatic hypotension. **GI:** anorexia, nausea, pancreatitis, hepatic encephalopathy. **Misc:** gout.

Nursing implications/Documentation

Possible nursing diagnoses: Fluid volume deficit; Altered patterns of urinary elimination; Potential for injury.

- Ascertain that baseline CBC, sodium, potassium, chloride, carbon dioxide, calcium, magnesium, BUN, creatinine, uric acid, and liver function studies have been obtained before giving first dose; report abnormalities and monitor closely thereafter.
- Document and monitor blood pressure, pulse, daily weight, and intake and output; report significant discrepancies.
- Monitor for hyperglycemia because of risk of thiazide diabetes.
- Observe for and report signs of fluid overload (auscultate lungs for rales; check feet, ankles, and sacrum for edema).
- Be aware that diuretics often induce hypokalemia, which predisposes individuals to cardiac arrhythmias, cramping, and digoxin toxicity.
- Check with physician to determine dietary restrictions; if a low-salt, high-potassium diet is recommended, consult with dietician to plan a low-salt diet that includes foods and juices high in potassium (orange juice; banana; green leafy vegetables).
- Observe the elderly for extreme diuresis (may require lower doses); monitor for ortho-

M

static hypotension; supervise ambulation until response is determined.

Patient & family teaching/Home care

Possible nursing diagnoses: Impaired home maintenance management; Knowledge deficit.

♦ Before giving first dose, explain that the drug will increase the amount and frequency of urination.

♦ Advise taking this drug with food to prevent GI symptoms.

♦ Emphasize the importance of taking this drug exactly as prescribed, and the importance of returning for medical follow-up.

♦ Explain that diuretics enhance the work of the kidney and reduce the workload of the heart.

♦ Recommend taking doses in early morning and early afternoon to prevent the need to disturb sleep to void.

♦ Explain that changing positions slowly helps prevent dizziness.

♦ Advise reporting dizziness, shortness of breath, swelling of hands and feet, or persistent sore throat; encourage daily monitoring of weight and reporting sudden weight gain.

♦ Provide a list of allowed foods and fluids; stress the need to stick to prescribed diet (explain the hazards of too much salt, or too little potassium).

♦ Warn against driving or activities that require alertness until response has been determined.

♦ Advise avoidance of OTC drugs unless approved by physician.

♦ Suggest using a (Number 15) sunscreen when outside because of photosensitivity (avoid products with PABA).

♦ *See Diuretics and Antihypertensives overviews for more information.*

metoprolol

me-toe'proe'lole

♦Apo-Metoprolol, ♦Betaloc, ♦Betaloc Durules, ♦Lopresor, ♦Lopresor SR, Lopressor, ♦Novometroprol

Class: Selective beta-1 adrenergic blocking agent, Antihypertensive, Antianginal

PEDS	PREG	GERI
♨	B	♨

Action Reduces blood pressure (precise mechanism is unknown), heart rate, and myocardial oxygen demand by blocking beta-1 receptors in the myocardium. Decreases SA- and AV-node conduction velocity, cardiac output, peripheral resistance, and renin secretion. Mechanism of action for its use as prophylaxis during acute myocardial infarction (MI) is not established.

Use/Therapeutic goal/Outcome

Hypertension: Resolution of hypertension. **Outcome criteria:** Blood pressure within normal range.

Angina: Prevention of anginal attacks. **Outcome criteria:** Report of decreased episodes of angina; increased activity tolerance.

MI prophylaxis: Reduction of mortality associated with MI. **Outcome criteria:** Decreased incidence of cardiac-related death.

Dose range/Administration

Interaction alert: Do not use with MAO inhibitors. Barbiturates, phenothiazines, rifampin, and phenytoin may enhance metoprolol metabolism. Indomethacin may antagonize antihypertensive effect. Cimetidine, and calcium channel blockers, may increase metoprolol's effects. May alter antidiabetic agent requirements.

☛ **Give with or after meals to increase absorption.**

Hypertension or angina: Adult: PO: 100 mg/day, or in divided doses bid; may increase weekly prn. *Maintenance dose:* 100 mg bid. *Maximum dose:* 450 mg/day.

Myocardial reinfarction prophylactic: Adult: IV (for acute MI): Administer three 5 mg boluses at 2-min intervals. *If this dose is tolerated,* begin PO therapy 15 min after the last IV bolus: give 50 mg q6h for 48 hr. Maintain on 100 mg bid. *If full IV dose is not tolerated* begin PO therapy 15 min after last IV bolus (or when condition improves): give 25–50 mg q6h.

Clinical alert: Be aware that patients taking this drug may not exhibit tachycardia as a symptom of fever, hypoglycemia, or hyperthyroidism.

Contraindications/Precautions

PREG
B

Contraindicated in hypersensitivity to metoprolol, and in cardiogenic shock, sinus bradycardia (heart rate < 45) second- or third-degree heart block (PR interval > 0.24 seconds), overt CHF, right ventricular failure, or systolic blood pressure less than 100 mm

M

Hg. *Use with caution* in impaired hepatic or renal function, cardiomegaly, pulmonary pathology, AV conduction abnormalities, thyrotoxicosis, diabetes, peripheral vascular disease, or history of allergies.

♛ **Use with caution for the elderly. Safe use for children and pregnant or nursing mothers has not been established.**

Side effects/Adverse reactions

Hypersensitivity: rash. *CV:* bradycardia, hypotension, CHF, peripheral vascular disease. *Resp:* respiratory distress, laryngospasm, sore throat. *CNS:* fatigue, lethargy, insomnia, depression, nightmares, hallucinations, dizziness. *GI:* vomiting, diarrhea, nausea, constipation. *GU:* decreased sexual ability. *MS:* muscle aches, arthralgia. *Misc:* fever.

Nursing implications/Documentation

Possible nursing diagnoses: Activity intolerance; Fatigue; Potential for injury.

♦ Assess mental status, and record pulse and blood pressure (if possible, lying, sitting, and standing, in both arms) before administration, and frequently thereafter until response is determined.

♦ Consult with physician to determine desired therapeutic range for blood pressure and heart rate (parameters for withholding the medication should be written by physician).

♦ Ascertain that baseline CBC, electrolytes, BUN, creatinine, and liver function studies have been obtained before giving first dose; report abnormalities and monitor closely thereafter.

♦ If on a cardiac monitor, watch for prolonged PR intervals; report if greater than 0.2 seconds.

♦ Be aware that cardioselectivity is relevant only at low doses; daily doses greater than 100 mg should be used with great caution for patients with bronchospastic disease.

♦ Monitor for allergic reactions and signs of confusion, dizziness, bradycardia, CHF, and hypotension; hold drug and report immediately if these occur.

♦ Supervise ambulation until response is determined.

♦ Document and monitor daily weight, and intake and output; report significant negative or positive balance.

Patient & family teaching/Home care

Possible nursing diagnoses: Knowledge deficit; Impaired home maintenance management; Altered sexuality patterns.

♦ Explain that taking this drug with meals or after will enhance absorption.

♦ Explain the importance of taking this drug exactly as prescribed, even when feeling well; warn not to discontinue drug abruptly (may precipitate anginal attack or MI).

♦ Stress the importance of good medical follow-up, explain that this drug reduces "wear and tear" on blood vessels, reduces the workload of the heart, and improves longevity and health.

♦ Teach how to monitor pulse and blood pressure; emphasize that syncope, hypertension or hypotension, or persistent dizziness should be reported; provide pulse and blood pressure parameters for withholding medication.

♦ Advise changing positions slowly to avoid dizziness.

♦ Encourage daily monitoring of weight, and reporting sudden weight gain (frequently is fluid retention).

♦ Warn against drinking alcohol or taking *any* OTC drugs without physician approval (some interactions can cause severe reactions).

♦ Explain that this drug may alter sexual ability; explore concerns and seek consultation as needed.

♦ *See Beta Adrenergic Blockers, Antihypertensives, and Antianginal overviews for more information.*

metronidazole

me-troe-ni'da-zole

♣Apo-Metronidazole, Flagyl, Metizol, Metric 21, ♣Metrogyl, ♣Metrozine, Metryl, ♣Neo-Metric, ♣Novonidazol, ♣PMS-Metronidazole, Protostat

metronidazole hydrochloride: *Flagyl I.V., Flagyl I.V. RTU, Metro I.V.,* ♣*Novonidazol*

Class: Anti-infective, Antibiotic, Amebicide, Trichomonacide, Bacteriocide, Antiprotozoal

PEDS	PREG	GERI
♛	B	♛

Action Kills susceptible amoebas, trichomonads, and bacteria (amebicidal, trichomonacidal, and bactericidal) by disrupting their ability to synthesize proteins (effective against anaerobic bacteria, *Trichomonas vaginalis, Entamoeba histolytica,* and *Giardia lamblia*).

Use/Therapeutic goal/Outcome

Infections (trichomoniasis, intestinal and liver amebiasis, intra-abdominal infections, skin and skin structure infections, bone and joint infections, CNS infections, septicemia, endocarditis): Resolution of infection. *Outcome criteria:* Absence of pathogenic growth on cultures; absence of clinical manifestations of infection (pain, redness, swelling, heat, drainage, diarrhea).

Dose range/Administration

Interaction alert: Do not mix with any other drug IV. Alcohol causes disulfiram-like reaction. Disulfiram causes acute psychoses and confusion. Potentiates action of anticoagulants.

❦ **Give PO doses with meals to reduce GI symptoms and metallic taste.**

Anaerobic bacterial infections: Adult: IV: *Loading dose:* 15 mg/kg (about 1 g/70 kg) over 1 hr. *Maintenance dose:* 7.5 mg/kg (about 500 mg/70 kg) IV or PO q6h.

Prophylaxis of infection from potentially contaminated colo-rectal surgery: Adult: IV: 15 mg/kg over 30–60 min, completed 1 hr before surgery, followed by 7.5 mg/kg over 30–60 min 6 and 12 hr later.

Trichomoniasis: Adult: PO: 250 mg tid for 7 days, or 2 g in a single dose if there is a problem with compliance. (Treat both female and male, even if male has negative cultures.) *For refractory trichomoniasis:* Additional 250 mg bid for 10 days.

Intestinal amoebas: Adult: PO: 500–750 mg tid for 5–10 days. *Child:* PO: 35–50 mg/kg/day in 3 divided doses for 10 days.

Giardiasis: Adult: PO: 250 mg tid for 5 days. *Child:* PO: 5 mg/kg/day in 3 divided doses for 5 days.

Amoebic liver abscess: Adult: PO: 500–700 mg tid for 5–10 days. *Child:* PO: 35–50 mg/kg/day in 3 divided doses for 10 days.

Clinical alert: Never give as an IV bolus. Administer by slow infusion over 1 hour. Follow the instructions precisely for reconstitution in the manufacturer's package insert.

Contraindications/Precautions

PREG B

Contraindicated in hypersensitivity to metronidazole. *Use with caution* in kidney or liver disease, contracted visual or color fields, blood dyscrasia, and CNS disorders.

✋ **Contraindicated in the first trimester of pregnancy and for nursing mothers. Use with caution for children and the elderly.**

Safe use for other pregnant mothers has not been established.

Side effects/Adverse reactions

Hypersensitivity: itching, rashes, hives, fever, chills. *GI:* dry mouth, anorexia, cramping, nausea, vomiting, diarrhea, constipation, epigastric discomfort, gastritis, anal itching or irritation. *CNS:* weakness, vertigo, malaise, headache, nervousness, confusion, depression, insomnia, drowsiness, peripheral neuropathy. *CV:* pain, redness, swelling, thrombophlebitis at injection site, flattened T waves on EKG. *GU:* dysuria, polyuria, darkened urine, incontinence, cystitis, decreased libido, dyspareunia, dryness of the vulva and vagina, sense of pelvic pressure. *Misc:* superinfection (especially Candida).

Nursing implications/Documentation

Possible nursing diagnoses: Potential for infection; Diarrhea; Constipation.

♦ Ensure that accurate height and weight are recorded to calculate drug dosage.

♦ Obtain necessary cultures (stool specimens should go to the lab while still warm) and baseline lab studies (CBC, electrolytes, BUN, creatinine, liver function) before starting metronidazole; monitor closely thereafter if therapy is prolonged.

♦ Provide preferred fluids; monitor and document stools, and intake and output, to ensure adequate hydration.

♦ Monitor bowel elimination: report diarrhea; treat constipation before problem is severe.

♦ Observe for and report symptoms of superinfection (vaginal or anal irritation, foul-smelling drainage, mouth lesions, sudden fever).

Patient & family teaching/Home care

Possible nursing diagnoses: Knowledge deficit; Impaired home maintenance management.

♦ Advise to take oral doses with food to reduce GI irritation.

♦ Teach the need to report symptoms of allergy or new symptoms of illness (sore throat, fever, diarrhea, genital itching); medication may need to be changed.

♦ Stress the importance of good handwashing after bowel movements and of daily cleansing of toilets.

♦ For trichomoniasis, discourage sex unless a condom is worn; advise that sexual partner

M

may also require treatment, even though symptoms may not be present.

♦ For intestinal amoebas, emphasize the importance of returning for follow-up cultures for at least 3 months.

♦ Point out the importance of taking metronidazole for the entire time prescribed, even if symptoms abate.

♦ Warn that drinking alcohol while taking this drug may result in a violent reaction.

♦ *See Anti-infectives overview for more information.*

metyrosine
me-tye'roe-seen

Demser

Class: Antihypertensive, Enzyme inhibitor

PEDS	PREG	GERI
☙	C	☙

Action Reduces blood pressure by inhibiting the enzyme tyrosine hydroylase which is involved in catecholamines synthesis.

Use/Therapeutic goal/Outcome

Hypertension in patients with pheochromocytoma: Reduction of blood pressure. **Outcome criteria:** Blood pressure within normal limits.

Dose range/Administration

Interaction alert: Use with alcohol, CNS depressants, and tricyclic antidepressants may increase sedative effects.

Adult: PO: 250 mg qid; may increase by 250 mg/day. *Maximum dose:* 4 g/day.

Clinical alert: Give with a full glass of water to prevent crystalluria. Be aware that peak effect of this drug usually occurs 2–3 days after treatment is initiated.

Contraindications/Precautions
PREG C

Contraindicated in hypersensitivity to metyrosine, and in essential hypertension. **Use with caution** in renal or hepatic disease.

☙ Use with caution for the elderly. Safe use for children and pregnant or nursing mothers has not been established.

Side effects/Adverse reactions

Hypersensitivity: rash, urticaria. **CNS:** sedation, extrapyramidal symptoms. **GI:** nausea, vomiting, abdominal pain, diarrhea. **GU:** hematuria, crystalluria, impotence.

Nursing implications/Documentation

Possible nursing diagnoses: Activity intolerance; Fatigue; Potential for injury; Fluid volume deficit.

♦ Assess mental status, and record pulse and blood pressure (lying, sitting, and standing, in both arms) prior to administration, and frequently thereafter until response is determined.

♦ Consult with physician to determine desired therapeutic range for blood pressure (be aware that some patients may require a slightly elevated blood pressure to perfuse vital organs).

♦ Ascertain that baseline urinalysis (to check for crystalluria and catecholamine measurements), CBC, electrolytes, BUN, creatinine, and liver function studies have been obtained before giving first dose; report abnormalities and monitor closely thereafter.

♦ Monitor for allergic reactions, and for confusion, dizziness, bradycardia, arrhythmias, hypotension; hold drug and report immediately if these occur.

♦ Supervise ambulation until response is determined.

♦ Document and monitor daily weight, and intake and output (intake goal should be 2 liters; urinary output should be 2 L/day).

♦ Be aware that increased IV fluids may be necessary to avoid hypotension and decreased organ perfusion caused by vasodilation and expanded volume capacity.

Patient & family teaching/Home care

Possible nursing diagnoses: Knowledge deficit; Impaired home maintenance management; Altered sexuality patterns.

♦ Explain the importance of taking medication exactly as prescribed, even when feeling well; stress the importance of taking medication with a full glass of water.

♦ Teach how to monitor pulse and blood pressure; emphasize that syncope, hypertension or hypotension, palpitations, tachycardia, or persistent dizziness should be reported.

♦ Advise changing positions slowly to avoid dizziness; warn that fatigue may be experienced at beginning of therapy, but should subside.

♦ Encourage daily monitoring of weight and reporting sudden weight gain (frequently fluid retention).

- Explain that driving should be avoided until response is determined (may cause drowsiness); use with alcohol may increase drowsiness.
- Warn against taking *any* OTC drugs without physician approval (some interactions can cause severe reactions).
- Counsel individuals with sexual concerns.
- *See Antihypertensives overview for more information.*

mexiletine
mex-il'e-teen

mexiletine hydrochloride: *Mexitil*
Class: Antiarrhythmic (Class IB)

PEDS	PREG	GERI
✋	C	✋

Action Suppresses ventricular ectopy by decreasing the duration of the action potential and increasing the electrical stimulation in the ventricle and in the His-Purkinje system (by inhibiting inward sodium current). Has a membrane-stabilizing effect. Structure and electrophysiologic properties are similar to lidocaine.

Use/Therapeutic goal/Outcome
Refractory ventricular arrhythmias, including premature ventricular contractions (PVCs) and ventricular tachycardia: Prevention of ventricular arrhythmias and promotion of effective heartbeat. *Outcome criteria:* Absence of ventricular ectopy on EKG; palpable regular pulses.

Dose range/Administration
Interaction alert: Phenytoin has been shown to decrease mexiletine serum levels. Cimetidine may increase serum drug levels.

✊ **Give with food to minimize GI upset.**
Adult: PO: *Loading dose:* 400 mg for rapid control of ventricular arrhythmias. *Maintenance dose:* 150–400 mg q6-8h, or q12h. Dose adjustments in 50–100 mg increments. *Maximum dose:* 1200 mg/day.

Contraindications/Precautions
PREG
C

Contraindicated in hypersensitivity to amide-type anesthetics, and in cardiogenic shock or second- or third-degree heart block. *Use with caution* in presence of congestive heart failure or sick sinus syndrome.

✋ **Use with caution for the elderly. Safe use for children and pregnant or nursing mothers has not been established.**

Side effects/Adverse reactions
Hypersensitivity: itching, rashes. **CV:** hypotension, bradycardia, chest pain, exacerbation of ventricular arrhythmias. **CNS:** tremor, dizziness, paresthesias, ataxia, confusion, headache, anxiety. **GI:** nausea, vomiting, dyspepsia. **Eye:** visual disturbances, nystagmus.

Nursing implications/Documentation
Possible nursing diagnoses: Potential for injury; Activity intolerance.

- Be sure to check baseline chest X-ray, EKG, and laboratory studies (CBC, sodium, potassium, chloride, carbon dioxide, magnesium, BUN, creatinine, SGPT, and LDH) before giving first dose; monitor closely thereafter as indicated by clinical condition.
- Remember that oxygen requirements must be met, and that electrolyte imbalances (especially potassium and magnesium) and abnormal blood pH must be corrected, before expected antiarrhythmic effect can be seen; report abnormalities immediately.
- Document baseline vital signs, lung sounds, and cardiac monitor strip (measure and record PR and QRS segments) before giving first dose and at least every 8 hr; monitor closely until response is determined; report if prolongation in PR or QRS segment is noted.
- Monitor for and report signs of CHF, hypotension, tachycardia, and bradycardia (drug may have to be discontinued).
- Observe mental status closely; report confusion or ataxia and institute measures to prevent injury (keep patient in bed with side rails up).
- Coordinate care to provide frequent rest periods.

Patient & family teaching/Home care
Possible nursing diagnoses: Fear; Knowledge deficit; Impaired home maintenance management.

- Explain that the purpose of this drug is to prevent arrhythmias and promote an effective heartbeat.
- Stress the need to follow dose regimen closely (the drug should be taken at the same time each day) and the need to return for med-

M

ical follow-up for early detection of adverse reactions.

♦ Teach how to assess pulse for irregularities in rhythm and rate; stress that irregularities be reported.

♦ Emphasize the need to pace activities, avoid stress, and plan for rest periods.

♦ Warn against driving or operating machinery until response is determined.

♦ Stress that dizziness or "weird feelings" be reported (may be related to mexiletine).

♦ Encourage learning CPR; reinforce that survival rate of cardiac arrest is greatly increased when CPR is initiated immediately.

♦ *See Antiarrhythmics overview for more information.*

mezlocillin
mez-loe-sill'in

mezlocillin sodium: *Mezlin*

Class: Anti-infective, Antibiotic, Extended-spectrum penicillin

PEDS	PREG	GERI
☝	B	☝

Action Extended-spectrum, usually bactericidal antibiotic; kills bacteria by inhibiting cell wall synthesis.

Use/Therapeutic goal/Outcome

Systemic infections (lower respiratory tract, urinary, GI, GYN, septicemia): Resolution of infection. *Outcome criteria:* Absence of pathogenic growth on cultures, absence of clinical manifestations of infection (fever, pain, redness, heat, swelling, odor, dysuria, drainage), normal WBC count, improvement of X rays.

Dose range/Administration

Interaction alert: Inactivates aminoglycosides (e.g., tobramycin and gentamicin); do not mix in solution. Give at least 1 hour after bacteriostatic antibiotics or aminoglycosides for optimal effect. Probenecid inhibits excretion of mezlocillin and may be given to increase serum levels of the drug. Increases effect of anticoagulants (because of anti-platelet effect).

Adult: IM, IV: 200–300 mg/kg/day, in divided doses q4-6h. *Maximum dose:* 350 mg/kg/day in severe cases. *Child > 1 mo:* IM, IV: 50 mg/kg, in divided doses q4h.

Clinical alert: Almost always given with another antibiotic.

Contraindications/Precautions
PREG
B

Contraindicated in allergy to penicillin. *Use with caution* in cephalosporin sensitivity, history of allergic responses (e.g., other drugs, hay fever, asthma), and renal insufficiency.

☝ Use with caution for pregnant or nursing mothers and for children and the elderly. Safe use for infants under 1 month has not been established.

Side effects/Adverse reactions

Hypersensitivity: itching, rashes, urticaria, fever, difficulty breathing, anaphylaxis. *GI:* nausea, vomiting, diarrhea, pseudomembranous colitis. *CV:* pain, redness, swelling, thrombophlebitis at injection site. *GU:* glomerulonephritis. *Hem:* thrombocytopenia, leukopenia, hypokalemia, hypernatremia, bleeding (with high doses), slight elevation in SGOT and SGPT. *CNS:* neuromuscular irritability. *Misc:* bone marrow depression, superinfection.

Nursing implications/Documentation

Possible nursing diagnoses: Potential for infection; Diarrhea.

♦ Determine history of allergies, and (regardless of history) monitor closely for allergic reactions.

♦ Obtain baseline CBC, creatinine, liver function studies, sodium, and necessary cultures before administering first dose; monitor closely thereafter if therapy is prolonged.

♦ Be aware that mezlocillin may cause a false-positive urine protein test.

♦ Encourage fluids, and record and monitor intake and output, to ensure adequate hydration; report significant negative or positive balance.

♦ Monitor for and report signs of superinfection (sore throat, fever, fatigue, thrush, vaginal discharge, diarrhea).

♦ For patients on anticoagulants, monitor for unusual bruising or bleeding.

Patient & family teaching/Home care

Possible nursing diagnoses: Knowledge deficit; Impaired home maintenance management.

♦ Teach the importance of reporting allergic symptoms, diarrhea, signs and symptoms that do not abate, or *any* new signs and symptoms of discomfort that might indicate superinfection (medication regimen may have to be changed).

◆ Advise drinking 2–3 L of fluids daily to maintain adequate hydration (especially important if fever exists).

◆ Stress the importance of taking antibiotics for the entire time prescribed, even if signs and symptoms abate.

◆ *See Anti-infectives overview for more information.*

miconazole (parenteral)   *mi-kon'a-zole*

Monistat I.V.

Class: Anti-infective, Antifungal

PEDS	PREG	GERI
🖐	C	🖐

Action Kills fungi (fungicidal) or limits fungal growth (fungistatic) by inhibiting ergosterol syntheses, which increases cell membrane permeability and allows leakage of intracellular components.

Use/Therapeutic goal/Outcome

Fungal infections (candidiasis, chronic mucocutaneous candidiasis, fungal meningitis, paracoccidioidomycosis, cryptococcosis, coccidioidomycosis): Resolution of infection. *Outcome criteria:* Absence of pathogenic growth on culture; absence of clinical manifestations of infection (redness, pain, swelling, fever, drainage, increased WBC count).

Dose range/Administration

Interaction alert: Do not use with rifampin or isoniazid (decreases antifungal effect). Metabolism of oral anticoagulants and antibiotic agents may be decreased.

Adult: IV: 200–3600 mg/day (depending upon diagnosis and causative organism) divided in 3 doses, q8h. Dilute each 20 mg ampule in at least 200 ml of NS and infuse at 10 mg/hr (rapid infusion may produce arrhythmias). D5W may be used if necessary. *Intrathecal:* As an adjunct to IV therapy, 20 mg q 3–7 days. *Child 1–12 yrs:* IV: 20–40 mg/kg/day slowly, not over 15 mg/kg per infusion.

Clinical alert: For IV administration, have epinephrine ready and monitor patient *closely* during administration of first dose (anaphylaxis and cardiorespiratory arrest has occurred with first dose). To reduce adverse GI symptoms, avoid administering at mealtime or reduce IV rate (sometimes an antiemetic will be given before doses).

Contraindications/Precautions   PREG C

Contraindicated in hypersensitivity to miconazole or paraben preservative. *Use with caution* in impaired kidney or liver function.

🖐 **Contraindicated in the first trimester of pregnancy and for children under 1 year. Use with caution for older children, pregnant women (second and third trimesters), and the elderly.**

Side effects/Adverse reactions

Hypersensitivity: itching, rashes, pruritus, anaphylaxis. *GI:* anorexia, nausea, vomiting, diarrhea. *CNS:* drowsiness, dizziness, headache. *CV:* tachycardia, arrhythmias with rapid IV infusion, thrombophlebitis at infusion site. *Hem:* hyponatremia, anemia, thrombocytopenia.

Nursing implications/Documentation

Possible nursing diagnoses: Potential for infection; Altered nutrition: less than body requirements.

◆ Obtain necessary cultures before starting miconazole.

◆ Monitor and record intake and output, and ensure adequate hydration (report excessive negative or positive balance).

◆ Monitor CBC and electrolytes at least weekly.

Patient & family teaching/Home care

Possible nursing diagnoses: Knowledge deficit; Impaired home maintenance management.

◆ Advise reporting unusual sensations during administration as they may be side effects that may require treatment.

◆ Stress the need to take miconazole for the entire time prescribed, even if symptoms abate (long-term treatment, from 2 wks to 3 mos may be required).

◆ *See Anti-infectives overview for more information.*

miconazole (topical)   *mi-kon'a-zole*

miconazole nitrate: **Micatin, Monistat-Derm Cream and Lotion, Monistat Vaginal Cream, Monistat 7 Vaginal Suppository, Monistat 3 Vaginal Suppository**

Class: Anti-infective, Antifungal

PEDS	PREG	GERI
OK	C	OK

Action Kills fungi (fungicidal) or limits fungal growth (fungistatic) by inhibiting ergosterol syntheses, which increases cell membrane permeability and allows leakage of intracellular components.

Use/Therapeutic goal/Outcome

Fungal infections (tinea pedis, tinea cruris, tinea corporis, tinea versicolor, cutaneous candidiasis, other common dermatophytes): Resolution of infection. ***Outcome criteria:*** After a fuil course of treatment, absence of signs and symptoms of infection (redness, itching, burning, scaling).

Vulvovaginal monilia (candidiasis): Resolution of infection. ***Outcome criteria:*** After a full course of treatment, absence of signs and symptoms of vaginitis (white "cheesy" drainage, itching, burning, redness of the vulva).

Dose range/Administration

Adult: *Topical:* Apply or spray sparingly bid for 2–4 weeks. *Vaginal suppository:* 1 qhs for 3 (Monistat 3) or for 7 (Monistat 7) consecutive nights. *Vaginal cream:* 1 applicatorful qhs for 7 nights.

Clinical alert: For vaginal route, insert high into the vagina with applicator provided (preferably at bedtime). This drug is available OTC.

PREG
C

Contraindications/Precautions

Contraindicated in hypersensitivity to miconazole. ***Use with caution*** in impaired kidney or liver function.

♨ **Contraindicated in first trimester of pregnancy. Use with caution in second and third trimesters.**

Side effects/Adverse reactions

Hypersensitivity: (rare) burning, maceration. ***GU:*** (with vaginal cream) vulvovaginal itching, burning, or irritation.

Nursing implications/Documentation

Possible nursing diagnoses: Potential for infection; Impaired tissue integrity.

♦ Obtain necessary cultures before starting miconazole (cultures are not *always* taken).

♦ Provide good perineal hygiene; monitor for and report chemical irritation.

Patient & family teaching/Home care

Possible nursing diagnoses: Knowledge deficit; Impaired home maintenance management; Altered sexuality patterns.

♦ Stress the importance of using the cream as ordered for the entire time prescribed, even if symptoms abate.

♦ Advise reporting if there is no improvement after 3 days or if new symptoms arise.

♦ Caution women to read package insert carefully; warn that cream form may damage diaphragms.

♦ Advise checking when intercourse may be resumed; for persistent infections, recommend that sexual partner be evaluated.

♦ Explore concerns about sexuality; refer for counseling as needed.

♦ *See Anti-infective overview for more information.*

midazolam
my-daz'owe-lam

midazolam hydrochloride: ***Versed***
Class: Benzodiazepine, Sedative-hypnotic

PEDS	PREG	GERI	CONTROLLED SUBSTANCE
♨	**D**	♨	**IV**

Action Produces relaxation and sleep and amnesia by causing CNS depression at limbic and subcortical levels. Has a rapid onset of action (within 1 1/2 to 3 min when given IV, and within 15 to 30 min when given IM).

Use/Therapeutic goal/Outcome

Sedation (pre-operative, pre-procedure, during procedure, or during induction to anesthesia): Promotion of relaxation and sleep (without complete loss of consciousness), reduction of sensitivity to discomfort, promotion of amnesia for uncomfortable events. ***Outcome criteria:*** Report of feeling comfortable, less anxious and more relaxed; observable drowsiness or sleep; inability to recall events of procedure.

Dose range/Administration

Interaction alert: Narcotics, analgesics, or other CNS depressants intensify respiratory and CNS depression (may require dosage adjustment).

Preoperative sedation: Adult: IM: 0.07–0.08 mg/kg deep into large muscle mass 1 hr preoperatively. May be given in conjunction with atropine, scopolamine, or reduced-dose narcotic. Mixes well in syringe with atropine, scopolamine, morphine, or meperidine.

Pre-procedure conscious sedation: Adult: IV: 0.1–0.15 mg/kg slowly (maximum of 0.2 mg/kg if given without narcotics).

M

Induction of general anesthesia: **Adult:** IV: 0.3–0.35 mg/kg over 20–30 seconds. May repeat 1/4 of initial dose (maximum dose of 0.6 mg/kg).

Clinical alert: Because initial response may be profound, keep patient in bed with side rails up and call bell in reach immediately after administration. Be aware that this drug should be given only in a facility where emergency drugs and equipment are readily available.

Contraindications/Precautions

PREG D

Contraindicated in hypersensitivity or intolerance to midazolam hydrochloride or other benzodiazepines, and in shock, coma, alcoholic intoxication, glaucoma. ***Use with caution*** in hepatic or renal impairment, neuromuscular disorders, or pulmonary disease.

🖑 **Use with caution for the elderly; those over 55 require fewer doses. Safe use for children and for pregnant or nursing mothers has not been established.**

Side effects/Adverse reactions

Hypersensitivity: itching, rashes, hives. ***CNS:*** profound drowsiness, hangover, headache, dizziness, ataxia. ***Resp:*** respiratory depression, apnea. ***CV:*** abnormal pulse rate or blood pressure. ***GI:*** vomiting, hiccups.

Nursing implications/Documentation

Possible nursing diagnoses: Potential for injury; Sensory, perceptual alterations (visual and auditory)

◆ Document mental status before administration, monitor patient activity closely following administration, and employ appropriate measures to ensure safety (i.e., side rails up, call bell within reach, and no unsupervised smoking).

◆ For IV route, document vital signs every 5–15 min during and after administration, until recovered; monitor closely for extravasation.

Patient & family teaching/Home care

Possible nursing diagnoses: Anxiety; Fear.

◆ Encourage voicing of questions and concerns; stress that this drug has been very successful in promoting comfort before and during procedures.

◆ Explain that amnesia of procedure may occur.

◆ Emphasize the need to remain in bed until recovered.

◆ *See Antianxiety Agents, Sedatives, and Hypnotics overview for more information.*

minocycline

mi-no-sye'kleen

minocycline hydrochloride: ***Minocin***, 🍁***Minomycin***, 🍁***Minomycin IV***

Class: Anti-infective, Broad-spectrum tetracycline antibiotic

PEDS	PREG	GERI
🖑	D	🖑

Action Limits bacterial growth (bateriostatic) by binding to the 30 S ribosomal subunit and inhibiting protein synthesis.

Use/Therapeutic goal/Outcome

Infections (acne, gonorrhea, syphilis, and infections caused by susceptible gram-negative and gram-positive pathogens, trachoma, amebiasis, and chlamydia): Prevention or resolution of infection. ***Outcome criteria:*** Absence of pathogenic growth on cultures, absence of clinical manifestations of infection (fever, pain, swelling, redness, heat, odor, drainage, productive cough, dysuria, frequency), normal WBC count, normal X rays.

Dose range/Administration

Interaction alert: Do not mix any other drug with IV minocycline. Antacids, milk, and other dairy products inhibit absorption. Give oral dose 2 hours before or 3 hours after iron products. Methoxyflurane increases risk of nephrotoxicity; avoid use. May decrease effectiveness of oral contraceptives and penicillins.

🍃 **Give with food to reduce GI symptoms.**

Adult: PO: 200 mg initially, then 100 mg q12h; or 100–200 mg, then 50 mg qid. IV: 200 mg initially, then 100 mg q12h. *Maximum dose:* 400 mg/24 hrs. **Child <45 kg, > 8 yrs:** PO, IV: 4 mg/kg initially, then 2 mg/kg given orally in divided doses q12h. If initial dose is IV, give in 500–1000 cc solution over 6 hrs.

Clinical alert: Monitor closely for thrombophlebitis and extravasation (minocycline is very irritating to tissues). Taking outdated tetracyclines has been associated with fatal nephrotoxicity.

Contraindications/Precautions

PREG D

Contraindicated in hypersensitivity to minocycline or other tetracyclines; oral route not intended for treatment of meningococcal infections. *Use with caution* in impaired renal or liver function.

🖐 **Contraindicated for children under 8 years (causes tooth discoloration and retards bone growth) and pregnant or nursing mothers. Use with caution for the elderly.**

Side effects/Adverse reactions

Hypersensitivity: (rare) itching, rashes, fever, anaphylaxis. *GI:* sore throat, glossitis, stomatitis, epigastric discomfort, nausea, cramps, diarrhea, enterocolitis, anogenital inflammation, hepatotoxicity. *CNS:* lightheadedness, headache, intracranial hypertension. *Skin:* photosensitivity. *CV:* pericarditis. *Hem:* blood dyscrasias; thrombophlebitis (with IV route). *Ear:* vestibular toxicity (causing dizziness).

Nursing implications/Documentation

Possible nursing diagnoses: Potential for infection; Potential fluid volume deficit.

♦ Determine history of allergies, and (regardless of history) monitor closely for allergic reactions.

♦ Weigh patient and obtain baseline CBC, BUN, creatinine, liver function studies, and necessary culture specimens before administering first dose; monitor closely thereafter if therapy is prolonged.

♦ Encourage fluids, and record and monitor intake and output, to ensure adequate hydration and urine output.

♦ Monitor for and report symptoms of superinfection (mouth lesions, thrush, vaginal irritation, diarrhea, respiratory symptoms).

♦ If there is no improvement within 3–5 days, consult with physician to determine if antibiotic regimen should be re-evaluated (and new cultures drawn).

Patient & family teaching/Home care

Possible nursing diagnoses: Knowledge deficit, Impaired home maintenance management.

♦ Advise taking minocycline with food if GI symptoms are experienced.

♦ Advise avoiding exposure to sunlight and warn that photosensitivity may continue for weeks after minocycline has been discontinued.

♦ Teach the need to report dizziness (may be due to vestibular toxicity), or persistent or new signs and symptoms of illness (e.g., fever, mouth lesions, vaginal irritation, respiratory symptoms, diarrhea); medication change may be necessary.

♦ Explain the importance of taking antibiotics for the entire time prescribed, even if symptoms abate.

♦ Caution women that this drug may decrease effectiveness of oral contraceptives.

♦ *See Anti-infectives overview for more information.*

minoxidil
mi-nox'-i-dil

Loniten

Class: Antihypertensive, Vasodilator

PEDS	PREG	GERI
🖐	C	🖐

Action Reduces blood pressure by relaxing arteriolar smooth muscle. Causes a reflex increase in heart rate and cardiac output.

Use/Therapeutic goal/Outcome

Hypertension: Reduction of blood pressure. *Outcome criteria:* Blood pressure within normal limits.

Dose range/Administration

Interaction alert: Epinephrine and norepinephrine may potentiate reflex cardiac stimulation. Use with guanethidine may cause severe hypotension.

Adult: PO: 5 mg. *Maintenance dose:* 10–40 mg/day. *Maximum dose:* 100 mg/day. *Child:* PO: 0.2 mg/kg/day. *Maintenance dose:* 0.25–1 mg/kg/day. *Maximum dose:* 50 mg/day.

Clinical alert: Monitor the elderly for increased hypotensive effects.

Contraindications/Precautions
PREG C

Contraindicated in hypersensitivity to minoxidil, and in pheochromocytoma. *Use with caution* in recent myocardial infarction, coronary artery disease and CHF.

🖐 **Use with caution for the elderly. Safe use for children and pregnant women has not been established.**

Side effects/Adverse reactions

Hypersensitivity: rash, urticaria. *CV:* tachycardia, pericardial effusion or tamponade, CHF, EKG changes. *Misc:* edema, Stevens-Johnson syndrome, breast tenderness, unusual hair growth (particularly in females), sodium and fluid retention.

M

Nursing implications/Documentation

Possible nursing diagnoses: Activity intolerance; Fatigue; Potential for injury.

• Assess mental status, and record pulse and blood pressure (lying, sitting, and standing in both arms) prior to administration, and frequently thereafter until response is determined.

• Consult with physician to determine desired therapeutic range for blood pressure (be aware that some patients may require a slightly elevated blood pressure to perfuse vital organs).

• Ascertain that baseline, CBC, electrolytes, BUN, creatinine, and liver function studies have been obtained before giving first dose; report abnormalities and monitor closely thereafter.

• Monitor for allergic reactions and for confusion, dizziness, rales, tachycardia, arrhythmias, and hypotension; hold drug and report immediately if these occur.

• Supervise ambulation until response is determined.

• Document and monitor daily weight, and intake and output; report significant negative or positive balance.

Patient & family teaching/Home care

Possible nursing diagnoses: Altered sexuality patterns; Knowledge deficit; Impaired home maintenance management.

• Explain the importance of taking antihypertensive medications exactly as prescribed, even when feeling well.

• Stress the importance of good medical follow-up, explain that this drug reduces "wear and tear" on blood vessels, and improves longevity and health.

• Teach how to monitor pulse and blood pressure; emphasize that syncope, palpitations, tachycardia, chest pains, hypertension or hypotension, or persistent dizziness should be reported immediately.

• Advise changing positions slowly to avoid dizziness.

• Encourage daily monitoring of weight and reporting sudden weight gain (frequently is fluid retention).

• Warn against taking *any* OTC drugs without physician approval (some interactions can cause severe reactions).

• Provide package insert for minoxidil (has been specifically written for lay people) for home use.

• Advise that this drug is likely to increase hair growth, which can be managed with a depilatory or shaving.

◆ *See Antihypertensives overview for more information.*

misoprostol
mye-soe-prost'ole

Cytotec

Class: Gastric mucosa protectant, Antiulcer agent

PEDS	PREG	GERI
✋	X	OK

Action Enhances natural gastromucosal defense mechanisms by increasing production of gastric mucus and mucosal secretion of bicarbonate; inhibits gastric acid secretion by direct action on parietal cells.

Use/Therapeutic goal/Outcome

Gastric ulcers induced by non-steroidal anti-inflammatory drugs (NSAIDs): Prevention of gastric ulcers in high-risk patients (elderly, seriously ill, or with previous history of ulcer). *Outcome criteria:* Stools negative for blood, stable hemoglobin and hematocrit; report of absence of epigastric pain.

Dose range/Administration

Interaction alert: Antacids containing magnesium increases risk of diarrhea.

🖐 **Give with meals and at bedtime to increase effectiveness.**

Adult: PO: 100–200 mcg qid.

Clinical alert: Misoprostol should be started with the initiation of NSAID therapy in high-risk patients.

Contraindications/Precautions
PREG
X

Contraindicated in hypersensitivity to prostaglandins. *Use with caution* in cerebral vascular disease, coronary artery disease, and epilepsy.

🖐 **Contraindicated for pregnant or nursing mothers. Use with caution for children.**

Side effects/Adverse reactions

Hypersensitivity: cough, dyspnea, wheezing, bronchospasm. *GI:* diarrhea, nausea, abdominal pain, flatulence. *CNS:* headache. *GU:*

▶

menstrual cramps, (in pregnancy) uterine contractions and incomplete abortion.

Nursing implications/Documentation

Possible nursing diagnoses: Diarrhea; Pain.

♦ For women of childbearing age, record negative results of pregnancy test within 2 weeks prior to beginning therapy; therapy should be initiated on second or third day of next normal menstrual cycle.

♦ Assess and document frequency and character of stools, especially early in therapy.

Patient & family teaching/Home care

Possible nursing diagnoses: Knowledge deficit; Impaired home maintenance management.

♦ Advise taking doses with meals and at bedtime to increase effectiveness.

♦ Caution that diarrhea may develop during initial period of therapy, but usually resolves in about 1 week; instruct to report prolonged diarrhea.

♦ Stress the need to avoid antacids containing magnesium.

♦ Warn women to use reliable contraception during therapy (misoprostol may cause abortion); teach the need to discontinue medication and notify physician if pregnancy is planned or suspected.

mitomycin
mye-toe-mey'sin

mitomycin-C: **Mutamycin**

Class: Antineoplastic (antibiotic) agent

PEDS	PREG	GERI
♨	D	♨

Action Kills rapidly growing cells (cancer, hair follicles, bone marrow, GI lining, ova, and sperm) by interfering with DNA replication and RNA transcription by alkylation (cross-linking of DNA occurs). Is cell-cycle–phase nonspecific.

Use/Therapeutic goal/Outcome

Disseminated adenocarcinoma of stomach and pancreas; cancer of the breast, colon, head, neck, and lung; malignant melanoma: Elimination or suppression of malignant cell proliferation. **Outcome criteria:** Tumor and disease regression or stabilization on radiologic and physical examination (usually evident within 2 courses of therapy).

Dose range/Administration

Interaction alert: Radiation and other antineoplastic agents may cause increased toxicity. Vinca alkaloids may cause severe bronchospasm in susceptible individuals.

Adult: IV: 2 mg/m^2/day for 5 days, stop drug for 2 days, then repeat dose for 5 days; or 10–20 mg/m^2 in one dose, then repeat in 6–8 weeks.

Clinical alert: This drug should be given only by nurses who are knowledgeable in the comprehensive management of the administration of antineoplastic agents. Doses may vary at physician's discretion. Repeat doses are held until it is ascertained that the patient has recovered sufficiently from toxicities of previous doses. Established protocols and policies for drug preparation, administration, and accidental skin contamination *must be followed closely* (gloves or double gloves are worn when handling drug; if the drug touches the skin, the area is washed immediately with plenty of soap and water). Mitomycin is given via bolus *slowly* or via diluted IV (mixed in 50–100 ml fluid) over 15–30 min to minimize inflammation and pain along the vein. This drug is a *potent* vesicant (can cause severe damage to tissues). *Prevention* of extravasation is essential. The drug is given by administering only when it is clear that the needle is in the vein (good blood return), and the infusion site is monitored *closely* for early signs of extravasation (pain and swelling at infusion site). If extravasation is suspected, the infusion is stopped *immediately*, the physician is notified, and protocols and policies for treatment are followed.

Contraindications/Precautions
**PREG
D**

Contraindicated in hypersensitivity to mitomycin or previous idiosyncratic reactions and in thrombocytopenia, coagulation disorders, increased bleeding tendencies, or serum creatinine > 1.7 mg dl. **Use with caution** in serious infections, impaired renal function, bone marrow depression, chickenpox or herpes, or previous radiation or chemotherapy.

♨ **Contraindicated for children and pregnant or nursing mothers.**

Side effects/Adverse reactions

Hypersensitivity: pruritus, fever, hypotension. **Hem:** anemia, leukopenia, thrombocytopenia. **GI:** anorexia, nausea, vomiting, diarrhea, stomatitis, hepatotoxicity. **Skin:** alopecia; purple coloration of nail beds; pain, inflammation, and induration at injection site; cellulitis, ulceration and sloughing if extravasation occurs. *GU:* edema, urinary retention, renal failure. *CV:* hypertension. *Resp:* dyspnea, pulmonary infiltrates, fibrosis, toxicity. *CNS:* headache, confusion, drowsiness, fatigue, syncope, paresthesias. *Eye:* blurred vision.

Nursing implications/Documentation

Possible nursing diagnoses: Potential for infection; Potential for injury; Fatigue; Altered oral mucous membrane; Fluid volume deficit; Diarrhea; Altered nutrition: less than body requirements.

◆ *See important Nursing implications in Antineoplastic agents overview on page 72.*

   ◆ Check for periodic chest X rays and pulmonary function studies (pulmonary fibrosis or infiltrate can occur with cumulative doses).

   ◆ Increase fluids to 2–3 L a day to prevent renal toxicity.

   ◆ Expect erythrocyte and especially WBC and platelet counts to drop to the nadir (lowest point) at 3–6 weeks after first dose; blood studies should continue for 7 weeks after therapy stops.

Patient & family teaching/Home care

Possible nursing diagnoses: Knowledge deficit; Ineffective coping (individual and family); Hopelessness; Impaired home maintenance management.

◆ *See important Patient & family teaching in Antineoplastic agents overview on page 72.*

   ◆ Stress that shortness of breath, nonproductive cough, chest pain, or rapid pulse should be reported immediately; they may require treatment (pulmonary toxicity can occur with cumulative doses).

   ◆ Explain that drinking 2–3 L per day can reduce risk of kidney complications.

◆ *See Antineoplastic agents overview for more information.*

mitotane

mye'toe-tane

Lysodren

Class: Antineoplastic agent, Antihormone

PEDS	PREG	GERI
♉	C	♉

Action Inhibits progression of adrenal cortical carcinoma by inhibiting corticosteroid synthesis without destroying cortical cells.

Use/Therapeutic goal/Outcome

Inoperable adrenal cortical carcinoma: Suppression of malignant cell proliferation. *Outcome criteria:* After 3 months, tumor and disease regression or stabilization on radiologic and physical examination; decreased plasma cortisol levels.

Dose range/Administration

Interaction alert: CNS depressants may produce additive depressant effects. May increase metabolism of heparin (requiring an increase in heparin dosage).

   Adult: PO: 2–6 g/day in 3–4 doses; increase dose to maximum of 10 g/day. *Child:* PO: 0.5 to 1 g/day in divided doses; increase dose gradually as tolerated.

Clinical alert: In case of shock or trauma, expect that mitotane will be stopped and corticosteroid replacement therapy will be ordered (stress causes an increased risk of adrenocortical insufficiency). Higher doses may be required for obese patients (mitotane is distributed primarily to body fat).

Contraindications/Precautions

PREG
C

Contraindicated in hypersensitivity to mitotane, or after shock or trauma. *Use with caution* in preexisting liver disease.

☙ **Contraindicated for pregnant or nursing mothers. Use with caution for children and the elderly.**

Side effects/Adverse reactions

Hypersensitivity: wheezing. *GI:* anorexia, nausea, vomiting, diarrhea. *CNS:* lethargy, somnolence, dizziness, vertigo; brain damage and functional impairment may result from prolonged administration of high doses. *Skin:* transient maculopapular rash. *Eye:* blurred vision, lens opacity, retinopathy, diplopia. *GU:* hematuria, albuminuria, hemorrhagic cystitis. *CV:* hypertension, orthostatic hypotension. *Misc:* adrenal insufficiency.

Nursing implications/Documentation

Possible nursing diagnoses: Fluid volume deficit; Self-esteem disturbance; Potential for injury; Altered nutrition: less than body requirements.

◆ *See important Nursing implications in Antineoplastic agents overview on page 72.*

▶

◆ Monitor for and report early signs of adrenocortical insufficiency (weakness, fatigue, lethargy, darkening skin, diarrhea, and weight loss); be aware that many need glucocorticoids during drug treatment (a large initial dose is given because the depressed adrenals may not be able to respond and produce sufficient amounts).

◆ Check results of early-morning plasma cortisol or 24 hr urinary 17 hydoxycorticosteroid on a routine basis to determine clinical response and evaluate need for supplemental steroid therapy.

◆ Report injuries or infection immediately because supplemental steroids may be required to avert adrenocortical insufficiency.

◆ Monitor mental status; report changes in behavior.

Patient & family teaching/Home care

Possible nursing diagnoses: Impaired home maintenance management; Knowledge deficit.

◆ *See important Patient & family teaching in Antineoplastic agents overview on page 72.*

◆ Explain that results are not usually seen for 3 months.

◆ Advise taking special precautions to avoid injury or infection and reporting immediately if these occur.

◆ Recommend wearing medical alert identification.

◆ *See Antineoplastic agents overview for more information.*

mitoxantrone

mye-toe-zan'trone

mitoxantrone hydrochloride: **Novantrone**
Class: Antineoplastic agent

PEDS	PREG	GERI
🖐	D	🖐

Action Kills rapidly growing cells (cancer, hair follicles, bone marrow, GI lining, ova, and sperm) by inhibiting DNA, RNA, and protein synthesis. Is cell-cycle–phase nonspecific.

Use/Therapeutic goal/Outcome

Acute nonlymphocytic and erythroid leukemias: Elimination or suppression of malignant cell proliferation. **Outcome criteria:** Absence of blasts in peripheral blood specimen.

Dose range/Administration

Interaction alert: Do not mix IV with other drugs. Use with radiation or any other antineoplastic drugs increases risk of toxicity.

Adult: IV: 12 mg/m^2 on days 1–3, then cytosine arabinoside 100 mg/m^2/day continuous infusion on days 1–7. Repeat if response is incomplete: with mitoxantrone for 2 days and cytosine arabinoside for 5 days. *Maintenance dose:* 6 wk after induction, give 12 mg/m^2 on days 1 and 2, then cytosine arabinoside 100 mg/m^2 as 24-hr infusion on days 1–5. A second maintenance dose may be given 4 wk later.

Clinical alert: This drug should be given only by nurses who are knowledgeable in the comprehensive management of the administration of antineoplastic agents. Doses may vary at physician's discretion. Repeat doses are held until it is ascertained that the patient has recovered sufficiently from toxicities of previous doses. Established protocols and policies for drug preparation, administration, and accidental skin contamination *must be followed closely* (gloves or double gloves are worn when handling drug; if the drug touches the skin, the area is washed immediately with plenty of soap and water). Mitoxantrone is given via bolus *slowly* over 3 min in a minimum of 50–100 ml fluid to minimize inflammation and pain along the vein (mitoxantrone is not a vesicant).

Contraindications/Precautions

PREG
D

Contraindicated in hypersensitivity to mitoxantrone, and in myelosuppression, or intrathecal use (may cause paralysis). **Use with caution** in decreased bone marrow reserve, heart disease, impaired hepatic function, or a history of hyperuricemia.

🖐 **Contraindicated for pregnant or nursing mothers. Use with caution for the elderly. Safe use for children has not been established.**

Side effects/Adverse reactions

Hypersensitivity: rash, dyspnea, urticaria. **GI:** nausea, vomiting, diarrhea, mucositis, GI bleeding, jaundice. **Hem:** leukopenia, thrombocytopenia. **CV:** cardiotoxicity, CHF, dysrhythmias. **Resp:** cough, dyspnea. **Skin:** alopecia; pain and erythema at injection site (drug is not a vesicant). **CNS:** headache, seizures. **GU:** renal failure, blue-green urine. **Eye:** conjunctivitis, bluish coloring of sclera.

Nursing implications/Documentation

Possible nursing diagnoses: Potential for infection; Potential for injury; Fatigue; Altered oral mucous membrane; Fluid volume deficit; Diarrhea; Altered nutrition: less than body requirements.

◆ *See important Nursing implications in Antineoplastic agents overview on page 72.*

 ◆ Monitor for and report early signs of cardiotoxicity (increased resting pulse rate, shortness of breath, activity intolerance, swelling of the ankles and feet); risk of cardiotoxicity increases with cumulative doses of 140–160 mg/m^2 (slightly less if there is preexisting heart disease).

 ◆ Increase fluids to 2–3 L a day to prevent renal tubular damage from hyperuricemia; record and monitor intake and output (report significant positive or negative balance).

 ◆ Expect WBC to drop to the nadir (lowest point) within 10 days, with recovery within 21 days.

Patient & family teaching/Home care

Possible nursing diagnoses: Knowledge deficit; Ineffective coping (individual and family); Hopelessness; Impaired home maintenance management.

◆ *See important Patient & family teaching in Antineoplastic agents overview on page 72.*

 ◆ Stress that shortness of breath, tachycardia, activity intolerance, or swelling of the ankles and feet should be reported immediately; they may require treatment (cardiotoxicity can occur with cumulative doses).

 ◆ Explain that drinking 2–3 L per day can reduce risk of kidney complications.

 ◆ Explain that urine and sclera of the eyes may be tinted blue for the first 24 hours of administration; point out that this is harmless.

◆ *See Antineoplastic agents overview for more information.*

molindone
moe-lin'done

molindone hydrochloride: ***Moban***

Class: Dihydroindolone antipsychotic

PEDS	PREG	GERI
🤚	C	🤚

Action Exact mechanism of action has not been determined. Believed to produce calmness and alleviate psychiatric symptoms (disorders of perception, thought, consciousness, mood, affect, and social interaction) by blocking dopamine receptors in the limbic system. Blocks peripheral muscarinic, adrenergic, and histamine receptors. Also has some effect on the hypothalamus and pituitary gland, causing changes in regulation of body temperature and endocrine function. A dose of 20 mg of molindone is therapeutically equivalent to 100 mg of chlorpromazine.

Use/Therapeutic goal/Outcome

Schizophrenia and psychotic disorders: Promotion of reality orientation, reduction in agitated hyperactivity. ***Outcome criteria:*** Demonstration of reality orientation and ability to problem solve and interact with others; absence of hyperactive and agitated behavior.

Dose range/Administration

Interaction alert: Alcohol and other CNS depressants may cause excessive sedation.

 Adult: PO: 50–75 mg/day; increase after several days prn. *Maximum dose:* 225 mg/day.

Clinical alert: Available in liquid form. May give entire dose at one time. Keep IV diphenhydramine available in case of side effect of acute dystonic reaction.

Contraindications/Precautions
PREG
C

Contraindicated in hypersensitivity to molindone or related drugs, and in CNS depression, comatose states. ***Use with caution*** in seizure disorders, hypertension, parkinsonism, narrow-angle glaucoma, cardiac disease, hypotension, paralytic ileus, liver damage, prostatic hypertrophy, and bone marrow depression.

🖐 **Contraindicated for nursing mothers. Use with caution for adolescents and the elderly or debilitated. Safe use for children under 12 years and pregnant women has not be established.**

Side effects/Adverse reactions

Hypersensitivity: rash. ***CNS:*** sedation, extrapyramidal reactions (pseudoparkinsonism, akathisia, [inability to sit down, need to keep moving] dystonia, tardive dyskinesia), neuroleptic malignant syndrome (fever, tachycardia, tachypnea, profuse diaphoresis), EEG changes, dizziness. ***CV:*** orthostatic hypotension, palpitations, dysrhythmias, EKG changes. ***GI:*** appetite changes, dry mouth, constipation, abnormal liver function. ***GU:*** urinary retention or hesitancy, impaired ejaculation, amen-

▶

orrhea. ***Eye:*** blurred vision. ***Hem:*** leukopenia, agranulocytosis, hyperglycemia. ***Skin:*** photosensitivity, jaundice. ***MS:*** weight gain. ***Misc:*** gynecomastia, galactorrhea.

Nursing implications/Documentation

Possible nursing diagnoses: Potential for injury; Constipation; Altered oral mucous membrane.

- Record mental status and vital signs before and 1–2 hr after administration during initial phase of treatment, then bid until response to therapy has been established, then periodically thereafter.
- Be sure that PO doses are swallowed (not hoarded).
- Monitor for orthostatic hypotension, dizziness, and drowsiness; supervise ambulation until response is established.
- Provide special mouth care; observe for and report oral ulcers.
- Prevent constipation by monitoring bowel movements and encouraging adequate fiber and fluid intake; offer laxatives or stool softeners before problem becomes severe.
- Report persistent sore throat, fever, and malaise, because these may indicate agranulocytosis.
- Monitor for (and report immediately) signs of neuroleptic malignant syndrome (muscle rigidity, tremors, high fever, tachycardia); this is a rare, but potentially fatal, side effect.

Patient & family teaching/Home care

Possible nursing diagnoses: Sleep pattern disturbance; Impaired home maintenance management.

- Emphasize the need to continue medication, even when feeling well.
- Warn to change positions slowly to prevent dizziness.
- Stress that the effects of alcohol, sedatives and other CNS depressants, and tranquilizers may be potentiated.
- Caution to consult with physician before using OTC drugs; stress the need for ongoing medical follow-up.
- Provide a list of side effects that should be reported: involuntary movements, muscular rigidity, tremors, fever, respiratory distress, tachycardia, persistent sore throat.
- Caution to wear a sunscreen (number 15), and sunglasses when out in the sun.
- Advise avoidance of driving and other potentially hazardous activities until response has been established.
- Suggest using ice chips, hard candy, or gum to relieve side effect of dry mouth; stress the need for good mouth care.
- Warn women to report if pregnancy is planned or suspected.

◆ *See Antipsychotics overview for more information.*

morphine

mor'feen

morphine hydrochloride: ***Morphine hydrochloride, ✤Morphitec, ✤M.O.S., ✤M.O.S.-SR***

morphine sulfate: ***Astramorph, Astramorph PF, Duramorph PF, ✤Epimorph, ✤Morphine HP, MS Contin, MSIR, RMS Uniserts, Roxanol, Roxanol SR, ✤Statex***

Class: **★Narcotic analgesic prototype,** Opiate agonist

Antidote: naloxone hydrochloride (Narcan)

PEDS ✋ PREG C GERI ✋

CONTROLLED SUBSTANCE II

Action Alters both the perception of and response to pain through an unclear mechanism. Believed to act by binding with opioid receptors at many CNS sites and altering the release of neurotransmitters from afferent nerves sensitive to painful stimuli.

Use/Therapeutic goal/Outcome

Moderate to severe pain: Relief of pain. ***Outcome criteria:*** Report of increased comfort; absence of signs of pain (grimacing, frowning, restlessness, reluctance to move or cough) with increase in signs of comfort (relaxed facial expression, decreased restlessness); blood pressure and pulse within normal limits when compared to baseline.

Ventilator phasing: Tolerance of mechanical ventilation. ***Outcome criteria:*** Respirations synchronized with mechanical ventilation; absence of signs of fighting, bucking, or attempting to override ventilator.

Dose range/Administration

Interaction alert: Tranquilizers, sedatives, hypnotics, general anesthetics, alcohol, CNS depressants, tricyclic antidepressants, and MAO inhibitors increase CNS depression.

Moderate to severe pain: ***Adult:*** PO: 10–20 mg diluted in juice q4-6h prn or around the clock.

Short-acting tablets: 15–30 mg q4-6h (crushed and mixed with food if patient has difficulty swallowing). *Sustained-release tablets:* 30 mg q8-12h. IM, SC: 5–20 mg (10 mg/70 kg) q4-6h. *Rectal:* 5–20 mg q4-6h. IV: 2–10 mg diluted in 4–5 ml sterile water for injection, given slowly over 4–5 min; then q1-4h, adjust doses based on response. *Continuous IV drip:* Loading dose 1–5 mg via bolus; then mix 125–250 mg MS in 250 cc D5W for a concentration 0.5–1 mg/ml and titrate according to physician's orders. *Epidural:* (By physician or anesthetist only.) *Initial dose:* 5 mg, then 1–2 mg prn. *Continuous epidural drip:* 2–4 mg/24 hr. *Maximum epidural dose:* 10 mg/24 hr. *Intrathecal:* (By physician only.) 0.2 to 1 mg/24 hr. **Child:** SC, IM: 0.1–0.2 mg/kg q4-6h prn.

Ventilator phasing: Adult: IV: 1–5 mg q1h prn. (Doses as great as 20 mg have been given to reduce respiratory drive.)

Clinical alert: Expect decreased dosage for children and the elderly or debilitated. Be aware that patient-controlled analgesia (PCA) via PCA pump may give best pain relief for terminally ill patients and for immediate postoperative period. Check respirations and blood pressure before giving morphine. Hold drug and report if respirations < 12 or if hypotension is noted. Keep naloxone readily available in case of respiratory depression.

Contraindications/Precautions

PREG C

Contraindicated in hypersensitivity to morphine or opiates, in acute bronchial asthma and upper-airway obstruction, and for epidural or intrathecal administration during labor. **Use with caution** in head injury, increased intracranial pressure, convulsive disorders, chronic pulmonary diseases, severe respiratory depression, acute alcoholism, hypothyroidism, acute abdominal conditions, acute ulcerative colitis, severe renal or hepatic disease, Addison's disease, severe obesity, urethral stricture, cardiac arrhythmias, toxic psychosis, or reduced blood volume.

☙ **Contraindicated for pregnant or nursing mothers. Use with caution for children and the elderly or debilitated.**

Side effects/Adverse reactions

Hypersensitivity: rash, hives, itching, swelling of face. **Resp:** respiratory depression, suppression of cough reflexes. **CNS:** mood changes, sedation, euphoria, convulsions (with large IV doses), physical dependence. **CV:** hypotension.

GI: nausea, vomiting, constipation. **GU:** urinary retention. **Skin:** flushing.

Nursing implications/Documentation

Possible nursing diagnoses: Pain; Anxiety; Potential for injury; Constipation.

◆ Have patient rate pain on a scale of 1–10 before and after medication is given; report and record inadequate pain control.

◆ Determine whether a less potent analgesic might effectively relieve pain (narcotic analgesics should be used in the smallest effective dose compatible with the patient's needs).

◆ Give analgesics before pain is severe for best effects.

◆ Document pulse, respirations, and blood pressure immediately before and 1 hr after administration until response is determined.

◆ Monitor closely for risk factors for injury; keep side rails up and supervise ambulation if allowed out of bed.

◆ Record and monitor bowel function to detect constipation; provide adequate fluid and fiber; give laxatives before problem becomes severe.

◆ Monitor those with abdominal pain carefully (morphine may mask or worsen gallbladder pain).

◆ Be aware of potential developing tolerance (requiring increased dose for same relief) and for psychic and physical dependence with prolonged use.

◆ After prolonged use, avoid abrupt withdrawal by reducing dosage by 50% every 3 days (abrupt withdrawal may result in abstinence symptoms such as chills, nausea, irritability, abdominal cramps, insomnia within 24–48 hr after last dose).

◆ For chronic pain, consider using sustained-release tablets, which last 8 hr; be sure that sustained-release tablets are not chewed or crushed.

◆ For ventilator phasing, auscultate lungs and be sure there is no obstruction before giving dose (once lungs are clear, mechanical ventilation may be better tolerated).

Patient & family teaching/Home care

Possible nursing diagnoses: Fear; Sensory/perceptual alterations; Impaired home maintenance management.

◆ Explain the rationale for taking analgesics before pain is severe.

M

♦ Advise those who are ambulatory to refrain from activities that require alertness and to seek assistance if there is any question about ability to get out of bed (e.g., if there is weakness or light headedness).

♦ Stress the need to adhere to the prescribed dose regimen because of risk of overdose, dependence, and abuse potential (instead of increasing dose regimen, unsatisfactory pain relief should be reported).

♦ If there is concern about prolonged use, explain that problems with tolerance, dependence, and addiction can be managed medically later, and that the need for pain control is more important at present.

♦ Warn that alcohol and other CNS depressants may cause excessive sedation.

♦ *See Narcotic and non-narcotic analgesics overview for more information.*

moxalactam
mox'a-lak-tam

moxalactam disodium (latamoxef disodium): ◆*Moxalactam, Moxam*

Class: Anti-infective, Antibiotic, Cephalosporin (third generation)

PEDS	PREG	GERI
🖐	C	🖐

Action Broad-spectrum, usually bactericidal, antibiotic; kills bacteria by inhibiting cell wall synthesis.

Use/Therapeutic goal/Outcome

Serious infections (lower respiratory and urinary tract, CNS, intraabdominal, GYN, skin, ear, blood): Prevention or resolution of infection. *Outcome criteria:* Absence of pathogenic growth on cultures, absence of clinical manifestations of infection (fever, pain, swelling, redness, heat, odor, drainage, productive cough, dysuria), normal WBC count, normal X rays.

Dose range/Administration

Interaction alert: Aspirin and anticoagulants increase risk of bleeding. Ingestion of alcohol within 48 hours of moxalactam administration may cause nausea, vomiting, hypotension, tachycardia, flushing, severe headache.
Adult: IV, Deep IM: 2–4 g/day divided q8h. *Maximum dose:* 12 g/day, depending on severity of infection. *Child:* IV, Deep IM: 50 mg/kg q6-8h. *Neonate:* IV, Deep IM: 50 mg/kg q8-12h.

Clinical alert: Expect that 10 mg Vitamin K may be given weekly to reduce risk of bleeding disorders associated with this drug.

Contraindications/Precautions   PREG C

Contraindicated in allergy to moxalactam or to cephalosporins. *Use with caution* in penicillin allergy, impaired renal function, and history of bleeding disorders.

🖐 **Contraindicated for pregnant or nursing mothers. Use with caution for children and the elderly.**

Side effects/Adverse reactions

Hypersensitivity: itching, erythema, rashes, urticaria, fever, eosinophilia, difficulty breathing, anaphylaxis, thrombocytopenia with serious bleeding. *GI:* nausea, vomiting, anorexia, abdominal pain, diarrhea, pseudomembranous colitis. *CV:* pain, redness, swelling, thrombophlebitis at injection site. *Hem:* anemia, bleeding tendencies, positive direct Coombs' test, slight elevation in SGOT, SGPT, BUN, and alkaline phosphatase. *GU:* vaginitis. *CNS:* headache, dizziness, fatigue. *Misc:* superinfection.

Nursing implications/Documentation

Possible nursing diagnoses: Potential for infection; Diarrhea.

♦ Determine history of allergies, and (regardless of history) monitor closely for allergic reactions.

♦ Obtain baseline CBC, creatinine, liver function studies, and necessary cultures before administering first dose; monitor closely thereafter if therapy is prolonged.

♦ Encourage fluids, and record and monitor intake and output, to ensure adequate hydration; report significant negative or positive balance.

♦ Monitor for and report signs of superinfection (sore throat, fever, persistent diarrhea, fatigue, thrush, vaginal discharge) or *bleeding* (check gums, urine, skin).

♦ Give IM doses deep into large muscle mass.

Patient & family teaching/Home care

Possible nursing diagnoses: Knowledge deficit; Impaired home maintenance management.

♦ Teach the importance of reporting allergic symptoms, persistent diarrhea, unusual bruising or bleeding, signs and symptoms that do not abate, or *any* new signs and symptoms of

M

discomfort that might indicate superinfection (medication regimen may have to be changed).

◆ Advise drinking 2–3 L of fluids daily to maintain adequate hydration (especially important if fever exists).

◆ Stress the importance of taking antibiotics for the entire time prescribed, even if signs and symptoms abate.

◆ *See Anti-infectives overview for more information.*

mupirocin
moo'purr-owe-sin

Bactroban

Class: Anti-infective, Local antibiotic

PEDS	PREG	GERI
OK	C	OK

Action Local antibiotic that eliminates bacterial growth (bacteriostatic) by inhibiting synthesis of DNA and RNA.

Use/Therapeutic goal/Outcome

Impetigo (due to *Staphylococcus aureus, Staphylococcus epidermidis, Staphylococcus saprophyticus, Streptococcus pyogenes*): Resolution of infection. **Outcome criteria:** After 3–5 days, improvement or absence of clinical manifestations of skin infection; absence of pathogenic growth on cultures.

Dose range/Administration

Adult and Child: *Topical:* Using clean or sterile gloves, apply a small amount to affected areas bid to tid.

Clinical alert: Be aware that local reactions are likely to be from the vehicle, polyethylene glycol. Do not use on burns.

Contraindications/Precautions
PREG
C

Contraindicated in hypersensitivity to mupirocin, or any components of the preparation.

✋ **Contraindicated for nursing mothers. Use with caution for pregnant women.**

Side effects/Adverse reactions

Hypersensitivity: itching, rashes. **Skin:** (rare) stinging, burning, tenderness, contact dermatitis, increased exudate. **GI:** (rare) nausea.

Nursing implications/Documentation

Possible nursing diagnoses: Altered skin integrity; Potential altered tissue integrity; Potential for infection.

◆ If culture for sensitivities test is ordered, obtain specimen before giving first dose.

◆ Monitor and record skin status; report deterioration in condition.

◆ If used over prolonged period of time, monitor for overgrowth of unsusceptible bacteria and fungi.

Patient & family teaching/Home care

Possible nursing diagnoses: Knowledge deficit; Impaired home maintenance management.

◆ Explain the importance of reporting new or deteriorating signs and symptoms of infection, and of continuing treatment for the entire time prescribed.

◆ Have the patient demonstrate method of applying mupirocin before discharge.

◆ Advise reporting if there is no improvement in 3–5 days.

◆ *See Anti-infectives overview for more information.*

muromonab-CD3
mur-oo-mone'ab

Orthoclone OKT3

Class: Immunosuppressant, Murine monoclonal antibody

PEDS	PREG	GERI
✋	C	✋

Action Suppresses immune response by reacting in the T-lymphocyte membrane with CD3 (needed for antigen recognition), thus depleting the blood of CD3-positive T-cells, reversing allograft rejection, and restoring kidney function.

Use/Therapeutic goal/Outcome

Acute allograft (kidney) rejection: Reversal of rejection, restoration of kidney function. **Outcome criteria:** Decrease in serum creatinine.

Dose range/Administration

Adult: IV: 5 mg bolus (given by physician) over 1 min qd for 10–14 days. **Child:** IV: 0.1 mg/kg bolus (given by physician) over 1 min qd for 10–14 days.

Clinical alert: First dose should not be given until chest X-ray report (within 24 hours) verifies that lungs are clear (because of increased risk of pulmonary edema), and temperature is less than 100° F. (37.8° C). This drug should be administered only in facilities equipped and staffed to monitor the patient closely, and to

▶

Muromonab-CD3   507

treat adverse effects promptly (most adverse effects occur within 30 minutes to 6 hours of the first dose, but patient should be monitored closely for 48 hours [follow hospital protocols for giving muromonab-CD3]).

Contraindications/Precautions

PREG
C

Contraindicated in hypersensitivity to murine products, infection, CHF, 3% weight gain in week before treatment, chest X-ray evidence of lung congestion. **Use with extreme caution** in fever, chickenpox exposure, and herpes zoster.

⚕ **Use with caution for children under 2 years, for pregnant or nursing mothers, and the elderly.**

Side effects/Adverse reactions

Hypersensitivity: fever, chills, wheezing, dyspnea, hypotension, anaphylaxis. **CNS:** tremors, malaise. **Resp:** pulmonary edema. **CV:** tachycardia, chest pain. **GI:** stomatitis, nausea, vomiting, diarrhea, hepatotoxicity. **Misc:** increased susceptibility to infection (cytomegalovirus, herpes, Pneumocystis carinii, Serratia organisms, Cryptococcus, Legionella and gram-negative bacteria).

Nursing implications/Documentation

Possible nursing diagnoses: Potential for infection; Altered oral mucous membrane.

◆ Expect that an antipyretic, antihistamine, and methylprenisolone sodium succinate (1 mg/kg IV) will be ordered before injection, and that hydrocortisone sodium succinate (100 mg IV) will be ordered to be given 30 minutes after injection to reduce severity of side effects.

◆ Monitor and document intake and output and daily weights; report positive balance or weight gain.

◆ Monitor hemoglobin, WBC, and platelet count closely (*hold drug* and report if leukocytes < 3000 mm³); also report increase in BUN, creatinine, and liver function studies (alkaline phosphatase, AST, ALT, bilirubin).

◆ Avoid giving IM injections to reduce risk of infection.

◆ Report signs and symptoms of infection immediately; avoid assigning health care workers with respiratory symptoms.

◆ Provide frequent mouth care.

◆ Be aware that patients often develop antibodies to this drug, therefore it is usually only given for one course of therapy.

Patient & family teaching/Home care

Possible nursing diagnoses: Knowledge deficit, Impaired home maintenance management.

◆ Teach that meticulous oral hygiene can help reduce incidence of oral inflammation.

◆ Reassure patient that although side effects are likely, they should diminish after the first 2 doses.

◆ Stress the need to report signs and symptoms of infection early to ensure prompt treatment (explain that the patient is at risk for opportunistic infections, such as herpes and cytomegalovirus).

◆ Warn women to use contraceptives for 12 weeks after completing therapy.

◆ *See Immunosuppressants overview for more information.*

nadolol

nay-doe'lole

Corgard

Class: Nonselective beta-adrenergic blocking agent, Antihypertensive, Antianginal

PEDS	PREG	GERI
⚕	C	⚕

Action Reduces heart rate, myocardial excitability, AV-node conduction velocity, blood pressure, and myocardial oxygen demand by blocking beta-1 (cardiac) and beta-2 adrenergic receptors, thereby reducing response to catecholamines. Reduces renin release.

Use/Therapeutic goal/Outcome

Hypertension: Reduction of blood pressure. **Outcome criteria:** Blood pressure within normal limits.

Angina: Prevention of angina. **Outcome criteria:** Report of decreased anginal attacks with increased activity tolerance.

Dose range/Administration

Interaction alert: Monitor for excessive bradycardia if given with cardiac glycosides or epinephrine. Other antihypertensives may potentiate hypotensive effects. Indomethacin may decrease antihypertensive effect. May alter antidiabetic agent requirements.

Adult: PO: 40 mg/day; may increase by 40–80 mg every 3 days to 1 week. *Maximum dose:* 320 mg/day for hypertension; 240 mg/day for angina.

Clinical alert: When discontinuing, wean over 1–2 weeks to avoid precipitating thyroid storm or myocardial infarction. Be aware that patients taking this drug may not exhibit tachycardia as a symptom of fever, hypoglycemia, or hyperthyroidism.

Contraindications/Precautions

PREG
C

Contraindicated in hypersensitivity to nadolol, and in cardiogenic shock, sinus bradycardia, second- or third-degree heart block (PR interval > 0.24 seconds), CHF, COPD, and bronchial asthma. **Use with caution** in diabetes, hyperthyroidism, or renal impairment.

☙ **Use with caution for the elderly. Safe use for children and pregnant women has not been established.**

Side effects/Adverse reactions

Hypersensitivity: rash, pruritis. **CV:** bradycardia, hypotension, CHF, peripheral vascular disease. **Resp:** increased airway resistance. **GI:** nausea, vomiting, diarrhea, constipation. **GU:** decreased sexual activity. **CNS:** mental depression, insomnia, nightmares, dizziness, hallucinations. **MS:** cold hands and feet, weakness, fatigue.

Nursing implications/Documentation

Possible nursing diagnoses: Activity intolerance; Fatigue; Potential for injury.

◆ Assess mental status, and record pulse and blood pressure (if possible, lying, sitting, and standing, in both arms) before administration, and frequently thereafter until response is determined.

◆ Consult with physician to determine desired therapeutic range for blood pressure and heart rate (parameters for withholding the medication should be written by physician).

◆ Ascertain that baseline CBC, electrolytes, BUN, creatinine, and liver function studies are obtained before giving first dose; report abnormalities and monitor closely thereafter.

◆ Monitor for allergic reactions and signs of confusion, dizziness, bradycardia, CHF, and hypotension; hold drug and report immediately if these occur.

◆ Supervise ambulation until response is determined.

◆ Document and monitor daily weight, and intake and output; report significant negative or positive balance.

Patient & family teaching/Home care

Possible nursing diagnoses: Knowledge deficit; Impaired home maintenance management; Altered sexuality patterns.

◆ Explain the importance of taking this drug exactly as prescribed, even when feeling well; warn not to discontinue drug abruptly.

◆ Stress the importance of good medical follow-up; explain that this drug reduces "wear and tear" on blood vessels, reduces the workload of the heart, and improves longevity and health.

◆ Teach how to monitor pulse and blood pressure; emphasize that syncope, hypertension or hypotension, or persistent dizziness should be reported; provide pulse and blood pressure parameters for withholding medication.

◆ Advise changing positions slowly to avoid dizziness.

◆ Encourage daily monitoring of weight and reporting sudden weight gain (frequently is fluid retention).

◆ Advise against excessive exposure to cold; advise reporting cold or painful hands or feet.

◆ Warn against drinking alcohol or taking *any* OTC drugs without physician approval (some interactions can cause severe reactions).

◆ Explain that this drug may alter sexual ability; explore concerns and seek consultation as needed.

◆ *See Beta Adrenergic Blockers, Antihypertensives, and Antianginals overviews for more information.*

nafcillin

naf-sill'in

nafcillin sodium: **Nafcil, Nallpen, Unipen**
Class: Anti-infective, Antibiotic, Penicillin (penicillinase–resistant)

PEDS	PREG	GERI
☙	B	☙

Action Broad-spectrum, usually bactericidal antibiotic; kills bacteria by inhibiting cell wall synthesis. Resistant to bacterial penicillinases (enzymes that degrade some penicillins).

Use/Therapeutic goal/Outcome

Systemic infections (caused by penicillinase-producing staphylococci): Resolution of infection. **Outcome criteria:** Absence of pathogenic growth on cultures, absence of clinical manifestations of infection (fever, pain, redness, heat, swelling, odor, drainage), normal WBC count, improvement of X rays.

Dose range/Administration

Interaction alert: Probenecid inhibits excretion of nafcillin and may be given to increase serum levels of the drug. Give at least 1 hour before bacteriostatic antibiotics for optimal effects.

▯ **Give oral dose with a full glass of water 1 hour before or 2–3 hours after meals; food may interfere with absorption.**
   Adult: PO: 250 mg to 1 g q4-6h. IM, IV: 500 mg to 1 g q4-6h. *Child:* PO: 50–100 mg/kg/day, in divided doses q4-6h. IM, IV: 100–200 mg/kg/day, in divided doses q12h. (IV route not recommended for neonates).

Clinical alert: IM route is extremely painful and not recommended (except for neonates). Dilute IV doses in 100–250 cc diluent and infuse slowly over a minimum of 30 minutes; monitor closely for thrombophlebitis.

Contraindications/Precautions
PREG
B

Contraindicated in allergy to penicillin. *Use with caution* in cephalosporin sensitivity, history of allergic responses (e.g., other drugs, hay fever, asthma), and renal insufficiency.

✋ **Use with caution for pregnant or nursing mothers and for children and the elderly. Safe use of IV route for neonates and infants has not been established.**

Side effects/Adverse reactions

Hypersensitivity: itching, rashes, urticaria, fever, difficulty breathing, anaphylaxis. *GI:* nausea, vomiting, diarrhea, pseudomembranous colitis, hepatitis. *CV:* pain, redness, swelling, thrombophlebitis at injection site. *GU:* acute interstitial nephritis. *Hem:* thrombocytopenia, leukopenia, slight elevation in SGOT and SGPT. *Misc:* superinfection.

Nursing implications/Documentation

Possible nursing diagnoses: Potential for infection; Diarrhea.

◆ Determine history of allergies, and (regardless of history) monitor closely for allergic reactions.

◆ Obtain baseline CBC, creatinine, liver function studies, and necessary cultures before administering first dose; monitor closely thereafter if therapy is prolonged.

◆ Encourage fluids, and document and monitor intake and output, to ensure adequate hydra-

tion; report significant negative or positive balance.

◆ Expect change to oral route as soon as possible (because IV and IM routes are irritating to tissues).

◆ Monitor for and report signs of superinfection (sore throat, fever, fatigue, thrush, vaginal discharge, diarrhea).

Patient & family teaching/Home care

Possible nursing diagnoses: Knowledge deficit; Impaired home maintenance management.

◆ Teach the importance of reporting allergic symptoms, diarrhea, signs and symptoms that do not abate, or *any* new signs and symptoms of discomfort that might indicate superinfection (medication regimen may have to be changed).

◆ Advise drinking 2–3 L of fluids daily to maintain adequate hydration (especially important if fever exists).

◆ Stress the importance of taking antibiotics for the entire time prescribed, even if signs and symptoms abate.

◆ *See Anti-infectives overview for more information.*

naftifine   *naf'te-feen*

naftifine hydrochloride: *Naftin*
Class: Topical broad spectrum antifungal

PEDS	PREG	GERI
✋	B	✋

Action Inhibits fungal growth by blocking enzyme activity.

Use/Therapeutic goal/Outcome

Fungal infections (tinea cruris, tinea pedia, and tinea corporis): Resolution of infection. *Outcome criteria:* After 4 weeks, absence of fungal growth on culture and absence of clinical manifestations of infection.

Dose range/Administration

Adult and Child: *Topical:* Using sterile gloves, apply generous amount of 1% cream to affected area and surrounding skin morning and evening; massage in gently. Continue 1–2 wk after symptoms subside.

Clinical alert: Cultures should be done before treatment to confirm diagnosis. Avoid the use of occlusive dressings (may intensify drug absorption and skin irritation) unless prescribed by physician.

Contraindications/Precautions
PREG B

Contraindicated in hypersensitivity to naftifine.

🖐 **Contraindicated for nursing mothers. Use with caution for children, pregnant or nursing mothers, and the elderly (monitor application carefully; observe for new lesions).**

Side effects/Adverse reactions

Hypersensitivity: local pain, itching, burning, stinging. ***Skin:*** excessive skin dryness, erythema.

Nursing implications/Documentation

Possible nursing diagnoses: Potential for infection; Impaired skin integrity.

♦ Record appearance of lesions daily.

♦ Report if there is no improvement after 4 weeks of therapy.

Patient & family teaching/Home care

Possible nursing diagnoses: Knowledge deficit; Impaired home maintenance management.

♦ Warn to keep ointment away from mouth, eyes, and nose (local irritation can be severe).

♦ Demonstrate procedure for cleansing and applying medication; observe return demonstration.

♦ Warn not to cover area with an occlusive dressing (unless otherwise ordered).

♦ Point out that this medication must be applied for 1–2 weeks after clinical manifestations have disappeared to prevent recurrence.

♦ Inform that increase in inflammation or failure to improve after 4 weeks should be reported.

♦ *See Anti-infectives overview for more information.*

nalbuphine
nal'byoo-feen

nalbuphine hydrochloride: ***Nubain***

Class: Non-narcotic analgesic, Opiate agonist (partial)

Antidote: naloxone hydrochloride (Narcan)

PEDS	PREG	GERI
🖐	C	🖐

Action Alters both perception of and response to pain through an undefined mechanism. Believed to act by binding with opiate receptors at many CNS sites.

Use/Therapeutic goal/Outcome

Moderate to severe pain, pre-procedural sedation: Relief of pain; promotion of relaxation. ***Outcome criteria:*** Report of feeling comfortable and relaxed; absence of observable signs of pain (grimacing, frowning, restlessness, reluctance to move or cough) with increase in signs of comfort (relaxed facial expression, decreased restlessness); blood pressure and pulse within normal limits when compared to baseline.

Dose range/Administration

Interaction alert: Alcohol, CNS depressants, narcotic analgesics, tranquilizers, sedatives, and hypnotics may increase CNS depression.

Adult: SC, IM, IV: 10–20 mg q3-6h prn or around the clock. *Maximum dose:* 160 mg/24 hr.

Clinical alert: Expect decreased dosage for the elderly or the debilitated. Check respirations and blood pressure before giving nalbuphine hydrochloride. Hold drug and report if respirations < 12 or if hypotension is noted. Keep naloxone readily available in case of respiratory depression.

Contraindications/Precautions
PREG C

Contraindicated in known hypersensitivity to nalbuphine hydrochloride or sulfites. ***Use with caution*** in emotional instability, drug abuse, head injury, increased intracranial pressure, hepatic or renal disease, myocardial infarction, biliary tract surgery, and impaired respirations.

🖐 **Contraindicated for children and for pregnant or nursing mothers. Use with caution for the elderly.**

Side effects/Adverse reactions

Hypersensitivity: itching, burning sensation, rash, urticaria (nalbuphine contains sodium metabisulfite; may cause allergic reaction in sulfite-sensitive individuals). ***CNS:*** sedation, vertigo, dizziness, nervousness, depression, crying, euphoria, unusual dreams, hallucinations. ***CV:*** hypertension, hypotension, bradycardia, tachycardia. ***Resp:*** respiratory depression. ***GI:*** nausea, vomiting. ***GU:*** urinary urgency. ***Skin:*** sweaty, clammy skin.

Nursing implications/Documentation

Possible nursing diagnoses: Pain; Anxiety; Potential for injury.

♦ Have patient rate pain on a scale of 1–10 before and after medication is given; report and record inadequate pain control.

♦ Give analgesics before pain is severe for best effects.

♦ Document pulse, respirations, and blood pressure immediately before and 1 hr after administration until response is determined (then qid if hospitalized).

♦ Monitor closely for risk factors for injury; keep side rails up and supervise ambulation if allowed out of bed.

♦ Monitor those with history of narcotic dependence for signs of withdrawal (this drug has narcotic antagonist properties); give 25% of usual dose initially, then increase if no withdrawal symptoms are noted.

♦ Be aware of potential for abuse and psychological and physiologic dependence if used for long term.

Patient & family teaching/Home care

Possible nursing diagnoses: Sensory/perceptual alterations; Impaired home maintenance management.

♦ Explain the rationale for taking analgesics before pain is too severe.

♦ Advise those who are ambulatory to refrain from activities that require alertness and to seek assistance if there is any question about ability to get out of bed (e.g., if there is weakness or light headedness).

♦ Stress the need to adhere to the prescribed dose regimen because of risk of overdose, dependence, and abuse potential (instead of increasing dosage regimen, unsatisfactory pain relief should be reported).

♦ Warn that alcohol and other CNS depressants may cause excessive sedation.

♦ *See Narcotic and non-narcotic analgesics overview for more information.*

nalidixic acid

nal-i-dix'ik

NegGram

Class: Urinary tract anti-infective

PEDS	PREG	GERI
♨	B	♨

Action Kills most gram-negative urinary tract bacteria (bactericidal) by inhibiting DNA synthesis. Not effective against Pseudomonas or bacteria outside the urinary tract.

Use/Therapeutic goal/Outcome

Treatment of acute and chronic urinary tract infection caused by susceptible gram-negative organisms (*Proteus, Klebsiella, Enterobacter* and *E. coli*): Elimination of bacterial growth. *Outcome criteria:* Absence of growth on urine culture; report of absence of dysuria, frequency.

Dose range/Administration

Interaction alert: Increases effect of oral anticoagulants. Nitrofurantoin interferes with therapeutic effect.

🗓 **Give one hour before or 2 hours after meals unless GI symptoms are noted.**
Adult: PO: 1 g qid for 7–14 days. *Long-term use:* 2 g/day. *Child > 3 mos:* PO: 55 mg/kg/day in divided doses qid for 7–14 days. *Long-term use:* 33 mg/kg/day.

Clinical alert: Report if symptoms persist or worsen after 48 hours (resistant bacteria may have emerged). Monitor the elderly for septic shock.

Contraindications/Precautions

PREG B

Contraindicated in hypersensitivity or intolerance to nalidixic acid or other quinolones, and in history of seizure disorders. *Use with caution* in kidney or liver disease, cerebral arteriosclerosis, or respiratory insufficiency.

♨ **Contraindicated for infants under 3 months and in the first trimester of pregnancy. Use with caution for prepubertal children, in the third trimester of pregnancy, and for the elderly.**

Side effects/Adverse reactions

Hypersensitivity: photosensitivity, itching, rashes, angioedema, fever, chills, arthralgia, hypersensitivity, pneumonia, increased intracranial pressure, bulging fontanelles in infants, anaphylaxis (rare). *GI:* nausea, vomiting, abdominal pain, diarrhea. *CNS:* drowsiness, headache, malaise, dizziness, vertigo, weakness, seizures (in epileptics), confusion, hallucinations. *Eye:* blurred or double vision, difficulty focusing, change in color perception.

Nursing implications/Documentation

Possible nursing diagnoses: Altered patterns of urinary elimination; Fluid volume deficit.

• Obtain urine for culture and sensitivity, and ensure that necessary lab studies (e.g., CBC, BUN, creatinine, liver function) are done before administering first dose; monitor closely thereafter if therapy is prolonged.

• Provide acidic juices (cranberry, plum, prune), and document and monitor intake and output, to maintain adequate hydration (at least 2 L not more, or urine will be too dilute).

• Observe closely for CNS reactions (especially in infants, children, and the elderly) until 3 consecutive doses have been taken.

• Report arthralgia in children immediately.

Patient & family teaching/Home care

Possible nursing diagnoses: Knowledge deficit; Impaired home maintenance management.

• Encourage taking doses one hour before meals or two hours after meals unless GI distress is noted.

• Advise reporting symptoms that do not abate after 48 hours, new symptoms of illness (respiratory symptoms, fever, sore throat), symptoms of allergy (itching, rashes), visual disturbances.

• Stress the importance of taking this drug without missing doses for the entire time prescribed, even if symptoms disappear.

• Advise against exposure to the sun (number 15 sunscreen should be worn), and warn that photosensitivity may persist for up to 3 months after drug is discontinued.

• *See Anti-infectives overview for more information.*

naloxone
na-lox'one

naloxone hydrochloride: ***Narcan***

Class: ★**Narcotic antagonist prototype**

PEDS	PREG	GERI
ṿ	B	ṿ

Action Precise mechanism of actions of narcotic antagonists is unclear. Believed to reverse effects of narcotics by displacing them from opiate receptor sites (competitive antagonism). When given alone, not as an antidote to narcotic analgesics, it has no pharmacologic activity. Produces an abstinence syndrome when administered to addicts who are taking a narcotic.

Use/Therapeutic goal/Outcome

Narcotic-induced respiratory depression: Reversal of respiratory depression. ***Outcome criteria:*** Respiratory rate and function re-established to that prior to depression; improved consciousness and response to pain; vital signs within normal limits when compared to baseline.

Dose range/Administration

Known or suspected narcotic-induced depression: ***Adult:*** IM, SC, IV: 0.4–2 mg (IV preferred), may repeat q 2–3 min prn. If no response after 10 mg, question diagnosis of narcotic-induced toxicity. ***Child:*** SC, IM, IV: 0.01 mg/kg (IV preferred), may repeat q 2–3 min. ***Neonate:*** IV: 0.1 mg/kg in umbilical vein, may repeat q 2–3 min for 3 doses.

Postoperative narcotic depression: ***Adult:*** IV: 0.1–0.2 mg q 2–3 min prn.

Clinical alert: If initial dose of 0.01 mg/kg does not result in clinical improvement, up to 10 times this dose (0.1 mg/kg) may be needed to be effective. Adult concentration of drug is 0.4 mg/ml. Child and neonate concentration of drug is 0.02 mg/ml. For neonatal use, may mix 0.5 ml adult concentration with 9.5 ml sterile water or saline solution. Naloxone is available in 1-ml prefilled disposable syringes, 10-ml vials, and 1-ml ampules.

Contraindications/Precautions

PREG
B

N

Contraindicated in hypersensitivity to drug. ***Use with caution*** in cardiac irritability and narcotic addiction (including newborns of addicted mothers).

ṿ **Use with caution for pregnant women, children, and the elderly.**

Side effects/Adverse reactions

Hypersensitivity: (with too rapid reversal) nausea, vomiting, sweating, tachycardia, increased blood pressure. ***CV:*** hypotension, ventricular tachycardia. ***Misc:*** withdrawal symptoms in narcotic addicts.

Nursing implications/Documentation

Possible nursing diagnoses: Potential for aspiration; Potential for injury; Pain.

• Monitor closely for airway obstruction and keep suction at bedside until patient is recovered; document vital signs, particularly respirations, every 3–5 min after administration until stable (respiratory rate should increase within 1–2 min, and effect lasts 1–4 hr; however, duration of action of narcotic may last

▶

longer than naloxone, with relapse into respiratory depression).

♦ Be prepared to provide airway support (have resuscitative equipment and suction and oxygen ready for use).

♦ Report respirations < 10/min immediately.

♦ Watch closely for potential for injury; position extremities and head carefully; keep side rails up.

♦ When used to reverse postoperative opioid depression, titrate dose carefully to avoid interfering with pain control.

Patient & family teaching/Home care

Possible nursing diagnoses: Fear; Sensory/perceptual alterations.

♦ Explain procedures briefly and in simple terms (even if the patient is not awake, he or she may be able to hear).

♦ Reassure that things are going well and measures are being taken to ensure safety (even if the patient is not awake).

naltrexone

nal-trex'one

naltrexone hydrochloride: *Trexan*

Class: Narcotic antagonist

PEDS	PREG	GERI
🖐	C	🖐

Action Weakens or completely reverses the subjective effects (the "high") of IV opioids and analgesics by competitively occupying opioid receptor sites in the brain.

Use/Therapeutic goal/Outcome

Adjunct for maintenance of opioid-free state in detoxified addicts: Continuation of opioid-free status. *Outcome criteria:* Report of desire to remain narcotic-free, reduced euphoria and drug craving; absence of signs of narcotic use (e.g., pinpoint pupils).

Dose range/Administration

Interaction alert: Do not give with opioid analgesics.

Adult: PO: *Initial dose:* 25 mg, then 25 mg in 1 hr if no withdrawal signs are evident. When 50 mg q24h is tolerated, implement a flexible maintenance schedule (e.g., 100 mg Monday, 150 mg Friday).

Clinical alert: A Narcan (naloxone) challenge test is administered prior to the use of this drug. If signs of opioid withdrawal persist after nalox-

one is given, naltrexone should not be given because the individual is most likely still taking narcotics. This drug should be used only as an adjunct to a *comprehensive* psychotherapeutic rehabilitation program.

Contraindications/Precautions

PREG
C

Contraindicated in hypersensitivity to the drug, and in use with opioid analgesics, those who are opioid-dependent, acute opioid withdrawal, acute hepatitis, liver failure, positive urine screen for opioids, and in anyone who fails the Narcan challenge. *Use with caution* in mild liver disease or history of recent liver disease.

🖐 **Contraindicated for children and pregnant women. Use with caution for the elderly.**

Side effects/Adverse reactions

Hypersensitivity: rash. *CNS:* insomnia, nightmares, anxiety, headache, irritability. *GI:* anorexia, nausea, vomiting, diarrhea, hepatoxicity. *MS:* muscle and joint pain. *Eye:* blurred vision.

Nursing implications/Documentation

Possible nursing diagnoses: Anxiety, Ineffective individual coping; Ineffective denial.

♦ Ascertain that the individual is completely opioid free before giving drug (may cause severe withdrawal symptoms if narcotics are being taken).

♦ Recognize that those addicted to short-acting opioids (heroin, meperidine) must wait at least 7 days after the last opioid dose before taking naltrexone; those addicted to longer-acting opioids (methadone) must wait at least 10 days.

♦ If an emergency occurs requiring opioid analgesia, consult with physician concerning use of higher doses (must be higher than usual to surmount the effect of naltrexone).

Patient & family teaching/Home care

Possible nursing diagnoses: Ineffective family coping; Knowledge deficit; Impaired home maintenance management.

♦ Advise carrying a medical identification card to alert medical treatment personnel to the fact that naltrexone is being taken.

♦ Warn that administration of large doses of heroin or other narcotics may cause serious injury or death.

♦ Point out the need to maintain a high motivation for being drug free because this drug

N

does not suppress the desire to experience a "high."

♦ Stress that the individual must return monthly for liver-function studies for the first 6 months, then as directed by physician; teach that signs of liver toxicity (dark urine, yellow skin, nausea, vomiting, and fatigue) should be reported immediately.

♦ Provide a list of non-opioid medications that may be taken to relieve discomfort.

nandrolone
nan'droe-lone

nandrolone decanoate: **Anabolin LA, Androlone-D, Deca-Durabolin, Decolone, Hybolin Decanoate, Kabolin, Nandrobolic L.A., Neo-Durabolic**

nandrolone phenpropionate: **Anabolin IM, Androlone, Durabolin, Hybolin Improved, Nandrobolic**

Class: Anabolic steroid, Antianemic, Antineoplastic agent

PEDS	PREG	GERI
✋	X	✋

Action Promotes body tissue-building processes and reverses catabolic processes by promoting protein anabolism and stimulating appetite; increases hemoglobin and red cell volume by stimulating erythropoiesis and heme formation; provides palliation of metastatic breast cancer.

Use/Therapeutic goal/Outcome

Anemia related to renal insufficiency: Stimulation of erythropoietin production resulting in stimulation of RBC production in bone marrow. **Outcome criteria:** Increase in hemoglobin, hematocrit, and red blood cell count.

Breast cancer: Palliation of inoperable metastatic disease. **Outcome criteria:** Evidence of decrease in tumor and metastatic activity.

Dose range/Administration

Interaction alert: Increases effect of insulin, oral hypoglycemics, and anticoagulants. Corticosteroids increase possibility of edema and severe acne. Avoid other hepatotoxic medications.

Anemia: **Adult:** IM: 50–100 mg q 1–4 wks. **Child:** IM: 25–50 mg q 3–4 wks.

Breast cancer: **Adult:** IM: 25–100 mg/wk.

Clinical alert: In treatment of anemia, adequate intake of iron is required for maximum response to nandrolone decanoate.

Contraindications/Precautions

Contraindicated in hypersensitivity to anabolic steroids, and in men with cancer of breast or prostate, women with hypercalcemia associated with breast cancer; hypercalcemia, and severe hepatic or renal impairment. **Use with caution** in cardiac, hepatic, or renal impairment; coronary artery disease; history of MI, diabetes mellitus, and prostatic hypertrophy.

✋ **Contraindicated for pregnant or nursing mothers. Use with caution for children and elderly men.**

Side effects/Adverse reactions

Hypersensitivity: rashes, anaphylaxis. **GU:** virilism of females (enlarged clitoris, deepening of voice, menstrual irregularities, unnatural hair growth or loss); virilism of prepubertal males (acne, enlarging penis, increased frequency of erections, unnatural hair growth); in older men, bladder irritability, breast soreness, gynecomastia, priapism, prostatic hypertrophy, prostatic carcinoma, testicular atrophy, suppression of spermatogenesis; decreased libido in both men and women. **Hem:** iron deficiency anemia, leukemia, suppression of clotting factors, hypercalcemia, decreased high-density lipoproteins (HDL), and increased low-density lipoproteins (LDL). **GI:** nausea, vomiting, diarrhea; hepatic dysfunction, carcinoma, or necrosis. **MS:** muscle cramps, premature epiphyseal closure in children. **Skin:** unexplained darkening, acne, edema.

Nursing implications/Documentation

Possible nursing diagnoses: Body image disturbance; Fluid volume excess.

♦ Administer deep into gluteal muscle; rotate sites.

♦ Assess IM sites for signs of inflammation.

♦ Record baseline blood pressure and weight.

♦ Assess for and report increased blood pressure, weight gain, or evidence of edema or congestive failure.

♦ Monitor serum calcium levels; assess, report, and document symptoms of hypercalcemia (nausea, vomiting, constipation, lethargy, muscle weakness).

♦ Monitor for changes in liver function tests, cholesterol levels, and iron and total iron-binding capacity.

♦ For diabetics, monitor glucose levels and assess for symptoms of hypoglycemia.

N

▶

Patient & family teaching/Home care

Possible nursing diagnoses: Knowledge deficit; Impaired home maintenance management; Sexual dysfunction.

♦ Advise restricting sodium intake to decrease edema.

♦ Caution women of child-bearing age to use reliable birth control and to stop drug and report any suspicion of pregnancy.

♦ For females, stress the importance of reporting the occurrence of masculinizing effects (abnormal growth of facial hair, deepening of voice, menstrual irregularities, enlarged clitoris).

♦ For males, advise reporting priapism, gynecomastia, or bladder irritability.

♦ For diabetics, caution about possible lowering of blood sugar and need for adjustment of doses of insulin or oral antidiabetic agents.

♦ Inform parents of prepubertal children that X rays will be taken periodically to determine effect on bone growth.

♦ Caution to maintain close medical supervision for early detection of adverse reactions.

♦ Stress that using anabolic steroids for improvement of athletic performance may result in serious side effects that outweigh any advantages.

naproxen

na-prox'en

Naprosyn, ♣*Apo-Naproxen,* ♣🍁*Naxen,* ♣*Novonaprox*

naproxen sodium: *Anaprox, Anaprox D.S. ,* 🍁*Naprogesic*

Class: Nonsteroidal anti-inflammatory drug (NSAID), Analgesic, Antipyretic, Antirheumatic, Antigout agent, Antidysmenorrheal

PEDS	PREG	GERI
🖐	🖐	🖐

Action Exact mechanism of action is unclear. Believed to reduce inflammation by inhibiting prostaglandin synthesis. Decreases uterine contractility by inhibiting intrauterine prostaglandin. Prostaglandin is a naturally occurring mediator in the inflammatory process which is found throughout body tissue.

Use/Therapeutic goal/Outcome

Pain and inflammation: Promotion of comfort and mobility; suppression of inflammation. **Outcome criteria:** Report of increased comfort with increased range of motion and ability to perform activities of daily life; reduction in or absence of joint stiffness, swelling, redness, and warmth.

Primary dysmenorrhea: Reduction of uterine hyperactivity (cramping). **Outcome criteria:** Report of pain relief and increased activity levels.

Dose range/Administration

Interaction alert: Coumarin-type anticoagulants prolong prothrombin time, increasing chance of bleeding; aspirin also increases risk of bleeding. Hydantoins, sulfonamides, or sulfonylureas increase risk of toxicity. Probenecid may reduce plasma clearance of naproxen.

🖐 **Give with food or milk to reduce GI symptoms.**

Arthritis: Adult: PO: 250–500 mg bid; n. sodium 275 mg bid. Dosage individualized. RECT: 500 mg at bedtime, with oral doses during the day. **Child > 14 yr:** PO: 10 mg/kg/day in divided doses bid.

Acute gout: Adult: PO: *Initial dose:* 750 mg, then 250 mg q8h; n. sodium 825 mg, then 275 mg q8h.

Primary dysmenorrhea, tendonitis, bursitis: Adult: PO: *Initial dose:* 500 mg, then 250 mg q6-8h. *Maximum dose:* 1250 mg/day; n. sodium 1375 mg/day.

Clinical alert: See maximum dose just above. Do not give naproxen sodium to patients on salt-restricted diet. Give doses in the morning and evening for optimum results.

Contraindications/Precautions

PREG
🖐

Contraindicated in hypersensitivity to naproxen, aspirin, or other NSAIDs and in active GI disease, severe renal or hepatic impairment, asthma, and nasal polyps. **Use with caution** in history of GI tract disorders; compromised renal, hepatic, or cardiac function; and angioedema.

🖐 **Use with caution for the elderly. Safe use for children under 14 years and pregnant women has not been established.**

Side effects/Adverse reactions

Hypersensitivity: rash, urticaria, asthma, dyspnea, bronchospasm, and anaphylaxis. **Ear:** tinnitus. **Skin:** pruritus. **GI:** GI distress, occult blood loss, nausea. **CNS:** headache, dizziness, drowsiness. **Eye:** blurred vision. **Hem:** elevated liver enzymes. **CV:** peripheral edema. **GU:** nephrotoxicity.

Nursing implications/Documentation

Possible nursing diagnoses: Pain; Impaired physical mobility.

♦ Establish a baseline for CBC, electrolytes, prothrombin time, BUN, creatinine, and liver function studies; if therapy is prolonged, monitor closely thereafter.

♦ Monitor for and report GI symptoms that may indicate peptic ulcer (nausea, pain, black stools).

♦ Record weight every other day; report edema or sudden weight gain.

♦ For diabetics, monitor blood sugar closely since insulin requirements may change.

Patient & family teaching/Home care

Possible nursing diagnoses: Altered health maintenance; Knowledge deficit.

♦ Advise taking doses with food to reduce GI symptoms.

♦ Explain the importance of watching for symptoms of GI bleeding (black stools, persistent GI distress).

♦ Explain the importance of taking doses in the morning and the evening for optimal effect; stress that full effect of drug may not be realized for up to 2 weeks.

♦ Stress the need to avoid aspirin, alcohol, and other OTC drugs (unless approved by physician) because of increased risk of GI bleeding.

♦ Instruct individuals to hold dose and report if any of the following side effects are experienced: vertigo, rashes, blood in urine, hearing or visual changes, sudden weight gain, edema.

♦ Warn against driving or activities that require alertness until response is determined.

♦ Reinforce the need for ongoing medical follow-up; advise telling dentist that naproxen is being taken.

♦ For diabetics, explain the importance of monitoring blood sugars with a blood glucose meter.

♦ *See Nonsteroidal anti-inflammatory drugs overview for more information.*

neomycin

nee-oh-mye'sin

neomycin sulfate: **Mycifradin, Myciguent, ♠Neosulf**

Class: Anti-infective, Aminoglycoside antibiotic

PEDS	PREG	GERI
✋	C	✋

Action Kills bacteria (bactericidal) by binding to ribosomes, thereby disrupting bacterial protein synthesis.

Use/Therapeutic goal/Outcome

Infectious diarrhea (caused by enteropathogenic *Escherichia coli*): Resolution of infection. **Outcome criteria:** Absence of pathogenic *Escherichia coli* on stool culture; absence of diarrhea.

Preoperative bowel preparation: Suppression of pathogenic bacteria. **Outcome criteria:** Not measured; ensure that all neomycin doses have been taken as prescribed.

Adjunctive treatment of hepatic coma: Reduction of ammonia-producing bacteria in the GI tract. **Outcome criteria:** Decreased serum ammonia levels.

Skin infections, wounds, and burns: Prevention or resolution of infection/promotion of healing. **Outcome criteria:** Absence of growth on cultures, evidence of healing.

Dose range/Administration

Infectious diarrhea caused by enteropathogenic *Escherichia coli*: Adult: PO: 50 mg/kg/day in 4 divided doses for 2–3 days. **Child:** PO: 50–100 mg/kg/day in divided doses q4-6h for 2–3 days.

Preoperative bowel preparation: Adult: PO: 1 g qh x 4 doses, then 1q q4h x 5 doses. **Child:** PO: 40–100 mg/kg/day in divided doses q4-6h.

Adjunctive treatment of hepatic coma: Adult: PO: 1–3 g qid for 5–6 days. *Enema:* 200 cc of 1% solution, or 100 cc of 2% solution q6h, retained for 20–60 min.

Skin infection, wounds, and burns: Adult and Child: *Topical:* Rub in a small amount bid, tid, or as ordered.

Clinical alert: A saline enema should be given before beginning preoperative oral neomycin. Doses greater than 4 g/day may lead to nephrotoxicity (although neomycin is poorly absorbed and has little systemic effect).

Contraindications/Precautions

PREG
C

Contraindicated in hypersensitivity to neomycin, and in intestinal obstruction. **Use with caution** in impaired kidney function, and in ulcerative bowel lesions.

▶

⚘ Contraindicated for pregnant or nursing mothers. Use with caution for children and the elderly.

Side effects/Adverse reactions

Hypersensitivity: itching, rashes, hives. *GI:* anorexia, nausea, vomiting, diarrhea, intestinal malabsorption. *GU:* nephrotoxicity (oliguria, proteinuria, decreased creatinine clearance, increased BUN and creatinine). *CNS:* confusion, depression, headache, lethargy. *Ear:* ototoxicity (ringing of the ears, vertigo, hearing loss). *Misc:* superinfection.

Nursing implications/Documentation

Possible nursing diagnoses: Potential for infection; Fluid volume deficit.

♦ Weigh patient and obtain baseline renal function studies and necessary cultures before administering first dose.

♦ Encourage fluid intake, and document and monitor intake and output, to ensure adequate hydration (report excessive negative or positive balance).

♦ If given in doses of greater than 4 g/day, monitor for and report signs of nephrotoxicity and ototoxicity; also monitor for signs of superinfection (fever, sore throat, oral thrush).

♦ If given as a preoperative bowel preparation, expect that a low residue diet, and a cathartic will be ordered before starting doses.

Patient & family teaching/Home care

Possible nursing diagnoses: Knowledge deficit.

♦ Stress the importance of taking the drug for the entire time prescribed, even if symptoms abate.

♦ For preoperative bowel preparation, explain that the drug is given to suppress pathogenic growth in the bowel.

♦ Teach the need to report ear symptoms (ringing, full feeling, hearing loss) and symptoms of superinfection (mouth sores, fever, new infections).

♦ *See Anti-infectives overview for more information.*

neostigmine
nee-oh-stig' meen

neostigmine bromide: *Prostigmin Bromide*
neostigmine methylsulfate: *Prostigmin*

Class: ★Cholinergic (parasympathomimetic) prototype, ★Anticholinesterase prototype

Antidote: Atropine

PEDS	PREG	GERI
⚘	C	⚘

Action When given in appropriate doses, promotes impulse transmission from nerve cells to muscle cells by inhibiting the action of cholinesterase, the enzyme that destroys acetylcholine. Acetylcholine is responsible for facilitating impulse transmission from nerve cells to muscle cells. *Excessive or deficient* acetylcholine may cause *neuromuscular blockade.* Onset of action for oral route is 2–4 hr with a duration of 2½–4 hr; for parenteral route, onset is 10–30 min, duration 2½–4 hr.

Use/Therapeutic goal/Outcome

Postoperative abdominal distention, ileus, and urinary retention: Promotion of intestinal and skeletal muscle tone and normal patterns of urinary elimination. *Outcome criteria:* Bowel sounds present; ability to pass flatus and void in normal amounts.

Anesthesia recovery: Reversal of effects of nondepolarizing muscle relaxants (tubocurarine, gallamine, pancuronium, etc.). *Outcome criteria:* Spontaneous respirations; ability to move arms and legs; return of muscle strength.

Myasthenia gravis: Improvement of muscle strength and function. *Outcome criteria:* Respirations within normal range; normal vital capacity; improved ability to chew, swallow, talk, and perform activities of daily life; absence of ptosis; report of absence of double vision.

Dose range/Administration

Interaction alert: Procainamide and quinidine may inhibit cholinergic effect on muscle. Other cholinergics should be discontinued before starting neostigmine.

🥄 Give PO doses with milk or food to reduce side effects by slowing absorption and reducing serum peaks.

Postoperative abdominal distention, ileus, and urinary retention: Adult: SC, IM: 0.25 mg–1 mg q4-6h.

Reversal of neuromuscular blocking agents:
Adult: IV: 0.5–2 mg slowly, after 0.6 mg–1.2 mg atropine; may repeat prn. *Maximum total dose:* 5 mg.

Myasthenia gravis: Adult: PO: 15–30 mg tid, 15–375 mg/day. IM, IV: 0.5–2 mg q1-3h. **Child:** PO: 7.5–15 mg tid tc qid.

Clinical alert: Doses individualized depending upon neurological response and incidence of side effects. For treatment of myasthenia gravis, expect larger doses to be given before periods of increased activity (e.g., 30 min before meals, if the patient has dysphagia). There is a fine line between inadequate dosage and overdosage, requiring careful monitoring of response. Keep atropine, suction, and resuscitative equipment readily available.

Contraindications/Precautions

PREG
C

Contraindicated in hypersensitivity to cholinergics or to bromides, and in intestinal or urinary obstruction and urinary tract infection.
Use with caution in asthma, cardiac disease, peptic ulcer, peritonitis, epilepsy, and hypotension.

🖐 **Contraindicated for nursing mothers. Use with caution for children and the elderly. Safe use for pregnant women has not been established (fetal problems have not been documented, but transient muscle weakness has occurred in 20% of neonates).**

Side effects/Adverse reactions

Hypersensitivity: rash, exaggeration of side effects. **GI:** nausea, vomiting, abdominal cramps, diarrhea, excessive salivation. **Eye:** miosis, blurred vision. **MS:** muscle weakness. **CV:** bradycardia, hypotension. **CNS:** restlessness, dizziness, confusion. **Resp:** respiratory depression and paralysis, restlessness. **Skin:** sweating. **Misc:** cholinergic crisis (increase in severity of side effects).

Nursing implications/Documentation

Possible nursing diagnoses: Activity intolerance; Potential for aspiration; Impaired swallowing; Constipation.

◆ Closely monitor ability to chew, swallow, and talk for 45–60 min after dosage, especially during periods of dose adjustment; record variations in strength and pulse, respirations, and blood pressure every 4 hr.

◆ Once the individual with myasthenia has demonstrated ability to manage dose regimen, check with physician to see if a supply of med-

ication can be kept at the bedside for self-medication (those with long-standing disease often insist on this).

◆ Monitor bowel sounds and encourage activity to promote gastric motility.

◆ Report rashes (may require discontinuation of drug).

◆ For urinary retention, catheterize 1 hr after neostigmine dose if urination has not occurred.

◆ With use in pregnancy, monitor neonates for transient muscle weakness.

Patient & family teaching/Home care

Possible nursing diagnoses: Impaired home maintenance management; Noncompliance.

◆ For those with myasthenia gravis, explain that taking this drug is vital to promote normal muscle function, and that this may be a life-long requirement; stress the need for ongoing medical follow-up because some individuals develop resistance to this drug.

◆ Point out that taking this drug with food helps reduce side effects; emphasize that doses must be taken on time exactly as prescribed, without missing doses.

◆ Advise reporting side effects or increased muscle weakness immediately, especially during periods of dose adjustment.

◆ For patients with postoperative distension, stress the need to increase activity to promote GI motility.

◆ Recommend wearing medical alert identification that states that the patient is taking neostigmine.

◆ *See Cholinergics overview for more information.*

niacin

nye'a-sin

nicotinic acid: *Niac, Nico-400, Nicobid, Nicolar, Ni-Span*

Class: Vitamin B3, Water-soluble vitamin, Antihyperlipemic

PEDS   PREG   GERI
🖐   🖐   OK

Action Needed for tissue respiration, carbohydrate, protein, lipid metabolism, and conversion of glycogen to glucose; lowers serum cholesterol and triglycerides by inhibiting synthesis of very-low-density lipoproteins (VLDL); causes peripheral vasodilation by direct effect on vascular smooth muscle.

Use/Therapeutic goal/Outcome

Niacin deficiency/Pellagra: Provides adequate blood levels of niacin. **Outcome criteria:** Absence or improvement in symptoms of niacin deficiency (dermatitis, diarrhea, dementia).

Hyperlipidemia: Reduction of elevated serum cholesterol and triglycerides. **Outcome criteria:** Serum triglyceride levels less than 1 g/dl.

Dose range/Administration

Interaction alert: Antihypertensive drugs (sympathetic blockers) increase vasodilatory effect and risk of postural hypotension. Decreases effectiveness of chenodiol (used to dissolve gallstones). Isoniazid increases niacin requirements.

🖐 **Give with meals to minimize gastric distress.**

Deficiency/Pellagra: Adult: PO, IM, IV: *Maximum dose:* 500 mg/day. **Child:** PO, IV: *Maximum dose:* 300 mg/day.

Hyperlipidemia: Adult: PO: 1–2 gm tid.

Clinical alert: Niacin therapy for hyperlipidemia should be discontinued if no response is seen after 1–2 months.

Contraindications/Precautions

PREG
🖐

Contraindicated in hypersensitivity to niacin (or to tartrazine if present in tablets), and in severe hepatic impairment, severe hypotension, active bleeding, and active peptic ulcer. **Use with caution** in gall bladder or liver disease, diabetes mellitus, gout, glaucoma, or peptic ulcer.

🖐 **Extended-release form contraindicated for children. Use with caution for nursing mothers. May be used safely in recommended daily allowances (RDA) for pregnant women (preg A); safe use in doses greater than RDA has not been established (preg C).**

Side effects/Adverse reactions

Hypersensitivity: skin rash, itching, wheezing. **CV:** excessive peripheral vasodilation, postural hypotension, dysrhythmias. **Skin:** flushing, dryness, itching. **CNS:** headache and dizziness. **Hem:** hyperglycemia, hyperuricemia. **GI:** nausea, vomiting, diarrhea, activation of peptic ulcer, hepatotoxicity.

Nursing implications/Documentation

Possible nursing diagnoses: Potential for injury; Pain; Impaired skin integrity.

* For IV administration, do not exceed rate of 2 mg/min.
* Monitor liver function test results.
* For diabetics, monitor glucose levels closely because requirements of insulin or oral hypoglycemics may change.
* Assess for orthostatic hypotension, especially when antihypertensives are also being administered.

Patient & family teaching/Home care

Possible nursing diagnoses: Knowledge deficit; Impaired home maintenance management.

* Instruct to take drug with meals to minimize GI side effects.
* Caution not to crush or chew extended-release preparations; however, capsule may be emptied into jam or jelly and swallowed without chewing.
* Explain that there is a possibility of dizziness or faintness; recommend to change position slowly to prevent hypotension and dizziness.
* Caution against driving or operating dangerous equipment until response is determined.
* Inform that skin flushing will last for 30 minutes to 1 hour after dose, that flushing usually diminishes within 2 weeks, and that 300 mg (1 tablet) of aspirin 30 minutes before dose may help reduce flushing.
* For niacin deficiency, identify important food sources of niacin (meats, eggs, and milk and dairy products).
* Advise not taking doses larger than RDA recommendation, except on physician's advice.
* For treatment of hyperlipidemia, stress importance of dietary management, weight reduction, and avoidance of alcohol (point out that excessive nausea and vomiting after drinking alcohol may indicate impaired liver function and should be reported).

nicardipine

nye-car'de-peen

Cardene

Class: Antihypertensive, Antianginal, Calcium channel blocking agent

PEDS	PREG	GERI
🖐	C	🖐

Action Reduces blood pressure and myocardial oxygen demand by decreasing total peripheral resistance and afterload, and by relaxing coronary artery smooth muscle. Inhibits calcium ion influx across the cell membrane.

Use/Therapeutic goal/Outcome

Antihypertensive: Reduction of blood pressure; reduction of total peripheral resistance and afterload. *Outcome criteria:* blood pressure within normal limits.

Angina pectoris: Promotion of myocardial oxygenation, prevention of anginal (ischemic) attacks. *Outcome criteria:* Patient report of decreased frequency and severity of anginal attacks; increased exercise tolerance.

Dose range/Administration

Interaction alert: Cimetidine may increase nicardipine serum levels. Nicardipine may elevate cyclosporine serum levels. Beta-blockers may increase cardiodepressant effects. Enhances theophylline effect.

Adult: PO: 20–40 mg tid.

Clinical alert: Allow 3 days between dose adjustments to achieve stable plasma levels. Check blood pressure prior to giving dose; hold dose and report if hypotension is present. Record blood pressure 1 hour after dose, when peak effects are likely.

Contraindications/Precautions

PREG
C

Contraindicated in hypersensitivity to nicardipine, and in hypotension and advanced aortic stenosis. *Use with caution* in patients with impaired renal or hepatic function.

✋ Use with caution for the elderly. Safe use for pregnant or nursing mothers and for children is unknown.

Side effects/Adverse reactions

Hypersensitivity: rash. *CNS:* dizziness, weakness, fatigue. *CV:* hypotension, pedal edema, palpitations, tachycardia. *GI:* nausea, dyspepsia. *Skin:* flushing.

Nursing implications/Documentation

Possible nursing diagnoses: Potential for injury; Activity intolerance.

◆ Keep a record of pulse and blood pressure before and after drug administration.

◆ Be aware that an increase in frequency or severity of angina may occur while initiating therapy or titrating dose; treat as ordered.

◆ Observe for postural hypotension; take blood pressure in both arms, and with patient sitting and standing if possible.

◆ Supervise ambulation until response is determined.

◆ Coordinate care to provide frequent rest periods.

Patient & family teaching/Home care

Possible nursing diagnoses: Fear; Knowledge deficit; Impaired home maintenance management.

◆ Explain that this drug controls blood pressure and reduces the workload of the heart.

◆ Stress the need to follow dose regimen closely (the drug should be taken at the same time each day) and the need to return for medical follow-up.

◆ Advise changing positions slowly to avoid dizziness.

◆ Warn against taking any other drugs without checking with primary physician.

◆ If possible, teach self-monitoring of blood pressure and pulse; stress that persistent hypotension, hypertension, pulse irregularities, or dizziness should be reported.

◆ Encourage keeping a record of angina attacks to observe pattern, and reporting an increase in frequency or severity (explain that angina episodes may increase when starting nicardipine, and that these should be treated as ordered).

◆ Warn not to drive or operate machinery until response is determined (may cause dizziness).

◆ *See Calcium Channel Blockers, Antihypertensives, and Antianginals overviews for more information.*

nifedipine

nye-fed'i-peen

Adalat, ♣Aldalat PA, Apo-Nifed, Novo-Nifedin, Procardia, Procardia-XL

Class: Antianginal, Calcium channel blocking agent

PEDS   PREG   GERI
✋   C   ✋

Action Inhibits calcium ion influx across the cell membrane, which results in increased availability of oxygen to the myocardium (by dilating coronary arteries) and decreased workload and oxygen demand of the heart (by reducing heart rate and force of contraction). Vasodilation causes blood pressure (and afterload) to drop, which may result in reflex tachycardia.

Use/Therapeutic goal/Outcome

Angina pectoris: Promotion of myocardial oxygenation, prevention of anginal (ischemic) attacks, improved activity tolerance. **Outcome criteria:** Patient reports decreased frequency and severity of angina, and demonstrates improved activity tolerance.

Hypertension: Reduction in blood pressure. **Outcome criteria:** Blood pressure within normal limits.

Raynaud's phenomenon: Improved peripheral perfusion. **Outcome criteria:** Patient reports and demonstrates a decrease in peripheral vascular symptoms (numbness, blanching, and cooling of skin).

Dose range/Administration

Interaction alert: Use with beta-blockers may cause heart block and CHF. Cimetidine and ranitidine may decrease nifedipine metabolism.

Adult: PO: 10 mg tid. May be increased as necessary. Range is 10–30 mg tid or qid (not to exceed 180 mg/day). Tell the patient not to chew, swallow or crush capsules. SL: puncture capsule with a needle and squirt fluid under tongue (use same dose as above).

Clinical alert: Check blood pressure before giving drug; hold dose and report if hypotension is present.

Contraindications/Precautions

PREG
C

Contraindicated in hypersensitivity to nifedipine. **Use with caution** in CHF or hypotension.

🖐 **Use with caution for pregnant and nursing mothers and for the elderly. Safe use for children has not been established.**

Side effects/Adverse reactions

Hypersensitivity: dermatitis, urticaria. **CNS:** dizziness, lightheadedness, headache, weakness, fatigue. **CV:** hypotension, congestive heart failure, pulmonary edema, palpitations, tachycardia, shortness of breath. **Resp:** nasal congestion. **GI:** nausea, vomiting, diarrhea, heartburn, constipation. **MS:** joint stiffness. **Eye:** transient blindness. **Misc:** fever, sweating, chills.

Nursing implications/Documentation

Possible nursing diagnoses: Potential for injury; Activity intolerance.

◆ Keep a record of pulse and blood pressure, before and after drug administration.

◆ Monitor for and report early signs of CHF.

◆ Be aware that increased episodes of angina may be experienced at the beginning of therapy; treat as ordered by physician.

◆ Observe for postural hypotension; take blood pressure in both arms, and sitting and standing if possible.

◆ Supervise ambulation until response to drug is determined.

◆ Coordinate care to provide frequent rest periods.

Patient & family teaching/Home care

Possible nursing diagnoses: Fear; Knowledge deficit; Impaired home maintenance management.

◆ Explain that nifedipine decreases blood pressure, reduces the workload of the heart and improves coronary blood supply.

◆ Stress the need to follow dose regimen closely (the drug should be taken at the same time each day), and the need to return for medical follow-up.

◆ Emphasize the need to pace activities, avoid stress (emotional and physical), and plan for rest periods.

◆ Explain that an extra sublingual dose of nitroglycerin may be necessary during stress, or at bedtime if angina is nocturnal.

◆ Warn against taking other drugs without consulting with primary physician.

◆ Advise changing positions slowly to avoid dizziness.

◆ Encourage keeping a record of angina attacks to determine pattern; stress that an increase in frequency or severity should be reported.

◆ Warn that drinking alcohol may cause fainting and hypotension.

◆ *See Calcium Channel Blockers, Antihypertensives, and Antianginals overviews for more information.*

nimodipine

ni-mode'i-peen

Nimotop
Class: Calcium channel blocking agent

PEDS	PREG	GERI
🖐	C	🖐

Action Inhibits contractions of vascular smooth muscle by inhibiting calcium ion influx across the cell membrane. Because it crosses the blood/brain barrier, its greatest effect is prevention of cerebral arterial spasm.

Use/Therapeutic goal/Outcome

Subarachnoid hemorrhage: Improvement of neurological deficits caused by vasospasms after subarachnoid hemorrhage. **Outcome criteria:** Increased level of consciousness and improved motor function.

Dose range/Administration

Interaction alert: Other calcium channel blockers may have additive cardiovascular effects. Cimetidine decreases metabolism of nimodipine.

Adult: PO: 60 mg q4h for 21 days. If capsule cannot be swallowed, aspirate contents of capsule with an 18-gauge needle and administer orally.

Clinical alert: Therapy should begin within 96 hours of subarachnoid hemorrhage and continue for 21 days. Dose should be reduced to 30 mg q4h in patients with severe liver disease.

Contraindications/Precautions

PREG C

Contraindicated in hypersensitivity to calcium channel blockers, and in lactation, second- or third-degree heart block, hypotension, and renal failure. **Use with caution** in patients with liver disease.

👋 **Use with caution in the elderly. Safe use for pregnant women and for children has not been established.**

Side effects/Adverse reactions

Hypersensitivity: rash. **CV:** hypotension, edema, EKG abnormalities, tachycardia. **CNS:** headache, depression, fatigue. **GI:** nausea, vomiting, diarrhea, abnormal liver function tests. **Resp:** dyspnea. **MS:** muscle pain or cramps.

Nursing implications/Documentation

Possible nursing diagnoses: Activity intolerance; Fatigue; Potential for injury.

◆ Assess neurological status and document pulse and blood pressure in both arms (with patient lying, sitting, and standing, if possible) prior to administration, and frequently thereafter until response is determined.

◆ Consult with physician to determine desired therapeutic range for blood pressure and heart rate (parameters for withholding the medication should be written by physician).

◆ Ascertain that results of baseline CBC, electrolytes, BUN, creatinine, and other liver function studies have been obtained before giving the first dose; report abnormalities and monitor closely thereafter.

◆ Monitor for allergic reactions, confusion, dizziness, bradycardia, congestive heart failure or hypotension; hold drug and report immediately if these occur.

◆ Document and monitor daily weight, and intake and output; report significant negative or positive balance.

◆ Supervise ambulation until response is determined.

Patient & family teaching/Home care

Possible nursing diagnoses: Knowledge deficit; Impaired home maintenance management.

◆ Explain the importance of taking this drug exactly as prescribed for 21 days, even when feeling well.

◆ Teach how to monitor pulse and blood pressure; emphasize that syncope, hypertension or hypotension, deterioration in neurological symptoms, or persistent dizziness should be reported; provide pulse and blood pressure parameters for withholding medication.

◆ Advise changing positions slowly, to avoid dizziness.

◆ *See Calcium Channel Blockers overview for more information.*

N

nitrofurantoin
nye-tro-fyoor'an-toyn

♣**Apo-Nitrofurantoin, Furadantin, Furalan, Furan, Furanite, Macrodantin,** ♣**Nephronex, Nitrofan,** ♣**Novofuran**

nitrofurantoin macrocrystals: **Macrodantin**

Class: Urinary tract anti-infective

PEDS	PREG	GERI
👋	B	👋

Action Bacteriostatic in low concentration, limits growth of a wide variety of gram-negative and gram-positive bacteria, presumably by damaging DNA. May kill bacteria (bactericidal) in high concentrations.

Use/Therapeutic goal/Outcome

Treatment or prophylaxis of pyelonephritis, pyelitis, and cystitis caused by susceptible organisms (*Escherichia coli, Staphylococcus aureus,* enterococci, certain strains of *Klebsiella, Proteus,* and *Enterobacter*): Prevention or resolution of infection. *Outcome criteria:* Absence of growth on urine culture; report of absence of dysuria, frequency.

Dose range/Administration

Interaction alert: Separate doses of nitrofurantoin from doses of magnesium-containing antacids by 1 hour. Probenicid and sulfinpyrazone increase blood levels of nitrofurantoin (monitor for toxicity).

🍴 **Give with food to reduce GI distress.**

Adult/Child > 12 yrs: PO: *Prophylaxis:* 50–100 mg qid. *Long-term suppression therapy:* 50–100 mg/day at bedtime. *Child 3 mos to 12 yrs:* PO: 5–7 mg/kg/day, in divided doses qid. If using suspension or crushed tablets, avoid direct contact with teeth (may cause staining).

Clinical alert: If nausea occurs after administration, it may be relieved by using *macrocrystalline* preparation. Monitor the elderly for septic shock.

Contraindications/Precautions

PREG
B

Contraindicated in hypersensitivity to nitrofurantoin or nitrofuran derivatives, and in anuria, oliguria, creatinine clearance < 40 ml/min, and G6PD deficiency. *Use with caution* in history of asthma, anemia, diabetes, Vitamin B deficiency, and electrolyte imbalance.

🖐 **Contraindicated for infants under 3 months. Use with caution for the elderly or debilitated. Safe use for pregnant or nursing mothers has not been determined.**

Side effects/Adverse reactions

Hypersensitivity: itching, rashes, angioedema, eosinophilia, fever, chills, arthralgia, allergic pneumonitis, asthma (with history of asthma), arthralgia, cholestatic jaundice, anaphylaxis. *GI:* anorexia, nausea, vomiting, abdominal pain, diarrhea, hepatitis. *Resp:* pneumonitis (chest pain, chills, cough, fever, dyspnea). *CNS:* drowsiness, headache, dizziness, peripheral neuropathy, ascending polyneuropathy (with renal impairment or high doses). *Hem:* granulocytosis, leukopenia, anemia, hemolysis (in patients with G6PD deficiency—reversed after drug is discontinued).

Nursing implications/Documentation

Possible nursing diagnoses: Altered patterns of urinary elimination; Fluid volume deficit.

◆ Obtain urine for culture and sensitivity, and ensure that necessary lab studies (e.g., CBC, BUN, creatinine, liver function) are done before administering first dose; monitor closely thereafter if therapy is prolonged.

◆ Monitor for and report pulmonary or flu-like symptoms (because of risk of allergic pneumonitis); infections caused by nonsusceptible organisms (especially *Pseudomonas*); symptoms of peripheral neuropathy (e.g., weakness, tingling, numbness; may be severe and irreversible).

◆ Watch for delayed-onset hypersensitivity.

◆ Provide acidic juices (cranberry, plum, prune), and document and monitor intake and output, to maintain adequate hydration (at least 2 L a day, not more, or urine will be too dilute).

Patient & family teaching/Home care

Possible nursing diagnoses: Knowledge deficit; Impaired home maintenance management.

◆ Encourage taking doses with meals to reduce GI symptoms.

◆ Explain that acidic juices (cranberry, plum, prune) enhance drug action, that the patient should drink 2 L of fluid daily (not more), and that intake of alkaline food (vegetables, milk, peanuts) should be limited.

◆ Advise reporting any symptoms that do not abate after 3 days, symptoms of allergy (itching, rashes, respiratory symptoms), muscle weakness, numbness, tingling, new symptoms of illness (e.g., fever, sore throat, joint pain); explain that medications may have to be changed.

◆ Warn that urine may be colored brown, but that this is harmless.

◆ *See Anti-infectives overview for more information.*

nitrofurazone

nye-tro-fyoor'a-zone

Furacin

Class: Local anti-infective

PEDS	PREG	GERI
🖐	C	🖐

Action Exact mechanism of action is unknown. Believed to limit bacterial growth (bactericidal action) by inhibiting bacterial enzymes that are necessary for bacterial metabolism. Effective against many bacteria that have developed resistance to other antibiotics and sulfonamides.

Use/Therapeutic goal/Outcome

Adjunctive therapy to prevent infection in patients with second- and third-degree burns and those with skin grafts or donor sites when bacterial resistance to other anti-infectives is suspected or has developed: Prevention, suppression, or elimination of bacterial growth, promotion of healing. *Outcome criteria:* Absence of growth on culture; absence of clinical manifestations of infection (redness, heat, pain, swelling, drainage); observable viable, healthy tissue.

Dose range/Administration

Adult and Child: Topical: Using sterile gloves, apply soluble 0.2% ointment or cream directly to lesion or onto gauze qd or less. May also use 0.2% solution. Spray saturated dressings (diluted 1:1 with sterile water or 0.9% NS).

Clinical alert: Frequency of application depends on condition being treated. If solution is cloudy, warm to 55–60 degrees. Persistent cloudiness suggests microbial contamination. Consult with physician for procedure for cleansing before application and for dressing after application. Usually petrolatum or zinc oxide is applied to normal skin surrounding wound for protection (contact dermatitis is common).

Contraindications/Precautions

PREG C

Contraindicated in hypersensitivity to nitrofurazone. *Use with caution* in renal impairment (contains polyethylene glycols that may not be excreted).

🖐 **Use with caution for children, pregnant or nursing mothers, and the elderly.**

Side effects/Adverse reactions

Hypersensitivity: allergic contact dermatitis, anaphylaxis. *Skin:* erythema, pruritus, burning, edema, vesiculation, denudation, ulceration, superinfections, and autosensitization. *GU:* renal impairment.

Nursing implications/Documentation

Possible nursing diagnoses: Potential for infection; Impaired skin integrity.

♦ Record appearance of skin with each dressing change.

♦ Report failure to heal or increase in signs of infection (superinfection and sensitization is possible).

♦ If used over large areas, monitor serum creatinine and BUN (polyethylene glycols from this drug can accumulate through denuded skin and compromise renal function).

Patient & family teaching/Home care

Possible nursing diagnoses: Knowledge deficit; Impaired home maintenance management.

♦ Demonstrate procedure for cleansing area, applying medication, and changing dressings; observe return demonstration.

♦ Advise reporting new symptoms of irritation or inflammation immediately.

♦ Warn that contact dermatitis is common if this drug comes in contact with normal skin.

♦ *See Anti-infectives overview for more information.*

nitroglycerin
nye-troe-gli'ser-in

Carabid, Corobid, Deponit NTG Film, Klavikordal, Niong, ♠Nitradisc, Nitro-Bid, Nitrocap, Nitrocap TD, Nitrocine, Nitrodisc, Nitro-Dur, Nitro-Dur II, Nitrogard, Nirtogard SR, Nitrol, Nitroglyn, ♠Nitrolate Ointment, Nitrolin, Nitrolingual, Nitrol Ointment, Nitronet, Nitrong, Nitron SR, Nitrospan, Nitrostat, Nitrostat IV, NTS, Transderm-Nitro, Tridil

Class: ★Antianginal prototype, Organic nitrate

PEDS	PREG	GERI
🖐	C	🖐

Action Decreases cardiac workload and myocardial oxygen demand by reducing left ventricular end-diastolic pressure (preload) and, to a lesser extent, by reducing systemic vascular resistance (afterload). Relaxes smooth muscle, particularly peripheral vascular smooth muscle, and has a vasodilating effect on the large systemic arteries and veins, which decreases blood pressure. Also improves myocardial oxygen perfusion by promoting collateral circulation.

Use/Therapeutic goal/Outcome

Angina pectoris: Promotion of myocardial oxygenation, resolution or prevention of angina, improvement in activity tolerance. *Outcome criteria:* Patient reports relief of chest discomfort and decreased frequency of angina attacks, and demonstrates increased activity tolerance.

▶

ST segments on the EKG return to normal.

Preoperative hypertension: Control of perioperative hypertension: prevention of hypertensive response during surgery, especially during anesthesia induction and intubation. **Outcome criteria:** Blood pressure within normal limits during surgery.

Congestive heart failure (CHF): Resolution of signs of CHF symptoms. **Outcome criteria:** Clearing of lung fields; urine output > 30 cc/hr; pulmonary artery pressure, pulmonary wedge pressure, and cardiac output within normal limits.

Dose range/Administration

Interaction alert: Antihypertensives and alcohol potentiate nitroglycerin action. When using IV nitroglycerine, do not mix with any other drugs. Decreases effect of heparin.

Give oral doses 30 minutes before or 2–3 hours after meals.

Adult: PO: (sustained release): *Loading Dose:* 1.3, 2.6, or 6.5 mg tid to qid. *Maintenance dose:* 2.6–9 mg q8-12h. SL: Dissolve one tablet of 0.15 mg, 0.3 mg, 0.4 mg, or 0.6 mg (1/400, 1/200, 1/150, or 1/100 grain) under tongue or in buccal pouch (tell the patient not to chew it or swallow it). May be repeated every 3–5 min for 15 min. TRANSDERMAL (ointment): Usual starting dosage is 1/2 inch q8h, which is then increased by 1/2-inch increments until desired response is achieved. (Frequency of administration may also be increased.) Use dose-measuring paper supplied with ointment. Avoid getting ointment on fingers. Do not rub in. Cover with plastic to aid absorption. Keep nitroglycerin ointment tube tightly closed. If using the Tape Surrounded Appli- Ruler system, keep ointment on skin area of applicator, not on Appli-Tape. TRANSDERMAL (patch): Apply to nonhairy areas once daily (avoid distal extremities; use chest, shoulders, arms, thighs, or abdomen). To prevent tolerance, apply patch only during the day, or while awake. Rotate transdermal sites to avoid irritation. IV: Must be diluted: *Not for direct injection.* Dilute in D5W or NS. Use a glass IV bottle. Avoid using a filter or PVC (polyvinyl) tubing (dosage adjustment may be necessary with PVC tubing). Dilutions range from 25–500 mcg/ml. Recommended initial rate: 5 mcg/min using an infusion pump. Titrate dose according to situation (comfort state and blood pressure response must be specified in writing by physician). Increments of 5 mcg/min every 3–5 min may be made while blood pressure is closely monitored until desired response is

achieved. Larger increments (10–20 mcg/min) may also be necessary. No fixed maximum dose has been established. TRANSLINGUAL: Spray 1–2 metered doses onto oral mucosa. Do not exceed 3 doses within 15 min. Tell patient not to inhale through mouth or swallow for 10 seconds after dose.

Clinical alert: Record blood pressure immediately before administering dose, and 5 min after dose, until desired response is achieved (with IV administration, record blood pressure every 5–10 min while dosage is being titrated). Check physician's orders for blood pressure parameters that indicate when the drug should be withheld. Have the patient use a scale of 1 to 10 to rate pain before and after dose.

Contraindications/Precautions

PREG C

Contraindicated in hypersensitivity to nitrates, and in myocardial infarction accompanied by hypotension, severe anemia, and the presence of increased intracranial pressure. Intravenous preparation should not be given in the presence of hypovolemia, increased intracranial pressure (cerebral hemorrhage, head trauma), pericardial tamponade or pericarditis. Topical preparation is contraindicated in contact dermatitis, or topical allergic reactions.

Use with caution in the elderly. Safe use for pregnant or nursing mothers and for children has not been established.

Side effects/Adverse reactions

Hypersensitivity: rash, contact dermatitis. **CNS:** headache, dizziness, weakness, fainting, apprehension, restlessness. **CV:** orthostatic hypotension, tachycardia, palpitations, circulatory collapse. **GI:** dry mouth, nausea, vomiting, sublingual burning. **Skin:** flushing, cutaneous vasodilation. **Eye:** blurred vision.

Nursing implications/Documentation

Possible nursing diagnoses: Potential for injury; Activity intolerance.

◆ Give sublingual doses at the first sign of angina; have the patient use a scale of 1 to 10 to rate pain immediately before and 5 minutes after administration; report unrelieved pain immediately.

◆ Keep a record of pulse and blood pressure, before and after drug administration.

◆ Monitor for and report headache (a side effect usually treated with mild analgesics; tolerance of headache usually occurs with long-term use).

- Observe for postural hypotension; take blood pressure in both arms, and with patient sitting and standing if possible.
- Supervise ambulation until response is determined.
- Coordinate care to provide frequent rest periods.
- Be aware that this drug is inactivated when exposed to heat, moisture, and air (bottle should be discarded and replaced 6 months after opening).
- Discontinuation of transdermal administration should be tapered over 4–6 weeks.
- Remove nitroglycerin patch before defibrillation—patch may explode.

Patient & family teaching/Home care

Possible nursing diagnoses: Fear; Knowledge deficit; Impaired home maintenance management.
- Explain that antianginals help reduce the workload of the heart and improve coronary blood supply.
- Stress the need to follow dose regimen closely (scheduled doses should be taken at the same time each day), and the need to return for medical follow-up.
- Advise taking oral doses 30 minutes before meals or 2–3 hours after meals; stress that sustained-release preparations not be chewed.
- Teach to take sublingual doses at the first sign of angina: wet tablet with saliva and place it under the tongue until completely dissolved.
- Assure that tolerance to headache develops with long-term use.
- Emphasize the need to pace activities, avoid stress (emotional and physical), and plan for rest periods.
- Explain that an extra sublingual dose may be necessary during stress, or at night time if angina is nocturnal; teach that dose may be repeated every 10–15 minutes for 3 doses. If angina is unrelieved, the paramedics should be called.
- Advise changing positions slowly to avoid dizziness.
- Encourage keeping a record of angina attacks to observe pattern; stress that an increase in frequency or severity should be reported.
- Advise reporting blurred vision or dry mouth.
- Stress that discontinuing this drug abruptly could precipitate coronary vasospasm.
- Warn that drinking alcohol may cause fainting and hypotension.
- Emphasize that this drug could be ineffective if exposed to moisture, heat, or air (keep in a cool dark place).
- *See Antianginals overview for more information.*

nitroprusside

nye-troe-pruss'ide

nitroprusside sodium: **Nipride, Nitropress**
Class: ★Antihypertensive crisis prototype, Vasodilator

PEDS	PREG	GERI
✋	C	✋

Action Reduces blood pressure by causing vasodilation of arteriolar and venous smooth muscle, thereby decreasing peripheral resistance (PVR) cardiac output (CO), and pulmonary capillary wedge pressure (PCWP).

Use/Therapeutic goal/Outcome

Hypertensive emergencies: Reduction of blood pressure. **Outcome criteria:** Blood pressure within normal limits.

Congestive heart failure: Resolution of congestive heart failure. **Outcome criteria:** Blood pressure within normal limits.

Dose range/Administration

Adult: IV: Add 2–3 cc of D5W only to a 50 mg vial, and further dilute in 250, 500, or 1000 cc D5W only. Begin infusion at 0.5 mcg/kg/min. Increase rate by 0.2 mcg/kg/min every 5 min as needed, while closely monitoring blood pressure. *Maximum dose:* 10 mcg/kg/min. *Average dose:* 3 mcg/kg/min. **Child:** IV: 1.4 mcg/kg/min. Adjust slowly according to response.

Clinical alert: Protect from light by wrapping IV bag in package provided. IV tubing need not be wrapped. Infuse with a pump or controller. Use solution within 4 hours of preparation. Reconstituted solution has a brownish tint; discard if strongly colored. Do not add other medications to solution.

Contraindications/Precautions

PREG
C

Contraindicated in hypersensitivity, compensatory hypertension (coarction of aorta, arteriovenous shunt), hepatic failure, inadequate cerebral circulation. *Use with caution* in coronary insufficiency, impaired renal function, and hypothyroidism.

🖐 **Use with caution for the elderly. Safe use for children and pregnant women has not been established.**

Side effects/Adverse reactions

Hypersensitivity: rash, urticaria. *CV:* palpitations, tachycardia, distant heart sounds, weak pulse, rebound hypertension. *CNS:* headache, dizziness, restlessness, loss of consciousness, coma, absent reflexes, muscle twitching. *Resp:* diaphoresis, dyspnea, shallow breathing. *GI:* vomiting, nausea, abdominal pain. *Misc:* metabolic acidosis.

Nursing implications/Documentation

Possible nursing diagnoses: Activity intolerance; Fatigue; Potential for injury.

♦ Assess mental status, and record pulse and blood pressure (lying and sitting and in both arms) prior to administration, every 5 minutes during initiation of therapy, then every 15 minutes, then every 30 minutes, then every hour when stable.

♦ Consult with physician to determine desired therapeutic range for blood pressure (be aware that some patients may require a slightly elevated blood pressure to perfuse vital organs).

♦ Ascertain that baseline, CBC, electrolytes, BUN, creatinine, and liver function studies have been obtained before giving first dose; report abnormalities and monitor closely thereafter.

♦ Monitor for allergic reactions and for confusion, dizziness, rales, tachycardia, arrythmias, and hypotension; hold drug (or decrease IV rate) and report immediately if these occur.

♦ Also watch for symptoms of thiocyanate poisoning (nausea, disorientation, muscle spasms, absent reflexes, metabolic acidosis). Thiocyanate levels should be checked every 3 days, levels greater than 10 mg/dl are toxic.

♦ Keep side rails up with call bell in reach.

♦ Document and monitor daily weight, and intake and output; report significant negative or positive balance.

Patient & family teaching/Home care

Possible nursing diagnoses: Knowledge deficit; Anxiety; Fear.

♦ Instruct the patient to remain in bed; advise changing positions slowly, to avoid dizziness.

♦ Explain the rationale for monitoring blood pressure frequently; ask the patient to report new symptoms or unusual feelings, in case they indicate a need for adjustment in medication rate.

♦ *See Antihypertensives overview for more information.*

nizatidine   *ni-zat'ih-dine*

Axid

Class: Histamine (H$_2$) receptor antagonist, Antiulcer agent, Gastric acid secretion inhibitor

PEDS	PREG	GERI
🖐	C	🖐

Action Decreases basal and nocturnal secretion of gastric acid by inhibiting the action of histamine at the H$_2$ receptors in the gastric parietal cells; decreases gastric acid secretion in response to food or chemical stimulus.

Use/Therapeutic goal/Outcome

Peptic ulcers: Promotion of healing and relief of pain. *Outcome criteria:* Report of absence of pain; hemoglobin and hematocrit within normal range; vital signs stable; stools negative for occult blood; endoscopic evidence of healing.

Prophylaxis of ulcer recurrence: Prevention. *Outcome criteria:* Report of absence of gastric pain; stable hemoglobin and hematocrit; stool and gastric secretions free of blood.

Dose range/Administration

Interaction alert: Do not give antacids within 1 hr to avoid interference with absorption of nizatidine. With large doses of aspirin, high serum salicylate levels may be seen.

🖐 **Give with food.**

Adult: PO: 300 mg/day at bedtime, or 150 mg bid. *Maintenance dose:* 150 mg at bedtime.

Clinical alert: In moderate to severe renal failure, reduced doses should be used.

Contraindications/Precautions   PREG C

Contraindicated in hypersensitivity to histamine (H$_2$) receptor antagonists. *Use with caution* in hepatic or renal impairment.

🖐 **Use with caution for pregnant or nursing mothers and the elderly. Safe use for children has not been established.**

Side effects/Adverse reactions

Hypersensitivity: rash, swelling of eyelids, bronchospasm. **CNS:** somnolence. **GI:** diarrhea. **MS:** joint or muscle pain. **Misc:** sweating, fever.

Nursing implications/Documentation

Possible nursing diagnoses: Potential for injury.

♦ Administer single dose at bedtime; with twice daily dosing, last dose should be at bedtime.

♦ Assess for and report excessive drowsiness.

♦ Record color and character of stools.

Patient & family teaching/Home care

Possible nursing diagnoses: Knowledge deficit.

♦ Teach that single daily dose should be taken at bedtime.

♦ Point out the need to avoid taking antacids within 1 hr of nizatidine.

♦ Advise smokers not to smoke after the bedtime dose to provide optimal suppression of nocturnal gastric acid secretion.

♦ Inform those being treated for active ulcer disease that this medication should be taken as prescribed for 4 to 8 weeks to ensure healing of the ulcer, even though symptoms usually subside earlier.

♦ Stress that the primary physician should be notified if somnolence or rash develop, or if "coffee grounds" vomit or tarry stools occur.

♦ Counsel smokers with active ulcer disease to stop smoking and to avoid the use of caffeine.

♦ *See Histamine₂ Antagonists overview for more information.*

norepinephrine

nor-ep-i-nef'rin

norepinephrine bitartrate: **Levophed**

Class: ★Direct-acting alpha adrenergic (sympathomimetic) prototype, Vasopressor agonist, Catecholamine

PEDS	PREG	GERI
🤚	**D**	🤚

Action Increases systemic blood pressure, coronary artery blood flow, and venous return by stimulating alpha and beta receptors in the sympathetic nervous system (acts as a powerful vasoconstrictor on arterial and venous beds and produces a positive inotropic stimulation of the heart). As a result of vasoconstriction there is a reduction in blood flow to the kidneys, other vital organs, skin, and skeletal muscle.

Use/Therapeutic goal/Outcome

Acute hypotension and shock: Improvement of blood pressure and coronary artery blood flow. **Outcome criteria:** Blood pressure > 90–100 systolic; absence of clinical signs of shock (confusion, restlessness, rapid weak pulse, urine output < 25 ml/hr).

Dose range/Administration

Interaction alert: Parenteral ergot alkaloids, guanethidine, methyldopa, tricyclic antidepressants, and some antihistamines increase effects. Alpha-adrenergic blocking agents may reduce effects. Do not use within 14 days of MAOI therapy (may cause hypertensive crisis). **Adult:** IV: 8–12 mcg/min. Dose highly individualized, titrated according to blood pressure. *Maintenance dose:* 2–4 mcg/min. **Child:** IV: 2 mcg/min. Titrate to maintain desired blood pressure.

Clinical alert: Ascertain that hypotension is not a result of hypovolemia (volume deficits should be corrected before starting vasopressors). Use a large vein and monitor closely for infiltration. If infiltration occurs, stop infusion immediately and notify physician. Expect that phentolamine (Regitine) 5–10 mg in 10–15 ml of normal saline may be injected with a fine hypodermic syringe into affected areas to minimize extravasation ischemia. Keep emergency drugs and equipment readily available.

Contraindications/Precautions

PREG
D

Contraindicated in hypersensitivity to norepinephrine and sulfites, and in mesenteric or peripheral vascular thrombosis, during cyclopropane or halothane anesthesia, profound hypoxia, or hypercapnia.

🤚 **Use with caution for children and the elderly. Use for pregnant women only if benefits outweigh risks (norepinephrine crosses placenta, causes uterine contractions).**

Side effects/Adverse reactions

Hypersensitivity: bluish coloration of skin; dizziness; flushing or redness of skin; rash; hives; itching; swelling of face, lips, or eyelids; wheezing or difficulty breathing; exaggeration of side effects. **CV:** palpitations, hypertension, bradycardia (reflex), fatal arrhythmias. **CNS:** restlessness, headache, anxiety, tremors, dizziness, weakness, insomnia. *Skin:* pallor, tissue necrosis with extravasation.

Nursing implications/Documentation

Possible nursing diagnoses: Potential for injury; Activity intolerance.

♦ Record and monitor pulse, blood pressure, and respirations every 2–5 min until stable, then every 15 min, then every 1/2–1 hr.

♦ Record urine output hourly; report persistent urine output less than 30 ml/hr.

♦ Keep head of the bed down and place side rails up; report changes in mental status.

♦ When weaning off norepinephrine bitartrate, taper dose slowly, while closely monitoring blood pressure.

Patient & family teaching/Home care

Possible nursing diagnoses: Knowledge deficit; Fear; Ineffective family coping.

♦ Stress that frequent monitoring of vital signs is needed to "fine tune" medication dose for optimum results; stress the need to remain in bed.

♦ Stress that the nurses need to be told of new symptoms or uncomfortable feelings in case they indicate a need for medication adjustment.

♦ *See Adrenergics (sympathomimetics) overview for more information.*

norfloxacin

nor-flox'a-sin

Noroxin

Class: Urinary tract anti-infective

PEDS	PREG	GERI
🖐	C	🖐

Action Potently bactericidal, kills virtually all urinary tract bacteria by inhibiting DNA synthesis.

Use/Therapeutic goal/Outcome

Urinary tract infection caused by susceptible organisms: Resolution of infection. *Outcome criteria:* Absence of growth on urine culture; report of absence of dysuria, frequency.

Dose range/Administration

Interaction alert: Do not use with nitrofurantoin (decreases effect). Separate doses of antacids from doses of norfloxacin as far as possible (antacids reduce and delay effects).

🥤 **Give with a full glass of water one hour before meals and at bedtime.**

Adult: PO: *Uncomplicated infections:* 400 mg bid for 7–10 days. *Complicated infections:* Continue for 10–20 days.

Clinical alert: Schedule doses on a strict 12-hour schedule (taking norfloxacin at erratic intervals may encourage emergence of resistant bacteria). Monitor the elderly closely for septic shock.

Contraindications/Precautions
PREG C

Contraindicated in hypersensitivity to norfloxacin, nalidixic acid, cinoxacin, or other quinolones, and history of seizure disorder. *Use with caution* in kidney or liver disease.

🖐 Use with caution for the elderly. Safe use for children and pregnant or nursing mothers has not been established.

Side effects/Adverse reactions

Hypersensitivity: itching, rashes. *GI:* nausea, constipation, heartburn, flatulence. *CNS:* drowsiness, headache, fatigue, dizziness. *Hem:* transient elevation in SGOT and SGPT.

Nursing implications/Documentation

Possible nursing diagnoses: Altered patterns of urinary elimination; Fluid volume deficit.

♦ Obtain urine for culture and sensitivity, and ensure that necessary lab studies (e.g., CBC, BUN, creatinine, liver function studies) are done before administering first dose; monitor closely thereafter if therapy is prolonged.

Patient & family teaching/Home care

Possible nursing diagnoses: Knowledge deficit; Impaired home maintenance management.

♦ Point out that norfloxacin should be taken on a strict 12-hour schedule, and on an empty stomach.

♦ Advise reporting any symptoms that do not abate after 3 days, new symptoms of illness (fever, sore throat), symptoms of allergy (itching, rashes).

♦ Stress the importance of taking this drug without missing doses for the entire time prescribed, even if symptoms disappear.

♦ *See Anti-infectives overview for more information.*

nortriptyline

nor-trip'ti-leen

nortriptyline hydrochloride: ***Aventyl, Pamelor***
Class: Tricyclic antidepressant (TCA)

PEDS	PREG	GERI
✋	**D**	✋

Action Improves mood by increasing levels of the neurotransmitters norepinephrine and serotonin in the CNS. (Blocks neurotransmitter reuptake into presynaptic neurons by inhibiting the "amine pump." Reuptake normally terminates the action of neurotransmitters.)

Use/Therapeutic goal/Outcome

Major depressive disorders: Promotion of sense of well-being, ability to cope with daily living. ***Outcome criteria:*** After 2–4 weeks, report of feeling less depressed, less anxious, and more energetic and able to cope; return of normal sleeping and eating habits; demonstration of improved ability to problem solve and perform activities of daily living.

Dose range/Administration

Interaction alert: Barbiturates may reduce antidepressant blood levels and effects. Cimetidine may increase levels. If given with epinephrine and norepinephrine, monitor for increased risk of hypertension. Avoid use with MAOIs (risk of excitation, hyperpyrexia, and seizures). Give cautiously with thyroid drugs because it may increase CNS stimulation and cardiac arrhythmias.

🐾 **Give with (or immediately after) food to reduce GI symptoms.**

Adult: PO: 25 mg tid or qid or 75–100 at hs, may gradually increase to a maximum of 150 mg/day.

Clinical alert: Whenever possible give entire dose at bedtime to reduce daytime sedation. This drug is available in liquid form.

Contraindications/Precautions
PREG
D

Contraindicated in hypersensitivity to TCAs, and in acute recovery period of myocardial infarction. ***Use with caution*** in renal or hepatic disease, convulsive disorders, hyperthyroidism, glaucoma, prostatic hypertrophy, urinary retention, and suicidal tendency.

✋ **Contraindicated for children under 6 years and pregnant or nursing mothers. Use with caution for adolescents and the elderly or debilitated.**

Side effects/Adverse reactions

Hypersensitivity: rash, sensitivity to sunlight. ***CNS:*** drowsiness, dizziness, anxiety, headache, fatigue, nervousness, agitation, extrapyramidal symptoms, sedation. ***CV:*** orthostatic hypotension, palpitations, tachycardia, hypertension. ***GI:*** anorexia, dry mouth, nausea, constipation, paralytic ileus. ***GU:*** urinary retention, decreased libido. ***Eye:*** blurred vision. ***Ear:*** tinnitus. ***Misc:*** (after abrupt withdrawal of long-term therapy) nausea, headache, malaise. ***Hem:*** agranulocytosis.

Nursing implications/Documentation

Possible nursing diagnoses: Potential for injury; Constipation; Altered oral mucous membrane.

◆ Document mental status and vital signs daily until response to therapy has been established.

◆ Be sure that doses are swallowed (not hoarded).

◆ Monitor for orthostatic hypotension, dizziness, and drowsiness; supervise ambulation until response is established.

◆ Record intake and output, and observe for dehydration or urinary retention; provide special mouth care.

◆ Monitor for and report suicidal tendencies, increased depression, or excessive drowsiness (may require change in medication).

◆ Prevent constipation by monitoring bowel movements and encouraging adequate fiber and fluid intake; offer laxatives or stool softeners before the problem becomes severe.

Patient & family teaching/Home care

Possible nursing diagnoses: Ineffective coping (family and individual); Sleep pattern disturbance; Impaired home maintenance management.

◆ Stress that this medication helps reduce the depression that inhibits ability to make decisions and cope effectively (once the individual feels less depressed, it will be easier to take steps toward making healthy changes).

◆ Explain that side effects are often noted immediately, but they usually diminish after a few weeks; on the other hand, it is likely to take 2–4 weeks before *beneficial* effects are noted (the patient may feel worse before feeling better).

◆ Warn to change positions slowly to prevent dizziness.

- Point out the role of adequate nutrition, exercise, and sleep in combating depression.

- Emphasize that the effects of alcohol, sedatives, and tranquilizers may be potentiated.

- Caution to consult with physician before using OTC drugs; stress the need for ongoing medical follow-up.

- Recommend reporting continued depression; stress that doses should not be increased or stopped without checking with physician because this may cause severe problems.

- Advise avoidance of driving and other potentially hazardous activities until response is established.

- Suggest using ice chips, hard candy, or gum to relieve side effect of dry mouth; stress the need for good mouth care.

- Warn women to report if pregnancy is planned or suspected.

- *See Antidepressants overview for more information.*

nylidrin

nye′li-drin

nylidrin hydrochloride: *Adrin, Arlidin, ✦Arlidin Forte, ✦PMS Nylidrin*

Class: Vasodilator, peripheral; Beta-adrenergic agonist; Sympathomimetic

PEDS	PREG	GERI
🤚	C	🤚

Action Stimulates peripheral vascular beta receptors, thus dilating arteriole smooth muscle and decreasing circulatory resistance. Increases cardiac output and systolic blood pressure. Decreases diastolic pressure.

Use/Therapeutic goal/Outcome

Peripheral vasospastic disorders (Raynaud's disease, acrocyanosis, diabetic vascular disease, and nocturnal leg cramps): Promotion of peripheral circulation. *Outcome criteria:* Improved pulse quality, skin color and temperature.

Meniere's disease: Promotion of circulation to middle ear. *Outcome criteria:* Report of decreased dizziness and nausea.

Dose range/Administration

Adult: PO: 3–12 mg tid or qid.

Contraindications/Precautions

Contraindicated in hypersensitivity to nylidrin, acute myocardial infarction, angina pectoris, and tachycardia. *Use with caution* in hypertension, peptic ulcer, or cardiac disorders.

🖐 **Use with caution for the elderly. Safe use for children and pregnant women has not been established.**

Side effects/Adverse reactions

Hypersensitivity: rash. *CNS:* nervousness, weakness, dizziness (not associated with labyrinthine artery insufficiency), trembling. *CV:* palpitations, hypotension. *GI:* nausea, vomiting.

Nursing implications/Documentation

Possible nursing diagnoses: Activity intolerance; Potential for injury.

- Document baseline mental status and circulatory status (presence and quality of peripheral pulses, skin color and temperature); monitor periodically thereafter.

- Monitor for dizziness and hypotension; supervise ambulation until response is determined.

Patient & family teaching/Home care

Possible nursing diagnoses: Knowledge deficit; Impaired home maintenance management.

- If GI symptoms are experienced, advise eating small frequent meals.

- Stress the need to change positions slowly to reduce dizziness; point out that alcohol may increase vasodilation and dizziness.

- Warn that response to therapy is gradual.

- Explain that side effect of palpitations should subside as therapy progresses.

- Discourage smoking and long periods of standing; stress the need for good skin care.

- Warn against driving or performing hazardous activities until response is determined.

nystatin

nye-stat′in

Mycostatin, ✦Nadostine, Nilstat, Nystex

Class: Anti-infective, Antifungal

PEDS	PREG	GERI
🤚	B	OK

Action Kills fungi (fungicidal) or limits fungal growth (fungistatic), depending upon drug concentration and susceptibility of the organisms, probably by binding to sterols in the cell membrane, altering cell permeability and allowing leakage of intracellular components.

Use/Therapeutic goal/Outcome

Oral, GI, vaginal, and skin infections caused by *Candida albicans* (Monilia) and other *Candida* species: Resolution of infection. **Outcome criteria:** Absence of pathogenic growth on culture; absence of clinical manifestations of infection (redness, itching, burning, pain, swelling, fever, drainage).

Dose range/Administration

Oral infection: Adult and Child: PO: *Suspension:* 4–6 cc (400,000–600,000 units) swished about mouth and swallowed qid. *Pastille:* Dissolve one 200,000 unit pastille slowly in mouth qid.

GI infection: Adult: PO: 1–2 tablets (500,000–1,000,000 units) tid. **Child > 3 mos:** PO: 250,000–500,000 units of suspension qid. **Newborns/premature infants:** 100,000 units of suspension qid. Swab medication on oral mucosa.

Vaginal/vulva infection: Adult: *Vaginal:* One vaginal tablet (100,000 units) inserted high into vagina qhs or bid for 2 weeks; *or* one 100,000–unit applicatorful, daily or bid for 2 weeks; *or* one 500,000–unit applicatorful daily for 2 weeks. Wash applicator thoroughly after each dose. Continue during menstruation. *Topical:* Cleanse vulva and apply cream bid for 2 wks.

Infant eczema/localized skin candidiasis: Adult and Child: *Topical:* Apply to affected area bid for 2 wks.

Clinical alert: For vaginal use, insert high into the vagina, preferably at bedtime.

Contraindications/Precautions

PREG B

Contraindicated in hypersensitivity to nystatin.

🖐 **Lozenges contraindicated in children under 5 years. Use with caution for pregnant women.**

Side effects/Adverse reactions

Hypersensitivity: itching, rashes (often occur within the first 24–72 hr; continuing problem may be hypersensitivity reaction). **GI:** (with large oral doses) nausea, vomiting, diarrhea.

Nursing implications/Documentation

Possible nursing diagnoses: Potential for infection; Altered oral mucous membrane; Impaired tissue integrity.

◆ Provide special mouth care as needed.

◆ Monitor affected areas for chemical irritation; report failure to improve after 3–5 days.

◆ For topical use, avoid occlusive dressings.

Patient & family teaching/Home care

Possible nursing diagnoses: Knowledge deficit; Impaired home maintenance management.

◆ Stress the importance of taking the drug for the entire time prescribed, even if symptoms abate (may need nystatin for 1–2 wks after being asymptomatic).

◆ For oral candidiasis, advise the person to avoid mouthwash (it may alter flora and promote infection).

◆ Point out the importance of good hygiene for moist areas of the body (feet, vulva, perineal area).

◆ *See Anti-infectives overview for more information.*

octreotide
oc-tree'oh-tide

octreotide acetate: *Sandostatin*

Class: Antidiarrheal

PEDS	PREG	GERI
🖐	**B**	**OK**

Action Prolongs intestinal transit time and stimulates fluid and electrolyte absorption from gastrointestinal tract by inhibiting secretion of gastroentero-pancreatic peptides; blocks carcinoid flush by suppressing secretion of serotonin; suppresses growth hormone, glucagon, and insulin.

Use/Therapeutic goal/Outcome

Carcinoid tumor: Reduction in associated symptoms. **Outcome criteria:** Decreased frequency of bowel movements, reduced water content of stools, and decreased episodes of facial flushing.

Vasoactive Intestinal Peptide tumor (VIPoma): Reduction in associated symptoms. **Outcome criteria:** Decreased frequency of bowel movements and reduced water content of stools.

Dose range/Administration

Interaction alert: May alter antidiabetic dose requirements; may reduce cyclosporine blood levels.

Carcinoid Tumor: Adult: SC: 100–600 mcg/day in 2–4 doses for 2 wk, then adjust based on response. **Child:** SC: 1–10 mcg/kg/day.

VIPoma: Adult: SC: 200–300 mcg/day in 2 to 4 doses for 2 wk, then adjust based on response. ***Child:*** SC: 1–10 mcg/kg/day.

Clinical alert: Administer between meals and at bedtime to reduce gastrointestinal side effects. Warm solution to room temperature and give slowly to reduce local reactions.

Contraindications/Precautions

PREG B

Contraindicated in hypersensitivity to octreotide. ***Use with caution*** in diabetes mellitus, severe renal impairment, and gallbladder disease.

🖐 **Use with caution for children and pregnant or nursing mothers.**

Side effects/Adverse reactions

Hypersensitivity: rare. ***GI:*** diarrhea, nausea and vomiting, abdominal discomfort, decreased absorption of fats, cholelithiasis, acute hepatitis. ***CNS:*** transient dizziness, headache. ***Hem:*** hyperglycemia, hypoglycemia, hyperbilirubinemia. ***Skin:*** pain, burning, or irritation at injection site. ***Misc:*** hypothyroidism.

Nursing implications/Documentation

Possible nursing diagnoses: Diarrhea; Potential for injury; Pain.

◆ Rotate injection sites, using hip, thigh, or abdomen.

◆ Assess and record symptoms of gastrointestinal distress.

◆ Monitor serum electrolyte levels for return to normal values as diarrhea decreases.

◆ For diabetic patients, monitor blood glucose levels and observe for symptoms of hyper- or hypoglycemia.

◆ Assess bowel sounds and document frequency and character of stools.

◆ Monitor for presence of undigested fat in stools (steatorrhea).

Patient & family teaching/Home care

Possible nursing diagnoses: Knowledge deficit; Potential for injury; Impaired home maintenance management.

◆ Teach subcutaneous injection technique, using hip, thigh, or abdomen; emphasize need to rotate sites.

◆ Explain the need to check ampules for particles or discoloration.

◆ Point out that warming the solution to room temperature and injecting slowly helps reduce local reaction.

◆ Advise that transient dizziness may occur but usually wears off with continued therapy; caution to avoid dangerous situations until dizziness is resolved.

◆ For diabetic patients, stress the need to monitor blood glucose levels.

◆ Advise reporting increased diarrhea or symptoms of gastrointestinal distress.

◆ Emphasize that close medical supervision is necessary.

ofloxacin

oh-flox'a-sin

Floxacin, Floxin

Class: Antibiotic, Anti-infective, Quinolone

PEDS	PREG	GERI
🖐	C	OK

Action Broad-spectrum antibiotic which is bactericidal (kills bacteria) by inhibiting bacterial DNA gyrase, an enzyme necessary for bacterial DNA replication.

Use/Therapeutic goal/Outcome

Infections (urinary tract, sexually transmitted diseases, prostate, respiratory, skin and skin structures, intestines): Resolution of infection. ***Outcome criteria:*** Absence of pathogenic growth on cultures, absence of clinical manifestations of infection (fever, pain, redness, heat, swelling, odor, drainage, dysuria, urinary frequency).

Dose range/Administration

Interaction alert: Separate doses of minerals (or vitamins with minerals) and antacids containing magnesium hydroxide or aluminum hydroxide from doses of ofloxacin by at least 2 hours (reduces risk of decreased antibiotic absorption). Probenecid may increase blood levels of ofloxacin. Ofloxacin may increase plasma concentration of theophylline and prolong theophylline half-life.

🖐 **Give 2 hours after meals for best absorption (food inhibits absorption).**

Adult: PO: 200–400 mg q12h (expect the higher dose range for more severe infections).

Clinical alert: Recognize that those with decreased kidney function may require reduced dosage.

Contraindications/Precautions

PREG
C

Contraindicated in allergy to ofloxacin or to quinolone antibiotics. **Use with caution** in CNS disorders, risk of seizures, and impaired renal function.

🖐 **Contraindicated for children less than 18 years and for pregnant or nursing mothers.**

Side effects/Adverse reactions

Hypersensitivity: rashes. **GI:** nausea, vomiting, diarrhea, abdominal discomfort. **CNS:** insomnia, headache, dizziness. **Misc:** photosensitivity, superinfection.

Nursing implications/Documentation

Possible nursing diagnoses: Potential for infection; Diarrhea.

◆ Determine history of allergies and monitor closely for allergic reactions, regardless of negative history. Hold dose and report if rash is noted.

◆ Obtain baseline CBC, BUN, creatinine, liver function studies, and necessary culture specimens before beginning ofloxacin; monitor closely thereafter if therapy is prolonged.

◆ Provide preferred fluids and encourage drinking at least 2 L/day.

◆ Monitor for and report symptoms of superinfection (mouth lesions, thrush, vaginal irritation, diarrhea, respiratory symptoms).

Patient & family teaching/Home care

Possible nursing diagnoses: Knowledge deficit; Impaired home maintenance management.

◆ Explain that, because food inhibits absorption, taking ofloxacin 2 hours after meals is most effective; point out that antacids containing magnesium hydroxide or aluminum hydroxide, or minerals (or vitamins with minerals) should not be taken for 2 hours before or after ofloxacin.

◆ Advise that ofloxacin is a very effective antibiotic that has few side effects.

◆ Teach the need to report if symptoms persist or if new signs and symptoms of illness appear (fever, mouth lesions, vaginal irritation, respiratory symptoms, diarrhea).

◆ Point out the importance of maintaining adequate hydration; encourage drinking at least 2 L of fluid a day.

◆ Teach the need to hold dose and report if rash develops.

◆ Explain the importance of taking antibiotics for the entire time prescribed, even if symptoms abate.

◆ Caution that sun exposure should be avoided; moderate to severe photosensitivity reactions have been reported.

◆ *See Anti-infectives overview for more information.*

omeprazole

o-mep'ra-zole

✦Losec, Prilosec

Class: Gastric acid pump inhibitor, Antiulcer agent

PEDS 🖐 PREG C GERI 🖐

Action Inhibits gastric acid secretion by binding irreversibly to an enzyme system at the secretory surface of parietal cells; this system is regarded as the acid pump of the gastric mucosa.

Use/Therapeutic goal/Outcome

Gastroesophageal reflux: Symptomatic treatment. **Outcome criteria:** Report of decrease or absence of epigastric burning and pain.

Gastric hypersecretory conditions (Zollinger-Ellison syndrome, systemic mastocytosis, multiple endocrine adenoma): Control of hypersecretion of acid. **Outcome criteria:** Report of relief of epigastric pain; decreased diarrhea/steatorrhea; decreased acidity of gastric secretions.

Duodenal or gastric ulcer: Promotion of healing and relief of pain. **Outcome criteria:** Report of absence of pain; hemoglobin and hematocrit within normal range; vital signs stable; stools negative for occult blood; endoscopic evidence of healing.

Dose range/Administration

Interaction alert: Reduces absorption of ampicillin, iron salts and ketoconazole. May increase serum levels of anticoagulants, diazepam and phenytoin by slowing their metabolism.

🖥 **Give before meal, preferably in morning.**

Gastroesophageal reflux: Adult: PO: 20–40 mg/day for 4–8 wk.

Gastric hypersecretory conditions: Adult: PO: 60 mg/day.

Duodenal or gastric ulcers: Adult: PO: 20–40 mg/day.

Clinical alert: For the elderly, daily dose should not exceed 20 mg.

Contraindications/Precautions

PREG C

Contraindicated in hypersensitivity to omeprazole. **Use with caution** in chronic liver disease.

🖐 Use with caution for pregnant or nursing mothers and for the elderly. Safe use for children has not been established.

Side effects/Adverse reactions

Hypersensitivity: rash, itching. **GI:** abdominal pain or colic, constipation, diarrhea, flatulence, nausea, vomiting. **CNS:** dizziness, headache, somnolence. **Hem:** anemia, thrombocytopenia, neutropenia. **GU:** hematuria, proteinuria, urinary tract infection.

Nursing implications/Documentation

Possible nursing diagnoses: Pain; Altered oral mucous membrane; Altered patterns of urinary elimination.

♦ Be aware that capsules are delayed-release preparation and must not be crushed or opened.

♦ Assess oral mucous membrane for signs of infection.

♦ Monitor for urinary frequency or urgency and observe urine for cloudiness or presence of blood.

♦ Record bowel elimination patterns.

Patient & family teaching/Home care

Possible nursing diagnoses: Knowledge deficit; Impaired home maintenance management.

♦ Teach the need to take dose immediately before a meal, preferably in the morning.

♦ Explain that capsules should be swallowed whole, without crushing, chewing, breaking, or opening.

♦ Inform that antacids may be taken for pain relief, since there is no problem with interaction.

♦ Caution to report if urinary frequency or urgency develop or if urine becomes cloudy or bloody.

♦ With active ulcer disease, advise to continue taking medication as prescribed for 4–8 weeks, although symptoms usually subside earlier.

♦ Counsel smokers to stop smoking and to avoid the use of caffeine.

orphenadrine

or-fen'a-dreen

orphenadrine citrate: **Banflex, Flexoject, Flexon, K-Flex, Marflex, Myolin, Neocyten, Noradex, Norflex, O-Flex, Orflagen, Orphenate**

orphenadrine hydrochloride: **Disipal**

Class: Skeletal-muscle relaxant (centrally acting), Antispasmodic

PEDS	PREG	GERI
🖐	C	🖐

Action
Relaxes skeletal muscle by producing analgesic response and by atropine-like central action. Does not act directly on skeletal muscle.

Use/Therapeutic goal/Outcome

Acute, painful musculoskeletal conditions: Promotion of comfort and mobility. **Outcome criteria:** Increased range of motion and ability to perform activities of daily life; report of decreased pain, anxiety, and tension.

Dose range/Administration

Interaction alert: The CNS effects may be additive to those of other CNS depressants and alcohol. Phenothiazines or propoxyphene may produce hypoglycemia, anxiety, tremors, or confusion. Decreases phenothiazine level.

🖐 Give with food to prevent gastric distress.

Orphenadrine citrate: Adult: PO: 100 mg bid. IM, IV: 60 mg, may repeat q12h.

Orphenadrine hydrochloride: Adult: PO: 50 mg tid, up to 250 mg/day.

Clinical alert: Orphenadrine citrate and orphenadrine hydrochloride are not interchangeable.

Contraindications/Precautions

PREG C

Contraindicated in hypersensitivity to orphenadrine, and in narrow-angle glaucoma, prostatic hypertrophy, pyloric, duodenal or bladder neck obstruction; cardiospasm, myasthenia gravis, stenosing peptic ulcer, severe hepatic or renal disease, ulcerative colitis. **Use with caution** in tachycardia, cardiac disease, or dysrhythmias.

🖐 Contraindicated for the elderly. Safe use for children and pregnant or nursing mothers has not been established.

Side effects/Adverse reactions

Hypersensitivity: pruritus, urticaria, and rash. **CNS:** drowsiness, headache, agitation, confusion, syncope, tremors. *GI:* dry mouth, constipation, nausea, abdominal cramps. *CV:* tachycardia. *GU:* urinary retention. *Eye:* ocular tension, dilated pupils, blurred vision. *Hem:* aplastic anemia.

Nursing implications/Documentation

Possible nursing diagnoses: Constipation; Altered oral mucous membrane; Potential for injury; Urinary retention.

♦ Monitor bowel elimination and food and fluid intake to prevent constipation.

♦ If dry mouth develops, relieve with mouth care, sips of liquids, and sugarless gum or candy. (This side effect indicates a need for dosage reduction.)

♦ Supervise out-of-bed activities, especially if drowsiness is present.

♦ Monitor for and report abnormal laboratory studies (blood, renal and liver studies), especially in long-term use.

♦ Observe the elderly carefully for anticholinergic effects of this drug (urine retention, constipation, dry mouth).

Patient & family teaching/Home care

Possible nursing diagnoses: Knowledge deficit; Impaired home maintenance management.

♦ Advise taking doses with food to reduce GI symptoms.

♦ Explain the importance of reporting dry mouth, urinary hesitency or retention, constipation, and palpitations to physician immediately.

♦ Teach to count pulse and notify physician if bradycardia or tachycardia develop.

♦ Encourage relieving mouth dryness by brushing teeth, rinsing mouth, using sugarless gum or candy, or using a saliva substitute.

♦ Stress the need to increase fluids and high-fiber foods to prevent constipation.

♦ Warn against operating machinery, driving, or taking alcohol or other CNS depressants, especially if drowsiness or dizziness is present (early therapy response should be determined).

♦ Emphasize importance of continuing with total treatment plan, including rest and physical therapy.

♦ *See Skeletal-muscle relaxants overview for more information.*

oxacillin
ox-a-sill'in

oxacillin sodium: ***Bactocill, Prostaphlin***
Class: Anti-infective, Antibiotic, Penicillin (penicillinase-resistant)

PEDS	PREG	GERI
🤚	B	🤚

Action Broad-spectrum, usually bactericidal antibiotic; kills bacteria by inhibiting cell wall synthesis. Resistant to bacterial penicillinases (enzymes that degrade some penicillins).

Use/Therapeutic goal/Outcome

Systemic infections (caused by penicillinase-producing staphylococci and streptococci): Resolution of infection. **Outcome criteria:** Absence of pathogenic growth on cultures, absence of clinical manifestations of infection (fever, pain, redness, heat, swelling, odor, drainage), normal WBC count, improvement of X rays.

Dose range/Administration

Interaction alert: Probenecid inhibits excretion of oxacillin and may be given to increase serum levels of the drug.

💊 **Give oral doses on an empty stomach with a full glass of water 1 hour before or 2–3 hours after meals; food may interfere with absorption.**

Adult: PO: 2–4 g/day, in divided doses q6h. IM, IV: 1.5 to 6 g/day, in divided doses q4-6h.
Child: PO: 50–100 mg/kg/day, in divided doses q4-6h. IM, IV: 100–200 mg/kg/day, in divided doses q4-6h.

Clinical alert: Give at least 1 hour before bacteriostatic antibiotics for optimal effect.

Contraindications/Precautions
PREG
B

Contraindicated in allergy to penicillin. **Use with caution** in cephalosporin sensitivity, history of allergic responses (e.g., other drugs, hay fever, asthma), and renal insufficiency.

🤚 **Use with caution for children, the elderly, and pregnant or nursing mothers.**

Side effects/Adverse reactions

Hypersensitivity: itching, rashes, urticaria, fever, difficulty breathing, anaphylaxis. *GI:* nausea, vomiting, diarrhea, hepatic dysfunction, pseudomembranous colitis. *CV:* pain, redness, swelling, thrombophlebitis at injection site. *GU:* glomerulonephritis, acute interstitial nephritis. *CNS:* neurotoxicity, seizures.

Hem: anemia, granulocytopenia, thrombocytopenia, leukopenia, neutropenia, slight elevation in SGOT and SGPT. **Misc:** superinfection, bone marrow depression.

Nursing implications/Documentation

Possible nursing diagnoses: Potential for infection; Diarrhea.

♦ Determine history of allergies, and (regardless of history) monitor closely for allergic reactions.

♦ Obtain baseline CBC, creatinine, liver function studies, and necessary cultures before administering first dose; monitor closely thereafter if therapy is prolonged.

♦ Encourage fluids, and record and monitor intake and output, to ensure adequate hydration; report significant negative or positive balance.

♦ Monitor for and report signs of superinfection (sore throat, fever, fatigue, thrush, vaginal discharge, diarrhea).

Patient & family teaching/Home care

Possible nursing diagnoses: Knowledge deficit; Impaired home maintenance management.

♦ Advise to take oral doses with a full glass of water 1 hour before meals or 2 hours after meals to enhance drug absorption.

♦ Teach the importance of reporting allergic symptoms, diarrhea, signs and symptoms that do not abate, or *any* new signs and symptoms of discomfort that might indicate superinfection (medication regimen may have to be changed).

♦ Advise drinking 2–3 L of fluids daily to maintain adequate hydration (especially important if fever exists).

♦ Stress the importance of taking antibiotics for the entire time prescribed, even if signs and symptoms abate.

♦ *See Anti-infectives overview for more information.*

oxandrolone
ox-an'droe-lone

Anavar, ♠*Lonavar*

Class: Anabolic steroid

PEDS	PREG	GERI
♥	X	♥

Action Promotes body tissue-building processes and reverses catabolic processes by promoting protein anabolism and stimulating appetite.

Use/Therapeutic goal/Outcome

Catabolic state: Reversal of negative nitrogen balance and increase in protein synthesis. **Outcome criteria:** Increased appetite, increased energy level, and weight gain.

Dose range/Administration

Interaction alert: Increases effect of insulin, oral hypoglycemics, and anticoagulants. Corticosteroids increase possibility of edema and severe acne. Avoid other hepatotoxic medications.

🥄 **Give with food or milk to minimize GI symptoms.**

Adult: PO: 2.5 mg 2–4 times daily. **Child:** PO: 0.25 mg/kg/day.

Clinical alert: Two to four weeks of therapy are usually adequate for adults. Treatment may be repeated intermittently for both adults and children.

Contraindications/Precautions
PREG X

Contraindicated in hypersensitivity to anabolic steroids, and in men with cancer of breast or prostate, women with hypercalcemia associated with breast cancer; hypercalcemia, and severe hepatic or renal impairment. **Use with caution** in cardiac, hepatic or renal impairment; coronary artery disease; history of MI; diabetes mellitus; and prostatic hypertrophy.

🤰 **Contraindicated for pregnant or nursing mothers. Use with caution for children and elderly men.**

Side effects/Adverse reactions

Hypersensitivity: rashes, anaphylaxis. **GU:** virilism of females (enlarged clitoris, deepening of voice, menstrual irregularities, unnatural hair growth or loss); virilism of prepubertal males (acne, enlarging penis, increased frequency of erections, unnatural hair growth); in older men, bladder irritability, breast soreness, gynecomastia, priapism, prostatic hypertrophy, prostatic carcinoma, testicular atrophy, suppression of spermatogenesis; decreased libido in both men and women. **Hem:** iron deficiency anemia, leukemia, suppression of clotting factors, hypercalcemia, decreased high-density lipoproteins (HDLs), and increased low-density lipoproteins (LDLs). **GI:** nausea, vomiting, diarrhea; hepatic dysfunction, carcinoma or necrosis. **MS:** muscle cramps, premature epiphyseal closure in children. *Skin:* unexplained darkening, acne, edema.

Nursing implications/Documentation

Possible nursing diagnoses: Body image disturbance; Fluid volume excess.

♦ Record baseline blood pressure and weight.

♦ Assess for and report increased blood pressure, weight gain, or evidence of edema or congestive failure.

♦ Monitor serum calcium levels; assess, report, and document symptoms of hypercalcemia (nausea, vomiting, constipation, lethargy, muscle weakness).

♦ Monitor for change in liver function tests and cholesterol levels.

♦ For diabetics monitor glucose levels and assess for symptoms of hypoglycemia.

Patient & family teaching/Home care

Possible nursing diagnoses: Knowledge deficit; Impaired home maintenance management; Sexual dysfunction.

♦ Advise taking with food or milk to reduce gastric irritation.

♦ Suggest restriction of sodium intake to decrease fluid retention.

♦ Encourage a diet high in protein and calories to obtain maximum anabolic benefit.

♦ Caution women of child-bearing age to use reliable birth control and to stop drug and report any suspicion of pregnancy.

♦ For females, stress importance of reporting the occurrence of masculinizing effects (abnormal growth of facial hair, deepening of voice, menstrual irregularities, enlarged clitoris).

♦ For males, advise reporting development of priapism, gynecomastia, or bladder irritability.

♦ For diabetics, caution about possible lowering of blood sugar and need for adjustment of doses of insulin or oral antidiabetic agents.

♦ Advise parents of prepubertal children that X rays will be taken periodically to determine effect on bone growth.

♦ Caution to maintain close medical supervision for early detection of adverse reactions.

♦ Stress that using anabolic steroids for improvement of athletic performance may result in serious side effects that outweigh any advantages.

oxazepam

ox-a'ze-pam

♣Apo-Oxazepam, ♣Novoxapam, ♣Ox-Pam, Serax, ♣Zapex

Class: Antianxiety agent, Sedative-hypnotic, Benzodiazepine

PEDS	PREG	GERI
🤚	D	🤚

CONTROLLED SUBSTANCE IV

Action Produces CNS depression and relaxation, and increases seizure threshold by potentiating the action of gamma-aminobuteric acid (GABA), which reduces neuronal activity in all regions of the CNS. Promotes muscle relaxation by inhibiting spinal motor reflex pathways. Decreases anxiety by inhibiting cortical and limbic arousal.

Use/Therapeutic goal/Outcome

Short-term treatment of anxiety: Alleviation of symptoms of apprehension, muscle tension, and insomnia. *Outcome criteria:* Report of feeling calmer, sleeping better, and coping better; observable signs of decreased anxiety (decreased motor activity, reduced muscle tension, decrease in pulse and blood pressure).

Dose range/Administration

Interaction alert: Alcohol and other CNS depressants may cause excessive sedation.

Adult: PO: 10–30 mg tid or qid, depending on severity. *If associated with alcohol withdrawal:* 15–30 mg tid or qid.

Clinical alert: When discontinuing drug, taper doses gradually, rather than withdrawing abruptly.

Contraindications/Precautions

PREG D

Contraindicated in hypersensitivity or intolerance to oxazepam or other benzodiazepines, and in narrow-angle glaucoma, psychosis, and depression. *Use with caution* in suicidal tendencies, or impaired liver or kidney function.

🤚 **Contraindicated for pregnant or nursing mothers. Use with caution for the elderly or debilitated. Safe use for children has not been established.**

Side effects/Adverse reactions

Hypersensitivity: rash, exaggeration of side effects. *CNS:* lethargy, drowsiness, headache, dizziness, confusion, tremors, ataxia, depression, paradoxical excitement. *CV:* hypotension, transient tachycardia and bradycardia. *Resp:* respiratory depression. *GI:* dry mouth,

►

nausea, vomiting, constipation, diarrhea, liver dysfunction. *GU:* urinary retention. *Eye:* blurred vision, mydriasis. *Misc:* drug tolerance and dependence.

Nursing implications/Documentation

Possible nursing diagnoses: Potential for injury; Constipation.

♦ Record baseline blood pressure; monitor closely if dizziness is experienced. Supervise ambulation until response is determined.

♦ Be sure that doses are swallowed (not hoarded).

♦ Provide a quiet environment that is conducive to rest.

♦ Monitor bowel elimination and provide adequate fluids and fiber to prevent constipation; offer laxatives before the problem is severe.

Patient & family teaching/Home care

Possible nursing diagnoses: Anxiety; Fear; Ineffective individual coping; Impaired home maintenance management.

♦ Help the individual identify stressors that contribute to anxiety and ways of coping effectively; stress that effective coping strategies can reduce the need for medication.

♦ Explain the importance of daily exercise in relieving stress, and encourage establishing a plan for getting enough exercise (e.g., daily walks).

♦ Point out that drug tolerance and dependence can occur, and that the drug should be used only on a short-term basis.

♦ Emphasize that the effects of alcohol, other sedatives and CNS depressants, and tranquilizers may be potentiated (these should be avoided).

♦ Advise avoidance of driving and other potentially hazardous activities until response is established.

♦ *See Antianxiety agents/Sedatives/Hypnotics overview for more information.*

oxybutynin

ox-i-byoo'ti-nin

oxybutynin chloride: *Ditropan*

Class: Urinary antispasmotic (spasmolytic), Antienuretic

Antidote: physostigmine

PEDS	PREG	GERI
🖐	C	🖐

Action Inhibits bladder spasms and increases bladder capacity by relaxing smooth muscles of the urinary tract.

Use/Therapeutic goal/Outcome

Bladder spasms associated with neurogenic bladder or urethral surgery: Promotion of normal patterns of urinary elimination, and relief of associated discomfort. *Outcome criteria:* Demonstration of normal patterns of urinary elimination; report of relief of symptoms.

Dose range/Administration

Adult: PO: 5 mg bid or tid, to a maximum of 5 mg qid. *Child > 5 yrs:* PO: 5 mg bid to a maximum of 5 mg tid.

Contraindications/Precautions

PREG
C

Contraindicated in hypersensitivity to oxybutynin, and for the debilitated with intestinal atony, in increased ocular pressure and glaucoma, myasthenia gravis, gastrointestinal obstruction, paralytic ileus, megacolon, ulcerative or severe colitis, or obstruction of the lower urinary tract. *Use with caution* in reflux esophagitis, autonomic neuropathy, with liver or kidney disease, hypertension, coronary artery disease, CHF, hyperthyroidism, tachycardia, arrhythmias, prostatic hypertrophy.

🖐 **Contraindicated for the elderly with intestinal atony. Use with caution for other elderly and in pregnancy. Safe use for children under 5 years has not been established.**

Side effects/Adverse reactions

Hypersensitivity: itching, rash, fever, anaphylaxis. *CNS:* drowsiness, headache, dizziness, nervousness, insomnia. *CV:* palpitations, tachycardia. *Eye:* visual disturbances, mydriasis, cycloplegia. *GI:* constipation, dry mouth, nausea, vomiting, abdominal bloating. *GU:* urinary hesitance (or retention), impotence. *Skin:* suppression of sweating. *Misc:* suppression of lactation.

Nursing implications/Documentation

Possible nursing diagnoses: Altered patterns of urinary elimination; Constipation.

♦ Monitor and document time and amount of urination.

♦ Provide favorite fluids to maintain adequate hydration.

♦ For patients with neurogenic bladders, be sure there has been diagnosis by cystometry before starting drug; be aware that drug should be stopped periodically to see if normal urinary patterns have been established.

♦ Monitor bowel elimination and ensure adequate fiber and fluids to prevent constipation.

♦ Monitor those with colostomies or ileostomies closely for abdominal distention (diarrhea may indicate partial intestinal obstruction and should be reported).

Patient & family teaching/Home care

Possible nursing diagnoses: Knowledge deficit; Impaired home maintenance management.

♦ Explain the importance of drinking at least 2 quarts of fluid a day, even if it causes more frequent urination.

♦ Advise that constipation, a common side effect, can be prevented by adequate fluids, fiber intake, and exercise.

♦ Warn that drowsiness, dizziness, and blurred vision may be experienced at the beginning of therapy; caution to avoid driving and activities that require mental alertness until effects are known.

♦ Explain that suppressed sweating may predispose the individual to heat stroke on hot days.

♦ Reinforce the importance of reporting new or persistent symptoms.

oxycodone
ox-i-koe'done

oxycodone hydrochloride: *♠Endone, Oxycodone Oral Solution, Roxicodone, ♣Supeudol.*

Oxycodone pectinate: *♣Proladone*

Combinations with acetaminophen: *Percocet, Percocet-Demi, Tylox.*

Combinations with aspirin: *Codoxy, Percodan, Percodan-Demi*

Class: Narcotic analgesic, Opiate agonist

Antidote: Naloxone hydrochloride (Narcan)

PEDS	PREG	GERI	CONTROLLED SUBSTANCE
🖐	C	🖐	II

Action Alters the perception of and response to pain via an unclear mechanism. Believed to act by binding with opiate receptors at various CNS sites. Its potency is equivalent to morphine and is 10–12 times more potent than codeine. This drug is available in the United States only in combination with other drugs.

Use/Therapeutic goal/Outcome

Moderate to severe pain: Relief of pain. **Outcome criteria:** Report of relief of pain; absence of signs of pain (grimacing, frowning, restlessness, reluctance to move or cough) with increase in signs of comfort (relaxed facial expression, decreased restlessness); blood pressure and pulse within normal limits when compared to baseline.

Dose range/Administration

Interaction alert: General anesthetics, tranquilizers, sedatives, hypnotics, other narcotic analgesics, alcohol, tricyclic antidepressants, or MAO inhibitors increase CNS depression (use reduced dose).

Adult: PO: 1–2 tablets q6h prn or around the clock; or 5 mg (5 ml) of oral solution. *Rectal:* 1–3 suppositories/day prn or around the clock. **Child > 6 yrs:** PO: (Percodan-Demi only) 1/4 tablet q6h prn.

Clinical alert: Expect decreased dosage for the elderly and debilitated. Count respirations before giving oxycodone; hold drug and report if respirations are less than 12. Do not give Tylox to children of any age. For children over 6 years, may give Percodan-Demi, but keep in mind that it contains aspirin and should not be given in the presence of flu symptoms (because of risk of Reye's syndrome).

PREG
C

Contraindications/Precautions

Contraindicated in hypersensitivity to oxycodone or principal drugs in combination preparations (aspirin or acetaminophen). **Use with caution** in head injury, increased intracranial pressure, seizures, asthma, COPD, alcoholism, renal or hepatic disease, viral infections, prostatic hypertrophy, Addison's disease, cardiac arrhythmias, acute abdominal conditions, chronic ulcerative colitis, urethral stricture, gallbladder disease, hypothyroidism, history of drug dependency or abuse, reduced blood volume, toxic psychosis, peptic ulcer, or (for combination preparations with aspirin) coagulation abnormalities.

🖐 **Contraindicated for children under 6 years and pregnant or nursing mothers. Use with caution for older children and the elderly or debilitated.**

Side effects/Adverse reactions

Hypersensitivity: rashes, hives, itching, wheezing, respiratory depression, extreme somnolence, coma, skeletal-muscle flaccidity, circulatory collapse. **CNS:** sedation, lightheadedness, dizziness, euphoria, convulsions with large doses. **GI:** nausea, vomiting, constipation. **Resp:** respiratory depression. **CV:** hypotension. **GU:** urinary retention. **Misc:** physical dependence.

Nursing implications/Documentation

Possible nursing diagnoses: Pain; Anxiety; Potential for injury; Constipation.

♦ Have patient rate pain on a scale of 1–10 before and after medication is given; report and record inadequate pain control.

♦ Determine whether a less potent analgesic might effectively relieve pain (narcotic analgesics should be used in the smallest effective dose compatible with the patient's needs).

♦ Consider alternating oxycodone hydrochloride with a non-narcotic analgesic (ASA, ibuprofen, acetaminophen) to improve pain control while requiring lower narcotic doses.

♦ Give analgesics before pain is severe for best effects.

♦ Document and monitor bowel elimination to detect constipation; provide adequate fluids and fiber; give laxatives before problem becomes severe.

♦ Monitor closely for risk factors for injury; keep side rails up and, if allowed out of bed, supervise ambulation until response is determined.

♦ Be aware that large doses of Percodan and Percodan-Demi may result in salicylate intoxication; overdose of Tylox or Percocet could result in acetaminophen poisoning.

♦ Monitor hepatic function and hematological studies periodically if therapy is prolonged.

♦ Be aware of potential for psychic and physical dependence after prolonged use.

Patient & family teaching/Home care

Possible nursing diagnoses: Sensory/perceptual alterations; Impaired home maintenance management.

♦ Explain the rationale for taking analgesics before **pain** is too severe.

♦ Advise those who are ambulatory to refrain from activities that require alertness and to seek assistance if there is any question about ability to get out of bed (e.g., if there is weakness or light headedness).

♦ If nausea, vomiting, dizziness, or drowsiness is noted, advise to lie down (if these symptoms persist beyond 1–2 days, they should be reported).

♦ Warn that this drug may cause constipation; suggest increasing fluid and fiber intake and using mild laxatives if necessary.

♦ Stress the need to adhere to the prescribed dose regimen because of risk of overdose, liver damage, dependence, and abuse (instead of increasing dosage regimen, unsatisfactory pain relief should be reported).

♦ Teach not to take Percodan if it has a vinegar-like odor (due to aspirin breakdown).

♦ Warn that alcohol and other CNS depressants may cause excessive sedation.

♦ *See Narcotic and non-narcotic analgesics overview for more information.*

oxymetholone
ox-i-meth'oh-lone

Anadrol-50, ♣Anapolon, ♣ ♠Anapolon 50

Class: Anabolic steroid, Antianemic, Angioedema prophylactic

PEDS	PREG	GERI
🤚	X	🤚

Action Promotes body tissue-building processes and reverses catabolic processes by promoting protein anabolism and stimulating appetite; increases hemoglobin and red cell volume by stimulating bone marrow to increase erythropoiesis; increases serum levels of complement system components.

Use/Therapeutic goal/Outcome

Anemia related to bone marrow failure and aplastic anemia: Stimulation of red blood cell production. **Outcome criteria:** Increased hemoglobin, hematocrit, and red blood cell count.

Hereditary angioedema: Prophylaxis. **Outcome criteria:** Decreased frequency or severity of episodes of cutaneous, abdominal, and laryngeal edema.

Dose range/Administration

Interaction alert: Increases effect of insulin, oral hypoglycemics, and anticoagulants; decreases effect of barbiturates. Corticosteroids increase potential for edema and severe acne. Avoid other hepatotoxic medications.

🖐 **Give with food or milk to minimize GI symptoms.**

Adult and Child: PO: 1–5 mg/kg/day.
Neonates: PO: 175 mcg/kg/day.

Clinical alert: Should be used for minimum of 3–6 months because a response is not always immediately observed; lifetime administration may be necessary for congenital aplastic anemia.

Contraindications/Precautions

PREG X

Contraindicated in hypersensitivity to anabolic steroids, and in men with cancer of breast or prostate, women with hypercalcemia associated with breast cancer; hypercalcemia, and severe hepatic or renal impairment. *Use with caution* in cardiac, hepatic, or renal impairment; coronary artery disease; history of MI, diabetes mellitus, and prostatic hypertrophy.

☞ **Contraindicated for pregnant or nursing mothers. Use with caution for children and elderly men.**

Side effects/Adverse reactions

Hypersensitivity: rashes, anaphylaxis. *GU:* virilism of females (enlarged clitoris, deepening of voice, menstrual irregularities, unnatural hair growth or loss); virilism of prepubertal males (acne, enlarging penis, increased frequency of erections, unnatural hair growth); in older men, bladder irritability, breast soreness, gynecomastia, priapism, prostatic hypertrophy, prostatic carcinoma, testicular atrophy, suppression of spermatogenesis; decreased libido in both men and women. *Hem:* iron deficiency anemia, leukemia, suppression of clotting factors, hypercalcemia, decreased high-density lipoproteins, and increased low-density lipoproteins. *GI:* nausea, vomiting, diarrhea; hepatic dysfunction, carcinoma, or necrosis. *MS:* muscle cramps, premature epiphyseal closure in children. *Skin:* unexplained darkening, acne, edema.

Nursing implications/Documentation

Possible nursing diagnoses: Body image disturbance; Fluid volume excess.

♦ Record baseline blood pressure and weight.

♦ Assess for and report increased blood pressure, weight gain or evidence of edema or congestive failure.

♦ Monitor serum calcium levels; assess, report, and document symptoms of hypercalcemia (nausea, vomiting, constipation, lethargy, muscle weakness).

♦ Monitor for changes in liver function tests, cholesterol levels, and iron and total iron-binding capacity.

♦ For diabetics monitor glucose levels and assess for symptoms of hypoglycemia.

Patient & family teaching/Home care

Possible nursing diagnoses: Knowledge deficit; Impaired home maintenance management; Sexual dysfunction.

♦ Advise taking with food or milk to reduce gastric irritation.

♦ Suggest restriction of sodium intake to decrease fluid retention.

♦ Caution women of child-bearing age to use reliable birth control and to stop drug and report any suspicion of pregnancy.

♦ For females, stress the importance of reporting the occurrence of masculinizing effects (abnormal growth of facial hair, deepening of voice, menstrual irregularities, enlarged clitoris).

♦ For males, advise reporting development of priapism, gynecomastia, or bladder irritability.

♦ For diabetics, caution about possible lowering of blood sugar and need for adjustment of doses of insulin or oral antidiabetic agents.

♦ Inform parents of prepubertal children that X rays will be taken periodically to determine effect on bone growth.

♦ Caution to maintain close medical supervision for early detection of adverse reactions.

♦ Stress that using anabolic steroids for improvement of athletic performance may result in serious side effects that outweigh any advantages.

oxymorphone

ox-i-mor'fone

oxymorphone hydrochloride: **Numorphan**
Class: Narcotic analgesic, Opiate agonist
Antidote: naloxone hydrochloride (Narcan)

PEDS	PREG	GERI	CONTROLLED SUBSTANCE
☜	B	☜	II

Action Alters both perception of and response to pain by an unclear mechanism. Believed to act by binding with opiate receptors at many CNS sites.

Use/Therapeutic goal/Outcome

Moderate to severe pain, pre-procedure sedation: Relief of pain; promotion of relaxation. *Outcome criteria:* Report of feeling comfortable and more relaxed; absence of signs of pain (grimacing, frowning, restlessness, reluc-

▶

tance to move or cough) with increase in signs of comfort (relaxed facial expression, decreased restlessness); blood pressure and pulse within normal limits when compared to baseline.

Dose range/Administration

Interaction alert: General anesthetics, tranquilizers, sedatives or hypnotics, alcohol, tricyclic antidepressants, or MAO inhibitors increase CNS depression (use reduced dose).

Adult: SC, IM: 1–1.5 mg q4-6h prn or around the clock. IV: 0.5 mg q4-6h prn or around the clock. *Rectal:* 2.5–5mg q4-6h prn or around the clock.

Clinical alert: Expect decreased dosage for the elderly and the debilitated. Be aware that this drug is well absorbed rectally, offering an alternative to parenteral administration. Check respirations and blood pressure before giving oxymorphone. Hold dose and report if respirations < 12 or if hypotension is noted. Keep naloxone readily available in case of respiratory depression.

Contraindications/Precautions

Contraindicated in hypersensitivity to morphine analogs. *Use with caution* in increased intracranial pressure, head injury, seizures, asthma, COPD, alcoholism, acute abdominal conditions, prostatic hypertrophy, severe hepatic or renal disease, urethral stricture, CNS or respiratory depression, hypothyroidism, Addison's disease, cardiac arrhythmias, reduced blood volume, and toxic psychosis.

✋ **Contraindicated for children under 12 years and pregnant or nursing mothers. Use with caution for the elderly or debilitated.**

Side effects/Adverse reactions

Hypersensitivity: (rare) skin rash, hives, itching, swelling of face. *CNS:* drowsiness, convulsions with large doses. *Resp:* respiratory depression. *CV:* hypotension, bradycardia. *GI:* nausea, vomiting, constipation. *GU:* urinary retention. *Eye:* miosis. *MS:* skeletal-muscle flaccidity. *Misc:* physical dependence.

Nursing implications/Documentation

Possible nursing diagnoses: Pain; Anxiety; Potential for injury.

◆ Have patient rate pain on a scale of 1–10 before and after medication is given; report and record inadequate pain control.

◆ Determine whether a less potent analgesic might effectively relieve pain (narcotic analgesics should be used in the smallest effective dose compatible with the patient's needs).

◆ Give analgesics before pain is severe for best effects.

◆ Document pulse, respirations, and blood pressure immediately before and 1 hr after administration until response is determined.

◆ Monitor closely for risk factors for injury; keep side rails up and supervise ambulation if allowed out of bed.

◆ Provide adequate fluids and fiber to prevent constipation; monitor bowel elimination to detect constipation, and provide laxative before problem is severe.

◆ Report if gallbladder pain is suspected (this drug may make it worse).

◆ Be aware of potential for psychic and physical dependence after prolonged use.

Patient & family teaching/Home care

Possible nursing diagnoses: Sensory/perceptual alterations; Impaired home maintenance management.

◆ Explain the rationale for taking analgesics before pain is too severe.

◆ Advise ambulatory patients to refrain from activities that require alertness and to seek assistance if there is any question about ability to get out of bed (e.g., if there is weakness or light headedness).

◆ Stress the need to adhere to the prescribed dose regimen because of risk of overdose, dependence, and abuse (instead of increasing dose regimen, unsatisfactory pain relief should be reported); advise using non-narcotic analgesics as soon as possible.

◆ Warn that alcohol and other CNS depressants may cause excessive sedation.

◆ *See Narcotic and non-narcotic analgesics overview for more information.*

oxyphenbutazone   *ox-i-fen-byoo'ta-zone*

Oxalid, Oxybutazone, Tandearil

Class: Nonsteroidal anti-inflammatory drug (NSAID), Specific analgesic, Antipyretic, Mild uricosuric

PEDS   PREG   GERI
✋   D   ✋

Action Exact mechanism of action is unclear. Believed to reduce inflammation by inhibiting prostaglandin synthesis, leukocyte migration, and lysosomal enzyme involvement. Prostaglandin is a naturally occurring mediator of the inflammatory process which is found throughout body tissue.

Use/Therapeutic goal/Outcome

Pain and inflammation: Promotion of comfort and mobility; suppression of inflammation. *Outcome criteria:* Report of increased comfort with increased range of motion and ability to perform activities of daily life; reduction in or absence of joint stiffness, swelling, redness, and warmth.

Acute gouty arthritis: Reduction of uric acid crystals and inflammation in affected joints. *Outcome criteria:* Report of pain relief and increased ability to perform ADLs; decreased redness, warmth, and swelling of joints.

Dose range/Administration

Interaction alert: Aspirin and coumarin-type anticoagulants increase risk of bleeding. May increase the action of insulin, anti diabetics, phenytoin and sulfonamides.

🖐 **Give with food, milk, or antacid to prevent GI irritation.**

Arthritis, spondylitis, painful shoulder: Adult: PO: *Initial dose:* 300–600 mg in divided doses tid to qid. *Maintenance dose:* < 400 mg/day.

Gouty arthritis: Adult: PO: *Initial dose:* 400 mg, then 100 mg q4h.

Clinical alert: For gouty arthritis and the elderly give no longer than 1 week. Because this drug increases sodium retention, monitor for weight gain, edema, and increase in blood pressure.

Contraindications/Precautions

PREG D

Contraindicated in hypersensitivity to oxyphenbutazone, phenylbutazone, or tartrazine, and in history of or active GI ulcer, blood dyscrasias (especially coagulation defect), and renal, hepatic, cardiac, or thyroid disease.

🖐 **Contraindicated for the elderly. Safe use for children under 14 years and pregnant women has not been determined.**

Side effects/Adverse reactions

Hypersensitivity: urticaria, pruritus, rash, drug fever, arthralgia, angiitis, vasculitis, serum sickness, and anaphylaxis. *CNS:* drowsiness, lethargy, dizziness. *GI:* nausea, vomiting, diarrhea, hepatic failure, dyspepsia. *CV:* hypertension, edema, pericarditis. *Eye:* optic neuritis, blurred vision. *Ear:* hearing loss. *GU:* proteinuria, renal failure, hematuria. *Resp:* respiratory alkalosis. *Hem:* hyperglycemia, bone marrow depression. *Misc:* metabolic acidosis, goiter.

Nursing implications/Documentation

Possible nursing diagnoses: Pain; Impaired physical mobility.

♦ Establish a baseline for CBC, electrolytes, prothrombin time, BUN, creatinine, and liver function studies; if therapy is prolonged, monitor periodically thereafter.

♦ Monitor for and report GI symptoms that may indicate peptic ulcer (nausea, pain, black stools).

♦ Report immediately any of the following side effects: rash, fever, sore throat, bleeding, or bruising.

♦ Record weight every other day; report edema or sudden weight gain.

♦ For diabetics, monitor blood sugar closely since insulin requirements may change.

Patient & family teaching/Home care

Possible nursing diagnoses: Altered health maintenance; Knowledge deficit.

♦ Advise taking doses with food to reduce GI symptoms.

♦ Explain the importance of watching for symptoms of GI bleeding (black stools, persistent GI distress).

♦ Inform that a favorable response should be noted within 4 days of therapy, and no improvement after 4 weeks should be reported (drug should be discontinued).

♦ Stress the need to avoid aspirin, alcohol, and other OTC drugs (unless approved by physician) because of increased risk of GI bleeding.

♦ Instruct individuals to hold dose and report if any of the following side effects are experienced: vertigo, rashes, blood in urine, hearing or visual changes, sudden weight gain, edema (this drug may increase sodium retention).

♦ Warn against driving or activities that require alertness until response is determined.

♦ Reinforce the need for ongoing medical follow-up; advise telling dentist that oxyphenbutazone is being taken.

- For diabetics, explain the importance of monitoring blood sugars with a blood glucose meter.
- *See Nonsteroidal anti-inflammatory drugs overview for more information.*

oxytetracycline

ock-see-te-tra-sye'kleen

oxytetracycline hydrochloride: *E.P. Mycin, Terramycin*

Class: Anti-infective, Broad spectrum tetracycline antibiotic

PEDS	PREG	GERI
✋	**D**	✋

Action Limits bacterial growth (bateriostatic) by binding to the 30S ribosomal subunit and inhibiting protein synthesis.

Use/Therapeutic goal/Outcome

Infections (caused by susceptible gram-negative and gram-positive pathogens, trachoma, rickettsia): Resolution of infection. *Outcome criteria:* Absence of pathogenic growth on cultures, absence of clinical manifestations of infection (fever, pain, swelling, redness, heat, odor, drainage, productive cough, dysuria, frequency), normal WBC count, normal X rays.

Dose range/Administration

Interaction alert: Do not mix IV with any other drugs. Give oral dose 2 hours before or 3 hours after antacids or iron products. Methoxyflurane increases risk of nephrotoxicity; avoid use. May decrease effectiveness of oral contraceptives and penicillins.

🥄 **Give oral doses with a full glass of water on an empty stomach 1 hour after or 2 hours before meals for best absorption. However, may give with food if GI symptoms are experienced.**

Infections (caused by susceptible gram-negative and gram-positive pathogens, trachoma, rickettsia): **Adult:** PO: 250 mg q6h. IM: 100 mg q8-12h; *or* 250 mg as a single dose. **Child < 45 kg, > 8 yrs:** PO: 25–50 mg/kg/day in divided doses q6h. IM: 15–25 mg/kg/day in divided doses q8-12h.

Brucellosis: **Adult:** PO: 500 mg q6h for 3 wks (with streptomycin 1 g IM q12h in first wk, then qd in second wk).

Syphilis: **Adult:** PO: 2–3 g/day in divided doses for 10–15 days (30–40 g total dose).

Gonorrhea: **Adult:** PO: 1.5 g initially, then 0.5 g q6h (9 g total dose).

Clinical alert: IM injection form contains 2% lidocaine—do not give IV. Taking outdated tetracyclines has been associated with fatal nephrotoxicity.

Contraindications/Precautions

PREG D

Contraindicated in allergy to oxytetracycline or other tetracyclines. *Use with caution* in impaired renal or liver function and (for IM route) allergy to "caines."

✋ **Contraindicated for children under 8 years (causes tooth discoloration and retards bone growth) and pregnant or nursing mothers. Use with caution for the elderly.**

Side effects/Adverse reactions

Hypersensitivity: (rare) itching, rashes, fever, anaphylaxis. *GI:* sore throat, dysphagia, glossitis, stomatitis, epigastric discomfort, nausea, vomiting, cramps, diarrhea, enterocolitis, anogenital inflammation. *Skin:* photosensitivity. *CNS:* dizziness, lightheadedness, headache, intracranial hypertension. *CV:* pericarditis. *Hem:* blood dyscrasias.

Nursing implications/Documentation

Possible nursing diagnoses: Potential for infection; Potential fluid volume deficit.

- Determine history of allergies, and (regardless of history) monitor closely for allergic reactions.
- Weigh patient and obtain baseline CBC, BUN, creatinine, liver function studies, and necessary culture specimens before administering first dose; monitor closely thereafter if therapy is prolonged.
- Encourage fluids, and record and monitor intake and output, to ensure adequate hydration and urine output.
- Monitor for and report symptoms of superinfection (mouth lesions, thrush, vaginal irritation, diarrhea, respiratory symptoms).
- If there is no improvement within 3–5 days, consult with physician to determine if antibiotic regimen should be re-evaluated (and new cultures drawn).

Patient & family teaching/Home care

Possible nursing diagnoses: Knowledge deficit, Impaired home maintenance management.

- Advise taking oxytetracycline with food *only* if GI symptoms are experienced.
- Advise avoiding exposure to sunlight; warn that photosensitivity may continue for weeks after oxytetracycline has been discontinued.

- Teach the need to report new signs and symptoms of illness (e.g., fever, mouth lesions, vaginal irritation, respiratory symptoms, diarrhea); medication change may be necessary.

- Explain the importance of taking antibiotics for the entire time prescribed, even if symptoms abate.

- Caution women that this drug may reduce effectiveness of oral contraceptives.

- *See Anti-infectives overview for more information.*

oxytocin   *ox-i-toe'sin*

oxytocin synthetic, injection: **Pitocin, Syntocinon**

oxytocin synthetic, nasal: **Syntocinon**

Class: Oxytocic, Hormone

Antidote: Magnesium sulfate (20% solution), Terbutaline sulfate.

PEDS	PREG	GERI
✋	X	✋

Action Promotes labor (increases force and frequency of contractions) by stimulating uterine muscle contractions (not effective before the third trimester of pregnancy); promotes initial lactation by causing mammary-gland smooth-muscle contraction.

Use/Therapeutic goal/Outcome

Induction or stimulation of labor and incomplete or inevitable abortion: Promotion of effective uterine contractions and vaginal delivery of infant. **Outcome criteria:** Increase in frequency and force of contractions, progression of cervical effacement to 100% and cervical dilatation to 10 cm (and ultimate birth of infant).

Postpartum bleeding after expulsion of placenta: Control of bleeding. **Outcome criteria:** Increase in uterine tone with reduction in bleeding.

Breastfeeding: Promotion of lactation; prevention of engorgement. **Outcome criteria:** Visible letdown of milk; absence of breast engorgement.

Dose range/Administration

Interaction alert: Severe hypertension may occur if oxytocin is given 3–4 hours after a vasoconstrictor is given to patients receiving a caudal block. When oxytocin is used with cyclopropane anesthesia, severe maternal hypotension and cardiac dysrhythmias have occurred. Thiopental anesthetics may reduce oxytoxic effects.

Induction or stimulation of labor: Adult: IV: Mix 10 units (1 ampule) in 1000 ml D5W or 0.9% NaCl and begin infusion at 1 milliunit/min; increase rate by 1–2 milliunits/min q 15–30 min until adequate response. *Maximum dose:* 20 milliunits/min (1–2 ml/min).

Postpartum bleeding after delivery of placenta: Adult: IV: 10–40 units/1000 ml of D5W or 0.9% NaCl at 20–40 milliunits/min to promote uterine tone. IM: 10 units immediately after delivery of placenta.

Incomplete or inevitable abortion: Adult: IV: 10 units/500 ml of D5W or 0.9% NaCl at 20–100 milliunits/min, depending on uterine response.

Promotion of milk letdown: Adult: *Nasal:* 1 spray or 3 gtt in 1 or both nostrils 2–3 min before breastfeeding or pumping breasts.

Clinical alert: Never give IV doses via bolus, always use a controller. Monitor and document maternal vital signs, fetal heart rate, vaginal blood loss, and uterine contractions every 15 min. Stop infusion, turn patient on her left side, and report immediately if contractions are less than 2 min apart and monitor shows contractions of 50 mm Hg or greater, or resting uterine tone of 15–20 mm Hg or greater; if contractions last longer than 80–90 sec; or if there is a significant change in fetal heart rate. Oxytocin infusions given over a 24-hr period may cause convulsions, coma, and death due to water intoxication (secondary to antidiuretic effect of oxytocin); a physician should be available during entire infusion process.

Contraindications/Precautions

PREG
X

Contraindicated in hypersensitivity to oxytocin, and in unfavorable fetal positions or presentations that require conversion, cephalopelvic disproportion, fetal distress without imminent delivery, prematurity, placenta previa, severe toxemia, obstetric emergencies that favor surgical intervention, and for nasal route during labor. **Use with extreme caution** during first and second stage of labor (cervical laceration, uterine rupture, and maternal and fetal death have been reported). **Use with caution** in history of cervical or uterine surgery, grand multiparity, uterine sepsis, traumatic delivery, or overdistended uterus: in conjunction with vasopressors or cyclopropane anesthesia; and in women over 35 years with first pregnancy.

- **Contraindicated for children, in certain stages of pregnancy and labor (see above), and for the elderly. Use with great caution at other stages of labor.**

Side effects/Adverse reactions

In mother: Hypersensitivity: itching, rashes, anaphylaxis, uterine hypertonicity, tetanic contractions, uterine rupture. **CV:** hypotension, hypertension, increased heart rate and systemic venous return, increased cardiac output, dysrhythmias, decreased utero-placental perfusion. **CNS:** subarachnoid hemorrhage, seizures, or coma (secondary to water intoxication). **Hem:** afibrinogenemia (may be related to increased postpartum bleeding). **GI:** nausea, vomiting. **Misc:** for nasal route, mild uterine cramping.

In fetus: CV: bradycardia, tachycardia, premature ventricular contractions, decreased utero-placental perfusion. **Resp:** asphyxia, anoxia. **Eye:** retinal hemorrhage.

Nursing implications/Documentation

Possible nursing diagnoses: Pain; Potential for injury; Impaired physical mobility; Potential for infection.

♦ Have magnesium sulfate readily available in case of tetanic uterine contraction (it relaxes uterus).

♦ Record progression of labor (check hospital protocols and see Clinical alert).

♦ Have patient rate pain on a scale of 1–10, assist in relaxation techniques, and medicate as ordered; report immediately if the pain is severe and associated with hard abdomen or change in maternal or infant vital signs.

♦ Keep mother in bed with side rails up and call-bell within reach.

♦ Assist mother in turning and changing positions frequently; massage back and pressure points every 2 hours.

♦ Monitor intake and output closely; report fluid overload immediately (may lead to seizures and coma).

♦ Report foul-smelling lochia or fever; discontinue drug and report if uterine hyperactivity or fetal distress is noted.

Patient & family teaching/Home care

Possible nursing diagnoses: Fear; Knowledge deficit.

♦ Explain that this drug is intended to expedite labor; stress that both mother and child will be closely monitored to "fine tune" medication.

♦ Encourage both mother and labor coach to ask questions and verbalize fears or concerns; encourage labor coach to provide physical and emotional comfort (backrubs, foot massages, verbal coaching during contractions).

♦ For nasal route, stress the need to clear nasal passages and inhale spray while sitting (not lying down); explain that a quiet, private environment assists in promoting letdown; warn that mild menstrual cramping and increase in lochia may be noted after dose is taken.

pancrelipase

pan-cre-li'pase

Cotazym, Cotazym-S, Creon, Festal II, Ilozyme, Ku-Zyme HP, Pancrease, Pancrease MT4, Pancrease MT10, Pancrease MT16, Viokase

Class: Pancreatic enzyme replenisher, Digestant

PEDS	PREG	GERI
✋	C	OK

Action Enhances digestion of proteins: Starches, and fats in gastrointestinal tract by supplying enzymes (protease, amylase, and lipase).

Use/Therapeutic goal/Outcome

Pancreatic insufficiency or steatorrhea: Promotion of digestion and absorption of essential nutrients. **Outcome criteria:** Decreased number of bowel movements and improved stool consistency; maintenance or attainment of adequate body weight.

Dose range/Administration

Interaction alert: Calcium and magnesium antacids may decrease effectiveness of pancrelipase. Absorption of oral iron supplements may be decreased.

Adult and Child: PO: 1–3 tablets or capsules, or 1–2 powder packs, with meals.

Clinical alert: Pancrelipase should be taken with each meal and snack, with the dose adjusted as needed and tolerated. With dosage forms that are not enteric coated, H_2 antagonists or antacids may be administered with meals to prevent destruction of pancrelipase by gastric acid.

Contraindications/Precautions

PREG
C

Contraindicated in hypersensitivity to pork protein and in acute pancreatitis. Use with caution in hyperuricemia, or hyperuricosuria.

⚜ Use with caution for children under 6 year and pregnant or nursing mothers.

Side effects/Adverse reactions

Hypersensitivity: rash, hives. **Resp:** with powdered form, shortness of breath, wheezing, or stuffy nose. **Hem:** hyperuricemia. **GI:** irritation of mouth, diarrhea, nausea, cramps. **GU:** bloody urine, hyperuricosuria. **MS:** joint pain, swelling of hands or feet.

Nursing implications/Documentation

Possible nursing diagnoses: Diarrhea; Pain.

♦ When administering to children, open capsules and sprinkle contents on food; with enteric coated spheres, administer with non-alkaline liquids or soft foods that do not require chewing.

♦ Assess and record frequency and character of stools.

♦ Weigh three times weekly and document.

♦ Assess for symptoms of hyperuricemia and hyperuricosuria (bloody urine, joint pain, or swelling of hands or feet).

Patient & family teaching/Home care

Possible nursing diagnoses: Knowledge deficit; Altered oral mucous membrane; Impaired home maintenance management.

♦ Teach the need to take pancrelipase with each meal or snack.

♦ Advise not to crush or chew capsules containing enteric coated spheres.

♦ Caution against mixing enteric coated spheres with alkaline foods such as milk or ice cream.

♦ For tablet form, explain the need to swallow tablets quickly with liquid and to avoid chewing to lessen possibility of mouth irritation.

♦ Warn of the possibility of sensitization from repeated inhalation of powder from opened capsules or powdered form.

♦ Stress the importance of following prescribed diet.

pancuronium

pan-kyoo-roe'nee-um

pancuronium bromide: **Pavulon**

Class: Skeletal-muscle relaxant, Nondepolarizing neuromuscular blocker

Antidote: Neostigmine methylsulfate

PEDS	PREG	GERI
⚜	C	⚜

Action Relaxes or paralyzes skeletal muscles (depending on dose) by competing with acetylcholine for cholinergic receptor sites, thereby inhibiting neuromuscular transmission. Does not alter consciousness, pain threshold, or thought processes.

Use/Therapeutic goal/Outcome

Endotracheal intubation, adjunct to general anesthesia, during mechanical ventilation, and during pharmacologically or electrically induced seizures: Facilitation of endotracheal tube and mechanical ventilation tolerance; relaxation or paralysis of skeletal muscle. **Outcome criteria:** Tolerance of endotracheal intubation and mechanical ventilation; diminished or absent voluntary and reflexive movement.

Dose range/Administration

Interaction alert: Succinylcholine, aminoglycoside, and polysyxin antibiotics, magnesium salts, quinidine, lithium, narcotic analgesics and inhalation agents, (halothane, diethyl ether, fluothane, methoxyflurane) enhance the neuromuscular blockade. Cardiac glycosides may have additive cardiotoxic effects. Acetylcholine, anticholinesterase, and potassium antagonize pancuronium bromide effect.

Surgery: Adult: IV: 0.04–0.1 mg/kg. May repeat 0.01 mg/kg q 30–60 min.

Endotracheal intubation: Adult and Child: IV: 0.06–0.1 mg/kg. **Neonate:** IV: give a test dose of 0.02 mg/kg; then individualize dose.

Clinical alert: Do not use plastic syringe to prepare pancuronium bromide other than immediately prior to administration. This drug should be given only by physicians and nurses who are familiar with its use, and in the presence of a physician, nurse anesthetist, or respiratory therapist who is qualified to manage endotracheal intubation.

P

Contraindications/Precautions

PREG
C

Contraindicated in hypersensitivity to pancuronium or bromides, and in tachycardia. **Use with caution** in myasthenia gravis, pulmonary, renal or hepatic impairment, electrolyte imbalance, dehydration, thyroid disorders, and collagen diseases.

👋 **Contraindicated for the elderly or debilitated. Use with caution for neonates. Safe use for pregnant women has not been established.**

Side effects/Adverse reactions

Hypersensitivity: tachycardia. **Resp:** respiratory depression, prolonged dose-related apnea. **CV:** flushing, elevated blood pressure, ventricular extrasystoles. **GI:** increased salivation. **MS:** skeletal muscle weakness. **Skin:** transient rash.

Nursing implications/Documentation

Possible nursing diagnoses: Impaired communication; Pain; Potential for aspiration; Potential for injury.

♦ Ascertain that baseline CBC, electrolytes, BUN, creatinine, liver function, chest X ray, and EKG studies are posted on chart before drug administration (report abnormalities).

♦ Protect airway, position for drainage of oropharyngeal secretions (if possible), and keep suction at bedside until the patient is fully alert; have emergency equipment and drugs available.

♦ Monitor and record vital signs every 15 min until stable; report abnormalities that might indicate potential complications.

♦ Recognize that this drug may *paralyze*, but does not relieve pain (provide analgesics if pain is suspected, anticipate human needs).

♦ Monitor for potential for injury: protect eyes if there is no blink reflex (tape shut); watch positioning of all extremities (provide range of motion exercises if therapy is prolonged).

♦ Monitor and document intake and output every 2–4 hours for 24 hours after administration.

♦ Be aware that pancuronium may decrease serum cholinesterase.

Patient & family teaching/Home care

Possible nursing diagnoses: Anxiety; Fear.

♦ Explain all procedures, even if the person seems unconscious (the ability to hear may be present).

♦ Reassure individual that muscle weakness or stiffness will subside.

♦ For use with mechanical ventilation, stress that you are aware that the patient cannot move, and that this drug is being given to control breathing; reassure that breathing is being closely monitored to be sure that the lungs are being adequately oxygenated, and that ability to move will return as soon as drug is stopped. Also reassure that medication for pain and anxiety will be given to help tolerate the endotracheal tube.

papaverine

pa-pa'ver-een

papaverine hydrochloride: **Cerespan, Genabid, Pavabid, Pavabid HP, Pavabid Plateau Caps, Pavarine Spancaps, Pavasule, Pavatine, Pavatym, Paverolan Lanacaps**

Class: Vasodilator, peripheral

PEDS	PREG	GERI
👋	C	👋

Action Produces vasodilation by relaxing smooth muscles directly, independent of autonomic innervation. Depresses myocardial conduction and irritability, and prolongs the refractory period. Clinical effectiveness has not been conclusively determined.

Use/Therapeutic goal/Outcome

Peripheral and cerebral ischemia associated with arterial vascular spasm; myocardial ischemia with arrhythmias; and smooth muscle spastic conditions, such as biliary, ureteral, or GI colic: Relaxation smooth muscle spasms/improved tissue perfusion. **Outcome criteria:** Patient report of decreased pain; improved mental alertness.

Dose range/Administration

Interaction alert: May reduce the efficacy of levodopa. Do not mix with Lactated Ringer's solution (forms a precipitate).

🖐 **Give with food or milk.**

Adult: PO: 60–300 mg 1 to 5 times/day. *Sustained release form:* 150–300 mg q8-12h. IM, IV: 30–120 mg q3h as needed. For cardiac extrasystoles, 2 doses may be given 10 min

P

apart. *Child:* IM, IV: 6 mg/kg/day divided into 4 doses.

Clinical alert: Give IV doses slowly over 1–2 min. Rapid infusion may cause arrythmias, respiratory arrest, and death.

Contraindications/Precautions

PREG
C

Contraindicated in hypersensitity to papaverine and in parkinsonism and (for IV route) complete AV block. *Use with caution* in the presence of glaucoma, coronary insufficiency and recent stroke.

⚠ Use with caution for children and the elderly. Safe use for pregnant women has not been established.

Side effects/Adverse reactions

Hypersensitivity: rash, pruritis. *GI:* constipation, nausea, dry mouth and throat, liver toxicity. *CNS:* dizziness, drowsiness, headache. *Skin:* facial flushing, sweating. *Misc:* rapid IV administration may cause arrhythmias, respiratory distress, fatal apnea.

Nursing implications/Documentation

Possible nursing diagnoses: Activity intolerance; Potential for injury.

♦ Document baseline mental status and circulatory status (presence and quality of peripheral pulses, skin color and temperature); monitor periodically thereafter.

♦ For parenteral route (used only when immediate response is needed) record pulse and blood pressure, before and after administration.

♦ Observe for dizziness and hypotension; supervise ambulation until response is determined.

♦ Monitor liver function studies periodically.

Patient & family teaching/Home care

Possible nursing diagnoses: Knowledge deficit; Impaired home maintenance management.

♦ Advise taking this drug with milk or food.

♦ Stress the need to change positions slowly to reduce dizziness; point out that alcohol may increase vasodilation and dizziness.

♦ Discourage smoking and long periods of standing; stress the need for good skin care.

♦ Warn against driving or performing hazardous activities until response is determined.

paraldehyde
pa-ral'de-hide

Paral

Class: Anticonvulsant, Sedative, Hypnotic

PEDS	PREG	GERI
⚠	C	⚠

CONTROLLED SUBSTANCE
IV

Action Limits seizure activity and produces CNS depression and sedation through an unknown mechanism. Action is believed to be similar to that of alcohol, barbiturates, and chloral hydrate.

Use/Therapeutic goal/Outcome

Status epilepticus and grand mal seizures unresponsive to other anticonvulsants: Limitation of seizure activity. *Outcome criteria:* Marked decrease or absence of seizures.

Sedation: Promotion of relaxation and sleep. *Outcome criteria:* Patient reports feeling less agitated and more relaxed; observable signs of relaxation (more quiet, less restless).

Dose range/Administration

Interaction alert: Alcohol and disulfiram may cause excessive sedation.

Adult: PO or Rectal: 5–10 cc. IM: 2–5 ml deep into large muscle mass. IV: (Sometimes not available, and used only in emergencies because it is very dangerous) 5 cc diluted in 100 cc sodium chloride infused at a rate of 1 cc/min. *Child:* PO, IM or Rectal: 0.15 cc/kg.

Clinical alert: Hold drug and report if respirations are less than 12/min. Use glass syringes and containers for administration (paraldehyde reacts with plastic). Because oral or rectal doses may cause severe corrosion of the stomach or rectum, give PO doses well diluted in juice or milk and rectal doses diluted 1:2 with olive or cottonseed oil or 200 cc normal saline. Protect drug from air; do not use if it has a brown color or vinegary odor or if container has been open longer than 24 hr.

Contraindications/Precautions

PREG
C

Contraindicated in hypersensitivity to paraldehyde and in bronchopulmonary disease, hepatic insufficiency, GI ulceration, or concomitant disulfiram therapy.

⚠ Use with caution for children and the elderly. Safe use for pregnant women has not been established.

P

Side effects/Adverse reactions

Hypersensitivity: skin rashes. **GI:** gastric or rectal irritation, unpleasant breath odor and taste. **CNS:** hangover, ataxia, confusion. **Skin:** necrosis or sterile abscess at injection site. **GU:** toxic nephrosis. **Signs of overdosage** include respiratory depression, pulmonary edema, hypotension, gastritis, renal and hepatic damage, right-sided heart failure, cardiovascular collapse.

Nursing implications/Documentation

Possible nursing diagnoses: Potential for injury; Sensory/perceptual alterations.

♦ Initiate seizure precautions upon admission.

♦ Hold drug and report if there is excessive sedation or respiratory depression.

♦ Keep side rails up and supervise ambulation until response is determined.

♦ Ventilate room to remove exhaled drug.

♦ Do not allow unsupervised smoking.

♦ Be alert for coughing, which may be a sign of early pulmonary toxicity.

Patient & family teaching/Home care

Possible nursing diagnoses: Fear; Knowledge deficit; Impaired home maintenance management.

♦ Stress the need to remain in bed and to call for assistance.

♦ Explain to family that paraldehyde causes a strong breath odor that may permeate the room.

♦ Warn that stopping anticonvulsants suddenly can cause an increase in severity and frequency of seizures.

♦ *See Antianxiety Agents, Sedatives, and Hypnotics, and Anticonvulsants overviews for more information.*

paramethadione
par-a-meth-a-dye'one

Paradione

Class: Anticonvulsant

PEDS	PREG	GERI
♨	D	♨

Action Limits seizure activity by elevating the threshold for seizure discharge in the thalamus. Prolongs the recovery period of postsynaptic neurons where repetitive discharges produce absence (petit mal) attacks.

Use/Therapeutic goal/Outcome

Absence (petit mal) seizures resistant to other drugs: Limitation of seizure activity. **Outcome criteria:** Marked decrease or absence of seizure activity.

Dose range/Administration

🍴 **Give with food or milk to reduce GI symptoms.**

Adult: PO: 300 mg tid for the first week; may increase weekly prn by 300 mg increments, to a maximum of 600 mg qid. **Child > 6 yrs:** PO: 300 mg tid or qid. **Child 2–6 yrs:** PO: 200 mg tid. **Child < 2 yrs:** PO: 100 mg tid.

Clinical alert: Available in capsules or liquid. Warn against chewing or crushing capsule (liquid is an oily). Measure oral solution with dropper provided by manufacturer, and dilute with water or juice before giving (65% alcohol in undiluted solution).

Contraindications/Precautions

PREG D

Contraindicated in hypersensitivity to oxazolidinedione anticonvulsants, and in severe blood dyscrasias, and renal or hepatic dysfunction. **Use with caution** in retinal or optic nerve disease.

🖐 **Use with caution for children and the elderly. Safe use for pregnant or nursing mothers has not been established.**

Side effects/Adverse reactions

Hypersensitivity: itching, swollen lymph glands, enlarged liver. **CNS:** sedation, drowsiness, ataxia, headache, dizziness. **CV:** hypotension, hypertension. **Eye:** photophobia, diplopia. **GI:** nausea, vomiting, weight loss, bleeding gums, hepatitis. **GU:** albuminuria, vaginal bleeding. **Hem:** agranulocytosis, aplastic anemia, leukopenia, neutropenia.

Nursing implications/Documentation

Possible nursing diagnoses: Potential for injury; Potential for aspiration.

♦ Document history of seizures (type, frequency, duration, usual time they occur, precipitating factors, presence of an aura); initiate seizure precautions as indicated.

♦ Monitor for and report signs of blood dyscrasias, hepatitis, lymphadenopathy (persistent sore throat, fever, malaise, easy bruising, bleeding gums, nausea, vomiting, fatigue, lumps in arms or groin).

• Obtain baseline liver function studies and urinalysis, and monitor monthly thereafter. Check CBC every 3 months; hold drug and report if neutrophils drop below 3000.

Patient & family teaching/Home care

Possible nursing diagnoses: Fear; Self-esteem disturbance; Knowledge deficit; Impaired home maintenance management.

• Advise taking this drug with food or milk to reduce GI symptoms.

• Stress the need for close medical follow-up; advise reporting persistent sore throat, fever, malaise, easy bruising, bleeding gums, nausea, vomiting, fatigue, or lumps in arms or groin.

• Warn that stopping anticonvulsants suddenly can cause an increase in severity and frequency of seizures.

• Caution against driving until response is determined (may cause drowsiness).

◆ *See Anticonvulsants overview for more information.*

pemoline
pem'oh-leen

Cylert, Cylert Chewable

Class: Cerebral stimulant

PEDS	PREG	GERI
♆	B	♆

CONTROLLED SUBSTANCE IV

Action *In hyperactive children,* decreases hyperactivity and prolongs attention span by increasing storage or synthesis of dopamine, and excitatory neurotransmitter.

Use/Therapeutic goal/Outcome

Attention Deficit Disorders with Hyperactivity (ADDH): Promotion of ability to concentrate and pay attention. **Outcome criteria:** Demonstration of increased attention span and increased ability to sit quietly.

Dose range/Administration

Interaction alert: CNS stimulation may be increased by decongestants and other CNS stimulants. May alter insulin and antidiabetic agent requirements.

Child 6 yrs and older: PO: 37.5 mg in the morning, with weekly increments of 18.75 mg prn (maximum of 112.5 mg/day). Usual effective dose range is 56.25–75 mg/day.

Clinical alert: Be aware that full therapeutic effects may not be observed until the third or fourth week of therapy.

Contraindications/Precautions

Contraindicated in hypersensitivity to pemoline and in liver impairment.

♆ **Contraindicated for children under 6 years, pregnant or nursing mothers, and other adults. Use with caution for children with renal impairment or Tourette's syndrome.**

Side effects/Adverse reactions

Hypersensitivity: itching, rashes. **CNS:** insomnia, seizures, tremors, hyperactivity, irritability, headache, dizziness, depression. **CV:** tachycardia. **GI:** anorexia, constipation, hepatitis, weight loss. **Misc:** suppression of growth, weight loss.

Nursing implications/Documentation

Possible nursing diagnoses: Altered thought processes; Sleep pattern disturbance; Constipation; Altered nutrition: less than body requirements.

• Question about the use of beverages and OTC drugs that contain caffeine.

• Monitor attention span and ability to concentrate, and report and document changes in status (dosage may need to be adjusted).

• Provide decaffeinated beverages; document daily weights, and keep a record of food intake to ensure adequate nutrition.

• Prevent side effect of constipation by monitoring bowel movements, ensuring adequate hydration, and providing fruits, juices, and vegetables (use laxatives only when necessary).

Patient & family teaching/Home care

Possible nursing diagnoses: Knowledge deficit; Impaired home maintenance management.

• Explain that CNS stimulants have a high potential for abuse, and should be taken only as prescribed.

• Explain the importance of checking labels for caffeine content and avoiding caffeine (may increase drug effects).

• Teach the family to monitor physical and mental growth, and to report growth failure and behavior extremes (dosage may have to be adjusted).

• Explain that dosage will probably be reduced as child progresses to puberty, and that periodic "drug holidays" may be planned to determine if the drug is still necessary.

◆ *See Cerebral Stimulants overview for more information.*

penbutolol sulfate
pen-bu'toe-lole

Levatol

Class: Nonselective beta adrenergic blocking agent, Antihypertensive, Antianginal

PEDS	PREG	GERI
🖐	C	🖐

Action Reduces blood pressure and heart rate by blocking beta-1 (cardiac) and beta-2 adrenergic receptors. Also reduces myocardial excitability and conduction velocity in the atria and AV-node. Reduces plasma renin activity. Has moderate intrinsic sympathomimetic activity (ISA).

Use/Therapeutic goal/Outcome

Hypertension: Reduction of blood pressure. *Outcome criteria:* Blood pressure within normal limits.

Dose range/Administration

Interaction alert: Other antihypertensives may potentiate hypotensive effects. Nonsteroidal anti-inflammatory agents may decrease antihypertensive effects. Concurrent use with clonidine may cause paradoxical hypertension. May alter antidiabetic agent requirements.

Adult: PO: 20 mg/day; may increase to 40–80 mg/day.

Clinical alert: When discontinuing, wean over a 1–2 week period to avoid precipitating thyroid storm or myocardial infarction. Be aware that patient receiving this drug may not exhibit tachycardia as a symptom of fever, hypoglycemia, and hyperthyroidism.

Contraindications/Precautions
PREG C

Contraindicated in hypersensitivity to penbutolol, and in cardiogenic shock, sinus bradycardia, second- or third-degree heart block (PR interval > 0.24 seconds), CHF, COPD, and bronchial asthma. *Use with caution* in diabetes, hyperthyroidism, and hepatic or renal impairment.

🖐 Use with caution for the elderly. Safe use for children and pregnant or nursing mothers has not been established.

Side effects/Adverse reactions

Hypersensitivity: rash, pruritis. *CNS:* headache, mental depression, fatigue, insomnia, nightmares, dizziness, hallucinations. *CV:* bradycardia, hypotension, CHF, peripheral vascular disease. *Resp:* increased airway resistance. *GI:* nausea, vomiting, diarrhea, constipation. *GU:* impotence, urinary retention. *MS:* cold hands and feet.

Nursing implications/Documentation

Possible nursing diagnoses: Activity intolerance; Fatigue; Potential for injury.

♦ Assess mental status and record pulse and blood pressure (if possible, lying, sitting, and standing, in both arms) before administration, and frequently thereafter until response is determined.

♦ Consult with physician to determine desired therapeutic range for blood pressure and heart rate (parameters for withholding the medication should be written by physician).

♦ Ascertain that baseline CBC, electrolytes, BUN, creatinine, and liver function studies have been obtained before giving first dose; report abnormalities and monitor closely thereafter.

♦ Monitor for allergic reactions and signs of confusion, dizziness, bradycardia, CHF, and hypotension; hold drug and report immediately if these occur.

♦ Supervise ambulation until response is determined.

♦ Document and monitor daily weight, and intake and output; report significant negative or positive balance.

Patient & family teaching/Home care

Possible nursing diagnoses: Knowledge deficit; Impaired home maintenance management; Altered sexuality patterns.

♦ Explain the importance of taking this drug exactly as prescribed, even when feeling well; warn not to discontinue drug abruptly (may precipitate angina).

♦ Stress the importance of good medical follow-up, explain that this drug reduces "wear and tear" on blood vessels, reduces the workload of the heart, and improves longevity and health.

♦ Teach how to monitor pulse and blood pressure; emphasize that syncope, hypertension or hypotension, or persistent dizziness should be reported; provide pulse and blood pressure parameters for withholding medication.

♦ Advise changing positions slowly, to avoid dizziness.

• Encourage daily monitoring of weight and reporting sudden weight gain (frequently is fluid retention).

• Warn against drinking alcohol or taking *any* OTC drugs without physician approval (some interactions can cause severe reactions).

• Advise against excessive exposure to cold; stress that persistent cold feet or hands should be reported.

• Explain that this drug may alter sexual activity; counsel about concerns.

◆ *See Adrenergic Beta Blockers, Antihypertensives, and Antianginals overviews for more information.*

penicillamine

pen-i-sill'a-meen

Cuprimine, Depen

Class: Chelating Agent, Antirheumatic (disease-modifying), Antiurolithic

PEDS	PREG	GERI
🖐	**D**	🖐

Action Chelates (binds together) heavy metals by forming stable, soluble complexes that are excreted in urine; reduces inflammation in joints by an unclear mechanism; reduces incidence of cystine renal stones by combining with cystine to form a soluble compound readily excreted in urine.

Use/Therapeutic goal/Outcome

Wilson's disease: Excretion of excess copper to prevent or resolve damage to brain, liver, kidneys and eyes. ***Outcome criteria:*** Upon examination of a 24-hour urine specimen, increased urinary copper excretion; absence or improvement in neurologic symptoms; liver and renal function studies within normal range; absence or improvement in copper-related eye pathology.

Severe rheumatoid arthritis not responsive to conventional therapy: Modification or suppression of disease and prevention of further damage to affected joints. ***Outcome criteria:*** Reduction in swelling of affected joints, decreased sedimentation rate, improved grip strength, decreased use of analgesics, decreased morning stiffness, and increased ability to ambulate.

Cystinuria when conventional prophylactic measures are not effective: Prevention or resolution of cystine renal stones. ***Outcome criteria:*** Urinary cystine excretion levels decreased to 100–200 mg/day.

Dose range/Administration

Interaction alert: Antimalarial or cytotoxic drugs, gold salts, oxyphenbutazone or phenylbutazone increase potential for hematologic and renal adverse reactions. Iron or mineral supplements and antacids may decrease effects of penicillamine. Digoxin serum levels may be reduced.

📧 **Give 1 hour before or 2 hours after meals.**

Wilson's disease: Adult: PO: 250 mg qid. **Child:** PO: 250 mg/day.

Rheumatoid arthritis: Adult: PO: 125–250 mg/day, increased q 1 to 3 months as needed and tolerated. *Maximum dose:* 1.5 g/day.

Cystinuria: Adult: PO: 250–500 mg qid. **Child:** PO: 7.5 mg/kg qid.

Clinical alert: If surgery is needed during penicillamine therapy, dosage will be decreased to permit wound healing. After interruption of therapy for any reason, restart penicillamine at small dosage to minimize sensitivity reactions.

Contraindications/Precautions

PREG
D

Contraindicated in hypersensitivity to penicillin and in lactose intolerance, or with history of agranulocytosis or aplastic anemia. ***Use with caution*** in renal impairment and with history of toxic reaction to gold salt therapy.

🖐 **Contraindicated for pregnant women unless used for Wilson's disease. Use with caution for children and the elderly.**

Side effects/Adverse reactions

Hypersensitivity: pruritus, rashes, hives, fever, joint pain, or swelling of lymph glands. **GI:** anorexia, epigastric pain, nausea, vomiting or diarrhea, altered taste perception, stomatitis, colitis. **Hem:** bone-marrow depression, aplastic anemia, agranulocytosis, leukopenia, thrombocytopenia. **GU:** proteinuria, hematuria, nephrotic syndrome. **Ear:** tinnitus. **Eye:** eye pain, blurred vision. **Skin:** delayed wound healing, increased friability, excessive wrinkling, white papules at venipuncture and surgical sites.

Nursing implications/Documentation

Possible nursing diagnoses: Altered nutrition: less than body requirements; Potential for infection; Potential for injury; Altered oral mucous membrane.

P

- Monitor results of hematologic, renal, and hepatic tests for signs of clinical response and adverse reactions.
- Anticipate toxic effects to be more common in the elderly.
- Monitor for and report signs of pyridoxine deficiency (eye pain, blurring or change in vision); daily supplements may be necessary.

Patient & family teaching/Home care

Possible nursing diagnoses: Knowledge deficit; Impaired home maintenance management.

- Teach the need to take doses on an empty stomach, 1 hour before or 2 hours after meals, and at least 1 hour apart from any other medication, food, or milk.
- With cystinuria, stress the importance of adhering to a prescribed diet and maintaining a high fluid intake; encourage drinking 500 ml at bedtime and 500 ml during the night.
- With rheumatoid arthritis, advise that improvement in symptoms may require 2–3 months of therapy; if no improvement occurs in 3–4 months, drug will be discontinued.
- With Wilson's disease, emphasize the importance of adhering to a low-copper diet (no chocolate, nuts, shellfish, mushrooms, liver, molasses, broccoli, or cereals enriched with copper); caution not to take vitamin preparations containing copper and to use distilled or demineralized water if drinking water contains > 0.1 mg of copper per liter. Advise that improvement may require 1–3 months of therapy.
- Caution women regarding dangers of pregnancy and advise reporting suspected pregnancy promptly.
- Advise avoiding iron supplements; if prescribed, point out that doses should not be taken within two hours of penicillamine.
- Teach that fever, sore throat, chills, bleeding, or bruising should be reported.
- Stress the need to remain under close medical supervision and to have blood and urine testing done as frequently as recommended; warn not to discontinue drug without consulting physician.

penicillin G

pen-i-sill'in

penicillin G benzathine (benzylpenicillin benzathine): **Bicillin L-A, Megacillin**

penicillin G potassium (benzylpenicillin potassium): ❦**Megacillin,** ❦**NovoPen-G,** ❦**P-50, Pentids, Pfizerpen**

penicillin G procaine (benzylpenicillin procaine): ❦**Ayercillin, Crysticillin A.S., Duracillin A.S., Pfizerpen–A.S., Wycillin**

penicillin G sodium: **Crystapen**

Class: ★**Anti-infective (natural penicillin) prototype,** Antibiotic

PEDS	PREG	GERI
🖑	B	🖑

Action Broad-spectrum, usually bactericidal antibiotic; kills bacteria by inhibiting cell wall synthesis.

Use/Therapeutic goal/Outcome

- **Benzathine/procaine**

Systemic infections (caused by susceptible gram-negative and gram-positive bacteria): Prevention or resolution of infection. **Outcome criteria:** Absence of pathogenic growth on cultures, absence of clinical manifestations of infection (fever, pain, redness, heat, swelling, odor, drainage), normal WBC count, improvement of X rays.

- **Potassium/sodium**

Moderate to severe systemic infections or prophylaxis: Prevention or resolution of infection. **Outcome criteria:** Absence of pathogenic growth on cultures, absence of clinical manifestations of infection (fever, pain, redness, heat, swelling, odor, drainage), normal WBC count, improvement of X rays.

Dose range/Administration

Interaction alert: Probenecid inhibits excretion of penicillin G and may be given to increase serum levels of the drug. Use of potassium or sodium form with anticoagulants or aspirin may cause bleeding tendency.

- **Penicillin G benzathine**

Group A streptococcal upper respiratory infections: Adult: IM: 1.2 million units in a single dose. **Child > 27 kg:** IM: 900,000 units in a single dose. **Child < 27 kg:** 300,000–900,000 units in a single dose.

Syphilis: Adult: IM: *Duration of disease < 1 yr:* 2.4 million units in a single dose. *Duration of disease > 1 yr:* 2.4 million units/wk for 3 wks. **Child < 2 yrs:** IM: 50,000 units/kg in a single dose.

Prophylaxis of poststreptococcal rheumatic fever: Adult and Child: IM: 1.2 million units/month in 1 or 2 doses.

◆ **Penicillin G potassium**

Moderate to severe systemic infections: Adult: PO: 1.6–3.2 million units/day in divided doses q6h. IM, IV: 1.2–24 million units/day in divided doses q4h. **Child:** PO: 25,000–100,000 units/kg/day in divided doses q6h. IM, IV: 25,000–300,000 units/kg/day in divided doses q4h.

◆ **Penicillin G procaine**

Moderate to severe systemic infections: Adult: IM: 600,000 to 1.2 million units qd. **Child:** IM: 300,000 units qd.

Uncomplicated gonorrhea: Adult/Child > 12 yrs: IM: 4.8 million units, divide and inject in 2 sites, 30 min after administering 1 g probenecid orally.

◆ **Penicillin G sodium**

Moderate to severe systemic infections: Adult: IM, IV: 1.2–24 million units/day, in divided doses q4h. **Child:** IM, IV: 25,000–300,000 units/kg/day, in divided doses q4h.

Endocarditis prophylaxis for dental surgery: Adult: IM, IV: 2 million units 30–60 min before procedure, then 1 million units 6 hr after.

Clinical alert: For benzathine and procaine forms, always aspirate IM injections carefully to avoid injecting into a vessel (inadvertant IV or intra-arterial administration can cause cardiac arrest and death); recognize that IM absorption is prolonged, resulting in more sustained therapeutic levels and more difficulty in treating allergic reactions.

Contraindications/Precautions

PREG
B

Contraindicated in allergy to penicillin or (procaine form) procaine. **Use with caution** in cephalosporin sensitivity, history of allergic responses (e.g., other drugs, hay fever, asthma), and renal insufficiency.

✋ **Use all forms with caution for pregnant or nursing mothers. Also use benzathine and procaine forms with caution for children and the elderly.**

Side effects/Adverse reactions

Hypersensitivity: itching, rashes, urticaria, fever, difficulty breathing, anaphylaxis, (benzathine and procaine forms) exfoliative dermati-

tis. **GI:** nausea, vomiting, diarrhea, flatulence. **Hem:** hyperkalemia, increased bleeding time, eosinophilia, hemolytic anemia, thrombocytopenia, leukopenia. **Skin:** pain, redness, swelling, sterile abscess or (IV route) thrombophlebitis at injection site. **CNS:** neurotoxicity, (with high doses) seizures. **MS:** (procaine form) arthralgia. **Misc:** superinfection, bone marrow depression.

Nursing implications/Documentation

Possible nursing diagnoses: Potential for infection; Diarrhea.

◆ Determine history of allergies, and (regardless of history) monitor closely for allergic reactions.

◆ Obtain baseline CBC, electrolytes, and necessary cultures before administering first dose.

◆ Encourage fluids, and record and monitor intake and output, to ensure adequate hydration.

◆ With benzathine and procaine forms, give deep IM (never IV) into large muscle mass.

◆ Monitor for and report signs of superinfection (sore throat, fever, fatigue, thrush, vaginal discharge, diarrhea).

◆ With potassium and sodium forms, observe for unusual bruising or bleeding (check urine, gums).

Patient & family teaching/Home care

Possible nursing diagnoses: Knowledge deficit; Impaired home maintenance management.

◆ Teach importance of reporting allergic symptoms, diarrhea, signs and symptoms that do not abate, or *any* new signs and symptoms of discomfort that might indicate superinfection (medication regimen may have to be changed).

◆ Advise drinking 2–3 L of fluids daily to maintain adequate hydration (especially important if fever exists).

◆ Stress the importance of taking antibiotics for the entire time prescribed, even if signs and symptoms abate.

◆ *See Anti-infectives overview for more information.*

P

penicillin V

pen-i-sill'in

penicillin V potassium (phenoxymethyl penicillin): *Abbocillin VK, Abo-Pen-VK, Beepen-VK, Betapen-VK, Cilicane VK, Ledercillin VK, Nadopen-V, NovoPen-VK, Penarpar VK, Pen-Vee-K, PVF K, PVK, Robicillin VK, V-Cillin K, VC-K, Veetids*

Class: Anti-infective, Antibiotic, Natural penicillin

PEDS	PREG	GERI
🖐	B	🖐

Action Broad-spectrum, usually bactericidal antibiotic; kills bacteria by inhibiting cell wall synthesis.

Use/Therapeutic goal/Outcome

Mild to moderate systemic infections or prophylaxis: Resolution or prevention of infection. **Outcome criteria:** Absence of pathogenic growth on cultures, absence of clinical manifestations of infection (fever, pain, redness, heat, swelling, odor, drainage), normal WBC count, improvement of X rays.

Dose range/Administration

Interaction alert: Probenecid inhibits excretion of penicillin V and may be given to increase serum penicillin levels.

🗓 **Give with a full glass of water, with or without food.**

Mild to moderate infection: Adult: PO: 125–500 mg (400,000–800,000 units) q6-12h. **Child:** PO: 15–50 mg/kg/day (25,000–90,000 units/kg/day) in divided doses q6-8h.

Endocarditis prophylaxis for dental surgery: Adult: PO: 2 g 30–60 min before procedure, then 500 mg 6 hr later. **Child < 30 kg:** PO: 1/2 adult dose.

Clinical alert: Give at least 1 hour before bacteriostatic antibiotics for optimal effects.

Contraindications/Precautions

PREG
B

Contraindicated in allergy to penicillin. **Use with caution** in cephalosporin sensitivity, history of allergic responses (e.g., other drugs, hay fever, asthma), and renal insufficiency.

🖐 **Use with caution for children, the elderly, and pregnant or nursing mothers.**

Side effects/Adverse reactions

Hypersensitivity: itching, rashes, urticaria, fever, difficulty breathing, anaphylaxis. **GI:** epigastric distress, nausea, vomiting, diarrhea, flatulence. **Hem:** increased bleeding time, eosinophilia, hemolytic anemia, thrombocytopenia, leukopenia. **CNS:** neurotoxicity. **Misc:** superinfection, bone marrow depression.

Nursing implications/Documentation

Possible nursing diagnoses: Potential for infection; Diarrhea.

♦ Determine history of allergies, and (regardless of history) monitor closely for allergic reactions.

♦ Obtain baseline CBC and necessary cultures before giving first dose.

♦ Encourage fluids, and record and monitor intake and output, to ensure adequate hydration.

♦ Monitor for and report signs of superinfection (sore throat, fever, fatigue, thrush, vaginal discharge, diarrhea).

♦ Observe for unusual bruising or bleeding (check urine, gums).

Patient & family teaching/Home care

Possible nursing diagnoses: Knowledge deficit; Impaired home maintenance management.

♦ Teach the importance of reporting allergic symptoms, diarrhea, signs and symptoms that do not abate, or *any* new signs and symptoms of discomfort that might indicate superinfection (medication regimen may have to be changed).

♦ Advise drinking 2–3 L of fluids daily to maintain adequate hydration (especially important if fever exists).

♦ Stress the importance of taking antibiotics for the entire time prescribed, even if signs and symptoms abate.

♦ *See Anti-infectives overview for more information.*

pentaerythritol

pen-ta-er-ith'ri-tole

pentaerythritol tetranitrate: *Dilar, Duotrate, Naptrate, Pentritol, Pentylan Peritrate, Peritrate Forte, Peritrate SA, PETN*

Class: Antianginal, Organic nitrate

PEDS	PREG	GERI
🖐	C	🖐

Action Decreases cardiac workload and myocardial oxygen demand by reducing left ventricular end-diastolic pressure (preload) and, to a lesser extent, by reducing systemic vascular resistance (afterload). Relaxes smooth muscle, particularly peripheral vascular smooth muscle, and has a vasodilating effect on the large systemic arteries and veins, which decreases blood pressure. Also improves myocardial oxygen perfusion by promoting collateral circulation.

Use/Therapeutic goal/Outcome

Angina pectoris: Prophylactic therapy, promotion of myocardial oxygenation, prevention of anginal (ischemic) attacks, improved activity tolerance. *Outcome criteria:* Patient reports decreased frequency and severity of angina, and demonstrates increased activity tolerance.

Dose range/Administration

Interaction alert: Antihypertensives and other vasodilators may potentiate hypotensive effect.

⬙ **Give 30 minutes before or 2–3 hours after meals for faster absorption.**

Adult: PO: 10–20 mg tid or qid. May gradually increase to 40 mg qid as tolerated. Sustained-release preparations (for maintenance) 30–80 mg q12h.

Clinical alert: Check blood pressure before giving dose; **hold dose and report** if hypotension is noted.

Contraindications/Precautions

PREG
C

Contraindicated in hypersensitivity to nitrates, and in myocardial infarction accompanied by hypotension, severe anemia, head trauma, cerebral hemorrhage, and increased intracranial pressure. *Use with caution* in presence of glaucoma.

🖐 **Use with caution for the elderly. Safe use for pregnant or nursing mothers and for children has not been established.**

Side effects/Adverse reactions

Hypersensitivity: rash. *CNS:* headache, dizziness, weakness, fainting. *CV:* orthostatic hypotension, tachycardia, palpitations. *GI:* nausea, vomiting. *Skin:* flushing, vasodilation.

Nursing implications/Documentation

Possible nursing diagnoses: Potential for injury; Activity intolerance.

♦ Keep a record of pulse and blood pressure before and after drug administration.

♦ Monitor for and report headache (a side effect usually treated with mild analgesics; tol-

erance of headache usually occurs with long-term use).

♦ Observe for postural hypotension; take blood pressure in both arms, and with patient sitting and standing if possible.

♦ Supervise ambulation until response is determined.

♦ Coordinate care to provide frequent rest periods.

♦ Be aware that this drug is inactivated when exposed to heat or moisture (should be discarded and replaced 6 months after opening).

Patient & family teaching/Home care

Possible nursing diagnoses: Fear; Knowledge deficit; Impaired home maintenance management.

♦ Explain that antianginals help reduce the workload of the heart and improve coronary blood supply.

♦ Stress the need to follow drug regimen closely (the drug should be taken at the same time each day) and the need to return for medical follow-up.

♦ Advise taking doses 30 minutes before meals or 2–3 hours after meals. Teach to swallow sustained-release capsules without chewing.

♦ Emphasize the need to pace activities, avoid stress (emotional and physical), and plan for rest periods.

♦ Advise changing positions slowly to avoid dizziness.

♦ Explain the tolerance to headache will develop with long-term use.

♦ Encourage keeping a record of angina attacks to observe pattern; stress that an increase in frequency or severity should be reported.

♦ Stress that discontinuing this drug abruptly could precipitate coronary vasospasm.

♦ Warn that drinking alcohol may cause fainting and hypotension.

♦ Emphasize that this drug could be ineffective if exposed to moisture or heat (keep in a cool dark place).

♦ *See Antianginals overview for more information.*

P

pentamidine

pen-tam'i-deen

pentamidine isethionate: **NebuPent, Pentam 300**
Class: Anti-infective, Antibiotic, Antiprotozoal

PEDS	PREG	GERI
✋	C	✋

Action Limits growth (bacteriostatic) of *Pneumocystis carinii* (a sporozoan parasite which causes pneumonia in immunosuppressed individuals) probably by blocking biosynthesis of DNA, RNA, phospholipids, and proteins.

Use/Therapeutic goal/Outcome

Pneumocystis carinii pneumonia (usually in people with AIDS or in other immunosuppressed states): Resolution of pneumonia. **Outcome criteria:** Chest X ray that demonstrates improvement; absence of *Pneumocystis carinii* growth on culture; absence of clinical manifestations of pneumonia (fever, pain, cough, increased WBC count).

Dose range/Administration

Interaction alert: Zidovudine, vancomycin, amphoteracin B, cisplatin, and aminoglycosides increase risk of nephrotoxicity.

Adult and Child: IM, IV: 4 mg/kg/day for 14 days (infuse IV over 60 min via controller device to reduce risk of hypotension).

Prophylaxis: *Adult: Inhalation:* 300 mg via Respirgard II nebulizer q 4 wks.

Clinical alert: During IV administration, monitor closely for sudden hypotension (have the person lie down flat, check blood pressure every 10–15 minutes during administration, then every 2 hours after administration, until stable). Individual who is administering inhalation product (if not self-administered) should wear protective goggles.

Contraindications/Precautions

PREG C

Contraindicated in life-threatening adverse reactions to pentamidine isethionate; however, in *confirmed* diagnosis *of P. carinii,* there are no *absolute* contraindications. **Use with caution** for women of child-bearing age, and in hypertension, hypotension, diabetes, hyperglycemia, blood dyscrasias, impaired liver or kidney function.

✋ **Use with caution for children and the elderly. Safe use for pregnant or nursing mothers has not been established.**

Side effects/Adverse reactions

Hypersensitivity: itching, rashes. **CNS:** dizziness, confusion, hallucinations. **CV:** tachycardia, hypotension (can be sudden and severe), phlebitis at infusion site. **Hem:** anemia, leukopenia, thrombocytopenia, hypocalcemia, elevated creatinine, elevated liver enzymes. **GI:** anorexia, nausea, metallic taste. **GU:** acute kidney failure. **Skin:** flushing. **Resp:** (with inhalation) chest pain or congestion, cough, wheezing, dyspnea, pharyngitis. **Misc:** hyperglycemia or hypoglycemia (may be followed by permanent insulin-dependent diabetes); fever.

Nursing implications/Documentation

Possible nursing diagnoses: Potential for infection; Fluid volume deficit.

♦ Institute appropriate isolation procedures to protect yourself and the immunosuppressed patient (the patient may require *reverse isolation*).

♦ Obtain necessary cultures and baseline laboratory studies (CBC, electrolytes, BUN, creatinine, and liver function) before administering first dose.

♦ Provide preferred fluids, and record and monitor intake and output to ensure adequate hydration; report negative or positive balance.

♦ Monitor for and report symptoms of superinfection (vaginal or anal irritation, foul smelling drainage, diarrhea, mouth lesions, sudden fever).

♦ Report excessive coughing (especially nonproductive).

♦ Be aware that dosage adjustment may be necessary for patients with impaired kidney function.

Patient & family teaching/Home care

Possible nursing diagnoses: Knowledge deficit; Social isolation; Impaired home maintenance management.

♦ Stress the importance of taking the drug for the entire time prescribed, even if symptoms abate.

♦ Instruct the person to report new symptoms (sore throat, fever, vaginal or anal itching), which may indicate a need for change in medication regimen.

♦ *See Anti-infectives overview for more information.*

pentazocine

pen-taz'oh-seen

pentazocine hydrochloride: 🍁 ♣*Fortral,* 🍁*Talwin*

pentazocine lactate: *Talwin-NX*

Class: Narcotic analgesic

Antidote: naloxone hydrochloride (Narcan)

PEDS	PREG	GERI		CONTROLLED SUBSTANCE
🖐	C	🖐		**IV**

Action Alters both perception of and response to pain through an unclear mechanism. Believed to act by binding with opiate receptors at many CNS sites.

Use/Therapeutic goal/Outcome

Moderate to severe pain, pre-procedural sedation: Relief of pain; promotion of relaxation. ***Outcome criteria:*** Report of feeling comfortable and more relaxed; absence of signs of pain (grimacing, frowning, restlessness, reluctance to move or cough) with increase in signs of comfort (relaxed facial expression, decreased restlessness); blood pressure and pulse within normal limits when compared to baseline.

Dose range/Administration

Interaction alert: Alcohol and CNS depressants increase effects. Other narcotic analgesics may decrease effects. Do not mix in same syringe with soluble barbiturates because precipitate will form.

Adult: PO: 50–100 mg q3-4h prn or around the clock. *Maximum dose:* 600 mg/day. SC, IM, IV: 30 mg q3-4h prn. *Maximum dose:* 360 mg/day. *Not recommended:* single doses > 60 mg SC or IM, or > 30 mg IV.

Clinical alert: Expect decreased dosage for the elderly or debilitated. Use IM route (not SC) if repeated injections are necessary (less irritating). Check respirations and blood pressure before giving pentazocine; hold drug and report if respirations are less than 12 or if hypotension is noted. Keep naloxone readily available in case of respiratory depression.

Contraindications/Precautions

PREG C

Contraindicated in hypersensitivity to pentazocine and in emotional instability, head injury, increased intracranial pressure, and history of drug abuse. ***Use with caution*** in hepatic or renal disease, biliary surgery, respiratory depression, post myocardial infarction, nausea, and vomiting.

🖐 **Contraindicated for children under 12 years and pregnant or nursing mothers (except during labor). Use with caution for the elderly.**

Side effects/Adverse reactions

Hypersensitivity: rash, hives, itching, swelling of face. ***Resp:*** respiratory depression. ***GI:*** nausea, vomiting. ***GU:*** urinary retention. ***CNS:*** dizziness or lightheadedness, euphoria. ***Skin:*** local tissue damage at injection sites (induration, nodules, sloughing, sclerosis). ***Misc:*** physical and psychological dependence. *When administered in high doses:* ***CNS:*** confusion, bizarre thoughts and dreams, hallucinations, anxiety. ***CV:*** hypertension, palpitation, tachycardia.

Nursing implications/Documentation

Possible nursing diagnoses: Pain; Anxiety; Potential for injury.

♦ Have patient rate pain on a scale of 1–10 before and after medication is given; report and record inadequate pain control.

♦ Determine whether a less potent analgesic might effectively relieve pain (narcotic analgesics should be used in the smallest effective dose compatible with the patient's needs).

♦ Give analgesics before pain is severe for best effects.

♦ Document pulse, respirations, and blood pressure immediately before and 1 hr after administration until response is determined.

♦ Monitor closely for risk factors for injury; keep side rails up and supervise ambulation if allowed out of bed.

♦ For those with history of narcotic dependence, monitor for withdrawal symptoms (this drug has antagonistic properties).

♦ Be aware of potential for psychic and physical dependence after prolonged use; avoid abrupt discontinuation of drug because it may cause chills, abdominal pain, tearing, rhinorrhea, anxiety, itching, and drug-seeking behavior.

Patient & family teaching/Home care

Possible nursing diagnoses: Sensory/perceptual alterations; Impaired home maintenance management.

♦ Explain the rationale for taking analgesics before pain is too severe.

- Advise those who are ambulatory to refrain from activities that require alertness and to seek assistance if there is any question about ability to get out of bed (e.g., if there is weakness or light headedness).

- Stress the need to adhere to the prescribed dose regimen because of risk of overdose, dependence, and abuse (instead of increasing dose regimen, unsatisfactory pain relief should be reported).

- Warn that alcohol and other CNS depressants may cause excessive sedation.

- *See Narcotic and non-narcotic analgesics overview for more information.*

pentobarbital   *pen-toe-bar'bi-tal*

pentobarbital: *Nembutal*

pentobarbital sodium: *Nembutal Sodium, ✦Novopentobarb*

Class: Short-acting barbiturate, sedative-hypnotic

PEDS	PREG	GERI		CONTROLLED
🖐	D	🖐		SUBSTANCE
				II

Action Produces relaxation or sleep, probably by interfering with transmission of impulses from the thalamus to the cortex of the brain. Exact mechanism of action is unknown.

Use/Therapeutic goal/Outcome

Sedation and sleep: Promotion of relaxation and sleep. *Outcome criteria:* Report of feeling less anxious and more relaxed; report of having slept well; observations of drowsiness or sleep.

Dose range/Administration

Interaction alert: Alcohol, narcotics, analgesics, or other CNS depressants intensify respiratory and CNS depression. MAO inhibitors may prolong effects.

Sedation: Adult: PO: 20–40 mg bid to qid. *Child:* PO: 6 mg/kg/day in divided doses.

Insomnia: Adult: PO: 100–200 mg at bedtime. IM: 150–200 mg at bedtime. IV: 100 mg given at rate not to exceed 50 mg/min. Rectal: 100–200 mg at bedtime. *Child:* IM: 3–5 mg/kg, not to exceed 100 mg. Rectal: 12–14 yrs, give 60–120 mg; 5–12 yrs, give 60 mg; 1–4 yrs, give 30–60 mg; 2–12 mos, give 30 mg.

Pre-procedure sedation: Adult: PO: 100–150 mg, 1 hr before procedure. IM: 150–200 mg, 1 hr before procedure. *Child:* IM: 2-6 mg/kg 1 hr before procedure (maximum of 100 mg).

Clinical alert: Use reduced dosage for elderly clients. Hold dose and report if the patient has respiratory depression or shows signs of overdosage (constricted pupils, somnolence, hypotension, clammy skin, cyanosis).

Contraindications/Precautions   PREG D

Contraindicated in hypersensitivity or intolerance to barbiturates, and in marked respiratory problems, uncontrolled severe pain, previous addiction to barbiturates, porphyria. *Use with caution* for people with liver or kidney impairment.

🖐 **Contraindicated in pregnancy, lactation, labor, and delivery. Use with caution for children and the elderly.**

Side effects/Adverse reactions

Hypersensitivity: itching, rashes, hives, fever, angioneurotic edema. *CNS:* drowsiness, lethargy, headache, neuralgia, paradoxical excitement in children and the elderly. *GI:* nausea, vomiting, diarrhea, constipation. *MS:* myalgia, arthralgia. *Resp:* (IV route): laryngospasm, bronchospasm. *CV:* (IV route): hypotension. *Misc:* exacerbation of porphyria.

Nursing implications/Documentation

Possible nursing diagnoses: Potential for injury; Sensory/perceptual alterations (visual and auditory).

- Document mental status before administration, monitor patient activity closely following administration, and employ appropriate measures to ensure safety (i.e., side rails up, call bell within reach, and no unsupervised smoking).

- Be sure that PO doses are swallowed (not hoarded).

- Be aware that sedatives and hypnotics *do not provide pain relief* (patient may need an analgesic as well).

- Monitor for and report signs of overdosage (slurred speech, continued somnolence, respiratory depression, confusion) and tolerance (increased anxiety and/or increased wakefulness).

Patient & family teaching/Home care

Possible nursing diagnoses: Sleep pattern disturbance; Ineffective coping (family and individual); Impaired home maintenance management.

- ◆ Explore problems that may contribute to insomnia.
- ◆ Reinforce that drug addiction and tolerance can occur, and that this drug should be for short-term use only, when other safer medications have failed.
- ◆ Emphasize that the effects of alcohol, other sedatives, tranquilizers, and OTC medications may be potentiated, and that these should be avoided.
- ◆ Warn not to drive while under effects of pentobarbital.
- ◆ *See Antianxiety Agents, Sedatives, and Hypnotics overview for more information.*

pentoxifylline
pen-tox-i'fi-leen

Trental

Class: Hemorrhealogic agent, Antiplatelet agent

PEDS	PREG	GERI
🖐	C	🖐

Action Improves capillary blood flow by increasing erythrocyte flexibility and lowering blood viscosity.

Use/Therapeutic goal/Outcome

Intermittent claudication associated with peripheral vascular disease: Increased tissue perfusion. **Outcome criteria:** (After 8 weeks) Report of increased walking tolerance with decreased episodes of leg pain.

Dose range/Administration

Interaction alert: Use with antihypertensives can increase risk of hypotension. Anticoagulants or drugs that inhibit platelet aggregation can prolong prothrombin times.

🖐 **Give with meals to minimize gastric irritation.**

Adult: PO: 400 mg tid for at least 8 weeks to determine efficacy.

Clinical alert: Do not crush or allow chewing of tablets.

Contraindications/Precautions
PREG
C

Contraindicated in hypersensitivity or intolerance to pentoxifylline or to methylxanthines (caffeine, theophylline, and theobromine). **Use with caution** for those with cardiac or cerebrovascular disease or bleeding tendencies.

🖐 **Contraindicated in nursing mothers. Use with caution for the elderly. Safe use for children and for pregnant women has not been established.**

Side effects/Adverse reactions

Hypersensitivity: rash, pruritus, urticaria. **GI:** dyspepsia, anorexia, nausea, vomiting, belching, flatus, bloating, abdominal discomfort, constipation, diarrhea, dry mouth. **CNS:** dizziness, headache, tremors, nervousness, drowsiness, insomnia. **CV:** angina, dysrhythmias, tachycardia, palpitations, flushing, dyspnea, edema, hypotension. **Eye:** conjunctivitis, blurred vision. **Ear:** earache. **Misc:** brittle fingernails, swollen neck glands.

Nursing implications/Documentation

Possible nursing diagnoses: Activity intolerance; Potential for injury.

- ◆ Assess for allergies to methylxanthines (caffeine, theophylline, theobromide) before giving pentoxifylline; hold dose and report if these are present.
- ◆ Establish a baseline of symptom severity against which to measure improvement; obtain a health history.
- ◆ Establish and record baseline ability to walk without pain before starting pentoxifylline; monitor exercise tolerance every 2–3 weeks for 8 weeks.
- ◆ Examine for signs of abnormal bruising or bleeding before giving drug; record pulse quality and leg color and temperature prior to first dose and every 2–3 weeks thereafter.
- ◆ Review PT and PTT to verify safe range of anticoagulation before giving drug.
- ◆ Monitor blood pressure periodically, especially if patient is receiving concurrent antihypertensive drug therapy.

Patient & family teaching/Home care

Possible nursing diagnoses: Knowledge deficit; Impaired home maintenance management.

- ◆ Explain that clinical effects may not be seen until after 2–8 weeks of therapy (stress that drug should be continued even if no immediate effect is noted).
- ◆ Point out the need to avoid smoking (nicotine constricts blood vessels).
- ◆ Advise reporting GI or CNS side effects (dosage may need adjustment).
- ◆ Warn against driving if dizziness or blurred vision is experienced.

P

- ◆ Suggest routine blood pressure measurements, especially if light-headedness is experienced.
- ◆ Stress the importance of routine follow-up with physician.

pergolide mesylate   *per'go-lyde me-sy-late*

Permax

Class: Antiparkinsonian, Dopaminergic agent

Antidote: Metoclopramide

PEDS	PREG	GERI
👋	B	👋

Action Controls symptoms of Parkinson's disease by directly stimulating and activating postsynaptic dopamine receptors in the CNS. (Clinical studies to date reveal that pergolide either decreases the levodopa requirements or improves a patient's response to it, although effects do wear off.)

Use/Therapeutic goal/Outcome

Parkinsonism (for those who have been on long-term levodopa therapy with deterioration in symptoms): Control of parkinsonian symptoms and promotion of mobility. **Outcome criteria:** Absence of (or decrease in) tremors, rigidity, akinesia and drooling; improvement in gait, balance, posture, and speech.

Dose range/Administration

Interaction alert: Can potentiate the effects of antihypertensive agents. Tricyclic antidepressants may decrease its effectiveness.

👋 **Give with meals to reduce GI symptoms.**
Parkinsonism: Adult: PO: Begin with 0.05 mg daily for 2 days, then increase as needed by 0.1 or 0.15 mg every third day for 12 days. Usual dose range is 3 mg daily. Efficacy of doses greater than 5 mg is questionable.

Clinical alert: Dose should be titrated to minimal effective dose.

Contraindications/Precautions

PREG
B

Contraindicated in hypersensitivity to pergolide mesylate or other ergot derivatives and in severe ischemic heart disease or peripheral vascular disease. **Use with caution** in hypotension, epilepsy, psychoses, arrhythmias, and impaired hepatic or renal function.

👋 **Contraindicated for nursing mothers. Use with caution for pregnant women and the** elderly. **Safe use for children has not been established.**

Side effects/Adverse reactions

Hypersensitivity: skin rash and ergotism (numbness and tingling in extremities, cold feet, muscle cramping, and Raynaud's phenomenon). **GI:** nausea, vomiting, diarrhea, constipation, dry mouth. **GU:** urinary tract infections. **CNS:** abnormal involuntary movements (dyskinesias), drowsiness, hallucinations, confusion, mental disturbances, sleep disorders. **Resp:** nasal congestion, shortness of breath. **CV:** postural hypotension, chest pain, atrial premature contractions, sinus tachycardia. **Eye:** glaucoma, diplopia. **MS:** bursitis.

Nursing implications/Documentation

Possible nursing diagnoses: Potential for injury; Impaired physical mobility.

- ◆ For use in Parkinson's, establish a baseline profile of patient's ability to differentiate between desired responses and drug-induced side effects.
- ◆ Monitor vital signs closely during periods of dose adjustment; record at least daily (or at each visit).
- ◆ Have patient dangle legs before ambulating (because of risk of postural hypotension); supervise ambulation until response is determined.
- ◆ Monitor mental status periodically (psychotic symptoms have been reported).

Patient & family teaching/Home care

Possible nursing diagnoses: Self-care deficit; Impaired home maintenance management.

- ◆ Point out the need to take this drug with food to reduce GI symptoms.
- ◆ Caution that there is a high incidence of side effects, especially at the beginning of therapy (lifestyle may have to change until side effects subside); advise reporting persistent side effects.
- ◆ Teach the need to report persistent CNS effects, chest pain, and urinary symptoms (burning, frequency).
- ◆ Warn that dizziness is common early during treatment and that position changes should be made slowly; caution against driving until response is determined.
- ◆ *See Antiparkinsons overview for more information.*

perphenazine

per-fen'a-zeen

♣Apo-Perphenazine, ♣Phenazine, Trilafon
Class: Phenothiazine antipsychotic, Antiemetic

PEDS	PREG	GERI
🖐	C	🖐

Action Exact mechanism of action has not been determined. Believed to produce calmness and alleviate psychiatric symptoms (disorders of perception, thought, consciousness, mood, affect, and social interaction) by blocking dopamine receptors in the limbic system. As an antiemetic, it acts by inhibiting the medullary chemoreceptor trigger zone. Blocks peripheral muscarinic, adrenergic, and histamine receptors. Also has some effect on the hypothalamus and pituitary gland, causing changes in regulation of body temperature and endocrine function. A dose of 8 mg of perphenazine is therapeutically equivalent to 100 mg of chlorpromazine.

Use/Therapeutic goal/Outcome

Schizophrenia, psychosis, agitated behavior: Promotion of reality orientation, elimination of hyperactivity. **Outcome criteria:** Demonstration of reality orientation, and ability to problem solve and interact with others; absence of agitated behavior.

Severe nausea and vomiting: Elimination of nausea and vomiting. **Outcome criteria:** Report of absence of nausea and vomiting.

Dose range/Administration

Interaction alert: Antacids may reduce absorption; separate doses of antacid and phenothiazines by at least 2 hr. Alcohol and other CNS depressants may cause excessive sedation. Barbiturates may decrease phenothiazine effects.

Psychiatric disorders: Adult: PO: *For hospitalized patients:* 8–18 mg bid to qid, gradually increasing. *Maximum dose:* 64 mg/day. *For outpatients:* 4–8 mg tid. IM: 5 mg q6h. *Maximum dose:* 30 mg/day. **Child > 12 yrs:** PO: 6–12 mg/day in divided doses.

Severe nausea and vomiting: Adult/Child > 12 yrs: PO: 8–16 mg/day in divided doses. *Maximum dose:* 24 mg/day. IM: 5–10 mg prn. *Maximum dose: For hospitalized patients:* 30 mg/day. *For outpatients:* 15 mg/day.

Clinical alert: Dilute liquid concentrate in milk, fruit juice, carbonated beverage, or soft food just before giving dose; do not mix with caffeine-containing soft drinks, coffee, grape juice, apple juice, or tea because it will precipitate. Avoid skin contact with liquid and parenteral forms (may cause contact dermatitis). Before IM doses, count respirations and check blood pressure; hold dose and report if respirations are less than 12 or if the patient is hypotensive. Keep IV diphenhydramine available in case of side effect of acute dystonic reaction.

Contraindications/Precautions

PREG
C

Contraindicated in hypersensitivity to perphenazine or phenothiazines, and in CNS depression, comatose states. **Use with caution** in seizure disorders, hypertension, Parkinson's disease, poorly controlled diabetes mellitus, asthma, emphysema, narrow-angle glaucoma, cardiac disease, hypotension, paralytic ileus, liver damage, prostatic hypertrophy, bone marrow depression, and subcortical brain damage.

🖐 **Contraindicated for nursing mothers. Use with caution for adolescents and the elderly or debilitated. Safe use for children under 12 years and pregnant women has not been established.**

Side effects/Adverse reactions

Hypersensitivity: rash, contact dermatitis. **CNS:** sedation, extrapyramidal reactions (pseudoparkinsonism, akathisia [restless need to keep moving], dystonia, tardive dykinesia), neuroleptic malignant syndrome (fever, tachycardia, tachypnea, profuse diaphoresis), EEG changes, dizziness. **CV:** orthostatic hypotension, palpitations, dysrhythmias, EKG changes. **GI:** appetite changes, dry mouth, constipation, abnormal liver function. **GU:** urinary retention or hesitancy, dark urine, priapism, impaired ejaculation, amenorrhea. **Eye:** blurred vision. **Skin:** photosensitivity, jaundice. **MS:** weight gain. **Hem:** hyperglycemia, transient leukopenia, agranulocytosis. **Misc:** gynecomastia, galactorrhea. **After abrupt withdrawal of long-term therapy:** gastritis, nausea, vomiting, lightheadedness, tremors, feeling of warmth or cold, diaphoresis, tachycardia, headache, insomnia.

Nursing implications/Documentation

Possible nursing diagnoses: Potential for injury; Constipation; Altered oral mucous membrane.

♦ Record mental status and vital signs before and 1 hr after administration during initial phase of treatment, then bid until response to

▶

therapy has been established, then periodically thereafter.

◆ Check CBC, liver function, BUN, and creatinine before giving first dose and periodically thereafter.

◆ Be sure that doses are swallowed (not hoarded).

◆ Monitor for orthostatic hypotension, dizziness, and drowsiness; supervise ambulation until response is established.

◆ Record weight every 2 weeks; report significant weight gain. Provide special mouth care; observe for and report oral ulcers.

◆ Prevent constipation by monitoring bowel movements and encouraging adequate fiber and fluid intake; offer laxatives or stool softeners before problem becomes severe.

◆ Report persistent sore throat, fever, and malaise, because these may indicate agranulocytosis (drug may have to be discontinued).

◆ Monitor for (and report immediately) signs of neuroleptic malignant syndrome (muscle rigidity, tremors, high fever, tachycardia); this is a rare, but potentially fatal, side effect.

◆ *For antiemetic use, see Nursing implications and Patient & family teaching sections in Antiemetics overview.*

Patient & family teaching/Home care

Possible nursing diagnoses: Sleep pattern disturbance; Impaired home maintenance management.

◆ Emphasize the need to continue medication, even when feeling well.

◆ Warn to change positions slowly to prevent dizziness.

◆ Stress that the effects of alcohol, sedatives and CNS depressants, and tranquilizers may be potentiated.

◆ Caution to consult with physician before using OTC drugs; stress the need for ongoing medical follow-up.

◆ Teach the need to report persistent sore throat, fever, and fatigue.

◆ Point out that doses should not be increased or stopped without checking with physician.

◆ Caution to wear a sunscreen (number 15), protective clothing, and sunglasses when out in the sun.

◆ Advise avoidance of driving and other potentially hazardous activities until response is determined.

◆ Suggest using ice chips, hard candy, or gum to relieve side effect of dry mouth; stress the need for good mouth care.

◆ Warn women to report if pregnancy is planned or suspected.

◆ *See Antipsychotics and Antiemetics overviews for more information.*

phenacemide

fen-nass'e-mide

Phenurone

Class: Anticonvulsant, Hydantoin

PEDS	PREG	GERI
✋	D	✋

Action Limits the spread of seizure activity and reduces abnormal excitability, stabilizing neuronal membranes in the motor cortex, probably by an effect on sodium ion flux across neuronal cell membranes. This drug is a potent structural analog of the hydantoins with a higher risk of severe toxic effects (used as a last resort).

Use/Therapeutic goal/Outcome

Severe epileptic states, usually mixed forms of psychomotor seizures that do not respond to other drugs: Limitation of seizure activity. **Outcome criteria:** Marked decrease or absence of seizure activity.

Dose range/Administration

Interaction alert: Other anticonvulsants, especially ethotoin, increase risk of toxic effects. Use with ethotoin may cause paranoia.

Adult: PO: 500 mg tid; may increase daily dosage weekly by 500 mg increments, to a maximum of 5g/day in divided doses (usual range is 1.5 to 5 g/day). **Child 5–10 yrs:** PO: 250 mg tid; may increase daily dosage weekly by 250 mg increments to a maximum of 1.5 g/day.

Clinical alert: Because of potential for extreme toxicity, this drug should be used when other anticonvulsants are ineffective. When switching from other anticonvulsants to phenacemide, increase dose of phenacemide gradually while slowly reducing dose of other drug.

Contraindications/Precautions

PREG
D

Contraindicated in hypersensitivity to phenacemide and in severe personality disorders. **Use with caution** in liver impairment, allergies, and concomitant use of other anticonvulsants.

⚘ Use with caution for children and the elderly. Safe use in childbearing years, especially for pregnant or nursing mothers, has not been established.

Side effects/Adverse reactions

Hypersensitivity: rash. *GI:* anorexia, weight loss, hepatitis. *CNS:* ataxia, drowsiness, dizziness, weakness, headache, paresthesia, depression, and suicidal tendencies. *Hem:* aplastic anemia, agranulocytosis, leukopenia. *GU:* nephritis.

Nursing implications/Documentation

Possible nursing diagnoses: Potential for injury; Potential for aspiration.

◆ Document history of seizures (type, frequency, duration, usual time they occur, precipitating factors, presence of an aura); initiate seizure precautions as indicated.

◆ Check baseline CBC, urinalysis, and liver function studies; monitor monthly thereafter; hold drug and report abnormalities.

◆ Report signs of hematological side effects (persistent fatigue, sore throat, fever, infections).

◆ Monitor for and report personality changes.

Patient & family teaching/Home care

Possible nursing diagnoses: Fear; Self-esteem disturbance; Knowledge deficit; Impaired home maintenance management.

◆ Stress the need for close medical follow-up; emphasize that persistent nausea, vomiting, fatigue, weakness, fever, sore throat or infections should be reported.

◆ Warn that stopping anticonvulsants suddenly can cause an increase in severity and frequency of seizures.

◆ Warn that drinking alcohol may reduce drug effectiveness.

◆ Advise reporting personality changes.

◆ Caution against driving until response is determined (may cause drowsiness at first).

◆ *See Anticonvulsants overview for more information.*

phenazopyridine   *fen-az-oh-peer'i-deen*

phenazopyridine hydrochloride: *Azo-Standard, Baridium, Di-Azo, Diridone, Eridium, Geridium, Phen-Azo, ♣Phenazo, Phenazodine, Pyridiate, Pyridin, Pyridium, ♣Pyronium, Urodine Urogesic, Viridium*

Class: Analgesic (urinary tract)

Antidote: Methylene blue

PEDS	PREG	GERI
⚘	B	⚘

Action Exact mechanism of action is unclear. Produces analgesic effect (through urinary excretion) on urinary tract; has little or no antibacterial action.

Use/Therapeutic goal/Outcome

Pain associated with urinary tract infection or irritation: Relief of pain. *Outcome criteria:* Report of relief of pain, burning, frequency, and urgency.

Dose range/Administration

🖢 **Give after meals to reduce GI upset.**

Adult: PO: 100–200 mg tid. Discontinue after 2 days if being given with antibacterial. *Child:* PO: 12 mg/kg/day in 3 divided doses.

Contraindications/Precautions

PREG
B

Contraindicated in hypersensitivity to phenazopyridine hydrochloride, and in renal and hepatic insufficiency, glomerulonephritis, and severe hepatitis.

⚘ **Use with caution for pregnant women, children, and the elderly.**

Side effects/Adverse reactions

Hypersensitivity: rash, renal and hepatic impairment and occasional failure. *CNS:* headache, vertigo. *GI:* infrequent GI distress; hepatic toxicity at overdose levels. *GU:* renal toxicity at overdose levels. *Hem:* methemoglobinemia, hemolytic anemia.

Nursing implications/Documentation

Possible nursing diagnoses: Altered patterns of urinary elimination; Fluid volume deficit.

◆ Document and monitor intake and output to monitor for dehydration.

◆ Provide favorite fluids to increase urinary flow.

◆ Report persistent fever immediately, especially in the elderly (they are more susceptible to septic shock with urinary-tract infections).

▶

P

Patient & family teaching/Home care

Possible nursing diagnoses: Knowledge deficit; Impaired home maintenance management.

• Stress that doses should be taken after meals.

• Explain that this drug colors urine red or orange, and that this is not blood.

• Advise that this drug is often discontinued after 3 days when pain subsides (should not be used on a long-term basis).

• Warn to hold dose and report immediately if there is yellowing of the skin (rare, but indicates toxicity).

◆ *See Narcotic and non-narcotic analgesics overview for more information.*

phenelzine
fen'el-zeen

phenelzine sulfate: **Nardil**

Class: Monoamine oxidase inhibitor (MAOI), Antidepressant

PEDS	PREG	GERI
🖐	C	🖐

Action Improves mood by promoting accumulation of the neurotransmitters norepinephrine, serotonin, and dopamine in the CNS (inhibits monoamine oxidase, the major enzyme responsible for the breakdown of neurotransmitters).

Use/Therapeutic goal/Outcome

Major depressive disorders that have not responded to other forms of treatment including other antidepressants: Promotion of sense of well-being, ability to cope with daily living. *Outcome criteria:* After 2–4 weeks, patient report of feeling less depressed, less anxious, and more energetic and able to cope; return of normal sleeping and eating habits; demonstration of improved ability to problem solve and perform activities of daily living.

Dose range/Administration

Interaction alert: MAOIs such as this have a strong potential for severe and unpredictable side effects when taken with other medications: check with pharmacist to ascertain most recent information on interactions. It is known that use with alcohol, barbiturates, sedatives, narcotics, dextromethorphan, and TCAs have produced a variety of problems; use with amphetamines, ephedrine, levodopa, meperidine, metaraminol, phenylephrine, and phenylpropanolamine can cause severe hypertension.

Monitor diabetics for altered hypoglycemic requirements. There is a potential for fatal hypertensive crisis if taken with tryptophan or food or beverages containing tyramine (aged cheese or wine, beer, avocados, chicken livers, chocolate, bananas, soy sauce, meat tenderizers, salami, or bologna).

Adult: PO: Begin with 45 mg/day in divided dose, increasing rapidly to 60–90 mg/day until benefits are maximized. Then decrease to 15 mg/day. *Elderly:* PO: 15 mg in the morning, then gradually increase to a maximum of 60 mg/day.

Clinical alert: Because of the *many* unpredictable food and drug interactions (see Interaction alert), monitor diet and medication regimen closely. Hold drug and report if hypertension is noted. Keep phentolamine (Regitine) available to treat hypertension.

Contraindications/Precautions
**PREG
C**

Contraindicated in hypersensitivity to MAOIs, and in cardiac, renal, or hepatic disease, alcoholism, hypertension, and pheochromocytoma. *Use with caution* in suicidal tendency, seizure disorders, psychosis, diabetes mellitus, and hyperactive behavior.

🖐 **Contraindicated for children under 16 years and pregnant or nursing mothers. Use with caution for the elderly.**

Side effects/Adverse reactions

Hypersensitivity: rash. *CNS:* insomnia, dizziness, anxiety, headache, restlessness, hyperreflexia, tremors, muscle twitching, mania, confusion, memory impairment, fatigue, sedation. *CV:* orthostatic hypotension, palpitations, dysrhythmias, hypertensive crisis. *GI:* anorexia, dry mouth, nausea, diarrhea, constipation. *GU:* urinary frequency, decreased libido. *Eye:* blurred vision. *MS:* weight gain.

Nursing implications/Documentation

Possible nursing diagnoses: Potential for injury; Diarrhea; Constipation; Altered oral mucous membrane.

◆ Document mental status and vital signs daily until response to therapy has been established; then periodically thereafter.

◆ Check CBC, liver function, BUN, and creatinine before giving first dose and periodically thereafter.

◆ Be sure that doses are swallowed (not hoarded).

- Monitor for orthostatic hypotension, dizziness, and drowsiness; supervise ambulation until response is established.

- Record weight every 2 weeks; report significant weight gain.

- Monitor for and report suicidal tendencies, increased depression, or excessive hyperactivity.

- Prevent constipation by monitoring bowel movements and encouraging adequate fiber and fluid intake; offer laxatives or stool softeners before the problem becomes severe. Report diarrhea.

- Check with pharmacy and dietary department to determine dietary restrictions for MAOI; continue restrictions for 10 days after stopping drug because effects last a long time.

Patient & family teaching/Home care

Possible nursing diagnoses: Ineffective coping (family and individual); Sleep pattern disturbance; Impaired home maintenance management.

- Stress that this medication helps reduce the depression that inhibits ability to make decisions and cope effectively (once the individual feels less depressed, it will be easier to take steps toward making healthy changes).

- Provide a list of foods that must be avoided; emphasize the need to stick to restrictions.

- Explain that side effects are often noted immediately, but they usually diminish after a few weeks; on the other hand, it is likely to take 2–4 weeks before *beneficial* effects are noted (the patient may feel worse before feeling better).

- Warn to change positions slowly to prevent dizziness.

- Point out the role of adequate nutrition, exercise, and sleep in combating depression.

- Advise against taking any doses in the evening to avoid interference with sleep.

- Emphasize that the effects of alcohol, sedatives, and tranquilizers may be potentiated.

- Caution to consult with physician before using OTC drugs; stress the need for ongoing medical follow-up.

- Recommend reporting continued depression; stress that doses should not be increased or stopped without checking with physician (may cause severe problems).

- Advise avoidance of driving and other potentially hazardous activities until response is established.

- Suggest using ice chips, hard candy, or gum to relieve side effect of dry mouth; stress the need for good mouth care.

- Warn women to report if pregnancy is planned or suspected.

- *See Antidepressants overview for more information.*

phenobarbital

fe-noe-bar'bi-tal

phenobarbital: *Barbita, ✦Gardenal, ✦Luminal, Solfoton*

phenobarbital sodium: *✦Luminal sodium*

Class: ★**Sedative and hypnotic prototype**, Anticonvulsant, Barbiturate

PEDS	PREG	GERI	CONTROLLED SUBSTANCE
✋	D	✋	IV

Action Exact mechanism of action is unclear. Believed to produce CNS depression, sedation and sleep by depressing the reticular activating system, which is concerned with both the sleep and arousal mechanisms. Limits seizures by increasing the threshold for motor cortex stimulation. Lowers blood levels of bilirubin by increasing production of glucuronyl transferase and by increasing the flow of bile salts. This is a long-acting barbiturate, and is absorbed slowly when administered orally or intramuscularly (peak serum concentrations after 8–12 hr).

Use/Therapeutic goal/Outcome

Insomnia, sedation, preoperative sedation: Promotion of relaxation and sleep. **Outcome criteria:** Report of feeling relaxed or having slept well; observable relaxation or sleep (relaxed facial expression, decreased activity, closing of eyes).

Seizures and status epilepticus: Limitation of seizure activity. **Outcome criteria:** Marked decrease or absence of seizures.

Neonatal hyperbilirubinemia: Reduction of serum bilirubin. **Outcome criteria:** Serum bilirubin within normal range (1–12 mg/dl).

Dose range/Administration

Interaction alert: Alcohol, antihistamines, narcotics, benzodiazepines, MAO inhibitors, methylphenidate, isoniazid, and CNS depressants may cause excessive sedation. Decreases the

▶

absorption of griseofulvin. May increase metabolism of **oral anticoagulants** (dosage may need adjustment), estrogens, oral contraceptives, doxycycline, and corticosteroids (monitor for diminished effects of these drugs). Inhibits metabolism of tricyclic antidepressants. If given with valproic acid, monitor for increased phenobarbital levels and toxicity. Use with primidone should be avoided.

Sedation: Adult: PO: 30–120 mg/day in divided doses bid or tid. *Child:* PO: 6 mg/kg/day in divided doses tid.

Preoperative sedation: Adult: IM: 100–200 mg, 60–90 min before procedure. *Child:* IM: 16–100 mg, 60–90 min before procedure.

Insomnia (hypnotic): Adult: PO or IM: 60–320 mg hs. *Child:* PO: 3–6 mg/kg hs.

Seizures (maintenance therapy): Adult: PO: 100–200 mg/day in divided doses tid, or as a single dose hs. *Child:* PO: 4–6 mg/kg/day in divided doses q12h, or as a single dose hs.

Status epilepticus or emergency treatment of seizures: Adult: IV: 10 mg/kg given no faster than 60 mg/min. In severe situations, may be repeated to a maximum total of 20 mg/kg. *Child:* IV: 5–10 mg/kg given no faster than 60 mg/min. In severe situations, may be repeated every 10–15 min to a maximum total of 20 mg/kg.

Neonatal hyperbilirubinemia: Neonates: PO: 7 mg/kg/day from the first to the fifth day of life. IM: 5 mg/kg on the first day of life, followed by 5 mg/kg/day orally on the second to seventh days.

Clinical alert: Hold dose and report if respirations are less than 12 and in the presence of hypotension. Expect lower dosages for the elderly. Children and the elderly may experience paradoxical excitement. Because of risk of cardiovascular collapse and apnea, give IV only in the presence of a professional qualified to perform intubation (physician or nurse anesthetist); monitor closely for infiltration (may cause tissue necrosis); and keep resuscitative drugs and equipment nearby.

Contraindications/Precautions

PREG D

Contraindicated in hypersensitivity to barbiturates, and in acute intermittent porphyria, porphyria variegata, and uncontrolled pain. *Use with caution* in renal or hepatic disease, diabetes mellitus, or borderline hypoadrenal function. The benefits and risks should be weighed carefully when considering the use of phenobarbital in a patient with a history of drug abuse.

☟ **Use with caution for children and the elderly or debilitated. Safe use for pregnant or nursing mothers has not be established.**

Side effects/Adverse reactions

Hypersensitivity: rash, angioneurotic edema, fever, serum sickness, urticaria, laryngospasm. *CNS:* somnolence, agitation, confusion, hyperkinesia, ataxia, vertigo, residual sedation. *CV:* bradycardia, hypotension. *GI:* nausea, vomiting, cramps, diarrhea, liver damage. *Hem:* agranulocytosis, thrombocytopenia. *MS:* ricketts and osteomalacia with prolonged use. *Misc:* Psychological and physical dependence.

Nursing implications/Documentation

Possible nursing diagnoses: Potential for injury; Sensory-perceptual alterations; Potential for aspiration.

◆ Document mental status *before* administration, monitor patient activity closely *following* administration, and employ appropriate measures to ensure safety (i.e., side rails up, call bell within reach, and no unsupervised smoking).

◆ Be sure that PO doses are swallowed (not hoarded).

◆ Recognize that sedatives and hypnotics *do not provide pain relief*, and that doses greater than 400 mg/day are likely to cause some degree of physical dependence.

◆ For anticonvulsant use, document history of seizures (type, frequency, duration, usual times they occur, precipitating factors, presence of an aura); initiate seizure precautions as indicated.

◆ After 2–3 weeks of therapy, check serum drug levels periodically to assure therapeutic range (15–40 mcg/ml); also check CBC, and renal and hepatic function studies.

◆ For IV route, document pulse and blood pressure before and after administration.

◆ Monitor for and report signs of overdosage or toxicity (slurred speech, continued somnolence, respiratory depression, confusion, asthmatic breathing).

Patient & family teaching/Home care

Possible nursing diagnoses: Sleep pattern disturbance; Ineffective coping (family and individual); Impaired home maintenance management).

- Stress that drug tolerance and dependence can occur; warn that stopping phenobarbital suddenly can cause an increase in severity and frequency of seizures.

- Emphasize that the effects of alcohol, other sedatives, and tranquilizers may be potentiated, and that these should be avoided.

- Reinforce the importance of consulting with physician before using OTC drugs, and of returning for medical follow-up.

- Stress that driving and other potentially hazardous activities be avoided while the medication is still causing drowsiness (tolerance to drowsiness usually develops after prolonged use).

- When phenobarbital is being used as an anticonvulsant, teach significant others—and have them demonstrate—how to protect the individual should a seizure occur.

- *See Antianxiety Agents, Sedatives, and Hypnotics, and Anticonvulsants overviews for more information.*

phenoxybenzamine *fen-ox-ee-benz'a-meen*

phenoxybenzamine hydrochloride: *Dibenzyline,* *Dibenyline*

Class: Antihypertensive, Alpha-adrenergic blocking agent

PEDS	PREG	GERI
✋	C	✋

Action Reduces blood pressure by decreasing vascular resistance and promoting vasodilation. (Combines with postganglionic alpha-adrenergic receptors to block the effects of catecholamine stimulation.)

Use/Therapeutic goal/Outcome

Hypertension associated with pheochromocytoma: Reduction of blood pressure. *Outcome criteria:* Blood pressure within normal limits.

Frostbite/Raynaud's acrocyanosis: Improvement of circulation to affected area. *Outcome criteria:* Return of capillary refill, skin color, palpable pulses, and warmth to affected area, patient reports return of sensation.

Dose range/Administration

Interaction alert: Do not give with epinephrine (may cause excessive hypotension).

🖐 **Give with food to reduce GI irritation.**

Hypertension: Adult: PO: 10 mg bid; may increase by 10 mg every other day as toler-

ated. *Maintenance dose:* 20–40 mg/day in divided doses. *Child:* PO: 1–2 mg/kg/day as single dose. *Maintenance dose:* 400 mcg (0.4 mg)/kg/day.

Frostbite/Raynaoud's acrocyanosis: Adult: PO: 10 mg/day. Increase by 10 mg every 4 days. *Maximum dose:* 60 mg/day.

Contraindications/Precautions
PREG
C

Contraindicated in hypersensitivity to phenoxybenzamine. *Use with caution* in cerebral or coronary arteriosclerosis, renal damage, respiratory disease, and in situations where hypotension would be detrimental.

🖐 **Use with caution for children and the elderly. Safe use for pregnant women has not been established.**

Side effects/Adverse reactions

Hypersensitivity: rash, urticaria, contact dermatitis. *CV:* orthostatic hypotension, tachycardia, shock. *CNS:* lethargy, drowsiness. *GI:* dry mouth, abdominal distress, vomiting. *Resp:* nasal stuffiness. *GU:* impotence, inhibition of ejaculation.

Nursing implications/Documentation

Possible nursing diagnoses: Activity intolerance; Fatigue; Potential for injury.

- Assess mental status, and record pulse and blood pressure (lying, sitting, and standing, in both arms) prior to administration, and frequently thereafter until response is determined.

- Consult with physician to determine desired therapeutic range for blood pressure (be aware that some patients may require a slightly elevated blood pressure to perfuse vital organs).

- Ascertain the baseline CBC, electrolytes, BUN, creatinine, and liver function studies have been obtained before giving first dose; report abnormalities and monitor closely thereafter.

- Monitor for allergic reactions and for confusion, dizziness, bradycardia or hypotension; hold drug and report immediately if these occur.

- If used for frostbite or Raynaud's acrocyanosis, monitor circulation to affected area.

- Supervise ambulation until response is determined.

- Document and monitor daily weight, and intake and output; report significant negative or positive balance.

- ◆ Provide frequent mouth care.

Patient & family teaching/Home care

Possible nursing diagnoses: Knowledge deficit; Impaired home maintenance management; Altered sexuality patterns.

- ◆ Explain the importance of taking medication exactly as prescribed, even when feeling well.
- ◆ Stress the importance of good medical follow-up, explain that this drug reduces "wear and tear" on blood vessels and improves longevity and health.
- ◆ Teach how to monitor pulse and blood pressure; emphasize that syncope, hypertension or hypotension, or persistent dizziness should be reported.
- ◆ Advise changing positions slowly to avoid dizziness.
- ◆ Encourage daily monitoring of weight and reporting sudden weight gain (frequently is fluid retention).
- ◆ Warn against taking *any* OTC drugs without physician approval (some interactions can cause *severe* reactions).
- ◆ Advise avoiding driving or hazardous activities until response is determined (may cause drowsiness); point out the need to avoid alcohol.
- ◆ Explain that dry mouth is a common side effect that can be managed by using ice chips, chewing gum, or sucking on hard candy.
- ◆ Explain that this drug may alter sexual ability; explore concerns and seek consultation as needed.
- ◆ *See Antihypertensives overview for more information.*

phensuximide

fen-sux'i-mide

Milontin

Class: Anticonvulsant

PEDS	PREG	GERI
✋	**D**	✋

Action Limits seizure activity by elevating CNS threshold to convulsive stimuli. This drug is less effective than other anticonvulsants.

Use/Therapeutic goal/Outcome

Absence seizures (petit mal): Limitation of seizure activity. **Outcome criteria:** Marked decrease or absence of seizures.

Dose range/Administration

Adult and Child: PO: 500 mg to 1 g bid to tid.

Clinical alert: May increase incidence of tonic-clonic seizures if used alone to treat mixed seizures.

Contraindications/Precautions

PREG
D

Contraindicated in hypersensitivity to succinimides and in intermittent porphyria.

- ✋ **Use with caution for children and the elderly. Safe use for pregnant women has not been established.**

Side effects/Adverse reactions

Hypersensitivity: pruritis, flushing, skin rash. **CNS:** muscular weakness, drowsiness, dizziness, insomnia, ataxia, headache. **GI:** anorexia, nausea, vomiting. **Hem:** agranulocytosis. **GU:** urinary frequency, hematuria.

Nursing implications/Documentation

Possible nursing diagnoses: Potential for injury; Potential for aspiration.

- ◆ Document history of seizures (type, frequency, duration, usual times they occur, precipitating factors, presence of an aura); initiate seizure precautions as indicated.
- ◆ Monitor serum drug levels periodically to assure therapeutic range (40–80 mcg/ml).
- ◆ Monitor CBC every 3 months, and liver function studies and urinalysis every 6 months.

Patient & family teaching/Home care

Possible nursing diagnoses: Fear; Self-esteem disturbance; Knowledge deficit; Impaired home maintenance management.

- ◆ Stress the need for close medical follow-up; emphasize that persistent fatigue, weakness, fever, sore throat, joint pains, mouth ulcers, and infections should be reported.
- ◆ Warn that stopping anticonvulsants suddenly can cause an increase in severity and frequency of seizures.
- ◆ Advise that this drug may make urine a harmless pink or red-brown color.
- ◆ Caution against driving until response is determined.
- ◆ *See Anticonvulsants overview for more information.*

phentolamine mesylate

fen-tole'a-meen

Regitine, ✛Rogitine

Class: Antihypertensive, Alpha-adrenergic blocking agent

PEDS	PREG	GERI
✋	C	✋

Action Reduces blood pressure by causing vasodilation of arteriolar and venous smooth muscle (competitively blocks catecholamines at presynaptic and postsynaptic alpha-receptors).

Use/Therapeutic goal/Outcome

Hypertension associated with pheochromocytoma: Control of blood pressure. **Outcome criteria:** Blood pressure within normal limits.

Extravasation: Prevention or treatment of tissue necrosis. **Outcome criteria:** Absence of signs of tissue necrosis at intravenous site.

Dose range/Administration

Interaction alert: Do not use with epinephrine (may cause excessive hypotension).

Blood pressure control before and during pheochromocytomectomy: Adult: IM, IV: 2–5 mg, 1–2 hr preop. Repeat intraop with 1 mg IV or 3 mg IM. **Child:** IV: 1 mg preop. IM: 3 mg; repeat with 1 mg IV prn.

Treatment of extravasation: Adult and Child: Dissolve 5–10 mg in 10 ml NS, and inject subcutaneously into the affected area within 12 hr.

Clinical alert: IM route is preferred. Document blood pressure every 10 minutes for 30 minutes prior to administration; do not administer unless blood pressure is stable within that period. Have norepinephrine (*not epinephrine*) readily available to treat excessive hypotension.

Contraindications/Precautions

PREG C

Contraindicated in hypersensitivity to phentolamine or related compounds, and in recent or prior myocardial infarction and cardiac disease. **Use with caution** in patients with ulcer disease.

✋ Use with caution for children and the elderly. Safe use for pregnant or nursing mothers has not been established.

Side effects/Adverse reactions

Hypersensitivity: rash, urticaria. **CV:** hypotension, arrhythmias, tachycardia, angina pectoris, palpitations, shock. **CNS:** dizziness, weakness, flushing. **GI:** diarrhea, nausea, vomiting, hyperperistalsis, abdominal pain. **Resp:** nasal stuffiness. **Hem:** hypoglycemia.

Nursing implications/Documentation

Possible nursing diagnoses: Activity intolerance; Fatigue; Potential for injury; Diarrhea.

◆ Assess mental status, as well as vital signs, before administration: expect maximum effect within 2 minutes of injection and return of pre-injection blood pressure within 30 minutes (a 60 mm Hg reduction in systolic blood pressure is common).

◆ After IM injection (preferred route), record blood pressure every 5 minutes for 30 minutes, then every 15 minutes until stable, then as ordered.

◆ After IV injection, record blood pressure every 30 seconds for 3 minutes, then every minute for 7 minutes, then every 15 minutes until stable, then as ordered.

◆ Monitor for allergic reactions, and for confusion, dizziness, tachycardia, arrythmias, hypotension, or chest pain; report immediately if these occur.

◆ Keep patient flat in bed with siderails up until condition is stable; supervise ambulation, when able.

Patient & family teaching/Home care

Possible nursing diagnoses: Anxiety; Fear; Knowledge deficit.

◆ Explain that blood pressure will be monitored frequently to control reactions.

◆ Encourage the patient to verbalize concerns, questions, or unusual feelings during therapy.

◆ Reinforce the need to remain flat in bed until stable.

◆ *See Antihypertensives overview for more information.*

phenylbutazone

fen-ill-byoo'ta-zone

✛ApoPhenylbutazone, Azolid, Butazolidin, Butazone, ✛Intrabutazone, ✛Novobutazone

Class: Nonsteroidal anti-inflammatory drug (NSAID), Specific analgesic, Antipyretic, Mild uricosuric

PEDS	PREG	GERI
✋	D	✋

Action Exact mechanism of action is unclear. Believed to reduce inflammation by inhibiting

▶

prostaglandin synthesis, leukocyte migration, and lysosomal enzyme involvement. Prostaglandin is a naturally occurring mediator of the inflammatory process which is found throughout body tissue.

Use/Therapeutic goal/Outcome

Pain and inflammation: Promotion of comfort and mobility; suppression of inflammation. *Outcome criteria:* Report of increased comfort with increased range of motion and ability to perform activities of daily life; reduction in or absence of joint stiffness, swelling, redness, and warmth.

Acute gouty arthritis: Reduction of inflammation in affected joints. *Outcome criteria:* Report of pain relief and increased ability to perform activities of daily life; decreased redness, warmth, and swelling of joints.

Dose range/Administration

Interaction alert: Aspirin and coumarin-type anticoagulants increase risk of bleeding. May increase the action of insulin, antidiabetics, phenytoins, and sulfonamides. Barbiturates may antagonize the effect of phenylbutazone.

🍎 **Give with food to reduce gastric irritation.**

Arthritis, spondylitis: Adult: PO: *Initial dose:* 300–600 mg in divided doses tid to qid. *Maintenance dose:* < 400 mg/day.

Acute gouty arthritis: Adult: PO: *Initial dose:* 400 mg, then 100 mg q4h.

Clinical alert: For acute gouty arthritis and the elderly, do not give longer than 1 week. Monitor for increased serum sodium and fluid retention since this drug increases sodium retention.

Contraindications/Precautions

PREG
D

Contraindicated in hypersensitivity to phenylbutazone, or tartrazine and in history of or active GI ulcer, blood dyscrasias (especially coagulation defect), renal, hepatic, cardiac, or thyroid disease; and use with chemotherapeutic agents. *Use with caution* in asthma and glaucoma. Safe use in dementia has not been established.

✋ **Contraindicated for nursing mothers. Use with caution for the elderly. Safe use for children under 14 years and pregnant women has not been established.**

Side effects/Adverse reactions

Hypersensitivity: urticaria, pruritus, rash, drug fever, arthralgia, angiitis, vasculitis, serum sickness, anaphylaxis. *Hem:* bone marrow

depression, hyperglycemia. *CNS:* drowsiness, dizziness, lethargy. *GI:* nausea, vomiting, diarrhea, dyspepsia. *CV:* edema, hypertension, fluid retention, pericarditis. *GU:* renal failure, hepatic failure, proteinuria, hematuria. *Eye:* optic neuritis, blurred vision. *Ear:* hearing loss. *Resp:* respiratory alkalosis. *Misc:* goiter, metabolic acidosis.

Nursing implications/Documentation

Possible nursing diagnoses: Pain; Impaired physical mobility.

♦ Establish a baseline for CBC, electrolytes, prothrombin time, BUN, creatinine, and liver function studies; if therapy is prolonged, monitor periodically thereafter.

♦ Monitor for and report GI symptoms that may indicate peptic ulcer (nausea, pain, black stools).

♦ Report visual or auditory changes immediately.

♦ Record weight every other day; report edema or sudden weight gain.

♦ For diabetics, monitor blood sugar closely since insulin requirements may change.

Patient & family teaching/Home care

Possible nursing diagnoses: Anxiety; Knowledge deficit.

♦ Advise taking doses with food to reduce GI symptoms.

♦ Explain the importance of watching for symptoms of GI bleeding (black stools, persistent GI distress).

♦ Stress the need to avoid aspirin, alcohol, and other OTC drugs (unless approved by physician) because of increased risk of GI bleeding.

♦ Explain that a favorable response should occur within 4 days; advise reporting if no improvement is seen after 1 week (the drug should be discontinued).

♦ Instruct individuals to hold dose and report if any of the following side effects are experienced: vertigo, rashes, blood in urine, hearing or visual changes, sudden weight gain, edema.

♦ Warn against driving or activities that require alertness until response is determined.

♦ Encourage limiting salt intake (this drug may cause sodium retention).

- ◆ Reinforce the need for medical follow-up; advise telling dentist that phenylbutazone is being taken.

- ◆ Teach smokers that smoking will decrease effects of this drug.

- ◆ For diabetics, explain the importance of monitoring blood sugars with a blood glucose meter.

- ◆ *See Nonsteroidal anti-inflammatory drugs overview for more information.*

phenylephrine

fen-ill-ef´rin

phenylephrine hydrochloride: *AK–Dilate, AK–Nefrin Opthalmic, Alconefrin (12, 25, and 50), Doktors, Duration, I–Phrine 2.5%, IsoptoFrin, Mydfrin, Synephrine, Prefrin Liquifilm, Rinall, Rinall 10, Sinex, St. Joseph Measured Dose Nasal Decongestant*

Class: ★"Pure" alpha adrenergic (sympathomimetic) prototype, Vasoconstrictor

PEDS	PREG	GERI
🖐	C	🖐

Action Elevates blood pressure by stimulating the alpha-adrenergic receptors, resulting in arteriolar constriction and increased venous return to the heart. Reduces intraocular pressure by producing prompt dilation of pupils and short duration of vasoconstriction. Acts as a potent decongestant when used topically for rhinitis (common cold), allergic rhinitis, and sinusitis.

Use/Therapeutic goal/Outcome

Acute hypotensive states: Improvement of blood pressure. *Outcome criteria:* Blood pressure > 90–100 systolic, absence of clinical signs of shock (confusion, restlessness, rapid weak pulse, urine output less than 25 ml/hr).

Rhinitis, sinusitis: Symptomatic relief of nasal congestion. *Outcome criteria:* Report of decreased nasal stuffiness and discharge, and easier breathing.

Eye refraction: Pupillary dilation. *Outcome criteria:* Upon measurement with tonometer, decreased intraocular pressure, dilated pupils.

Dose range/Administration

Interaction alert: Ergot alkaloids, guanethidine, reserpine, and tricyclic antidepressants may increase the vasopressor effects. Phentolamine may reverse severe hypertensive effects of phenylephrine hydrochloride. Halothane, digitalis, and mercurial diuretics may cause

arrhythmias. Do not give with MAOI therapy or oxytocics (may produce hypertensive crisis).

Mild to moderate hypotension: **Adult:** SC, IM: 2–5 mg, then repeat once prn. *Maximum dose:* 10 mg. Should raise blood pressure in 1–2 hr. IV: 0.2 mg, then repeat once or twice prn.

Acute hypotension, severe shock: **Adult:** IV: 100–180 mcg/min. *Maintenance dose:* 40–60 mcg/min. **Child:** SC, IM: 0.04–0.088 mg/kg.

Mydriasis (without cycloplegia): **Adult and Child:** *Ophthalmic:* 1 drop 2.5% or 10% solution before examination. Do not use 10% solution for infants or small children.

Adhesion of the iris (posterior synechia): **Adult and Child:** *Ophthalmic:* 1 drop 10% solution. Do not use for infants and small children.

Nasal constriction: **Adult:** *Nasal:* 1–2 sprays or drops 0.25–0.5% solution, or a small amount of jelly or spray on nasal mucosa, q4h prn. **Child 6–12 yr:** *Nasal:* 1–2 sprays or drops 0.25% solution on nasal mucosa q4h prn. **Child < 6 yr:** *Nasal:* 2–3 sprays or drops 0.125% solution on nasal mucosa q4h prn.

Clinical alert: For IV route, ascertain that hypotension is not due to hypovolemia before starting phenylephrine hydrochloride (volume deficit should be corrected before starting vasopressors). Place patient on continuous cardiac monitor and keep emergency drugs and equipment readily available. Obtain written parameters from physician for regulating rate according to blood pressure (usually maintained at slightly below patient's normotensive state).

Contraindications/Precautions

PREG
C

Contraindicated in hypersensitivity to phenylephrine and sulfites, and in severe hypertension, ventricular tachycardia, severe arteriosclerosis, narrow-angle glaucoma, severe coronary disease; (ophthalmic route) in narrow-angle glaucoma and with soft contact lenses. *Use with caution* (10% solution) in marked hypertension and cardiac disorders.

🖐 **Contraindicated (10% solution) for infants and small children. Use with caution for heavier children and the elderly. Safe use for pregnant or nursing mothers has not been established; do not use in late pregnancy or during labor.**

Side effects/Adverse reactions

Hypersensitivity: bluish coloration of skin; dizziness; flushing or redness of skin; rash; hives; itching; swelling of face, lips, or eyelids; wheezing or difficulty breathing; exaggeration of side

▶

effects. **CV:** reflex bradycardia, ventricular tachycardia, hypertension, palpitations. **CNS:** trembling, sweating, pallor, tingling of the extremities. **Resp:** (intranasal use) rebound congestion, nasal stinging, burning, dryness, sneezing. **Eye:** (ophthalmic use) transient stinging, lacrimation, headache, browache, blurred vision, conjunctival allergy (itching, redness), sensitivity to light.

Nursing implications/Documentation

Possible nursing diagnoses: Potential for injury; Activity intolerance; Sleep pattern disturbance.

♦ For ophthalmic route, have the individual apply gentle pressure to lacrimal duct for 1 min after application to prevent systemic absorption.

♦ **IV route**

♦ Record and monitor pulse, blood pressure, and respirations every 5 min until stable, then every 15 min, then every 1/2 hr.

♦ Record urine output hourly; report persistent urine output < 30 ml/hr.

♦ Monitor for and report decreased mental status; keep patient in bed with side rails up.

♦ When weaning off phenylephrine hydrochloride, taper dose slowly, while closely monitoring blood pressure.

Patient & family teaching/Home care

Possible nursing diagnoses: Knowledge deficit; Fear; Ineffective family coping.

♦ For hypotensive states, stress that frequent monitoring of vital signs is needed to "fine tune" medication dose for optimum results; stress the need to remain in bed.

♦ Stress that the nurses need to be told of new symptoms or uncomfortable feelings in case they indicate a need for medication adjustment.

♦ **Ophthalmic and nasal routes**

♦ Warn against exceeding prescribed dose (may result in systemic effects).

♦ Give written and verbal instructions on how to instill eye drops; have the patient or caregiver return demonstration.

♦ Stress that droppers and sprays should not be shared.

♦ Explain that this drug will widen pupils; caution not to drive until vision is sharp and light sensitivity reduced.

♦ See Adrenergics (sympathomimetics) overview for more information.

phenytoin
fen'i-toyn

phenytoin: **Dilantin, Dilantin Infatabs, Dilantin-30 Pediatric, Dilantin-125**

phenytoin sodium (extended): **Dialantin Kapseals**

phenytoin sodium (prompt): **Diphenylan**

Class: ★**Anticonvulsant prototype**, Hydantoin, Class IB antiarrhythmic

PEDS	PREG	GERI
🖐	D	🖐

Action Limits the spread of seizure activity and reduces abnormal excitability in the motor cortex without causing general CNS depression. Nerve impulses in the motor cortex are probably inhibited by an effect on sodium ion flux across cell membranes but exact mechanism of anticonvulsant action is unclear. Acts as an antiarrhythmic by slowing conduction in the His-Purkinje system and ventricles, and elevating electrical stimulation threshold of the ventricles during diastole (decreases sodium influx across the cell membranes of the Purkinje fibers in digitalis-induced dysrhythmias).

Use/Therapeutic goal/Outcome

Grand mal seizures and status epilepticus: Limitation of seizure activity. **Outcome criteria:** Marked decrease or absence of seizures.

Supraventricular and ventricular dysrhythmias unresponsive to lidocaine or procainamide, digitalis-induced supraventricular and ventricular dysrhythmias: Elimination of dysrhythmias; promotion of normal sinus rhythm. **Outcome criteria:** Marked decrease or absence of dysrhythmias; normal sinus rhythm.

Dose range/Administration

Interaction alert: Chronic alcohol use, dexamethasone carbamazepine, theophylline, and folic acid may decrease effectiveness. Oral anticoagulants, antihistamines, tolbutamide, chloramphenicol, cimetidine, some benzodiazepines, diazoxide, disulfiram, estrogens, isoniazid, phenothiazines, phenylbutazone, salicylates, and sulfonamides may increase risk of toxicity. The result of concurrent therapy with valproic acid, and with phenobarbital, is unpredictable. If given with tube feedings (Osmolite or Isocal), separate feedings as far apart from doses as possible (these may inhibit phenytoin absorption). Cardiac depression may be increased by lidocaine or propranolol.

🖐 **Give with meals (except tube feedings) if GI distress is noted.**

Seizures: *Adult:* PO: *Loading dose:* 900 mg to 1.5 g, divided into 3 doses over the first 24 hr. *Maintenance dose:* 100 mg tid or (Extended phenytoin sodium capsules, USA) 300 mg once daily. IV: *Loading dose:* 900 mg to 1.5 g, divided into 3 doses over the first 24 hr. *Maintenance dose:* 100 mg q8h. *Child:* PO or IV: *Loading dose:* 15 mg/kg/day in divided doses q8h or q12h. *Maintenance dose:* 5–7 mg/kg.

Dysrhythmias: *Adult:* PO: *Loading dose:* 1 g divided into 4 doses over the first 24 hr; then 500 mg daily in divided doses for 2 days. *Maintenance dose:* 300 mg daily, in divided doses q8h. IV: *Loading dose:* 250 mg over 5 min until dysrhythmia subsides, adverse effects develop, or 1 g has been given; or 100 mg every 15 min until dysrhythmia subsides, adverse effects develop, or 1 g has been given. *Child:* PO or IV: 3–8 mg/kg/day or 250 mg/m²/day. For IV route, give *IV push* slowly, over at least 5 min, as a single dose or in divided doses.

Clinical alert: Check phenytoin serum level of those on prolonged therapy before giving first dose (therapeutic level is 10–20 mcg/ml). Expect lower dose for the elderly. Give IV push doses at 50 mg/min (if glucose is running, flush with saline before and after, or a precipitate may form). Because of risk of severe tissue irritation, monitor closely for infiltration and avoid IV sites on hands. Avoid IM administration. Tablets may be crushed; capsules may be opened and mixed with food; suspension should be shaken well before pouring dose. Schedule doses of prompt-release forms as evenly as possible over a 24-hr period to maintain therapeutic levels.

Contraindications/Precautions

PREG D

Contraindicated in hypersensitivity to hydantoins, and in hypoglycemia-induced seizures, sinus bradycardia, all degrees of heart block, Adams-Stokes syndrome. *Use with caution* in impaired liver or kidney function, alcoholism, hypotension, myocardial insufficiency, heart failure, pancreatic adenoma, diabetes mellitus, hyperglycemia, respiratory depression.

🖐 **Use with caution for children and the elderly. Safe use for pregnant or nursing mothers has not been established (use only if benefits outweigh risk to fetus).**

Side effects/Adverse reactions

Hypersensitivity: itching, fever, arthralgia, rash, dermatitis, lymphadenopathy, acute renal failure, Stevens-Johnson syndrome. *CV:* hypotension and (less commonly) ventricular fibrillation with rapid IV infusion, bradycardia, cardiac depression, polyarteritis nodosa. *GI:* gingival hyperplasia, and (less commonly) nausea, vomiting, constipation, epigastric pain, dysphagia, weight loss, loss of taste, hepatitis, liver necrosis. *Skin:* hirsutism, and (less commonly) pain at IV site, tissue necrosis. *CNS:* lethargy, drowsiness, ataxia, dizziness, slurred speech, confusion, tremors, insomnia, headache, encephalopathy, peripheral neuropathy. *Eye:* nystagmus, decreased vision, diplopia, and (less commonly) photophobia, conjunctivitis. *Hem:* leukocytosis, agranulocytosis, eosinophilia, macrocytosis, megaloblastic anemia, pancytopenia, hyperglycemia, transient increase in serum thyrotropic hormone (TSH) level, elevated alkaline phosphatase. *GU:* glycosuria. *Resp:* (uncommon) respiratory depression with rapid IV infusion, pulmonary fibrosis. *Misc:* acute systemic lupus erythematosus, craniofacial abnormalities in young children on long-term therapy.

Nursing implications/Documentation

Possible nursing diagnoses: Potential for injury; Altered oral mucous membranes.

◆ *For anticonvulsant use,* document history of seizures (type, frequency, duration, usual time they occur, precipitating factors, presence of an aura); initiate seizure precautions as indicated.

◆ Provide special mouth care and observe for gum inflammation (especially children); report if this persists.

◆ Monitor serum drug levels periodically to assure therapeutic range (10–20 mcg/cc); expect steady state to occur after 7–10 days. Therapeutic and toxic range is narrow with IV route.

◆ Never inject a cloudy phenytoin solution (slightly yellow, clear solution is acceptable). A precipitate that develops during refrigeration may disappear when solution is warmed.

◆ Monitor pregnant women closely; they may require higher dosages. After delivery, monitor neonates for bleeding (increased risk).

◆ *For IV route,* document pulse and blood pressure before and after administration.

◆ *For antiarrhythmic use,* document monitor strip before and after IV administration.

P

▶

- Monitor CBC and liver function studies periodically if therapy is prolonged.
- Report signs of hematological side effects (persistent fatigue, sore throat, fever, infections).

Patient & family teaching/Home care

Possible nursing diagnoses: Fear; Self-esteem disturbance; Knowledge deficit; Impaired home maintenance management.

- Advise taking this drug with meals; point out the need for good oral hygiene (because of side effects of gum hyperplasia).
- Stress the need for close medical follow-up; emphasize that persistent fatigue, weakness, fever, sore throat, mouth ulcers, gum inflammation, and infections are signs of side effects that should be reported.
- Warn that stopping anticonvulsants suddenly can cause an increase in severity and frequency of seizures.
- *When phenytoin is being used as an anticonvulsant,* teach significant others—and have them demonstrate—how to protect the individual should a seizure occur.
- Advise that this drug may make urine a harmless pink or red-brown color.
- *If hirsutism occurs,* explore feelings, and discuss ways of coping (e.g., might use a depilatory).
- Warn that drinking alcohol may reduce drug effectiveness.
- Caution against driving until response is determined (may cause drowsiness at first).
- *See Anticonvulsants and Antiarrhythmics overviews for more information.*

physostigmine

fi-zoe-stig'meen

physostigmine salicylate (eserine): *Antilirium*

Class: Cholinergic, Anticholinesterase, Ophthalmic-miotic

Antidote: Atropine

PEDS	PREG	GERI
☜	C	☜

Action Counteracts the action of anticholinergic by inhibiting the destruction of acetylcholine by the enzyme cholinesterase. Reduces intraocular pressure by producing papillary constriction and increasing outflow of aqueous humor.

Use/Therapeutic goal/Outcome

Tricyclic antidepressant or anticholinergic overdose: Reversal of toxic CNS and cardiac effects. *Outcome criteria:* BP and pulse within normal range; return of normal neuromuscular function.

Wide-angle glaucoma: Reduction of intraocular pressure. *Outcome criteria:* Upon measurement with tonometer, intraocular pressure within normal range.

Dose range/Administration

Interaction alert: Antihistamines, antidepressants, atropine, phenothiazines, quinidine, and disopyramide may antagonize cholinergic effects. Physostigmine prolongs action of depolarizing muscle relaxers (succinylcholine).

Tricyclic or anticholinergic overdose: Adult: IM, IV: 0.5–2 mg (IV rate < 1 mg/min); repeat q 5–10 min if life-threatening signs return.

Wide-angle glaucoma: Adult: 0.25% ophthalmic ointment: 1 cm qd to tid. 0.25 or *0.5% ophthalmic solution:* 1–2 gtt qd to qid.

Clinical alert: Doses individualized depending upon clinical response and incidence of side effects. There is a fine line between inadequate dosage and overdosage, requiring careful monitoring of response. Keep atropine, suction, and resuscitative equipment readily available.

Contraindications/Precautions

PREG
C

Contraindicated in hypersensitivity to physostigmine or salicylates, and in asthma, diabetes, gangrene, cardiovascular disease, or intestinal or urinary obstruction. *Use with caution* in epilepsy, hyperthyroidism, parkinsonism, and peptic ulcer.

☜ **Contraindicated for children (except in emergency). Use with caution for the elderly. Safe use for pregnant or nursing mothers has not been established.**

Side effects/Adverse reactions

Hypersensitivity: rashes, exaggeration of side effects. *CNS:* restlessness, excitability, headache, muscle twitching and weakness, ataxia, convulsions. *Resp:* respiratory distress. *CV:* irregular pulse. *GI:* nausea, vomiting, diarrhea, excessive salivation, abdominal cramps. *Eye:* eyelid twitching, miosis, dimness and blurring of vision, conjunctivitis. *Misc:* cholinergic crisis (increase in severity of side effects).

Nursing implications/Documentation

Possible nursing diagnoses: Potential for aspiration; Impaired swallowing; Potential for injury.

• Closely monitor muscle strength and ability to chew, swallow, and talk until condition is stable (keep in mind that because of short duration of action, repeated doses may be required); document variations in strength and pulse, respirations, and blood pressure every 5–15 min until stable.

• Protect airway by positioning the patient on his or her side and clearing oral secretions.

• Discard darkened solutions (should be colorless and clear).

• Keep patient in bed with side rails up until response is determined.

• Recognize that this is the only cholinergic that crosses the blood-brain barrier, making it useful for treating CNS effects of anticholinergic or tricyclic antidepressant overdosage.

Patient & family teaching/Home care

Possible nursing diagnoses: Impaired home maintenance management.

• Reassure that the patient will be closely monitored to ensure safety, and that measures are being taken to reverse toxicity.

• Explore reasons for overdosage of medication; identify ways of avoiding overdosage in the future.

• For treatment of glaucoma, stress the need for ongoing medical supervision to monitor eye pressure; explain that eye drops may cause dimness of vision and lid twitches.

• *See Cholinergics overview for more information.*

phytonadione

fye-toe-na-dye'one

AquaMEPHYTON, Konakion, Mephyton

Class: Vitamin K1, Prothrombogenic, Antihemorrhagic

PEDS	PREG	GERI
✥	C	OK

Action Promotes blood clotting by promoting hepatic formation of essential clotting factors (II, VII, IX, and X).

Use/Therapeutic goal/Outcome

Hypoprothrombinemia: Prevention or control of bleeding. **Outcome criteria:** Absence or control of bleeding; prothrombin time within 2 seconds of control.

Hemorrhagic disease of newborn: Prevention or control of bleeding. **Outcome criteria:** Absence of signs and symptoms of bleeding; decreased prothrombin time within 2–4 hours.

Dose range/Administration

Interaction alert: Antacids, sucralfate, cholestyramine, colestipol, and mineral oil may decrease oral absorption. Broad spectrum antibiotics, sufonamides, quinidine, and salicylates may increase dose requirements. Decreases effect of oral anticoagulants.

Hypoprothrombinemia: Adult: PO: 2.5 to 10 mg; repeat after 12–48 hr if necessary. IM, SC: 2.5 to 25 mg; repeat after 6–8 hr if necessary. **Child:** PO, IM, SC: 5–10 mg. **Infants:** IM, SC: 1–2 mg.

Hemorrhagic disease of the newborn: neonate: IM, SC: 0.5 to 1 mg immediately after delivery; repeat after 6–8 hr if necessary.

Clinical alert: Phytonadione is the Vitamin K preparation of choice for oral anticoagulant–induced hypoprothrombinemia. The smallest effective dose is used to avoid decreased response to subsequent anticoagulation therapy. Phytonadione does not affect anticoagulant action of heparin.

Contraindications/Precautions

PREG C

Contraindicated in hypersensitivity to phytonadione. **Use with caution** by IV route and in glucose-6-phosphate dehydrogenase (G6PD) deficiency, and impaired liver function.

✥ **Preparations containing benzyl alcohol are contraindicated for neonates. Use with caution for neonates and pregnant women.**

Side effects/Adverse reactions

Hypersensitivity: pruritus, urticaria, rash; anaphylaxis and death after rapid IV administration. **Hem:** hemolysis in G6PD deficiency, hyperbilirubinemia in neonates. **GI:** unusual taste. **Skin:** redness, pain, or swelling at injection site. **Misc:** flushing of face.

Nursing implications/Documentation

Possible nursing diagnoses: Impaired tissue integrity; Knowledge deficit.

• IV route is for emergency use; infusion rate should be no more than 1 mg/min. Observe for flushing, tightness of chest, weakness, tachycardia, and hypotension; have resuscitation equipment available.

• Administer only freshly prepared IV solutions and wrap infusion container with foil to protect from light.

• Be aware that therapeutic effect may take 3–6 hours and that fresh plasma or blood transfusions may be needed initially.

• For patients receiving total parenteral nutrition, expect phytonadione to be administered weekly to maintain clotting ability.

• With IM/SC administration, assess for pain, swelling, and tenderness at injection site, and provide comfort measures.

• Patients with obstructive jaundice or biliary fistulas must be given bile salts to absorb PO phytonadione.

• Monitor prothrombin times; report significant changes to physician so that dosage can be regulated effectively.

Patient & family teaching/Home care

Possible nursing diagnosis: Knowledge deficit.

• Caution not to take other medications without consulting primary physician.

• Stress importance of follow-up medical exams and blood studies.

pilocarpine
pye-lo-kar'peen

pilocarpine hydrochloride: *Adsorbocarpine, Isopto Carpine, ♣Miocarpine, Ocusert Pilo, Pilocar, Pilocel, Pilomiotin, Pilopine HS, ♠Pilopt*

pilocarpine nitrate: *P.V. Carpine Liquifilm*

Class: Miotic, Cholinergic, Antiglaucoma agent

PEDS	PREG	GERI
✋	C	✋

Action Constricts the pupil and reduces intraocular pressure (IOP) by stimulating the ciliary and pupillary sphincter muscles (this pulls the iris away from the filtration angle, allowing for increased outflow of aqueous humor). Decreases production of aqueous humor.

Use/Therapeutic goal/Outcome

Primary open-angle glaucoma, acute-angle closure glaucoma, and lens protection during surgery: Reduction of intraocular pressure. **Outcome criteria:** Decreased intraocular pressure measured by physician with tonometer.

Dose range/Administration

Interaction alert: Avoid use with phenylephrine hydrochloride (decreases effects) and carbachol or echothiophate (increases effects).

Primary open-angle glaucoma: Adult and Child: *Ophthalmic:* Instill 1–2 drops q12h, q8h, or q6h, or apply ointment along the length of lower conjunctival sac qd at hs, or insert 1 Ocusert System/wk (20–40 mcg/hr) in cul-de-sac of eye at bedtime.

Acute-angle closure glaucoma: Adult and Child: *Ophthalmic:* Instill 1 drop 2% solution in the affected eye q5-10 min for 3–6 doses, then 1 drop q1-3h until pressure is controlled.

Clinical alert: Double check labels for correct concentration. Be sure that applicator tip does not touch the eyelid (may contaminate drops). To prevent *systemic absorption,* apply light finger pressure to lacrimal sac for 30–60 sec after instilling drops.

Contraindications/Precautions
PREG C

Contraindicated in hypersensitivity to pilocarpine, and in acute iritis, secondary glaucoma, or acute inflammatory disease of the anterior segment of the eye. **Use with caution** in coronary artery disease, hypertension, and bronchial asthma.

✋ **Use with caution for children, pregnant or nursing mothers, and the elderly.**

Side effects/Adverse reactions

Usually well tolerated. **Hypersensitivity:** itching, stinging, burning, lacrimation, conjunctivitis, keratitis, iritis, bronchospasm, pulmonary edema. **Eye:** myopia, blurred vision, ciliary spasm with transient browache, twitching of the eyelids, reduced visual acuity, eye pain. **GI:** nausea, vomiting, abdominal cramps, diarrhea. **CV:** hypotension, tachycardia.

Nursing implications/Documentation

Possible nursing diagnoses: Sensory/perceptual alterations (visual); Potential for injury.

• Wash hands thoroughly before and after administration.

• Ensure adequate light in the environment and monitor for risk of injury (blurred vision is common).

• Document and report tachycardia, hypotension, eye pain, tearing, or redness of the eye.

Patient & family teaching/Home care

Possible nursing diagnoses: Knowledge deficit; Impaired home maintenance management.

♦ Explain that without strict adherence to medication regimen and regular tonometry measurements by physician, vision could deteriorate without the patient realizing it.

♦ Teach the procedure for instilling medication, and observe return demonstration.

♦ Caution to report immediately if difficult breathing or vision changes are experienced (blurred vision, however, is common, especially during the first 2 weeks of treatment).

♦ Warn against driving until vision is accurate.

♦ Teach those using the Ocusert system how to insert system; observe return demonstration and advise that if it is lost during sleep, it should be rinsed under cold tap water and reinserted (unless it is deformed).

♦ *See Cholinergics overview for more information.*

pindolol

pin'doe-lole

♠*Barbloc, Visken*

Class: Nonselective beta-adrenergic blocking agent, Antihypertensive

PEDS	PREG	GERI
♨	**B**	♨

Action Reduces blood pressure (precise mechanism is unclear) possibly by blocking beta-1 (cardiac) and beta-2 adrenergic receptors. Has prominent intrinsic sympathomimetic activity (may have less effect on cardiac output, heart rate, bronchial constriction than other beta-blockers).

Use/Therapeutic goal/Outcome

Hypertension: Control of hypertension. *Outcome criteria:* Blood pressure within normal range.

Dose range/Administration

Interaction alert: With cardiac glycosides, monitor for severe bradycardia. Cimetidine may inhibit metabolism of pindolol, increasing its effect. Indomethacin may decrease pindolol effects. May alter antidiabetic agent requirements.

Adult: PO: 5 mg bid; may increase by 10 mg/day every 2–3 weeks. *Maximum dose:* 60 mg/day.

Clinical alert: Patients taking pindolol may not exhibit tachycardia as a symptom of fever, hypoglycemia, or hyperthyroidism.

Contraindications/Precautions

PREG
B

Contraindicated in hypersensitivity to pindolol, and in bronchial asthma, overt CHF, cardiogenic shock, second- or third-degree heart block (PR interval > 0.24 seconds), or marked sinus bradycardia. **Use with caution** in diabetes mellitus, hyperthyroidism, or impaired renal and hepatic function.

♨ **Use with caution for the elderly. Safe use for children and pregnant or nursing mothers has not been established.**

Side effects/Adverse reactions

Hypersensitivity: pruritis, rash, fever. **CV:** bradycardia, peripheral vascular disease, CHF, hypotension, cardiac-related chest pain, edema. **CNS:** fatigue, dizziness, lethargy, insomnia, nervousness, vivid dreams, hallucinations. **GU:** decreased sexual ability, priapism. **Resp:** increased airway resistance, pharyngitis, respiratory distress. **GI:** vomiting, nausea, diarrhea. **Skin:** cold extremities. **Eye:** visual disturbances.

Nursing implications/Documentation

Possible nursing diagnoses: Activity intolerance; Fatigue; Potential for injury.

♦ Assess mental status and record pulse and blood pressure (if possible, lying, sitting, and standing, in both arms) before administration, and frequently thereafter until response is determined.

♦ Consult with physician to determine desired therapeutic range for blood pressure and heart rate (parameters for withholding the medication should be written by physician).

♦ Ascertain that baseline CBC, electrolytes, BUN, creatinine, and liver function studies have been obtained before giving first dose; report abnormalities and monitor closely thereafter.

♦ Monitor for allergic reactions and signs of confusion, dizziness, bradycardia, CHF, and hypotension; hold drug and report immediately if these occur.

♦ Supervise ambulation until response is determined.

♦ Document and monitor daily weight, and intake and output; report significant negative or positive balance.

Patient & family teaching/Home care

Possible nursing diagnoses: Knowledge deficit; Impaired home maintenance management; Altered sexuality patterns.

• Explain the importance of taking this drug at the same time every day exactly as prescribed, even when feeling well; warn not to discontinue drug abruptly (may precipitate angina).

• Stress the importance of good medical follow-up; explain that this drug reduces "wear and tear" on blood vessels, reduces the workload of the heart, and improves longevity and health.

• Teach how to monitor pulse and blood pressure; emphasize that syncope, hypertension or hypotension, or persistent dizziness should be reported; provide pulse and blood pressure parameters for withholding medication.

• Advise changing positions slowly to avoid dizziness.

• Encourage daily monitoring of weight and reporting sudden weight gain (frequently is fluid retention).

• Warn against drinking alcohol or taking *any* OTC drugs without physician approval (some interactions can cause severe reactions).

• Explain that this drug may alter sexual ability; explore concerns and seek consultation as needed.

• *See Beta Adrenergic Blockers and Antihypertensives overviews for more information.*

piperacillin

pi-per'a-sill-in

piperacillin sodium: *Pipracil,* ⚫*Pipril*

Class: Anti-infective, Antibiotic, Extended-spectrum penicillin

PEDS	PREG	GERI
☟	B	☟

Action Extended-spectrum, usually bactericidal antibiotic; kills bacteria by inhibiting cell wall synthesis.

Use/Therapeutic goal/Outcome

Systemic infections: Resolution of infection. *Outcome criteria:* Absence of pathogenic growth on cultures, absence of clinical manifestations of infection (fever, pain, redness, heat, swelling, odor, drainage), normal WBC count, improvement of X rays.

Dose range/Administration

Interaction alert: Inactivates aminoglycosides (e.g., gentamicin, tobramycin); do not mix together in solution. Give at least 1 hour before bacteriostatic antibiotics for optimum effect. Probenecid inhibits excretion of piperacillin. May potentiate oral anticoagulants.

Systemic infection: **Adult:** IM, IV: 3–4 g q4-6h. *Maximum dose:* 24 g/day.

Prophylaxis of surgical infections: **Adult/Child > 12 yrs:** IM, IV: 2 g 30–60 min prior to procedure; may repeat during procedure, then 1–2 doses after procedure.

Clinical alert: Patients with cystic fibrosis are more prone to fever or rash.

Contraindications/Precautions

PREG B

Contraindicated in allergy to penicillin. *Use with caution* in cephalosporin sensitivity, history of allergic responses (e.g., other drugs, hay fever, asthma), and renal insufficiency.

☙ Use with caution for the elderly and for pregnant or nursing mothers. Safe use for children under 12 years has not been established.

Side effects/Adverse reactions

Hypersensitivity: itching, rashes, urticaria, fever, difficulty breathing, anaphylaxis. *GI:* nausea, vomiting, diarrhea, pseudomembranous colitis. *CV:* pain, redness, swelling, thrombophlebitis, sterile abscess at injection site. *CNS:* headache, dizziness, neuromuscular irritability, seizures. *Hem:* thrombocytopenia, leukopenia, hypokalemia, eosinophilia, increased bleeding time. *Misc:* superinfection.

Nursing implications/Documentation

Possible nursing diagnoses: Potential for infection; Diarrhea.

• Determine history of allergies, and (regardless of history) monitor closely for allergic reactions.

• Obtain baseline CBC, creatinine, liver function studies, and necessary cultures before administering first dose; monitor closely thereafter if therapy is prolonged.

• Give IM doses deep into large muscle mass.

• Encourage fluids, and record and monitor intake and output, to ensure adequate hydration; report significant negative or positive balance.

- Monitor for and report signs of superinfection (sore throat, fever, fatigue, thrush, vaginal discharge, diarrhea).

- Watch for unusual bruising or bleeding (check gums, urine).

Patient & family teaching/Home care

Possible nursing diagnoses: Knowledge deficit; Impaired home maintenance management.

- Teach the importance of reporting allergic symptoms, diarrhea, signs and symptoms that do not abate, or *any* new signs and symptoms of discomfort that might indicate superinfection (medication regimen may have to be changed).

- Advise drinking 2–3 L of fluids daily to maintain adequate hydration (especially important if fever exists).

- Stress the importance of taking antibiotics for the entire time prescribed, even if signs and symptoms abate.

- *See Anti-infectives overview for more information.*

pirbuterol

purr-byoo'ter-ole

Maxair

Class: Sympathomimetic (adrenergic) bronchodilator

PEDS	PREG	GERI
♨	C	♨

Action Produces bronchodilation by stimulating beta-2 adrenergic receptors, which relax bronchial smooth muscles.

Use/Therapeutic goal/Outcome

Prevention and reversal of acute bronchospasm (asthma): Reduction in airway resistance, improvement of air movement. **Outcome criteria:** Report of decrease or absence of episodes of asthma; improved forced expiratory volume (FEV).

Dose range/Administration

Interaction alert: Propranolol and other beta-blockers may reduce bronchodilation effect. Tricyclic antidepressants and monoamine oxidase inhibitors may produce undesired cardiovascular effects.

Adult/Child > 12 yrs: *Inhal:* 1–2 inhalations (0.2–0.4 mg) q4-6h, not to exceed 12 inhalations in 24 hr.

Clinical alert: Monitor for and report paradoxical bronchospasm.

Contraindications/Precautions

Contraindicated in hypersensitivity to adrenergics, pirbuterol acetate, or any of the preparation's ingredients. **Use with caution** in hyperthyroidism, diabetes mellitus, ischemic heart disease, arrhythmias, hypertension, and convulsive disorders. Tolerance to bronchodilator effect occurs over time.

♨ **Use with caution for the elderly. Safe use for children under 12 years and for pregnant or nursing mothers has not been established.**

Side effects/Adverse reactions

Hypersensitivity: excessive side effects. **CNS:** nervousness, tremor, headache, dizziness. **CV:** palpitations, tachycardia. **Resp:** chest pain, cough. **GI:** nausea, dry mouth.

Nursing implications/Documentation

Possible nursing diagnoses: Activity intolerance; Ineffective breathing pattern.

- Determine and record known allergies; provide an environment that is free from allergens (e.g., use air conditioning).

- Record lung sounds, respirations, pulse, and blood pressure, before and after dose administration, until response is determined.

- Provide favorite fluids, and monitor **intake** and **output** to ensure adequate hydration (at least 2 liters a day is recommended).

Patient & family teaching/Home care

Possible nursing diagnoses: Knowledge deficit; Impaired home maintenance management; Fear.

- Explain that this drug will enlarge air passages and make breathing easier.

- Warn that paradoxical bronchospasm can occur (instruct to stop using this drug and report bronchospasm immediately, rather than increase dose).

- Point out that stress and exercise can aggravate wheezing and bronchospasm, and that relaxation and controlled breathing techniques can help reduce severity and frequency of wheezing episodes.

- Give written and verbal instructions on how to use inhalers (shake container, exhale completely, hold mouthpiece to mouth, inhale deeply while pressing canister once, hold breath for a few seconds, remove canister and exhale slowly. Allow 2 minutes between inha-

P

lations, and at least 5 minutes before using a steroid inhalant).

♦ Warn against taking OTC drugs without physician's approval. Instruct to report deterioration in symptoms, instead of increasing dose.

♦ *See Adrenergics (Sympathomimetics) and Bronchodilators overviews for more information.*

piroxicam

peer-ox'i-kam

♣*Apo-Piroxicam, Feldene, Novopirocam*

Class: Nonsteroidal anti-inflammatory drug (NSAID), Analgesic, Antipyretic, Antirheumatic

PEDS	PREG	GERI
✋	C	✋

Action Exact mechanism of action is unclear. Believed to inhibit prostaglandin synthesis. Prostaglandin is a naturally occurring mediator of the inflammatory process which is found throughout body tissue.

Use/Therapeutic goal/Outcome

Pain and inflammation: Promotion of comfort and mobility; suppression of inflammation. *Outcome criteria:* Report of increased comfort with increased range of motion and ability to perform activities of daily life; reduction in or absence of joint stiffness, swelling, redness, and warmth.

Dose range/Administration

Interaction alert: May enhance the effects of coumarin-type anticoagulants. Aspirin may decrease therapeutic effect of NSAID and increase risk of bleeding.

🥄 **Give 30 min before or 2 hr after meals to enhance absorption, unless GI distress is experienced (then give with food).**

Adult: PO: 20 mg qd in single or divided doses. RECT: 20 mg qd bid.

Clinical alert: Give at the same time every day, in a single dose.

Contraindications/Precautions

PREG
C

Contraindicated in hypersensitivity to piroxicam, aspirin, or other NSAIDs. *Use with caution* in bleeding disorders, asthma, nasal polyps, GI disorders, angioedema, hepatic or renal disease, decreased cardiac function, hypertension, and peripheral edema.

🖐 **Use with caution for the elderly. Safe use for children and pregnant or nursing mothers has not been established.**

Side effects/Adverse reactions

Hypersensitivity: bronchospasm, urticaria, and rhinitis. *GI:* nausea, vomiting, indigestion, diarrhea, constipation, flatulence, dry mouth, peptic ulcer, GI bleeding, impaired liver function. *Skin:* rash, pruritus. *Eye:* photosensitivity. *CNS:* headache, dizziness, drowsiness. *CV:* peripheral edema. *GU:* nephrotoxicity. *Hem:* hyperglycemia, prolonged bleeding time.

Nursing implications/Documentation

Possible nursing diagnoses: Pain; Impaired physical mobility.

♦ Establish a baseline for CBC, electrolytes, prothrombin time, BUN, creatinine, and liver function studies; monitor periodically thereafter if therapy is prolonged.

♦ Monitor for and report GI symptoms that may indicate peptic ulcer (nausea, pain, black stools).

♦ Report visual and auditory changes immediately.

♦ Record weight every other day; report edema or sudden weight gain.

♦ For diabetics, monitor blood sugar closely since insulin requirements may change.

Patient & family teaching/Home care

Possible nursing diagnoses: Anxiety; Knowledge deficit.

♦ Advise taking doses with food to reduce GI symptoms.

♦ Explain the importance of watching for symptoms of GI bleeding (black stools, persistent GI distress).

♦ Stress the need to avoid aspirin, alcohol, and other OTC drugs (unless approved by physician) because of increased risk of GI bleeding.

♦ Encourage drinking 6–8 glasses of water a day to promote excretion of drug.

♦ Instruct individuals to hold dose and report if any of the following side effects are experienced: vertigo, rashes, blood in urine, jaundice, hearing or visual changes, sudden weight gain, edema.

♦ Warn that side effects may not occur for up to 7–10 days after therapy begins, and that full beneficial effects may not be noted for up to 4 weeks.

♦ Advise against driving or activities that require alertness until response is determined.

- Reinforce the need for ongoing medical follow-up; advise telling dentist that piroxicam is being taken.
- For diabetics, explain the importance of monitoring blood sugars with a blood glucose meter.
- *See Nonsteroidal anti-inflammatory drugs overview for more information.*

plasma

plazz'ma

plasma protein fraction (human): **Plasmanate, Plasma-Plex, Plasmatein, Protenate**

Class: Blood volume expander

PEDS	PREG	GERI
🖐	C	🖐

Action Replenishes plasma proteins (colloids) and expands circulating blood volume by exerting osmotic pull on tissue fluids.

Use/Therapeutic goal/Outcome

Hypovolemic shock: Promotion of adequate circulatory volume and tissue perfusion until whole blood is available. **Outcome criteria:** Reversal in signs and symptoms of shock (systolic blood pressure > 100 mm Hg; urine output > 25–30 cc/hr; heart rate < 100, with palpable peripheral pulses).

Hypoproteinemia: Replenishment of proteins in the blood. **Outcome criteria:** Total serum protein within normal limits (5.7–7.9 g/dl); serum albumin within normal limits (3.4–4.8 g/dl).

Dose range/Administration

Interaction alert: Do not administer with other solutions or through the same IV tubings as other fluids.

Hypovolemic shock: Adult: IV: 250–500 ml (12.5–25 g protein), maximum rate 10 ml/min, 500 ml in 50 min.

Hypoproteinemia: Adult: IV: 1000–1500 ml (50–75 g protein), maximum rate 8 ml/min, 480 ml/hr. **Child:** IV: 22–33 ml/kg, maximum rate 5–10 ml/min.

Clinical alert: Discard bottles that are not used within 4 hours (has no preservatives). Use only clear amber solutions.

Contraindications/Precautions

PREG C

Contraindicated in severe anemia and cardiac failure. **Use with caution** in low cardiac reserve, liver or kidney failure, in the absence of albumin deficiency, and in sodium restriction (contains 130–160 mEq sodium/liter).

🖐 **Use with caution for children, pregnant or nursing mothers, and the elderly.**

Side effects/Adverse reactions

Hypersensitivity: fever, chills, itching, erythema, rashes, tingling, chest tightness, backache, anaphylaxis. **CV:** (with rapid infusion) circulatory overload with pulmonary edema. **GI:** nausea, vomiting, increased salivation.

Nursing implications/Documentation

Possible nursing diagnosis: Potential for injury.

- Before infusing, record baseline assessment of lung and heart sounds, vital signs, and CVP or PAP (if available).
- Report presence of peripheral edema, sacral edema, or neck vein distension.
- During infusion, record vital signs every 15 minutes to every hour, depending on patient condition; record intake and output q1–2h.
- Stop infusion if signs and symptoms of congestive heart failure or pulmonary edema (cough, dyspnea, rales, cyanosis) become evident; notify physician immediately.
- For use in hypovolemic shock due to hemorrhage, monitor for new bleeding sites: higher blood pressure may cause hemorrhage of severed vessel that failed to bleed at a lower blood pressure.
- Keep patient in bed with side rails up.

Patient & family teaching/Home care

Possible nursing diagnoses: Anxiety; Fear; Knowledge deficit.

- Encourage voicing of questions and concerns; explain rationale for all actions.
- Explain that this solution replenishes deficient supplies of protein.
- Stress that vital signs will be monitored closely to ensure safety.

plicamycin

plik-a-mi'cin

mithramycin: **Mithracin**

Class: Antineoplastic (antibiotic) agent

PEDS	PREG	GERI
🖐	X	🖐

Action Kills rapidly growing cells (cancer, hair follicles, bone marrow, GI lining, ova, and sperm) by interfering with the synthesis of DNA, RNA, and protein, causing disruption of nucleic acid function. Is cell-cycle–phase non-

P

specific. Lowers calcium levels by interfering with osteocitic activity, blocking calcium and phosphorus reabsorption from bone.

Use/Therapeutic goal/Outcome

Testicular cancer and hypercalcemia associated with metastases that is nonresponsive to other chemotherapeutic agents: Suppression of malignant cell proliferation, reduction in hypercalcemia. **Outcome criteria:** Tumor and disease regression or stabilization on radiologic and physical examination; normal serum calcium.

Hypercalcemia associated with advanced cancer: Reduction of serum calcium levels. **Outcome criteria:** Serum calcium within normal levels.

Dose range/Administration

Testicular cancer: Adult: IV: 25–35 mcg/kg/day for 8–10 days; do not exceed 30 mg/kg/day. May repeat monthly.

Hypercalcemia: Adult: IV: 25 mcg/kg/day for 3–4 days; repeat at 1 wk intervals.

Clinical alert: This drug should be given only to hospitalized patients by nurses who are knowledgeable in the comprehensive management of the administration of antineoplastic agents. Doses may vary at physician's discretion. Repeat doses are held until it is ascertained that the patient has recovered sufficiently from toxicities of previous doses. Established protocols and policies for drug preparation, administration, and accidental skin contamination *must be followed closely* (gloves or double gloves are worn when handling drug; if the drug touches the skin, the area is washed immediately with plenty of soap and water). Plicamycin is given *slowly* over 4–6 hr in 50–100 ml fluid to minimize inflammation and pain along the vein. Rapid infusion can cause severe GI side effects.

Contraindications/Precautions

PREG X

Contraindicated in hypersensitivity to plicamycin, thrombocytopenia, impaired bone marrow function, and coagulation and bleeding disorders. **Use with caution** in renal or hepatic impairment or electrolyte imbalances and with previous radiation or chemotherapy.

✋ **Contraindicated for children under 15 and pregnant or nursing mothers. Use with caution for the elderly.**

Side effects/Adverse reactions

Hypersensitivity: rash, flushing. **GI:** anorexia, nausea, vomiting (within 6 hr and lasting for 24 hr), stomatitis, diarrhea, increased liver enzymes. **Hem:** hemorrhage secondary to thrombocytopenia; bleeding tendencies; decreased serum calcium, potassium, and phosphorus. **GU:** increased BUN and creatinine, proteinuria. **CNS:** drowsiness, lethargy, headache, depression. **Skin:** pain and erythema at injection site; cellulitis, ulceration, and sloughing if extravasation occurs; toxic epidermal necrolysis.

Nursing implications/Documentation

Possible nursing diagnoses: Potential for infection; Potential for injury; Fatigue; Altered oral mucous membrane; Fluid volume deficit; Diarrhea; Altered nutrition: less than body requirements.

♦ *See important Nursing implications in Antineoplastic agents overview on page 72, which apply to all neoplastics. The interventions that follow are additional and specific to this drug only.*

♦ Determine that dehydration and volume depletion are corrected before initial dose.

♦ If edema, hydrothorax, or ascites is present, use ideal body weight instead of actual body weight for dose calculation.

♦ Monitor calcium levels closely as they may drop quickly (effect usually seen within 24–48 hr and lasts for 3–15 days).

♦ Report facial flushing and epistaxis as it may be an early sign of toxic epidermal necrolysis.

♦ Increase fluids to 2–3 L a day to prevent dehydration.

Patient & family teaching/Home care

Possible nursing diagnoses: Knowledge deficit; Ineffective coping (individual and family); Hopelessness; Impaired home maintenance management.

♦ *See important Patient & family teaching in Antineoplastic agents overview on page 72, which apply to all neoplastics. The teachings that follow are additional and specific to this drug only.*

♦ Stress that signs of hypocalcemia (muscle spasms, spasms of the feet) should be reported immediately; it may require treatment. Facial flushing should also be reported; it may be an early sign of toxicity.

♦ Explain that drinking 2–3 L per day can reduce risk of kidney complications.

♦ *See Antineoplastic agents overview for more information.*

polythiazide

pol-i-thye'a-zide

Renese

Class: Thiazide diuretic, Antihypertensive

PEDS	PREG	GERI
🖐	**D**	🖐

Action Promotes sodium chloride, potassium, and water excretion by inhibiting the reabsorption of sodium in the early portion of the distal tubule. Lowers blood pressure by reducing plasma and extra-cellular volume.

Use/Therapeutic goal/Outcome

Hypertension: Promotion of diuresis, reduction of blood pressure. **Outcome criteria:** After 3–4 days, blood pressure within normal limits.
Edema: Promotion of diuresis, resolution of edema. **Outcome criteria:** Increased urinary output; weight loss; absence of rales and peripheral and sacral edema.

Dose range/Administration

Interaction alert: Cholestyramine and colestipol decreases intestinal absorption. Diazoxide potentiates the hyperuricemic, hyperglycemic, and antihypertensive effects. Nonsteroidal anti-inflammatory drugs may decrease effects. Do not give concomitantly with lithium. Give cautiously with corticosteroids, antidiabetics, lanoxin, and skeletal muscle relaxants.

🖐 **Give with meals to decrease GI upset.**
Adult: PO: 1–4 mg/day. **Child:** 0.02–0.08 mg/kg/day.
Clinical alert: Give in morning to avoid nocturnal diuresis.

Contraindications/Precautions

PREG D

Contraindicated in hypersensitivity to sulfonamides or thiazides, and in anuria. **Use with caution** in patients with renal or hepatic dysfunction, systemic lupus erythematosus, gout, diabetes, allergies, pancreatitis, arteriosclerosis, and debilitated states.

🖐 **Contraindicated for pregnant or nursing mothers. Use with caution for children and the elderly.**

Side effects/Adverse reactions

Hypersensitivity: rash, urticaria, dermatitis with photosensitivity, pneumonitis, vasculitis.
Hem: hypokalemia, hyperglycemia, azotemia, impaired glucose tolerance, asymptomatic hyperuricemia, electrolyte imbalances, metabolic alkalosis, hypercalcemia, lipid abnormalities, aplastic anemia, agranulocytosis, leukopenia, thrombocytopenia. **CV:** volume depletion, dehydration, orthostatic hypotension. **GI:** anorexia, nausea, pancreatitis, hepatic encephalopathy. **Misc:** gout.

Nursing implications/Documentation

Possible nursing diagnoses: Fluid volume deficit; Altered patterns of urinary elimination; Potential for injury.

♦ Ascertain that baseline CBC, sodium, potassium, chloride, carbon dioxide, calcium, magnesium, BUN, creatinine, uric acid, and liver function studies have been obtained before giving first dose; report abnormalities and monitor closely thereafter.

♦ Document and monitor blood pressure, pulse, daily weight, and intake and output; report significant discrepancies.

♦ Monitor for hyperglycemia because of risk of thiazide diabetes.

♦ Observe for and report signs of fluid overload (auscultate lungs for rales; check feet, ankles, and sacrum for edema).

♦ Be aware that diuretics often induce hypokalemia, which predisposes individuals to cardiac arrhythmias, cramping, and digoxin toxicity.

♦ Check with physician to determine dietary restrictions; if a low-salt, high-potassium diet is recommended, consult with dietician to plan a low-salt diet that includes foods and juices high in potassium (orange juice; banana; green leafy vegetables).

♦ Observe the elderly for extreme diuresis (may require lower doses); monitor for orthostatic hypotension; supervise ambulation until response is determined.

Patient & family teaching/Home care

Possible nursing diagnoses: Knowledge deficit; Impaired home maintenance management.

♦ Before giving first dose, explain that the drug will increase the amount and frequency of urination.

♦ Emphasize the importance of taking this drug exactly as prescribed, and the importance of returning for medical follow-up.

♦ Explain that diuretics enhance the work of the kidney and reduce the workload of the heart.

- ◆ Encourage monitoring weight daily.
- ◆ *See Diuretics and Antihypertensives overviews*

potassium supplements   *poe-tass'ee-um*

potassium acetate

potassium bicarbonate: *K+Care ET, Klor-Con/EF*

potassium chloride: *K-Dur, K-Lor, K-Lyte/Cl,
Kaochlor 10%, Kaochlor S-F 10%, Kaon-Cl,
Kaon-Cl 20%, Kato Powder, Kay Ciel, Klor-10%,
Klor-Con, Kloride, Klorvess, Klotrix, K-Tab,
Micro-K Extencaps, SK-Potassium Chloride,
Slow-K, Ten-K*

potassium gluconate: *Kaon Liquid, Kaon Tablets,
Kaylixer, K-G elixir, ♣Potassium Rougier*

Class: Electrolyte, antihypokalemic

*Antidote:*Sodium polystyrene sulfate (Kay exalate)

PEDS	PREG	GERI
🖐	A	🖐

Action Increases serum potassium levels. Normal serum potassium levels are essential for acid-base balance and for cardiac, kidney, nervous system, and skeletal muscle function. Abnormal levels may be life threatening.

Use/Therapeutic goal/Outcome

Hypokalemia: Prevention or correction of hypokalemia. **Outcome criteria:** Serum potassium level of 3.5–5.5 mEq/L.

Dose range/Administration

Interaction alert: Other potassium products, potassium-sparing diuretics, enalapril, captopril, lisinopril, cyclosporine, low-salt milk, salt substitutes, and foods high in potassium may cause hyperkalemia. Steroids may reduce effectiveness of potassium supplements. Heparin, anticholinergics, and NSAIDS may increase risk of GI ulceration.

🍎 **Give with or after food to reduce GI upset.**

potassium acetate: Adult: IV: Up to 3 mEq/kg/day. Dose and infusion rate is based on individual needs. *Maximum daily dose:* 400 mEq. **Child:** IV: Up to 3 mEq/kg or 40 mEq/square meter of body surface. Volume of administered fluid is adjusted to body size.

potassium bicarbonate: Adult: PO: 25–50 mEq dissolved in 4–8 ounces of water daily or bid. *Maximum daily dose:* 100 mEq.

potassium chloride: Adult: PO: 20–100 mEq daily in divided doses. IV: 10–40 mEq per liter of IV fluid. Dose and infusion rate is based on individual needs (rate should not exceed 20 mEq/h). *Maximum daily dose:* 400 mEq/day. Child: PO: (oral *solution* only) 15–40 mEq per square meter of body surface or 2–3 mEq/kg given in divided doses daily. IV: Up to 3 mEq/kg or 40 mEq per square meter of body surface. Volume of administered fluid is adjusted to body size.

potassium gluconate: Adult: PO: 20–100 mEq daily in divided doses. **Child:** PO: (elixir only) 20–40 mEq per square meter of body surface or 2–3 mEq/kg given in divided doses daily.

Clinical alert: To reduce risk of life-threatening hyperkalemia, before giving first dose, ascertain that the patient has voided and that serum BUN, creatinine, and potassium levels are not elevated. Do not substitute one potassium product for another without a physician's order. Mix liquid or powdered doses in 4–8 ounces of cold water or juice to reduce bitter taste and gastric irritation. Never give undiluted potassium IV push (can be fatal); concentrated potassium injection must be mixed in a large volume (preferably 1000 ml, but in critical situations, the volume may be less). Administer high concentrations via a central venous catheter, using an infusion control device.

Contraindications/Precautions

PREG
D

Contraindicated in hypersensitivity to tartrazine dye that is in some liquid solutions, and in hyperkalemia. **Use with Caution** in impaired renal function; oliguria, anuria, acute dehydration; metabolic acidosis; prolonged severe diarrhea; GI obstruction, ulceration, or abnormal motility; complete or severe heart block; potassium intolerance; trauma-related problems such as burns, crushing injuries, extensive infections, major surgery within the previous 24 hours, massive hemolysis.

🖐 **Safe use for children of potassium gluconate tablets, potassium chloride suspension and tablets, and all forms of potassium bicarbonate has not been established. Use with caution for children and the elderly because kidney function may be limited.**

Side effects/Adverse reactions

Hypersensitivity: rash. **GI:** nausea, vomiting, abdominal distress, diarrhea, bowel ulceration, chest or throat pain with swallowing. **Hem:** hyperkalemia (slow or irregular heart beat, severe leg weakness or heaviness, confusion, tingling or numbness of the lips or extremities, difficulty breathing, unexplained anxiety, fatigue; with severe hyperkalemia, cardiovascular collapse and cardiac arrest).

Nursing implications/Documentation

Possible nursing diagnoses: Altered health maintenance.

◆ Establish a baseline serum potassium; monitor closely thereafter as indicated by condition.

◆ Administer parenteral doses into a large vein only and monitor closely for inflammation and infiltration; stop IV and report immediately if these are suspected.

◆ Record intake and output until condition is stable; report decreasing urinary output immediately.

Patient & family teaching/Home care

Possible nursing diagnoses: Knowledge deficit; Impaired home maintenance management.

◆ Stress the need to take doses as prescribed and to return for lab work as ordered (especially important for those taking diuretics or digoxin). Oral doses must be taken with or immediately after meals; if a dose is missed, it should be taken as soon as possible with food, milk, or juice. If GI distress is noted, suggest sipping liquid form slowly (enteric-coated tablets are *not* recommended).

◆ Provide a list of foods that may increase serum potassium (bananas, orange juice, whole grains, broccoli, carrots, prunes, low-salt milk, salt substitutes); caution to check labels of all low-salt products for high potassium content.

◆ Caution against taking OTC analgesics without physician's approval.

pralidoxime

pra-li-dox'eem

pralidoxime chloride: *Proptopam chloride*
Class: Cholinesterase reactivator

PEDS	PREG	GERI
☙	C	☙

Action Restores normal neuromuscular transmission by reactivating cholinesterase that has been inactivated by organophosphorus pesticides and related compounds, permitting degradation of accumulated acetycholine.

Use/Therapeutic goal/Outcome

Antidote for overdosage of anticholinesterase drugs and organophosphate insecticide and pesticide poisoning: Reduction of nicotinic effects such as twitching, cramping, weakness, seizures, respiratory arrest. **Outcome criteria:** Increased voluntary muscle relaxation, muscle strength, and coordination; report of relief of cramping.

Dose range/Administration

Interaction alert: For use in organophosphate poisoning, avoid use of morphine, theophyllines, succinylcholine, reserpine, and phenothiazines. Use cautiously with barbiturates.

Anticholinesterase overdose: **Adult:** IV: 1–2 g, then 250 mg q 5 min prn.

Organophosphate poisoning: **Adult:** IV: 1–2 g in 100 ml NS infused over 15–30 min or (in pulmonary edema) IV push over 5 min; may repeat in 1 hr prn. SC, IM: Only if IV is not feasible. PO: If no GI distress, 1–3 g q5h. **Child:** IV: 20–40 mg/kg.

Clinical alert: IV route is recommended. Use sterile water without preservatives to reconstitute. Ascertain that serum cholinesterase levels are drawn before giving pralidoxime. If there is respiratory or autonomic nervous system involvement, concomitant administration of atropine is recommended. Start atropine and pralidoxime at same time if both are to be used.

Contraindications/Precautions

PREG C

Contraindicated in hypersensitivity to pralidoxime, and in asthma, peptic ulcer, and severe cardiac disease. **Use with caution** in myasthenia gravis and renal insufficiency.

☙ Use with caution for children and the elderly. Safe use for pregnant or nursing mothers has not been established.

Side effects/Adverse reactions

Hypersensitivity: none listed. **CNS:** dizziness, headache. **Resp:** hyperventilation, laryngospasm. **CV:** tachycardia, hypertension. **Eye:** blurred vision, impaired accommodation. **MS:** muscular weakness, muscle rigidity. **GI:** nausea.

Nursing implications/Documentation

Possible nursing diagnoses: Potential for aspiration; Potential for injury.

- Maintain airway, respirations, and other supportive therapy as needed.
- Ascertain chemical or drug causing overdose; contact poison control for up-to-date definitive treatment.
- Anticipate excitement and manic behavior upon recovery of consciousness (protect from injury).
- Monitor closely for cardiac, blood pressure, and respiratory changes for 48–72 hr, especially if poison was ingested.
- Record and monitor intake and output; report oliguria.
- Observe those with myasthenia gravis closely (may rapidly reverse to myasthenic crisis during or immediately post treatment; have Tensilon available for rapid treatment).

Patient & family teaching/Home care

Possible nursing diagnoses: Fear; Knowledge deficit; Impaired home maintenance management.

- Reassure that measures are being taken to reverse symptoms (even if the patient appears comatose, he or she may be able to hear).
- Stress that chest discomfort or difficulty breathing should be reported immediately.
- Explore how overdose occurred; discuss how to prevent its reoccurrence.
- If used as an antidote for poisoning, advise avoiding use of organophosphate pesticide compounds for several weeks following episode.

P

prazepam
pray'ze-pam

Centrax

Class: Antianxiety agent, Benzodiazepine

PEDS	PREG	GERI	CONTROLLED SUBSTANCE
✋	D	✋	IV

Action Produces CNS depression and relaxation, and increases seizure threshold by potentiating the action of gamma-aminobuteric acid (GABA), which reduces neuronal activity in all regions of the CNS. Promotes muscle relaxation by inhibiting spinal motor reflex pathways. Decreases anxiety by inhibiting cortical and limbic arousal.

Use/Therapeutic goal/Outcome

Short-term treatment of anxiety: Alleviation of symptoms of apprehension, muscle tension, and insomnia. **Outcome criteria:** Report of feeling more calm, sleeping better, and coping better; observable signs of decreased anxiety (decreased motor activity, reduced muscle tension, decrease in pulse and blood pressure).

Dose range/Administration

Interaction alert: Alcohol and other CNS depressants may cause excessive sedation. Cimetidine increases blood levels.

Adult: PO: 30 mg/day in divided doses (dependent on severity of symptoms; usual range is 20–60 mg/day). **Elderly:** 10–15 mg/day in divided doses.

Clinical alert: May give entire daily dose at bedtime. When discontinuing drug, taper doses gradually, rather than withdrawing abruptly.

Contraindications/Precautions
PREG D

Contraindicated in hypersensitivity or intolerance to prazepam or other benzodiazepines, and in narrow-angle glaucoma, psychosis, and depression. **Use with caution** in suicidal tendencies, or impaired liver or kidney function.

✋ **Contraindicated for pregnant or nursing mothers. Use with caution for the elderly or debilitated. Safe use for children has not been established.**

Side effects/Adverse reactions

Hypersensitivity: rash, exaggeration of side effects. **CNS:** lethargy, drowsiness, headache, dizziness, confusion, ataxia, tremors, depression, paradoxical excitement. **CV:** hypotension, transient tachycardia and bradycardia. **Eye:** blurred vision. **Resp:** respiratory depression. **GI:** dry mouth, nausea, vomiting, diarrhea, constipation. **GU:** urinary retention. **Misc:** drug tolerance and dependence.

Nursing implications/Documentation

Possible nursing diagnoses: Potential for injury; Constipation.

- Record baseline blood pressure; monitor closely if dizziness is experienced. Supervise ambulation until response is determined.
- Be sure that doses are swallowed (not hoarded).
- Provide a quiet environment that is conducive to rest.
- Monitor bowel elimination and provide adequate fluids and fiber to prevent constipation; offer laxatives before the problem is severe.

Patient & family teaching/Home care

Possible nursing diagnoses: Anxiety; Fear; Ineffective individual coping; Impaired home maintenance management.

♦ Help the individual identify stressors that contribute to anxiety and ways of coping effectively; stress that effective coping strategies can reduce the need for medication.

♦ Explain the importance of daily exercise in relieving stress, and encourage establishing a plan for getting enough exercise (e.g., daily walks).

♦ Point out that drug tolerance and dependence can occur, and that the drug should be used on a short-term basis.

♦ Emphasize that the effects of alcohol, other sedatives and CNS depressants, and tranquilizers may be potentiated (these should be avoided).

♦ Advise avoidance of driving and other potentially hazardous activities until response is established.

♦ *See Antianxiety agents/Sedatives/Hypnotics overview for more information.*

prazosin   *pra'zos-sin*

Minipress

Class: Antihypertensive, Alpha adrenergic blocking agent

PEDS	PREG	GERI
♦	C	♦

Action Reduces blood pressure by causing vasodilation of arteriolar and venous smooth muscle by blocking postsynaptic alpha-adrenergic receptors. Decreases systemic resistance and reduces preload and afterload.

Use/Therapeutic goal/Outcome

Hypertension: Reduction of blood pressure. ***Outcome criteria:*** After 4–6 weeks, blood pressure within normal limits.

Congestive heart failure: Resolution of CHF. ***Outcome criteria:*** Clear lung sounds, increased activity tolerance; central venous pressure and pulmonary capillary wedge pressure measurements within normal range; urine output > 30 cc/hr.

Dose range/Administration

Interaction alert: Use with other antihypertensive may cause additive hypotensive effects (particularly propranolol and other beta-blockers). When adding other antihypertensives or diuretics to therapeutic regimen, dose should be decreased to 1–2 mg tid and retitrated.

Adult: PO: 1 mg at bedtime (to avoid first-dose syncope). If tolerated, increase to 1 mg tid and increase slowly as needed. *Maintenance dose:* 6–15 mg/day in 3 divided doses. *Maximum dose:* 20 mg/day in divided doses.

Clinical alert: Be aware of first-dose phenomena (dizziness, weakness, lightheadedness). Monitor for these symptoms 30 minutes to 2 hours after administration. Expect lower doses for the elderly.

Contraindications/Precautions   PREG C

Contraindicated in hypersensitivity to prazosin. ***Use with caution*** in chronic renal failure.

🖐 **Use with caution for the elderly. Safe use for children and pregnant women has not been established.**

Side effects/Adverse reactions

Hypersensitivity: rash, urticaria. ***CV:*** first-dose syncope (very common), orthostatic hypotension, palpitations, fluid retention. ***CNS:*** dizziness, weakness, lightheadedness, drowsiness, headache, depression. ***GI:*** vomiting, diarrhea, abdominal cramps, constipation, nausea. ***Eye:*** blurred vision. ***GU:*** priapism, impotence.

Nursing implications/Documentation

Possible nursing diagnoses: Activity intolerance; Fatigue; Potential for injury.

♦ Assess mental status, and record pulse and blood pressure (lying, sitting, and standing, in both arms) before administration, and frequently thereafter until response is determined.

♦ Consult with physician to determine desired therapeutic range for blood pressure (be aware that some patients may require a slightly elevated blood pressure to perfuse vital organs).

♦ Ascertain that baseline CBC, electrolytes, BUN, uric acid, creatinine, and liver function studies have been obtained before giving first dose; report abnormalities and monitor closely thereafter.

♦ Monitor for allergic reactions and for confusion, dizziness, bradycardia, or hypotension; hold drug and report immediately if these occur.

- Supervise ambulation until response is determined.
- Document and monitor daily weight, and intake and output; report significant negative or positive balance.

Patient & family teaching/Home care

Possible nursing diagnoses: Altered sexuality patterns; Knowledge deficit; Impaired home maintenance management.

- Explain the importance of taking medication exactly as prescribed, even when feeling well; warn about first-dose phenomenon, which is common (see clinical alert).
- Warn that this drug should not be discontinued abruptly.
- Emphasize the importance of good medical follow-up, explain that this drug reduces "wear and tear" on blood vessels, and improves longevity and health.
- Teach how to monitor pulse and blood pressure; stress that syncope, hypertension or hypotension, or persistent dizziness should be reported.
- Advise changing positions slowly to avoid dizziness.
- Encourage daily monitoring of weight and reporting sudden weight gain (frequently is fluid retention).
- Warn against taking *any* OTC drugs without physician approval (some interactions can cause severe reactions); point out that alcohol should be avoided.
- Advise avoiding driving or hazardous activities until response is determined (may cause drowsiness).
- Explain that this drug may affect sexual activity; counsel about concerns.
- *See Antihypertensives overview for more information.*

prednisolone
pred-niss'oh-lone

prednisolone: **Cortalone, Delta-Cortef, ◣Delta-solone, ✦Novoprednisolone, ◣Panafcortelone, Prelone, ◣Solone**

prednisolone acetate: **Articulose, Econopred Ophthalmic, Econopred Plus Ophthalmic, Key-Pred, Niscort, Ocu-Pred A, Predaject, Predalone, Predate, Predcor, Pred-Forte, Predicort, Pred Mild Ophthalmic**

prednisolone sodium phosphate: **Ak-Pred, Codesol, Hydeltrasol, Hydeltrasol Ophthalmic, Inflamase Forte, Inflamase Ophthalmic, Key-Pred-SP, Ocu-Pred, Pediapred, Predate-S, Predicort RP, ◣Predsol Eye Drops, ◣Predsol Retention Enema, ◣Predsol Suppositories**

prednisolone steaglate: **◣Sintisone**

prednisolone tebutate: **Hydeltra-TBA, Metalone-TBA, Nor-Pred TBA, Predalone TBA, Predate TBA, Predcor TBA, Prednisol TBA**

Class: Synthetic adrenocorticosteroid, Intermediate-acting glucocorticoid, Steroidal anti-inflammatory, Immunosuppressant

PEDS	PREG	GERI
✋	C	✋

Action Suppresses inflammation by inhibiting accumulation of inflammatory cells, reducing dilatation and permeability of capillaries, and inhibiting release of chemical mediators of inflammation. Modifies immune response by suppressing cell-mediated immune reactions. Provides physiologic glucocorticoid and mineralocorticoid activity when endogenous hormones are diminished.

Use/Therapeutic goal/Outcome

Adrenal insufficiency: Replacement of deficient endogenous hormones. **Outcome criteria:** Improved appetite, decreased fatigue, normal blood pressure, normal skin color and turgor, report of improved sense of well-being.

Inflammatory or allergic conditions: Symptomatic relief. **Outcome criteria:** Decreased symptoms associated with condition being treated.

Dose range/Administration

Interaction alert: May reduce effectiveness of anticoagulants and antidiabetics. Vaccines may lead to diminished antibody response and serious infection. Potassium-depleting diuretics may cause severe hypokalemia. Alcohol or medications known to cause gastric irritation may cause gastric bleeding. Drugs that increase metabolism of corticosteroids (e.g., phenytoin, barbiturates, ephedrine, and rifampin) and those that decrease its absorption (e.g., cholestyramine, colestipol, and antacids) may decrease prednisolone levels, requiring an increase in prednisolone dosage.

🖐 **Give oral doses with food or milk to minimize gastric irritation.**

Adult: PO: 5–60 mg/day. IM, IV: 4–60 mg/day. *Rectal:* 1 suppository bid or 1 retention enema hs for 2–4 weeks. **Child:** PO: 0.14–2 mg/kg/ day in divided doses tid to qid. IM: 0.14–1 mg/kg q12-24h. **Adult and Child:** *Ophthalmic:* 1–2 gtt bid to q4h. *Otic:* 3–4 gtt bid to tid.

Clinical alert: Give single daily or alternate-day doses in the morning to reduce adrenal suppression. Give IM doses deep into gluteal muscle to lessen muscle atrophy. Give retention enema (available in Australia only) at bedtime. May also be injected directly into joints, soft tissues, or lesions.

Contraindications/Precautions

PREG
C

Contraindicated in hypersensitivity to corticosteroids or to parabens, sulfites, or tartrazine (present in some preparations); and in active peptic ulcer disease, active tuberculosis or fungus infections, and herpes of eyes, lips, or genitals. **Use with caution** in acquired immunodeficiency syndrome (AIDS), hypertension, thrombophlebitis, congestive heart failure, diabetes mellitus, hypothyroidism, glaucoma, osteoporosis, myasthenia gravis, and history of bleeding ulcers, seizure disorder, or mental illness.

🖐 **Use with caution for children, pregnant or nursing mothers, and the elderly.**

Side effects/Adverse reactions

Hypersensitivity: rash, hives, hypotension, respiratory distress, anaphylaxis. **CNS:** euphoria, restlessness, insomnia, hallucinations, depression, psychosis. **Eye:** glaucoma, cataracts. **MS:** impaired growth in children. **CV:** thrombophlebitis, embolism, irregular heartbeat. **GI:** increased appetite, oral candidiasis. **Misc:** hyperglycemia, withdrawal syndrome.

With prolonged use: Skin: acne; increased hair growth; thin, shiny skin; ecchymosis or petechiae; delayed wound healing. **GI:** nausea or vomiting, GI bleeding, pancreatitis. **MS:** osteoporosis; pain in hip, back, ribs, arms, or legs; muscle wasting. **CV:** hypertension, edema, hypokalemia. **GU:** menstrual irregu-

larity. **Misc:** increased susceptibility to infection; Cushingoid appearance (moon-face and buffalo hump); withdrawal syndrome or acute adrenal insufficiency.

Nursing implications/Documentation

Possible nursing diagnoses: Potential for infection; Impaired skin integrity; Impaired physical mobility; Fluid volume excess.

♦ Assess for hypersensitivity reactions, especially with parenteral administration.

♦ Record baseline weight, blood pressure, and electrolyte levels.

♦ Assess and document improvement in condition being treated so dosage can be decreased as early as possible.

♦ Monitor electrolyte levels to detect sodium retention and potassium loss; assess for development of edema and/or muscle weakness and document findings.

♦ Observe for signs of infection and delayed wound healing.

♦ During dose reduction, monitor for signs and symptoms of adrenal insufficiency (hypotension, hypoglycemia, weight loss, vomiting, and diarrhea).

Patient & family teaching/Home care

Possible nursing diagnoses: Knowledge deficit; Impaired home maintenance management; Body image disturbance.

♦ Explain the need to take oral doses with food or milk to minimize gastric irritation.

♦ Advise reporting unusual weight gain, swelling of lower extremities; muscle weakness; black tarry stools; vomiting of blood; epigastric burning; puffing of face; menstrual irregularities; prolonged sore throat, fever, cold, or infections; also caution to report symptoms of adrenal insufficiency (fatigue, anorexia, nausea, vomiting, diarrhea, weight loss, weakness, dizziness, depression, mood swings).

♦ Warn against taking OTC or prescription drugs without consulting primary physician.

♦ Advise against drinking alcohol while taking prednisolone to decrease ulcer potential.

♦ For long-term therapy, advise wearing a medical alert medal indicating need for additional systemic steroids in case of trauma or surgery.

♦ For rectal route (Australia only), demonstrate administration technique; caution to report signs of rectal irritation or infection.

▶

prednisolone 593

- Counsel to adhere to prescribed dose schedule and not to discontinue medication against medical advice.

- Stress the importance of medical follow-up for evaluation of therapy.

- *See Adrenocorticosteroids overview for more information.*

prednisone

pred'ni-sone

♣Apo-Prednisone, Deltasone, Liquid Pred, Meticorten, ♣Novo-prednisone, Orasone, ♠Panafcort, Panasol, Prednicen-M, Prednisone Intensol, ♠Sone, Sterapred, ♣Winpred

Class: Synthetic adrenocorticosteroid, Intermediate-acting glucocorticoid, Steroidal anti-inflammatory, Immunosuppressant

PEDS	PREG	GERI
🖐	C	🖐

Action Suppresses inflammation by inhibiting accumulation of inflammatory cells, reducing dilatation and permeability of capillaries, and inhibiting release of chemical mediators of inflammation. Modifies immune response by suppressing cell-mediated immune reactions.

Use/Therapeutic goal/Outcome

Inflammatory, allergic, and immune conditions: Symptomatic relief. **Outcome criteria:** Decreased symptoms associated with condition being treated.

Dose range/Administration

Interaction alert: May decrease effectiveness of anticoagulants and antidiabetics. Vaccines may lead to diminished antibody response and serious infection. Potassium-depleting diuretics may cause severe hypokalemia. Alcohol or medications known to cause gastric irritation may cause gastric bleeding. Drugs that increase metabolism of corticosteroids (e.g., phenytoin, barbiturates, ephedrine, and rifampin) and those that decrease its absorption (e.g., cholestyramine, colestipol, and antacids) may decrease prednisone levels, requiring an increase in prednisone dosage.

🖐 **Give with food or milk to reduce gastric irritation.**

Inflammatory, allergic, and immune conditions: Adult: PO: 5–60 mg/day. **Child:** PO: 0.14–2 mg/kg/day in divided doses qid.

Multiple sclerosis, acute exacerbations: Adult: PO: 200 mg/day for 1 wk, then 80 mg qod for 1 mo.

Clinical alert: Give single daily or alternate-day doses early in the morning to reduce adrenal suppression. If there is a problem with swallowing, use solution or syrup preparations.

Contraindications/Precautions
PREG
C

Contraindicated in hypersensitivity to corticosteroids and in active peptic ulcer disease, active tuberculosis or fungus infections, and herpes of eyes, lips, or genitals. **Use with caution** in acquired immunodeficiency syndrome (AIDS), hypertension, thrombophlebitis, congestive heart failure, diabetes mellitus, hypothyroidism, glaucoma, osteoporosis or myasthenia gravis and history of bleeding ulcers, seizure disorder, or mental illness.

🖐 **Use with caution for children, pregnant or nursing mothers, and the elderly.**

Side effects/Adverse reactions

Hypersensitivity: rash, hives, hypotension, respiratory distress, anaphylaxis. **CNS:** euphoria, restlessness, insomnia, hallucinations, depression, or psychosis. **Eye:** glaucoma, cataracts. **MS:** impaired growth in children. **CV:** thrombophlebitis, embolism, irregular heartbeat. **GI:** increased appetite, oral candidiasis. **Misc:** hyperglycemia, withdrawal syndrome.

With prolonged use: Skin: acne; increased hair growth; thin, shiny skin; ecchymosis or petechiae; delayed wound healing. **GI:** nausea or vomiting, GI bleeding, pancreatitis. **MS:** osteoporosis; pain in hip, back, ribs, arms, or legs; muscle wasting. **CV:** hypertension, edema, hypokalemia. **GU:** menstrual irregularity. **Misc:** increased susceptibility to infection; Cushingoid appearance (moon-face and buffalo hump); withdrawal syndrome or acute adrenal insufficiency.

Nursing implications/Documentation

Possible nursing diagnoses: Impaired tissue integrity; Body image disturbance; Impaired physical mobility.

- Assess for hypersensitivity reactions, especially with parenteral administration.

- Record baseline weight, blood pressure, and electrolyte levels.

- Assess and document improvement in condition being treated, so dosage can be decreased as early as possible.

- Monitor laboratory findings; and report and record signs of sodium and fluid retention or potassium depletion.
- Observe for signs of infection or delayed wound healing.
- Assess for withdrawal symptoms (hypotension, hypoglycemia, weight loss, vomiting, and diarrhea) while tapering or discontinuing drug.

Patient & family teaching/Home care

Possible nursing diagnoses: Knowledge deficit; Impaired home maintenance management; Fluid volume excess; Potential for infection.

- Explain the need to take oral doses with food or milk.
- Advise reporting unusual weight gain; swelling of lower extremities; muscle weakness; black tarry stools; vomiting of blood; epigastric burning; puffing of face; menstrual irregularities; prolonged sore throat, fever, cold, or infections.
- Advise against taking OTC or prescription drugs without consulting primary physician.
- For long-term therapy, encourage to wear medical alert identification indicating need for supplemental systemic steroids in case of trauma or surgery.
- With dose reduction or withdrawal of drug, teach how to recognize symptoms of adrenal insufficiency (fatigue, anorexia, nausea, vomiting, diarrhea, weight loss, weakness, dizziness, depression, and mood swings); stress that these should be reported.
- Counsel adhering to prescribed dose schedule and not discontinuing medication against medical advice.
- *See Adrenocorticosteroids overview for more information.*

primidone

pri'mi-done

Apo-Primidone, Myldone, Mysoline, Sertan
Class: Anticonvulsant

PEDS	PREG	GERI
✋	**D**	✋

Action Limits the spread of seizure activity and increases the threshold for nerve cell stimulation. Precise anticonvulsant mechanism of action is unknown; may block the active transport of ions across the cell membrane. Phenobarbital is an active metabolite and may contribute to primidone's action.

Use/Therapeutic goal/Outcome

Grand mal and psychomotor seizures: Prevention and limitation of seizure activity. **Outcome criteria:** Marked decrease or absence of, seizure activity.

Dose range/Administration

Interaction alert: Alcohol and other CNS depressants may cause excessive sedation. If given with valproic acid, MAO inhibitors, or carbamazepine, monitor for increased toxicity. If given with phenytoin, monitor for increased phenobarbital effect (phenytoin stimulates metabolism of primidone).

🥄 Give with food if GI symptoms are noted.

Adult/Child > 8 yrs: PO: 125–250 mg daily. May increase by 125 mg weekly, to a maximum of 2 g/day in divided doses qid. **Child < 8 yrs:** PO: 50 mg daily. May increase by 50 mg weekly, to a maximum of 1 g/day in divided doses qid.

Clinical alert: Give single doses or larger doses at bedtime.

Contraindications/Precautions

PREG **D**

Contraindicated in hypersensitivity to phenobarbital or barbiturates, and in porphyria. **Use with caution** in chronic lung disease, and liver or kidney disease.

🖐 Use with caution for children (especially hyperactive children) and the elderly. Safe use for pregnant women has not been established (risks must be weighed against benefits). Mothers taking this drug should not nurse their infants.

Side effects/Adverse reactions

Hypersensitivity: rash, lupus-like syndrome. **CNS:** lethargy, ataxia, vertigo, irritability, headache, excitability in children, confusion, emotional disturbances, and acute psychosis. **GI:** nausea and vomiting. **Hem:** leukopenia, eosinophilia. **Eye:** diplopia, nystagmus, periorbital edema. **Skin:** alopecia. **GU:** impotence.

Nursing implications/Documentation

Possible nursing diagnoses: Potential for injury; Potential for aspiration.

- Document history of seizures (type, frequency, duration, usual time they occur, precipitating factors, presence of an aura); initiate seizure precautions as indicated.

- Monitor serum drug levels periodically to assure therapeutic range (5–15 mcg/ml of primidone, and 15–40 mcg/ml of phenobarbital).

- Check CBC and serum chemistries at least every 6 months.

- Monitor for excessive drowsiness and hemorrhage in newborns of mothers taking primidone.

Patient & family teaching/Home care

Possible nursing diagnoses: Fear; Self-esteem disturbance; Knowledge deficit; Impaired home maintenance management.

- Advise taking this drug with meals if GI symptoms are noted.

- Explain that full therapeutic effect may not be seen for several weeks.

- Stress the need for close medical follow-up; emphasize that persistent fatigue, weakness, fever, sore throat, mouth ulcers, gum inflammation, and infections are signs of side effects that should be reported.

- Warn that stopping anticonvulsants suddenly can cause an increase in severity and frequency of seizures.

- Advise wearing a medic alert bracelet and notifying dentist and other physicians that primidone is being taken.

- Teach significant others—and have them demonstrate—how to protect the individual should a seizure occur.

- Caution against driving until response is determined.

- *See Anticonvulsants overview for more information.*

probenecid

pro-ben'e-sid

Benemid, Benn, ✦Benuryp, Probalan, Robenecid

Class: ★**Uricosuric prototype**, Antigout, Antihyperuricemic, Anti-inflammatory

PEDS	PREG	GERI
🖐	B	🖐

Action Reduces serum levels of uric acid by inhibiting its reabsorption in renal tubules. Inhibits renal excretion of penicillins and other antibiotics.

Use/Therapeutic goal/Outcome

Gouty arthritis: Prevention or reduction of urate deposits in joints. **Outcome criteria:** Decreased serum uric acid levels; reduced frequency and severity of gout attacks; decreased joint deformities.

Adjunct to antibiotic therapy: Increased and prolonged concentrations of antibiotic. **Outcome criteria:** Absence of signs and symptoms of infection; absence of pathogenic growth on cultures; antibiotic serum levels within therapeutic range.

Dose range/Administration

Interaction alert: Aspirin, other salicylates, thiazide diuretics, ethacrynic acid, and antineoplastic agents may decrease effectiveness. Probenecid may increase the effects of sulfonylurea-type oral hypoglycemic drugs, acyclovir, anti-inflammatory agents, penicillins, cephalosporins, clofibrate, heparin, indomethacin, methotrexate, rifampin, and sulfonamides.

🍴 **Give with food or milk.**

Gout: Adult: PO: 250 mg bid for 1 wk, then 500 mg bid.

Antibiotic adjunct: Adult: PO: 500 mg qid. **Child:** PO: 25 mg/kg, then 10 mg/kg qid.

Clinical alert: Colchicine may be administered prophylactically during the first 3–6 months of treatment with probenecid because of the increased possibility of acute attacks of gout.

Contraindications/Precautions

PREG
B

Contraindicated in hypersensitivity to probenecid, and in acute gout attacks, blood dyscrasias, uric acid kidney stones, and neoplastic disease (especially with radiation or chemotherapy). **Use with caution** in history of peptic ulcer and in impaired renal function.

🖐 **Contraindicated for children under 2 years and nursing mothers. Use with caution for older children, pregnant women, and the elderly.**

Side effects/Adverse reactions

Hypersensitivity: dermatitis, pruritus, fever, sweating, hypotension, and anaphylactic reaction. **GI:** nausea, vomiting, diarrhea, sore throat. **GU:** painful or bloody urination, uric acid renal stones, scanty urine. **Hem:** blood dyscrasias. **CNS:** headache.

Nursing implications/Documentation

Possible nursing diagnoses: Pain; Altered urinary elimination.

- Encourage fluid intake to produce urinary output of at least 2 L daily to prevent uric acid stone formation.

- Monitor and record intake and output.
- Expect that medications to maintain urine alkalinity (e.g., sodium bicarbonate or potassium citrate) will be ordered to prevent urinary stone formation.
- Monitor results of renal function studies since probenecid is not effective in decreased renal function.
- Assess for flank pain, blood in urine, or decreased urine volume, which may indicate stone formation (the elderly are especially prone to this).

Patient & family teaching/Home care

Possible nursing diagnoses: Knowledge deficit; Impaired home maintenance management; Pain.

- Inform that use of probenecid may increase the frequency of acute attacks of gout during the first 6–12 months of therapy, but that eventually attacks will become less severe and of shorter duration.
- Advise that probenecid has no effect on pain and inflammation of gout, and to continue anti-inflammatory drug therapy while symptoms are present.
- Stress the need to drink at least 8–12 8-oz glasses of fluids daily.
- Advise avoidance of Vitamin C preparations and cranberry juice, which acidify urine and encourage renal stone formation.
- Encourage to have scheduled blood tests done as ordered.
- Warn against using alcoholic beverages, aspirin, and caffeine, which increase the amount of uric acid in the blood.
- Explain that probenecid may be taken for an indefinite period to maintain low uric acid levels.
- Advise that flank pain or bloody or darkened urine should be reported.
- Inform diabetics that probenecid may cause false positive results with Clinitest, but will not interfere with Clinistix.
- Warn those taking oral hypoglycemics that probenecid may increase hypoglycemic effects.

probucol

proe-byoo'kole

Lorelco, ♣*Lurselle*

Class: Antilipemic

PEDS	PREG	GERI
✋	C	✋

Action Reduces serum cholesterol levels by interfering with cholesterol transport from intestine; may also decrease cholesterol synthesis. Increases excretion of bile acids in feces. Reduces levels of high-density lipoproteins (HDL) and low-density lipoproteins (LDL).

Use/Therapeutic goal/Outcome

Primary hypercholesterolemia (type): Reduction of serum cholesterol levels. **Outcome criteria:** Decreased serum cholesterol levels within 1 to 3 months of the initiation of therapy.

Dose range/Administration

Interaction alert: Use with clofibrate not recommended.

🥄 **Give with morning and evening meals to enhance absorption.**

Adult: PO: 500 mg bid.

Clinical alert: Hold drug and report if EKG shows prolonged QT interval. Discontinue if there is no improvement after 3 months.

Contraindications/Precautions

PREG
C

Contraindicated in hypersensitivity to the drug. **Avoid use** with antiarrhythmics that may prolong QT interval and in patients whose baseline QT interval is long. **Use with caution** in the presence of recent myocardial damage, unexplained syncope, or liver disease.

✋ **Contraindicated for pregnant or nursing mothers. Use with caution for the elderly. Safe use for children has not been established.**

Side effects/Adverse reactions

Hypersensitivity: dizziness and palpitations. **GI:** GI bleeding, indigestion, flatulence, anorexia, bloating, diarrhea, nausea, vomiting, stomach pain. **CV:** prolonged QT interval on EKG, palpitations, chest pain, arrhythmias. **CNS:** headache, dizziness, paresthesias. **Hem:** eosinophilia, thrombocytopenia, decreased hemoglobin and hematocrit. **Eye:** visual disturbances. **GU:** impotence, nocturia. **Skin:** rash. **Misc:** diminished sense of taste and smell.

▶

Nursing implications/Documentation

Possible nursing diagnoses: Diarrhea; Altered nutrition: more than body requirements.

◆ Monitor for and report persistent GI symptoms or diarrhea.

◆ Observe for and report pulse irregularities or unexplained syncope; drug may have to be discontinued.

◆ Establish a baseline EKG (measure PR, QRS, and ST segments) and monitor periodically during therapy, especially for prolongation of QT interval.

Patient & family teaching/Home care

Possible nursing diagnoses: Altered health maintenance; Knowledge deficit; Impaired home maintenance management.

◆ Explain that the purpose of this drug is to reduce serum cholesterol and to decrease the risk of cardiovascular disease.

◆ Stress the need to take this drug with morning and evening meal for increased absorption.

◆ Emphasize the need to reduce other cardiac risk factors (obesity, smoking, high cholesterol diet, sedentary lifestyle), and help develop a plan to reduce these.

◆ Reinforce that this drug will have to be taken for a long time, and that ongoing medical follow-up of cholesterol level and liver function studies is essential.

◆ Stress that dizziness or fainting should be reported immediately.

◆ *See Antilipemics overview for more information.*

procainamide   *pro-kay'na-mide*

procainamide hydrochloride: *Procamide, Procan, Procan SR, Promine, Pronestyl, Pronestyl SR, Rhythmin, Sub-Quin*

Class: Antiarrhythmic (Class IA)

PEDS	PREG	GERI
🖐	C	🖐

Action Suppresses atrial and ventricular ectopy by increasing the effective refractory period, decreasing conduction velocity, and depressing excitability in the atria, His-Purkinje system, and ventricles. Has vagolytic and peripheral vasodilating properties. Myocardial contractility and cardiac output is not affected except when myocardial damage exists.

Use/Therapeutic goal/Outcome

PVCs, ventricular tachycardia, atrial fibrillation and tachycardias: Suppression of atrial and ventricular ectopy and promotion of effective heartbeat. *Outcome criteria:* Absence of or decrease in atrial and ventricular ectopy; regular palpable pulse.

Dose range/Administration

Interaction alert: Monitor for toxicity if given with cimetidine or amiodarone. May enhance action of neuromuscular blocking agents.

🍴 **Give with meals if GI distress is noted.**

PVCs and ventricular tachycardia: **Adult:** PO: Begin with 1–1.25 g, then 6.25 mg/kg q3h. *Maintenance dose:* 250–500 mg q3-4h, not to exceed 3.0 g in 24 hr. *Sustained release preparation:* 500 mg to 1 g q6h. IV: 50–100 mg q 5 min, at a rate not exceeding 50 mg/min until arrhythmia subsides, side effects develop, or a total of 1 g is given. *To prepare IV infusion,* add 1 g procainamide to 250 cc D5W. Recommended infusion rate is 2–6 mg/min via IV pump.

Atrial fibrillation and supraventricular tachycardia: **Adult:** PO: Begin with 1.25 g; then 750 mg in 1 hr if no EKG changes, then 500 mg to 1 g q2h until arrhythmia subsides. *Maintenance dose:* 500 mg to 1 g q6h. IM: 500 mg to 1 g q4-8h. IV: Use dose for PVCs and ventricular tachycardia.

Clinical alert: Continuous cardiac monitoring is recommended when intravenous route is used. Watch for and report widening of QRS complex or hypotension (the elderly are especially at risk; occurrence of hypotension increases with rapid injection). Have resuscitative equipment nearby.

Contraindications/Precautions   PREG C

Contraindicated in hypersensitivity to procainamide and amide-type anesthetics, and in advanced heart blocks (unless a pacemaker is present), torsades de pointes, and history or presence of systemic lupus erythematosus (SLE). *Use with caution* in myasthenia gravis, and reduce dose in CHF (may significantly affect contractility), and renal impairment.

🖐 **Reduce dose in the elderly (hypotension more likely). Safe use for children and pregnant or nursing mothers has not been established.**

Side effects/Adverse reactions

Hypersensitivity: itching, rash, lupus-like syndrome (fever, cough, joint pain, presence of antinuclear antibodies). *Hem:* blood dyscrasias, including neutropenia and agranulocytosis. *CV:* hypotension, bradycardia, widening of the QRS complex and prolongation of QT and PR intervals, ventricular arrhythmias. *GI:* nausea, vomiting, anorexia, diarrhea, bitter taste. *CNS:* giddiness, psychosis, hallucinations, depression and syncope.

Nursing implications/Documentation

Possible nursing diagnoses: Potential for injury; Activity intolerance.

♦ Be sure to check baseline chest X ray, EKG, and laboratory studies (CBC, sodium, potassium, chloride, carbon dioxide, magnesium, BUN, creatinine, SGPT, and LDH) before giving first dose; monitor closely thereafter as indicated by clinical condition.

♦ Remember that oxygen requirements must be met, and that electrolyte imbalances (especially potassium and magnesium) and abnormal blood pH must be corrected, before expected antiarrhythmic effect can be seen; report abnormalities immediately.

♦ Document baseline vital signs, lung sounds, and cardiac monitor strip (measure and record PR, and QRS segments) before giving first dose and at least every 8 hr; monitor closely until response is determined; report if prolongation in PR or QRS segment is noted (drug should be stopped or dosage decreased if QRS complex widens greater than 25 percent of if PR interval is prolonged greater than 50 percent).

♦ When therapy is prolonged, be aware that periodic blood work (ANA titer, CBC, and hepatic and renal profiles) is necessary.

♦ When giving IV, monitor closely for hypotension; report a blood pressure reductions of 15 mm Hg or more.

♦ Be aware that the procainamide metabolite N-acetylprocainamide (NAPA) is also an antiarrhythmic, and that it has a longer half-life than procainamide.

♦ Coordinate care to provide frequent rest periods.

Patient & family teaching/Home care

Possible nursing diagnoses: Fear; Knowledge deficit; Impaired home maintenance management.

♦ Explain that the purpose of this drug is to prevent arrhythmias and promote an effective heartbeat.

♦ Advise taking oral doses with meals if GI symptoms are noted.

♦ Stress the need to follow dose regimen closely (the drug should be taken at the same time each day), and the need to return for medical follow-up for early detection of adverse reactions.

♦ Teach how to assess pulse for irregularities in rhythm and rate; stress that these irregularities be reported.

♦ Advise that symptoms of fever, joint pain or stiffness, chest pain, and sore mouth, gums, or throat should be reported immediately.

♦ Emphasize the need to pace activities, avoid stress, and plan for rest periods.

♦ Encourage learning CPR; reinforce that survival rate of cardiac arrest is greatly increased when CPR is initiated immediately.

♦ *See Antiarrhythmic overview for more information.*

procaine
proe'kane

procaine hydrochloride: *Novocain*
Class: Local anesthetic (ester-type)

PEDS	PREG	GERI
✋	C	✋

Action Produces local anesthesia by inhibiting sodium flux across the nerve cell membrane, thus preventing depolarization and generation and conduction of nerve impulses. Procaine has a rapid onset (2–5 min), is short-acting (60 min), and has low potency and toxicity. When combined with epinephrine, action is prolonged.

Use/Therapeutic goal/Outcome

Local infiltration, and spinal and epidural anesthesia when short duration is desired: Prevention of pain during surgical procedures. *Outcome criteria:* Patient report of numbness and absence of pain in anesthetized area. Patients receiving epidural anesthesia will demonstrate temporary loss of motor function in the anesthetized area.

Dose range/Administration

Adult: *Epidural block*: Up to 375 mg (25 cc) 1.5% solution. *Local infiltration*: 250–600 mg 0.25–0.5% solution. Maximum first dose is 1 g, dose and interval may be increased with epinephrine. *Perineal block*: Inject 0.5 cc 10% solution diluted with an equal volume of diluent. *Perineal and lower extremity block*: Inject 1 cc 10% solution diluted with an equal volume of diluent. *Peripheral nerve block*: Up to 500 mg 1% solution *or* 2% solution. *Spinal block*: Up to 11 mg/kg, 14 mg/kg with epinephrine. Dilute 10% solution with NS or sterile water for injection or CSF. If using hyperbaric technique, use dextrose solution.

Clinical alert: This drug should be administered only by clinicians thoroughly familiar with its use. Dose is highly individualized, depending on the procedure, method of administration, area to be anesthetized, vascularity of tissues, patient condition, tolerance, and response. Preparations with epinephrine may result in angina, tachycardia, tremors, headache, restlessness, palpitations, dizziness, and hypertension. Have oxygen and resuscitative drugs and equipment readily available.

Contraindications/Precautions

PREG
C

Contraindicated in hypersensitivity to procaine, other ester-type anesthetics or to PABA, and in generalized septicemia, inflammation or sepsis at proposed injection site; cerebrospinal disease, heart block, hypotension, hypertension, bowel pathology, and GI hemorrhage. *Use with caution* for debilitated or acutely ill patients; increased intra-abdominal pressure, known drug allergies and sensitivities, dysrhythmias, and shock.

🖐 Use with caution for the elderly. Safe use in women with childbearing potential and in early pregnancy has not been established.

Side effects/Adverse reactions

Hypersensitivity: rashes, cutaneous lesions of delayed onset, urticaria, pruritis, angioneurotic edema, sweating, syncope, anaphylaxis. *CNS:* anxiety, nervousness, dizziness, tinnitus, circumoral paresthesia, blurred vision, tremors, drowsiness, sedation, convulsions, respiratory arrest. *CV:* myocardial depression, arrhythmias, bradycardia, fetal bradycardia, hypotension. *GI:* nausea, vomiting.

Nursing implications/Documentation

Possible nursing diagnoses: Pain; Potential for injury.

♦ Be sure that history of allergies and accurate height and weight are recorded before procedure.

♦ Record vital signs according to protocol, and monitor for and report immediately signs of systemic or hypersensitivity reactions.

♦ Report blood pressure reduction of 25% of preanesthetic measurement immediately (requires intervention of putting in head-down position with legs raised to promote venous return, and administration of fluids and medications to increase cardiac output).

♦ If epinephrine has been added, monitor for arrhythmias.

♦ Determine with anesthesiologist or anesthetist whether there are any restrictions on patient positioning; post these at bedside.

♦ Monitor anesthetized area for level of sensation and motor function; watch for poor positioning and protect area from injury.

♦ Give prescribed pain medication as sensation begins to return, **before pain is too severe**.

Patient & family teaching/Home care

Possible nursing diagnoses: Anxiety; Fear.

♦ Stress the need to protect areas of the body that have lost sensation.

♦ Explain rationale for taking prescribed pain medication before pain becomes too uncomfortable.

♦ *See Local anesthetics overview for more information.*

procarbazine
pro-kar' ba-zeen

procarbazine hydrochloride: *Matulane,* ✦ ✦*Natulan*

Class: Antineoplastic agent, Monoamine oxidase (MAO) inhibitor

PEDS PREG GERI
🖐   D   🖐

Action Kills rapidly growing cells (cancer, hair follicles, bone marrow, GI lining, ova, and sperm) by interfering with the synthesis of DNA, RNA, and protein, causing disruption of nucleic acid function. Is cell-cycle–phase specific for S phase of cell division.

Use/Therapeutic goal/Outcome

Hodgkin's disease and non-Hodgkin's lymphomas, brain and lung tumors, and mycosis fungoides: Elimination or suppression of malignant cell proliferation. *Outcome criteria:* Tumor and disease regression or stabilization on radiologic and physical examination.

Dose range/Administration

Interaction alert: Barbiturates, antihistamines, antihypertensives, phenothiazines, and narcotics may increase CNS depression. Avoid use with meperidine hydrochloride (may cause severe hypotension and death). Lowers plasma digoxin levels. Tricyclic antidepressants, tyramine foods, alcohol, sympathomimetics, and local anesthetics may cause disulfiram-like reactions (respiratory depression, chest pains, palpitations, shock, convulsions, and death). Antidiabetics may cause increased hypoglycemia. Do not give with other MAOIs.

🖐 **Give with food or fluids if GI distress is present.**

Adult: PO: 2–4 mg/kg/day for 7 days, then 4–6 mg/kg/day until WBC < 4000/mm^3 or platelets < 100,000/mm^3, or maximum response is obtained. *Maintenance dose:* (after bone marrow recovery) 1–2 mg/kg/day. *Child:* PO: 50 mg/m^2/day for 1 week, then 100 mg/m^2 until desired response or toxicity occurs. *Maintenance dose:* (after bone marrow recovery) 50 mg/m^2/day.

Clinical alert: To reduce nausea, give in divided doses or at bedtime. **This drug is a potent carcinogen and may cause acute leukemia.** It is almost always used in combination chemotherapy with nitrogen mustard, vincristine, and prednisone. Recognize that this drug is an MAO inhibitor and can cause serious or fatal hypertensive crisis if taken with foods high in tyramine or tryptophan (aged cheese, wine, beer, chicken livers, avocados, chocolate, bananas, soy sauce, meat tenderizer, bologna, salami). These foods must be avoided during therapy and for 14 days after discontinuation of therapy.

Contraindications/Precautions

PREG
D

Contraindicated in hypersensitivity to procarbazine, and in inadequate bone marrow reserve, low CBC, and concurrent use with MAOIs. *Use with caution* in leukopenia, thrombocytopenia, anemia, hepatic and renal impairment, diabetes, or infection.

✋ **Contraindicated for pregnant or nursing mothers. Use with caution for children and the elderly.**

Side effects/Adverse reactions

Hypersensitivity: rash, urticaria, wheezing, hypotension, tachycardia. *Hem:* bone marrow depression 2–3 weeks after drug is stopped (leukopenia, anemia, thrombocytopenia, bleeding tendencies). *GI:* severe nausea and vomiting, stomatitis, dry mouth, dysphagia, diarrhea, hepatotoxicity, constipation. *CV:* orthostatic hypotension. *CNS:* paresthesia, neuropathies, hallucinations, depression, confusion, convulsions, insomnia, nightmares. *Resp:* pneumonitis, pleural effusion. *GU:* azoospermia, amenorrhea. *Skin:* hyperpigmentation, dermatitis, alopecia. *Eye:* retinal hemorrhage, photophobia, nystagmus.

Nursing implications/Documentation

Possible nursing diagnoses: Potential for infection; Potential for injury; Fatigue; Altered oral mucous membrane; Fluid volume deficit; Diarrhea; Altered nutrition: less than body requirements.

♦ *See important Nursing implications in Antineoplastic agents overview on page 72, which apply to all neoplastics. The interventions that follow are additional and specific to this drug only.*

♦ Monitor for and report early signs of CNS toxicity (muscle weakness, numbness or tingling of the lower extremities, wristdrop, footdrop, coordination problems).

♦ Prevent constipation by increasing activity and intake of fluid and fiber (give stool softeners and/or laxatives before problem is severe).

♦ Document and monitor intake and output; prevent kidney complications by maintaining adequate hydration.

♦ Expect that WBC, platelet, and erythrocyte counts should drop to the nadir (lowest point) in 2–8 weeks.

Patient & family teaching/Home care

Possible nursing diagnoses: Knowledge deficit; Ineffective coping (individual and family); Hopelessness; Impaired home maintenance management.

♦ *See important Patient & family teaching in Antineoplastic agents overview on page 72, which apply to all neoplastics. The teachings that follow are additional and specific to this drug only.*

♦ Provide a list of foods and beverages that must be avoided (see Clinical alert).

♦ Warn that constipation should be prevented by adequate activity and intake of fluid and fiber (and use of laxatives if necessary).

♦ Advise reporting muscle weakness, wristdrop, footdrop, numbness or tingling of the legs and feet, or problems with coordination.

- Stress that alcohol and CNS depressants may cause excessive drowsiness.
- Warn against driving or other hazardous activities until response is established.
- *See Antineoplastic agents overview for more information.*

prochlorperazine
proe-klor-per'a-zeen

prochlorperazine: *Compazine,* ♠ ♣*Stemetil*

prochlorperazine edisylate: *Compazine*

prochlorperazine maleate: ♠*Anti-Naus, Chlorpazine, Compazine,* ♠ ♣*Stemetil*

Class: Antiemetic, Psychotropic, Antipsychotic, Phenothiazine

PEDS	PREG	GERI
🖐	B	🖐

Action Relieves and prevents nausea and vomiting by acting on the chemoreceptor trigger zone in the brain.

Use/Therapeutic goal/Outcome

Nausea or vomiting: Prevention or resolution. *Outcome criteria:* Report of absence of, or reduction in, feelings of nausea; absence of vomiting.

Dose range/Administration

Interaction alert: Never mix in a syringe with another drug. Because of CNS depressant effects, may increase effects of other CNS depressants and alcohol. Increases the effects of anticholinergic drugs (may increase parkinson-like side effects). Separate antacid doses and prochlorperazine doses by at least 2 hr (antacid may inhibit absorption).

📙 **Give doses 30 min before meals.**

Adult: PO: *Tablet, oral solution:* 5–10 mg tid or qid. *Extended release:* 10 mg bid or 15 mg/day upon arising. IM: 5–10 mg q4h prn. *Maximum dose:* 40 mg. RECT: 25 mg bid. *Child:* RECT, PO: *For weight 9–13 kg:* 2.5 mg qd or bid (not over 7.5 mg/day). *For weight 14–17 kg:* 2.5 mg bid or tid (not over 10 mg/day). *For weight 18–19 kg:* 2.5 mg tid (not over 15 mg/day). *Child > 2 yrs:* IM: 0.13 mg/kg in a single dose.

Clinical alert: Dermatitis may result from skin contact with liquid forms. Give the elderly lower dose range because they are very sensitive to effects. Since drug has a long duration of action, there is little advantage to using time release form.

Contraindications/Precautions

Contraindicated in hypersensitivity to prochlorperazine or other phenothazines, and in narrow-angle glaucoma, coma, CNS depression, subcortical damage, bone marrow depression, during pediatric surgery, in conjunction with spinal or epidural anesthetic or adrenergic blockers, and in use with alcohol. *Use with caution* in liver disease, cardiovascular disease (may cause hypotension), CNS depression, respiratory disorders, hypocalcemia, prostatic hypertrophy, or intestinal obstruction.

🖐 **Contraindicated for children who may have Reye's syndrome (because of hepatotoxicity). Use with caution for other children and the elderly or debilitated. Safe use for pregnant or nursing mothers has not been established.**

Side effects/Adverse reactions

Hypersensitivity: extrapyramidal reactions, tardive dyskinesia (slow rhythmical, automatic stereotyped muscle movements, particularly in the elderly), rashes, exfoliative dermatitis. *CNS:* drowsiness, pseudoparkinsonism, dizziness, EEG changes. *CV:* tachycardia, EKG changes, orthostatic hypotension. *Eye:* ocular changes, dry eyes, blurred vision. *GI:* dry mouth, constipation, ileus, hepatitis. *GU:* dark urine, urinary retention, irregular menses, inhibited ejaculation. *Hem:* hyperprolactinemia. *Skin:* photosensitivity with pigment changes. *Misc:* gynecomastia.

Nursing implications/Documentation

Possible nursing diagnoses: Potential for injury; Constipation; Fluid volume deficit; Altered oral mucous membrane.

- Assess for presence of bowel sounds, pain, nausea, or vomiting before and after administering antiemetics; hold drug and report if bowel sounds are absent.
- Determine cause of symptoms before giving prochlorperazine; ascertain that nausea and vomiting symptoms are not due to intestinal obstruction, increased intracranial pressure, or drug overdosage before giving first dose.
- Give IM doses deep into large muscle mass, never give SC.
- Dilute oral solution with fruit juice, milk, pudding, or other beverage.
- If therapy is prolonged, monitor CBC and liver function studies.
- Observe for orthostatic hypotension, tachycardia, drowsiness, and eye problems, until response is determined.

• Notify physician if person experiences extrapyramidal side effects or tardive dyskinesia (slow, rhythmic, automatic, stereotyped movements), or if more than 4 doses are required in a 24 hr period.

• Offer frequent mouth care.

• Supervise ambulation until response is determined.

• Document and monitor intake and output to detect dehydration.

• Monitor bowel movements to detect constipation; provide adequate fluids and fiber.

• When able to tolerate liquids, begin with small amount of ice chips, then water, then clear liquids, then full liquids, then food.

Patient & family teaching/Home care

Possible nursing diagnoses: Knowledge deficit; Impaired home maintenance management.

• Teach that doses should be taken 30 min before meals and at bedtime.

• Stress that slow rhythmic movements, difficulty with coordination, or persistent nausea, vomiting, or abdominal discomfort should be reported.

• Explain that avoiding fatty foods and eating smaller and more frequent meals may reduce nausea.

• Advise against use of alcohol or other CNS depressants; warn against driving or activities that require mental alertness until response is determined.

• Emphasize the need to maintain good mouth care, especially when not taking liquids by mouth; suggest that chewing sugarless gum may relieve symptoms of dry mouth.

• *See Antiemetics overview for more information.*

procyclidine   *proe-sye'kli-deen*

procyclidine hydrochloride: *Kemadrin, ♥PMS Procyclidine, ♥Procyclid*

Class: Anticholinergic, Cholinergic blocker (parasympatholytic)

Antidote: Physostigmine

PEDS	PREG	GERI
♨	C	♨

Action Reduces muscle rigidity by blocking excess CNS cholinergic activity associated with dopamine deficiency in basal ganglia. Also has some peripheral anticholinergic action.

Use/Therapeutic goal/Outcome

Parkinsonism: Reduction of muscle rigidity, promotion of mobility. *Outcome criteria:* Absence of or decrease in rigidity, akinesia, and drooling; improvement in gait, balance, and posture.

Dose range/Administration

🍴 **Give with or after meals to minimize GI side effects.**

Adult: PO: 2–2.5 mg tid; increase prn. *Maximum dose:* 60 mg/day.

Contraindications/Precautions
PREG
C

Contraindicated in hypersensitivity to procyclidine and in narrow-angle glaucoma. *Use with caution* in tachycardia, hypotension, and prostatic hypertrophy.

🖐 **Use with caution for the elderly. Safe use for children and pregnant or nursing mothers has not been established.**

Side effects/Adverse reactions

Hypersensitivity: rash. *GI:* dry mouth, constipation, nausea, vomiting, epigastric distress. *CNS:* lightheadedness, mental confusion. *Eye:* blurred vision, mydriasis. *CV:* palpitations. *GU:* urinary retention.

Nursing implications/Documentation

Possible nursing diagnoses: Potential for injury; Urinary retention; Constipation.

• Have patient void before doses; monitor intake and output because this drug can cause voiding difficulties.

• Record status of Parkinson symptoms daily.

• Monitor the elderly and debilitated for increased incidence of side effects; document and report changes in mental status.

• Relieve dry mouth by providing frequent mouth care and keeping ice chips at the bedside.

• Monitor for constipation; provide adequate fluids and fiber (laxatives and/or stool softeners should be given before problem is severe).

Patient & family teaching/Home care

Possible nursing diagnoses: Knowledge deficit; Impaired home maintenance management.

• Stress that taking this drug with food helps reduce GI symptoms.

• Explain that as spasticity resolves, tremors may increase.

- Warn that this drug may cause drowsiness and dizziness; caution to change position slowly.

- Advise against driving until response is determined.

◆ *See Anticholinergics overview for more information.*

promethazine

pro-meth'a-zeen

promethazine hydrochloride: *Anergan 25, Anergan 50,* ♥*Histanil, K-Phen, Mallergan, Pentazine, Phenameth, Phenazine 25, Phenazine 50, Phencen-50, Phenergan, Phenergan-Fortis, Phenergan-Plain, Phenoject-50,* ♥*PMS-Promethazine, Prometh-25, Prometh-50, Promethegan,* ♠*Prothazine, Prothazine-25, Prothazine-50, Prothazine Plain, Remsed, V-Gan-25, V-Gan-50*

Class: Antihistamine (H₁ receptor antagonist), Antiemetic, Phenothiazine, Antivertigo agent, Sedative-hypnotic

PEDS	PREG	GERI
✋	C	✋

Action Prevents but does not reverse histamine-mediated allergic responses by competing with histamine for H₁ receptor sites on effector cells. Antiemetic action is probably due to depression of the chemoreceptor trigger zone. Produces sedation by depressing the CNS.

Use/Therapeutic goal/Outcome

Sedation: Promotion of relaxation or sleep. *Outcome criteria:* Report of feeling relaxed or having rested well; observable signs of relaxation or sleep (eyes closed, decreased restlessness, relaxed facial expression).

Nausea, motion sickness: Prevention of nausea. *Outcome criteria:* Report of absence of nausea.

Allergic conditions: Decrease in allergic response. *Outcome criteria:* Report and demonstration of an absence or decrease in allergic symptoms (nasal secretions, sneezing, itching).

Dose range/Administration

Interaction alert: CNS depressants and alcohol may cause excessive drowsiness and sedation. Do not give with other phenothiazines because of additive effects. Do not give with MAOIs because of potentially severe side effects.

🖤 **Give with milk or food to avoid GI upset.**

Sedation: **Adult:** PO, RECT, IM, IV: 25–50 mg q4-6h prn, at bedtime, or before procedure. May be given with an analgesic to enhance pain relief. **Child:** PO, RECT, IM, IV: 12.5–25 mg q4-6h prn, at bedtime, or before procedure. May be given with an analgesic to enhance pain relief.

Nausea: **Adult:** PO, RECT, IM: 12.5–25mg q4-6h prn. **Child:** RECT, IM: 0.25–0.5 mg/kg q4-6h prn.

Motion Sickness: **Adult:** PO, RECT: 25 mg bid. **Child:** PO, RECT: 12.5–25 mg bid.

Allergic Conditions: **Adult:** PO, RECT: 12.5 mg qid, or 25 mg at bedtime. **Child:** PO, RECT: 6.25–12.5 mg tid or 25 mg at bedtime.

Clinical alert: Expect reduced dosage for children and the elderly, and monitor for excessive drowsiness or dizziness. Be aware that tablets may be crushed and mixed with food. Give IM doses deep into large muscle mass (never give SC). IV concentration should be no greater that 25 mg/cc, and injection should be given slowly over at least one min.

Contraindications/Precautions

PREG
C

Contraindicated in hypersensitivity to promethazine or other phenothiazines, and in acute asthma, narrow-angle glaucoma, stenosing peptic ulcer, pyloroduodenal obstruction, epilepsy, bone marrow depression, comatose or severely depressed states, concomitant use with MAOI. *Use with caution* in impaired hepatic function, cardiovascular disease, history of asthma, acute or chronic respiratory impairment (particularly in children), hypertension, and for debilitated patients.

🤚 **Contraindicated for nursing mothers and dehydrated children. Use with caution for the elderly. Safe use in pregnancy and children under 2 years has not been established.**

Side effects/Adverse reactions

Hypersensitivity: rash. *CNS:* sedation, drowsiness, confusion, dizziness, disturbed coordination, restlessness, tremors, stimulation (especially in children). *CV:* transient and mild hypotension or hypertension. *GI:* anorexia, dry mouth, nausea, vomiting, constipation. *Hem:* leukopenia, agranulocytosis. *Resp:* irregular respiration, dry nose, throat. *Eye:* blurred vision, photosensitivity. *GU:* urinary retention.

Nursing implications/Documentation

Possible nursing diagnoses: Potential for injury; Fluid volume deficit.

- When used for bedtime sedation, explore reasons for insomnia and explore holistic measure for promoting sleep (see Antianxiety Agents, Sedatives, and Hypnotics classification overview).

◆ Before giving for nausea, ascertain that nausea is not related to increased intracranial pressure, overdose, or an acute abdominal condition (may mask important symptoms).

◆ When used for allergic conditions, determine and record known allergies; provide an environment that is free from allergens (especially sleeping areas).

◆ For parenteral routes, keep in bed or supervise ambulation (may cause marked sedation, dizziness); when given together with an analgesic for pain relief, be aware that the patient may develop involuntary movements, which should subside after pain is controlled.

◆ Record intake and output, and monitor closely for dehydration (especially in children); offer sips of clear liquids when nausea is reduced.

Patient & family teaching/Home care

Possible nursing diagnoses: Knowledge deficit; Impaired home maintenance management.

◆ Advise taking this drug with food or milk if GI symptoms are experienced.

◆ Warn that alcohol and other CNS depressants may cause excessive drowsiness; advise against driving while taking this drug.

◆ If used for allergies, point out that avoiding pollens and staying in an air-conditioned environment may help reduce seasonal rhinitis.

◆ If used for motion sickness, advise taking 30–60 min before travel, and q8-12h as needed.

◆ Suggest that coffee or tea may reduce drowsiness, and that sugarless gum or hard candy may relieve dry mouth.

◆ Explain that antihistamines should be stopped for 4 days before allergy testing to ensure accurate results.

◆ *See Antianxiety agents, Sedatives, and Hypnotics, Antiemetics, and Antihistamines overviews for more information.*

propantheline
pro-pan'the-leen

propantheline bromide: *Norpanth, ✦Pantheline, Pro-Banthine, ✿Propanthel*

Class: Anticholinergic, Antimuscarinic

PEDS	PREG	GERI
✋	C	✋

Action Decreases GI motility and inhibits gastric secretion by blocking the action of acetylcholine at neuroeffector sites.

Use/Therapeutic goal/Outcome

Peptic ulcer: As adjunct for promotion of healing and relief of pain. *Outcome criteria:* Report of absence of pain; hemoglobin and hematocrit within normal range; stable vital signs; stools negative for occult blood.

Dose range/Administration

Interaction alert: Do not give antacids or antidiarrheals within 1 hr of propantheline (interferes with absorption).

▯ **Give 30–60 minutes before meals for maximum effects.**

Adult: PO: 15 mg before meals and 30 mg at bedtime.

Clinical alert: For elderly or debilitated, half the usual dose may be prescribed.

Contraindications/Precautions
PREG C

Contraindicated in hypersensitivity to anticholinergics, and in glaucoma and myasthenia gravis. *Use with caution* in prostatic hypertrophy, obstructive disorders of the GI tract, hyperthyroidism, and cardiac arrhythmias.

🖐 **Contraindicated for pregnant or nursing mothers. Use with caution for the elderly. Safe use for children has not been established.**

Side effects/Adverse reactions

Hypersensitivity: rash or hives. *CNS:* headache, dizziness, confusion, excitement, agitation, drowsiness. *CV:* palpitations, rapid heart rate. *GI:* constipation, dry mouth. *GU:* urinary hesitancy and retention, impotence. *Misc:* fever, decreased sweating, heat stroke. *Eye:* blurred vision, eye pain.

Nursing implications/Documentation

Possible nursing diagnoses: Urinary retention; Constipation; Hyperthermia.

◆ Do not administer antacids or antidiarrheals within 1 hr of propantheline.

◆ Assess and document bowel elimination pattern; institute measures to avoid constipation.

◆ Monitor urinary output and assess for retention.

◆ Assess, report, and record mental changes, especially in the elderly.

Patient & family teaching/Home care

Possible nursing diagnoses: Knowledge deficit; Potential for injury; Impaired maintenance management.

♦ Explain the need to take propantheline 30–60 min before meals.

♦ Caution against chewing or crushing tablets because of very bitter taste.

♦ Advise reporting rash, inability to void, difficulty in initiating urination, or bladder distention.

♦ Suggest chewing gum or hard candy to alleviate the discomfort of dry mouth.

♦ Stress the importance of monitoring bowel elimination and increasing intake of fluids and fiber to avoid constipation.

♦ Advise against using alcohol or other CNS depressants.

♦ Explain the need to avoid hot baths, saunas, and excessive activity in hot, humid weather.

♦ Caution against driving and operating dangerous machinery until response has been determined.

♦ Advise family to report confusion or excitement, especially in elderly patients, and to keep propantheline out of reach of children since overdose is very dangerous in this age group.

♦ *See Anticholinergics overview for more information.*

P

propoxyphene

pro-pox'i-feen

propoxyphene hydrochloride: ***Darvon, Dolene, Doraphen, Doxaphene, ♣Novopropoxyn, Profene, Propoxyphene, Propoxycon 642, Pro-Pox***

propoxyphene napsylate: ***Darvocet-N, Darvon-N, ♠Doloxene, ♠Doloxene Co***

Class: Narcotic analgesic, Opiate agonist

Antidote: naloxone hydrochloride (Narcan)

PEDS	PREG	GERI	CONTROLLED SUBSTANCE
♛	C	♛	IV

Action Alters both perception of and response to pain through an unclear mechanism. Believed to act by binding with opiate receptors at many CNS sites.

Use/Therapeutic goal/Outcome

Mild to moderate pain: Relief of pain. *Outcome criteria:* Report of feeling comfortable; absence of signs of pain (grimacing, frowning, restlessness, reluctance to move or cough) with increase in signs of comfort (relaxed facial expression, decreased restlessness); blood pressure and pulse within normal limits when compared to baseline.

Dose range/Administration

Interaction alert: Alcohol and CNS depressants may cause excessive sedation.

Propoxyphene hydrochloride: *Adult:* PO: One 65-mg capsule q4h prn.

Propoxyphine napsylate: *Adult:* PO: 100 mg (tablet or suspension) q4h prn.

Clinical alert: 65 mg p. hydrochloride is equal to 100 mg p. napsylate. Capsules may be emptied and given with a small amount of food or water (food in stomach may delay absorption). Expect reduced doses for the elderly or debilitated.

Contraindications/Precautions

PREG C

Contraindicated in hypersensitivity to propoxyphene and in suicidal potential, addiction-prone individuals, dependence on opiates, and alcoholism. *Use with caution* in renal or hepatic disease, and concomitant use with antidepressants, tranquilizers, or alcohol.

✋ **Contraindicated for children and pregnant or nursing mothers. Use with caution for the elderly.**

Side effects/Adverse reactions

Hypersensitivity: rash, hives, itching, swelling of face. *CNS:* dizziness, sedation, somnolence, insomnia, stupor, coma, psychological and physical dependence. *GI:* nausea, vomiting.

Nursing implications/Documentation

Possible nursing diagnoses: Pain; Anxiety; Potential for injury.

♦ Have patient rate pain on a scale of 1–10 before and after medication is given; report and record inadequate pain control.

♦ Give analgesics before pain is severe for best effects.

♦ Be aware of potential for psychic and physical dependence after prolonged use.

♦ Report if there is suspected propoxyphene abuse; propoxyphene in excessive doses ranks second to barbiturates as a cause of drug-related deaths.

Patient & family teaching/Home care

Possible nursing diagnoses: Sensory/perceptual alterations; Impaired home maintenance management.

- Explain the rationale for taking analgesics before pain is too severe.
- Advise those who are ambulatory to refrain from activities that require alertness until response is determined.
- Stress the need to adhere to prescribed dose regimen because of risk of overdose, dependence, and abuse (instead of increasing dose regimen, unsatisfactory pain relief should be reported).
- Advise using a less potent analgesic as soon as possible to avoid developing tolerance and dependence.
- Suggest lying down if dizziness, drowsiness, nausea, or vomiting are experienced (these should be reported if persistent).
- Warn that alcohol and other CNS depressants may cause excessive sedation.
- *See Narcotic and non-narcotic analgesics overview for more information.*

propranolol
proe-pran'oh-lole

propranolol hydrochloride: ✤Apo-Propranolol, ◆Deralin, ✤Detensol, Inderal, Inderal LA, Ipran, ✤Novopranol, ✤PMS-Propranolol

Class: ★Nonselective beta-adrenergic blocking agent prototype, Antihypertensive, Antianginal, Antiarrhythmic

PEDS	PREG	GERI
🖐	C	🖐

Action Reduces heart rate, myocardial irritability, force of contraction, atrioventricular and intraventricular conduction velocity by blocking beta-1 (cardiac) adrenergic receptors. Decreases myocardial oxygen demand and increases exercise tolerance by blocking catecholamine-induced increases in heart rate and blood pressure. Reduces blood pressure by an unclear mechanism. Prevents vasodilation of cerebral arteries. Decreases plasma renin activity.

Use/Therapeutic goal/Outcome

Hypertension: Reduction of blood pressure. **Outcome criteria:** Blood pressure within normal limits.

Arrhythmias: Resolution of arrhythmias. **Outcome criteria:** Absence of supraventricular and ventricular tachyarrhythmias on EKG.

Angina: Prevention of angina. **Outcome criteria:** Report of decreased anginal attacks, increased exercise tolerance.

Pheochromocytoma: Control of tachycardia. **Outcome criteria:** Heart rate less than 100 beats per minute.

Myocardial infarction: Reduced mortality following MI; prevention of reinfarction. **Outcome criteria:** Decreased incidence of sudden death following MI.

Migraine headaches: Resolution or prevention of migraine headaches. **Outcome criteria:** Report of reduced incidence of migraine attacks.

Dose range/Administration

Interaction alert: Aminophylline antagonizes effect of propranolol. Cardiac glycosides and verapamil may cause excessive bradycardia. Cimetidine inhibits metabolism of propranolol. Isoproterenol and glucagon antagonize propranolol effect and may be given as an antidote. NSAIDs, especially indomethacin, may decrease the antihypertensive effect. May alter antidiabetic agent requirement. Stopping smoking may increase therapeutic effects by decreasing metabolism, thereby increasing serum concentrations; dosage adjustment may be necessary.

🗩 **Give with meals to increase absorption.**

Hypertension: *Adult:* PO: 40 mg bid; gradually increase as needed until desired response is attained. *Maintenance dose:* 120–240 mg/day.

Arrhythmias: *Adult:* PO: 10–30 mg tid or qid. IV: 1–3 mg injected at a rate not to exceed 1 mg/min. Administer second dose after 2 min; then in 4 hrs (if needed).

Angina: *Adult:* PO: 10–20 mg tid or qid. Dose may be increase every 3–7 days. Usual dose is 160 mg/day; may need to be as high as 320 mg/day.

Pheochromocytoma: *Adult:* PO: 60 mg/day in divided doses, for 3 days preop.

Myocardial infarction: *Adult:* PO: 180–240 mg/day in divided doses (bid, tid, or qid).

Clinical alert: Use IV route only for life-threatening arrhythmias, and monitor closely for sudden and severe hypotension. Be aware that patients taking this drug may not exhibit tachycardia as a symptom of fever, hypoglycemia, or hyperthyroidism. When discontinuing, wean over a 1–2 week period to avoid precipitating tachycardia or myocardial infarction.

Contraindications/Precautions

PREG C

Contraindicated in hypersensitivity to propranolol, and in cardiogenic shock, sinus bradycardia, second- or third-degree heart block (PR interval > 0.24 seconds), CHF, COPD and bronchial asthma. *Use with caution* in aortic or mitral valvular disease, peripheral arterial insufficiency, renal or hepatic impairment, major surgery, diabetes, myasthenia gravis, Wolff-Parkinson-White syndrome, chronic bronchitis or emphysema.

☙ **Use with caution for the elderly. Safe use for children and pregnant women has not been established.**

Side effects/Adverse reactions

Hypersensitivity: rash, pruritus. *CV:* bradycardia, hypotension, CHF, peripheral vascular disease. *CNS:* fatigue, lethargy, depression, vivid dreams, insomnia, hallucinations. *Resp:* increased airway resistance. *GI:* nausea, vomiting, diarrhea, constipation. *GU:* decreased sexual ability. *MS:* arthralgia, cold hands and feet. *Hem:* hypoglycemia.

Nursing implications/Documentation

Possible nursing diagnoses: Activity intolerance; Fatigue; Potential for injury.

♦ Assess mental status, and record pulse and blood pressure (if possible, lying, sitting, and standing, in both arms) before administration, and frequently thereafter until response is determined.

♦ Consult with physician to determine desired therapeutic range for blood pressure and heart rate (be aware that parameters for withholding the medication should be written by physician).

♦ Ascertain that baseline CBC, electrolytes, BUN, creatinine, and liver function studies have been obtained before giving first dose; report abnormalities and monitor closely thereafter.

♦ Monitor for allergic reactions and signs of confusion, dizziness, bradycardia, CHF, and hypotension; hold drug and report immediately if these occur.

♦ Supervise ambulation until response is determined.

♦ Document and monitor daily weight, and intake and output; report significant negative or positive balance.

Patient & family teaching/Home care

Possible nursing diagnoses: Knowledge deficit; Impaired home maintenance management; Altered sexuality patterns.

♦ Explain the importance of taking this drug exactly as prescribed, even when feeling well; warn not to discontinue drug abruptly.

♦ Stress the importance of good medical follow-up, explain that this drug reduces "wear and tear" on blood vessels, reduces the workload of the heart, and improves longevity and health.

♦ Teach how to monitor pulse and blood pressure; emphasize that syncope, hypertension or hypotension, or persistent dizziness should be reported; provide pulse and blood pressure parameters for withholding medication.

♦ Advise changing positions slowly, to avoid dizziness.

♦ Encourage daily monitoring of weight, and reporting sudden weight gain (frequently is fluid retention).

♦ Warn against drinking alcohol or taking *any* OTC drugs without physician approval (some interactions can cause severe reactions).

♦ Warn that discontinuing drug may precipitate cardiac problems.

♦ Explain that this drug may alter sexual ability; explore concerns and seek consultation as needed.

♦ *See Beta Adrenergic Blockers, Antiarrhythmics, and Antihypertensives overviews for more information.*

propylthiouracil   *proe-pill-thye-oh-yoor′a-sill*

propylthiouracil (PTU): ✦*Propyl-Thyracil*
Class: Thyroid hormone antagonist

PEDS   PREG   GERI
☙   **D**   ☙

Action Interferes with synthesis of thyroid hormones (T_3 and T_4) by blocking oxidation of iodine, thus inhibiting its ability to combine with tyrosine to form thyroxin. Also blocks peripheral conversion of T_4 to T_3.

Use/Therapeutic goal/Outcome

Severe hyperthyroidism and thyrotoxic crisis: Suppression of circulating thyroid hormones, promotion of normal metabolism. *Outcome criteria:* After 3 weeks, decreased T_4 levels; weight gain; normal pulse rate; decreased sweating.

Preparation for thyroidectomy: Reduction of vascularity of the thyroid gland (reduced risk of bleeding) and promotion of normal metabolism. ***Outcome criteria:*** Decrease in thyroid size.

Dose range/Administration

Interaction alert: Increases the effect of anticoagulants (monitor for hypothrombinemia, manifested by increased bruising, bleeding). Lithium may be synergistic (monitor for hypothyroidism).

🖐 **Give with meals to reduce GI distress.**

Severe hyperthyroidism: Adult: PO: 100–300 mg q8h (maximum 900 mg/day), depending upon severity of hyperthyroidism; continue until euthyroid, then maintenance dose 100–150 mg/day to tid. ***Child > 10 yrs:*** PO: 100 mg tid; continue until euthyroid, then maintenance dose 25 mg tid to 100 mg bid. ***Child 6–10 yrs:*** 50–150 mg/day in divided doses q8h.

Preparation for thyroidectomy: Adult and Child: PO: With iodine for 10 days.

Thyrotoxic crisis: Adult and Child: PO: Give hyperthyroidism dose with iodine and propranolol.

Clinical alert: Give dose at the same time every day to maintain therapeutic levels. Hold drug and report if any of the following are noted: rashes, cough or shortness of breath (may be interstitial pneumonitis), enlarged cervical lymph nodes, peripheral nonpitting edema, petechiae, ecchymosis, persistent fatigue, or signs of bone marrow depression (fever, chills, sore throat). This is the drug of choice for pregnancy because of decreased risk to the fetus.

Contraindications/Precautions

PREG
D

Contraindicated in hypersensitivity to propylthiouracil. ***Use with caution*** in infection, bone marrow depression, and liver disease.

🖐 **Contraindicated for nursing mothers. Use with caution for children, pregnant women, and the elderly.**

Side effects/Adverse reactions

Hypersensitivity: itching, rashes, drug fever, coughing with shortness of breath (may indicate interstitial pneumonitis). Other effects are usually dose related. ***GI:*** nausea, vomiting, decreased appetite, loss of taste, diarrhea, salivary gland enlargement, hepatotoxicity. ***CNS:*** headache, drowsiness, dizziness. ***Hem:*** agranulocytosis, leukopenia, thrombocytopenia. ***Eye:*** visual problems. ***Skin:*** jaundice, hyperpigmentation. ***CV:*** vasculitis. ***MS:*** muscle and joint pain. ***Misc:*** lymphadenopathy, lupus-like syndrome.

Nursing implications/Documentation

Possible nursing diagnoses: Altered nutrition: less than body requirements; Altered nutrition: more than body requirements.

♦ Observe for and report signs of hypothyroidism (fatigue, weight gain, drowsiness, dry skin, constipation), overdose (peripheral edema, heat intolerance, sweating, palpitations, tachycardia, CNS irritability, vomiting), or blood dyscrasias (sore throat, chills, fever, mouth sores).

♦ Document and monitor vital signs and weights at least daily during initial treatment.

♦ Monitor T_3 and T_4 levels for therapeutic range; report abnormalities (level below or above normal range indicates need for dose adjustment).

♦ For prolonged treatment, periodically monitor CBC, prothrombine time, serum alkaline phosphatase, SGOT, SGPT, and liver function tests.

Patient & family teaching/Home care

Possible nursing diagnoses: Knowledge deficit; Impaired home maintenance management.

♦ Explain the need to take this drug with food to reduce GI symptoms.

♦ Stress the importance of taking this drug daily exactly as prescribed (not skipping or increasing dosage, taking it at the same time every day with meals).

♦ Advise reporting signs and symptoms of hypothyroidism, hypersensitivity, or overdose (see Nursing implications).

♦ Suggest checking with physician whether iodized salt and foods (seafood, some breads) should be avoided.

♦ Stress the importance of returning for medical follow-up (blood work).

♦ Advise wearing a medical alert bracelet stating that propylthiouracil is being taken (injuries, myocardial infarction, surgery, and other illnesses may precipitate thyrotoxicosis).

♦ *See Thyroid Hormone Antagonists overview for more information.*

protamine

pro'ta-meen

protamine sulfate

Class: Antidote

PEDS	PREG	GERI
✋	C	✋

Action Neutralizes heparin (which is acidic) by forming an inactive salt. If given alone, high dose protamine sulfate also acts as an anticoagulant.

Use/Therapeutic goal/Outcome

Heparin overdose: Counteraction of anticoagulant effect. **Outcome criteria:** PTT within normal limits; stable hemoglobin and hematocrit.

Dose range/Administration

Adult: IV: Dosage is guided by coagulation studies and must be administered by physician or under direct supervision of a physician. Usual dose is 1 mg per 78–100 units of heparin. *Maximum dose:* 100 mg over 2 hours. Dilute protamine sulfate to 1% solution (10 mg/cc) and give *slowly* (maximum rate 50 mg/10 min).

Clinical alert: If protamine sulfate is given too rapidly, it can cause severe hypotension and anaphylactoid-like reactions. Be aware that as protamine is metabolized, heparin rebound may occur (increased bleeding, hypotension) necessitating additional doses of protamine.

Contraindications/Precautions

PREG
C

Contraindicated in previous intolerance to protamine sulfate, and for hemorrhage not induced by heparin overdosage. **Use with caution** in cardiovascular disease, prior exposure to protamine, and fish allergy.

✋ Use with caution for the elderly. Safe use for children and pregnant women has not been established.

Side effects/Adverse reactions

Hypersensitivity: itching, rashes, hives, anaphylaxis. **CV:** abrupt fall in blood pressure, bradycardia. **Resp:** dyspnea. **Misc:** transient flushing with feeling of warmth, nausea, vomiting, lassitude. Decreasing administration rate may alleviate these effects.

Nursing implications/Documentation

Possible nursing diagnosis: Potential for injury.

♦ Document baseline vital signs before administration and every 5 minutes during administration.

♦ Monitor PTT closely, observing for heparin rebound (as evidenced by increase in PTT).

Patient & family teaching/Home care

Possible nursing diagnosis: Knowledge deficit.

♦ Recognize that protamine sulfate is given to hospitalized patients only.

♦ Explain that this drug helps to prevent bleeding, and that blood studies will be drawn to ensure desired effects.

♦ If side effects occur, reduce IV rate and reassure patient that symptoms should subside.

protriptyline

pro-trip'tie-leen

protriptyline hydrochloride: ♦*Triptil, Vivactil*

Class: Tricyclic antidepressant (TCA)

PEDS	PREG	GERI
✋	C	✋

Action Improves mood by increasing levels of the neurotransmitters norepinephrine and serotonin in the CNS. (Blocks neurotransmitter reuptake into presynaptic neurons by inhibiting the "amine pump." Reuptake normally terminates the action of neurotransmitters.) Has high anticholinergic effects.

Use/Therapeutic goal/Outcome

Depressive disorders, particularly associated with social withdrawal: Promotion of sense of well-being and ability to interact with others and cope with daily living. **Outcome criteria:** After 2–4 weeks, report of feeling less depressed, less anxious, more energetic and able to cope; return of normal sleeping and eating habits; demonstration of improved ability to problem solve, interact socially, and perform activities of daily living.

Dose range/Administration

Interaction alert: Barbiturates may reduce antidepressant blood levels and effects. Cimetidine may increase levels. If given with epinephrine and norepinephrine, monitor for increased risk of hypertension. Avoid use with MAOIs (risk of excitation, hyperpyrexia, and seizures). Give cautiously with thyroid medications, because of increased CNS stimulation and cardiac arrhythmias.

👉 **Give with (or immediately after) food to reduce GI symptoms.**

Adult: PO: 15–40 mg/day in divided doses, may gradually increase to a maximum of 60 mg/day. *For the elderly or adolescent:* 3–5 mg tid.

Clinical alert: Give doses during the day to prevent the common side effect of insomnia. Monitor for tachycardia and orthostatic hypotension, which are more common with this TCA than others.

Contraindications/Precautions

PREG C

Contraindicated in hypersensitivity to TCAs, concomitant use with electroconvulsive therapy, and in acute recovery period of myocardial infarction. **Use with caution** in renal or hepatic disease, hyperthyroidism, glaucoma, prostatic hypertrophy, urinary retention, hypomania, mania, and suicidal tendencies.

✋ **Contraindicated for children under 12 years and pregnant or nursing mothers. Use with caution for adolescents and the elderly or debilitated.**

Side effects/Adverse reactions

Hypersensitivity: rash, sensitivity to sunlight. **CNS:** drowsiness, dizziness, anxiety, headache, fatigue, nervousness, agitation, extrapyramidal symptoms. **CV:** orthostatic hypotension, palpitations, tachycardia, hypertension. **GI:** anorexia, dry mouth, nausea, constipation, paralytic ileus. **GU:** urinary retention, decreased libido. **Eye:** blurred vision. **Ear:** tinnitus. **Skin:** sweating. **Hem:** agranulocytosis. **Misc:** (after abrupt withdrawal of long-term therapy) nausea, headache, malaise.

Nursing implications/Documentation

Possible nursing diagnoses: Potential for injury; Constipation; Altered oral mucous membrane.

♦ Document mental status and vital signs daily until response to therapy has been established.

♦ Be sure that doses are swallowed (not hoarded).

♦ Monitor for orthostatic hypotension, dizziness, and drowsiness; supervise ambulation until response is established.

♦ Record intake and output, and observe for dehydration or urinary retention; provide special mouth care.

♦ Monitor for and report suicidal tendencies, increased depression, or excessive drowsiness (may require change in medication).

♦ Prevent constipation by monitoring bowel movements and encouraging adequate fiber and fluid intake; offer laxatives or stool softeners before the problem becomes severe.

Patient & family teaching/Home care

Possible nursing diagnoses: Ineffective coping (family and individual); Sleep pattern disturbance; Impaired home maintenance management.

♦ Stress that this medication helps reduce the depression that inhibits ability to make decisions and cope effectively (once the individual feels less depressed, it will be easier to take steps toward making healthy changes).

♦ Explain that side effects are often noted immediately, but they usually diminish after a few weeks; on the other hand, it is likely to take 2–4 weeks before *beneficial* effects are noted (the patient may feel worse before feeling better).

♦ Warn to change positions slowly to prevent dizziness.

♦ Point out the role of adequate nutrition, exercise, and sleep in combating depression.

♦ Emphasize that the effects of alcohol, sedatives, and tranquilizers may be potentiated.

♦ Caution to consult with physician before using OTC drugs; stress the need for ongoing medical follow-up.

♦ Recommend reporting continued depression; stress that doses should not be increased or stopped without checking with physician because this may cause severe problems.

♦ Advise avoidance of driving and other potentially hazardous activities until response is established.

♦ Suggest using ice chips, hard candy, or gum to relieve side effect of dry mouth; stress the need for good mouth care.

♦ Warn women to report if pregnancy is planned or suspected.

♦ *See Antidepressants overview for more information.*

P

pseudoephedrine
soo-doe-e-fed'rin

pseudoephedrine hydrochloride: *Cenafed, Children's Sudafed Liquid, ♣Eltor, Genaphed, Novafed, ♣Ornex Cold, Robidrine, Sudafed, Sudafed SA, Sufedrin*

pseudoephedrine sulfate: *Afrinol Repetabs*

Class: Direct- and indirect-acting sympathomimetic, Adrenergic agent, Nasal decongestant

PEDS	PREG	GERI
♨	C	♨

Action Produces vasoconstriction and nasal decongestion by stimulating alpha-adrenergic receptors.

Use/Therapeutic goal/Outcome

Congestion: Symptomatic relief of nasal and eustachian tube congestion. *Outcome criteria:* Report of easier nasal breathing and reduction in nasal discharge.

Dose range/Administration

Interaction alert: Do not give within 14 days of MAOI therapy.

p. hydrochloride: Adult/Child > 12 yr: PO: 60 mg q4-6h. *Sustained-release tablets or capsules:* 120 mg q12h. *Maximum dose:* 240 mg/day. *Child 6–12 yr:* PO: 30 mg q6h, not over 120 mg/day. *Child 2–5 yr:* PO: 15 mg q6h, not over 60 mg/day.

p. sulfate: Adult/Child > 12 yr: PO: 120 mg q12h.

Clinical alert: To prevent insomnia, avoid giving within 2 hr of bedtime.

Contraindications/Precautions

PREG
C

Contraindicated in hypersensitivity to pseudoephedrine hydrochloride and sympathomimetics, and in severe hypertension, severe coronary artery disease, dysrhythmias, tachycardia, MAO inhibitor therapy, and angle-closure glaucoma. *Use with caution* in diabetes and prostatic hypertrophy.

♨ **Contraindicated for children under 12 years (sulfate or sustained release form). Use with caution for children and the elderly. Safe use for pregnant or nursing mothers has not been established; use not recommended.**

Side effects/Adverse reactions

Hypersensitivity: rash, itching, exaggeration of side effects. *CNS:* restlessness, fear, anxiety, tension, tremor, headache. *Skin:* flushing, pallor, sweating. *GI:* nausea, vomiting. *CV:* hypertension, palpitations, arrhythmias, anginal pain, precordial distress.

Nursing implications/Documentation

Possible nursing diagnoses: Potential for injury; Sleep pattern disturbance.

♦ Record presence of nasal stuffiness, discharge, or ear pain before and after administration.

♦ Hold drug and report if excessive restlessness or excitement occurs.

Patient & family teaching/Home care

Possible nursing diagnoses: Knowledge deficit; Impaired home maintenance management.

♦ Explain that this drug should not be given within 2 hr of bedtime to prevent insomnia.

♦ Stress that this drug should be taken only when necessary on a short-term basis to prevent rebound rhinitis; failure to improve in 5 days should be reported.

♦ Warn against use of OTC drugs without physician's approval.

♦ Point out that excessive restlessness should be reported because it may be drug related.

♦ *See Adrenergics (sympathomimetics) overview for more information.*

psyllium
sill'i-um

Cillium, Konsyl, Metamucil, Metamucil Instant Mix, Metamucil Sugar Free, Naturacil, Perdiem Plain, Siblin, Syllact

Class: Bulk-forming laxative

PEDS	PREG	GERI
♨	C	♨

Action Promotes normal peristalsis and bowel motility by increasing bulk and moisture content of stool.

Use/Therapeutic goal/Outcome

Constipation: Promotion of regular evacuation of soft stool. *Outcome criteria:* Passage of soft, formed stool without straining (usually within 12–24 hr after initial dose, but may take up to 3 days).

Dose range/Administration

Interaction alert: Oral anticoagulants, digitalis glycosides, and salicylates should be separated

P

from psyllium by a 2-hr interval to prevent decreased absorption of these medications due to physical binding.

Adult: PO: 1 to 2 rounded tsp or one packet/day to tid. **Child:** PO: 1/2 to 1 tsp or 1/2 packet/day to tid.

Clinical alert: Mix in 8-oz glass of water or juice and give immediately, before congealing takes place.

Contraindications/Precautions
PREG
C

Contraindicated in hypersensitivity to any bulk-forming laxative, and in dysphagia, symptoms of appendicitis, undiagnosed rectal bleeding, and intestinal obstruction.

♨ **Use with caution for children under 6 years and the elderly.**

Side effects/Adverse reactions

Hypersensitivity: rash, itching, difficulty breathing. **GI:** esophageal blocking, intestinal impaction.

Nursing implications/Documentation

Possible nursing diagnoses: Constipation.

• Administer each dose with 8-oz glass of water and encourage increased fluid intake.

• Avoid giving before meals to prevent interference with appetite.

• With sodium restriction, avoid use of effervescent powders that are high in sodium content; for diabetics, monitor the amount of sugar in preparations used.

• Assess abdomen for bowel sounds and distention.

• Monitor and record character, frequency, and amount of stool evacuated.

Patient & family teaching/Home care

Possible nursing diagnoses: Knowledge deficit; Impaired home maintenance management.

• Caution not to swallow psyllium in the dry form to prevent obstruction of the GI tract.

• Stress the importance of drinking 6–8 glasses of liquid daily, and taking each dose of psyllium with 8-oz glass of water or juice to provide enough fluid for the desired action to take place.

• Warn against taking psyllium at bedtime, to reduce risk of intestinal obstruction.

• Advise not to take other oral medicines within 2 hr of psyllium to avoid decreased absorption due to binding.

• Make patient aware of the sodium, sugar, and carbohydrates in bulk-forming laxatives if these substances must be limited in diet.

• Stress the importance of dietary bulk, fluids, and exercise to prevent constipation; caution that high intake of bran, when combined with psyllium, increases the risk of impaction.

• Point out that daily bowel movements are not necessary for each individual; regular evacuation of soft stool that does not require straining is an appropriate goal.

• *See Laxatives overview for more information.*

pyrantel
pi-ran'tel

pyrantel embonate: ♠*Anthel,* ♠*Combantrin,* ♠*Early Bird*

pyrantel pamoate: *Antiminth,* ♣*Combantrin*

Class: Anti-infective, Anthelmintic

PEDS	PREG	GERI
♨	C	OK

Action Eliminates helminths (intestinal worms) in an infected host by paralyzing them and allowing their expulsion through normal peristalsis.

Use/Therapeutic goal/Outcome

Pinworm and roundworm: Elimination of intestinal helminths. **Outcome criteria:** Expulsion of worms followed by 3 negative stool samples after completion of treatment; for pinworms, perianal swabs negative for 7 days.

Dose range/Administration

Interaction alert: Piperazine antagonizes action.

👊 **Give with milk, juice, or food.**

Adult/Child > 2 yrs: PO: 11 mg/kg in a single dose. *Maximum dose: 1 g. For pinworms:* Repeat dose in 2 wks in case pinworm eggs survived initial treatment.

Clinical alert: This drug is now available without prescription.

Contraindications/Precautions
PREG
C

Contraindicated in hypersensitivity to pyrantel. **Use with caution** in malnutrition, severe anemia, dehydration, or liver disease.

♨ **Safe use for children under 2 years and pregnant or nursing mothers has not been established.**

Side effects/Adverse reactions

Hypersensitivity: (rare) rash. **GI:** abdominal discomfort or cramping, diarrhea, nausea, vomiting. **CNS:** headache, dizziness. **Misc:** fever.

Nursing implications/Documentation

Possible nursing diagnoses: Potential for infection; Diarrhea; Situational low self-esteem.

◆ Practice meticulous handwashing before and after contact with the patient or changing of bed linens or clothing.

◆ Record character of all stools and inspect them closely for worms before and during therapy (stool specimens must go to the lab while still warm).

◆ Determine close contacts (family members, playmates, babysitters with long-term contact), who should also be treated.

Patient & family teaching/Home care

Possible nursing diagnoses: Knowledge deficit; Impaired home maintenance management.

◆ Explore feelings and concerns, and explain that this common childhood illness is not associated with "dirtiness" of the child or family.

◆ Teach how to recognize pinworms, roundworms, and ova.

◆ Stress the importance of preventing reinfection or spread of infection by treating all family members and close contacts, taking the medication exactly as prescribed, washing foods especially carefully, meticulously washing hands after bowel movements, cutting nails short, changing clothing every day, keeping fingers out of mouth, having infected individuals sleep alone, eliminating ova by washing all linens daily in hot water (without shaking them), vacuuming and damp-mopping the house daily, cleaning the toilet with disinfectant daily.

◆ Warn that if dizziness is experienced, hazardous activities and driving should be avoided.

◆ *See Anti-infectives overview for more information.*

pyrazinamide

peer-a-zin' a-mide

♣PMS Pyrazinamide, ♣Tebrazid, ▲Zinamide

Class: Anti-infective, Antitubercular

PEDS	PREG	GERI
✋	C	✋

Action
Kills tubercle bacilli (bactericidal action) or limits their growth (bacteriostatic action). Exact mechanism of action is unknown.

Use/Therapeutic goal/Outcome

Treatment of tuberculosis and other mycobacterium diseases: Resolution of infection. **Outcome criteria:** Absence of acid-fast bacilli on sputum culture, decreased productive cough, normal temperature, improvement of X rays.

Dose range/Administration

Interaction alert: May alter insulin requirements.

🍽 **Give with meals.**

Adult: PO: 20–35 mg/kg/day in 3–4 divided doses to a maximum of 3 g/day.

Clinical alert: Document and report temperature greater than 101°F (dose should be adjusted).

Contraindications/Precautions   PREG C

Contraindicated in hypersensitivity to pyrazinamide, and in pre-existing liver disease. **Use with caution** in gout and diabetes.

🖐 **Use with caution for the elderly. Safe use for children under 13 yrs and for pregnant or nursing women has not been established.**

Side effects/Adverse reactions

Hypersensitivity: itching, rash. **GI:** nausea, vomiting, dry mouth, liver tenderness and enlargement (with jaundice). **GU:** dysuria. **Hem:** disturbances in blood clotting, hyperuricemia. **MS:** joint pain, gout. **Misc:** splenomegaly, malaise, fever.

Nursing implications/Documentation

Possible nursing diagnoses: Potential for infection; Fatigue; Activity intolerance; Fluid volume deficit.

◆ Ascertain that baseline CBC, BUN, creatinine, and liver function studies are obtained, and that necessary culture specimens are collected, before starting pyrazinamide; monitor periodically thereafter, depending on clinical symptoms.

◆ Allow for a balance between rest and activity.

◆ Monitor and record intake and output and provide favorite fluids to ensure adequate hydration.

- For diabetic patients, monitor serum glucose levels closely (pyrazinamide affects sugar metabolism).

Patient & family teaching/Home care

Possible nursing diagnoses: Knowledge deficit; Impaired home maintenance management.

- Advise taking with food.
- Stress the importance of taking this drug as prescribed without missing doses, and the importance of long-term medical follow-up to avoid relapses or complications.
- Advise avoiding alcohol to prevent liver toxicity.
- Encourage drinking at least 2 L of fluid a day to maintain adequate hydration.
- See *Anti-infectives overview* for more information.

pyridostigmine
peer-id-oh-stig'meen

pyridostigmine bromide: ***Mestinon, ✦Mestinon Supraspan, Mestinon Timespan, Regonol***

Class: Cholinergic, Anticholinesterase

Antidote: Atropine

PEDS	PREG	GERI
🖐	C	🖐

Action When given in appropriate doses, promotes impulse transmission from nerve cells to muscle cells by inhibiting the destruction of acetylcholine by the enzyme cholinesterase. Acetylcholine is responsible for facilitating impulse transmission from nerve cells to muscle cells. *Excessive or deficient* acetylcholine may cause *neuromuscular blockade.* Onset of action for PO route is 2–4 hr, with a duration of 2½–4 hr. Onset for IV route is within 10–30 min, and duration is 2½–4 hr.

Use/Therapeutic goal/Outcome

Myasthenia gravis: Improvement of muscle strength and function. **Outcome criteria:** Respirations within normal range; normal vital capacity; improved ability to chew, swallow, talk, and perform activities of daily life; absence of ptosis; report of absence of double vision.

Anesthesia recovery: Reversal of nondepolarizing neuromuscular blocking agents and return of muscle strength and function. **Outcome criteria:** Spontaneous respirations; ability to move arms and legs; return of muscle strength.

Dose range/Administration

Interaction alert: Quinidine and anticholinergics may antagonize cholinergic effects. Other cholinergic drugs should be discontinued before giving pyridostigmine.

🍴 **Give with food or milk to minimize side effects by slowing absorption and reducing serum peaks.**

Myasthenia gravis: **Adult:** PO: 60–120 mg q3-4h (600 mg/day in divided doses). *Maximum dose:* 1500 mg/day. *Timed release tablets:* 1–3 tablets (180–540 mg) bid, at least 6 hr between doses. IM, IV: ⅓₀ oral dose. **Child:** PO: 7 mg/kg/day in 5–6 doses.

Reversal of neuromuscular blocker: **Adult:** IV: 10–20 mg, after 0.6–1.2 mg IV atropine.

Clinical alert: Must be given on a strict, exact time schedule to maintain muscle strength. Doses are individualized depending upon neurological response and incidence of side effects. There is a fine line between inadequate dosage and overdosage, requiring careful monitoring of response. Keep atropine, suction, and resuscitative equipment readily available.

Contraindications/Precautions
PREG
C

Contraindicated in hypersensitivity to anticholinesterase agents or to bromides, and in intestinal or urinary obstruction, hypotension, and bradycardia. **Use with caution** in bronchial asthma, peumonia, urinary tract infections, and dysrhythmias.

🖐 **Use with caution for children and the elderly. Safe use for pregnant women has not been established, but 20% of neonates have transient muscle weakness.**

Side effects/Adverse reactions

Hypersensitivity: rash (may be acneiform), exaggeration of side effects. **Resp:** increased bronchial secretions, weakness or paralysis of respiratory muscles. **Eye:** lacrimation, diplopia. **MS:** cramps, dysarthria. **CV:** dysrhythmias (especially bradycardia), hypotension. **GI:** increased salivation, dysphagia, abdominal cramps, nausea, vomiting, diarrhea. **GU:** urinary frequency. **Skin:** sweating. **Misc:** cholinergic crisis (increase in severity of side effects).

Nursing implications/Documentation

Possible nursing diagnoses: Activity intolerance; Potential for aspiration; Impaired swallowing; Fear.

P

◆ Closely monitor ability to chew, swallow, and talk, especially during periods of dose adjustment; document variations in strength and pulse, respirations, and blood pressure every 4 hours.

◆ Report presence of rash (may require discontinuation of drug).

◆ Once the individual has demonstrated ability to manage dose regimen, check with physician to see if a supply of medication can be kept at the bedside for self-medication (those with long-standing disease often insist on this).

◆ For use in pregnancy, monitor neonates for transient muscle weakness.

Patient & family teaching/Home care

Possible nursing diagnoses: Knowledge deficit; Impaired home maintenance management.

◆ Explain that taking this drug on a strict time schedule is vital to promote normal muscle function, and that this may be a life-long requirement.

◆ Point out that taking this drug with food helps reduce side effects.

◆ Stress the need for ongoing medical follow-up because some individuals develop a resistance to this drug.

◆ Advise reporting side effects or increased muscle weakness immediately, especially during periods of dose adjustment.

◆ Recommend wearing medical alert identification that states that the patient has myasthenia gravis and is taking this drug.

◆ *See Cholinergics overview for more information.*

quinacrine

kwin'a-kreen

quinacrine hydrochloride: *Atabrine*

Class: Anti-infective, Anthelmintic, Antiparasitic

PEDS	PREG	GERI
♨	C	✋

Action Eliminates tapeworms and giardia protozoa by detaching the *scolex* (attachment organ) from intestinal tract. Rapidly absorbed from GI tract.

Use/Therapeutic goal/Outcome

Tapeworms: Elimination. *Outcome criteria:* Expulsion of worms followed by 3 negative stool samples after completion of treatment.

Giardiasis: Elimination of giardia protozoa. *Outcome criteria:* Absence of diarrhea, cramp-

ing, nausea. Absence of giardia in stool sample.

Dose range/Administration

Interaction alert: Do not give with primaquine (greatly enhances its toxicity). Drinking alcohol, may cause disulfiram-like reaction.

🖐 **Give after meals with a full glass of water or juice to reduce GI distress.**

Giardiasis: Adult: PO: 100 mg tid for 5–7 days. *Child:* PO: 7 mg/kg/day in divided doses tid pc for 5 days. *Maximum dose:* 300 mg/day. May be necessary to repeat in 2 wks.

Tapeworm: Adult/Child > 14 yrs: PO: 200 mg q 10 min for 4 doses. *Child 11–14 yrs:* PO: 600 mg divided in 3–4 doses, one dose q 10 min. *Child 5–10 yrs:* PO: 400 mg divided in 3–4 doses, one dose q 10 min.

Clinical alert: To ensure therapeutic effect with tapeworms, the patient should avoid fat and eat bland, semi-soft foods the day before treatment, and then fast the night before treatment (after the last meal). Taking sodium bicarbonate with each large dose will reduce incidence of nausea and vomiting. Follow treatment with a saline cathartic to expel worms.

Contraindications/Precautions

PREG
C

Contraindicated in hypersensitivity to quinacrine hydrochloride, and in concomitant primaquine antimalarial therapy. *Use with caution* in liver disease, alcoholism, history of psychosis, psoriasis, porphyria, or G6PD deficiency.

🖐 **Use with caution for children under 1 year and the elderly. Safe use for pregnant or nursing mothers has not been established.**

Side effects/Adverse reactions

Hypersensitivity: rashes, skin eruptions, visual disturbances (halos, blurring). *GI:* abdominal discomfort or cramping, diarrhea, anorexia, nausea, vomiting. *CNS:* nervousness, dizziness, headache, mood shifts, nightmares, transitory toxic psychoses, seizures. *GU:* profoundly yellow urine. *Skin:* yellow discoloration of the skin. *Misc:* black nails.

Nursing implications/Documentation

Possible nursing diagnoses: Potential for infection; Situational low self-esteem.

◆ If tablets must be crushed, mix with jam or honey to disguise bitter taste.

◆ Collect all stools for 48 hrs, and observe for worms and *scolex*, which will be stained yellow from drug. Stools should be sent to the lab while still warm.

♦ Determine close contacts (family/significant others), who should be evaluated for treatment as well.

Patient & family teaching/Home care

Possible nursing diagnoses: Knowledge deficit; Impaired home maintenance management.

♦ Explore feelings and concerns, and explain that intestinal worms or parasites are not associated with "dirtiness."

♦ Emphasize the need to continue taking quinacrine for full course of treatment.

♦ Stress the importance of preventing reinfection or spread of infection by treating all family members and close contacts, taking the medication exactly as prescribed, washing foods especially carefully, meticulously washing hands after bowel movements, cutting nails short, changing clothing every day, keeping fingers out of mouth, having infected individuals sleep alone, eliminating ova by washing all linens daily in hot water (without shaking them), vacuuming and damp-mopping the house daily, cleaning the toilet with disinfectant daily, and, for giardiasis, returning for a second treatment in 2 weeks.

♦ Explain that skin and urine may turn yellow, but that this is harmless and will subside.

♦ Warn that if dizziness is experienced, hazardous activities and driving should be avoided.

♦ Point out that rashes or visual disturbances should be reported.

♦ Inform that lactose intolerance caused by the infection may persist for months, causing symptoms similar to the infection.

♦ *See Anti-infectives overview for more information.*

quinethazone

kwin-eth'a-zone

♣Aquamox, Hydromox

Class: Thiazide-like diuretic, Antihypertensive

PEDS	PREG	GERI
♨	D	✋

Action Promotes the excretion of sodium chloride, potassium, and water by inhibiting reabsorption of sodium in the early portion of the distal tubule. Lowers blood pressure by reducing plasma and extra-cellular volume.

Use/Therapeutic goal/Outcome

Hypertension: Promotion of diuresis, reduction of blood pressure. **Outcome criteria:** After 3–4 days, blood pressure within normal limits. **Edema:** Promotion of diuresis, resolution of edema. **Outcome criteria:** Increased urine output; weight loss; absence of rales and peripheral edema.

Dose range/Administration

Interaction alert: Cholestyramine and colestipol inhibit intestinal absorption. Diazoxide increases hypotensive, hyperglycemic, and hyperuricemic effects.

Adult: PO: 50–100 mg/day. *Maximum dose:* 200 mg/day.

Clinical alert: Give in morning to avoid nocturnal diuresis. Antihypertensive response may not occur for 3–4 days.

Contraindications/Precautions

PREG
D

Contraindicated in hypersensitivity to sulfonamides, thiazides, and quinethazones, and in anuria. **Use with caution** in allergies, renal or hepatic disease, gout, diabetes, and sympathectomy.

♨ **Contraindicated for pregnant or nursing mothers. Use with caution for the elderly. Safe use in children has not been established.**

Side effects/Adverse reactions

Hypersensitivity: rash, urticaria, dermatitis with photosensitivity, pneumonitis, vasculitis. **Hem:** hypokalemia, hyperglycemia, azotemia, impaired glucose tolerance, asymptomatic hyperuricemia, electrolyte imbalance, metabolic alkalosis, hypercalcemia, lipid abnormalities, aplastic anemia, agranulocytosis, leukopenia, thrombocytopenia. **CV:** volume depletion, dehydration, orthostatic hypotension. **GI:** anorexia, nausea, pancreatitis, hepatic encephalopathy. **Misc:** gout.

Nursing implications/Documentation

Possible nursing diagnoses: Fluid volume deficit; Altered patterns of urinary elimination; Potential for injury.

♦ Ascertain that baseline CBC, sodium, potassium, chloride, carbon dioxide, calcium, magnesium, BUN, creatinine, uric acid, and liver function studies have been obtained before giving first dose; report abnormalities and monitor closely thereafter.

- Document and monitor blood pressure, pulse, daily weight, and intake and output; report significant discrepancies.
- Monitor for hyperglycemia because of risk of thiazide diabetes.
- Observe for and report signs of fluid overload (auscultate lungs for rales; check feet, ankles, and sacrum for edema).
- Be aware that diuretics often induce hypokalemia, which predisposes individuals to cardiac arrhythmias, cramping, and digoxin toxicity.
- Check with physician to determine dietary restrictions; if a low-salt, high-potassium diet is recommended, consult with dietician to plan a low-salt diet that includes foods and juices high in potassium (orange juice; banana; green leafy vegetables).
- Observe the elderly for extreme diuresis (may require lower doses); monitor for orthostatic hypotension; supervise ambulation until response is determined.

Patient & family teaching/Home care

Possible nursing diagnoses: Knowledge deficit; Impaired home maintenance management.

- Before giving first dose, explain that the drug will increase the amount and frequency of urination.
- Emphasize the importance of taking this drug exactly as prescribed, and the importance of returning for medical follow-up.
- Explain that diuretics enhance the work of the kidney and reduce the workload of the heart.
- Recommend taking doses in early morning and early afternoon to prevent the need to disturb sleep to void.
- Explain that changing positions slowly helps prevent dizziness.
- Advise reporting dizziness, shortness of breath, swelling of hands and feet, or persistent sore throat; encourage daily monitoring of weight and reporting sudden weight gain.
- Warn that hyperglycemia is common; advise reporting thirst, fatigue, or weight loss.
- Provide a list of allowed foods and fluids; stress the need to stick to prescribed diet (explain the hazards of too much salt, or too little potassium).

- Warn against driving or activities that require alertness until response has been determined.
- Advise avoidance of OTC drugs unless approved by physician.
- Suggest using a (Number 15) sunscreen when outside because of photosensitivity (avoid products with PABA).
- *See Diuretics and Antihypertensives overviews for more information.*

quinidine

kwin'i-deen

quinidine gluconate (62% quinidine alkaloid): **Duraquin, Quinaglute DURA-TABS, Quinalan, ♦Quinate**

quinidine polygalacturonate (60.5% quinidine alkaloid): **Cardioquin**

quinidine sulfate (83% quinidine alkaloid): **♦Apo-Quinidine, Cin-Quin, ♦Novoquindin, Quine, Quinidex, Extentabs, Quinora**

Class: Antiarrhythmic (Class IA)

PEDS	PREG	GERI
✋	C	✋

Action Has an overall myocardial depressant effect. Decreases impulse conduction by depressing excitability, conduction velocity, and contractility of the myocardium. Stabilizes cell membrane and prolongs effective refractory period of both atria and ventricles. Has anticholinergic action which inhibits vagal tone on SA and AV nodes. Larger doses may decrease peripheral vascular resistance.

Use/Therapeutic goal/Outcome

Atrial arrhythmias (flutter, fibrillation, paroxysmal atrial tachycardia [PAT]), nodal tachycardia, ventricular ectopy (PVCs), and tachycardia: Suppression of ventricular and atrial ectopy and promotion of effective heartbeat. **Outcome criteria:** Absence of atrial and ventricular ectopy on EKG; regular palpable pulses.

Dose range/Administration

Interaction alert: Antacids, sodium bicarbonate, thiazide diuretics, acetazolamide, or other urinary alkalizers may increase serum quinidine levels. May increase serum digoxin level (monitor closely). Phenobarbital, phenytoin, and rifampin may decrease serum quinidine. Give cautiously with calcium channel blocking agents (can increase hypotensive effect) and neuromuscular blocking agents (increases neuromuscular blockade). May potentiate hypotensive effects of thiazide diuretics, antianginals, and other antihypertensive agents. Cimetidine may increase serum quinidine levels.

🍂 **Give with meals to minimize GI upset.**

PACs or PVCs (premature atrial or ventricular contractions): *Adult:* PO: 200–300 mg tid or qid.

PAT, PNT (paroxysmal nodal tachycardia), and ventricular tachycardia: *Adult:* PO: 400–600 mg q2-3h until arrhythmias are terminated.

Atrial fibrillation/flutter: *Adult:* PO: *Quinidine sulfate:* 200 mg q2-3h for 5–8 doses; maintenance dose is 200–300 mg tid to qid. *Quinidine gluconate* (maintenance and prophylaxis): 324–660 mg q8-12h. *Quinidine polygalacturonate:* 275–825 mg q3-4h for 3–4 doses; may be increased by 137.5–275 mg every third or fourth dose until fibrillation or flutter subsides, or until toxic effects or serum levels are noted. IM: *Quinidine gluconate:* Loading dose of 600 mg, followed by 400 mg repeated as often as q2h. IV: *Quinidine gluconate:* Dilute 800 mg in 40 cc D5W and inject slowly at a rate of 1 cc/min. *Child:* PO: *Quinidine sulfate:* 6 mg/kg/day in 5 divided doses.

Clinical alert: Be aware that a 50–200 mg test dose may be given. Quinidine should be started after digitalization to reduce risk of AV conduction failure. Dose varies depending upon clinical response and therapeutic drug levels. These should be monitored closely because of risk of severe toxic effects.

Contraindications/Precautions

PREG
C

Contraindicated in hypersensitivity to quinidine, and in AV block, intraventricular conduction defects, myasthenia gravis, and suspected digitalis toxicity. *Use with caution* in congestive heart failure and hypotension.

🖐 Use with caution for children and the elderly. Safe use for pregnant or nursing mothers has not been established.

Side effects/Adverse reactions

Hypersensitivity: thrombocytopenia, skin eruptions, fever, hepatotoxicity, lupus-like syndrome (fever, chills, rash, itching, joint pain and swelling, wheezing, shortness of breath). *GI:* nausea, vomiting, diarrhea, excessive salivation. *CV:* severe hypotension, EKG changes (widening of the QRS complex and prolongation of the QT interval), asystole, arrhythmias. *Hem:* hemolytic anemia, agranulocytosis.

CNS: vertigo, lightheadedness, restlessness, headache, apprehension, excitability, confusion, syncope. *Eye:* visual disturbances. *Ear:* hearing disturbances.

Nursing implications/Documentation

Possible nursing diagnoses: Potential for injury; Activity intolerance; Diarrhea.

♦ Be sure to check baseline chest X-ray, EKG, and laboratory studies (CBC, sodium, potassium, chloride, carbon dioxide, magnesium, BUN, creatinine, SGPT, and LDH) before giving first dose; monitor closely thereafter as indicated by clinical condition.

♦ Remember that oxygen requirements must be met, and that electrolyte imbalances (especially potassium and magnesium) and abnormal blood pH must be corrected, before expected antiarrhythmic effect can be seen; report abnormalities immediately.

♦ Document baseline vital signs, lung sounds, and cardiac monitor strip (measure and record PR, QRS, and QT segments) before giving first dose and at least every 8 hr; monitor closely until response is determined; report if prolongation in PR, QRS, or QT segment is noted.

♦ Monitor for and report "quinidine syncope," which can result from tachyarrhythmias (especially common when quinidine is given for atrial fibrillation or flutter).

♦ Monitor serum quinidine for therapeutic levels (greater than 8 mcg/cc is toxic).

♦ Report GI disturbances (especially diarrhea), which may be early signs of toxicity.

♦ When giving IV, monitor for hypotension and cardiovascular collapse (oral route is preferred).

♦ Coordinate care to provide frequent rest periods.

Patient & family teaching/Home care

Possible nursing diagnoses: Fear; Knowledge deficit; Impaired home maintenance management.

♦ Explain that the purpose of this drug is to prevent arrhythmias and promote an effective heartbeat.

♦ Advise taking oral doses with meals to reduce GI symptoms.

♦ Stress the need to follow dose regimen closely (the drug should be taken at the same time each day), and the need to return for medical follow-up for early detection of adverse reactions.

◆ Teach how to assess pulse for irregularities in rhythm and rate; stress that irregularities be reported.

◆ Advise that diarrhea, sore throat, sore mouth and gums, bruising, or bleeding should be reported immediately.

◆ Emphasize the need to pace activities, avoid stress, and plan for rest periods.

◆ Encourage learning CPR; reinforce that survival rate of cardiac arrest is greatly increased when CPR is initiated immediately.

◆ *See Antiarrhythmics overview for more information.*

radioactive iodine

(sodium iodide) ^{131}I: *Iodotope Therapeutic, Sodium Iodide ^{131}I Therapeutic*

Class: Radiopharmaceutical antineoplastic agent, Antihyperthyroid agent

PEDS	PREG	GERI
🖑	X	🖑

Action Destroys thyroid tissue (thus limiting thyroid hormone secretion); converts to protein bound iodine, and binds to cancerous thyroid tissue that has metastasized to other sites in the body (thus destroying the metastatic tissue).

Use/Therapeutic goal/Outcome

Hyperthyroidism: Suppression of circulating thyroid hormones, promotion of normal metabolism. *Outcome criteria:* After 3 weeks, decreased T_4 levels; weight gain; normal pulse rate.

Thyroid cancer: Destruction of cancerous tissue. *Outcome criteria:* X-ray evidence of decrease in thyroid tumor size, decrease in numbers and size of metastatic tumors on total body scan.

Dose range/Administration

Interaction alert: Avoid stable iodine, thyroid, or antithyroid drugs (they decrease uptake of radioactive iodine). Lithium carbonate may be synergistic (monitor for hypothyroidism).

Hyperthyroidism, Graves' disease: Adult: PO: 4–10 millicuries (dose based on estimated weight of thyroid gland and thyroid uptake). Repeat treatment in 6 wks if indicated by serum thyroxine levels and clinical status.

Thyroid cancer: Adult: PO: 50–150 millicuries (dose based on estimated malignant thyroid tissue and metastatic tissue as determined by

total body scan); may repeat depending upon clinical status. Usually not given to patients < 30 yrs unless there is no other choice.

Clinical alert: Follow hospital policies for caring for individuals taking a radioactive substance (isolate patient, prohibit pregnant women from entering room, use disposable utensils and linen, save all urine). After dose for hyperthyroidism, implement full radiation precautions for 24 hours (urine and saliva are slightly radioactive for 24 hours, and vomitus is highly radioactive for 8 hours). After dose for cancer, implement full radiation precautions for 3 days and expect course of SSKI.

Contraindications/Precautions PREG X

Contraindicated in hypersensitivity to iodine, and in recent MI, large nodular goiter, age under 30 years, vomiting, diarrhea, acute hyperthyroidism, and use of thyroid drugs. *Use with caution* in the presence of cardiac or kidney disease.

🖑 **Contraindicated for pregnant and nursing mothers. Use with caution for children and the elderly.**

Side effects/Adverse reactions

Hypersensitivity: itching, rashes, angioedema, fever. Other effects are usually dose-related. *GI:* stomatitis, nausea, vomiting, diarrhea, decreased appetite, metallic taste, salivary gland enlargement, hepatotoxicity, small bowel lesions, abdominal pain. *CNS:* headache, drowsiness, dizziness. *Hem:* agranulocytosis, leukopenia, thrombocytopenia. *Eye:* visual problems, periorbital edema. *Skin:* acne, hair loss, petechiae, jaundice, hyperpigmentation. *CV:* vasculitis. *MS:* muscle and joint pain, weakness. *Misc:* hypothyroidism, transient thyroiditis, hyperthyroid adenoma, mucosal hemorrhage, radiation sickness, chromosomal abnormalities.

Nursing implications/Documentation

Possible nursing diagnoses: Altered nutrition: less than body requirements; Altered nutrition: more than body requirements; Altered oral mucous membrane.

◆ Have the patient fast all night before dose; stop all antithyroid drugs, thyroid drugs, and iodine-containing preparations one week before ^{131}I dose; if drugs have not been stopped, may give thyroid-stimulating hormone 3 days before ^{131}I dose.

◆ Monitor T_3, T_4, and serum thyroxine levels.

- Provide favorite fluids and encourage drinking 3–4 L a day for 48 hr after treatment (helps flush radioactive iodine from body).
- Document and monitor daily weights.
- Institute radiation precautions (see Clinical alert).
- Offer frequent mouth care.

Patient & family teaching/Home care

Possible nursing diagnoses: Knowledge deficit; Impaired home maintenance management.

- If patient is discharged less than 7 days after treatment, advise the person to sleep alone and to avoid close contact with small children for 7 days (due to increased risk of thyroid cancer for those exposed to ^{131}I).
- Stress that good oral hygiene can prevent gum problems.
- Reinforce the importance of returning for medical follow-up.
- Advise to increase fluid intake to promote frequent voiding and decrease radiation exposure to urinary bladder; double-flush toilet.
- *See Thyroid Hormone Antagonists overview for more information.*

ranitidine

ra-nit'ih-deen

Zantac

Class: Histamine (H_2) receptor antagonist, Antiulcer agent, Gastric acid secretion inhibitor

PEDS	PREG	GERI
🖐	B	🖐

Action Decreases basal and nocturnal secretion of gastric acid by inhibiting the action of histamine at the H_2 receptors in the gastric parietal cells; decreases gastric acid secretion in response to food or chemical stimulus.

Use/Therapeutic goal/Outcome

Peptic ulcers: Promotion of healing and relief of pain. **Outcome criteria:** Report of absence of pain; hemoglobin and hematocrit within normal range; vital signs stable; stools negative for occult blood; endoscopic evidence of healing.

Ulcer recurrence and stress induced ulcers: Prevention. **Outcome criteria:** Report of absence of gastric pain; stable hemoglobin and hematocrit; stool and gastric secretions free of blood.

Gastroesophageal reflux disease: Symptomatic treatment. **Outcome criteria:** Report of

decrease or absence of epigastric burning and pain.

Hypersecretory conditions (e.g., Zollinger-Ellison syndrome): Control of hypersecretion of acid. **Outcome criteria:** Report of relief of epigastric pain; decreased diarrhea/steatorrhea; decreased acidity of gastric secretions.

Dose range/Administration

Interaction alert: Give antacids 1 hr before or after ranitidine to avoid interference with absorption. May markedly reduce absorption of ketoconazole. With high doses of ranitidine, metabolism of oral anticoagulants, metoprolol, phenytoin, cyclosporine, disulfiram, oral contraceptives, isoniazid, and procainamide may be decreased, leading to higher blood levels and toxicity.

Adult: PO: 150 mg bid, or 300 mg at bedtime. IM, IV: 50 mg q6-8h. *Maintenance dose:* 150 mg at bedtime. *Maximum dose:* 400 mg (may be greater for treatment of hypersecretion).

Clinical alert: In moderate to severe renal failure, reduced doses should be used.

Contraindications/Precautions

PREG B

Contraindicated in hypersensitivity to histamine (H_2) receptor antagonists. **Use with caution** in renal and hepatic impairment.

🖐 **Use with caution for pregnant or nursing mothers and the elderly. Safe use for children has not been established.**

Side effects/Adverse reactions

Hypersensitivity: rash, fever, bronchospasm. **CNS:** headache, confusion (especially in the elderly with hepatic and renal impairment). **GI:** nausea, constipation.

Nursing implications/Documentation

Possible nursing diagnoses: Constipation; Potential for injury.

- Give doses without regard to meals; single daily dose should be given at bedtime.
- Crush tablets for NG administration since they are highly soluble.
- Document and report changes in mental state, especially in the elderly and in patients with hepatic and renal impairment.

Patient & family teaching/Home care

Possible nursing diagnoses: Knowledge deficit; Constipation; Impaired home maintenance management.

R

- Point out the need to avoid taking antacids within 1 hr of ranitidine.

- Advise those who are ordered one daily dose to take that dose at bedtime.

- Teach smokers not to smoke cigarettes after the bedtime dose to obtain optimal suppression of nocturnal gastric acid secretion.

- Inform those being treated for active ulcer disease that medication should be taken as prescribed for 4 to 8 weeks to ensure healing of the ulcer, even though symptoms usually subside earlier.

- For nursing mothers, advise to wait 1 to 2 hr after dose of ranitidine before nursing infant.

- Counsel smokers with active ulcer disease to stop smoking and to avoid the use of caffeine.

- Stress need to advise primary physician if dizziness, somnolence, rash, or hallucinations develop or if "coffee grounds" vomit or tarry stools occur.

- *See Histamine₂ Antagonists overview for more information.*

rauwolfia

rah-wool'fee-a

rauwolfia serpentina: *Raudixin, Rauval, Rauverid, Wolfina*

Class: Antihypertensive, Antiadrenergic

PEDS	PREG	GERI
🖐	D	🖐

Action Reduces blood pressure by inhibiting the release of norepinephrine and depleting norepinephrine stores at peripheral adrenergic nerve endings (results in relaxation of smooth muscle of the blood vessels). This action within the CNS leads to tranquilization and sedation.

Use/Therapeutic goal/Outcome
Hypertension: Reduction of blood pressure. *Outcome criteria:* Blood pressure within normal limits.

Dose range/Administration
Interaction alert: Use with MAO inhibitors may potentiate sympathomimetic response, causing hyperexcitability and hypertension. Use with anesthetics, barbiturates, diuretics, and other antihypertensives may potentiate hypotensive effect. Use with digitalis or quinidine may cause cardiac arrhythmias. Use with anticholinergics, anticonvulsants, indirect-acting sympathomimetics, levodopa, morphine, salicy-

lates, and vasopressors can decrease their effects.

🍴 **Give with meals to reduce GI irritation.**
Adult: PO: 200–400 mg/day in single or divided doses; may increase after 1–3 weeks. *Maintenance dose:* 50–300 mg/day in single or divided doses.

Clinical alert: Drug effect may last for 10 days after withdrawal.

Contraindications/Precautions
PREG
D
Contraindicated in hypersensitivity to rauwolfia alkaloids, and in bronchial asthma, respiratory disturbances, depression, ulcer disease, and pheochromocytoma. *Use with caution* in impaired renal function, cerebrovascular disease or severe cardiac disease.

🖐 **Use with caution for the elderly. Safe use for children and pregnant women has not been established.**

Side effects/Adverse reactions
Hypersensitivity: rash, urticaria, pruritis. *CV:* orthostatic hypotension, bradycardia. *CNS:* syncope, drowsiness, sedation, confusion, depression, anxiety, nightmares, nervousness, extrapyramidal symptoms, headache. *GI:* dry mouth, nausea, vomiting, gastric distress, gastric bleeding. *Eye:* glaucoma. *GU:* impotence. *Resp:* nasal stuffiness. *Misc:* weight gain.

Nursing implications/Documentation
Possible nursing diagnoses: Activity intolerance; Fatigue; Potential for injury; Altered oral mucous membrane.

- Assess mental status, and record pulse and blood pressure (lying, sitting, and standing, in both arms) before administration, and frequently thereafter until response is determined.

- Consult with physician to determine desired therapeutic range for blood pressure (be aware that some patients may require a slightly elevated blood pressure to perfuse vital organs).

- Ascertain that baseline CBC, electrolytes, BUN, creatinine, and liver function studies have been obtained before giving first dose; report abnormalities and monitor closely thereafter.

- Monitor for signs of depression, confusion, dizziness, bradycardia, hypotension; hold drug and report immediately if these occur.

- Supervise ambulation until response is determined.
- Document and monitor daily weight, and intake and output; report significant negative or positive balance.
- Provide frequent mouth care.

Patient & family teaching/Home care

Possible nursing diagnoses: Knowledge deficit; Impaired home maintenance management; Altered sexuality patterns.

- Teach the person to take this drug with food to reduce GI symptoms.
- Explain the importance of taking medication exactly as prescribed, even when feeling well.
- Stress the importance of good medical follow-up, explain that this drug reduces "wear and tear" on blood vessels, and improves longevity and health.
- Teach how to monitor pulse and blood pressure; emphasize that syncope, hypertension or hypotension, or persistent dizziness should be reported.
- Advise changing positions slowly to avoid dizziness.
- Encourage daily monitoring of weight and reporting sudden weight gain (frequently fluid retention).
- Warn against drinking alcohol or taking *any* OTC drugs without physician approval (some interactions can cause severe reactions).
- Emphasize that the person should not drive or operate machinery until response is determined (may cause drowsiness).
- Explain that this drug may alter sexual activity; encourage the individual to voice concerns.
- *See Antihypertensives overview for more information.*

rescinnamine

re-sin'a-meen

Anaprel, Moderil

Class: Antihypertensive, Antiadrenergic

PEDS	PREG	GERI
✋	**D**	✋

Action Reduces blood pressure by inhibiting the release of norepinephrine and depleting norepinephrine stores at peripheral adrenergic nerve endings (results in relaxation of smooth muscles of the blood vessels). This action within the CNS leads to tranquilization and sedation.

Use/Therapeutic goal/Outcome

Hypertension: Reduction of blood pressure. **Outcome criteria:** Blood pressure within normal limits.

Dose range/Administration

Interaction alert: Use with MAO inhibitors may potentiate sympathomimetic response, causing excitability and hypertension. Anesthetics, barbiturates, diuretics, and other antihypertensives may potentiate hypotensive effect. Use with digitalis or quinidine may cause cardiac arrhythmias. Use with anticholinergics, anticonvulsants, indirect-acting sympathomimetics, levodopa, morphine, salicylates, and vasopressors can decrease their effects.

🖐 **Give with meals to reduce GI irritation.**
Adult: PO: 0.5 mg bid; increase gradually. *Maintenance dose:* 0.25–0.5 mg/day.

Clinical alert: Drug effect may last for 10 days after withdrawal. Discontinue 2 weeks before surgery and 1 week before exercise stress test.

Contraindications/Precautions

PREG D

Contraindicated in hypersensitivity to rauwolfia alkaloids, and in depression, ulcer disease, electroconvulsive therapy. **Use with caution** in cardiac disease, asthma, cerebrovascular disease, and with other antihypertensives.

🖐 **Use with caution for the elderly. Safe use for children and pregnant women has not been established.**

Side effects/Adverse reactions

Hypersensitivity: rash, urticaria, pruritis. **CV:** orthostatic hypotension, bradycardia. **CNS:** syncope, drowsiness, sedation, confusion, depression, anxiety, nightmares, nervousness, parkinsonism. **GI:** mouth dryness, nausea, vomiting, gastric distress. **Eye:** glaucoma. **GU:** impotence. **Resp:** nasal stuffiness. **Misc:** weight gain, fluid retention.

Nursing implications/Documentation

Possible nursing diagnoses: Activity intolerance; Fatigue; Potential for injury; Altered oral mucous membrane.

- Assess mental status, and record pulse and blood pressure (lying, sitting, and standing, in both arms) prior to administration, and fre-

R

quently thereafter until response is determined.

♦ Consult with physician to determine desired therapeutic range for blood pressure (be aware that some patients may require a slightly elevated blood pressure to perfuse vital organs).

♦ Ascertain that baseline CBC, electrolytes, BUN, creatinine, and liver function studies have been obtained before giving first dose; report abnormalities and monitor closely thereafter.

♦ Monitor for signs of depression, confusion, dizziness, bradycardia, hypotension; hold drug and report immediately if these occur.

♦ Supervise ambulation until response is determined.

♦ Document and monitor daily weight, and intake and output; report significant negative or positive balance.

♦ Provide frequent mouth care.

Patient & family teaching/Home care

Possible nursing diagnoses: Knowledge deficit; Impaired home maintenance management; Altered sexuality patterns.

♦ Teach the person to take this drug with food to reduce GI symptoms.

♦ Explain the importance of taking medication exactly as prescribed, even when feeling well.

♦ Stress the importance of good medical follow-up, explain that this drug reduces "wear and tear" on blood vessels and improves longevity and health.

♦ Teach how to monitor pulse and blood pressure; emphasize that syncope, hypertension or hypotension, or persistent dizziness should be reported.

♦ Advise changing positions slowly to avoid dizziness.

♦ Encourage daily monitoring of weight and reporting sudden weight gain (frequently fluid retention).

♦ Warn against taking *any* OTC drugs without physician approval (some interactions can cause severe reactions).

♦ Emphasize that the person should not drive or operate machinery until response is determined (may cause drowsiness).

♦ Explain that this drug may alter sexual activity; encourage individuals to voice concerns; consult a specialist if necessary.

♦ See *Antihypertensives overview* for more information.

reserpine

re-ser'peen

♣*Novoreserpine,* ♣*Reserfia, Serpalan, Serpasil*
Class: ★**Antiadrenergic antihypertensive prototype**, Antihypertensive

PEDS	PREG	GERI
🖐	C	🖐

Action Reduces blood pressure by depleting norepinephrine stores at peripheral adrenergic nerve endings (results in relaxation of smooth muscles of the blood vessels). This action in the CNS leads to tranquilization and sedation.

Use/Therapeutic goal/Outcome

Hypertension: Reduction of blood pressure. **Outcome criteria:** Blood pressure within normal limits.

Dose range/Administration

Interaction alert: Use with MAO inhibitors may potentiate sympathomimetic response causing excitation and hypertension. Use with anesthetics, barbiturates, diuretics, and other antihypertensives may potentiate hypotensive effect. Use with digitalis or quinidine may cause cardiac arrhythmias. Use with anticholinergics, anticonvulsants, indirect-acting sympathomimetics, levodopa, morphine, salicylates and vasopressors can decrease their effects.

🥄 **Give with meals to reduce GI irritation.**
Hypertension: Adult: PO: 0.25–0.5 mg/day for 1–2 weeks. *Maintenance dose:* 0.1–0.5 mg/day. **Child:** PO: 0.02 mg/kg/day. *Maximum dose:* 0.25 mg/day.

Clinical alert: Full effect begins in 2–3 weeks and may last for 4–6 weeks after withdrawal.

Contraindications/Precautions

PREG
C

Contraindicated in hypersensitivity to rauwolfia alkaloids, and in depression, peripheral vascular disease, severe cardiac disease, cerebrovascular disease, and heart failure. **Use with caution** in impaired renal function, cerebrovascular disease, or severe cardiac disease.

🖐 **Use with caution for the elderly. Safe use for children and pregnant women has not been established.**

Side effects/Adverse reactions

Hypersensitivity: rash, urticaria, pruritis, asthma. **CV:** orthostatic hypotension, bradycardia. **CNS:** syncope, drowsiness, depression, anxiety, sedation, nervousness, confusion, extrapyramidal symptoms, headache, nightmares. **GI:** dry mouth, nausea, vomiting, gastric distress, gastric bleeding. **Eye:** glaucoma. **GU:** impotence. **Resp:** nasal stuffiness. **Misc:** weight gain, fluid retention.

Nursing implications/Documentation

Possible nursing diagnoses: Activity intolerance; Fatigue; Potential for injury; Altered oral mucous membrane.

♦ Assess mental status, and record pulse and blood pressure (lying, sitting, and standing, in both arms) before administration, and frequently thereafter until response is determined.

♦ Consult with physician to determine desired therapeutic range for blood pressure (be aware that some patients may require a slightly elevated blood pressure to perfuse vital organs).

♦ Ascertain that baseline CBC, electrolytes, BUN, creatinine, and liver function studies have been obtained before giving first dose; report abnormalities and monitor closely thereafter.

♦ Monitor for signs of depression, confusion, dizziness, bradycardia, hypotension, visual problems; hold drug and report immediately if these occur.

♦ Supervise ambulation until response is determined.

♦ Document and monitor daily weight, and intake and output; report significant negative or positive balance.

♦ Provide frequent mouth care.

Patient & family teaching/Home care

Possible nursing diagnoses: Knowledge deficit; Impaired home maintenance management; Altered sexuality patterns.

♦ Teach the person to take this drug with food to reduce GI symptoms.

♦ Explain the importance of taking medication exactly as prescribed, even when feeling well.

♦ Stress the importance of good medical follow-up; explain that this drug reduces "wear and tear" on blood vessels and improves longevity and health.

♦ Teach how to monitor pulse and blood pressure; emphasize that syncope, hypertension or hypotension, or persistent dizziness should be reported.

♦ Advise changing positions slowly to avoid dizziness.

♦ Encourage daily monitoring of weight and reporting sudden weight gain (frequently is fluid retention).

♦ Warn against taking *any* OTC drugs without physician approval (some interactions can cause severe reactions).

♦ Emphasize that the person should not drive or operate machinery until response is determined (may cause drowsiness).

♦ Stress that the individual should have periodic eye exams.

♦ Explain that this drug may alter sexual activity; encourage individuals to voice concerns.

♦ *See Antihypertensives overview for more information.*

rifampin

ri-fam'pin

Rifadin, Rimactane, ♠Rimycin

Class: Anti-infective, Antitubercular

PEDS	PREG	GERI
🖐	C	🖐

Action Kills bacteria (bactericidal action) and limits their growth (bacteriostatic action) by inhibiting RNA synthesis in susceptible bacteria.

Use/Therapeutic goal/Outcome

Clinical tuberculosis: Resolution of tubercular infection. **Outcome criteria:** Absence of acid-fast bacilli on sputum culture, decreased productive cough, normal temperature, improvement of X rays.

Meningococcal carriers, prophylaxis for Hemophilus influenza Type B infection: Prevention of infection. **Outcome criteria:** Absence of signs and symptoms of meningococcal or *Hemophilus influenza* Type B infection.

Dose range/Administration

Interaction alert: Alcohol, isoniazid, and halothane increase risk of hepatotoxicity. Probenecid increases rifampin levels. Rifampin may decrease plasma concentrations of barbiturates, benzodiazapines, beta-blockers, chloramphenicol, clofibrate, corticosteroids, digitalis glycosides, cyclosporin, methadone and other narcotics, oral anticoagulants, oral antidiabetic agents, oral contraceptives, estrogens and progestins, theophylline and quinidine. Ketoconazole and aminosalicylic acid may delay absorption.

▯ **Give 1 hr before meals or 2 hrs after meals, unless GI symptoms are noted (then give with meals).**

Active tuberculosis: With at least one other antitubercular agent. *Adult:* PO, IV: 600 mg/day for 6–9 mos. *Child > 5 yrs:* PO, IV: 10–20 mg/kg/day. *Maximum dose:* 600 mg/day.

Meningococcal carriers: *Adult:* PO: 600 mg/day for 4 days. *Child 1–12 yrs:* PO: 10 mg/kg/day bid for 2 days. *Maximum dose:* 600 mg. *Child 3 mos–1 yr:* PO: 5 mg/kg bid for 2 days.

Prevention of Hemophilus influenza Type B: *Adult/Child:* PO: 20 mg/kg/day for 4 days. *Maximum dose:* 600 mg/day.

Clinical alert: If there is trouble swallowing, empty capsules into food or fluid, or use suspension.

Contraindications/Precautions

Contraindicated in hypersensitivity to rifampin, and in clinically active hepatitis.

☝ **Contraindicated for nursing mothers. Use with caution for the elderly, children under 13 yrs and during pregnancy (in last weeks of pregnancy, may cause bleeding in mother and infant).**

Side effects/Adverse reactions

Hypersensitivity: itching, rash. *GI:* anorexia, nausea, vomiting, epigastric distress, abdominal pain, diarrhea, flatulence, sore mouth and tongue, hepatotoxicity. *CNS:* drowsiness, headache, fatigue, dizziness, ataxia, confusion, generalized numbness. *Hem:* thrombocytopenia, transient leukopenia, hemolytic anemia, hyperuricemia. *Misc:* flu-like syndrome, discoloration of body fluids (red-orange).

Nursing implications/Documentation

Possible nursing diagnoses: Potential for infection; Potential for injury; Fatigue; Activity intolerance; Fluid volume deficit.

◆ Ascertain that baseline CBC, BUN, creatinine, and liver function studies are obtained, and that necessary culture specimens are collected before starting rifampin; monitor periodically thereafter, depending on clinical symptoms.

◆ Recognize that hepatotoxicity can be serious; monitor for and report persistent GI symptoms, jaundice, clay-colored stools.

◆ Allow for a balance between rest and activity.

◆ Monitor and record intake and output and provide favorite fluids to ensure adequate hydration.

◆ Monitor for drowsiness and ataxia until response is determined.

Patient & family teaching/Home care

Possible nursing diagnoses: Knowledge deficit; Impaired home maintenance management.

◆ Explain that drug should be taken on an empty stomach unless GI symptoms are experienced (then it should be taken *with* food).

◆ Stress the importance of taking this drug as prescribed without missing doses, and the importance of long-term medical follow-up to avoid relapses or complications.

◆ Advise avoiding alcohol to reduce risk of liver toxicity.

◆ Advise that rifampin may cause body fluids (tears, saliva, sputum, urine, stools) to turn a red-orange color; soft contact lenses may become permanently stained.

◆ Warn that drowsiness may occur, and that driving should be avoided, until response is determined.

◆ Advise women taking oral contraceptives to use alternative methods of birth control.

◆ Encourage drinking at least 2 quarts a day to maintain adequate hydration.

◆ *See Anti-infectives overview for more information.*

ritodrine

ri'toe-dreen

ritodrine hydrochloride: *Yutopar*

Class: Sympathomimetic, Uterine relaxant

PEDS	PREG	GERI
X	B	X

Action Decreases the frequency and intensity of uterine contractions by stimulating beta$_2$-adrenergic receptors in uterine smooth muscle.

R

Use/Therapeutic goal/Outcome

Preterm labor (after 20 weeks) in selected women: Inhibition of uterine contractions. *Outcome criteria:* Cessation of labor.

Dose range/Administration

Interaction alert: If given with corticosteroids, monitor closely for maternal pulmonary edema. Inhalation anesthetics may potentiate adverse cardiac effects (dysrhythmias, hypotension). Avoid use with beta-blockers because they may inhibit the action of ritodrine. If given with other sympathomimetics, monitor for additive effects.

▣ **Give oral doses 1 hour before or 2 hours after meals for best absorption.**

Adult: IV: Dilute 150 mg in 500 ml of D5W (concentration 0.3 mg/ml); infuse at 0.1 mg/min via IV controller. Increase if needed, by 0.05 mg/min q 10 min until effective. *Usual effective dose:* 0.15–0.35 mg/min. Continue infusion for 12–24 hrs after uterine contractions cease. PO: *Maintenance dose:* 10 mg 30 min before the termination of IV therapy, then 10 mg q2h for 24 hrs, then 10–20 mg q4-6h.

Clinical alert: Do not use IV solution if it is discolored or if a precipitate is present. Because of risk of fluid overload, avoid mixing with saline unless the patient is sensitive to glucose (e.g., diabetic). During IV administration, place mother in the left lateral position to minimize risk of positional hypotension and to promote circulation; monitor mother and fetus closely for cardiovascular effects (increase in maternal blood pressure and heart rate, increase in fetal heart rate), which are common. Stop IV and report immediately if mother's heart rate is 130–140 or if there is persistent tachypnea (may be a sign of impending pulmonary edema).

Contraindications/Precautions

PREG
B

Contraindicated in hypersensitivity to ritodrine or to components of preparation (contains sodium metabisulfites), and in use before 20 weeks gestation, cervical dilation of greater than 3–4 cm, severe preeclampsia, eclampsia, intrauterine fetal death, antepartum hemorrhage, chorioamnionitis, cardiac disease, pulmonary hypertension, uncontrolled diabetes mellitus, hyperthyroidism, pre-existing medical conditions seriously affected by a betamimetic drug (e.g., hypovolemia, cardiac dysrhythmias, uncontrolled hypertension, pheochromocytoma, bronchial asthma already treated by betami-

metics or steroids). *Use with caution* in preterm labor with premature rupture of membranes, diabetes mellitus, or history of migraine headaches.

✋ **Contraindicated in certain stages of pregnancy and labor (see above), for children, and for the elderly. Use with caution in preterm labor.**

Side effects/Adverse reactions

In mother: **Hypersensitivity:** erythema, rashes, anaphylaxis. **CV:** increased heart rate, increased systolic blood pressure, decreased diastolic blood pressure, palpitations, chest pain or tightness, heart murmur, supraventricular tachycardia, sinus bradycardia on withdrawal of drug, pulmonary edema. **CNS:** headache, anxiety, restlessness, agitation. **Hem:** transient hypokalemia, hyperglycemia. **GI:** severe nausea or vomiting, epigastric distress, diarrhea, ileus, constipation, bloating, glycosuria. **MS:** weakness.

In fetus and neonate: **CV:** hypotension. **Hem:** hyperglycemia, hypocalcemia. **GI:** ileus.

Nursing implications/Documentation

Possible nursing diagnoses: Pain; Potential for injury; Impaired physical mobility.

◆ Document vital signs, fetal and maternal heart rate, presence of contractions, and vaginal drainage every 15 min during IV administration (check hospital protocols and physician's orders; this may vary); record every 4 hours during oral administration.

◆ Monitor serum potassium and serum glucose for hypokalemia and hyperglycemia.

◆ Have patient rate pain on a scale of 1–10, assist in relaxation techniques, and medicate as ordered; report immediately if the pain is severe and associated with hard abdomen or change in maternal or infant vital signs.

◆ Keep mother in bed with side rails up and call-bell within reach during IV administration.

◆ Assist in changing positions; massage back and pressure points q2h while on bedrest.

◆ Monitor intake and output; report fluid retention.

Patient & family teaching/Home care

Possible nursing diagnoses: Fear; Ineffective individual coping; Knowledge deficit.

• Explain that this drug is intended to stop labor; stress that both mother and child will be closely monitored to fine tune medication for optimum results.

• Point out that taking this drug 1 hour before or 2 hours after meals enhances absorption.

• Stress the need to take ritodrine at the same time each day; missed doses can be taken within 3 hours of the scheduled time (doses should never be doubled).

• Encourage both mother and significant others to ask questions and verbalize fears or concerns; encourage significant others to provide physical and emotional comfort (backrubs, foot massages, verbal coaching).

• Stress the need to report palpitations, chest pain or tightness, dizziness, weakness, tremors, increase in discomfort, or feelings of having trouble breathing.

• Provide emotional support: prolonged hospitalization may be required and individuals may need assistance in coping with possibility of delivering prematurely or losing the baby.

• Advise that ambulation usually can begin 3–4 days after IV infusion has been stopped, but only if contractions do not recur.

• Reinforce the need not to take OTC medications without physician's approval.

• Caution to lie down immediately and call physician if uterine contractions begin, membranes rupture, or bleeding or spotting occurs.

salicylamide

sal-ee-sye'la-mide

Artritex, Lapidar, Uromide

Class: Analgesic, Nonsteroidal Anti-inflammatory Drug (NSAID), Salicylate

PEDS	PREG	GERI
🖐	C	🖐

Action Blocks pain impulses by an unclear mechanism. Believed to act by inhibiting prostaglandin synthesis.

Use/Therapeutic goal/Outcome

Mild to moderate pain: Relief of pain. **Outcome criteria:** After 2 weeks, report of feeling more comfortable; absence of signs of discomfort (frowning, restlessness, crying).

Dose range/Administration

Interaction alert: Antacids, steroids, and urinary alkalizers reduce effect. Heparin and alcohol increase risk of bleeding. Probenecid, spironolactone, sulfinpyrazone, and sulfonamides decrease effects. PABA may cause toxic effects.

🍮 **Give with food or milk to reduce GI symptoms.**

Adult: PO: 650 mg tid to qid prn. **Child:** PO: 65 mg/kg/day in 6 divided doses.

Clinical alert: Tablet may be taken crushed or whole.

Contraindications/Precautions

PREG C

Contraindicated in hypersensitivity to salicylamide, in bleeding disorders, and GI ulcers. **Use with caution** in hypoprothrombinemia, Vitamin K deficiency, and anemia.

🖐 **Contraindicated in children under 18 years with chickenpox or influenza-like symptoms (because of risk of Reye's syndrome). Use with caution for children, pregnant or nursing mothers, and the elderly.**

Side effects/Adverse reactions

Hypersensitivity: hives, rash, itching, bronchospasm, anaphylaxis. **CNS:** stimulation, drowsiness, dizziness, sedation in the elderly, confusion, convulsions, headache, flushing, hallucinations, coma. **GI:** nausea, vomiting, GI bleeding, diarrhea, heartburn, abnormal liver-function studies, hepatitis. **Ear:** tinnitus, hearing loss (high doses). **Skin:** bruising.

Nursing implications/Documentation

Possible nursing diagnoses: Pain; Impaired physical mobility; Diarrhea.

• Be aware that salicylamide is not officially classified as a salicylate, but is structurally and pharmacologically related and requires many of the same precautions.

• Schedule doses so that drug is given at least 1 hr before maximum effect is needed; document effectiveness.

• Monitor for and report GI symptoms that may indicate peptic ulcer (nausea, pain, black stools).

• If on long-term use, monitor prothrombin time, CBC, BUN, creatinine, AST, ALT, and bilirubin.

• Observe the elderly for toxicity.

Patient & family teaching/Home care

Possible nursing diagnoses: Knowledge deficit; Impaired home maintenance management.

• Stress the need to take salicylamide with food to reduce GI symptoms; explain the importance of watching for symptoms of GI bleeding (black stools, persistent GI distress).

• Explain that therapeutic response may not be seen until after 2 weeks of taking salicylamide.

• Caution about the danger of masking a serious illness by self-medicating for fever reduction; persistent fever lasting longer than 3 days should be reported.

• Stress that those under 18 years with flu-like symptoms or chicken pox should not receive salicylamide or aspirin (risk of developing Reye's syndrome).

• Point out that long-term use of salicylamide (or use in high doses) is likely to increase risk of bleeding and that those taking it on a long-term basis should be followed by a physician for monitoring of blood studies.

• Advise telling physician and dentist if salicylamide is taken on a regular basis.

• Stress that use with alcohol increases risk of bleeding.

• *See Narcotic and non-narcotic analgesics and Nonsteroidal anti-inflammatory drugs overviews for more information.*

salsalate

sal'sa-late

Artha-G, Mono-gesic, Disalcid, Salflex, Salgesic, Salsitab

Class: Analgesic, Nonsteroidal Anti-inflammatory Drug (NSAID), Salicylate

PEDS	PREG	GERI
🖐	C	🖐

Action **Relieves pain** by an ill-defined effect on the hypothalamus (central action) and by blocking generation of pain impulses (peripheral action), which may involve inhibition of prostaglandin synthesis. **Reduces inflammation** by inhibiting prostaglandin synthesis and may also inhibit synthesis or action of other mediators of the inflammatory response. **Reduces fever** by acting on the hypothalamic heat-regulating center to cause peripheral vasodilation, which increases peripheral blood supply, and promotes heat loss through sweating and cooling by evaporation. Does not appear to inhibit platelet aggregation.

Use/Therapeutic goal/Outcome

Inflammation: Relief of pain and inflammation. *Outcome criteria:* After 3–4 days, report and demonstration of reduced discomfort, stiffness, swelling of joints; increased mobility.

Dose range/Administration

Interaction alert: May increase effects of anticoagulants and heparin. Ammonium chloride and other urine acidifiers may cause toxicity. Antacids (high doses), other urine alkalinizers, and corticosteroids may decrease effects.

🖐 **Give with food, milk, low doses of antacid, or large glass of water to reduce GI symptoms.**

Adult: PO: 325 mg to 3 g/day in divided doses, depending on individual response.

Clinical alert: Monitor the elderly for increased risk of toxicity.

Contraindications/Precautions

PREG C

Contraindicated in hypersensitivity to salsalate or salicylates, and in GI bleeding. *Use with caution* in Vitamin K deficiency, bleeding disorders, and hypoprothrombinemia.

🖐 **Contraindicated for children and pregnant or nursing mothers. Use with caution for the elderly.**

Side effects/Adverse reactions

Hypersensitivity: rash, hives, itching, asthma, anaphylaxis. *Misc:* usually the result of overdosage (salicylism) — tinnitus, reversible hearing loss, vertigo, headache, confusion, drowsiness, hyperventilation, sweating, vomiting, and diarrhea; occasionally, nausea, and GI distress.

Nursing implications/Documentation

Possible nursing diagnoses: Pain; Impaired physical mobility.

• Monitor for and report GI symptoms that may indicate peptic ulcer (nausea, pain, black stools).

• Observe the elderly for toxicity.

Patient & family teaching/Home care

Possible nursing diagnoses: Knowledge deficit; Impaired home maintenance management.

• Stress the need to take salsalate with food to reduce GI symptoms; explain the importance of watching for symptoms of GI bleeding (black stools, persistent GI distress).

S

• Explain that it may take 3–4 days for effects to be noted.

• Point out that long-term use of salsalate (or use in high doses) is likely to increase risk of bleeding and that those taking salsalate on a long-term basis should be followed by a physician for monitoring of blood studies.

• Advise telling physician and dentist if salsalate is taken on a regular basis.

• Advise holding salsalate and reporting if rash appears.

• Warn against using aspirin or other salicylates with salsalate.

• Stress that those under 18 years with flu-like symptoms or chicken pox should not receive aspirin or this drug (risk of developing Reye's syndrome).

• *See Narcotic and non-narcotic analgesics and Nonsteroidal anti-inflammatory drugs overviews for more information.*

scopolamine
skoe-pol'a-meen

scopolamine (transdermal): ***Transderm-Scop,*** ❦ ***Transderm***

scopolamine hydrobromide (optic): ***Isopto-Hyoscine***

scopolamine hydrobromide (injection): ❦ ***Hyoscine***

scopolamine butylbromide: ❦ 🍁***Buscospan***

Class: Anticholinergic, Cholinergic blocker (parasympatholytic), Antiemetic

Antidote: Physostigmine

PEDS	PREG	GERI
✋	C	✋

Action Dilates pupils and reduces respiratory and GI secretions by inhibiting cholinergic (muscarinic) actions of acetylcholine at parasympathetic postganglionic sites. Produces memory loss by depressing the cerebral cortex. Prevents motion sickness by reducing nerve stumulation and conduction in the inner ear.

Use/Therapeutic goal/Outcome

Preoperative medication or obstetric analgesia: Reduction of respiratory secretions, promotion of amnesia and sedation ("twilight sleep"). ***Outcome criteria:*** Report of feeling dry and thirsty; amnesia of procedures.

Motion sickness: Prevention of nausea and vomiting. ***Outcome criteria:*** Report of absence of nausea and vomiting.

Ophthalmic: Promotion of mydriasis (dilation of pupil) and cycloplegia (paralysis of accommodation) for eye exam. ***Outcome criteria:*** Dilated pupils when checked with a flashlight.

Dose range/Administration

Interaction alert: Alcohol, narcotics, antihistamines, or phenothiazines increase anticholinergic effects. Do not mix with diazepam, chloramphenicol, pentobarbital, or sodium bicarbonate.

Preoperative medication, obstetric analgesia: Adult: SC, IM: 0.3–0.6 mg.

Motion sickness: Adult: PO: 0.25–0.6 mg 1 hr before travel. *Transdermal patch:* 0.5 mg applied postauricular 4–12 hr before travel (lasts for 3 days).

Ophthalmic exam: Adult: *Ophthalmic:* 1 to 2 gtts 0.25% solution 1 hr before refraction.

Clinical alert: When used for preoperative sedation or obstetrical procedures, be aware that initial response may be excitement, which is followed by sedation. Keep side rails up and monitor for risk of injury.

Contraindications/Precautions
PREG C

Contraindicated in hypersensitivity to scopolamine, and in narrow-angle glaucoma, asthma, hepatitis, and obstructive diseases of GI or urinary tract. ***Use with caution*** in hyperthyroidism, cardiac disease, hypertension, and hepatic or renal disease.

✋ **Contraindicated for nursing mothers. Use with caution for children under 3 years, pregnant women, and adults over 40 years.**

Side effects/Adverse reactions

Hypersensitivity: rash. ***GI:*** dry mouth, constipation. ***GU:*** urinary retention. ***CNS:*** fatigue, dizziness, drowsiness, amnesia, disorientation. ***CV:*** tachycardia, palpitations. ***Eye:*** dilated pupils, photophobia, increased intraocular pressure. ***Skin:*** decreases sweating.

Nursing implications/Documentation

Possible nursing diagnoses: Potential for injury; Urinary retention.

• Have patient void before doses; monitor intake and output because this drug can cause voiding difficulties.

• Monitor the elderly and debilitated for increased incidence of side effects and risk factors for injury.

• Relieve dry mouth by providing frequent mouth care.

Patient & family teaching/Home care

Possible nursing diagnoses: Knowledge deficit; Impaired home maintenance management.

♦ Warn that this drug may cause drowsiness and dizziness; caution to change position slowly.

♦ Explain that dry mouth and visual difficulties are common side effects.

♦ Advise against driving until response is determined (after use for eye exam, the patient should not drive until pupils are reactive).

♦ **Transdermal patch for motion sickness**

♦ Advise patient to apply disk the night before motion is experienced, or at least 4 hr before the aggravating motion.

♦ If smaller dose is desired, cut disk and apply reduced size.

♦ Advise to wash site before application of disk to improve adhesion and after removal to stop systemic absorption; wash hands after application and removal of disk to decrease chance of drug contact with eyes.

♦ *See Anticholinergics and Antiemetics overviews for more information.*

secobarbital sodium
see-koe-bar'bi-tal

♣*Novosecobark, Seconal Sodium*

Class: Short-acting barbiturate sedative, hypnotic

PEDS	PREG	GERI	CONTROLLED SUBSTANCE
✋	D	✋	II/III

Action Produces relaxation, sleep by inhibiting transmission of impulses in the reticular activating system. Limits acute seizure activity by increasing threshold for motor cortex stimuli.

Use/Therapeutic goal/Outcome

Sedation and sleep: Promotion of relaxation and sleep. *Outcome criteria:* Report of feeling less anxious and more relaxed; report of having slept well; visible drowsiness or sleep.

Dose range/Administration

Interaction alert: Alcohol, narcotics, analgesics, or other CNS depressants intensify respiratory and CNS depression. MAO inhibitors may prolong effects; rifampin may decrease effects. Injection is incompatible with bacteriostatic water for injection.

Adult: PO or IM: 100–200 mg at bedtime, or 100–300 mg 1–2 hr before procedure. *Child:* PO, IM or rect: 3–5 mg/kg at bedtime (maxi-

mum of 100 mg), or 50–100 mg orally, or 4–5 mg/kg rectally, 1–2 hr before procedure.

Clinical alert: Hold dose and report if respiratory depression or signs of overdosage (constricted pupils, somnolence, hypotension, clammy skin, cyanosis) are present. Use parenteral doses within 30 minutes of reconstitution and discard if solution is cloudy (to reconstitute, rotate ampule rather than shake).

Contraindications/Precautions
PREG **D**

Contraindicated in hypersensitivity or intolerance to barbiturates, and in marked respiratory problems, uncontrolled severe pain, severe trauma, history of addiction, patient or family history of porphyria, edema, or uncontrolled diabetes. *Use with caution* with toxemia or history of bleeding during pregnancy; compromised kidney, liver, or cardiac function; CNS depression, history of alcoholism, hypotension, fever, anemia, shock, asthenia, senile psychoses, and suicidal tendencies.

🖐 **Contraindicated in pregnancy, lactation, labor, and delivery. Use with caution for children and the elderly.**

Side effects/Adverse reactions

Hypersensitivity: itching, rash, hives, fever, angioneurotic edema, serum sickness. *CNS:* paradoxical excitement (most often in the elderly), drowsiness, lethargy, headache. *GI:* nausea, vomiting, liver damage. *Resp:* respiratory depression, coughing. *CV:* hypotension. *Misc:* exacerbation of porphyria.

Nursing implications/Documentation

Possible nursing diagnoses: Potential for injury; Sensory/perceptual alterations (visual and auditory).

♦ Document mental status before administration, monitor patient activity closely following administration, and employ appropriate measures to ensure safety (i.e., side rails up, call bell within reach, and no unsupervised smoking).

♦ Be sure that PO doses are swallowed (not hoarded).

♦ Be aware that sedatives and hypnotics *do not provide pain relief* (patient may need an analgesic as well).

♦ Monitor for and report signs of overdosage (slurred speech, continued somnolence, respiratory depression, confusion) and tolerance (increased anxiety and/or increased wakefulness).

♦ Inject IM doses deep into large muscle mass; use IV route for emergency or unusual situations only.

♦ For patients with renal insufficiency, do not use injection containing polyethylene glycol.

Patient & family teaching/Home care

Possible nursing diagnoses: Sleep pattern disturbance; Ineffective coping (family and individual); Impaired home maintenance management.

♦ Explore problems that may contribute to insomnia or anxiety and ways of coping effectively with the problems (stress that effective coping can promote restful sleep).

♦ Explain the importance of daily exercise in promoting rest, and encourage the person to establish a method for getting enough exercise (e.g., daily walks).

♦ Stress that drug tolerance and dependence can occur, and that the drug should be used only when holistic measures (e.g., quiet music, relaxation techniques) don't work.

♦ Emphasize that the effects of alcohol, other sedatives, and tranquilizers may be potentiated and should be avoided.

♦ Reinforce the importance of consulting with physician before using OTC drugs, and of returning for medical follow-up.

♦ Teach the person to avoid driving and other potentially hazardous activities while under the effects of the medication.

♦ Warn that secobarbital is a common street drug that has a high potential for abuse.

♦ *See Antianxiety Agents, Sedatives, and Hypnotics overview for more information.*

selegiline

se-leg′e-lean

Eldepryl

Class: Antiparkinsonian, Dopaminergic agent

PEDS	PREG	GERI
✋	C	✋

Action Helps control symptoms of parkinsonism by an unclear mechanism of action. May act primarily by inhibiting MAO beta-receptor activity, thereby increasing dopaminergic activity (dopamine is a neurotransmitter thought to be decreased in parkinsonism).

Use/Therapeutic goal/Outcome

Parkinsonism: Control of parkinsonian symptoms and promotion of mobility in patients receiving levodopa-carbidopa who have exhibited a deterioration in their response to therapy. **Outcome criteria:** Absence of (or decrease in) tremors, rigidity, akinesia and drooling; improvement in gait, balance, posture, and speech.

Dose range/Administration

Interaction alert: Should not be administered with meperidine or MAO inhibitors because fatal drug interactions have occurred.

💊 **Give with food or milk, preferably at breakfast and lunch.**

Adult: PO: 10 mg daily in two divided doses.

Contraindications/Precautions

PREG
C

Contraindicated in hypersensitivity to selegiline, and in patients receiving meperidine or MAO inhibitors. **Use with caution** in history of peptic ulcers.

✋ **Use with caution for the elderly. Safe use for pregnant or nursing mothers and for children has not been established.**

Side effects/Adverse reactions

Hypersensitivity: rashes. **GI:** nausea, diarrhea, abdominal pain, dry mouth. **CNS:** abnormal involuntary movements (dyskinesias), drowsiness, dizziness, lightheadedness, fainting, hallucinations, confusion, mental disturbances, vivid dreams, sleep disorders, headache, generalized ache, anxiety, lethargy. **CV:** palpitations, orthostatic hypotension, severe hypertension. **GU:** urinary retention. **MS:** leg pain, low back pain.

Nursing implications/Documentation

Possible nursing diagnoses: Potential for injury; Impaired physical mobility.

♦ Establish baseline profile of patient's abilities and disabilities to differentiate between desired responses to therapy and drug-induced adverse reactions; thereafter, monitor and record tolerance and response to drug.

♦ Monitor mental status frequently (CNS symptoms have been reported); identify methods to prevent injury.

Patient & family teaching/Home care

Possible nursing diagnoses: Knowledge deficit; Impaired home maintenance management.

- Advise that side effects of dizziness and drowsiness may occur early in therapy.
- Inform that levodopa-carbidopa dosage may be decreased after selegiline therapy begins.
- Caution to avoid tyramine-containing foods (cheese, beer, alcohol), caffeine, OTC cold medications.
- Stress the need to report signs of hypertensive crisis (severe headache, chest pain, nausea, and vomiting).
- *See Antiparkinsons overview for more information.*

senna

sen'nah

Black-Draught, Senokot, X-Prep Liquid
Class: Stimulant laxative

PEDS	PREG	GERI
🖑	C	🖑

Action Increases peristalsis by direct effect on the nerve supply of the smooth muscles of the intestine; promotes fluid and ion accumulation in colon.

Use/Therapeutic goal/Outcome

Constipation and preparation for surgery or diagnostic studies: Evacuation of fecal material from colon. *Outcome criteria:* Forceful bowel evacuation (within 6 to 12 hr).

Dose range/Administration

Interaction alert: May interfere with the effectiveness of potassium-sparing diuretics or potassium supplements by promoting potassium loss through intestinal tract.

Adult: PO: *X-Prep:* Contents of bottle at 2 to 4 PM on day prior to diagnostic procedure. *Granules:* 1 tsp. *Tablets:* 2 tablets. *Suppository:* 1 after meals. *Child:* PO: *Granules:* 1/2 tsp. *Syrup:* 5–10 ml. *Tablets:* 1 tablet. *Suppository:* 1/2 after meals.

Contraindications/Precautions

PREG
C

Contraindicated in hypersensitivity to stimulant laxatives, and in symptoms of appendicitis, intestinal obstruction, undiagnosed rectal bleeding, and for those with a colostomy or ileostomy.

🖑 **Contraindicated for infants under 2 years. Use with caution for children 2–6 years, pregnant or nursing mothers, and the elderly.**

Side effects/Adverse reactions

Hypersensitivity: rash, difficulty breathing. *GI:* nausea, abdominal cramping, diarrhea. *MS:* muscle weakness. *Skin:* irritation around rectal area. *Misc:* hypokalemia, fluid and electrolyte imbalance, laxative dependence.

Nursing implications/Documentation

Possible nursing diagnoses: Impaired skin integrity; Diarrhea; Pain.

- Give doses with a full glass of water at bedtime, unless directed otherwise.
- Monitor for abdominal distention and bowel sounds.
- Monitor and record frequency, appearance, and amount of stool evacuated.
- Assess perianal area and provide appropriate measures for good hygiene.
- Expect side effects to be more frequent and/or severe in elderly patients.

Patient & family teaching/Home care

Possible nursing diagnoses: Knowledge deficit; Impaired home maintenance management.

- Inform that urine and feces may become yellowish or reddish brown in color.
- For nursing mothers, advise that brown discoloration of breast milk may be seen and that diarrhea may occur in infant.
- Stress the importance of following directions and precautions printed on packaging.
- Teach that regular use of senna can cause laxative dependence and loss of essential electrolytes, especially in the elderly.
- Point out the importance of regular toileting routine, dietary bulk, fluids, and exercise in preventing constipation.
- *See Laxatives overview for more information.*

simethicone

si-meth'i-cone

Gas-X, Mylicon, Ovol-40, Ovol-80, Phazyme, Silain
Class: Antiflatulent

PEDS	PREG	GERI
🖑	C	OK

Action Facilitates elimination of gas by reducing surface tension of gas bubbles trapped in GI tract.

Use/Therapeutic goal/Outcome

Gastric or intestinal gas retention: Relief of painful symptoms. *Outcome criteria:* Belching, passing of flatus, and report of increased comfort.

Dose range/Administration

Adult: PO: 45–125 mg pc and hs. *Child:* PO: Individualize dose.

Clinical alert: Simethicone is an ingredient in several antacid products. Shake suspension form well and use packaged dropper for measuring dose.

Contraindications/Precautions ^{PREG C}

Contraindicated in treatment of infant colic.

☞ Use with caution for children (individualize dose).

Side effects/Adverse reactions

None reported of clinical significance.

Nursing implications/Documentation

Possible nursing diagnoses: Pain.

♦ Assess for abdominal pain, distention, and bowel sounds; record occurrence of belching and passing of flatus.

♦ Document color and character of stools.

Patient & family teaching/Home care

Possible nursing diagnoses: Pain; Impaired home maintenance management.

♦ Teach the need to chew chewable tablets well for faster and more complete results.

♦ Stress that simethicone does not prevent gas formation.

♦ Explain the importance of eliminating gas-forming foods and increasing exercise to reduce flatulence.

sodium bicarbonate

Baking soda, Citrocarbonate, Soda Mint
Class: Alkalinizer, Antacid, Electrolyte replenisher

PEDS	PREG	GERI
☞	C	☞

Action Reverses metabolic acidosis by buffering hydrogen ions with bicarbonate ions; alkalizes urine by increasing excretion of free bicarbonate ions; neutralizes existing stomach acid when administered orally.

Use/Therapeutic goal/Outcome

Metabolic acidosis/cardiac arrest: Reversal of clinical manifestations of acidosis without producing alkalosis. *Outcome criteria:* Arterial blood pH between 7.35 and 7.45.

Renal stones and urinary crystallization: Prevention of renal stone formation and crystallization in urinary tract. *Outcome criteria:* Urinary pH greater than 6 on freshly voided specimen.

Dose range/Administration

Interaction alert: Concurrent administration with enteric-coated drugs may cause coating to be dissolved too rapidly, leading to stomach or duodenal irritation. Affects the absorption of other drugs, causing increased blood levels of quinidine, amphetamines, and ephedrine; and decreased levels of phenobarbital, lithium, chlorpropramide, tetracycline, and methotrexate.

Cardiac arrest (doses should be based on frequent ABGs): Adult and Child: IV: 10 min after onset, give 1 mEq/kg; follow with 0.5 mEq/kg q10min during arrest.

Metabolic acidosis: Adult and Child: IV: Infuse 2–5 mEq/kg over 4–8 hr.

Renal stones and urinary crystallization: Adult: PO: 325 mg to 2 g qid. *Child:* PO: 12–120 mg/kg/day.

Clinical alert: During cardiac resuscitation, definitive measures (i.e., defibrillation, chest compression, hyperventilation) should be used to reverse acidosis before sodium bicarbonate is administered. Administer in separate IV line to avoid inactivating catecholemines (dopamine and epinephrine) that are frequently given during resuscitation.

Contraindications/Precautions ^{PREG C}

Contraindicated in hypochloremia, metabolic or respiratory alkalosis, and hypertension. *Use with caution* in patients with congestive heart failure, kidney impairment, edema, or arrhythmias.

☞ Contraindicated in children < 6 years. Use with caution for pregnant women and the elderly.

Side effects/Adverse reactions

CNS: twitching, hyperreflexia, tetany, convulsions. *GI:* gastric distention and belching. *Misc:* metabolic alkalosis, hypernatremia, hyperosmolality, hypercalcemia, hypokalemia, milk-alkali syndrome.

Nursing implications/Documentation

Possible nursing diagnoses: Fluid volume excess.

◆ Administer other oral medication 1 to 2 hr after sodium bicarbonate to avoid affecting their absorption.

◆ Assess for symptoms of alkalosis (mental changes, muscle twitching, restlessness, weakness).

◆ Weigh and assess for development of edema.

◆ Document results of ABGs during cardiac arrest, and keep code team informed of values.

Patient & family teaching/Home care

Possible nursing diagnoses: Knowledge deficit.

◆ Discourage use of sodium bicarbonate as an antacid because of risk of metabolic alkalosis and sodium overload; suggest an antacid without systemic effects.

◆ Encourage those on sodium-restricted diets to avoid using sodium bicarbonate.

◆ Advise avoiding prolonged use with calcium supplements, calcium antacids, or milk because of the danger of milk-alkali syndrome (headache, nausea, vomiting, and appetite loss; metabolic alkalosis, hypercalcemia, confusion, and renal insufficiency).

sodium polystyrene sulfonate

Kayexalate, Resonium A, SPS Suspension
Class: Potassium-removing resin, Antihyperkalemic

PEDS	PREG	GERI
OK	C	🖐

Action Reduces serum potassium levels by exchanging sodium ions for potassium ions in large intestine.

Use/Therapeutic goal/Outcome

Hyperkalemia: Reduction of elevated potassium level. **Outcome criteria:** Serum potassium level within 4–5 mEq/L.

Dose range/Administration

Interaction alert: Magnesium or calcium-containing antacids or laxatives may bind with oral doses reducing potassium-exchanging capability.

Adult: PO: 15 gm daily to qid. RECT: 30–50 g q6h. **Child:** PO: 1 g/kg/dose. RECT: 1 g/kg/dose.

Clinical alert: Chill oral preparation for improved palatability. Give rectal preparation at body temperature (heating resin will affect exchange

properties.) Rectal administration for the elderly may decrease incidence of fecal impaction.

Contraindications/Precautions

PREG
C

Use with caution in digitalis therapy, severe congestive heart failure, marked edema, and severe hypertension.

🖐 **Use with caution for pregnant or nursing mothers and the elderly.**

Side effects/Adverse reactions

Hypersensitivity: rare. **GI:** constipation, anorexia, nausea, vomiting, abdominal pain, fecal impaction. **CNS:** confusion. **CV:** irregular heartbeat. **MS:** severe muscle weakness. **Misc:** sodium retention, hypokalemia, hypocalcemia, digitalis toxicity.

Nursing implications/Documentation

Possible nursing diagnoses: Constipation; Fluid volume excess.

◆ Recognize that oral administration is more effective than rectal administration.

◆ For oral use

Mix in water, sorbitol, or any low-potassium beverage (sorbitol is usually ordered as a laxative with oral doses to prevent fecal impaction; it may be mixed with resin or given separately).

◆ Expect one or two watery stools per day.

◆ Assess the elderly for and report fecal impaction; document findings.

◆ Monitor serum potassium levels for return to normal range; testing will be done frequently since administration must be discontinued promptly to prevent hypokalemia.

◆ Assess for development of EKG abnormalities and clinical symptoms of hypokalemia (irritable confusion, irregular heartbeat, and severe muscle weakness).

◆ Monitor serum calcium and magnesium levels, which may also be decreased by resin; assess for fluid retention due to increased sodium intake.

◆ Additional guidelines for rectal use

◆ Administer cleansing enema before giving resin.

◆ Mix powder with water and sorbitol if not supplied as suspension; use 100–200-ml volume to provide adequate resin surface for effective exchange.

◆ Administer as high (20 cm) retention enema

▶

S

with rectal tube or catheter, stirring suspension gently during slow, gravity administration; follow with 50–100 ml flush of tepid water.

◆ Point out the need to retain suspension as long as possible (at least 30 to 45 min); if bowel elimination has not occurred within 8 to 10 hr, administer cleansing enema.

Patient & family teaching/Home care

Possible nursing diagnoses: Knowledge deficit.

◆ Stress the importance of lowering potassium to normal levels, and of need for frequent blood tests.

◆ With oral administration, inform that 1 or 2 watery stools per day is expected result.

sodium salicylate
so'dee-um sal-i'si-late

Uracel-5

Class: Analgesic, Nonsteroidal Anti-inflammatory Drug (NSAID), Salicylate

Antidote: Lavage, activated charcoal, monitor electrolytes and vital signs

PEDS 🖐 **PREG** C **GERI** 🖐

Action
Relieves pain by an ill-defined effect on the hypothalamus (central action) and by blocking generation of pain impulses (peripheral action, which may involve inhibition of prostaglandin synthesis). **Reduces inflammation** by inhibiting prostaglandin synthesis, and may also inhibit synthesis or action of other mediators of the inflammatory response. **Reduces fever** by acting on the hypothalamic heat-regulating center to cause peripheral vasodilation, which increases peripheral blood supply, and promotes heat loss through sweating and cooling by evaporation.

Use/Therapeutic goal/Outcome
Inflammation: Resolution of pain and inflammation. **Outcome criteria:** After 2 weeks, report and demonstration of reduced discomfort, stiffness, swelling of joints; increased mobility.

Dose range/Administration
Interaction alert: May increase action of anticoagulants. Ammonium chloride and other urine acidifiers may increase risk of toxicity. High antacid doses, other urine alkalinizers and corticosteroids may decrease effects.

🍴 **Give with food, milk, low doses of antacids, or full glass of water to reduce GI distress (do not take enteric-coated form with milk or antacids).**

Adult: PO: 325–650 mg q4-6h prn. IV: 500 mg slow infusion over 4–8 hr. *Maximum dose:* 1 g/day. **Child:** PO: 1.5 g/kg/day in 4–6 divided doses.

Clinical alert: Do not allow enteric-coated tablets to be crushed or chewed. Do not give salicylates to children < 18 years with chicken pox or influenza-like symptoms because of their association with Reye's syndrome. Monitor the elderly for increased risk of toxicity.

Contraindications/Precautions
PREG C

Contraindicated in hypersensitivity to aspirin or other salicylates, and in GI ulcer or bleeding and severe hepatic or renal damage. **Use with caution** in hyperprothrombinemia, Vitamin K deficiency, bleeding disorders, asthma with nasal polyps (may cause severe bronchospasm), congestive heart failure, and hypertension (increases sodium load).

🖐 **Contraindicated for pregnant or nursing mothers and for children under 18 years with chickenpox or influenza-like symptoms. Use with caution for children over 6 years and the elderly. Safe use for children under 6 years is not established.**

Side effects/Adverse reactions
Hypersensitivity: rash, hives, itching, anaphylaxis, asthma. **GI:** nausea, vomiting, GI distress, abnormal liver function, hepatitis. **Skin:** bruising, thrombophlebitis from IV administration. **Ear:** tinnitus, hearing loss.

Nursing implications/Documentation
Possible nursing diagnoses: Pain; Impaired physical mobility.

◆ Monitor for and report GI symptoms that may indicate peptic ulcer (nausea, pain, black stools).

◆ Observe the elderly for toxicity.

Patient & family teaching/Home care
Possible nursing diagnoses: Knowledge deficit; Impaired home maintenance management.

◆ Stress the need to take sodium salicylate with food to reduce GI symptoms; explain the importance of watching for symptoms of GI bleeding (black stools, persistent GI distress).

S

- Explain that it may take 2 weeks for effects to be noted.
- Point out that long-term use of sodium salicylate (or use in high doses) is likely to increase the risk of bleeding and that those taking it on a long-term basis should be followed by a physician for monitoring of blood studies.
- Advise telling physician and dentist if sodium salicylate is taken on a regular basis; warn against using OTC drugs without physician's approval.
- Advise holding sodium salicylate and reporting if rashes or ringing of the ears is noted.
- Warn against using aspirin or other salicylates with sodium salicylate.
- Stress that those under 18 years with flu-like symptoms or chicken pox should not receive aspirin or sodium salicylate (risk of developing Reye's syndrome).
- *See Narcotic and non-narcotic analgesics and Nonsteroidal anti-inflammatory drugs overviews for more information.*

sodium thiosalicylate   *thy-o-sal-i'si-late*

Asproject, Rexolate, Tusal

Class: Analgesic, Nonsteroidal Anti-inflammatory Drug (NSAID), Salicylate, Antipyretic

PEDS	PREG	GERI
✋	C	X

Action **Relieves pain** by an ill-defined effect on the hypothalamus (central action) and by blocking generation of pain impulses (peripheral action, which may involve inhibition of prostaglandin synthesis). **Reduces inflammation** by inhibiting prostaglandin synthesis, and may also inhibit synthesis or action of other mediators of the inflammatory response. **Reduces fever** by acting on the hypothalamic heat-regulating center to cause peripheral vasodilation, which increases peripheral blood supply and promotes heat loss through sweating and cooling by evaporation.

Use/Therapeutic goal/Outcome

Inflammation: Resolution of pain and inflammation. **Outcome criteria:** After 2 weeks, report and demonstration of reduced pain and decreased stiffness and swelling of joints; increased mobility.

Fever: Reduction of fever. **Outcome criteria:** Reduction in temperature.

Dose range/Administration

Interaction alert: Anticoagulants increase risk of bleeding. Ammonium chloride and other urine acidifiers increase risk of toxicity. Antacids (high doses), other urine alkalinizers, and corticosteroids may decrease effects.

Arthritis: Adult: IM: 50–100 mg/day.

Rheumatic fever: Adult: IM, IV: 100–150 mg q4-6h for 3 days, then 100 mg bid until asymptomatic.

Clinical alert: Do not give salicylates to children < 18 years with chicken pox or influenza-like symptoms because of their association with Reye's syndrome. Monitor the elderly for toxicity.

Contraindications/Precautions
PREG
C

Contraindicated in hypersensitivity to sodium thiosalicylate or aspirin, and in GI ulcer, and GI bleeding. **Use with caution** in hypoprothrombinemia, Vitamin K deficiency, bleeding disorders, and asthma with nasal polyps (may cause severe bronchospasm).

🖐 **Contraindicated for pregnant or nursing mothers and for children under 18 years with chickenpox or influenza-like symptoms. Use with caution for the elderly.**

Side effects/Adverse reactions

Hypersensitivity: rash, hives, itching, anaphylaxis. **Ear:** tinnitus and hearing loss. **GI:** nausea, vomiting, GI distress, occult bleeding, abnormal liver-function studies, hepatitis. **Skin:** bruising.

Nursing implications/Documentation

Possible nursing diagnoses: Pain; Impaired physical mobility.

- Monitor for and report GI symptoms that may indicate peptic ulcer (nausea, pain, black stools).
- Observe the elderly for toxicity.
- Report symptoms of mild toxicity (ringing of the ears, headache, dizziness, confusion, fever, sweating, thirst, drowsiness, dim vision, hyperventilation, tachycardia).

Patient & family teaching/Home care

Possible nursing diagnoses: Knowledge deficit; Impaired home maintenance management.

- Explain that long-term use of sodium thiosalicylate (or use in high doses) is likely to

S

increase risk of bleeding; stress the need for medical follow-up to monitor blood studies.

◆ Advise that therapeutic effects may not be seen for 2 weeks.

◆ Stress that those under 18 years with flu-like symptoms or chicken pox should not receive sodium thiosalicylate or aspirin (risk of developing Reye's syndrome).

◆ *See Narcotic and non-narcotic analgesics and Nonsteroidal anti-inflammatory drugs overviews for more information.*

spectinomycin

spek-ti-noe-mye'sin

spectinomycin dihydrochloride: *Trobicin*
Class: Anti-infective, Antibiotic

PEDS	PREG	GERI
🤚	**B**	**OK**

Action Usually bacteriostatic, limits bacterial growth by binding to the 30S ribosomal subunit and inhibiting protein synthesis.

Use/Therapeutic goal/Outcome

Penicillin-resistant gonorrhea: Resolution of infection. *Outcome criteria:* Absence of *Neisseria gonorrhoeae* growth on culture.

Dose range/Administration

Adult: IM: Using a 20-gauge needle, give 2–4 g deep into the ventrogluteal or dorsogluteal muscle (for 4 g dose, give 2 g in each buttock).

Contraindications/Precautions

PREG B

Contraindicated in hypersensitivity to spectinomycin. *Use with caution* for people with history of multiple allergies.

🤚 **Contains benzyl alcohol, which can be fatal in infants. Safe use for children and pregnant or nursing mothers has not been established.**

Side effects/Adverse reactions

Hypersensitivity: fever, itching, rashes. *CNS:* dizziness, insomnia. *GI:* nausea. *GU:* decreased urine output. *Misc:* chills.

Nursing implications/Documentation

Possible nursing diagnoses: Potential for infection.

◆ Obtain necessary cultures before giving first dose.

Patient & family teaching/Home care

Possible nursing diagnoses: Knowledge deficit; Situational low self-esteem; Altered sexuality patterns.

◆ Stress the importance of treatment of sexual partners, and of returning for medical follow-up.

◆ *See Anti-infectives overview for more information.*

spironolactone

speer-on-oh-lak'tone

Aldactone, ✦Novospiroton, ✦Sincomen, ✦Spiro-tone
Class: Potassium-sparing diuretic (aldosterone antagonist), Antihypertensive

PEDS	PREG	GERI
🤚	**D**	🤚

Action Produces mild diuresis of sodium and water while sparing potassium excretion by antagonizing aldosterone at receptors in the late distal tubule and by interfering with sodium reabsorption in the collecting system of the kidney.

Use/Therapeutic goal/Outcome

Hypokalemia and edema in CHF, cirrhosis of liver, and nephrotic syndromes: Promotion of diuresis while maintaining serum potassium levels within normal limits. *Outcome criteria:* Increased urine output; absence of rales; absence of peripheral and sacral edema; weight loss; potassium within normal limits.

Hypertension: Promotion of mild diuresis while maintaining serum potassium levels within normal limits. *Outcome criteria:* Increased urinary output; blood pressure within normal range; potassium within normal limits.

Primary aldosteronism: Antagonism of excessive levels of aldosterone. *Outcome criteria:* Increased urine output, increased sodium excretion, and decreased urinary potassium levels.

Dose range/Administration

Interaction alert: Aspirin and nonsteroidal anti-inflammatory drugs may interfere with action. Use cautiously with digitalis, lithium, and ACE inhibitors. Do not give with other potassium-sparing agents such as amiloride or triamterene.

🍷 **Give with food to reduce GI upset.**

Edema: **Adult:** PO: 25–200 mg/day in divided doses. *Range:* 25–400 mg/day. **Child:** PO: 1–3 mg/kg/day in single or divided doses.

Hypertension: **Adult:** PO: 50–100 mg/day in divided doses.

Primary aldosteronism: **Adult:** PO: 100–400 mg/day in divided doses prior to surgery; smaller maintenance doses for poor surgical risks.

Clinical alert: Give in early morning to avoid nocturnal diuresis. Antihypertensive response may not occur for 2 weeks.

Contraindications/Precautions

PREG
D

Contraindicated in hypersensitivity to the drug, hyperkalemia, and impaired renal and hepatic functions. *Use with caution* in presence of fluid and electrolyte imbalances.

✋ **Contraindicated for pregnant or nursing mothers. Use with caution for children and the elderly.**

Side effects/Adverse reactions

Hypersensitivity: **CNS:** lethargy, headache, confusion. **GI:** gastrointestinal upset, cramping, diarrhea, vomiting. **GU:** gynecomastia (especially in males), breast tenderness, irregular menses, impotency. **Skin:** cutaneous eruptions, urticaria. **Hem:** fluid and electrolyte imbalances, acidosis, increased BUN. **Misc:** hirsutism, voice deepening.

Nursing implications/Documentation

Possible nursing diagnoses: Fluid volume deficit; Altered patterns of urinary elimination; Potential for injury.

◆ Ascertain that baseline CBC, sodium, potassium, chloride, carbon dioxide, calcium, magnesium, BUN, creatinine, uric acid, and liver function studies have been obtained before giving first dose; report abnormalities and monitor closely thereafter.

◆ Watch for *hyper*kalemia, since this is a potassium-sparing diuretic.

◆ Document and monitor blood pressure, pulse, daily weight, and intake and output; report significant discrepancies.

◆ Observe for and report signs of fluid overload (auscultate lungs for rales; check feet, ankles, and sacrum for edema).

◆ Check with physician to determine dietary restrictions; consult with dietician to plan diet.

◆ Observe the elderly for extreme diuresis (may require lower doses); monitor for orthostatic hypotension; supervise ambulation until response is determined.

Patient & family teaching/Home care

Possible nursing diagnoses: Impaired home maintenance management; Altered patterns of sexuality.

◆ Before giving first dose, explain that the drug will increase the amount and frequency of urination.

◆ Advise taking this drug with food to prevent GI symptoms.

◆ Emphasize the importance of taking this drug exactly as prescribed, and the importance of returning for medical follow-up.

◆ Explain that diuretics enhance the work of the kidney and reduce the workload of the heart.

◆ Recommend taking doses in early morning and early afternoon to prevent the need to disturb sleep to void.

◆ Explain that changing positions slowly helps prevent dizziness.

◆ Advise reporting dizziness, shortness of breath, muscle weakness or spasms, swelling of hands and feet; encourage daily monitoring of weight and reporting sudden weight gain.

◆ Provide a list of allowed foods and fluids; stress the need to stick to prescribed diet (explain the hazards of too much salt or potassium).

◆ Warn against driving or activities that require alertness until response has been determined.

◆ Advise avoidance of OTC drugs unless approved by physician.

◆ *See Diuretics and Antihypertensives overviews for more information.*

streptokinase

strep-toe-kye'naze

Kabakinase, Streptase

Class: ★**Thrombolytic enzyme (fibrinolytic) prototype**

Antidote: Aminocaproic acid

PEDS	PREG	GERI
✋	C	✋

Action Directly dissolves existing clots (thrombi) by binding to plasminogen; the complex then

▶

S

converts free plasminogen to plasmin. (the enzyme that degrades fibrin).

Use/Therapeutic goal/Outcome

Emergency treatment of coronary artery thrombosis (not used more than 4 hr after onset of symptoms of coronary artery occlusion): Lysis of thrombi obstructing coronary arteries, reperfusion of ischemic cardiac tissue, prevention (or reduction in size) of acute myocardial infarction. *Outcome criteria:* Abrupt cessation of chest pain (often accompanied by sudden onset of hypotension and reperfusion arrhythmias); smaller Q waves, and return of ST segment to baseline on EKG; cardiac enzyme *washout* (cardiac enzymes peak faster than they do in untreated myocardial infarction); absence of coronary occlusion upon cardiac catheterization (may be performed days later when risk of bleeding has diminished).

Emergency treatment of venous thrombosis, pulmonary embolism, and arterial thrombosis and embolism: Lysis of thrombi obstructing blood vessels/reperfusion of ischemic tissue, prevention of tissue infarction. *Outcome criteria:* Signs of reperfusion of tissue (absence of pain; return of peripheral pulse quality, satisfactory capillary refill with improved temperature and color of skin; for pulmonary embolus, normal blood gases and absence of infarction on lung scan).

Dose range/Administration

Interaction alert: Do not mix any other IV drugs with streptokinase solution. Risk of bleeding increases with concurrent oral anticoagulants, heparin, other thrombolytics, or drugs that affect platelet function (salicylates, dipyridamole, nonsteroidal anti-inflammatories); however, concomitant IV heparin is common, as is therapy with aspirin and/or dipyridamole following heparin (check policy, some physicians believe that these should be avoided).

Coronary artery thrombosis: Adult: Intracoronary: Initial loading dose of 20,000 IU, followed by 2,000 IU/min via IV route for 60 min. IV: Initial bolus dose of 500,000 IU given slowly over 5 min, followed by 1 million (1,000,000) IU over 60 min via IV pump for a total of 1.5 million units.

Arterial or venous thrombosis: Adult: IV infusion: Using an IV pump, administer a loading dose of 250,000 IU over 30 min, followed by an infusion of 100,000 IU/hr for 72 hr.

Pulmonary embolism: Adult: IV infusion: Using an IV pump, administer a loading dose of 250,000 IU over 30 min, followed by an infusion of 100,000 IU/hr for 24–72 hr.

Clinical alert: This drug should be administered only by professionals who are well educated in all aspects of its administration. Follow package insert instructions for reconstituting streptokinase carefully to prevent precipitation of medication. Check hospital policy and procedure for administration (in some hospitals, diphenhydramine is routinely given before streptokinase because of the high incidence of allergic reactions). Be sure that three large-bore IV sites are established **before** administering streptokinase, and have the following at the patient's bedside:

- Electrocardiogram machine
- Emergency medications (including IV diphenhydramine, which may be ordered pre-infusion)
- Advanced cardiac life support (ACLS) cart (with defibrillator)
- IV pump.

Contraindications/Precautions
PREG
C

Contraindicated in hypersensitivity to streptokinase; and in active internal bleeding or known potential bleeding source (e.g., ulcer disease); recent cerebrovascular accident (CVA), intracranial neoplasm, arteriovenous malformation, intracranial aneurysm; bleeding diathesis; diabetic retinopathy; cranial or spinal surgery (or trauma), organ biopsy, or cavity aspiration within 8 weeks; surgery, trauma, or CPR (especially with rib fractures) within 10 days; traumatic endotracheal intubation; persistent hypertension (with systolic blood pressure greater than 180 mm Hg or diastolic greater than 110 mm Hg) after treatment; subacute bacterial endocarditis. Recent streptococcal infections or streptokinase administration may significantly decrease the effectiveness of streptokinase because of antibody formation. *Use with caution* for patient with recent puncture (within 10 days) of a noncompressible vessel, prothrombin time greater than 15 seconds, aspirin consumption within 72 hr, known (or suspected) left heart thrombus (risk of cerebral infarction).

🖐 **Contraindicated in known or suspected pregnancy. Use with caution for those over 75 years (physician may deem to be contraindicated). Safety for children has not been established.**

Side effects/Adverse reactions

Hypersensitivity: itching, rashes, nausea, flushing, fever, respiratory difficulties, angioneurotic edema. **CNS:** cerebral hemorrhage. **GI:** bleeding, nausea, vomiting. **CV:** bleeding, hypotension, dysrhythmias. **Misc:** bleeding of surgical or traumatic injury and of puncture sites, fever.

Nursing implications/Documentation

Possible nursing diagnoses: Potential for Injury; Pain.

♦ Obtain a careful history of pain, and closely monitor level of pain before, during, and after administration of streptokinase.

♦ Assess carefully for contraindications to streptokinase.

♦ For coronary artery thrombosis, attach patient to cardiac monitor and select the lead that shows the highest ST-segment elevation (also attach patient to a 12-lead EKG; periodic EKGs will be necessary during administration).

♦ Monitor closely for hypersensitivity reactions and report immediately if they occur; be prepared to treat anaphylactic reactions (bronchospasm, hypotension).

♦ *Check hospital policy and procedure to determine variations in the following interventions.*

♦ Be sure baseline and other "stat" lab studies are drawn before initiating alteplase (PT, PTT, CBC, fibrinogen level, renal lab studies, cardiac enzymes, type and crossmatch for 2 units of blood, and other routine coronary admission studies determined by hospital policy).

♦ Have the necessary equipment ready for three large-bore peripheral intravenous lines (one for streptokinase; another for other drugs, such as heparin and lidocaine, and the third for drawing blood samples; one of these may be needed for blood transfusion if hemorrhage occurs).

♦ Before, during, and after administration of streptokinase, document and report presence of abnormal pulses, abnormal neurological findings, or **skin lesions** (may indicate coagulation defects).

♦ Document vital signs every 15 min during infusion and for 1–2 hr after infusion, then every 30 min until ordered otherwise; also document EKG strips to have a record of changes in ST segments.

♦ Document neurological signs on a flow sheet every 30 min for at least 2 hr (check policy).

♦ Be prepared to treat reperfusion dysrhythmias (ventricular tachycardia or fibrillation; atrial tachycardia or fibrillation) according to hospital protocol or individual physician orders; have emergency drugs and defibrillator readily available (some protocols will include starting a lidocaine drip and a heparin drip when streptokinase is initiated).

♦ Keep all needle punctures to an absolute minimum; apply manual pressure for 10 min to all venous puncture sites, and for 30 min to arterial puncture sites; follow this with pressure dressing, and observe all intravenous and intra-arterial sites every 15 min for 1 hr, every 30 min for 2 hr, every hr for 4 hr, then every 2 hr until removed.

♦ Place a sign on door and over bed to alert staff and phlebotomist of bleeding precautions.

♦ Maintain patient on complete bedrest until otherwise ordered, and monitor closely for bleeding: hemoptysis, CVA, hematuria, hematemesis, melena, pain or swelling from closed space bleeding, and signs and symptoms of cardiac tamponade (distended neck veins and significant pulsus paradoxus). Report immediately if these are observed.

♦ Keep aminocaproic acid available as antidote in case of hemorrhage.

♦ Check for the following lab orders post infusion: CPK, CPK Isoenzymes (q4h × 3, then qd × 2); Hgb and Hct (q4h the first 24 hr, then once the next day); PTT (stat and q4h × 2, then daily throughout heparin therapy; should be maintained in the 80–120 second range.

Patient & family teaching/Home care

Possible nursing diagnoses: Anxiety; Fear; Knowledge deficit.

♦ Explain the rationale for prompt initiation of treatment, and for routine procedures that ensure patient safety.

♦ Encourage the person to voice questions and concerns, and to keep nurses informed of new symptoms (headache, dizziness, chest discomfort, abdominal discomfort).

♦ Explain that symptoms associated with hypotension and dysrhythmias are likely to be transient.

♦ Stress the need to remain in bed.

◆ See *Anticoagulants and Thrombolytic Enzymes* overview for more information.

streptomycin

strep-toe-mye'sin

streptomycin sulfate

Class: Anti-infective, Aminoglycoside antibiotic, Anti-tuberculosis agent

PEDS	PREG	GERI
🖐	D	🖐

Action Kills bacteria (bactericidal) by binding to ribosomes, thereby disrupting bacterial protein synthesis.

Use/Therapeutic goal/Outcome

Streptococcal and enterococcal endocarditis: Resolution of infection. *Outcome criteria:* Absence of pathogenic growth on cultures, absence of clinical manifestations of endocarditis.

Adjunctive treatment of tuberculosis: Elimination of tubercle bacilli. *Outcome criteria:* Absence of tubercular bacilli on 3 consecutive sputum cultures.

Dose range/Administration

Interaction alert: Cephalothin and loop diuretics (e.g., furosemide) increase risk of toxicity and nephrotoxicity. Dimenhydrinate may mask symptoms of ototoxicity. May potentiate neuromuscular blockade effect of general anesthetics.

Streptococcal endocarditis: **Adult:** IM: 10 mg/kg q12h for 2 weeks, concurrent with penicillin. *Maximum dose:* 0.5 g.

Enterococcal endocarditis: **Adult:** IM: 1 g q12h for 2 weeks, then 500 mg q12h for 4 weeks, concurrent with penicillin.

Tuberculosis: **Adult:** IM: 1 g/day for 2–3 months, then 1 g 2–3 times a week, concurrent with other antitubercular drugs. **Child:** IM: 20 mg/kg/day, concurrent with other antitubercular drugs (*not capreomycin*), until sputum cultures become negative.

Clinical alert: In impaired kidney function, give initial dose listed above; subsequent doses and frequency should be determined by examining serum levels and kidney function studies. Never give IV or SC, give deep IM into large muscle mass. Avoid direct contact with streptomycin because it can irritate the skin (wear gloves).

Contraindications/Precautions

Contraindicated in hypersensitivity or toxic reaction to streptomycin or other aminoglycosides, and in labyrinth disease, myasthenia gravis, concurrent use with other neurotoxic or nephrotoxic drugs. *Use with caution* in impaired renal function (reduce dosage).

🖐 **Contraindicated for pregnant or nursing mothers. Use with caution for infants and the elderly.**

Side effects/Adverse reactions

Hypersensitivity: itching, burning, rashes, drug fever, arthralgia, blood dyscrasias, angioneurotic edema, anaphylaxis. *Ear:* ototoxicity (hearing loss, tinnitus). *CNS:* neurotoxicity (dizziness, vertigo, headache, unsteady gait, nausea, vomiting), neuromuscular blockade. *GU:* nephrotoxicity (oliguria, proteinuria, cells in urine, hematuria, decreased creatinine clearance, increased serum BUN and creatinine). *Skin:* pain, sterile abscess at injection site.

Nursing implications/Documentation

Possible nursing diagnoses: Potential for infection; Fluid volume deficit.

◆ Determine history of allergies and (regardless of history) monitor closely for allergic reactions.

◆ Weigh patient, and obtain baseline renal function studies, hearing ability, and necessary culture specimens before administering first dose.

◆ Monitor renal function (urine output, specific gravity, serum BUN and creatinine, creatinine clearance) and report signs of decreased function.

◆ Encourage fluid intake, and document and monitor intake and output, to ensure adequate hydration and prevent renal damage from chemical irritation of renal tubules.

◆ Monitor for and report symptoms of hearing loss, tinnitus, vertigo, headache, nausea, vomiting and superinfection (mouth lesions, thrush, vaginal irritation, diarrhea, respiratory symptoms).

◆ Refer patients with tuberculosis to visiting nurse before discharge.

Patient & family teaching/Home care

Possible nursing diagnoses: Knowledge deficit; Impaired home maintenance management.

• Instruct the need to report ear symptoms (e.g., full feeling, ringing of the ears, hearing loss, dizziness) immediately.

• Advise reporting new signs and symptoms of illness (e.g., fever, mouth lesions, vaginal irritation, diarrhea, respiratory symptoms) since medications may have to be changed.

• Explain the importance of taking antibiotics for the entire time prescribed, regardless of absence of signs and symptoms and of maintaining hydration (drinking at least 2 L is recommended).

♦ *See Anti-infectives overview for more information.*

streptozocin

strep-toe-zo'sin

Zanosar

Class: Antineoplastic (alkylating) agent

PEDS	PREG	GERI
✋	C	✋

Action Kills rapidly growing cells (cancer, hair follicles, bone marrow, GI lining, ova, and sperm) by interfering with DNA replication and RNA transcription through alkylation (cross-linking of DNA occurs). Is cell-cycle–phase nonspecific, affecting actively dividing cells and dormant (resting) cells.

Use/Therapeutic goal/Outcome

Cancer (metastatic islet cell pancreatic carcinomas, metastatic carcinoid tumor, pancreatic adenocarcinomas, and colorectal cancer): Elimination or suppression of malignant cell proliferation. *Outcome criteria:* Tumor and disease regression or stabilization on radiologic and physical examination.

Dose range/Administration

Interaction alert: Phenytoin decreases drug effectiveness. Radiation therapy and other cytotoxic agents may cause severe myelosuppression. Aminoglycosides may increase the risk of renal toxicity.

Adult: IV: 500 mg/m^2/day for 5 days, q 6 wk until optimum benefit or toxicity occurs; or 1 g/m^2/wk for 2 weeks. *Maximum single dose:* 1.5 g/m^2.

Clinical alert: This drug should be given only by nurses who are knowledgeable in the comprehensive management of the administration of antineoplastic agents. Doses may vary at physician's discretion and are held until the patient has recovered sufficiently from toxicities of previous doses. Protocols for drug preparation, administration, and accidental skin contamination must be followed. Gloves or double gloves must be worn when handling streptozocin (skin contamination may cause a local reaction). Contaminated areas should be washed with large amounts of soap and water. Streptozocin is diluted in 50–100 ml D5W and given slowly over 1–2 hr. Careful assessment of the IV site is essential to prevent extravasation; if this is suspected the IV is stopped immediately, the physician notified, and protocols for treatment initiated.

Contraindications/Precautions

PREG
C

Contraindicated in hypersensitivity to streptozocin, and with other nephrotoxic drugs. **Use with caution** in impaired renal or liver function (increased incidence of nephrotoxicity or hepatotoxicity).

♕ **Contraindicated for pregnant or nursing mothers. Use with caution for the elderly. Safe use for children has not been established.**

Side effects/Adverse reactions

Hypersensitivity: itching, rashes. **GI:** nausea, vomiting, diarrhea, elevated liver enzymes. **Hem:** leukopenia, thrombocytopenia, hyperglycemia, hypoglycemia. **GU:** renal toxicity (noted by azotemia, glycosuria, renal tubular acidosis), mild proteinuria. **Skin:** pain, redness, swelling along injection site.

Nursing implications/Documentation

Possible nursing diagnoses: Potential for infection; Potential for injury; Fatigue; Altered oral mucous membrane; Fluid volume deficit; Diarrhea; Altered nutrition: less than body requirements.

♦ *See important Nursing implications in Antineoplastic agents overview on page 72, which apply to all antineoplastics. The interventions that follow are additional and specific to this drug only.*

• Keep 50% dextrose available to treat hypoglycemia (first dose may cause sudden insulin release).

• Monitor blood sugars carefully; this drug may cause irreversible damage to pancreatic beta cells.

• Test urine for protein and glucose every 8 hours; report proteinuria (early sign of renal toxicity).

• Increase fluid intake to 2–3 L a day to prevent renal tubular damage form hyperuricemia secondary to cell lysis.

• Be aware that therapeutic response is often accompanied by toxicity and that nausea and vomiting almost always occur.

Patient & family teaching/Home care

Possible nursing diagnoses: Knowledge deficit; Ineffective coping (individual and family); Hopelessness; Impaired home maintenance management.

◆ *See important Patient & family teaching in Antineoplastic agents overview on page 72, which apply to all antineoplastics. The teachings that follow are additional and specific to this drug only.*

• Point out that drinking 2–3 L a day helps prevent kidney complications; IV fluids may be necessary.

• Teach the need to test urine for protein.

◆ *See Antineoplastic agents overview for more information.*

succinylcholine

suk-sin-il-koe'leen

succinylcholine chloride: **Anectine, Quelicin, Sucostrin, ♠Scoline, Anectine Flo-Pak**

Class: ★**Depolarizing neuromuscular blocker prototype,** Skeletal-muscle relaxant

Antidote: Neostigmine methylsulfate

PEDS	PREG	GERI
OK	C	🖐

Action Relaxes or paralyzes skeletal muscles (depending on dose) by competing for cholinergic receptor sites at motor endplates, producing initial transient muscle contraction, followed by depolarization and flaccid paralysis. Ultra short-acting. Does not alter consciousness, pain threshold, or thought processes.

Use/Therapeutic goal/Outcome

Endotracheal intubation, adjunct to general anesthesia, during mechanical ventilation, endoscopy, or pharmacologically or electrically induced seizures: Facilitation of endotracheal tube and mechanical ventilation tolerance; relaxation of skeletal muscle. **Outcome criteria:** Tolerance of endotracheal intubation and mechanical ventilation; diminished or absent voluntary and reflexive movement.

Dose range/Administration

Interaction alert: Diazepam decreases effect of succinylcholine. The following drugs alter neuromuscular blockade: phenelzine, promazine, oxytocin, aminoglycoside, and polymyxin antibiotics, quinidine, cardiac glycosides, MAO inhibitors, beta blockers, procainamide, lidocaine, trimethaphan, lithium, magnesium salts, chloroquine, quinine, fluorane, acetylcholine, anticholinesterase, furosemide, and other depolarizing and nondepolarizing relaxants.

Adult: IV: 2.5–4 mg/kg. *Maximum dose:* 150 mg. *Intermittent dose:* 0.3–1.1 mg/kg. **Child:** IV: 1–2 mg/kg. IM: (Only when suitable IV site not available). 2.5 mg/kg, not to exceed 150 mg.

Clinical alert: Succinylcholine should be given only by physicians and nurses who are familiar with its use, and in the presence of a physician, nurse anesthetist, or respiratory therapist who is qualified to manage endotracheal intubation.

Contraindications/Precautions

PREG
C

Contraindicated in hypersensitivity to succinylcholine and in family history of malignant hypertension or hyperthermia. **Use with caution** in hepatic, renal, or pulmonary impairment; severe burns; electrolyte imbalance; penetrating eye injuries; fractures; cardiac depression; acute narrow-angle glaucoma; degenerative or dystrophic neuromuscular disease; myasthenia gravis; dehydration; thyroid disorders; and collagen disease.

🖐 **Use with caution for children and the elderly or debilitated. Safe use for pregnant or nursing mothers has not been established.**

Side effects/Adverse reactions

Hypersensitivity: rash, anaphylaxis. **MS:** muscle fascilculations, postoperative muscle pain. **Resp:** prolonged respiratory depression, bronchospasm, apnea. **CNS:** malignant hyperthermia. **CV:** pulse and blood pressure changes, dysrhythmias, cardiac arrest. **Hem:** hyperkalemia. **Eye:** increased intraocular pressure. **GI:** excessive salivation.

Nursing implications/Documentation

Possible nursing diagnoses: Impaired communication; Pain; Potential for aspiration; Potential for injury.

• Ascertain that baseline CBC, electrolytes, BUN, creatinine, liver function, chest X ray, and EKG studies are posted on chart before drug administration (report abnormalities).

♦ Protect airway, position for drainage of oropharyngeal secretions (if possible), and keep suction at bedside until the patient is fully alert; have emergency equipment and drugs available.

♦ Monitor and record vital signs every 15 min until stable; report abnormalities that might indicate potential complications.

♦ Recognize that this drug may *paralyze*, but does not relieve pain (provide analgesics if pain is suspected, anticipate human needs).

♦ Monitor for potential for injury: protect eyes if there is no blink reflex (tape shut); watch positioning of all extremities (provide range of motion exercises if therapy is prolonged).

♦ Monitor and document intake and output frequently, every 2–4 hr for 24 hr.

Patient & family teaching/Home care

Possible nursing diagnoses: Anxiety; Fear.

♦ Explain all procedures, even if the person seems unconscious (the ability to hear may be present).

♦ Reassure that muscle weakness or stiffness will subside.

♦ For use with mechanical ventilation, stress that you are aware that the patient cannot move, and that this drug is being given to control breathing; reassure that breathing is being closely monitored to be sure that the lungs are being adequately oxygenated, and that the ability to move will return as soon as drug is stopped. Also reassure that medication for pain and anxiety will be given to help tolerate the endotracheal tube.

sucralfate
soo-kral'fate

Carafate, ✦Sulcrate
Class: Antiulcer agent

PEDS	PREG	GERI
✋	B	✋

Action Combines with proteins at ulcer site to form a protective coating resistant to hydrochloric acid, pepsin, and bile salts.

Use/Therapeutic goal/Outcome

Duodenal ulcers: Promotion of healing. **Outcome criteria:** Report of reduction of epigastric pain; healing of ulcers on endoscopic examination.

Stress-induced ulcers: Prevention. **Outcome criteria:** Report of absence of epigastric pain.

Mouth ulcers: Promotion of healing and relief of discomfort associated with eating. **Outcome criteria:** Visible healing of ulcers; report of increased comfort.

Dose range/Administration

Interaction alert: Do not give antacids for 1/2 hr before or after sucralfate since they will interfere with binding at ulcer site. Do not give sucralfate within 2 hr of tetracycline, digoxin, phenytoin, or cimetidine to prevent these drugs from being bound by sucralfate in the GI tract.

🥤 **Administer on empty stomach.**

Adult: PO: 1 g qid 1 hr before meals and at hs. *Topical:* Apply prepared suspension (8 g in 120 ml water-sorbitol solution) to mouth ulcers before meals and at bedtime.

Clinical alert: For **NG route**, place sucralfate tablet in barrel of 30 ml syringe and draw up 15–20 ml warm water; wait 1 or 2 min; shake syringe well. Flush tube before and after administration.

Contraindications/Precautions
PREG
B

Contraindicated in hypersensitivity to sucralfate.

🖐 **Use with caution for pregnant or nursing mothers and the elderly. Safe use for children has not been established.**

Side effects/Adverse reactions

Hypersensitivity: rash, hives, itching. **GI:** constipation, indigestion, abdominal pain, nausea, vomiting. **CNS:** sleepiness and vertigo.

Nursing implications/Documentation

Possible nursing diagnoses: Constipation; Potential for injury.

♦ Monitor and record bowel elimination, especially in the elderly.

♦ Provide appropriate interventions to prevent or treat constipation.

♦ For mouth ulcers, use cotton-tipped applicator to coat lesions or have patient swish suspension around mouth and spit out excess.

♦ Recognize that sucralfate may be used to provide ulcer prophylaxis in the critically ill instead of antacids and/or histamine₂ antagonists.

Patient & family teaching/Home care

Possible nursing diagnoses: Knowledge deficit; Impaired home maintenance management.

♦ Advise taking sucralfate 1/2 hr before meals and at bedtime for best results; advise not to chew or crush tablets.

♦ Stress the importance of dietary bulk, ample fluids, and exercise to prevent constipation.

♦ Caution to avoid driving or operating dangerous equipment until response to drug is identified.

♦ Advise avoiding alcohol and other CNS depressants while taking sucralfate.

♦ Emphasize need to take sucralfate for 4 to 8 weeks, even though ulcer symptoms may have subsided; using longer than 8 weeks is not recommended.

sufentanil citrate

soo-fen'ta-nil

Sufenta

Class: Narcotic analgesic, Opiate agonist, Anesthetic

Antidote: naloxone hydrochloride

PEDS	PREG	GERI	CONTROLLED SUBSTANCE
✋	C	✋	II

Action Alters both perception of and response to pain through an unclear mechanism. Believed to act by binding with opiate receptors at many CNS sites. Inhibits sympathetic responses to surgical stress (e.g., excessive increase in blood pressure) by producing a dose-related decrease in catecholamine release, particularly norepinephrine.

Use/Therapeutic goal/Outcome

Adjunct to anesthesia or as a primary anesthetic: Promotion of comfort and relaxation. *Outcome criteria:* Absence of observable signs of pain (grimacing, frowning, restlessness, muscle tension at operative site); blood pressure and pulse within normal limits when compared to baseline.

Dose range/Administration

Interaction alert: Alcohol and other CNS depressants increase effects.

Adjunct to general anesthesia: Adult: IV: 1–8 mcg/kg based on duration of surgery, with oxygen and nitrous oxide.

Primary anesthetic: Adult: IV: 8–30 mcg/kg, with 100% oxygen and a muscle relaxant. **Child > 12 yrs:** IV: 10–25 mcg/kg, with 100% oxygen. *Maintenance dose:* up to 25–50 mcg/kg.

Clinical alert: This drug should be given only by those specifically qualified to manage the use of IV anesthetics. Expect reduced dosage for the elderly or debilitated. Keep narcotic antagonist (naloxone) and resuscitation equipment readily available.

Contraindications/Precautions
PREG C

Contraindicated in hypersensitivity to sufentanil citrate. **Use with caution** in pulmonary disease, lowered respiratory reserve, and impaired renal or hepatic function.

✋ **Contraindicated for children under 12 years and pregnant women. Use with caution for the elderly.**

Side effects/Adverse reactions

Hypersensitivity: rash, hives, itching, respiratory depression, skeletal-muscle rigidity. **CV:** tachycardia, bradycardia, hypotension, hypertension. **GI:** nausea, vomiting. **Resp:** apnea, bronchospasm. **CNS:** chills. **MS:** muscle rigidity, intraoperative muscle movement, chest-wall rigidity.

Nursing implications/Documentation

Possible nursing diagnoses: Potential for aspiration; Potential for injury; Pain.

♦ Monitor closely for airway obstruction and keep suction at bedside until patient is recovered; be prepared to use mechanical ventilation if doses higher than 8 mcg/kg have been given because of extended respiratory depression.

♦ Document vital signs as needed and according to recovery protocol.

♦ Watch closely for potential for injury; position extremities and head carefully; keep side rails up.

Patient & family teaching/Home care

Possible nursing diagnoses: Fear; Sensory/perceptual alterations.

♦ Explain procedures briefly and in simple terms (even if the patient is not awake, he or she may be able to hear).

♦ Explain the rationale for reporting pain before it is severe.

- ◆ Reassure that things are going well and measures are being taken to ensure safety (even if the patient is not awake).
- ◆ *See Narcotic and non-narcotic analgesics overview for more information.*

sulfacetamide

sul-fa-see'ta-mide

sulfacetamide sodium 10%: ***Bleph-10 Liquifilm-Opthalmic, Cetamide Opthalmic, Sodium Sulamyd 10% Opthalmic, Sulf-10 Opthalmic***

sulfacetamide sodium 15%: ***Isopto Cetamide Opthalmic, Sulfacel-15 Opthalmic***

sulfacetamide sodium 30%: ***Sodium Sulamyd 30% Opthalmic***

Class: Antibiotic, Sulfonamide, Opthalmic

PEDS	PREG	GERI
OK	C	OK

Action Usually bacteriostatic, limits gram-negative and gram-positive bacterial growth by interfering with bacterial folic acid biosynthesis (required for growth).

Use/Therapeutic goal/Outcome

Conjunctivitis, corneal ulcers, infections of the eye: Prevention or resolution of infection. ***Outcome criteria:*** Absence of signs and symptoms of infection following a full course of therapy.

Dose range/Administration

Interaction alert: Wait 30 minutes after instilling anesthetics or para-amino-benzoic acid derivatives (they decrease sulfacetamide sodium action) before instilling sulfacetamide. Wait 10 minutes after instilling sulfacetamide before instilling any other drops. Do not mix with silver preparations.

Adult and Child: *Solution:* Instill 1–2 drops in lower conjunctival sac q2-3h while awake; use ointment or instill drops less often at night. *10% ointment:* ½ to 1 inch in conjunctival sac.

Clinical alert: Read labels carefully to ascertain correct concentration. Remove as much exudate as possible from lids before instilling sulfacetamide (exudate interferes with drug action).

Contraindications/Precautions

PREG
C

Contraindicated in allergy to sulfonamides.

Side effects/Adverse reactions

Hypersensitivity: itching, burning. ***Eye:*** pain on instillation of eye drop, slowed corneal healing.

Nursing implications/Documentation

Possible nursing diagnoses: Potential for infection; Sensory/perceptual alterations: visual.

- ◆ Determine history of allergies, and (regardless of history) monitor closely for allergic reactions.
- ◆ Wash hands thoroughly before and after administration, and use correct procedure (see Guidelines for eye medications in Section I).
- ◆ Do not use if solution is brown or discolored.
- ◆ Monitor and record clinical status of infection (report deterioration immediately).

Patient & family teaching/Home care

Possible nursing diagnoses: Knowledge deficit; Impaired home maintenance management.

- ◆ Warn that the drops may burn and blur vision when instilled, but that this should improve within 10 minutes.
- ◆ Give verbal and written instructions for instilling eyedrops (see Section I for procedure for administering eye drops).
- ◆ Teach the need to report increased itching or burning (may be an allergic reaction) or lack of improvement in signs and symptoms (may indicate need for change in medication regimen).
- ◆ Warn of the dangers of sharing eye medications, wash cloths, and towels with other family members (if others develop symptoms, they should notify physician).
- ◆ Advise that wearing sunglasses may reduce sensitivity to light.
- ◆ Explain the importance of taking the drug for the entire time prescribed, even if symptoms abate.
- ◆ *See Anti-infectives overview for more information.*

sulfadiazine

sul-fa-dye'a-zeen

Microsulfon

Class: Anti-infective, Sulfonamide

PEDS	PREG	GERI
🖐	🖐	🖐

Action Usually bacteriostatic, limits bacterial growth by blocking bacterial folic acid biosynthesis.

S

Use/Therapeutic goal/Outcome

Infections (urinary tract, rheumatic fever, toxoplasmosis, meningitis, ulcerative colitis): Prevention or resolution of infection. **Outcome criteria:** Absence of pathogenic growth on cultures, absence of clinical manifestations of infection (fever, pain, swelling, redness, heat, odor, drainage, productive cough, dysuria), normal chest X rays, normal WBC count.

Dose range/Administration

Interaction alert: Para-aminobenzoic acid (PABA) may inhibit action. Ammonium chloride or ascorbic acid may cause sulfonamide precipitation with resultant crystalluria. Increases effects of methotrexate, phenytoin, anticoagulants and oral hypoglycemics. Decreases effects of oral contraceptives.

▯ **Give with full glass of water.**

Adult: PO: 2–4 g/day in 3–6 equal doses. **Child > 2 mos:** PO: 150 mg/kg/day in 4–6 equal doses. *Maximum dose: 6 g/day. For rheumatic fever prophylaxis:* 0.5 to 1 g/day.

Contraindications/Precautions

PREG
💮

Contraindicated in allergy to sulfonamides, and in megaloblastic anemia due to folate deficiency. **Use with caution** in impaired renal or hepatic function, with anticonvulsant therapy, in malabsorption syndrome or malnutrition, and in history of other allergic responses (e.g., other drugs, hay fever, asthma).

💮 **Contraindicated for infants under 2 months, pregnant women near term (preg B; preg D near term) and nursing mothers. Use with caution for the elderly.**

Side effects/Adverse reactions

Hypersensitivity: itching, rashes, fever, angioedema, difficulty breathing, anaphylaxis. **GI:** abdominal pain, stomatitis, nausea, vomiting, diarrhea, pseudomembranous colitis, hepatitis. **GU:** nephrotoxicity (oliguria, anuria, crystalluria, hematuria). **CNS:** headache, depression, seizures. **Hem:** agranulocytosis, aplastic anemia, eosinophilia, thrombocytopenia, leukopenia, hemolytic anemia, bleeding disorders. **Skin:** photosensitivity.

Nursing implications/Documentation

Possible nursing diagnoses: Potential for infection; Potential fluid volume deficit; Diarrhea.

◆ Determine history of allergies, and (regardless of history) monitor closely for allergic reactions.

◆ Obtain baseline CBC, BUN, urinalysis, creatinine, liver function studies, and necessary culture specimens before administering first dose; monitor closely thereafter if therapy is prolonged.

◆ Encourage fluids, and record and monitor input and output; 3000–4000 ml/day is advised (for urine output of 1500 ml/day).

◆ Document and report diarrhea.

◆ If there is no improvement within 3–5 days, consult with physician to determine if antibiotic regimen should be re-evaluated (and new cultures drawn).

Patient & family teaching/Home care

Possible nursing diagnoses: Knowledge deficit; Impaired home maintenance management.

◆ Stress the importance of drinking 3 to 4 quarts of fluids daily to optimize drug action and minimize side effects.

◆ Teach the need to report persistent diarrhea, or new signs and symptoms of illness (e.g., fever, mouth lesions, vaginal irritation, respiratory symptoms, diarrhea); medication change may be necessary.

◆ Explain the importance of taking antibiotics for the entire time prescribed, even if symptoms abate.

◆ Caution that this drug may cause increased sensitivity to the sun; warn women that effectiveness of oral contraceptives may be reduced.

◆ *See Anti-infectives overview for more information.*

sulfamethoxazole   *sul-fa-me-thox'a-zoal*

❧Apo-Sulfamethoxazole, Gantanol, Gantanol DS
Class: Anti-infective, Sulfonamide

PEDS	PREG	GERI
🖐	💮	🖐

Action Usually bacteriostatic, limits bacterial growth by blocking bacterial biosynthesis of folic acid.

Use/Therapeutic goal/Outcome

Urinary tract infections: Prevention or resolution of infection. **Outcome criteria:** Absence of pathogenic growth on urine cultures, absence of clinical manifestations of urinary tract infection (fever, dysuria, frequency), normal WBC count.

Dose range/Administration

Interaction alert: Para-aminobenzoic acid (PABA) may inhibit antibacterial action. Ammonium chloride or ascorbic acid may cause precipitation of sulfonamide with resultant crystalluria. Increases effects of oral hypoglycemics and anticoagulants. Decreases effects of oral contraceptives and may cause breakthrough bleeding.

Give with full glass of water.

Adult: PO: Initial dose 2 g, then 1 g bid, or tid for severe infections. *Child > 2 mo:* PO: Initial dose 50–60 mg/kg, then 25–30 mg/kg bid. *Maximum dose:* 75 mg/kg/day.

Contraindications/Precautions

PREG

Contraindicated in allergy to sulfonamides, and in porphyria. *Use with caution* in impaired renal or hepatic function, in conjunction with anticonvulsant therapy, in malabsorption syndrome or malnutrition, and in history of other allergic responses (e.g., other drugs, hay fever, asthma).

Contraindicated for infants under 2 months, pregnant women near term (Preg B; preg D near term), and nursing mothers. Use with caution for the elderly.

Side effects/Adverse reactions

Hypersensitivity: itching, rashes, drug fever, angioedema, difficulty breathing, serum sickness, anaphylaxis. *GI:* nausea, vomiting, diarrhea, abdominal pain, anorexia, stomatitis, pseudomembranous colitis, hepatitis. *GU:* nephrotoxicity (oliguria, anuria, crystalluria, hematuria). *CNS:* headache, dizziness, fatigue, seizures, hallucinations. *Hem:* agranulocytosis, aplastic anemia, eosinophilia, thrombocytopenia, leukopenia, hemolytic anemia, bleeding disorders. *Skin:* photosensitivity. *Misc:* superinfections.

Nursing implications/Documentation

Possible nursing diagnoses: Potential for infection; Potential fluid volume deficit; Diarrhea.

◆ Determine history of allergies, and (regardless of history) monitor closely for allergic reactions.

◆ Weigh patient and obtain baseline CBC, BUN, creatinine, liver function studies, and necessary culture specimens before administering first dose; monitor closely thereafter if therapy is prolonged.

◆ Encourage fluids, and record and monitor intake and output; 3000–4000 ml/day is advised (for urine output of 1500 ml/day).

◆ Document and report diarrhea.

◆ If there is no improvement within 3–5 days, consult with physician to determine if antibiotic regimen should be re-evaluated (and new cultures drawn).

◆ Monitor for bleeding tendencies (check gums, urine).

Patient & family teaching/Home care

Possible nursing diagnoses: Knowledge deficit; Impaired home maintenance management.

◆ Stress the importance of drinking 3 to 4 quarts of fluids daily to optimize drug action and minimize side effects.

◆ Teach the patient and family to report persistent diarrhea or new symptoms of illness (e.g., fever, mouth lesions, vaginal irritation, respiratory symptoms, diarrhea); medication change may be necessary.

◆ Explain the importance of taking antibiotics for the entire time prescribed, even if symptoms abate.

◆ If taking Azo-Gantanol (sulfamethoxazole combined with pyridium), explain that urine and perspiration may become orange-yellow.

◆ Caution that this drug may cause increased sensitivity to the sun; warn women that effectiveness of oral contraceptives may be reduced.

◆ *See Anti-infectives overview for more information.*

sulfasalazine

sul-fa-sal'a-zeen

Azulfidine, Azulfidine EN–Tabs, ♥PMS Sulfasalazine E.C., ♥ ♠Salazopyrin, ♥ ♠Salazoprine, ♥ ♠Salazoprin EN–Tabs, S.A.S., S.A.S.–Enteric

Class: Anti-infective, Sulfonamide

PEDS   PREG   GERI

Action Usually bacteriostatic, limits bacterial growth by blocking bacterial biosynthesis of folic acid. May also have an anti-inflammatory effect.

Use/Therapeutic goal/Outcome

Interaction alert: May increase effects of oral anticoagulants and oral hypoglycemics. May decrease effectiveness of oral contraceptives.

Give with or after food to reduce GI upset; encourage taking with a full glass of water.

Ulcerative colitis, collagenous colitis, and Crohn's disease: Prevention or resolution. *Outcome*

S

▶

criteria: Absence of diarrhea and blood in stool, report of absence of abdominal cramping, absence of inflammatory lesions upon proctoscopic exam.

Rheumatoid arthritis: Reduction in joint inflammation. *Outcome criteria:* Report of increased mobility with decreased pain; decrease in joint swelling.

Dose range/Administration

▣ **Give with full glass of water.**

Adult: PO: 2 g/day in divided doses q6h. *Maximum dose:* 8 g/day. *Child > 2 yr:* PO: 30–60 mg/kg/day in 3–6 equal doses.

Contraindications/Precautions

PREG
🖑

Contraindicated in allergy to sulfonamides or salicylates, and in intestinal or urinary obstruction, and porphyria. *Use with caution* in impaired renal or hepatic function, in conjunction with anticonvulsant therapy, in malabsorption syndrome or malnutrition, blood dyscrasias, G6PD deficiency, and in history of other allergic responses (e.g., other drugs, hay fever, asthma).

🖑 **Contraindicated for infants under 2 years, pregnant women near term (Preg b; preg D near term), and nursing mothers. Use with caution for the elderly.**

Side effects/Adverse reactions

Hypersensitivity: itching, rashes, fever, angioedema, exfoliative dermatitis, joint pain, erythema multiform, difficulty breathing, anaphylaxis. *GI:* abdominal pain, stomatitis, nausea, vomiting, diarrhea, pseudomembranous colitis, hepatitis. *GU:* nephrotoxicity (oliguria, anuria, crystalluria, hematuria, orange-yellow urine color. *CNS:* headache, dizziness, fatigue, seizures, hallucinations. *Hem:* agranulocytosis, aplastic anemia, eosinophilia, thrombocytopenia, leukopenia, hemolytic anemia, bleeding disorders. *Skin:* photosensitivity. *Misc:* superinfections.

Nursing implications/Documentation

Possible nursing diagnoses: Potential for infection; Potential fluid volume deficit; Diarrhea.

♦ Determine history of allergies, and (regardless of history) monitor closely for allergic reactions.

♦ Weigh patient and obtain baseline CBC, BUN, creatinine, liver function studies, and necessary culture specimens before administer-

ing first dose; monitor closely thereafter if therapy is prolonged.

♦ Encourage fluids, and document and monitor intake and output; 3000–4000 cc/day is advised (for urine output of 1500 cc/day).

♦ Document and report diarrhea.

♦ If there is no improvement within 3–5 days, consult with physician to determine if antibiotic regimen should be re-evaluated (and new cultures drawn); with enteric-coated tablets, there may be a problem with failure of tablets to dissolve.

♦ Monitor for bleeding tendencies (check gums, urine).

Patient & family teaching/Home care

Possible nursing diagnoses: Knowledge deficit; Impaired home maintenance management.

♦ Emphasize the importance of drinking 3 to 4 quarts of fluids daily to optimize drug action and minimize side effects.

♦ Teach the patient and family to report persistent diarrhea or new symptoms of illness (e.g., fever, mouth lesions, vaginal irritation, respiratory symptoms, diarrhea); medication change may be necessary.

♦ Explain the importance of taking antibiotics for the entire time prescribed, even if symptoms abate.

♦ Caution that this drug may cause increased sensitivity to the sun; warn women that effectiveness of oral contraceptives may be reduced.

♦ *See Anti-infectives overview for more information.*

sulfisoxazole

sul-fi-sox'a-zoal

sulfurazole: ✤ ⚕️*Azo-Sulfisoxazole, Gantrisin, Lipo Gantrisin,* ✤*Novosoxazole*

Class: ★**Anti-infective (sulfonamide) prototype**

PEDS	PREG	GERI
🖑	C	🖑

Action Usually bacteriostatic, limits bacterial growth by blocking bacterial biosynthesis of folic acid.

Use/Therapeutic goal/Outcome

Infections (urinary tract and systemic): Prevention or resolution of infection. *Outcome criteria:* Absence of pathogenic growth on cultures, absence of clinical manifestations of infection (fever, pain, swelling, redness, heat, odor, drainage, productive cough, dysuria), normal chest X rays, normal WBC count.

Dose range/Administration

Interaction alert: Para-aminobenzoic acid (PABA) may inhibit antibacterial action. Ammonium chloride or ascorbic acid may cause precipitation of sulfonamide with resultant crystalluria. Increases effects of oral hypoglycemics and oral anticoagulants. Decreases effects of oral contraceptives.

▯ **Give with full glass of water.**

Adult: PO: 2–8 g/day in divided doses. *Suspension:* 4–5 g q12h. **Child > 2 mo:** PO: 75–150 mg/kg/day in divided doses. *Maximum dose:* 6 g/day.

Contraindications/Precautions
PREG
C

Contraindicated in allergy to sulfonamides, and in porphyria. **Use with caution** in impaired renal or hepatic function, in conjunction with anticonvulsant therapy, in malabsorption syndrome or malnutrition, and in history of other allergic responses (e.g., other drugs, hay fever, asthma).

✋ **Contraindicated for infants under 2 months, pregnant women near term, and nursing mothers. Use with caution for the elderly.**

Side effects/Adverse reactions

Hypersensitivity: itching, rashes, drug fever, angioedema, serum sickness, difficulty breathing, erythema multiform, anaphylaxis. **GI:** nausea, vomiting, diarrhea, abdominal pain, stomatitis, pseudomembranous colitis, hepatitis. **GU:** nephrotoxicity (oliguria, anuria, crystalluria, hematuria). **CNS:** headache, mental depression, dizziness, fatigue, hallucinations, seizures. **Hem:** agranulocytosis, aplastic anemia, eosinophilia, thrombocytopenia, leukopenia, hemolytic anemia, bleeding disorders. **Skin:** photosensitivity. **Misc:** superinfection.

Nursing implications/Documentation

Possible nursing diagnoses: Potential for infection; Potential fluid volume deficit; Diarrhea.

♦ Determine history of allergies, and (regardless of history) monitor closely for allergic reactions.

♦ Weigh patient and obtain baseline CBC, BUN, creatinine, liver function studies, and necessary culture specimens before administering first dose; monitor closely thereafter if therapy is prolonged.

♦ Monitor for bleeding tendencies (check gums and urine).

♦ Encourage fluids, and document and monitor intake and output; 3000–4000 ml/day is advised (for urine output of 1500 ml/day).

♦ Document and report diarrhea.

♦ If there is no improvement within 3–5 days, consult with physician to determine if antibiotic regimen should be re-evaluated (and new cultures drawn).

Patient & family teaching/Home care

Possible nursing diagnoses: Knowledge deficit; Impaired home maintenance management.

♦ Emphasize the importance of drinking 3 to 4 quarts of fluids daily to optimize drug action and minimize side effects (advise taking sulfisoxazole with a full glass of water).

♦ Teach the patient and family to report persistent diarrhea or new symptoms of illness (e.g., fever, mouth lesions, vaginal irritation, respiratory symptoms, diarrhea); medication change may be necessary.

♦ Explain the importance of taking antibiotics for the entire time prescribed, even if symptoms abate.

♦ Caution that this drug may cause increased sensitivity to the sun; warn women that effectiveness of oral contraceptives may be reduced.

♦ *See Anti-infectives overview for more information.*

sulindac
sul-in'dak

♦**Apo-Sulin, Clinoril,** ♦**Novo-Sundac**

Class: Nonsteroidal anti-inflammatory drug (NSAID), Analgesic, Antipyretic

PEDS	PREG	GERI
✋	✋	✋

S

Action Exact mechanism of action is unclear. Believed to inhibit prostaglandin synthesis. Prostaglandin is a naturally occurring mediator of the inflammatory process which is found throughout body tissue. Structurally and pharmacologically related to indomethacin.

Use/Therapeutic goal/Outcome

Pain and inflammation: Promotion of comfort and mobility; suppression of inflammation. **Outcome criteria:** Report of increased comfort with increased range of motion and ability to perform activities of daily life; reduction in or absence of joint stiffness, swelling, redness, and warmth.

Dose range/Administration

Interaction alert: May alter anticoagulants and oral hypoglycemic agents requirements. Aspirin will suppress serum sulindac levels, increase GI side effects, and increase risk of bleeding.

🖐 **Give with food, milk, or antacid to prevent GI irritation.**

Arthritic joints: Adult: PO: *Initial dose:* 150 mg bid, then adjusted according to individual response.

Painful shoulder and gout: Adult: PO: 200 mg bid for 1–2 wk, then reduce as signs and symptoms subside.

Clinical alert: Do not exceed 400 mg/day.

Contraindications/Precautions

PREG
🖐

Contraindicated in hypersensitivity to sulindac, aspirin, or other NSAIDs. **Use with caution** in history of GI disorders, hypertension, coagulation defects, and impaired cardiac, renal, or hepatic function.

🖐 **Use with caution for the elderly. Safe use for children and pregnant women has not been established (first two trimesters, preg B; in third trimester, preg D).**

Side effects/Adverse reactions

Hypersensitivity: asthma, rash, pruritus, urticaria, rhinitis, Stevens-Johnson syndrome.
GI: diarrhea, GI irritation, dry mouth, occult blood loss, nausea, impaired liver function.
CV: edema. **CNS:** dizziness, headache, drowsiness. **Eye:** blurred vision. **Ear:** decreased hearing. **Hem:** hematologic changes, aplastic anemia.

Nursing implications/Documentation

Possible nursing diagnoses: Pain; Impaired physical mobility.

♦ Establish a baseline for CBC, electrolytes, prothrombin time, BUN, creatinine, and liver function studies; if therapy is prolonged, monitor periodically thereafter.

♦ Monitor for and report GI symptoms that may indicate peptic ulcer (nausea, pain, black stools).

♦ Record weight every other day; report edema or sudden weight gain.

♦ For diabetics, monitor blood sugar closely since insulin requirements may change.

Patient & family teaching/Home care

Possible nursing diagnoses: Altered health maintenance; Knowledge deficit.

♦ Advise taking doses with food to reduce GI symptoms.

♦ Explain the importance of watching for symptoms of GI bleeding (black stools, persistent GI distress).

♦ Explain that it may require up to 2 weeks for full effects of therapy to be seen.

♦ Encourage checking blood pressure at regular intervals; advise decreasing salt intake.

♦ Stress the need to avoid aspirin, alcohol, and other OTC drugs (unless approved by physician) because of increased risk of GI bleeding.

♦ Instruct individuals to hold dose and report if any of the following side effects are experienced: vertigo, rashes, blood in urine, hearing or visual changes, sudden weight gain, edema.

♦ Warn against driving or activities that require alertness until response is determined.

♦ Reinforce the need for medical follow-up; advise telling dentist that sulindac is being taken.

♦ For diabetics, explain the importance of monitoring blood sugars with a blood glucose meter.

♦ *See Nonsteroidal anti-inflammatory drugs overview for more information.*

tamoxifen

ta-mox'i-fin

tamoxifen citrate: **Nolvadex,** 🍁 **Nolvadex D, Tamofen**

Class: Antineoplastic agent, Antihormone

PEDS	PREG	GERI
🖐	C	🖐

Action Inhibits malignant cellular growth of estrogen-responsive tumors by blocking uptake of estradiol in breast tissue.

Use/Therapeutic goal/Outcome

Postmenopausal breast cancer: Suppression of malignant cell proliferation. **Outcome criteria:** Tumor and disease regression or stabilization on radiologic and physical examination.

Dose range/Administration

🖐 **Give with meals if GI distress occurs.**

Adult: PO: 10–20 mg bid, in morning and evening.

Clinical alert: Hold dose and report if early signs of hypercalcemia (insomnia, lethargy, nausea, vomiting, vascular collapse) are noted.

Contraindications/Precautions

PREG
C

Contraindicated in hypersensitivity to tamoxifen. *Use with caution* for women in their childbearing years, and in leukopenia, thrombocytopenia, and cataracts.

⚕ **Contraindicated for children and pregnant or nursing mothers. Use with caution for the elderly.**

Side effects/Adverse reactions

Hypersensitivity: hot flashes, rash, fever. *GI:* anorexia, nausea, vomiting, distaste for food. *CV:* chest pain, pulmonary embolism, thromboembolic disorders. *CNS:* hot flashes, depression, headache, dizziness. *GU:* vaginal bleeding or discharge, dysmenorrhea, pruritus vulvae. *Hem:* myelosuppression, hypercalcemia, transient thrombocytopenia, leukopenia. *Eye:* ocular lesions, retinopathy. *Skin:* alopecia. *MS:* bone pain. *Misc:* pain at tumor site.

Nursing implications/Documentation

Possible nursing diagnoses: Fluid volume deficit; Self-esteem disturbance; Potential for injury; Altered nutrition: less than body requirements.

◆ *See important Nursing implications in Antineoplastic agents overview.*

  ◆ Increase fluid to 2 L per day, unless contraindicated, to aid in calcium excretion.

  ◆ Observe for increased risk of thrombophlebitis.

Patient & family teaching/Home care

Possible nursing diagnoses: Impaired home maintenance management; Knowledge deficit.

◆ *See important Patient & family teaching in Antineoplastic agents overview.*

  ◆ Stress that doses should be taken exactly on schedule (without missing or doubling up on doses) to maintain therapeutic levels.

  ◆ Explain that bone pain may occur and that this is indicative of a positive drug response; advise consulting physician for recommended analgesics.

  ◆ Point out the need to drink at least 2 L per day.

  ◆ Advise reporting visual disturbances or signs of hypercalcemia (insomnia, lethargy, nausea,

vomiting, dizziness) or thrombophlebitis (pain and swelling of leg veins).

  ◆ Encourage bedridden patients to perform leg exercises to improve circulation and prevent thrombophlebitis.

  ◆ Encourage recording daily weights; advise to report edema or weight gain.

  ◆ Teach that daily exercise may help reduce hypercalcemia.

  ◆ Counsel women to use a nonhormonal method of contraception and to report suspected pregnancy immediately.

◆ *See Antineoplastic agents overview for more information.*

temazepam

te-maz′e-pam

Restoril, Temaz

Class: Sedative, hypnotic, benzodiazepine

PEDS ⚕ PREG X GERI ⚕

CONTROLLED SUBSTANCE
IV

Action Produces sleep by acting upon the limbic system, thalamus, and hypothalamus of the central nervous system. Onset of action may be as long as 2 to 2 1/2 hrs.

Use/Therapeutic goal/Outcome

Insomnia: Promotion of sleep. *Outcome criteria:* Report of having slept well.

Dose range/Administration

Interaction alert: Alcohol, narcotics, analgesics, antihistamines, and other CNS depressants intensify CNS depression.

Adult <65 yrs: PO: 15–30 mg at bedtime.
Adult >65 yrs: 15 mg at bedtime.

Clinical alert: Recognize that dose may need to be given 2 hr before sleep is desired because it may take as long as 2 to 2 1/2 hr before onset of action.

Contraindications/Precautions

PREG
X

Contraindicated in hypersensitivity or intolerance to benzodiazepines, narrow angle glaucoma, or psychoses. *Use with caution* for patients with depression, suicidal tendencies, and impaired liver or kidney function.

⚕ **Contraindicated for children under 18 years and for pregnant women. Use with caution for nursing mothers and for the elderly.**

T

Side effects/Adverse reactions

Hypersensitivity: rashes. **CNS:** lethargy, drowsiness, dizziness, confusion, daytime somnolence, coordination problems. **GI:** anorexia, diarrhea. **Misc:** drug tolerance and dependence.

Nursing implications/Documentation

Possible nursing diagnoses: Potential for injury; Sensory, perceptual alterations (visual and auditory)

♦ Document mental status before administration, monitor patient activity closely following administration, and employ appropriate measures to ensure safety (side rails up, call bell within reach, and no unsupervised smoking).

♦ Be sure that doses are swallowed (not hoarded).

♦ Be aware that sedatives and hypnotics do not provide pain relief (patient may need an analgesic as well).

♦ Monitor for and report signs of overdosage (slurred speech, continued somnolence, respiratory depression, confusion) and tolerance (increased anxiety and/or increased wakefulness).

Patient & family teaching/Home care

Possible nursing diagnoses: Sleep pattern disturbance; Ineffective coping (family and individual); Impaired home maintenance management.

♦ Explore problems that may contribute to insomnia or anxiety, and ways of coping effectively with the problems (stress that effective coping can promote restful sleep).

♦ Explain the importance of daily exercise in promoting rest, and encourage the person to establish a method for getting enough exercise (e.g., daily walks).

♦ Stress that drug tolerance and dependence can occur, and that the drug should be used only when holistic measures (e.g., quiet music, relaxation techniques) don't work.

♦ Emphasize that the effects of alcohol, other sedatives, and tranquilizers may be potentiated and should be avoided.

♦ Reinforce the importance of consulting with physician before using OTC drugs, and of returning for medical follow-up.

♦ Advise avoidance of driving and other potentially hazardous activities while under the effects of the medication.

♦ See Antianxiety Agents, Sedatives, and Hypnotics overview for more information.

teniposide

ten-ip'o-side

teniposide VM-26: ♣**Vumon**

Class: Antineoplastic agent

PEDS	PREG	GERI
♨	D	♨

Action Kills rapidly growing cells (cancer, hair follicles, bone marrow, GI lining, ova, and sperm) by arresting cell mitosis.

Use/Therapeutic goal/Outcome

Hodgkin's and non-Hodgkin's lymphomas; carcinoma of the brain, lung, bladder, and breast; malignant melanoma; myelogenous leukemia: Elimination or suppression of malignant cell proliferation. **Outcome criteria:** Tumor and disease regression or stabilization on radiologic and physical examination; for leukemias, absence of blasts in peripheral blood specimen.

Dose range/Administration

Adult: IV: 50–100 mg/m^2 once or twice a week, for 4–6 weeks; or 40–50 mg/m^2/day for 5 days, repeat every 3–4 weeks.

Clinical alert: This drug should be given only by nurses who are knowledgeable in the comprehensive management of the administration of antineoplastic agents. Doses may vary at physician's discretion. Repeat doses are held until it is ascertained that the patient has recovered sufficiently from toxicities of previous doses. Established protocols/policies for drug preparation, administration, and accidental skin contamination *must be followed closely* (gloves or double gloves are worn when handling drug; if the drug touches the skin, the area is washed immediately with plenty of soap and water). Teniposide is diluted in 100–150 ml saline and infused (*without* a membrane-type filter) over 45–90 min to prevent side effect of hypotension and minimize pain and inflammation. Avoid extravasation. Teniposide may also be instilled in the bladder for treatment of bladder cancer.

Contraindications/Precautions

PREG
D

Contraindicated in hypersensitivity to teniposide.

♨ **Contraindicated for pregnant or nursing mothers. Use with caution for the elderly. Safe use for children has not been established.**

Side effects/Adverse reactions

Hypersensitivity: fever, rash, wheezing, hypotension, anaphylaxis. **Hem:** myelosuppression, leukopenia, thrombocytopenia. **GI:** nausea, vomiting, diarrhea, stomatitis. **Skin:** alopecia, pain, and burning along injection site.

Nursing implications/Documentation

Possible nursing diagnoses: Potential for infection; Potential for injury; Fatigue; Altered oral mucous membrane; Fluid volume deficit; Diarrhea; Altered nutrition: less than body requirements.

◆ *See important Nursing implications in Antineoplastic agents overview on page 72, which apply to all antineoplastics. The interventions that follow are additional and specific to this drug only.*

 ◆ Record baseline blood pressure and then every 30 min during administration; stop infusion and report if blood pressure drops below 90 systolic.

 ◆ Monitor for and report early signs of anaphylaxis (restlessness, tachycardia, difficulty breathing); keep emergency drugs and equipment available.

Patient & family teaching/Home care

Possible nursing diagnoses: Knowledge deficit; Ineffective coping (individual and family); Hopelessness; Impaired home maintenance management.

◆ *See important Patient & family teaching in Antineoplastic agents overview on page 72, which apply to all antineoplastics. The teachings that follow are additional and specific to this drug only.*

 ◆ Stress the need to drink 2–3 L of fluid per day (if the patient can't keep fluids down, IV fluids may be necessary).

◆ *See Antineoplastic agents overview for more information.*

terazosin

te-ra′zoe-sin

Hytrin

Class: Antihypertensive, Alpha adrenergic blocking agent

PEDS	PREG	GERI
🖐	C	🖐

Action Reduces blood pressure by causing vasodilation of arteriolar and venous smooth muscle by blocking of postsynaptic alpha-adrenergic receptors.

Use/Therapeutic goal/Outcome

Hypertension: Reduction of blood pressure. **Outcome criteria:** Blood pressure within acceptable limits.

Dose range/Administration

Interaction alert: Use caution when giving with other antihypertensive agents. When the addition of other antihypertensives is necessary, dosage reduction and titration may be necessary.

Adult: PO: 1 mg at bedtime; increase slowly. *Maintenance dose:* 1–5 mg/day. *Maximum dose:* 20 mg/day in divided doses.

Contraindications/Precautions

PREG
C

Contraindicated in hypersensitivity to terazosin, and in hypotension.

🖐 **Use with caution for the elderly. Safe use for children and pregnant or nursing mothers has not been established.**

Side effects/Adverse reactions

Hypersensitivity: itching, rashes. **CNS:** dizziness, lightheadedness, syncope from orthostatic hypotension, headache, weakness, fatigue, drowsiness, somnolence. **Eye:** blurred vision. **CV:** palpitations, tachycardia, pulmonary edema. **GI:** nausea. **GU:** impotence. **Resp:** nasal congestion. **Misc:** weight gain, fluid retention.

Nursing implications/Documentation

Possible nursing diagnoses: Activity intolerance; Fatigue; Potential for injury.

◆ Assess mental status, and record pulse and blood pressure (lying, sitting, and standing, in both arms) prior to administration, and frequently thereafter until response is determined.

◆ Consult with physician to determine desired therapeutic range for blood pressure (be aware that some patients may require a slightly elevated blood pressure to perfuse vital organs).

◆ Ascertain that baseline CBC, electrolytes, BUN, creatinine, and liver function studies have been obtained before giving first dose; report abnormalities and monitor closely thereafter.

◆ Monitor for allergic reactions, and for confusion, dizziness, arrhythmias, or hypotension;

T

hold drug and report immediately if these occur.

♦ Supervise ambulation until response is determined.

♦ Document and monitor daily weight, and intake and output; report significant negative or positive balance.

Patient & family teaching/Home care
Possible nursing diagnoses: Knowledge deficit; Impaired home maintenance management; Altered sexuality patterns.

♦ Explain the importance of taking medication exactly as prescribed, even when feeling well.

♦ Stress the importance of good medical follow-up, explain that this drug reduces "wear and tear" on blood vessels and improves longevity and health.

♦ Teach how to monitor pulse and blood pressure; emphasize that syncope, hypertension or hypotension, or persistent dizziness should be reported.

♦ Advise changing positions slowly to avoid dizziness.

♦ Encourage daily monitoring of weight and reporting sudden weight gain (frequently is fluid retention).

♦ Warn against taking *any* OTC drugs without physician approval (some interactions can cause severe reactions).

♦ Advise avoiding driving or hazardous activities until response is determined (may cause drowsiness).

♦ Explain that this drug may alter sexual activity; explore concerns.

♦ *See Antihypertensives overview for more information.*

terbutaline
ter-byoo'te-leen

terbutaline sulfate: **Brethaire, Brethine, Bricanyl**
Class: Bronchodilator, Tocolytic, Adrenergic agonist, Sympathomimetic

PEDS	PREG	GERI
♛	B	♛

Action Causes relaxation of vascular smooth muscle, contraction of GI and urinary sphincters, and bronchodilation by stimulating beta-2 receptors.

Use/Therapeutic goal/Outcome
Asthma, bronchitis, emphysema, and reversible airway obstruction: Reduction of airway resistance, improved movement of air. **Outcome criteria:** Decreased wheezing, increased forced expiratory volume (FEV), increased ability to bring forth sputum; report of easier breathing, fewer episodes of wheezing.

Premature labor: Prevention of premature labor. **Outcome criteria:** Absence of uterine contractions.

Dose range/Administration
Interaction alert: Do not use within 14 days of MAOIs (may cause hypertensive crisis). Propranolol may reduce bronchodilating effects. Other sympathomimetics increase effects.

♥ Give with food if GI distress is noted.

Bronchospasm: **Adult/Child >11 yr:** PO: 5 mg tid q6h during waking hours. *Maximum dose:* 15 mg in 24 hr. *Inhalation:* 2 breaths 1-min apart q4-6h. SC: 0.25 mg may repeat once in 15–30 min.

Premature labor: **Adult:** IV: 10–80 mcg/min for up to 4 hr after contractions cease. PO: *Maintenance dose:* 2.5 mg q4-6h until term.

Clinical alert: Give SC injections to the lateral deltoid area. Oral tablets may be crushed.

Contraindications/Precautions
PREG B

Contraindicated in hypersensitivity to sympathomimetics and in coronary artery disease, hypertension, within 14 days of MAOI therapy, and in tachycardia with digitalis toxicity. **Use with caution** in cardiac disease, diabetes, and history of seizures.

✋ **Contraindicated for children under 12 years. Use with caution for older children, pregnant women, and the elderly.**

Side effects/Adverse reactions
Hypersensitivity: exaggeration of side effects. **CV:** tachycardia, hypotension, hypertension, palpitations. **GI:** nausea, vomiting, dry mouth, unusual taste. **CNS:** nervousness, tremor, lightheadedness, fatigue, drowsiness, dizziness, headache, insomnia, seizures, sweating. **MS:** muscle cramps.

Nursing implications/Documentation
Possible nursing diagnoses: Potential for injury; Activity intolerance: Ineffective breathing pattern.

- Record lung sounds, respirations, pulse, and blood pressure before and after dose administration until response is determined.
- Provide favorite fluids and monitor intake and output to ensure adequate hydration (at least 2 L a day is recommended).
- Hold drug and report immediately if paradoxical bronchospasm occurs.

Patient & family teaching/Home care

Possible nursing diagnoses: Knowledge deficit; Fear; Ineffective family coping.

- Explain that this drug will enlarge air passages and make breathing easier.
- Warn that paradoxical bronchospasm can occur (instruct to hold drug and report immediately if this should happen, rather than increase dose).
- Point out that stress and exercise can aggravate wheezing and bronchospasm, and that learning relaxation and controlled breathing techniques can help reduce severity and frequency of episodes of wheezing.
- Give written and verbal instructions on how to use inhalers (shake container, exhale slowly and completely through nose, inhale deeply through mouth while administering aerosol, hold breath for a few seconds, then exhale slowly; allow 1 min between inhalations). Have individual or caregiver demonstrate technique before going home.
- Explain that tolerance may develop with prolonged use, and therefore should only be used when necessary.
- Warn against taking OTC drugs without physician's approval.
- *See Adrenergics (sympathomimetics) overview for more information.*

terfenadine

ter-fen'a-deen

Seldane, ◆Teldane
Class: Antihistamine (H₁ receptor antagonist)

PEDS	PREG	GERI
👋	C	👋

Action Structurally unrelated to other currently available antihistamines. Prevents but does not reverse histamine-mediated allergic responses by competing with histamine for H_1 receptors on effector cells. Terfenadine dissociates slowly from H_1 receptor, providing prolonged action. Produces less drowsiness than other antihista-mines because it does not cross the blood-brain barrier.

Use/Therapeutic goal/Outcome

Allergic conditions: Decrease in allergic response. **Outcome criteria:** Within 1 hr, report and demonstration of an absence of or decrease in allergic symptoms (nasal secretions, sneezing, itching).

Dose range/Administration

🖐 **Give with milk or food to avoid GI upset.**
Adult/Child > 12 yrs: PO: 60 mg q8-12h. **Child 6–12 yrs:** PO: 30–60 mg q12h. **Child 3–5 yrs:** PO: 15 mg q12h.

Clinical alert: For child's dose, tablets must be broken.

Contraindications/Precautions

PREG C

Contraindicated in hypersensitivity to terfenadine. **Use with caution** in asthma or other lower airway disease.

🖐 **Contraindicated for nursing mothers. Use with caution for the elderly. Safe use for pregnant women and for children under 12 years has not been established.**

Side effects/Adverse reactions

Adverse reactions are rare. **Hypersensitivity:** urticaria. **CNS:** drowsiness, headaches, fatigue, dizziness, nervousness, weakness, insomnia. **GI:** increased appetite, GI distress, dry mouth.

Nursing implications/Documentation

Possible nursing diagnoses: Fluid volume deficit.

- Determine and record known allergies; provide an environment that is free from allergens (especially sleeping areas).
- Encourage fluids and monitor for dehydration.

Patient & family teaching/Home care

Possible nursing diagnoses: Knowledge deficit; Impaired home maintenance management.

- Stress that avoiding pollens and staying in an air-conditioned environment may help reduce seasonal rhinitis. Point out that prescribed dose should not be increased; advise reporting worsening symptoms or persistent symptoms.
- Suggest that coffee or tea may reduce drowsiness, and that sugarless gum or hard candy may relieve dry mouth.

♦ Explain that antihistamines should be stopped for 4 days before allergy testing to ensure accurate results.

♦ *See Antihistamines overview for more information.*

terpin hydrate

ter'pin

terpin hydrate
terpin hydrate with codeine
Class: Expectorant, Antitussive

PEDS	PREG	GERI
✋	C	✋

CONTROLLED SUBSTANCE II

Action A volatile oil derivative, terpin hydrate enhances ability to expectorate by directly stimulating respiratory tract secretory glands, which reduces the viscosity and adhesiveness of the secretions. Codeine suppresses the cough reflex, and the combination promotes controlled, productive coughing.

Use/Therapeutic goal/Outcome

Cough: Expectoration, removal of secretions. ***Outcome criteria:*** Patient reports and demonstrates increased ability to bring forth mucus.

Dose range/Administration

🖐 **Give after meals to reduce GI symptoms.**
Terpin hydrate: Adult: PO: 5–10 cc q3-4h prn.
Terpin hydrate with codeine: Adult: PO: 5 cc tid or qid.
Clinical alert: Do not dilute doses. Keep in mind that the elixir is 43% ethanol (86 proof), and that codeine is a narcotic.

Contraindications/Precautions

PREG C

Contraindicated in hypersensitivity to terpin hydrate or (for terpin hydrate with codeine) to codeine, and in peptic ulcer, severe diabetes mellitus, history of drug abuse, and in recovering alcoholics.
🖐 **Contraindicated for children under 12 years. Use with caution for the elderly. Use for pregnant or nursing mothers has not been established, and is not recommended.**

Side effects/Adverse reactions

Hypersensitivity: rash. ***GI:*** nausea, vomiting, epigastric pain.
♦ *See codeine for its side effects.*

Nursing implications/Documentation

Possible nursing diagnoses: Ineffective airway clearance; Fluid volume deficit.

♦ Document lung sounds and sputum production to monitor for effectiveness; report cough that lasts longer than a week.
♦ Provide preferred fluids to promote hydration.

Patient & family teaching/Home care

Possible nursing diagnoses: Knowledge deficit; Impaired home maintenance management.

♦ Advise reporting rash or increase in breathing problems; may indicate a need to stop this drug.
♦ Stress the importance of adequate hydration; advise taking doses with a full glass of water.
♦ Point out that increased environmental humidity with decreased environmental irritants (e.g., smoke) can minimize aggravating factors.
♦ Advise reporting a cough that persists longer than a week.
♦ Warn that this drug has a high alcohol content and should be taken in very small doses only, and that terpin hydrate with codeine has a potential for dependence and abuse.
♦ *See Antitussives, Expectorants, and Mucolytics overview for more information.*

testolactone

tess-toe-lak'tone

Teslac
Class: Antineoplastic agent, Hormone

PEDS	PREG	GERI
✋	C	✋

Action Inhibits malignant cellular growth by altering the tumor's hormonal environment (inhibits the synthesis of estrone).

Use/Therapeutic goal/Outcome

Advanced, disseminated breast cancer in postmenopausal women and in women who have had their ovaries removed: Suppression of malignant cell proliferation. ***Outcome criteria:*** Tumor and disease regression or stabilization on radiologic and physical examination.

Dose range/Administration

Interaction alert: May increase the effect of oral anticoagulants.
Adult: PO: 250 mg qid for at least 3 months.

Clinical alert: Hold dose and report if early signs of hypercalcemia (insomnia, lethargy, nausea, vomiting, vascular collapse) are noted.

Contraindications/Precautions

PREG
C

Contraindicated in hypersensitivity to testolactone in premenopausal women with intact ovaries, and in male breast cancer. **Use with caution** in impaired liver function, hypercalcemia, cardiac decompensation, nephritis, or nephrosis.

✋ **Contraindicated for children and pregnant or nursing mothers. Use with caution for the elderly.**

Side effects/Adverse reactions

Hypersensitivity: rash. **GI:** anorexia, nausea, vomiting; glossitis; diarrhea. **CNS:** paresthesia in fingers, toes, and face. **CV:** hypertension, peripheral edema. **Hem:** hypercalcemia. **Skin:** maculopapular erythema, alopecia, facial hair growth.

Nursing implications/Documentation

Possible nursing diagnoses: Fluid volume deficit; Self-esteem disturbance; Potential for injury; Altered nutrition: less than body requirements.

◆ *See important Nursing implications in Antineoplastic agents overview.*

♦ Increase fluid to 2 L per day, unless contraindicated, to aid in calcium excretion.

♦ Check blood pressure daily or every visit; report diastolic increase greater than 20 mm Hg.

Patient & family teaching/Home care

Possible nursing diagnoses: Impaired home maintenance management; Knowledge deficit.

◆ *See important Patient & family teaching in Antineoplastic agents overview.*

♦ Explain that it may take up to 3 months to see results from therapy.

♦ Point out the need to drink at least 2 L a day.

♦ Stress the need to report signs of hypercalcemia (insomnia, lethargy, nausea, vomiting).

♦ Teach that exercising daily may help reduce hypercalcemia.

◆ *See Antineoplastic agents overview for more information.*

testosterone

tess-toss'ter-ohne

Andro, Andronaq, Histerone, Malogen Testaqua, Testoject

testosterone cypionate: **Andro-Cyp, Andronaq-LA, Andronate, depAndro, Depotest, Depo-Testosterone, Duratest, T-Cypionate, Tesionate, Testa-C, Testaject-LA, Testred Cypionate, Virilon IM**

testosterone enanthate: **Android-T, Andro-LA, Andryl, Delatestryl, Durathate, Everone, ✦Malogex, Testone LA, Testrin PA**

testosterone propionate: **✦Malogen, Testex**

Class: Androgen, Antineoplastic agent

PEDS	PREG	GERI
✋	X	✋

Action Stimulates development and maintenance of male sex organs; induces development of male secondary sex characteristics; stimulates sperm production; increases body size by stimulating growth of skeletal muscles.

Use/Therapeutic goal/Outcome

Androgen deficiency and hypogonadism: Correction of deficiency. **Outcome criteria:** Absence or improvement of deficiency symptoms (delayed development of male secondary sex characteristics, impotence, or male climacteric).

Breast cancer: Palliation of inoperable metastatic disease for women 1–5 years postmenopause; suppression of hormone-responsive tumors. **Outcome criteria:** Evidence of decreased metastatic and tumor activity; decreased bone pain.

Dose range/Administration

Interaction alert: Increases effect of insulin, oral hypoglycemics, and anticoagulants. Corticosteroids increase possibility of edema and severe acne. Avoid other hepatotoxic medications.

◆ **testosterone, t. propionate:**

Androgen deficiency: Adult: IM: 25–50 mg 2–3 times a wk. **Child:** IM: 12.5–25 mg 2–3 times per week for 4–6 mos.

Antineoplastic: Adult: IM: 50–100 mg 3 times per week.

◆ **t. cypionate, t. enanthate:**

Androgen deficiency: Adult: IM: 50–400 mg q2-4 wks. **Child:** IM: 25–200 mg q2-4 wks.

Antineoplastic: Adult: IM: 200–400 mg q2-4 wks.

T

Clinical alert: Crystals in parenteral solution may be redissolved by warming and shaking vial; a wet needle or syringe may cause harmless clouding of solution. For oil-based suspensions, warm container and shake well to mix medication.

Contraindications/Precautions

Contraindicated in hypersensitivity to androgens, and in severe renal, hepatic, or cardiac disease, hypercalcemia, breast or prostatic cancer in men, and genital bleeding. *Use with caution* in diabetes mellitus, prostatic hypertrophy, gynecomastia, history of MI, and cardiac failure.

☙ **Contraindicated for pregnant or nursing mothers. Use with caution for children and elderly men.**

Side effects/Adverse reactions

Hypersensitivity: rashes and anaphylaxis. *GU:* virilism of females (enlarged clitoris, deepening of voice, menstrual irregularities, unnatural hair growth or loss); virilism of prepubertal males (acne, enlarging penis, increased frequency of erections, unnatural hair growth); in older men, bladder irritability, breast soreness, gynecomastia, priapism, prostatic hypertrophy, prostatic carcinoma, epididymitis, increased libido. *Hem:* polycythemia, hypercalcemia, decreased high-density lipoproteins, and increased low-density lipoproteins. *GI:* hepatic dysfunction, carcinoma, or necrosis. *MS:* premature epiphyseal closure in children. *Skin:* edema, unexplained darkening, acne, pain or swelling at injection site.

Nursing implications/Documentation

Possible nursing diagnoses: Impaired tissue integrity; Body image disturbance.

◆ Administer IM injections deep in gluteal muscle and rotate sites; assess site and record presence of inflammation.

◆ Monitor serum calcium levels; assess, report, and document symptoms of hypercalcemia (vomiting, constipation, polyuria, lethargy and muscle weakness).

◆ For elderly men, monitor for difficult or frequent urination.

◆ Record baseline blood pressure and weight.

◆ Assess for and report decreased urine output, edema, increased blood pressure, weight gain, and congestive failure.

◆ Monitor electrolyte and cholesterol levels and liver function tests.

◆ For diabetics, monitor glucose levels and assess for symptoms of hypoglycemia.

Patient & family teaching/Home care

Possible nursing diagnoses: Knowledge deficit; Impaired home maintenance management; Sexual dysfunction.

◆ Advise restricting sodium intake to decrease edema.

◆ Caution women of child-bearing age to use reliable birth control and to stop drug and report any suspicion of pregnancy.

◆ For women, stress the importance of reporting the occurrence of masculinizing effects (abnormal growth of facial hair, deepening of voice, menstrual irregularities, enlarged clitoris).

◆ For men, advise reporting development of priapism, gynecomastia, or bladder irritability.

◆ For diabetics, caution about possible lowering of blood sugar and need for adjustment of doses of insulin or oral antidiabetic agents.

◆ Inform parents of prepubertal children that X rays will be taken periodically to determine effect on bone growth.

◆ Caution to maintain close medical supervision for early detection of adverse reactions.

◆ Warn that using high doses of androgens for improvement of athletic performance may result in serious side effects that outweigh any advantages.

tetanus toxoid
tet'an-us

tetanus toxoid (adsorbed)
tetanus toxoid (fluid)
Class: Toxoid, Immunizing agent

PEDS	PREG	GERI
☙	C	OK

Action Promotes active immunity to tetanus by inducing protective antitoxin formation. Adsorbed form produces antitoxin titers for a longer period of time. Fluid form produces quicker effects as a booster in patients with previous active immunity.

Use/Therapeutic goal/Outcome

Primary immunization against tetanus in adults and children over 6 weeks: Promotion of immunity, prevention of tetanus. *Outcome criteria:* Absence of clinical symptoms and a documented course of tetanus toxoid immunization (laboratory antitoxin titers can demonstrate immunity, but this rarely done).

Dose range/Administration

Interaction alert: Chloramphenicol may interfere with response to tetanus toxoid.

Adult and Child: SC, IM: *Adsorbed toxoid:* 0.5 ml, followed by a second dose in 4–6 wks, then a third dose in 12 mos. *Fluid toxoid:* 0.5 ml q 4–8 wks, 3 doses followed by a fourth dose in 12 mos. *Booster:* 0.5 ml q 10 yr.

Clinical alert: Shake vigorously before withdrawing dose to ensure homogeneous suspension of antigen. Do not give if resuspension does not occur. Keep epinephrine available in case of anaphylaxis.

Contraindications/Precautions

PREG
C

Contraindicated in hypersensitivity to tetanus toxoid, in immunosuppression, immunoglobulin abnormalities, and active infections (excluding upper respiratory infections), except in an emergency.

🖐 **Contraindicated for infants under 6 weeks. Use with caution for older children (especially in history of febrile seizures, cerebral damage, or neurologic disorders) and pregnant or nursing mothers.**

Side effects/Adverse reactions

Hypersensitivity: itching, rashes, hives, fever, tachycardia, hypotension, anaphylaxis. *Skin:* pain, redness, swelling at injection site. *Misc:* flushing, chills, malaise, aches, and pains.

Nursing implications/Documentation

Possible nursing diagnosis: Potential for infection.

♦ Record date of last tetanus immunization and history of adverse reactions to immunization; if date of last immunization unknown, then the patient is considered to have had no previous immunization.

♦ Monitor for immediate reaction (anaphylaxis) after administration.

Patient & family teaching/Home care

Possible nursing diagnoses: Knowledge deficit; Altered health maintenance; Fear.

♦ Encourage asking questions and verbalizing fears and concerns; explain that there is no risk of developing tetanus from the vaccine.

♦ Recommend keeping personal record of date of immunizations. Advise that pain, redness, swelling, and tenderness at injection site may persist for 24–48 hours; caution not to apply cold or heat to site (may make it worse).

♦ For first-time administration, stress the need to return for follow-up doses.

♦ Point out that immunity lasts 10 years and that a booster is required every 10 years.

♦ Explain that transient fever and malaise may be noted for 2 days; fevers over 101°F, especially in young children, should be reported immediately.

tetracaine

tet'ra-kane

tetracaine hydrochloride: *Pontocaine*
Class: Local anesthetic (ester-type)

PEDS	PREG	GERI
🖐	C	🖐

Action Produces local anesthesia by inhibiting sodium flux across the nerve cell membrane, thus preventing depolarization and generation and conduction of nerve impulses. Tetracaine begins to act in 15 min, may last up to 3 hr, and has high potency and toxicity.

Use/Therapeutic goal/Outcome

Spinal anesthesia: Prevention of pain during surgical procedures. *Outcome criteria:* Patient report of numbness and absence of pain in anesthetized area; temporary loss of motor function in the anesthetized area.

Dose range/Administration

Adult: *Low spinal block (saddle block during vaginal delivery):* 2–5 mg in D10W solution as a hyperbaric (heavier than CSF) solution.

Clinical alert: This drug should be administered only by clinicians thoroughly familiar with its use. Dose is highly individualized, depending on the procedure, method of administration, area to be anesthetized, vascularity of tissues, patient condition, tolerance, and response. Keep resuscitative drugs and equipment readily available.

Contraindications/Precautions

PREG
C

Contraindicated in hypersensitivity to tetracaine, other ester-type anesthetics, or to PABA and derivatives, and for the debilitated. *Use with caution* in shock, cachexia, and cardiac decompensation.

T

☙ Contraindicated for the elderly. Use with caution for nursing mothers. Safe use for children and pregnant women has not been established.

Side effects/Adverse reactions

Hypersensitivity: anaphylaxis, convulsions, rashes, hives, itching, sneezing, syncope, hypotension, edema. *CNS:* postspinal headache, spinal nerve paralysis, anxiety, seizures, tremors. *Resp:* respiratory arrest. *CV:* vasodilatation, hypotension, myocardial depression, arrhythmias, hypertension, cardiac arrest. *GI:* nausea, vomiting. *Eye:* blurred vision. *Ear:* tinnitus.

Nursing implications/Documentation

Possible nursing diagnoses: Pain; Potential for injury.

♦ Be sure that history of allergies and accurate height and weight are recorded before procedure.

♦ Record vital signs according to protocol, and monitor for and report immediately signs of systemic or hypersensitivity reactions.

♦ Determine from anesthesiologist or anesthetist whether there are any restrictions on patient positioning; post these at bedside.

♦ Monitor anesthetized area for level of sensation and motor function; watch for poor positioning and protect area from injury.

♦ Encourage movement of legs as soon as motor function returns.

♦ Give prescribed pain medication as sensation begins to return, **before pain is too severe**.

Patient & family teaching/Home care

Possible nursing diagnoses: Anxiety; Fear.

♦ Stress the need to protect areas of the body that have lost sensation.

♦ Explain rationale for taking prescribed pain medication before pain becomes too uncomfortable.

♦ *See Local anesthetics overview for more information.*

tetracycline

te-tra-sye′kleen

tetracycline: *Achromycin Opthalmic*

tetracycline hydrochloride: *Achromycin V, ✦Apo-Tetra, ◢Austramycin V, Bristacycline, Cyclopar, ◢Hostacycline P, Kesso-Tetra, Nor-Tet, Novotetra, Panmycin, ◢Panmycin P, Robitet, Sarocycline, Sumycin, Tetracap, Tetracyn, Tetralan, ♣Tetralean, Topicycline*

Class: ★Anti-infective (broad-spectrum tetracycline) prototype, Antibiotic

PEDS	PREG	GERI
☙	D	☙

Action Limits bacterial growth (bateriostatic) by binding to the 30S ribosomal subunit and inhibiting protein synthesis.

Use/Therapeutic goal/Outcome

Infections (acne, gonorrhea, syphilis, and infections caused by susceptible gram-negative and gram-positive pathogens, trachoma, rickettsia, mycoplasma, and chlamydia): Prevention or resolution of infection. *Outcome criteria:* Absence of pathogenic growth on cultures, absence of clinical manifestations of infection (fever, pain, swelling, redness, heat, odor, drainage, productive cough, dysuria, frequency), normal WBC count, normal X rays.

Malignant pleural effusion (sclerosing agent): Prevention or resolution of effusion. *Outcome criteria:* Absence of pleural effusion on X ray.

Eye infections: Prevention/resolution of infection. *Outcome criteria:* Absence of pain, redness, tearing.

Acne: Resolution of acne. *Outcome criteria:* Absence of or reduction in pimples.

Dose range/Administration

Interaction alert: Do not mix any other drug with IV tetracycline. To prevent decreased antibiotic absorption, give 1 hour before or 2 hours after food, milk or dairy products, antacids (including sodium bicarbonate), or laxatives containing aluminum, magnesium, or calcium. Give 2 hours before or 3 hours after iron products. Methoxyflurane increases risk of nephrotoxicity; avoid use. May decrease effectiveness of oral contraceptives or penicillins.

▯ **Give with a full glass of water 1 hour before or 2 hours after meals.**

Infections caused by sensitive gram-negative and gram-positive pathogens, trachoma, rickettsia, mycoplasma, and chlamydia: Adult: PO: 250–

500 mg q6h. IM: 250 mg/day; or 150 mg q12h. IV: 250–500 mg q8-12h. *Child > 8 yrs:* PO: 25–50 mg/kg/day in divided doses q6h. IM: 15–25 mg/kg/day in a single dose or in divided doses q8h or q12h. *Maximum dose:* 250 mg. IV: 10–20 mg/kg/day in divided doses q12h.

Uncomplicated endocervical, urethral, or rectal infections: Adult: PO: 500 mg qid for at least 7 days.

Brucellosis: Adult: PO: 500 mg q6h for 3 wks (concurrent with streptomycin 1 g IM q12h in wk 1, then qd in wk 2).

Gonorrhea: Adult: PO: 1.5 g initially, then 500 mg q6h for 7 days.

Syphilis: Adult: PO: 2–3 g/day in divided doses for 10–15 days. *Duration > 1 yr:* Treat for 30 days.

Eye infections: Adult and Child: Ophthalmic: Instill 2 drops bid to qid.

Trachoma: Adult and Child: Ophthalmic: Instill 2 drops or ointment bid to qid for 30 days.

Ophthalmia neonatorum prophylaxis: Neonate: 1–2 drops in each eye shortly after delivery.

Acne: Adult: PO: *Initial dose:* 250 mg q6h. *Maintenance dose:* 125–500 mg qod. *Topical:* Apply generously to affected areas bid.

Clinical alert: Protect IV tetracycline from light and monitor closely for thrombophlebitis or extravasation (tetracycline is very irritating to tissues). IM tetracycline contains 40 mg procaine HCl per vial; check for allergy to local anesthetics before giving. Taking outdated tetracyclines has caused fatal nephrotoxicity.

Contraindications/Precautions

PREG
D

Contraindicated in allergy to tetracyclines, in common bile duct obstruction, and significant kidney or liver impairment. *Use with caution* in history of multiple allergies and in impaired renal or liver function.

✋ **Contraindicated for children under 8 years (causes tooth discoloration and retards bone growth) and pregnant or nursing mothers. Use with caution for the elderly or debilitated.**

Side effects/Adverse reactions

Hypersensitivity: (rare) itching, rashes, fever, anaphylaxis. *GI:* sore throat, glossitis, stomatitis, epigastric discomfort, nausea, vomiting, cramps, diarrhea, enterocolitis, anogenital inflammation, hepatotoxicity with large IV doses. *Skin:* photosensitivity. *CNS:* dizziness, lightheadedness, headache, intracranial hyper-

tension. *CV:* pericarditis. *Hem:* blood dyscrasias; thrombophlebitis (with IV route).

Nursing implications/Documentation

Possible nursing diagnoses: Potential for infection; Potential fluid volume deficit.

◆ Determine history of allergies, and (regardless of history) monitor closely for allergic reactions.

◆ Weigh patient and obtain baseline serum sodium, CBC, BUN, creatinine, liver function studies, and necessary culture specimens before administering first dose; monitor closely thereafter if therapy is prolonged.

◆ Encourage fluids, and record and monitor intake and output, to ensure adequate hydration and urine output.

◆ Monitor for and report symptoms of superinfection (mouth lesions, thrush, vaginal irritation, diarrhea, respiratory symptoms).

◆ If there is no improvement within 3–5 days, consult with physician to determine if antibiotic regimen should be re-evaluated (and new cultures drawn).

Patient & family teaching/Home care

Possible nursing diagnoses: Knowledge deficit, Impaired home maintenance management.

◆ Emphasize the importance of avoiding iron-containing products, and of taking tetracycline 1 hour before or 2 hours after milk or food to enhance drug absorption.

◆ Advise avoiding exposure to sunlight; warn that photosensitivity may continue for weeks after tetracycline has been discontinued.

◆ Teach the need to report persistent or new signs and symptoms of illness (e.g., fever, mouth lesions, vaginal irritation, respiratory symptoms, diarrhea) medication change may be necessary.

◆ Explain the importance of taking antibiotics for the entire time prescribed, even if symptoms abate.

◆ Caution women that this drug may reduce effectiveness of oral contraceptives.

◆ *See Anti-infectives overview for more information.*

theophylline

thee-off'i-lin

Immediate-release tablet and capsule: *Bronkodyl, Elixophyllin, ♠Nuelin, Slo-Phyllin, Somophyllin-T.*

Immediate-release liquid: *Accurbron, Aerolate, Aquaphyllin, Asmalix, Bronkodyl, Elixcon, Elixomin, Elixophyllin, Lanophyllin, Lixolin, Slo-Phyllin, Theolair, Theon, Theophyl.*

Timed-release capsule: *Aerolate, Bronkodyl S-R, Elixophyllin SR, Lodrane, ♠Nuelin-SR, Slo-bid Gyrocaps, Slo-Phyllin, Somophyllin-CRT, Theo-24, Theobid Durocaps, Theobid Jr., Theochron, Theo-Dur Sprinkle, Theophyl-SR, Theospan SR, Theovent Long Acting.*

Timed-release tablet: *Constant-T, Duraphyl, Quibron-T/SR, Respbid, Sustaire, Theo-Dur, Theolair-SR, Theo-Time, Uniphyl.*

theophylline sodium glycinate: *♣Acet-Am, Synophyllate*

Class: ★**Antiasthmatic prototype,** Smooth muscle relaxant, Bronchodilator, CNS stimulant, Respiratory stimulant, Xanthine

PEDS	PREG	GERI
🖐	C	🖐

Action Causes bronchial smooth muscle relaxation and bronchodilation by increasing tissue concentration of AMP. Also causes cardiac and CNS stimulation, diuresis, and increased gastric secretions.

Use/Therapeutic goal/Outcome

Bronchospasm associated with asthma, bronchitis, and COPD: Reduction in bronchiole obstruction with improved movement of air. ***Outcome criteria:*** Clearing of lung fields upon auscultation; forced expiratory volume (FEV) improved by 8%; patient reports breathing easier and having fewer wheezing episodes.

Apnea and bradycardia in premature infants (unlabeled use): Stimulation of respirations. ***Outcome criteria:*** Absence of episodes of apnea and bradycardia; respiratory and cardiac rate within normal limits.

Dose range/Administration

Interaction alert: Sympathomimetics may increase CNS and cardiovascular side effects. Erythromycin, beta-blockers, cimetidine, and large doses of allopurinol decrease theophylline metabolism (monitor for toxicity). Phenobarbital, phenytoin, rifampin, and carbamazepine increase theophylline metabolism (may need higher doses). Smoking diminishes effect.

🖐 Give on an empty stomach with a full glass of water, unless GI symptoms are experienced (then may give with food or antacids—absorption may be slower).

Theophylline: Adult: PO: *Loading dose:* 6 mg/kg, followed by 2–3 mg/kg q4h for 2 doses. *Maintenance dose:* Use 1–3 mg/kg q6h. ***Child 9–16 yrs:*** PO: *Loading dose:* 6 mg/kg, followed by 3 mg/kg q4h for 3 doses. *Maintenance dose:* Use 3 mg/kg q6h. ***Child 6 mos–9 yrs:*** PO: *Loading dose:* 4 mg/kg q4h for 3 doses. *Maintenance dose:* Use 4 mg/kg q6h.

Theophylline sodium glycinate: Adult: PO: 330–660 mg q6-8h. ***Child > 12 yrs:*** PO: 220–330 mg q6-8h. ***Child 6–12 yrs:*** PO: Use 330 mg q6-8h. ***Child 3–6 yrs:*** PO: Use 110–165 mg q6-8h. ***Child 1–3 yrs:*** PO: Use 55–110 mg q6-8h.

Clinical alert: Doses are highly individualized because theophylline is metabolized at varying rates. Children may need relatively high doses because of high clearance rate. Periodic theophylline levels should be obtained; therapeutic levels are between 10 and 20 mcg/ml (hold dose and report if level is more than 20 mcg/ml). Be aware that physician may order higher or more frequent loading doses, followed by lower or less frequent maintenance doses. Do not crush enteric-coated or sustained release form. Check with pharmacist for availability of sprinkle form of drug (may be sprinkled on food when there is difficulty swallowing pills).

Contraindications/Precautions

PREG
C

Contraindicated in hypersensitivity to the drug or to xanthine compounds (caffeine, theobromine), and in seizure disorders, and active peptic ulcer disease. ***Use with caution*** in CHF, cor pulmonale, liver, kidney or cardiac disease, history of ulcers or diabetes mellitus.

🖐 Contraindicated for nursing mothers. Use with caution for children and the elderly. Safe use during pregnancy has not been established.

Side effects/Adverse reactions

Hypersensitivity: itching, rash, angioedema. ***GI:*** anorexia, nausea, vomiting, indigestion, cramping, bitter taste in mouth, diarrhea. ***CV:*** flushing, palpitations, hypotension, ventricular arrythmias, circulatory collapse; with IV route: pain, redness, swelling, thrombophlebitis at injection site. ***Resp:*** increase in respiratory rate. ***CNS:*** headache, irritability, restlessness, nervousness, insomnia, dizziness, seizures, hyperexcitability.

Nursing implications/Documentation

Possible nursing diagnoses: Ineffective airway clearance; Potential for injury; Activity intolerance.

♦ During acute illness, record lung sounds and vital signs immediately before and 30 min after administration (a sudden, unexplained, sharp increase in pulse rate may indicate onset of toxicity; additional signs of toxicity include anorexia, nausea, vomiting, restlessness, tachycardia, seizures. Hold drug and report if these occur.

♦ Schedule doses around the clock; give single dose long-acting preparation upon arising in the morning.

♦ Monitor closely for tachycardia and ventricular arrythmias; hold drug and report if these are significant.

♦ Pace activity to allow for rest periods.

♦ Be aware that smokers are likely to need higher doses, because of increased elimination of theophylline.

♦ Monitor serum theophylline levels; report levels outside therapeutic range.

♦ Observe for potential for injury related to restlessness and dizziness, and take appropriate precautions.

Patient & family teaching/Home care

Possible nursing diagnoses: Knowledge deficit; Impaired home maintenance management; Fear.

♦ Explain that this drug helps reduce wheezing and makes breathing easier.

♦ If GI symptoms are experienced, advise taking theophylline after meals.

♦ Reinforce the importance of taking doses exactly as prescribed, without missing or "doubling up" doses (if a dose is skipped, it should be taken as soon as possible).

♦ Stress that a different brand should not be substituted without physician approval.

♦ Explore factors that cause asthma attacks (environmental, emotional), and teach holistic measures for reducing stress and coping with wheezing.

♦ Instruct the patient to report palpitations or increased dyspnea.

♦ Emphasize the need for medical follow-up; point out that the physician should be notified if usual dose fails to alleviate or prevent symptoms.

♦ Warn against taking OTC drugs without checking with physician, because there is a risk of drug interaction; advise to avoid caffeine.

♦ *See Bronchodilators overview for more information.*

thiabendazole
thye-a-ben'da-zole

Mintezol

Class: Anti-infective, Anthelmintic, Antibiotic

PEDS ✋ **PREG** C **GERI** OK

Action Vermicidal, kills helminths (intestinal worms) in an infected host by inhibiting their ability to produce enzymes necessary for life.

Use/Therapeutic goal/Outcome

Pinworm, roundworm, threadworm, whipworm, cutaneous larva migrans (creeping eruption), and trichinosis: Elimination of intestinal helminths. **Outcome criteria:** Expulsion of worms followed by 3 negative stool samples after completion of treatment.

Dose range/Administration

👆 **Give after meals to reduce incidence of GI distress.**

Adult/Child > 15 kg: PO: 25 mg/kg/day divided bid pc for 2–5 days. *Maximum dose:* 3 g/day.

Clinical alert: Have the person chew *tablets* before swallowing. Shake *suspension* before measuring.

Contraindications/Precautions
PREG C

Contraindicated in hypersensitivity to thiabendazole. **Use with caution** in malnutrition, dehydration (rehydrate first), impaired liver or kidney function, or anemia.

🖐 **Use with caution for children under 15 kg. Safe use for pregnant or nursing mothers has not been established.**

Side effects/Adverse reactions

Hypersensitivity: rashes, lymphadenophy. **GI:** epigastric distress, abdominal discomfort or cramping, diarrhea, anorexia, nausea, vomiting. **CNS:** impaired physical alertness or coordination, drowsiness, giddiness, hallucinations, headache, dizziness, seizures, numbness of hands and feet. *GU:* unusual urine odor (asparagus). *Misc:* flushing, chills, fever.

Nursing implications/Documentation

Possible nursing diagnoses: Potential for infection; Diarrhea.

◆ Observe stools for expulsion of worms (stool specimens should be sent to the lab while still warm).

◆ Determine close contacts (family/significant others), who should be evaluated for treatment as well.

Patient & family teaching/Home care

Possible nursing diagnoses: Knowledge deficit; Impaired home maintenance management; Situational low self-esteem.

◆ Explore feelings and concerns, and explain that intestinal worms are not associated with "dirtiness".

◆ Stress the need to continue taking drug for full course of treatment.

◆ Emphasize the importance of preventing reinfection or spread of infection by treating all family members and close contacts, taking the medication exactly as prescribed, washing foods especially carefully, meticulously washing hands after bowel movements, cutting nails short, changing clothing every day, keeping fingers out of mouth, having infected individuals sleep alone, eliminating ova by washing all linens daily in hot water (without shaking them), vacuuming and damp-mopping the house daily, cleaning the toilet with disinfectant daily.

◆ Caution that driving, or activities that require alertness, should be avoided until response is established (may cause drowsiness and dizziness).

◆ *See Anti-infectives overview for more information.*

thiamine

thye'-a-min

thiamine hydrochloride: *Apatate Drops, Betalin S, ♣Betamin, ♣Beta-Sol, Biamine, Thia*

Class: Vitamin B1, Water-soluble vitamin

PEDS	PREG	GERI
OK	☙	**OK**

Action Forms a coenzyme necessary for carbohydrate metabolism.

Use/Therapeutic goal/Outcome

Thiamine deficiency, beriberi, Wernicke's encephalopathy: Provides adequate blood levels of thiamine. *Outcome criteria:* Absence or improvement in deficiency symptoms (nausea and vomiting, anorexia, parathesias, tachycardia, disorientation, memory loss, depression, insomnia).

Dose range/Administration

Interaction alert: Alcohol inhibits absorption of thiamine.

🖐 **Give with food to increase absorption.**

Adult: PO: 5–40 mg/day. IM, IV: 5–100 mg tid.
Child: PO: 10–50 mg/day. IM/IV: 10–25 mg/day.

Clinical alert: Parenteral route is used only when oral administration is not possible or acceptable.

Contraindications/Precautions

PREG
☙

Contraindicated in known hypersensitivity to thiamine.

☙ **May be used safely in recommended daily allowances (RDA) for pregnant women (preg A); safe use in doses greater than RDA has not been determined (preg C).**

Side effects/Adverse reactions

Hypersensitivity: rash, itching, wheezing, anaphylaxis with large IV dose. *CV:* pulmonary edema, hypotension after rapid IV administration. *Skin:* tenderness and induration at IM site. *Misc:* feeling of warmth.

Nursing implications/Documentation

Possible nursing diagnoses: Impaired tissue integrity; Pain.

◆ With suspected sensitivity, skin test patient prior to administration.

◆ For IM injection, rotate sites to minimize pain and inflammation; apply cold compresses to decrease pain.

Patient & family teaching/Home care

Possible nursing diagnoses: Knowledge deficit; Impaired home maintenance management.

◆ Teach best dietary sources of thiamine (whole-grain and enriched cereals, meats).

◆ Advise against self-prescribed megadoses of thiamine.

◆ Caution that alcohol may decrease effectiveness of thiamine.

thioguanine

thye-oh-gwah'-neen

6-thioguanine, 6–T6: ♣*Lanvis*

Class: Antineoplastic (antimetabolite) agent

PEDS	PREG	GERI
♨	**D**	♨

Action Kills rapidly growing cells (cancer, hair follicles, bone marrow, GI lining, ova, and sperm) by inhibiting DNA and RNA synthesis and enzyme reactions (purine antagonist). Is cell-cycle specific in the S-phase.

Use/Therapeutic goal/Outcome

Nonlymphocytic leukemias (combination therapy), multiple myeloma, solid tumors, and chronic myelogenous leukemia: Elimination or suppression of malignant cell proliferation. *Outcome criteria:* Tumor and disease regression or stabilization on radiologic and physical examination for leukemias, absence of blasts in peripheral blood specimen.

Dose range/Administration

Interaction alert: Use with radiation therapy or other cytotoxic agents can cause severe myelosuppression.

▯ **Give on an empty stomach for best absorption and least toxicity.**

Adult and Child: PO: 2 mg/kg/day (compute dose to closest 20 mg); may increase to 3 mg/kg if no response or toxicity occurs. *Maintenance dose:* 2 mg/kg/day.

Clinical alert: Hold dose and report if platelets <100,000/mm^3 or WBC < 4000/mm^3.

Contraindications/Precautions

PREG **D**

Contraindicated in hypersensitivity to thioguanine or prior drug resistance. *Use with caution* in renal and hepatic impairment, bone marrow depression, infection, and recent radiation.

♨ **Contraindicated for pregnant or nursing mothers. Use with caution for children and the elderly.**

Side effects/Adverse reactions

Hypersensitivity: rash, urticaria, tachycardia. *Hem:* leukopenia, anemia, thrombocytopenia (usually in 2–4 weeks). *GI:* hyperuricemia, anorexia, nausea, vomiting, and diarrhea; stomatitis, hepatotoxicity, and jaundice. *GU:* oliguria, renal failure. *Skin:* dry skin.

Nursing implications/Documentation

Possible nursing diagnoses: Potential for infection; Potential for injury; Fatigue; Altered oral mucous membrane; Fluid volume deficit; Diarrhea; Altered nutrition: less than body requirements.

♦ *See important Nursing implications in Antineoplastic agents overview on page 72, which apply to all antineoplastics. The interventions that follow are additional and specific to this drug only.*

   ♦ Monitor CBC daily during induction, then weekly during maintenance therapy.

   ♦ Report abnormal lab studies immediately (early recognition of side effects is essential for successful treatment).

Patient & family teaching/Home care

Possible nursing diagnoses: Knowledge deficit; Ineffective family coping; Hopelessness; Impaired home maintenance management.

♦ *See important Patient & family teaching in Antineoplastic agents overview on page 72, which apply to all antineoplastics. The teachings that follow are additional and specific to this drug only.*

   ♦ Stress the need to drink 2–3 L a day to prevent kidney complications.

♦ *See Antineoplastic agents overview for more information.*

thioridazine

thye-or-id'a-zeen

thioridazine hydrochloride: ♠*Aldazine,* ♣*Apo-Thioridazine, Mellaril, Mellaril-S,* ♣*Novoridazine,* ♣*PMS Thioridazine*

Class: Phenothiazine antipsychotic

PEDS	PREG	GERI
♨	**C**	♨

Action Exact mechanism of action has not been determined. Believed to produce calmness and alleviate psychiatric symptoms (disorders of perception, thought, consciousness, mood, affect, and social interaction) by blocking dopamine receptors in the limbic system. Blocks peripheral muscarinic, adrenergic, and histamine receptors. Also has some effect on the hypothalamus and pituitary gland, causing changes in regulation of body temperature and endocrine function. A dose of 100 mg of thioridazine is therapeutically equivalent to 100 mg of chlorpromazine.

T

Use/Therapeutic goal/Outcome

Schizophrenia, psychosis, agitation: Promotion of reality orientation, reduction in agitation. *Outcome criteria:* Demonstration of reality orientation, and ability to problem solve and interact with others, with decrease in signs of agitation (pacing, hyperactivity).

Depressive neuroses and senile dementia: Elimination of symptoms associated with depression (anxiety, insomnia, fearfulness) promotion of sense of well-being. *Outcome criteria:* Report of having less anxiety, fearfulness and difficulty sleeping; demonstration of improved ability to interact with others and cope with daily activities.

Severe behavioral problems in children: Control of combative, hyperactive, explosive behavior. *Outcome criteria:* Absence of combative, hyperactive, explosive behavior.

Dose range/Administration

Interaction alert: Antacids may reduce absorption; separate doses of antacid and thioridazine by at least 2 hours. Alcohol and other CNS depressants may cause excessive sedation. May reduce effects of centrally acting antihypertensives. Barbiturates and lithium may decrease effects.

Psychoses: *Adult:* PO: 50–100 mg tid, gradually increasing to a maximum of 800 mg/day until response is established. *Maintenance dose:* 200–800 mg/day in divided doses. *For the elderly:* Initial dose of 25 mg tid. *Child 2–12 yrs:* PO: 0.5 to 3 mg/kg/day in divided doses.

Depressive neuroses and senile dementia: *Adult:* PO: 25 mg tid. Increase dose as needed, up to 200 mg/day. *Maintenance dose:* 20–200 mg/day.

Behavioral disturbances: *Child 2–12 yrs:* PO: 0.5 to 3 mg/kg/day in divided doses.

Clinical alert: Avoid skin contact with liquid forms (may cause contact dermatitis). Read labels of liquid preparations carefully (there are four different types of liquid thioridazine available: two suspensions and two concentrates). Dilute liquid concentrate in water or juice just before giving dose. Keep IV diphenhydramine available in case of side effect of acute dystonic reaction.

Contraindications/Precautions

PREG
C

Contraindicated in hypersensitivity to thioridazine or phenothiazines, and in CNS depression, comatose states. *Use with caution* in seizure disorders, hypertension, parkinsonism, poorly controlled diabetes mellitus, asthma, emphysema, narrow-angle glaucoma, cardiac disease, hypotension, paralytic ileus, liver damage, prostatic hypertrophy, and bone marrow depression.

✋ **Contraindicated for children under 2 years and nursing mothers. Use with caution for older children and the elderly or debilitated. Safe use for pregnant women has not been established.**

Side effects/Adverse reactions

Hypersensitivity: rash, contact dermatitis. *CNS:* sedation, dizziness, extrapyramidal reactions (pseudoparkinsonism, akathisia [restless need to keep moving], tardive dykinesia, dystonia). *CV:* orthostatic hypotension, palpitations, tachycardia, EKG changes. *GI:* appetite changes, dry mouth, constipation, diarrhea, abnormal liver function. *GU:* urinary retention or hesitancy, dark urine, priapism, impaired ejaculation, amenorrhea. *Eye:* blurred vision. *Skin:* photosensitivity, jaundice. *MS:* weight gain. *Hem:* hyperglycemia, transient leukopenia, agranulocytosis. *Misc:* galactorrhea, gynecomastia. *After abrupt withdrawal of long-term therapy:* gastritis, nausea, vomiting, lightheadedness, tremors, feeling of warmth or cold, diaphoresis, tachycardia, headache, insomnia.

Nursing implications/Documentation

Possible nursing diagnoses: Potential for injury; Constipation; Altered oral mucous membrane.

◆ Record mental status and vital signs before and 1–2 hours after administration during initial phase of treatment, then bid until response to therapy has been established, then periodically thereafter.

◆ Check CBC, liver function, BUN, and creatinine before giving first dose and periodically thereafter.

◆ Be sure that doses are swallowed (not hoarded).

◆ Monitor for orthostatic hypotension, dizziness, and drowsiness; supervise ambulation until response is established.

◆ Provide special mouth care; observe for and report oral ulcers.

◆ Prevent constipation by monitoring bowel movements and encouraging adequate fiber and fluid intake; offer laxatives or stool softeners before problem becomes severe.

T

• Report persistent sore throat, fever, and malaise, because these may indicate agranulocytosis.

Patient & family teaching/Home care

Possible nursing diagnoses: Sleep pattern disturbance; Impaired home maintenance management.

• Emphasize the need to continue medication, even when feeling well.

• Warn to change positions slowly to prevent dizziness.

• Stress that the effects of alcohol, sedatives and CNS depressants, and tranquilizers may be potentiated.

• Caution to consult with physician before using OTC drugs; stress the need for ongoing medical follow-up.

• Teach the need to report persistent sore throat, fever, and fatigue.

• Point out that doses should not be increased or stopped without checking with physician.

• Caution to wear a sunscreen (number 15), protective clothing, and sunglasses when out in the sun.

• Advise avoidance of driving and other potentially hazardous activities until response is determined.

• Suggest using ice chips, hard candy, or gum to relieve side effect of dry mouth; stress the need for good mouth care.

• Warn women to report if pregnancy is planned or suspected.

• *See Antipsychotics overview for more information.*

thiotepa
thye-oh-tep'a

Thiotepa

Class: Antineoplastic (alkylating) agent

PEDS	PREG	GERI
🖐	D	🖐

Action Kills rapidly growing cells (cancer, hair follicles, bone marrow, GI lining, ova, and sperm) by interfering with DNA replication and RNA transcription through alkylation (cross-linking of DNA occurs). Is cell-cycle–phase nonspecific, affecting both actively dividing cells and dormant (resting) cells.

Use/Therapeutic goal/Outcome

Ovarian, breast, and lung carcinomas; Hodgkin's disease; lymphomas; superficial bladder tumors; and neoplastic effusions: Elimination or suppression of malignant cell proliferation. **Outcome criteria:** Tumor and disease regression or stabilization on radiologic and physical exam.

Dose range/Administration

Interaction alert: Radiation therapy and other cytotoxic agents can cause severe myelosuppression. Concurrent use with succinylcholine can cause apnea.

Adenocarcinoma of breast and ovaries, Hodgkin's disease, lymphomas, bronchogenic carcinomas, and lymphosarcomas: Adult/Child > 12 yrs: IV: 0.2 to 0.4 mg/kg/day for 2–4 weeks or 0.2 mg/kg/day for 4–5 days q 2–4 wk.

Neoplastic effusions: Adult/Child > 12 yrs: *Intracavitary, Intratumor:* 0.6 to 0.8 mg/kg (by physician) weekly or prn.

Superficial papillary adenocarcinoma of the bladder: Adult/Child > 12 yr: *Intravesical:* 60–90 mg dissolved in 60–100 ml of sterile water, instilled by catheter into the bladder and held there for 2 hr, once a week for 4 weeks.

Clinical alert: This drug should be given only by nurses who are knowledgeable in the comprehensive management of the administration of antineoplastic agents. Protocols for drug preparation, administration, and accidental skin contamination must be followed. Gloves or double gloves must be worn when handling thiotepa (skin contamination may cause a local reaction). Contaminated areas should be washed with large amounts of soap and water. IV dose should be given directly into the vein (this drug is not a vesicant). For bladder instillation, the drug should be retained for 2 hr, while the patient is repositioned every 15 min so the bladder area will have maximum drug contact. The patient should be NPO for 6–8 hr to promote drug retention.

Contraindications/Precautions
PREG
D

Contraindicated in hypersensitivity to thiotepa and in preexisting hepatic, renal, or bone marrow damage (increased toxicity).

🖐 **Contraindicated for pregnant or nursing mothers. Use with caution for the elderly. Safe use for children has not been established.**

Side effects/Adverse reactions

Hypersensitivity: hives, rash, pruritus, anaphylaxis. **Hem:** hyperuricemia, leukopenia (within 5–30 days), anemia, thrombocytopenia, and pancytopenia. **GI:** anorexia; nausea and vomiting; stomatitis; ulceration of intestinal mucosa; hepatotoxicity. **GU:** hematuria; amenorrhea, and azoospermia. **CNS:** headache, dizziness. **Skin:** pain and erythema at injection site.

Nursing implications/Documentation

Possible nursing diagnoses: Potential for infection; Potential for injury; Fatigue; Altered oral mucous membrane; Fluid volume deficit; Diarrhea; Altered nutrition: less than body requirements.

◆ *See important Nursing implications in Antineoplastic agents overview on page 72, which apply to all antineoplastics.*

Patient & family teaching/Home care

Possible nursing diagnoses: Knowledge deficit; Ineffective coping (individual and family); Hopelessness; Impaired home maintenance management.

◆ *See important Patient & family teaching in Antineoplastic agents overview on page 72, which apply to all antineoplastics.*

◆ *See antineoplastic agents overview for more information.*

thiothixene

thye-oh-thix'een

thiothixene hydrochloride: **Navane**

Class: Thioxanthene antipsychotic

PEDS	PREG	GERI
✋	C	✋

Action Exact mechanism of action has not been determined. Believed to produce calmness and alleviate psychiatric symptoms (disorders of perception, thought, consciousness, mood, affect, and social interaction) by blocking dopamine receptors in the limbic system. Blocks peripheral muscarinic, adrenergic, and histamine receptors. Also has some effect on the hypothalamus and pituitary gland, causing changes in regulation of body temperature and endocrine function. A dose of 4 mg of thiothixene is therapeutically equivalent to 100 mg of chlorpromazine.

Use/Therapeutic goal/Outcome

Schizophrenia and psychotic disorders: Promotion of reality orientation, reduction in agitated hyperactivity. **Outcome criteria:** Demonstration of reality orientation and ability to problem solve and interact with others; absence of hyperactive and agitated behavior.

Dose range/Administration

Interaction alert: Alcohol and other CNS depressants may cause excessive sedation.

💋 **Give with food or milk to avoid GI upset.**

Adult: PO: Begin with 2–5 mg bid to qid, gradually increasing to 15–30 mg/day in divided doses. For severely disturbed persons, as high as 60 mg/day may be required. IM: 4 mg bid to qid, not to exceed 30 mg/day. Change to oral route as soon as possible.

Clinical alert: Dilute liquid concentrate in juice, milk, or semisolid food just before giving dose. Avoid skin contact with liquid and parenteral forms (may cause contact dermatitis). Keep patient lying down for 1 hour after IM administration and have IV diphenhydramine available in case of side effect of acute dystonic reaction.

Contraindications/Precautions

PREG C

Contraindicated in hypersensitivity to thiothixene or thioxanthenes, and in circulatory collapse, blood dyscrasias, CNS depression, and in comatose states, parkinsonism, asthma, emphysema, narrow-angle glaucoma, cardiac disease, hypotension, liver damage, prostatic hypertrophy, bone marrow depression, and Reye's syndrome. **Use with caution** in seizure disorders, alcoholism, peptic ulcers, and hypertension.

✋ **Contraindicated for nursing mothers. Use with caution for adolescents and the elderly and debilitated. Safe use for children under 12 years and pregnant women has not been established.**

Side effects/Adverse reactions

Hypersensitivity: rash, pruritis, contact dermatitis, urticaria, anaphylaxis. **CNS:** sedation, extrapyramidal reactions (pseudoparkinsonism, akathisia [restless need to keep moving], dystonia, tardive dykinesia), neuroleptic malignant syndrome (fever, tachycardia, tachypnea, profuse diaphoresis), EEG changes, dizziness. **CV:** orthostatic hypotension, palpitations, dysrhythmias, EKG changes. **GI:** appetite changes, dry mouth, constipation, abnormal liver function. **GU:** urinary retention or hesitancy, impaired ejaculation, amenorrhea. **Eye:** blurred vision. **Hem:** leukopenia, agranulocytosis, hyperglycemia. **Skin:** photosensitivity, jaundice. **MS:** weight gain. **Misc:** gynecomastia, galactorrhea. **After abrupt withdrawal of long-term therapy:** gastritis, nausea, vomiting, light-headedness, tremors, feeling of warmth or cold, sweating, tachycardia, headache, insomnia.

Nursing implications/Documentation

Possible nursing diagnoses: Potential for injury; Constipation; Altered oral mucous membranes.

◆ Check baseline CBC, BUN, creatinine and liver function before giving first dose, then monitor every 2 weeks during the first month, then periodically thereafter.

◆ Record mental status and vital signs before and 1–2 hours after administration during initial phase of treatment, then bid until response to therapy has been established, then periodically thereafter.

◆ Be sure that PO doses are swallowed (not hoarded).

◆ Monitor for orthostatic hypotension, dizziness, and drowsiness; supervise ambulation until response is established.

◆ Provide special mouth care; observe for and report oral ulcers.

◆ Prevent constipation by monitoring bowel movements and encouraging adequate fiber and fluid intake; offer laxatives or stool softeners before problem becomes severe.

◆ Report persistent sore throat, fever, and malaise, because these may indicate agranulocytosis.

◆ Monitor for (and report immediately) signs of neuroleptic malignant syndrome (muscle rigidity, tremors, high fever, tachycardia); this is a rare, but potentially fatal, side effect.

Patient & family teaching/Home care

Possible nursing diagnoses: Sleep pattern disturbance; Impaired home maintenance management.

◆ Emphasize the need to continue medication, even when feeling well.

◆ Warn to change positions slowly to prevent dizziness.

◆ Stress that the effects of alcohol, sedatives and CNS depressants, and tranquilizers may be potentiated.

◆ Caution to consult with physician before using OTC drugs; stress the need for ongoing medical follow-up.

◆ Provide a list of side effects that should be reported: involuntary movements, muscular rigidity, tremors, fever, respiratory distress, tachycardia, persistent sore throat.

◆ Caution to wear a sunscreen (number 15) and sunglasses when out in the sun.

◆ Advise avoidance of driving and other potentially hazardous activities until response has been established.

◆ Suggest using ice chips, hard candy, or gum to relieve side effect of dry mouth; stress the need for good mouth care.

◆ Warn women to report if pregnancy is planned or suspected.

◆ *See Antipsychotics overview for more information.*

thyroglobulin
thye-roe-glob'u-lin

Proloid

Class: Thyroid hormone

PEDS	PREG	GERI
✋	A	✋

Action Accelerates rate of cellular metabolism by increasing blood levels of thyroid hormone (resulting in increased metabolic rate, cardiac output, oxygen consumption, body temperature, and blood volume, and promotion of growth and development).

Use/Therapeutic goal/Outcome

Hypothyroidism, myxedema, and cretinism: Replacement of deficient circulating thyroid hormones, promotion of normal metabolism. **Outcome criteria:** Increased T_3 and T_4 levels, weight loss, increased appetite, decreased fatigue, normal skin and hair texture, normal growth and development.

Dose range/Administration

Interaction alert: Give at least 1 hour before or 4 hours after giving cholestyramine and colestipol (they impair thyroglobulin absorption). Increases effects of anticoagulants, and tricyclic antidepressants. Monitor those taking digoxin for digitalis toxicity. Catecholamines increase risk of coronary insufficiency (report chest pain). May alter insulin requirements.

📙 **Give 1 hour before meals or 2 hours after meals for best absorption.**

Hypothyroidism and myxedema: Adult: PO: 15–30 mg/day qAM, then increase by 15–30 mg q 2 wks prn. *Maintenance dose:* 60–180 mg/day. *For the elderly:* 7.5–15 mg/day qAM, then double dosage q6-8 wks prn.

Juvenile hypothyroidism and cretinism: Child > 1 yr: 60–180 mg/day qAM. *4–12 mos:* 60–80 mg/day qAM. *1–4 mos:* 15–30 mg/day qAM. Then increase dose q 2 wks prn. *Maintenance dose:* 30–45 mg.

Clinical alert: Do not substitute different brands or generic brands for this drug unless approved by physician (they may not be bio-equivalent). Individual response and dose requirement for thyroid hormones *vary greatly.*

Contraindications/Precautions

PREG A

Contraindicated in hypersensitivity to thyroglobulin, and in adrenal insufficiency, myocardial infarction, thyrotoxicosis. *Use with caution* in angina, ischemia, or hypertension.

🖐 **Use with caution for children, pregnant or nursing mothers, and the elderly.**

Side effects/Adverse reactions

Hypersensitivity: itching, rashes. Other side effects are usually dose related. *CNS:* headache, nervousness, insomnia, tremors. *CV:* palpitations, tachycardia, dysrhythmias, angina, hypertension. *GI:* increased appetite, nausea, abdominal cramps, diarrhea. *GU:* change in menstrual flow or cycle. *MS:* weight loss, leg cramps. *Misc:* sweating, heat intolerance.

Nursing implications/Documentation

Possible nursing diagnoses: Altered nutrition: less than body requirements; Altered nutrition: more than body requirements.

◆ Record and monitor pulse and blood pressure at least once a day during initial treatment; also document daily weights.

◆ Monitor T_4 and TSH levels for therapeutic range (level below normal indicates need for increase in dose).

◆ For patients over 40 or with a history of cardiovascular disease, monitor for and report symptoms of cardiovascular disease (chest pain, tachycardia, dyspnea).

◆ If radioactive iodine uptake tests are necessary, discontinue drug 4 weeks before test.

◆ For children, monitor growth and development every 3–6 months.

Patient & family teaching/Home care

Possible nursing diagnoses: Knowledge deficit; Impaired home maintenance management.

◆ Emphasize the importance of taking this drug daily as prescribed (avoid generic or different brands; take doses at the same time every day, preferably in the morning to prevent insomnia; do not skip or double up on doses).

◆ Explain that this medication is likely to be needed for life, and that medical follow-up is necessary to ensure health.

◆ Advise reporting signs and symptoms of increased fatigue or nervousness, palpitations or tachycardia, chest pain.

◆ Explain that symptoms of hypothyroidism may persist for several months.

◆ Stress that this drug is potentially dangerous and should not be used for simple weight loss or fatigue.

◆ Point out the need to advise other physicians that thyroid medication is being taken.

◆ *See Thyroid Hormones overview for more information.*

thyroid

thye'roid

THYROID USP (dessicated): *Armour Thyroid, S-P-T, Thyrar, Thyroid Strong, Thyroid USP Enseals, Thyro-Teric*

Class: Thyroid hormone

PEDS	PREG	GERI
🖐	A	🖐

Action. Accelerates rate of cellular metabolism by increasing blood levels of thyroid hormone (resulting in increased metabolic rate, cardiac output, oxygen consumption, body temperature, and blood volume, and promotion of growth and development).

Use/Therapeutic goal/Outcome

Hypothyroidism, myxedema, and cretinism: Replacement of deficient circulating thyroid hormones, promotion of normal metabolism. *Outcome criteria:* Increased T_3 and T_4 levels, weight loss, increased appetite, decreased fatigue, normal skin and hair texture, normal growth and development.

Dose range/Administration

Interaction alert: Give at least 1 hour before or 4 hours after giving cholestyramine and colestipol (they impair thyroid absorption). Increases effects of anticoagulants, and tricyclic antidepressants. Monitor those taking digoxin for digitalis toxicity. Catecholamines increase risk of coronary insufficiency (report chest pain). May alter insulin requirements.

⬚ **Give 1 hour before meals or 2 hours after meals for best absorption.**

Hypothyroidism: Adult: PO: 60 mg/day qAM, then increase by 60 mg q 30 days prn. *Maintenance dose:* 60–180 mg/day. *For the elderly:* 7.5–15 mg/day, then double dose q6-8 wks prn.

Myxedema: Adult: PO: 16 mg/day qAM, then double dose q 2 wks prn. *Maximum dose:* 120 mg.

Juvenile hypothyroidism and cretinism: Child > 1 yr: 60 mg/day qAM, then increase to 180 mg prn. *Child 4–12 mos:* 30–60 mg/day qAM. *Child 1–4 mos:* 15–30 mg/day qAM, then increase q 2 wks prn. *Maintenance dose:* 30–45 mg.

Clinical alert: Do not substitute different brands or generic brands for this drug unless approved by physician (they may not be bio-equivalent). Individual response and dose requirement for thyroid hormones *vary greatly.*

Contraindications/Precautions

PREG
A

Contraindicated in hypersensitivity to desiccated thyroid, and in adrenal insufficiency, myocardial infarction, thyrotoxicosis. *Use with caution* in angina, ischemia, or hypertension.

✋ **Use with caution for children, pregnant or nursing mothers, and the elderly.**

Side effects/Adverse reactions

Hypersensitivity: itching, rashes. Other side effects are usually dose related. *CNS:* headache, nervousness, insomnia, tremors. *CV:* palpitations, tachycardia, arrhythmias, angina, hypertension. *GI:* increased appetite, nausea, abdominal cramps, diarrhea. *GU:* change in menstrual flow or cycle. *MS:* weight loss, leg cramps. *Misc:* sweating, heat intolerance.

Nursing implications/Documentation

Possible nursing diagnoses: Altered nutrition: less than body requirements; Altered nutrition: more than body requirements.

♦ Record and monitor pulse and blood pressure at least once a day during initial treatment; also document daily weights.

♦ Monitor T_4 and TSH levels for therapeutic range (level below normal indicates need for increase in dose).

♦ For patients over 40 or with a history of cardiovascular disease, monitor for and report symptoms of cardiovascular disease (chest pain, tachycardia, dyspnea).

♦ If radioactive iodine uptake tests are necessary, discontinue drug 4 weeks before test.

♦ For children, monitor growth and development every 3–6 months.

Patient & family teaching/Home care

Possible nursing diagnoses: Knowledge deficit; Impaired home maintenance management.

♦ Emphasize the importance of taking this drug daily as prescribed (avoid generic or different brands; take doses at the same time every day, preferably in the morning to prevent insomnia; do not skip or double up on doses).

♦ Explain that this medication is likely to be needed for life, and that medical follow-up is necessary to ensure health.

♦ Advise reporting signs and symptoms of increased fatigue or nervousness, palpitations or tachycardia, chest pain.

♦ Explain that symptoms of hypothyroidism may persist for several months.

♦ Stress that this drug is potentially dangerous and should not be used for simple weight loss or fatigue.

♦ Point out the need to tell other physicians that thyroid medication is being taken.

♦ *See Thyroid Hormones overview for more information.*

ticarcillin

tye-kar-sill'in

ticarcillin disodium: *Ticar,* ◆*Ticillin*
ticarcillin disodium with clavulanate potassium: *Timentin*
Class: Anti-infective, Antibiotic, Extended-spectrum penicillin

PEDS	PREG	GERI
✋	B	✋

Action Extended-spectrum, bactericidal antibiotic; kills bacteria by inhibiting cell wall syn-

▶

thesis. Clavulanate potassium potentiates by inactivating bacterial beta-lactamose, the enzyme that destroys ticarcillin. Especially effective against gram-negative organisms.

Use/Therapeutic goal/Outcome

Severe systemic infections: Resolution of infection. *Outcome criteria:* Absence of pathogenic growth on cultures, absence of clinical manifestations of infection (fever, pain, redness, heat, swelling, odor, drainage), normal WBC count, improvement of X rays.

Dose range/Administration

Interaction alert: Probenecid inhibits excretion of ticarcillin and may be given to increase serum levels of the drug. Inactivates aminoglycosides (e.g., gentamicin, tobramycin); do not mix together in solution. Give at least 1 hour before bacteriostatic antibiotics for optimal effect. May potentiate oral anticoagulants (because of antiplatelet effect).

Adult: IM, IV: 1 g/day (up to 150–200 mg/kg) in divided doses q4-6h. *Maximum dose:* 24 g/day IV or 2 g IM. *Child:* IM, IV: 200–300 mg/kg/day, in divided doses q4-6h.

Clavulanate potassium form: Preparation dose is based on combined dose of each active component (3.1 g = 3 g ticarcillin plus 0.1 g [100 mg] clavulanate potassium). *Adult:* IV: 3.1 g q4-6h infused over 30 min (never give IV push).

Clinical alert: Never give clavulanate potassium form IM.

Contraindications/Precautions

PREG
B

Contraindicated in allergy to penicillin. *Use with caution* in cephalosporin sensitivity, history of allergic responses (e.g., other drugs, hay fever, asthma), and renal insufficiency.

🖐 Use with caution for children, the elderly, and for pregnant or nursing mothers. Safe use of clavulanate potassium form for children under 12 years has not been established.

Side effects/Adverse reactions

Hypersensitivity: itching, rashes, urticaria, fever, difficulty breathing, anaphylaxis. *GI:* nausea, vomiting, diarrhea. *CV:* pain, redness, swelling, thrombophlebitis, sterile abscess. *CNS:* headache, dizziness. *Hem:* thrombocytopenia, leukopenia, hypernatremia, eosinophilia, increased bleeding time. *Misc:* superinfection.

Nursing implications/Documentation

Possible nursing diagnoses: Potential for infection; Diarrhea.

♦ Determine history of allergies, and (regardless of history) monitor closely for allergic reactions.

♦ Obtain baseline CBC, electrolytes, creatinine, liver function studies, and necessary cultures before administering first dose; monitor closely thereafter if therapy is prolonged.

♦ Give IM doses deep into large muscle mass (limit dose to 2 g at any single injection site).

♦ Encourage fluids, and record and monitor intake and output, to ensure adequate hydration; report significant negative or positive balance.

♦ Monitor for and report signs of superinfection (sore throat, fever, fatigue, thrush, vaginal discharge, diarrhea).

♦ Watch for unusual bruising or bleeding (check gums, urine).

Patient & family teaching/Home care

Possible nursing diagnoses: Knowledge deficit; Impaired home maintenance management.

♦ Teach the importance of reporting allergic symptoms, diarrhea, signs and symptoms that do not abate, or *any* new signs and symptoms of discomfort that might indicate superinfection (medication regimen may have to be changed).

♦ Advise drinking 2–3 L of fluids daily to maintain adequate hydration (especially important if fever exists).

♦ Stress the importance of taking antibiotics for the entire time prescribed, even if signs and symptoms abate.

♦ *See Anti-infectives overview for more information.*

timolol

tye'moe-lole

♦Apo-Timolol, Blocadren, Timoptic

Class: Nonselective beta-adrenergic blocking agent, Antihypertensive

PEDS	PREG	GERI
🖐	C	🖐

Action Reduces blood pressure (precise mechanism in unclear), and decreases heart rate and cardiac output by blocking beta-1 (cardiac) and beta-2 adrenergic receptors. Decreases renin secretion. Thought to reduce intraocular pressure by decreasing the formation of aqueous humor; may also slightly increase outflow of intraocular aqueous humor.

Use/Therapeutic goal/Outcome

Hypertension: Reduction of blood pressure. **Outcome criteria:** Blood pressure within normal limits.

Prophylaxis following myocardial infarction: Prevention of reinfarction. **Outcome criteria:** Lack of enzymatic or cardiographic evidence of reinfarction.

Glaucoma (open angle, aphakic, and secondary/ocular hypertension): Reduction of intraocular pressure. **Outcome criteria:** Upon measurement with tonometer, intraocular pressure within normal limits.

Dose range/Administration

Interaction alert: If used with cardiac glycosides, monitor for excessive bradycardia and hypotension. Indomethacin may antagonize antihypertensive effects. May alter antidiabetic agent requirements.

Hypertension: Adult: PO: 10 mg bid; may increase or decrease, depending on response, at 7-day intervals. *Maintenance dose:* 20–40 mg/day in divided doses. *Maximum dose:* 60 mg/day.

Myocardial infarction prophylaxis: Adult: PO: 10 mg bid.

Glaucoma: Adult: 1 drop of 0.25 percent solution to affected eye(s) bid; use 0.5 percent solution if response is inadequate.

Clinical alert: Be aware that patients taking timolol may not exhibit tachycardia as a symptom of fever, hypoglycemia, or hyperthyroidism.

Contraindications/Precautions

PREG C

Contraindicated in hypersensitivity to timolol, and in cardiogenic shock, sinus bradycardia, second- or third-degree heart block (PR interval > 0.24 seconds), uncompensated CHF, right ventricular failure resulting from pulmonary hypertension, diabetes, severe COPD, asthma, allergic rhinitis, and during ethyl ether anesthesia. **Use with caution** in CHF or respiratory or liver disease.

⚕ **Use with caution for the elderly. Safe use for children and pregnant women has not been established.**

Side effects/Adverse reactions

Hypersensitivity: rash, pruritus. **CV:** bradycardia, hypotension, congestive heart failure, peripheral vascular disease. **CNS:** fatigue, lethargy, insomnia, vivid dreams, depression, dizziness. **GU:** decreased sexual ability. **Resp:** increased airway resistance. **GI:** nausea, vomiting, diarrhea. **MS:** cold hands and feet.

Nursing implications/Documentation

Possible nursing diagnoses: Activity intolerance; Fatigue; Potential for injury.

♦ Assess mental status, and record pulse and blood pressure prior to administration, and frequently thereafter until response is determined.

♦ Consult with physician to determine desired therapeutic range for blood pressure and heart rate (be aware that parameters for withholding the medication should be written by physician).

♦ Ascertain that baseline CBC, electrolytes, BUN, creatinine, and liver function studies are obtained prior to beginning first dose; report abnormalities and monitor closely thereafter.

♦ Monitor for allergic reactions and for symptoms of confusion, dizziness, bradycardia, congestive heart failure or hypotension; hold drug and report immediately if these occur.

♦ Supervise ambulation until response is determined.

♦ Document and monitor daily weight, and intake and output; report significant negative or positive balance.

Patient & family teaching/Home care

Possible nursing diagnoses: Knowledge deficit; Impaired home maintenance management; Altered sexuality patterns.

♦ Explain the importance of taking this drug exactly as prescribed, even when feeling well; warn not to discontinue drug abruptly.

♦ Stress that with good medical follow-up, taking timolol will help reduce "wear and tear" on blood vessels, reduce the workload of the heart, and improve longevity and health.

♦ Teach how to monitor pulse and blood pressure; emphasize that syncope, hypertension or hypotension, or persistent dizziness should be reported; provide pulse and blood pressure parameters for withholding medication.

♦ Advise changing positions slowly to avoid dizziness.

* Encourage monitoring of daily weights and reporting sudden weight gain (likely to be water weight gain).

* Warn against drinking alcohol or taking *any* OTC drugs without physician approval (some interactions can cause severe reactions).

* Warn that discontinuing drug may precipitate cardiac problems.

* Explain that this drug may alter sexual ability; explore concerns and seek consultation as needed.

* *See Adrenergic Beta-blockers and Antihypertensives overviews for more information.*

tobramycin
toe-bra-mye′sin

tobramycin sulfate: **Nebcin**

Class: Anti-infective, Aminoglycoside antibiotic

PEDS	PREG	GERI
🖑	**D**	🖑

Action Kills bacteria (bactericidal) by binding to the ribosomes, thereby disrupting bacterial protein synthesis.

Use/Therapeutic goal/Outcome

Serious infections (caused by susceptible strains of *Escherichia coli, Proteus, Klebsiella, Enterobacter, Serratia, Staphylococcus aureus, Pseudomonas, Citrobacter, Providencia*): Resolution of infection. *Outcome criteria:* Absence of pathogenic growth on cultures, absence of clinical manifestations of infection (pain, fever, redness, heat, swelling, drainage, productive cough, elevated WBC).

Dose range/Administration

Interaction alert: Do not mix IV with penicillins or cephalosporins. Loop diuretics (e.g., furosemide) increase risk of toxicity. Dimenhydrinate may mask symptoms of ototoxicity. Use cautiously with cephalosporins, other aminoglycosides, amphotericin B, cisplatin, methoxyflurane that increase risk of toxicity.

Adult and Child: IM, IV: 3 mg/kg/day in divided doses q8h; for life-threatening infections, up to 5 mg/kg/day in divided doses q6-8h. Dilute IV doses in 50–100 cc NS or D5W and infuse over 20–60 min. *Ophthalmic:* 1–2 drops in affected eye q4h. For severe infection, up to 2 drops qh. *Neonate:* IM, IV: Up to 4 mg/kg/day in divided doses q12h (infuse IV over 20–60 min).

Clinical alert: For patients with impaired kidney function, give same initial dose, then adjust according to kidney function studies. Schedule blood drawing for peak levels 1 hour after IM injection, or 30–60 minutes after IV administration. Schedule blood drawing for trough levels just before next dose. Peak levels over 12 mcg/ml and trough levels above 2 mcg/ml are associated with toxicity.

Contraindications/Precautions
PREG
D

Contraindicated in hypersensitivity or toxic reaction to tobramycin or other aminoglycosides, and in concurrent use with potent diuretics or other neurotoxic or nephrotoxic drugs. *Use with caution* in impaired renal function (reduce dosage).

🖑 **Contraindicated for pregnant or nursing mothers. Use with caution for infants and the elderly.**

Side effects/Adverse reactions

Hypersensitivity: itching, burning, rashes, drug fever, arthralgia, blood dyscrasias, angioneurotic edema, anaphylaxis. *Ear:* ototoxicity (hearing loss, tinnitus). *CNS:* neurotoxicity (dizziness, vertigo, headache, nausea, vomiting, unsteady gait, neuromuscular blockade). *GU:* nephrotoxicity (oliguria, proteinuria, cells in urine, hematuria, decreased creatinine clearance, increased serum BUN and creatinine). *Hem:* thrombophlebitis with IV infusion. *Eye:* burning, itching with ophthalmic use (if persistent, may be sign of hypersensitivity).

Nursing implications/Documentation

Possible nursing diagnoses: Potential for infection; Fluid volume deficit.

* Determine history of allergies and (regardless of history) monitor closely for allergic reactions.

* Weigh patient, and obtain baseline renal function studies, hearing ability, and culture specimens before administering first dose.

* Monitor renal function (urine output, specific gravity, serum BUN and creatinine, creatinine clearance) and report signs of decreased function.

* Encourage fluid intake, and document and monitor intake and output to ensure adequate hydration and prevent renal damage from irritation of renal tubules.

* Monitor for and report symptoms of hearing loss, tinnitus, vertigo, headache, nausea, vomiting and superinfection (mouth lesions, thrush,

vaginal irritation, diarrhea, respiratory symptoms).

♦ If symptoms do not improve within 2–3 days, consult with physician to re-evaluate antibiotic regimen (new cultures should be drawn).

Patient & family teaching/Home care

Possible nursing diagnoses: Knowledge deficit; Impaired home maintenance management.

♦ Advise reporting ear symptoms (e.g., full feeling, ringing of the ears, hearing loss, dizziness) immediately.

♦ Teach the need to report new signs and symptoms of illness (e.g., fever, mouth lesions, vaginal irritation, diarrhea, respiratory symptoms) since medications may have to be changed.

♦ Explain the importance of taking antibiotics for the entire time prescribed, regardless of absence of signs and symptoms, and of maintaining hydration (drinking at least 2 L is recommended).

♦ *See Anti-infectives overview for more information.*

tocainide

toe-kay'nide

tocainide hydrochloride: *Tonocard*
Class: Antiarrhythmic (Class IB)

PEDS	PREG	GERI
✋	C	✋

Action Suppresses ventricular ectopy by decreasing the duration of the action potential of Purkinje fibers. Decreases myocardial excitability of the AV node and ventricles.

Use/Therapeutic goal/Outcome

Ventricular arrhythmias, including premature ventricular contractions, couplets, and ventricular tachyarrhythmias (used when other antiarrhythmics fail): Suppression of ventricular ectopy and promotion of effective heartbeat. **Outcome criteria:** Absence of or decrease in ventricular ectopy on EKG; regular palpable pulses.

Dose range/Administration

Interaction alert: Concurrent use with betablockers may decrease myocardial contractility.

♥ **Give with food to minimize GI upset.**

Adult: PO: 400 mg q8h. Range is 1200–1800 mg/day in 3 divided doses. May be given q12h if tolerated by the patient.

Clinical alert: Place patient on continuous monitoring before initiating therapy. Monitor for tremor, which may indicate onset of CNS toxicity. Monitor WBC count for agranulocytopenia, bone marrow depression, thrombocytopenia.

Contraindications/Precautions

PREG
C

Contraindicated in hypersensitivity to lidocaine or other amide-type local anesthetics, and in second- or third-degree heart block unless an artificial pacemaker is in place. *Use with caution* with hepatic or renal impairment or congestive heart failure.

✋ **Use with caution for the elderly (may require lower doses). Safe use for children and pregnant or nursing mothers has not been determined.**

Side effects/Adverse reactions

Hypersensitivity: rash, exfoliative dermatitis, blistering, peeling skin, mouth ulcers. **CV:** hypotension, congestive heart failure, PVC's **CNS:** lightheadedness, tremor, paresthesias, numbness, confusion, dizziness. **Resp:** pneumonitis, pulmonary fibrosis, pneumonia. **GI:** nausea, vomiting, epigastric pain, diarrhea, and anorexia. **Skin:** sweating. **Hem:** aplastic anemia, agranulocytosis, thrombocytopenia. (CNS and GI adverse reactions are usually mild and transient, and may be reduced by decreasing the dosage.)

Nursing implications/Documentation

Possible nursing diagnoses: Potential for injury; Activity intolerance.

♦ Be sure to check baseline chest X-ray, EKG, and laboratory studies (CBC, sodium, potassium, chloride, carbon dioxide, magnesium, BUN, creatinine, SGPT, and LDH) before giving first dose; monitor closely thereafter as indicated by clinical condition.

♦ Remember that oxygen requirements must be met, and that electrolyte imbalances (especially potassium and magnesium) and abnormal blood pH must be corrected, before expected antiarrhythmic effect can be seen; report abnormalities immediately.

♦ Document baseline vital signs, lung sounds, and cardiac monitor strip (measure and record PR, and QRS segments) before giving first dose and at least every 8 hr; monitor closely until response is determined; report if prolongation in PR or QRS segment is noted.

T

♦ Monitor for and report early signs of CHF (tocainide may need to be discontinued).

♦ Supervise ambulation until response is determined.

♦ Coordinate care to provide frequent rest periods.

Patient & family teaching/Home care

Possible nursing diagnoses: Fear; Knowledge deficit; Impaired home maintenance management.

♦ Explain that the purpose of this drug is to prevent arrhythmias and promote an effective heartbeat.

♦ Advise taking this drug with meals to avoid GI problems.

♦ Stress the need to follow dose regimen closely (the drug should be taken at the same time each day), and the need to return for medical follow-up for early detection of adverse reactions.

♦ Teach how to assess pulse for irregularities in rhythm and rate; stress that irregularities be reported.

♦ Emphasize the need to pace activities, avoid stress, and plan for rest periods.

♦ Warn against driving or operating machinery until response is determined.

♦ Encourage learning CPR; reinforce that survival rate of cardiac arrest is greatly increased when CPR is initiated immediately.

♦ *See Antiarrhythmics overview for more information.*

tolazamide   *tole-az'a-mide*

Ronase, Tolamide, Tolinase

Class: Antidiabetic (oral hypoglycemic), First-generation sulfonylurea

Antidote: D$_{50}$W, glucagon

PEDS	PREG	GERI
☟	C	☟

Action Reduces serum glucose and promotes cellular nutrition by stimulating insulin release in beta cells of the pancreas (not effective if beta cells have ceased to function). Onset of action occurs within 1 hour; peak action is in 1–6 hours, and duration of action is 6–12 hours.

Use/Therapeutic goal/Outcome

Mild to moderately severe, stable, Type II (noninsulin-dependent) diabetes mellitus not controlled by diet or weight control alone: Normalization of blood glucose levels, glycemic control. **Outcome criteria:** Absence of clinical symptoms of hypoglycemia (confusion, shakiness, weakness, diaphoresis, apprehension) together with blood glucose studies that demonstrate glycemic control (fasting blood sugar: 100–140 mg/dl is good control; 140–200 mg/dl is fair control).

Dose range/Administration

Interaction alert: Alcohol, anabolic steroids, insulin, chloramphenicol, oral anticoagulants, salicylates, MAOIs, phenylbutazone, sulfonamides, guanethidine, and clofibrate may *increase* hypoglycemic activity. Glucocorticoids, rifampin, glucagon, calcium channel blockers, thyroid preparations, and thiazide diuretics may *decrease* hypoglycemic activity and exacerbate diabetic symptoms. Alcohol ingestion may cause a disulfiram-like reaction (facial reddening, headache, nausea, and vomiting). Beta-blockers and clonidine may mask and prolong hypoglycemic reactions.

Adult: PO: 100 mg/day before or with breakfast. May adjust dose by 100–250 mg q wk according to fasting blood sugars. *Maximum dose:* 500 mg bid, before or with breakfast and dinner. *For the elderly:* 100 mg/day before breakfast.

Clinical alert: Tolazamide is a first-generation sulfonylurea; assess for allergy to sulfa before giving first dose. Check blood glucose levels 3 times a day during transition from an insulin regimen to tolazamide. Recognize that dose requirements vary with age, food intake, activity levels, and concurrent medical problems. Monitor the elderly closely for hypoglycemic reactions; they are likely to require slightly higher fasting blood sugars to prevent clinical symptoms of hypoglycemia.

Contraindications/Precautions   PREG
                                           C

Contraindicated in hypersensitivity to tolazamide and in Type I diabetes mellitus, uncontrolled diabetes mellitus, and severe renal, hepatic, or endocrine impairment. **Use with caution** in allergy to sulfa, cardiac disease, and Type II diabetics who require surgery, experience trauma, or are compromised by an infection (may require insulin).

Contraindicated for children and pregnant women (insulin usually required). Use with caution for the elderly.

Side effects/Adverse reactions

Hypersensitivity: itching, erythema, urticaria, rash. **GI:** nausea, vomiting, abdominal cramps, constipation, diarrhea, heartburn, hepatotoxicity. **CNS:** headache, weakness, dizziness, fatigue, vertigo. **Hem:** leukopenia, thrombocytopenia, agranulocytosis, aplastic anemia, hypoglycemia, hyponatremia.

Nursing implications/Documentation

Possible nursing diagnoses: Potential for injury; Impaired skin integrity; Impaired tissue integrity; Altered nutrition: more than body requirements; Altered nutrition: less than body requirements.

♦ Keep a record of blood sugars taken upon rising in the morning and 30 minutes before each meal and before bedtime snack; report persistent trends or significant episodes of hyperglycemia or hypoglycemia.

♦ Monitor food intake; notify physician when the patient is not eating.

♦ Monitor daily weights, especially during periods of illness.

♦ If signs of hypoglycemia (tremors, sweating, sudden weakness, pale skin, anxiety, confusion, agitation) are noted, confirm by a capillary blood glucose test first, then give 15 g of a fast-acting carbohydrate (4 oz of fruit juice, 4–6 pieces of hard candy, 1 tablespoon of sugar or honey). If blood glucose monitoring equipment is not immediately available, then give carbohydrate and check glucose level later.

♦ If signs of hyperglycemia (extreme thirst, frequent urination, fatigue, blurred vision) are noted, confirm by blood glucose meter and report immediately.

Patient & family teaching/Home care

Possible nursing diagnoses: Knowledge deficit; Impaired home maintenance management.

♦ Explain that hypoglycemics control blood sugar but do not cure diabetes; stress that regular exercise, careful regulation of diet and medication, close monitoring of blood sugars, and medical supervision can help promote health and prevent the long-term complications of diabetes (heart, kidney, eyes).

♦ Advise taking doses in the earlier part of the day to avoid nighttime hypoglycemia.

♦ Point out that diet, activity, weight fluctuations, illness, and emotional stress can affect hypoglycemic medication requirements.

♦ Stress that everything on meal plan should be eaten, especially carbohydrates, but that concentrated sweets should be avoided.

♦ Teach the signs and symptoms of hypoglycemia and hyperglycemia; advise that a fast-acting carbohydrate (4 oz of fruit juice, 4–6 pieces of hard candy, 1 tablespoon of honey or sugar) should be given for suspected *hypo*glycemia (suspected *hyper*glycemia should be reported immediately).

♦ Advise reporting weight fluctuations over 10 pounds (5 kg) or persistent symptoms of nausea, vomiting, fatigue, thirst, and frequent urination.

♦ Suggest carrying some form of fast-acting carbohydrates (e.g., small box of raisins) for treatment of hypoglycemia.

♦ Warn against use of alcohol and OTC drugs without physician's approval.

♦ Recommend wearing a medical alert bracelet to alert others to hypoglycemics use.

♦ Point out the need for wearing a sunscreen (SPF #15) because of side effect of photosensitivity.

♦ *See Antidiabetics overview for more information.*

tolazoline
toe-laz'a-leen

tolazoline hydrochloride: *Priscoline, Tazol, Toloxan, Tolzol*

Class: Alpha-adrenergic blocker (sympatholytic), Peripheral vasodilator

PEDS	PREG	GERI
	C	

Action Decreases pulmonary hypertension by reducing pulmonary artery pressure and vascular resistance. Dilates peripheral blood vessels by direct action on vascular smooth muscle and by inhibiting the effect of sympathomimetic amines (epinephrine, norepinephrine) at alpha-adrenergic receptor sites. Action may also be related to effect on histamine receptors.

Use/Therapeutic goal/Outcome

Persistent pulmonary hypertension of newborn: Maintenance of systemic arterial oxygenation. **Outcome criteria:** Arterial blood gases within normal limits.

Dose range/Administration

Interaction alert: Antihypertensive drugs may increase hypotensive effect.

>*Persistent pulmonary hypertension:* **Neonate:** IV: 1–2 mg/kg over 10 min, then 2 mg/kg/hr.

Clinical alert: In newborns, response should be evident after 30 min; little is known about infusions lasting longer than 48 hr.

Contraindications/Precautions

PREG
C

Contraindicated in hypersensitivity to tolazoline and in systolic blood pressure < 40 mm Hg. *Use with caution* in acidosis and mitral stenosis.

Ⓦ Use with caution for the elderly. Safe use for children and pregnant or nursing mothers has not been established.

Side effects/Adverse reactions

Hypersensitivity: rash. *CV:* chills, flushing, tingling, or numbness in extremities; sweating; edema; tachycardia; dysrhythmias, chest pain, postural hypotension. *GI:* nausea, vomiting, diarrhea, GI hemorrhage, abdominal pain. *CNS:* headache. *Hem:* thrombocytopenia, acidosis. *GU:* renal failure.

Nursing implications/Documentation

Possible nursing diagnoses: Activity intolerance; Impaired skin integrity; Potential for injury.

♦ Follow NICU protocols and physician's orders for monitoring ABGs, oxygen saturation, electrolytes, and chest X rays.

♦ Document pulse, blood pressure, and neurovascular checks every 1–2 hr as indicated by condition.

♦ Provide a warm environment to enhance effectiveness of this drug.

Patient & family teaching/Home care

Possible nursing diagnoses: Knowledge deficit; Fear.

♦ Encourage parents to voice questions and concerns; counsel as indicated.

tolbutamide

tole-byoo-ta'mide

Apo-Tolbutamide, ✦Mobenol, ✦Novobutamide, Oramide, Orinase

Class: ★Antidiabetic (oral hypoglycemic) prototype, First-generation sulfonylurea

Antidote: D$_{50}$W, glucagon

PEDS	PREG	GERI
⍖	C	⍖

Action Reduces serum glucose and promotes cellular nutrition by stimulating insulin release in beta cells of the pancreas (not effective if beta cells have ceased to function). Increases blood pressure and blood volume by stimulating the release of antidiuretic hormone. Onset of action occurs within 1 hour; peak action is in 4–6 hours, and duration of action is 6–12 hours.

Use/Therapeutic goal/Outcome

Mild to moderately severe, stable, Type II (noninsulin-dependent) diabetes mellitus; for those not controlled by meal plan or weight control alone: Normalization of blood glucose levels, glycemic control. *Outcome criteria:* Absence of clinical symptoms of hypoglycemia (confusion, shakiness, weakness, diaphoresis, apprehension) together with blood glucose studies that demonstrate glycemic control (fasting blood sugar: 100–140 mg/dl is good control, 140–200 mg/dl is fair control).

Dose range/Administration

Interaction alert: Alcohol, anabolic steroids, insulin, chloramphenicol, oral anticoagulants, salicylates, NSAIDs, MAOIs, phenylbutazone, sulfonamides, guanethidine, and clofibrate may *increase* hypoglycemic activity. Glucocorticoids, rifampin, glucagon, calcium channel blockers, thyroid preparations, and thiazide diuretics may *decrease* hypoglycemic activity and exacerbate diabetic symptoms. Alcohol ingestion may cause a disulfiram-like reaction (facial reddening, headache). Beta-blockers and clonidine may mask and prolong hypoglycemic reactions.

Adult: PO: Dose is highly individualized. 1–2 g/day as a single dose or divided bid or tid, 30 min after meals. *Maximum dose:* 3 g/day.

Clinical alert: Because tolbutamide is a first-generation sulfonylurea, assess for allergy to sulfa before giving first dose. Check blood glucose levels 3 times a day during transition from chlorpropamide or an insulin regimen to tolbutamide. Recognize that dose requirements vary with age, food intake, activity levels, and concurrent medical problems. Monitor the elderly closely for hypoglycemic reactions; they are likely to require slightly higher fasting blood sugars to prevent clinical symptoms of hypoglycemia. Although tolbutamide is associated with more serious side effects than second-generation sulfonylureas, it is frequently the preferred oral hypoglycemic agent for those with impaired kidney function because it is primarily eliminated by the liver.

Contraindications/Precautions
PREG C

Contraindicated in hypersensitivity to tolbutamide and in Type I diabetes mellitus, uncontrolled diabetes mellitus, and severe renal, hepatic, or endocrine impairment. **Use with caution** in allergy to sulfa; cardiac disease, and in Type II diabetics who require surgery, experience trauma, or are compromised by an infection (may require insulin).

✋ **Contraindicated for children and pregnant women (insulin usually required). Use with caution for the elderly.**

Side effects/Adverse reactions

Hypersensitivity: itching, erythema, urticaria, rash. **Hem:** hypoglycemia, leukopenia, thrombocytopenia, agranulocytosis, aplastic anemia, dilutional hyponatremia. **GI:** nausea, vomiting, abdominal cramping, diarrhea, heartburn, epigastric fullness, hepatotoxicity. **CNS:** headache, weakness, dizziness, paresthesia. **GU:** renal sodium and water retention. **CV:** hypertension, heart failure. **MS:** joint pain.

Nursing implications/Documentation

Possible nursing diagnoses: Potential for injury; Impaired skin integrity; Impaired tissue integrity; Altered nutrition: more than body requirements; Altered nutrition: less than body requirements.

◆ Keep a record of blood sugar taken upon rising in the morning and 30 minutes before each meal and before bedtime snack; report persistent trends or significant episodes of hyperglycemia or hypoglycemia.

◆ Monitor food intake; notify physician when the patient is not eating.

◆ Monitor daily weights, especially during periods of illness.

◆ If signs of hypoglycemia (tremors, sweating, sudden weakness, pale skin, anxiety, confusion, agitation) are noted, confirm by a capillary

blood glucose test first, then give 15 g of a fast-acting carbohydrate (4 oz of fruit juice, 4–6 pieces of hard candy, 1 tablespoon of sugar or honey). If blood glucose monitoring equipment is not immediately available, then give carbohydrate and check glucose level later.

◆ If signs of hyperglycemia (extreme thirst, frequent urination, fatigue, blurred vision) are noted, confirm by blood glucose meter and report immediately.

Patient & family teaching/Home care

Possible nursing diagnoses: Knowledge deficit; Impaired home maintenance management.

◆ Explain that hypoglycemics control blood sugar but do not cure diabetes; stress that regular exercise, careful regulation of diet and medication, close monitoring of blood sugars, and medical supervision help promote health and prevent the long-term complications of diabetes (heart, kidney, eyes).

◆ Advise taking doses in the earlier part of the day to avoid nighttime hypoglycemia.

◆ Point out that diet, activity, weight fluctuations, illness, and emotional stress can affect hypoglycemic medication requirements.

◆ Stress that everything on meal plan should be eaten, especially carbohydrates, but that concentrated sweets should be avoided.

◆ Teach the signs and symptoms of hypoglycemia and hyperglycemia; advise that a fast-acting carbohydrate (4 oz of fruit juice, 4–6 pieces of hard candy, 1 tablespoon of honey or sugar) should be given for suspected *hypo*glycemia (suspected *hyper*glycemia should be reported immediately).

◆ Advise reporting weight fluctuations of over 10 pounds (5 kg) or persistent symptoms of nausea, vomiting, fatigue, thirst, and frequent urination.

◆ Suggest carrying some form of fast-acting carbohydrate (e.g., small box of raisins) for treatment of hypoglycemia.

◆ Warn against use of alcohol and OTC drugs without physician's approval.

◆ Recommend wearing a medical alert bracelet to alert others to hypoglycemics use.

◆ Point out the need to avoid driving or activities that require alertness until response is established (may cause dizziness).

◆ *See Antidiabetics overview for more information.*

T

tolmetin

tole'met-in

tolmetin sodium: *Tolectin, Tolectin DS*

Class: Nonsteroidal anti-inflammatory drug (NSAID), Analgesic, Antirheumatic

PEDS	PREG	GERI
⚐	⚐	⚐

Action Exact mechanism to reduce inflammation is unclear. Thought to inhibit prostaglandin synthesis and lower plasma levels of prostaglandin E.

Use/Therapeutic goal/Outcome

Pain and inflammation: Promotion of comfort and mobility; suppression of inflammation. *Outcome criteria:* Report of increased comfort with increased range of motion and ability to perform activities of daily life; reduction in or absence of joint stiffness, swelling, redness, and warmth.

Dose range/Administration

Interaction alert: Aspirin may increase incidence of ulcers and risk of bleeding. May alter insulin requirements. Do not give with sodium-bicarbonate–base antacids.

🌢 **Give with milk or food to reduce GI distress.**

Rheumatoid arthritis: Adult: PO: *Initial dose:* 400 mg tid. *Maintenance dose:* 600–1800 mg/day in divided doses tid to qid. *Maximum dose:* 2000 mg/day. *Child > 2 yr:* PO: *Initial dose:* 20 mg/kg/day in divided doses tid to qid. *Maintenance dose:* 15–30 mg/kg/day. *Maximum dose:* 30 mg/kg/day.

Osteoarthritis: Adult: PO: *Initial dose:* 400 mg tid. *Maintenance dose:* 600–1600 mg/day in divided doses tid to qid. *Maximum dose:* 1600 mg/day.

Clinical alert: For best results, give 1 dose on rising, 1 dose at bedtime, and intersperse other doses in between.

Contraindications/Precautions

PREG ⚐

Contraindicated in hypersensitivity to tolmetin, aspirin, tartrazine, or other NSAIDs. *Use with caution* in upper GI disease; impaired renal, hepatic, or cardiac function; and prolonged prothrombin time.

⚐ **Use with caution for the elderly. Safe use for children under 2 years and pregnant women has not been determined (first 2 trimesters, preg B; in third trimester, preg D).**

Side effects/Adverse reactions

Hypersensitivity: wheezing, dyspnea, rhinitis, rash, pruritus. *CNS:* dizziness, light-headedness, headache, drowsiness, insomnia. *GI:* dyspepsia, abdominal pain, nausea, diarrhea, constipation. *CV:* edema, hypertension. *Ear:* tinnitus. *Hem:* hyperglycemia.

Nursing implications/Documentation

Possible nursing diagnoses: Pain; Impaired physical mobility.

◆ Establish a baseline for CBC, electrolytes, prothrombin time, BUN, creatinine, and liver function studies; if therapy is prolonged, monitor periodically thereafter.

◆ Be aware that elevated BUN, alkaline phosphatase, and SGOT levels may be observed; also false-positive for proteinuria, increased bleeding time, and decreased hemoglobin and hematocrit.

◆ Do not give Tolmetin DS to tartrazine-sensitive people (it may contain the dye tartrazine).

◆ Monitor for and report GI symptoms that may indicate peptic ulcer (nausea, pain, black stools).

◆ Record weight every other day; report edema or sudden weight gain.

◆ For diabetics, monitor blood sugar closely since insulin requirements may change.

Patient & family teaching/Home care

Possible nursing diagnoses: Altered health maintenance; Knowledge deficit.

◆ Advise taking doses with food to reduce GI symptoms.

◆ Explain the importance of watching for symptoms of GI bleeding (black stools, persistent GI distress).

◆ Explain that benefits of therapy may take 3–7 days to be noted; then progressive improvement is expected.

◆ Encourage drinking 6–8 glasses of water a day to promote excretion of drug.

◆ Stress the need to avoid aspirin, alcohol, and other OTC drugs (unless approved by physician) because of increased risk of GI bleeding.

◆ Instruct individuals to hold dose and report if any of the following side effects are experienced: respiratory problems, rashes, blood in urine, hearing or visual changes, sudden weight gain, edema.

- ◆ Warn against driving or activities that require alertness until response is determined.

- ◆ Reinforce the need for medical follow-up; advise telling dentist that tolmetin is being taken.

- ◆ For diabetics, explain the importance of monitoring blood sugars with a blood glucose meter.

- ◆ *See Nonsteroidal anti-inflammatory drugs overview for more information.*

tranylcypromine
tran-ill-sip'ro-meen

tranylcypromine sulfate: *Parnate*

Class: Monoamine oxidase inhibitor (MAOI), Antidepressant

PEDS	PREG	GERI
🖐️	C	🖐️

Action Improves mood by promoting accumulation of the neurotransmitters norepinephrine, serotonin, and dopamine in the CNS (inhibits monoamine oxidase, the major enzyme responsible for the breakdown of neurotransmitters). This drug has a more rapid onset of action than phenelzine sulfate or isocarboxazid.

Use/Therapeutic goal/Outcome

Major depressive disorders that have not responded to other forms of treatment including other antidepressants: Promotion of sense of well-being, ability to cope with daily living. *Outcome criteria:* After 2–4 weeks, report of feeling less depressed, less anxious, and more energetic and able to cope; return of normal sleeping and eating habits; demonstration of improved ability to problem solve and perform activities of daily living.

Dose range/Administration

Interaction alert: MAOIs such as this have a strong potential for severe and unpredictable side effects when taken with other medications: check with pharmacist to ascertain most recent information on interactions. It is known that use with alcohol, barbiturates, sedatives, narcotics, dextromethorphan, and TCAs have produced a variety of problems; use with amphetamines, ephedrine, levodopa, meperidine, metaraminol, phenylephrine, and phenylpropanolamine can cause severe hypertension. Monitor diabetics for altered hypoglycemic requirements. There is a potential for fatal hypertensive crisis if taken with tryptophan or foods or beverages containing tyramine (aged

cheese or wine, beer, avocados, chicken livers, chocolate, bananas, soy sauce, meat tenderizers, salami, or bologna).

Adult: PO: Begin with 10 mg morning and afternoon. After 1–2 weeks, may increase to 30 mg/day in divided doses. When improvement occurs, decrease to maintenance dose of 10 mg daily or bid.

Clinical alert: Because of the many unpredictable food and drug interactions (see Interaction alert), monitor diet and medication regimen closely. Hold drug and report if hypertension is noted. Keep phentolamine (Regitine) available to treat hypertension. Tranylcypromine is associated with unusually severe side effects.

Contraindications/Precautions
PREG C

Contraindicated in hypersensitivity to MAOIs, and in cardiac, renal, or hepatic disease, alcoholism, hypertension, and pheochromocytoma. *Use with caution* in suicidal tendency, seizure disorders, psychosis, diabetes mellitus, and hyperactive behavior.

🖐️ **Contraindicated for children under 16 years, pregnant or nursing mothers, and the elderly.**

Side effects/Adverse reactions

Hypersensitivity: rash. *CNS:* insomnia, dizziness, anxiety, headache, restlessness, hyperreflexia, tremors, muscle twitching, mania, confusion, memory impairment, fatigue, sedation. *CV:* orthostatic hypotension, palpitations, dysrhythmias, hypertensive crisis. *GI:* anorexia, dry mouth, nausea, diarrhea, constipation. *GU:* urinary frequency, decreased libido. *Eye:* blurred vision. *MS:* weight gain.

Nursing implications/Documentation

Possible nursing diagnoses: Potential for injury; Diarrhea; Constipation; Altered oral mucous membrane.

- ◆ Document mental status and vital signs daily until response to therapy has been established; then periodically thereafter.

- ◆ Check CBC, liver function, BUN, and creatinine before giving first dose and periodically thereafter.

- ◆ Be sure that doses are swallowed (not hoarded).

- ◆ Monitor for orthostatic hypotension, dizziness, and drowsiness; supervise ambulation until response is established.

T

◆ Record weights every 2 weeks; report significant weight gain.

◆ Monitor for and report suicidal tendencies, increased depression, or excessive hyperactivity.

◆ Prevent constipation by monitoring bowel movements and encouraging adequate fiber and fluid intake; offer laxatives or stool softeners before the problem becomes severe. Report diarrhea.

◆ Check with pharmacy and dietary department to determine dietary restrictions for MAOI; continue restrictions for 2 weeks after stopping drug because effects last a long time.

Patient & family teaching/Home care

Possible nursing diagnoses: Ineffective coping (family and individual); Sleep pattern disturbance; Impaired home maintenance management.

◆ Stress that this medication helps reduce the depression that inhibits ability to make decisions and cope effectively (once the individual feels less depressed, it will be easier to take steps toward making healthy changes).

◆ Explain that side effects are often noted immediately, but they usually diminish after a few weeks; on the other hand, it is likely to take 2–4 weeks before *beneficial* effects are noted (the patient may feel worse before feeling better).

◆ Provide a list of foods that must be avoided; emphasize the need to stick to restrictions.

◆ Warn to change positions slowly to prevent dizziness.

◆ Point out the role of adequate nutrition, exercise, and sleep in combating depression.

◆ Advise against taking any doses in the evening to avoid disturbing sleep.

◆ Emphasize that the effects of alcohol, sedatives, and tranquilizers may be potentiated.

◆ Caution to consult physician before using OTC drugs; stress the need for ongoing medical follow-up.

◆ Recommend reporting continued depression; stress that doses should not be increased or stopped without checking with physician (may cause severe problems).

◆ Advise avoidance of driving and other potentially hazardous activities until response is established.

◆ Suggest using ice chips, hard candy, or gum to relieve side effect of dry mouth; stress the need for good mouth care.

◆ Warn women to report if pregnancy is planned or suspected.

◆ *See Antidepressants overview for more information.*

trazodone
tray'zoe-done

trazodone hydrochloride: ***Desyrel, Trazon, Trialodine***

Class: Antidepressant

PEDS	PREG	GERI
✋	C	✋

Action Improves mood by increasing levels of the neurotransmitter serotonin in the CNS (selectively blocks serotonin reuptake). This drug is not chemically related to tricyclic antidepressants or MAOIs and has minimal anticholinergic and adverse cardiac effects.

Use/Therapeutic goal/Outcome

Major depressive disorders: Promotion of sense of well-being, ability to cope with daily living. **Outcome criteria:** After 2–4 weeks, report of feeling less depressed, less anxious, and more energetic and able to cope; return of normal sleeping and eating habits; demonstration of improved ability to problem solve and perform activities of daily living.

Dose range/Administration

Interaction alert: Alcohol and other CNS depressants may cause excessive sedation. Antihypertensive drug doses may need to be decreased because of hypotension, especially orthostatic hypotension. May increase digoxin and phenytoin levels (monitor for toxicity). Use extreme caution if given with MAOIs because there is no clinical experience with using these two drugs together.

🖐 **Give after meals or with a snack for best absorption and to reduce incidence of dizziness.**

Adult: PO: Begin with 50 mg tid, may gradually increase. *Maximum dose:* for hospitalized patients, 600 mg/day; for outpatients, 400 mg/day. *For the elderly and adolescents:* Begin with 50 mg/day, increase as needed to 100 mg/day.

Clinical alert: Report complaints of prolonged erections immediately. This drug has caused priapism, which may require surgical intervention.

Contraindications/Precautions

Contraindicated in hypersensitivity to trazodone hydrochloride, and for concomitant use with electroconvulsive therapy, and in acute recovery period of myocardial infarction. **Use with caution** for those with suicidal tendencies.

👆 **Contraindicated for children under 12 years and for pregnant or nursing mothers. Use with caution for adolescents and the elderly or debilitated.**

Side effects/Adverse reactions

Hypersensitivity: rash, sensitivity to sunlight. **CNS:** drowsiness, dizziness, fatigue, nervousness, agitation, confusion, tremors, weakness. **CV:** orthostatic hypotension, palpitations, tachycardia, hypertension. **GI:** anorexia, dry mouth, nausea, constipation, paralytic ileus. **GU:** urinary retention, priapism (may lead to impotence). **Eye:** blurred vision. **Ear:** tinnitus. **Skin:** sweating.

Nursing implications/Documentation

Possible nursing diagnoses: Potential for injury; Constipation; Altered oral mucous membrane.

♦ Document mental status and vital signs daily until response to therapy has been established.

♦ Be sure that doses are swallowed (not hoarded).

♦ Monitor for orthostatic hypotension, dizziness, and drowsiness; supervise ambulation until response is established.

♦ Record intake and output, and observe for dehydration or urinary retention; provide special mouth care.

♦ Monitor for and report suicidal tendencies, increased depression, or excessive drowsiness (may require change in medication).

♦ Prevent constipation by monitoring bowel movements and encouraging adequate fiber and fluid intake; offer laxatives or stool softeners before the problem becomes severe.

Patient & family teaching/Home care

Possible nursing diagnoses: Ineffective coping (family and individual); Sleep pattern disturbance; Impaired home maintenance management.

♦ Teach that doses should be taken with food.

♦ Stress that this medication helps reduce the depression that inhibits ability to make decisions and cope effectively (once the individual feels less depressed, it will be easier to take steps toward making healthy changes).

♦ Explain that side effects are often noted immediately, but they usually diminish after a few weeks; on the other hand, it is likely to take 2–4 weeks before *beneficial* effects are noted.

♦ Warn to change positions slowly to prevent dizziness.

♦ Point out the role of adequate nutrition, exercise, and sleep in combating depression.

♦ Emphasize that the effects of alcohol, sedatives, and tranquilizers may be potentiated.

♦ Caution to consult with physician before using OTC drugs; stress the need for ongoing medical follow-up.

♦ Advise avoidance of driving and other potentially hazardous activities until response is established.

♦ Suggest using ice chips, hard candy, or gum to relieve side effect of dry mouth; stress the need for good mouth care.

♦ Warn women to report if pregnancy is planned or suspected.

♦ *See Antidepressants overview for more information.*

tretinoin

tret'i-noyn

Retin-A, ✦StieVAA

Class: Antiacne agent (topical)

PEDS	PREG	GERI
OK	B	OK

Action Facilitates the removal of existing comedones and inhibits formation of new comedones by increasing epidermal cell mitosis and epidermal cell turnover.

Use/Therapeutic goal/Outcome

Acne vulgaris: Marked improvement, clearing of skin condition. **Outcome criteria:** Decrease in number and size of acneiform lesions.

Dose range/Administration

Interaction alert: Isotretinoin or with other topical acne preparations may cause cumulative irritant or drying effect. Not compatible with benzoyl peroxide.

T

Adult and Child: *Topical:Cream:* 0.01–0.1% hs. *Gel:* 0.01–0.1% hs. *Solution:* 0.025–0.1% hs.

Contraindications/Precautions

PREG
B

Contraindicated in hypersensitivity to tretinoin. **Use with caution** in eczema or sunburn.

✋ Use with caution for pregnant or nursing mothers.

Side effects/Adverse reactions

Hypersensitivity: rash. **Skin:** hyperpigmentation or hypopigmentation; rash, blistering, crusting, severe burning, redness, or swelling of skin.

Nursing implications/Documentation

Possible nursing diagnoses: Impaired skin integrity.

• Before therapy is begun, assess for recovery of skin from effects of other peeling agents.

• Monitor for severe blistering or swelling of treated areas.

Patient & family teaching/Home care

Possible nursing diagnoses: Knowledge deficit; Impaired home maintenance management; Impaired skin integrity; Body image disturbance.

• Stress the importance of using tretinoin only once daily (at bedtime) and avoiding contact with eyes, mouth, and nose.

• Teach how to wash skin with mild soap and warm water and pat dry; wait 20–30 min before applying tretinoin.

• With cream or gel, demonstrate how to apply enough to cover affected areas and to rub in gently.

• With solution, show how to use fingertips, gauze pad, or cotton swab, being careful not to oversaturate applicator.

• Caution that acne may appear to worsen during first 2 or 3 weeks of treatment.

• Advise against applying to windburned or sunburned skin or to open wounds.

• Stress the need to avoid using skin cleansers, medicated soaps, cosmetics with drying effects, or alcohol-containing preparations (e.g., shaving lotions, shaving creams, perfumed toiletries).

• Advise to wash face only 2–3 times daily with bland soap, especially before applying (nonmedicated) cosmetics.

• Warn to wear sunscreen (SPF #15) preparation or protective clothing over treated areas during exposure to sunlight; caution about increased sensitivity to wind and cold temperatures.

• Explain that improvement will be seen in about 6 weeks, but treatment should continue for at least 3 months.

• Acknowledge that acne is difficult for all young people; recognize the impact on body image, and encourage verbalizing feelings, frustrations, and concerns.

triamcinolone

trye-am-sin'oh-lone

triamcinolone: **Aristocort, Atolone, Kenacort, Tricilone**

triamcinolone acetonide: **Aristocort, Azmacort, Cenocort A, Cinonide, Flutex, Kenaject, Kenalog, ✦Kenalone, Tramacort, Triam-A, Triamonide, Triderm, Tri-Kort, Trilog**

triamcinolone diacetate: **Amcort, Aristocort Forte, Aristocort Intralesional, Articulose-L.A., Cinalone, Kenacort, Triam-Forte, Trilone, Tristoject**

triamcinolone hexacetonide: **Aristospan Intraarticular, Aristospan Intralesional**

Class: Synthetic adrenocorticosteroid, Intermediate-acting glucocorticoid, Steroidal anti-inflammatory, Immunosuppressant

PEDS	PREG	GERI
✋	C	✋

Action Suppresses inflammation by inhibiting accumulation of inflammatory cells, reducing dilatation and permeability of capillaries, and inhibiting release of chemical mediators of inflammation. Modifies immune response by suppressing cell-mediated immune reactions. Inhibits bronchoconstriction and enhances effects of bronchodilators.

Use/Therapeutic goal/Outcome

Inflammatory, immune, and allergic conditions: Symptomatic relief. **Outcome criteria:** Decreased symptoms associated with condition being treated.

Bronchial asthma: Improved air movement. **Outcome criteria:** Improved forced expiratory volume (FEV); decreased wheezing, coughing, and dyspnea.

Dose range/Administration

Interaction alert: May decrease effectiveness of anticoagulants and antidiabetics. Vaccines may lead to diminished antibody response and serious infection. Potassium-depleting diuretics may cause severe hypokalemia. Alcohol or medications known to cause gastric irritation may cause gastric bleeding. Drugs that increase metabolism of corticosteroids (e.g., phenytoin, barbiturates, ephedrine, and rifampin) and those that decrease its absorption (e.g., cholestyramine, colestipol, and antacids) may decrease triamcinolone levels, requiring an increase in triamcinolone dosage.

🖐 **Give oral doses with food or milk to reduce gastric irritation.**

Inflammatory, immune, and allergic conditions: **Adult:** PO: 4–48 mg/day. IM: 40–80 mg, repeat q 1–4 wk prn. *Topical:* Apply sparingly bid to qid. **Child:** PO: 0.4–1.7 mg/kg/day. IM: 40 mg, repeat q 1–4 wk prn. *Topical:* Apply sparingly qd to bid.

Asthma: **Adult:** *Inhalation:* 2 puffs tid to qid. *Maximum dose:* 16 puffs/day. **Child:** *Inhalation:* 1–2 puffs tid to qid. *Maximum dose:* 2 puffs/day.

Clinical alert: Give single daily or alternate-day doses in the morning to reduce adrenal suppression. Give IM doses deep into gluteal muscle to lessen muscle atrophy. With inhalation, give prescribed bronchodilator inhalation 5 minutes before triamcinolone to increase bronchial penetration. May also be injected directly into joints, soft tissues, or lesions.

Contraindications/Precautions

PREG C

Contraindicated in hypersensitivity to corticosteroids or to parabens or fluorocarbons (present in some preparations) and in active peptic ulcer disease, active tuberculosis or fungus infections, and herpes of eyes, lips, or genitals. *Use with caution* in acquired immunodeficiency syndrome (AIDS), hypertension, thrombophlebitis, congestive heart failure, diabetes mellitus, hypothyroidism, glaucoma, osteoporosis, myasthenia gravis, and history of bleeding ulcers, seizure disorder, or mental illness.

🖐 **Use with caution for children, pregnant or nursing mothers, and the elderly.**

Side effects/Adverse reactions

Hypersensitivity: rash, hives, hypotension, respiratory distress, anaphylaxis. *CNS:* euphoria, restlessness, insomnia, hallucinations, depression, psychosis. *Eye:* glaucoma, cataracts. *MS:* impaired growth in children. *CV:* thrombophlebitis, embolism, irregular heartbeat.

GI: increased appetite, oral candidiasis. *Misc:* hyperglycemia, withdrawal syndrome.

With prolonged use: *Skin:* acne; increased hair growth; thin, shiny skin; ecchymosis or petechiae; delayed wound healing. *GI:* nausea, vomiting, GI bleeding, pancreatitis. *MS:* osteoporosis; pain in hip, back, ribs, arms, or legs; muscle wasting. *CV:* hypertension, edema, hypokalemia. *GU:* menstrual irregularity. *Misc:* increased susceptibility to infection; Cushingoid appearance (moon-face and buffalo hump); withdrawal syndrome or acute adrenal insufficiency.

Nursing implications/Documentation

Possible nursing diagnoses: Impaired skin integrity; Impaired physical mobility; Fluid volume excess; Altered oral mucous membrane.

♦ Assess for hypersensitivity reactions, especially with parenteral administration.

♦ Record baseline weight, blood pressure, and electrolyte levels.

♦ Apply topical cream sparingly to clean, moist skin; occlusive dressing increases absorption.

♦ Assess for proper use of inhalation therapy; suggest use of spacer device if unable to coordinate inhalation with activation of inhaler.

♦ With oral inhalation, assess oral mucous membrane for signs of fungal infection; report and record abnormal findings.

♦ Assess and document improvement in condition being treated so dosage can be decreased as early as possible.

♦ Monitor for signs of infection and delayed wound healing.

♦ With prolonged use or high-dose therapy, assess for withdrawal symptoms (hypotension, hypoglycemia, weight loss, vomiting, and diarrhea) while tapering or discontinuing drug.

Patient & family teaching/Home care

Possible nursing diagnoses: Knowledge deficit; Impaired home maintenance management; Potential for infection; Body image disturbance.

♦ Explain the need to take oral doses with food or milk.

♦ Advise against taking OTC medications without consulting primary physician.

♦ Stress the need to adhere to prescribed dose schedule and not to discontinue medication against medical advice.

• Teach proper inhalation technique; advise to use prescribed bronchodilator inhalations 5 minutes before triamcinolone to increase bronchial penetration.

• With oral inhalation, advise to gargle and rinse mouth (without swallowing) after inhalation to help prevent fungal infection in mouth or throat.

• Teach the need to assess oral mucosa for creamy white patches indicating fungal infection; point out these should be reported.

• For long-term therapy, advise wearing a medical alert medal indicating need for supplemental systemic glucocorticoids in case of trauma or surgery.

• Caution to report unusual weight gain, swelling of lower extremities, muscle weakness, black tarry stools, vomiting of blood, epigastric burning, puffing of face, menstrual irregularities, prolonged sore throat, fever, cold, or infections; also advise reporting symptoms of adrenal insufficiency (fatigue, anorexia, nausea, vomiting, diarrhea, weight loss, weakness, dizziness, depression, and mood swings).

• During withdrawal from long-term systemic therapy, emphasize the need to follow prescribed schedules for gradual reduction of medication.

• Stress importance of medical follow-up for periodic evaluation of therapy.

• *See Adrenocorticosteroids overview for more information.*

triamterene
trye-am'ter-een

Dyrenium, ◆Dytac

Class: ★**Potassium-sparing diuretic prototype**

PEDS	PREG	GERI
✋	D	✋

Action Promotes excretion of sodium, chloride, and water, while sparing potassium, by inhibiting reabsorption of sodium in the distal tubule and collecting system of the kidney.

Use/Therapeutic goal/Outcome

Edema: Promotion of excretion of sodium and water, while sparing potassium. *Outcome criteria:* Increased urine output; weight loss; absence of peripheral and sacral edema.

Dose range/Administration

Interaction alert: Other potassium-sparing agents such as spironolactone or amiloride may increase risk of hyperkalemia.

🖐 **Give with meals to minimize GI upset.**
Adult: PO: 100 mg bid. *Maximum dose:* 300 mg/day. **Child:** PO: 2–4 mg/kg/day on alternate days in divided doses.

Clinical alert: Give doses in early morning and early afternoon to avoid nocturnal diuresis.

Contraindications/Precautions
PREG
D

Contraindicated in hypersensitivity to drug, hyperkalemia, hyperuricemia, gout, impaired renal or hepatic function. *Use with caution* in presence of fluid and electrolyte imbalances.

🖐 **Contraindicated for pregnant women. Use with caution for the elderly. Safe use for children and nursing mothers has not been established.**

Side effects/Adverse reactions

Hypersensitivity: anaphylaxis, rash, photosensitivity. *CNS:* headache, drowsiness, dizziness. *GI:* nausea, vomiting, thirst, dry mouth, metallic taste, sore throat. *Hem:* hyperkalemia, hyponatremia, hyperuricemia, thrombocytopenia, acidosis, increase in BUN. *CV:* dehydration, hypotension, leg cramps. *GU:* nephritis.

Nursing implications/Documentation

Possible nursing diagnoses: Fluid volume deficit; Altered patterns of urinary elimination; Potential for injury.

• Ascertain that baseline CBC, sodium, potassium, chloride, carbon dioxide, calcium, magnesium, BUN, creatinine, uric acid, and liver function studies have been obtained before giving first dose; report abnormalities and monitor closely thereafter.

• Watch for hyperkalemia, since this is a potassium-sparing diuretic.

• Document and monitor blood pressure, pulse, daily weight, and intake and output; report significant discrepancies.

• Observe for and report signs of fluid overload (auscultate lungs for rales; check feet, ankles, and sacrum for edema).

• Check with physician to determine dietary restrictions; consult with dietician to plan diet.

• Observe the elderly for extreme diuresis (may require lower doses); monitor for ortho-

T

static hypotension; supervise ambulation until response is determined.

Patient & family teaching/Home care

Possible nursing diagnoses: Knowledge deficit; Impaired home maintenance management.

◆ Before giving first dose, explain that the drug will increase the amount and frequency of urination.

◆ Advise taking this drug with food to prevent GI symptoms.

◆ Emphasize the importance of taking this drug exactly as prescribed, and the importance of returning for medical follow-up.

◆ Explain that diuretics enhance the work of the kidney and reduce the workload of the heart.

◆ Recommend taking doses in early morning and early afternoon to prevent the need to disturb sleep to void.

◆ Inform that triamterene may cause discoloration of urine.

◆ Advise reporting dizziness, shortness of breath, muscle weakness or spasms, swelling of hands and feet; encourage daily monitoring of weight and reporting sudden weight gain.

◆ Provide a list of allowed foods and fluids; stress the need to stick to prescribed diet (explain the hazards of too much salt or potassium).

◆ Warn against driving or activities that require alertness until response has been determined.

◆ Advise avoidance of OTC drugs unless approved by physician.

◆ Advise use of sun block preparations when exposed to sunlight.

◆ *See Diuretics and Antihypertensives overviews for more information.*

triazolam

try-az'oh-lam

Halcion

Class: Hypnotic, benzodiazepine

PEDS	PREG	GERI
✋	X	✋

CONTROLLED SUBSTANCE IV

Action Produces sleep by acting upon the limbic system, thalamus, and hypothalamus of the central nervous system. Onset of action is in 30 to 45 min, with a duration of 6 to 8 hr.

Use/Therapeutic goal/Outcome

Short-term insomnia: Promotion of sleep. ***Outcome criteria:*** Report of having slept well.

Dose range/Administration

Interaction alert: Use with cimetidine, alcohol, narcotics, analgesics, antihistamines, and other CNS depressants may intensify CNS depression.

Adult <65 yrs: PO: 0.125–0.5 mg at bedtime.
Adult >65 yrs: 0.125–0.25 mg at bedtime.

Clinical alert: Be aware that triazolam is rapid acting and potent. Overdosage may occur at 2 mg (four times highest recommended dose).

Contraindications/Precautions

PREG X

Contraindicated in hypersensitivity or intolerance to triazolam or other benzodiazepines. ***Use with caution*** for patients with depression, suicidal tendencies, and impaired liver or kidney function.

✋ **Contraindicated during pregnancy. Use with caution for nursing mothers and for the elderly. Safe use for children has not been established.**

Side effects/Adverse reactions

Hypersensitivity: rashes. ***CNS:*** lethargy, drowsiness, dizziness, confusion, coordination problems, amnesia, rebound insomnia. ***GI:*** anorexia, diarrhea. ***Misc:*** drug tolerance and dependence.

Nursing implications/Documentation

Possible nursing diagnoses: Potential for injury; Sensory/perceptual alterations (visual and auditory)

◆ Document mental status before administration, monitor patient activity closely following administration, and employ appropriate measures to ensure safety (i.e., side rails up, call bell within reach, and no unsupervised smoking).

◆ Be sure that doses are swallowed (not hoarded).

◆ Be aware that sedatives and hypnotics *do not provide pain relief* (patient may need an analgesic as well).

◆ Monitor for and report signs of overdosage (slurred speech, continued somnolence, respiratory depression, confusion) and tolerance (increased anxiety and/or increased wakefulness).

Patient & family teaching/Home care

Possible nursing diagnoses: Sleep pattern disturbance; Ineffective coping (family and individual); Impaired home maintenance management.

♦ Explore problems that may contribute to insomnia or anxiety and ways of coping effectively with the problems (stress that effective coping can promote restful sleep).

♦ Explain the importance of daily exercise in promoting rest and encourage the person to establish a method for getting enough exercise (e.g., daily walks).

♦ Stress that drug tolerance and dependence can occur, and that the drug should be used only when holistic measures (e.g., quiet music, relaxation techniques) don't work.

♦ Emphasize that the effects of alcohol, other sedatives, and tranquilizers may be potentiated, and that these should be avoided.

♦ Warn the patient that rebound insomnia can occur for 1–2 nights after stopping therapy; advise that coping through a few nights of insomnia without medication will help reestablish normal sleep pattern.

♦ Reinforce the importance of consulting with physician before using OTC drugs, and of returning for medical follow-up.

♦ Teach person to avoid driving and other potentially hazardous activities while under the effects of the medication.

♦ *See Antianxiety Agents, Sedatives, and Hypnotics overview for more information.*

trichlormethiazide   *trye-klor-meth-eye′a-zide*

Aquazide, Diurese, Metahydrin, Naqua

Class: Thiazide diuretic, Antihypertensive

PEDS	PREG	GERI
♛	B	♛

Action Promotes sodium, chloride, potassium, and water excretion by inhibiting sodium reabsorption in the early portion of the distal tubule. Lowers blood pressure by reducing plasma and extra-cellular volume.

Use/Therapeutic goal/Outcome

Hypertension: Promotion of diuresis, reduction of blood pressure. **Outcome criteria:** After 3–4 days, blood pressure within normal limits.
Edema: Promotion of diuresis, resolution of edema. **Outcome criteria:** Increased urine out-put; weight loss; absence of rales and peripheral edema.

Dose range/Administration

Interaction alert: Cholestyramine and colestipol decreases intestinal absorption. Diazoxide potentiates the hyperglycemic, hyperuricemic, and hypotensive effects. Nonsteroidal anti-inflammatory drugs may decrease effects. Do not give concomitantly with lithium. Give cautiously with corticosteroids, antidiabetics, lanoxin, and skeletal muscle relaxants.

Adult: PO: 1–4 mg/day or divided bid. **Child > 6 mos:** PO: 0.07 mg/kg/day.

Clinical alert: Give in morning to avoid nocturnal diuresis. Antihypertensive response may not occur for 3–4 days.

Contraindications/Precautions

PREG
B

Contraindicated in hypersensitivity to thiazides or sulfonamides, and in anuria and oliguria. **Use with caution** in patients with allergic history, bronchial asthma, renal or hepatic dysfunction, gout, diabetes, pancreatitis, arteriosclerosis, systemic lupus erythematosus, and debilitated states.

♛ **Contraindicated for pregnant or nursing mothers. Use with caution for children and the elderly.**

Side effects/Adverse reactions

Hypersensitivity: rash, urticaria, dermatitis with photosensitivity, pneumonitis, vasculitis. **Hem:** hypokalemia, hyperglycemia, impaired glucose tolerance, asymptomatic hyperuricemia, electrolyte imbalances, metabolic alkalosis, hypercalcemia, lipid abnormalities, aplastic anemia, agranulocytosis, leukopenia, thrombocytopenia. **CV:** volume depletion, orthostatic hypotension, dehydration. **GI:** anorexia, nausea, pancreatitis, hepatic encephalopathy. **Misc:** gout.

Nursing implications/Documentation

Possible nursing diagnoses: Fluid volume deficit; Altered patterns of urinary elimination; Potential for injury.

♦ Ascertain that baseline CBC, sodium, potassium, chloride, carbon dioxide, calcium, magnesium, BUN, creatinine, uric acid, and liver function studies have been obtained before giving first dose; report abnormalities and monitor closely thereafter.

- Document and monitor blood pressure, pulse, daily weight, and intake and output; report significant discrepancies.

- Monitor for hyperglycemia because of risk of thiazide diabetes.

- Observe for and report signs of fluid overload (auscultate lungs for rales; check feet, ankles, and sacrum for edema).

- Be aware the diuretics often induce hypokalemia, which predisposes individuals to cardiac arrhythmias, cramping, and digoxin toxicity.

- Check with physician to determine dietary restrictions; if a low-salt, high-potassium diet is recommended, consult with dietician to plan a low-salt diet that includes foods and juices high in potassium (orange juice; banana; green leafy vegetables).

- Observe the elderly for extreme diuresis (may require lower doses); monitor for orthostatic hypotension; supervise ambulation until response is determined.

Patient & family teaching/Home care

Possible nursing diagnoses: Knowledge deficit; Impaired home maintenance management.

- Before giving first dose, explain that the drug will increase the amount and frequency of urination.

- Emphasize the importance of taking this drug exactly as prescribed, and the importance of returning for medical follow-up.

- Explain that diuretics enhance the work of the kidney and reduce the workload of the heart.

- Recommend taking doses in early morning and early afternoon to prevent the need to disturb sleep to void.

- Explain that changing positions slowly helps prevent dizziness.

- Advise reporting dizziness, shortness of breath, swelling of hands and feet, or persistent sore throat; encourage daily monitoring of weight and reporting sudden weight gain.

- Warn that hyperglycemia is common; advise reporting thirst, fatigue, or weight loss.

- Provide a list of allowed foods and fluids; stress the need to stick to prescribed diet (explain the hazards of too much salt, or too little potassium).

- Warn against driving or activities that require alertness until response has been determined.

- Advise avoidance of OTC drugs unless approved by physician.

- Suggest using a (Number 15) sunscreen when outside because of photosensitivity (avoid products with PABA).

- *See Diuretics and Antihypertensives overviews for more information.*

trifluoperazine

try′floo-oh-per′a-zeen

trifluoperazine hydrochloride: **♥Apo-Trifluoperazine, ♠Calmazine, ♥Novo-Flurazine, ♥Solazine, Stelazine, Suprazine, ♥Terfluzine**

Class: Phenothiazine antipsychotic

PEDS	PREG	GERI
🖐	C	🖐

Action Exact mechanism of action has not been determined. Believed to produce calmness and alleviate psychiatric symptoms (disorders of perception, thought, consciousness, mood, affect, and social interaction) by blocking dopamine receptors in the limbic system. Blocks peripheral muscarinic, adrenergic, and histamine receptors. Also has some effect on the hypothalamus and pituitary gland, causing changes in regulation of body temperature and endocrine function. A dose of 5 mg of trifluoperazine is therapeutically equivalent to 100 mg of chlorpromazine.

Use/Therapeutic goal/Outcome

Schizophrenia, psychosis, agitation: Promotion of reality orientation, reduction in agitation. **Outcome criteria:** Demonstration of reality orientation, and ability to problem solve and interact with others, with decrease in signs of agitation (pacing, hyperactivity).

Extreme anxiety: Reduction in anxiety, promotion of sense of well-being. **Outcome criteria:** Report of less anxiety and improved sense of well-being and ability to cope.

Dose range/Administration

Interaction alert: Antacids reduce absorption; separate doses of antacid and trifluoperazine by at least 2 hours. Alcohol and other CNS depressants may cause excessive sedation. May reduce effects of centrally acting antihypertensives. Lithium may decrease effects. Concurrent use with beta blockers may result in increased concentration of both drugs.

▶

Schizophrenia, psychosis, agitation: *Adult:* PO: *For hospitalized patients:* 2–5 mg bid. *Maximum dose:* 15–20 mg/day. *For outpatients:* 1–2 mg bid. *Maximum dose:* 4 mg/day. IM: 1–2 mg q4-6h. *Child* > *6 yrs:* PO: 1 mg/day or bid. IM: not recommended.

Anxiety: *Adult:* PO: 1–2 mg bid. *Maximum dose:* 5 mg/day. Do not use longer than 12 wks.

Clinical alert: Avoid skin contact with liquid and parenteral forms (may cause contact dermatitis). Dilute liquid concentrate in at least 60 cc of juice, carbonated beverage, milk, or water just before giving dose. Before IM doses, count respirations and check blood pressure; hold dose and report if respirations are less than 12/min or if the patient is hypotensive. Keep patient lying down for 1 hour after injection. Keep IV diphenhydramine available in case of side effect of acute dystonic reaction.

Contraindications/Precautions

PREG C

Contraindicated in hypersensitivity to trifluoperazine or phenothiazines, severe CNS depression, and comatose states. *Use with caution* in seizure disorders, hypertension, Parkinson's disease, poorly controlled diabetes mellitus, asthma, emphysema, narrow-angle glaucoma, cardiac disease, hypotension, paralytic ileus, liver damage, prostatic hypertrophy, and bone marrow depression.

☝ **Contraindicated for nursing mothers. Use with caution for children over 6 years and the elderly or debilitated. Safe use for pregnant women and children under 6 years has not been established.**

Side effects/Adverse reactions

Hypersensitivity: rash, contact dermatitis. *CNS:* extrapyramidal reactions (pseudoparkinsonism, akathisia [restless need to keep moving], dystonia, tardive dykinesia), sedation, EEG changes, dizziness, neuroleptic malignant syndrome (fever, tachycardia, tachypnea, profuse diaphoresis). *CV:* orthostatic hypotension, palpitations, tachycardia, EKG changes. *GI:* appetite changes, dry mouth, constipation, abnormal liver function. *GU:* urinary retention or hesitancy, dark urine, priapism, impaired ejaculation, amenorrhea. *Eye:* blurred vision. *Skin:* photosensitivity, jaundice. *MS:* weight gain. *Hem:* hyperglycemia, transient leukopenia, agranulocytosis. *Misc:* galactorrhea, gynecomastia. *After abrupt withdrawal of long-term therapy:* gastritis, nausea, vomiting, lightheadedness, tremors, feeling of warmth or cold, diaphoresis, tachycardia, headache, insomnia.

Nursing implications/Documentation

Possible nursing diagnoses: Potential for injury; Constipation; Altered oral mucous membranes.

◆ Record mental status and vital signs before and 1–2 hours after administration during initial phase of treatment, then bid until response to therapy has been established, then periodically thereafter.

◆ Check CBC, liver function, BUN, and creatinine before giving first dose and periodically thereafter.

◆ Be sure that doses are swallowed (not hoarded).

◆ Monitor for orthostatic hypotension, dizziness, and drowsiness; supervise ambulation until response is established.

◆ Provide special mouth care; observe for and report oral ulcers.

◆ Prevent constipation by monitoring bowel movements and encouraging adequate fiber and fluid intake; offer laxatives or stool softeners before problem becomes severe.

◆ Report persistent sore throat, fever, and malaise, because these may indicate agranulocytosis.

◆ Monitor for (and report immediately) signs of neuroleptic malignant syndrome (muscle rigidity, tremors, high fever, tachycardia); this is a rare, but potentially fatal, side effect.

Patient & family teaching/Home care

Possible nursing diagnoses: Sleep pattern disturbance; Impaired home maintenance management.

◆ Emphasize the need to continue medication, even when feeling well.

◆ Warn to change positions slowly to avoid dizziness.

◆ Stress that the effects of alcohol, sedatives and CNS depressants, and tranquilizers may be potentiated.

◆ Caution to consult with physician before using OTC drugs; stress the need for ongoing medical follow-up.

◆ Teach the need to report persistent sore throat, fever, and fatigue.

◆ Point out that doses should not be increased or stopped without checking with physician.

◆ Caution to wear a sunscreen (number 15), protective clothing, and sunglasses when out in the sun.

◆ Advise avoidance of driving and other potentially hazardous activities until response is determined.

◆ Suggest using ice chips, hard candy, or gum to relieve side effect of dry mouth; stress the need for good mouth care.

◆ Warn women to report if pregnancy is planned or suspected.

◆ *See Antipsychotics overview for more information.*

triflupromazine
try-flew-proe'ma-zeen

triflupromazine hydrochloride: *Vesprin*

Class: Phenothiazine, Antipsychotic, Antiemetic

PEDS	PREG	GERI
🖐	C	🖐

Action Believed to promote calmness by blocking dopamine receptors in the limbic system. Reduces nausea and vomiting by inhibiting the chemoreceptor trigger zone in the brain. A dose of 25 mg is therapeutically equivalent to 100 mg of chlorpromazine.

Use/Therapeutic goal/Outcome

Agitation: Elimination of agitation and hyperactivity and promotion of reality orientation. *Outcome criteria:* Absence of agitation, hyperactivity.

Nausea and Vomiting: Relief of nausea and vomiting. *Outcome criteria:* Reports absence of nausea and demonstrates absence of vomiting.

Dose range/Administration

Interaction alert: Separate doses of antacid and phenothiazines by at least 2 hours or absorption may be reduced. Use with alcohol and other CNS depressants may cause excessive sedation. Barbiturates and lithium may decrease phenothiazine effects. May decrease antihypertensive effects of centrally acting antihypertensives. Propranolol may increase levels of both drugs. May decrease the effect of anticoagulants.

Agitation: Adult: IM: 60–150 mg in 2 or 3 divided doses. *Child > 2 1/2 yrs:* IM: 0.2 mg/kg in divided doses. Maximum daily dose is 10 mg.

Nausea and Vomiting: Adult: IM: 5–15 mg q4h. Maximum daily dose is 60 mg. IV: 1–3 mg daily. *Child > 2 1/2 yrs:* IM: 0.2 mg/kg in divided doses. Maximum dose is 10 mg.

Clinical alert: Expect reduced dosage for the elderly or debilitated. Give IM only in buttocks. Injection may sting.

Contraindications/Precautions
PREG
C

Contraindicated in hypersensitivity to phenothiazines, in withdrawal from alcohol, barbiturates, or other nonbarbiturate sedatives, and in CNS depression, comatose states, Parkinson's disease, asthma, emphysema, narrow-angle glaucoma, cardiac disease, hypotension. *Use with caution* in paralytic ileus, liver disease, prostatic hypertrophy, bone marrow depression, myasthenia gravis, Reye's syndrome.

🖐 **Contraindicated for children 2 1/2 years or younger, and for pregnant or nursing mothers. Use with caution for children and the elderly or debilitated.**

Side effects/Adverse reactions

Hypersensitivity: rash. *CNS:* sedation, extrapyramidal reactions including pseudoparkinsonism, akathisia (inability to sit down, need to keep moving) and dystonia, tardive dyskinesia; sedation, EEG changes, dizziness. *CV:* orthostatic hypotension, dysrhythmias, EKG changes. *GI:* appetite changes, dry mouth, susceptibility to oral thrush, constipation, abnormal liver function. *GU:* urinary retention, urinary hesitancy, dark urine, impaired ejaculation, amenorrhea. *Eye:* blurred vision, photophobia. *Skin:* photosensitivity. *MS:* weight gain. *Hem:* hyperglycemia, transient leukopenia, agranulocytosis. *Misc:* galactorrhea, gynecomastia, neuroleptic malignant syndrome (rare, and produces symptoms of fever, tachycardia, tachypnea, profuse diaphoresis); after abrupt withdrawal of long-term therapy, gastritis, nausea, vomiting, light-headedness, tremors, feeling of warmth or cold, diaphoresis, tachycardia, headache, insomnia.

Nursing implications/Documentation

Possible nursing diagnoses: Potential for injury; Constipation; Altered oral mucous membranes.

◆ Document mental status and vital signs before and 1 hour after administration during initial phase of treatment; then bid until response to therapy has been established; periodically thereafter.

T

• Check CBC, liver function, BUN, and creatinine before giving first dose, and periodically thereafter.

• Monitor for orthostatic hypotension, dizziness, and drowsiness; supervise ambulation until response is established.

• Record weights every 2 weeks; report significant weight gain.

• Provide special mouth care and observe for signs of oral candidiasis (may require medication).

• Prevent constipation by monitoring bowel movements and providing adequate fiber and fluid intake; offer laxatives or stool softeners before problem becomes severe.

• Report persistent sore throat, fever, and malaise because these may indicate agranulocytosis (drug may have to be discontinued).

Patient & family teaching/Home care

Possible nursing diagnoses: Sleep pattern disturbance; Noncompliance; Impaired home maintenance management.

• Warn to change positions slowly to prevent dizziness and falls.

• Explain that meticulous brushing and flossing can help to prevent side effect of oral infection.

• Stress that the effects of alcohol, sedatives, and tranquilizers may be potentiated.

• Caution to consult with physician before using OTC drugs; stress the need for ongoing medical follow-up.

• Teach the need to report persistent sore throat, fever, and fatigue.

• Point out that doses should not be increased or stopped without checking with physician.

• Advise to avoid driving and other potentially hazardous activities while under the effects of the medication.

• Suggest using ice chips, hard candy, or gum to relieve side effect of dry mouth.

• Teach that this drug may cause urine to be red or brown (due to a metabolite, not blood).

• Warn women to report if pregnancy is planned or suspected.

• *See Antipsychotics and Antiemetics overviews for more information.*

trihexyphenidyl   *trye-hex-ee-fen'i-dill*

trihexyphenidyl hydrochloride: ✿*Aparkane,* ✿*Apo-Trihex, Artane, Artane Sequels, Hexophen,* ✿*Novohexidyl, Trihexane, Trihexy-2, Trihexy-5*
Class: Anticholinergic, Cholinergic blocker (parasympatholytic)
Antidote: Physostigmine

PEDS	PREG	GERI
🖑	C	🖑

Action Reduces abnormal motor activity by blocking excess CNS cholinergic activity associated with dopamine deficiency in basal ganglia. Also has some peripheral anticholinergic actions.

Use/Therapeutic goal/Outcome

Drug-induced parkinsonism or parkinsonism: Control of symptoms of parkinsonism; promotion of mobility. **Outcome criteria:** Absence of or decrease in tremors, rigidity, akinesia, and drooling; improvement in gait, balance, posture, and speech.

Dose range/Administration

Interaction alert: Reduce dosage when administering with amantadine (may cause confusion and hallucinations). Antihistamines, tricyclic antidepressants, antipsychotics, narcotics, and MAOIs may increase effects.

🥄 **Give with or after meals (causes nausea if given on an empty stomach).**

Adult: PO: 1 mg tid to qid (last dose hs), then increase by 2 mg q 3–5 days. *Maximum dose:* 6–10 mg/day for elixir and 10–15 mg/day for tablets. *Extended release:* (after stabilized on conventional forum) 5 mg with breakfast and 5 mg 12h later.

Clinical alert: Available in extended-release form and in elixir. Report deterioration in symptoms (some patients develop a tolerance and require an increase in dosage).

Contraindications/Precautions   PREG
                                           C

Contraindicated in hypersensitivity to trihexyphenidyl hydrochloride, and in narrow-angle glaucoma. **Use with caution** in hypertension, cardiac, hepatic or renal disease, obstructive diseases of GI or urinary tract, and prostatic hypertrophy.

🖑 **Use with caution for the elderly. Safe use for children and pregnant or nursing mothers has not been established.**

Side effects/Adverse reactions

Hypersensitivity: rash. **GI:** dry mouth, constipation, nausea. **CNS:** dizziness, nervousness, confusion, insomnia. **CV:** tachycardia, hypotension. **Eye:** increased intraocular pressure, blurred vision. **GU:** urinary retention.

Nursing implications/Documentation

Possible nursing diagnoses: Potential for injury; Urinary retention; Constipation.

◆ Have patient void before doses; monitor intake and output because this drug can cause voiding difficulties.

◆ Record status of Parkinson symptoms daily (or every visit).

◆ Monitor the elderly or debilitated for increased incidence of side effects; document and report changes in mental status.

◆ Relieve dry mouth by providing frequent mouth care and keeping ice chips at the bedside.

◆ Monitor for constipation; provide adequate fluids and fiber (laxatives and/or stool softeners should be given before problem is severe).

Patient & family teaching/Home care

Possible nursing diagnoses: Knowledge deficit; Impaired home maintenance management.

◆ Stress that taking this drug on an empty stomach is likely to cause nausea.

◆ Warn that this drug may cause drowsiness and dizziness; caution to change position slowly.

◆ Point out that constipation is a common side effect; stress the need for adequate fluids, fiber, and exercise.

◆ Advise having an eye exam and to inform eye doctor that this drug is being taken (intraocular pressure and eye motility should be monitored).

◆ Caution against driving until response is determined.

◆ *See Anticholinergics overview for more information.*

trilostane

trye-loss'tane

Modrastane

Class: Antineoplastic agent, Hormone

PEDS	PREG	GERI
✋	X	✋

Action Suppresses adrenal cortex by blocking synthesis of adrenal steroids.

Use/Therapeutic goal/Outcome

Adrenal cancer, and suppression of adrenal cortical hyperfunction in Cushing's syndrome: Suppression of malignant cell proliferation; decreased synthesis of adrenal steroids. **Outcome criteria:** Tumor and disease regression or stabilization on radiologic and physical examination; decreased circulating levels of adrenocortical hormones.

Dose range/Administration

Interaction alert: Aminoglutethimide and mitotane may cause severe adrenocortical hypofunction.

Adult: PO: 30 mg qid; may increase to 480 mg/day.

Clinical alert: In case of severe trauma or stress, expect that trilostane will be stopped and corticosteroid replacement therapy will be ordered (stress causes an increased risk of adrenocortical insufficiency).

Contraindications/Precautions

PREG
X

Contraindicated in hypersensitivity to trilostane, and in hypothyroidism, and severe renal or hepatic disease. **Use with caution** with other drugs that suppress adrenal function.

✋ **Contraindicated for children and pregnant or nursing mothers. Use with caution for the elderly.**

Side effects/Adverse reactions

Hypersensitivity: rash, fever. **GI:** anorexia, nausea, vomiting, flatulence, bloating, diarrhea, hepatotoxicity. **CNS:** dizziness, headache. **CV:** orthostatic hypotension, tachycardia. **Misc:** adrenocortical insufficiency.

Nursing implications/Documentation

Possible nursing diagnoses: Fluid volume deficit; Altered patterns of urinary elimination; Self-esteem disturbance; Potential for injury; Altered nutrition: less than body requirements.

◆ *See important Nursing implications in Antineoplastic agents overview.*

◆ Check baseline and periodic early morning cortisol levels.

◆ Monitor blood pressure for orthostatic hypotension (trilostane suppresses aldosterone and can cause hypotension); supervise ambulation until response is determined.

T

Patient & family teaching/Home care

Possible nursing diagnoses: Impaired home maintenance management; Knowledge deficit.

♦ *See important Patient & family teaching in Antineoplastic agents overview.*

  ♦ Advise that this drug may be discontinued if no results are seen within 2 weeks.

  ♦ Explain that steroid supplements may be required during periods of stress.

♦ *See Antineoplastic agents overview for more information.*

trimeprazine tartrate
try-mep'ra-zeen

♦Panectyl, Temaril

Class: Phenothiazine, Antihistamine (H₁ receptor antagonist), Antipruritic

PEDS	PREG	GERI
👎	C	✋

Action Prevents but does not reverse histamine-mediated allergic responses by competing with histamine at H₁ receptors. Actually a phenothiazine, it has prominent antipruritic activity. Exerts anticholinergic and antiserotonin effects. Suppresses cough reflex.

Use/Therapeutic goal/Outcome

Pruritus: Relief of itching. **Outcome criteria:** Report and demonstration of an absence of itching and scratching.

Dose range/Administration

Interaction alert: CNS depressants and alcohol may cause excessive drowsiness and sedation.

🖐 **Give with milk or food to reduce GI symptoms.**

Adult/Child > 12 yrs: PO: *Tablet, syrup:* 2.5 mg hs, or 2.5 mg tid prn. *Sustained-release capsule:* 5 mg q12h. **Child > 6 yrs:** PO: *Sustained-release capsule:* 5 mg/day. **Child 3–6 yrs:** PO: *Tablet, syrup:* 2.5 mg hs, or 2.5 mg tid, if needed. **Child 6 mos–3 yrs:** PO: *Syrup:* 1.25 mg hs, or 1.25 mg tid, if needed.

Clinical alert: Do not give sustained-release capsules to children under 6 years.

Contraindications/Precautions

PREG C

Contraindicated in hypersensitivity to trimeprazine or phenothiazines, in coma, and drug-induced CNS depression. **Use with extreme caution** in acute asthma, narrow-angle glaucoma, prostatic hypertrophy, stenosing peptic ulcer, bladder-neck obstruction, and MAOI therapy. **Use with caution** in upper respiratory infections, impaired hepatic function, history of ulcer disease, history of convulsive disorder, and for debilitated patients.

🖐 **Contraindicated for premature infants, newborns, and nursing mothers. Use with caution for the elderly. Safe use in pregnancy and children under 6 months has not been established.**

Side effects/Adverse reactions

Hypersensitivity: skin rash. **CNS:** drowsiness, dizziness, extrapyramidal reactions; (occasionally in children) paradoxical hyperactivity, irritability, insomnia, hallucinations. **GI:** GI upset, cholestatic jaundice.

Nursing implications/Documentation

Possible nursing diagnoses: Potential for injury; Impaired skin integrity.

♦ Determine and record known allergies; provide an environment that is free from allergens (e.g., use nonallergic linens).

♦ Observe skin closely for signs of increased inflammation; report open areas to physician.

♦ Keep fingernails clipped as short as possible (especially children).

♦ Monitor for drowsiness until response is established.

♦ If therapy is prolonged, monitor for blood dyscrasias (toxic effects are most likely to occur in first 4–10 weeks of therapy).

Patient & family teaching/Home care

Possible nursing diagnoses: Knowledge deficit; Impaired home maintenance management.

♦ Advise taking this drug with food or milk if GI symptoms are experienced.

♦ Assess for environmental allergens at home, and help identify ways of avoiding contact (e.g., use nonallergenic linen); teach holistic methods of reducing itching (e.g., applying cool compresses, avoiding moisture and heat).

♦ Stress the need to use a sunscreen when outside.

♦ Explain that side effect of drowsiness should diminish after a few days of treatment; advise not to drive until response is determined.

♦ Warn that alcohol and other CNS depressants may cause excessive drowsiness.

* Explain that antihistamines should be stopped for 4 days before allergy testing to ensure accurate results.

◆ *See Antihistamines overview for more information.*

trimethaphan *trye-meth'a-fan*

Arfonad

Class: Antihypertensive, ganglionic blocking agent

PEDS	PREG	GERI
✋	C	✋

Action Profoundly lowers blood pressure by reducing autonomic stimulation of the heart and blood vessels (blocks the effects of acetylcholine on all nicotinic receptors in the ganglia; also has a direct vasodilatory action on peripheral blood vessels). Promotes release of histamine.

Use/Therapeutic goal/Outcome

Hypertensive emergencies: Reduction of blood pressure. **Outcome criteria:** Blood pressure within normal limits.

Dose range/Administration

Interaction alert: Other antihypertensives, diuretics, and anesthetics may potentiate hypotensive effects. Do not mix with any other drugs in IV solution.

Adult: IV: Dilute 500 mg in 500 cc D5W. Begin infusion at 3–4 mg/min, and titrate to desired blood pressure. Administer with an infusion pump or controller. **Child:** IV: 50–100 mcg/min, adjusted according to response.

Clinical alert: Document vital signs every 2 minutes until stable; every 5 minutes thereafter during infusion; every 30 minutes for 2 hours after infusion, and then every 4 hours. It may take 48 hours of administration before significant response is seen.

Contraindications/Precautions
PREG
C

Contraindicated in hypersensitivity to trimethaphan, and with history of allergy (drug liberates histamine); in hypovolemia, shock, respiratory insufficiency, asphyxia, anemia, and glaucoma. **Use with caution** for debilitated patients, and in cardiac disease, arteriosclerosis, hepatic or renal disease, degenerative CNS disease, diabetes, Addison's disease, and patients taking steriods.

✋ **Contraindicated for pregnant women. Use with caution for children and the elderly.**

Side effects/Adverse reactions

Hypersensitivity: rash, pruritis, histamine reaction at site of venous injection. **CV:** severe orthostatic hypotension, tachycardia. **Resp:** respiratory depression. **GI:** nausea, vomiting, anorexia. **GU:** urinary retention. **CNS:** weakness, depression. **Eye:** dilated pupils.

Nursing implications/Documentation

Possible nursing diagnoses: Activity intolerance; Fatigue; Potential for injury.

◆ Assess mental status before administration, and frequently thereafter until response is determined; monitor for confusion, dizziness, respiratory distress, bradycardia, hypotension (report immediately if these occur).

◆ Consult with physician to determine desired therapeutic range for blood pressure (be aware that some patients may require a slightly elevated blood pressure to perfuse vital organs).

◆ Ascertain that baseline CBC, electrolytes, BUN, creatinine, and liver function studies have been obtained before giving first dose; report abnormalities and monitor closely thereafter.

◆ Document and monitor intake and output; report significant negative or positive balance (be aware that ganglionic blockade may reduce ability to void).

Patient & family teaching/Home care

Possible nursing diagnoses: Knowledge deficit; Impaired home maintenance management.

◆ Explain that vital signs will be taken frequently to fine-tune medication to optimum dose.

◆ Encourage reporting of new symptoms (e.g., dizziness, breathing difficulties), which may indicate a need for dose adjustment.

◆ *See Antihypertensives overview for more information.*

T

trimethobenzamide *try-meth-oh-ben'za-mide*

trimethobenzamide hydrochloride: **Tebamide, Tegamide, Ticon, Tigan, Tiject-20**

Class: Antiemetic

PEDS	PREG	GERI
✋	C	✋

Action Treats and prevents nausea and vomiting by acting on the chemoreceptor trigger zone.

▶

Use/Therapeutic goal/Outcome

Nausea and vomiting: Prevention or resolution. *Outcome criteria:* Report of absence of, or reduction in, feelings of nausea; absence of vomiting.

Dose range/Administration

Interaction alert: Because of CNS depressant effects, may increase effects of other CNS depressants (antihistamines, narcotics, sedatives) and alcohol.

Adult: PO: 250 mg tid or qid. Capsules may be opened and mixed with liquid or food if swallowing is difficult. IM, RECT: 200 mg tid or qid, or q3-4h prn. *Child:* Do not use if viral illness is suspected because it may contribute to Reye's syndrome. RECT, PO: *For weight < 13 kg:* Use only for prolonged vomiting of unknown origin; 100 mg tid or qid. *For weight 13–40 kg:* 100–200 mg tid or qid.

Clinical alert: Give IM doses deep into well-developed muscle mass to minimize tissue irritation; never give SC.

Contraindications/Precautions

PREG
C

Contraindicated in hypersensitivity to this drug, and (for suppository form) in the presence of hypersensitivity to benzocaine hydrochloride or similar local anesthetics.

✋ Contraindicated for children (if viral illness is suspected). Use with caution for the elderly. Safe use for pregnant or nursing mothers has not been determined.

Side effects/Adverse reactions

Hypersensitivity: rashes. *CNS:* drowsiness, dizziness. *CV:* hypotension. *GI:* diarrhea, increase in nausea (in large doses), hepatitis.

Nursing implications/Documentation

Possible nursing diagnoses: Potential for injury; Altered nutrition: less than body requirements; Fluid volume deficit; Altered oral mucous membranes.

♦ Assess for presence of bowel sounds, pain, nausea, or vomiting before and after administering antiemetics; hold drug and report if bowel sounds are absent.

♦ Determine cause of symptoms before giving antiemetics; ascertain that nausea and vomiting symptoms are not due to intestinal obstruction, increased intracranial pressure, or drug overdosage before giving first dose.

♦ Monitor for orthostatic hypotension, tachycardia, or drowsiness.

♦ Offer frequent mouth care.

♦ Supervise ambulation until response is determined.

♦ Document and monitor intake and output to detect dehydration.

♦ When able to tolerate liquids, begin with small amount of ice chips, then water, then clear liquids, then full liquids, then food.

Patient & family teaching/Home care

Possible nursing diagnoses: Knowledge deficit; Impaired home maintenance management.

♦ Stress that persistent nausea, vomiting, or abdominal discomfort should be reported.

♦ Explain that avoiding fatty foods and eating smaller and more frequent meals may reduce nausea.

♦ Advise against using alcohol or other CNS depressants; warn against driving or activities that require mental alertness.

♦ Point out the need to maintain good mouth care, especially when not taking liquids by mouth; suggest that chewing sugarless gum may relieve symptoms of dry mouth.

♦ *See Antiemetics overview for more information.*

trimethoprim
trye-meth'oh-prim

➡*Alprin, Proloprim, Trimpex,* ➡*Triprim*
Class: Urinary tract anti-infective, Antibiotic, Folic acid inhibitor, Enzyme inhibitor

PEDS	PREG	GERI
✋	C	OK

Action Kills bacteria (bactericidal) by blocking synthesis of folic acid.

Use/Therapeutic goal/Outcome

Uncomplicated urinary tract infections (caused by susceptible strains of *Escherichia coli, Proteus mirabilis, Klebsiella,* and *Enterobacter:* Resolution of infection. *Outcome criteria:* Absence of pathogenic growth on culture; report of absence of dysuria, frequency.

Dose range/Administration

Adult/Child > 12 yrs: PO: 100 mg q12h for 10 days.

Clinical alert: Monitor for and report for signs of side effect of blood dyscrasias (sore throat, fever, pallor, purpura).

Contraindications/Precautions

Contraindicated in hypersensitivity to tri-methoprim, with creatinine clearance less than 15 ml/min. *Use with caution* in liver or kidney impairment and megaloblastic anemia due to folic acid deficiency.

✋ **Contraindicated for children under 12 years and pregnant or nursing mothers.**

Side effects/Adverse reactions

Hypersensitivity: itching, rashes. *GI:* nausea, vomiting, epigastric discomfort, inflamed tongue. *Skin:* photosensitivity. *Hem:* (secondary to bone marrow depression) thrombocytopenia, leukopenia, megaloblastic anemia, methemoglobinemia. *Misc:* fever.

Nursing implications/Documentation

Possible nursing diagnoses: Potential for infection; Altered patterns of urinary elimination.

◆ Obtain necessary cultures and baseline lab studies (CBC, BUN, creatinine, and liver function) before giving first dose; monitor closely thereafter if therapy is prolonged.

◆ Provide preferred fluids (2 L/day), and document and monitor intake and output, to ensure adequate hydration.

Patient & family teaching/Home care

Possible nursing diagnoses: Knowledge deficit; Impaired home maintenance management.

◆ Stress the importance of taking the drug for the entire time prescribed, even if symptoms abate.

◆ Teach the need to report new symptoms (sore throat, fever); medication change may be necessary.

◆ Advise maintaining fluid intake of 2 L of fluid daily to ensure adequate hydration.

◆ *See Anti-infectives overview for more information.*

trimipramine

tri-mip'ra-meen

trimipramine maleate ✦*Apo-Trimip, Surmontil*

Class: Tricyclic antidepressant (TCA)

PEDS	PREG	GERI
✋	C	✋

Action Improves mood by increasing levels of the neurotransmitter norepinephrine in the CNS. (Blocks neurotransmitter reuptake into presynaptic neurons by inhibiting the "amine pump."

Reuptake normally terminates the action of neurotransmitters.) Has a strong sedative effect.

Use/Therapeutic goal/Outcome

Major depressive disorders: Promotion of sense of well-being, ability to cope with daily living. *Outcome criteria:* After 2–4 weeks, report of feeling less depressed, less anxious, and more energetic and able to cope; return of normal sleeping and eating habits; demonstration of improved ability to problem solve and perform activities of daily living.

Dose range/Administration

Interaction alert: Barbiturates may reduce antidepressant blood levels and effects. Cimetidine may increase blood levels. If given with epinephrine and norepinephrine, monitor for increased risk of hypertension. Avoid use with MAOIs (risk of excitation, hyperpyrexia, and seizures). Give cautiously with thyroid drugs because of increased CNS stimulation and cardiac arrhythmias.

👍 **Give with (or immediately after) food to reduce GI symptoms.**

Adult: PO: 75 mg/day in divided doses or entire dose at hs, may gradually increase to a maximum of 300 mg/day. *For the elderly and adolescents:* Begin with 50 mg/day and increase as needed to 150 mg/day.

Clinical alert: When possible, give entire dose at hs to reduce daytime sedation.

Contraindications/Precautions

Contraindicated in hypersensitivity to TCAs, for concomitant use with electroconvulsive therapy, and in acute recovery period of myocardial infarction. *Use with caution* in renal or hepatic disease, glaucoma, prostatic hypertrophy, urinary retention, hypomania, mania, and suicidal tendencies.

✋ **Contraindicated for children under 12 years and pregnant or nursing mothers. Use with caution for adolescents and the elderly or debilitated.**

Side effects/Adverse reactions

Hypersensitivity: rash, sensitivity to sunlight. *CNS:* drowsiness, dizziness, anxiety, headache, fatigue, nervousness, agitation, extrapyramidal symptoms, sedation. *CV:* orthostatic hypotension, palpitations, tachycardia, hypertension. *GI:* anorexia, dry mouth, nausea, constipation, paralytic ileus. *GU:* urinary retention,

T

decreased libido. *Eye:* blurred vision. *Ear:* tinnitus. *Hem:* agranulocytosis. *Misc:* (after abrupt withdrawal of long-term therapy) nausea, headache, malaise.

Nursing implications/Documentation

Possible nursing diagnoses: Potential for injury; Constipation; Altered oral mucous membrane.

♦ Document mental status and vital signs daily until response to therapy has been established.

♦ Be sure that doses are swallowed (not hoarded).

♦ Monitor for orthostatic hypotension, dizziness, and drowsiness; supervise ambulation until response is established.

♦ Record intake and output, and observe for dehydration or urinary retention; provide special mouth care.

♦ Monitor for and report suicidal tendencies, increased depression, or excessive drowsiness (may require change in medication).

♦ Prevent constipation by monitoring bowel movements and encouraging adequate fiber and fluid intake; offer laxatives or stool softeners before the problem becomes severe.

Patient & family teaching/Home care

Possible nursing diagnoses: Ineffective coping (family and individual); Sleep pattern disturbance; Impaired home maintenance management.

♦ Stress that this medication helps reduce the depression that inhibits ability to make decisions and cope effectively (once the individual feels less depressed, it will be easier to take steps toward making healthy changes).

♦ Explain that side effects are often noted immediately, but they usually diminish after a few weeks; on the other hand, it is likely to take 2–4 weeks before *beneficial* effects are noted (the patient may feel worse before feeling better).

♦ Warn to change positions slowly to prevent dizziness.

♦ Point out the role of adequate nutrition, exercise, and sleep in combating depression.

♦ Emphasize that the effects of alcohol, sedatives, and tranquilizers may be potentiated.

♦ Caution to consult with physician before using OTC drugs; stress the need for ongoing medical follow-up.

♦ Recommend reporting continued depression; stress that doses should not be increased or stopped without checking with physician because this may cause severe problems.

♦ Advise avoidance of driving and other potentially hazardous activities until response is established.

♦ Suggest using ice chips, hard candy, or gum to relieve side effect of dry mouth; stress the need for good mouth care.

♦ Warn women to report if pregnancy is planned or suspected.

♦ *See Antidepressants overview for more information.*

tripelennamine   *try-pel-een'a-min*

tripelennamine citrate: *PBZ*

tripelennamine hydrochloride: *PBZ, PBZ-SR, Pelamine, Pynbenzamine*

Class: Antihistamine (H_1 receptor antagonist), Enzyme inhibitor

PEDS	PREG	GERI
✋	B	✋

Action Prevents but does not reverse histamine-mediated allergic responses by competing with histamine at H_1 receptors. Has antiemetic, antitiussive, and mild CNS depressant effects.

Use/Therapeutic goal/Outcome

Allergic conditions: Decrease in allergic response. *Outcome criteria:* Patient demonstrates and reports relief of allergic symptoms (nasal secretions, sneezing, itching).

Dose range/Administration

Interaction alert: Use with CNS depressants or alcohol may cause excessive drowsiness. Do not give with MAOIs or anticholinergics.

🍂 **Give with food or milk to reduce GI distress, unless given for motion sickness.**

Adult: PO: 25 to 50 mg q4-6h (as much as 600 mg daily in divided doses, if necessary). Long-acting tablets and sustained relief form: 100 mg morning and evening or q8-12h, not to exceed 600 mg/24h. *Child:* PO: 5 mg/kg/24h divided into 4–6 doses, not to exceed 300 mg/24h.

Clinical alert: Do not give sustained release form to children. Expect reduced dosage for the elderly and monitor closely for drowsiness, dizziness.

Contraindications/Precautions

Contraindicated in hypersensitivity to antihistamines of similar structure, and in narrow-angle glaucoma, symptomatic prostatic hypertrophy, bladder-neck obstruction, GI obstruction or stenosis, and in use within 14 days of MAOIs. *Use with caution* in history of asthma, convulsive disorders, increased intraocular pressure, hyperthyroidism, cardiovascular disease, hypertension, diabetes mellitus.

☙ **Do not give sustained-release form to children. Use with caution for the elderly. Safe use for pregnant or nursing mothers and for neonates and premature infants has not been established.**

Side effects/Adverse reactions

Hypersensitivity: rash. *CNS:* moderate sedation, paradoxical excitation, hyperirritability. *GI:* GI distress.

Nursing implications/Documentation

Possible nursing diagnoses: Potential for injury; Fluid volume deficit.

◆ Determine and record known allergies; provide an environment that is free from allergens.

◆ Provide favorite fluids and ensure adequate hydration (2 L/day).

Patient & family teaching/Home care

Possible nursing diagnoses: Knowledge deficit; Impaired home maintenance management.

◆ Advise taking this drug with food or milk if GI symptoms are experienced; warn not to chew sustained-release tablets.

◆ Stress that dosage should not be increased without physician's approval; explain that tolerance may occur, requiring a change in medication.

◆ Warn that combining with alcohol or other CNS depressants may cause excessive drowsiness; advise against driving until response is determined.

◆ Point out that avoiding pollens and staying in an air-conditioned environment may help reduce seasonal rhinitis.

◆ Suggest that coffee or tea may reduce drowsiness and that sugarless gum or hard candy may relieve dry mouth.

◆ Explain that antihistamines should be stopped for 4 days before allergy testing to ensure accurate results.

◆ See *Antihistamines overview* for more information.

triprolidine

trye-poe'li-deen

triprolidine hydrochloride: *Actidil, Myidyl*

Class: Antihistamine (H$_1$ receptor antagonist)

PEDS	PREG	GERI
☙	C	☙

Action Prevents but does not reverse histamine-mediated allergic responses by competing with histamine for H$_1$ receptors on effector cells.

Use/Therapeutic goal/Outcome

Colds and allergy symptoms: Relief of symptoms. *Outcome criteria:* Patient reports and demonstrates absence of (or decrease in) nasal symptoms (sneezing, stuffiness, excessive secretions).

Dose range/Administration

Interaction alert: Alcohol and CNS depressants may cause excessive drowsiness. Do not give with MAOIs or anticholinergics.

☙ **Give with milk or food to avoid GI upset.**

Adult: PO: 2.5 mg q4-6h to a maximum of 10 mg/day. *Child > 6 yrs:* PO: 1.25 mg q4-6h to a maximum of 5 mg/day. *Child 4–6 yrs:* PO: 0.9 mg q4-6h to a maximum of 2.5 mg/day. *Child 4 mos–6 yrs:* PO: 0.3 mg q4-6h to a maximum of 1.25 mg/day.

Clinical alert: For children under 12 years, give only under the direction of a physician. Monitor children and the elderly for excessive CNS side effects.

Contraindications/Precautions

Contraindicated in hypersensitivity to H$_1$ receptor antagonists, and in acute asthma and lower respiratory tract disease. *Use with caution* in increased intraocular pressure, cardiac disease, hypertension, kidney disease, bronchial asthma, seizure disorders, diabetes, stenosed gastric ulcers, hyperthyroidism, prostatic hypertrophy, and bladder-neck obstruction.

☙ **Use with caution for children and the elderly. Avoid use for pregnant or nursing mothers (use only if benefits outweigh risk; safe use is not established).**

Side effects/Adverse reactions

Hypersensitivity: exaggeration of side effects, itching, rashes. *CNS:* drowsiness, dizziness,

T

coordination problems, fatigue, confusion, paresthesia, neuritis. *GI:* constipation, dry mouth and throat, anorexia, nausea, vomiting, diarrhea. *GU:* retention, dysuria, frequency. *Resp:* nasal stuffiness, thick secretions, wheezing, chest tightness.

Nursing implications/Documentation

Possible nursing diagnoses: Potential for injury; Constipation; Fluid volume deficit; Urinary retention.

♦ Determine and record known allergies; provide an environment that is free from allergens (especially sleeping areas).

♦ Provide favorite fluids to ensure adequate hydration.

♦ Monitor for urinary retention; if this is a problem, have patient void before doses (if this does not work, may have to change medication).

♦ Monitor bowel elimination for constipation; provide adequate fluid and fiber intake, and give mild laxatives before problem is severe.

Patient & family teaching/Home care

Possible nursing diagnoses: Knowledge deficit; Impaired home maintenance management.

♦ Advise taking this drug with milk or food to reduce GI symptoms.

♦ Stress the need to drink at least 2 quarts a day; point out that constipation is a side effect and may be avoided by adequate exercise and fluid and fiber intake.

♦ Point out that avoiding pollens and staying in an air-conditioned room may help reduce symptoms of seasonal allergies.

♦ Caution family members that children and the elderly are more likely to experience excessive side effects (children under 12 years should be given this drug only under the direction of a physician).

♦ Recommend avoiding driving or activities that require alertness until response is determined.

♦ Warn that alcohol and other CNS depressants cause excessive drowsiness.

♦ Suggest that coffee or tea may help reduce drowsiness, and that hard candy or sugarless gum may help relieve dry mouth.

♦ Explain that this drug should not be taken for 4 days before allergy testing.

♦ See *Antihistamines* overview for more information.

tubocurarine   *too-boe-kyoo-ar'een*

tubocurarine chloride: ✦*Tubarine, D-Tubocurarine*
Class: ★**Nondepolarizing neuromuscular blocker prototype**, Skeletal-muscle relaxant
Antidote: Neostigmine methylsulfate

PEDS	PREG	GERI
OK	**C**	🖐

Action Relaxes or paralyzes skeletal muscles (depending on dose) by competing with acetylcholine at cholinergic receptor sites at the myoneural junction, thereby blocking neuromuscular transmission and producing paralysis. Cumulative effect may occur. Does not alter consciousness, pain threshold, or thought processes.

Use/Therapeutic goal/Outcome

Adjunct to general anesthesia, maintenance during mechanical ventilation, orthopedic manipulations, pharmacologically or electrically induced seizures, and tetanus: Facilitation of endotracheal tube and mechanical ventilation tolerance; relaxation of skeletal muscles. *Outcome criteria:* Tolerance of endotracheal intubation and mechanical ventilation; diminished or absent voluntary and reflexive movement.

Dose range/Administration

Interaction alert: Do not mix with alkaline solutions such as barbiturates. Cyclopane, ether, halothane, methoxyflurane, aminoglycosides, bacitracin, polymyxin B, colistin, sodium colistimethate, tetracyclines, quinine, quinidine, calcium and magnesium salts, propanolol, trimethophan, and succinylcholine may potentiate or prolong the action of tubocurarine. Antagonists to this drug include potassium, acetylcholine, and anticholinesterase. Diazepam may cause episodes of malignant hyperthermia.

Adjunct to surgery: *Adult and Child:* IV: 1 U/kg (avg 40–60 U), then 20–30 U in 3–5 min prn.

Electroshock therapy: *Adult:* IV: 1 U/kg over 60–90 sec.

Mechanical ventilation: *Adult:* IV: 0.0165 mg/kg (average of 1 mg to 7 U), then adjust repeated doses to patient's response.

Clinical alert: Tubocurarine should be given only by physicians and nurses who are familiar with its use, and in the presence of a physician, nurse anesthetist, or respiratory therapist who is qualified to manage endotracheal intubation.

Contraindications/Precautions

PREG
C

Contraindicated in hypersensitivity to curare preparations and in those whom release of histamine is hazardous (asthma). *Use with caution* in renal, hepatic, or cardiovascular impairment; dehydration; thyroid disorders; collagen diseases; carcinomatosis; acid/base imbalance; neuromuscular disease; and myasthenia gravis.

🖐 **Use with caution for the elderly or debilitated. Safe use for pregnant or nursing mothers has not been established.**

Side effects/Adverse reactions

Hypersensitivity: excessive bronchial secretions, flushing, itching, wheezing occurs rarely. *Resp:* respiratory depression to point of apnea, bronchospasm. *CNS:* dizziness. *MS:* profound or prolonged muscle relaxation, residual muscle weakness. *CV:* circulatory collapse. *GI:* decreased GI motility.

Nursing implications/Documentation

Possible nursing diagnoses: Impaired communication; Pain; Potential for aspiration; Potential for injury.

◆ Ascertain that baseline CBC, electrolytes, BUN, creatinine, liver function, chest X ray, and EKG studies are posted on chart before drug administration (report abnormalities).

◆ Protect airway, position for drainage of oropharyngeal secretions (if possible), and keep suction at bedside until the patient is fully alert; have emergency equipment and drugs available.

◆ Monitor and record vital signs every 15 min until stable; report abnormalities that might indicate potential complications.

◆ Recognize that this drug may *paralyze*, but does not relieve pain (provide analgesics if pain is suspected, anticipate human needs).

◆ Monitor for potential for injury: protect eyes if there is no blink reflex (tape shut); watch positioning of all extremities (provide range of motion exercises if therapy is prolonged).

◆ Be aware that complete recovery from effects of this drug may take several hours.

◆ Monitor those with myasthenia gravis for risk of aspiration.

◆ Monitor intake and ouput every 2–4 hr for 24 hr.

◆ Report prolonged muscle weakness.

Patient & family teaching/Home care

Possible nursing diagnoses: Anxiety; Fear.

◆ Explain all procedures, even if the person seems unconscious (the ability to hear may be present).

◆ Reassure individual that muscle weakness or stiffness will subside.

◆ For use with mechanical ventilation, stress that you are aware that the patient cannot move, and that this drug is being given to control breathing; reassure that breathing is being closely monitored to be sure that the lungs are being adequately oxygenated, and that the ability to move will return as soon as drug is stopped. Also reassure that medication for pain and anxiety will be given to help tolerate the endotracheal tube.

uracil mustard

yoor'a-sill

Uracil Mustard Capsules

Class: Antineoplastic (nitrogen mustard alkylating) agent

PEDS	PREG	GERI
🖐	X	🖐

Action Kills rapidly growing cells (cancer, hair follicles, bone marrow, GI lining, ova, and sperm) by interfering with DNA replication and RNA transcription through alkylation (cross-linking of DNA occurs). Is cell-cycle–phase nonspecific, affecting both actively dividing cells and dormant (resting) cells.

Use/Therapeutic goal/Outcome

Chronic leukemias (myelocytic and lymphocytic); Hodgkin's disease; non-Hodgkin's lymphomas (lymphocytic and histiocytic); mycosis fungoides; polycythemia vera: Elimination or suppression of malignant cell proliferation.
Outcome criteria: Tumor and disease regression or stabilization on radiologic and physical examination; for leukemias, absence of blasts in peripheral blood specimen.

U

Dose range/Administration

Interaction alert: Radiation therapy and other cytotoxic agents can cause severe myelosuppression.

🔔 **Give doses at bedtime to reduce nausea.**

Adult: PO: 0.15 mg/kg/wk for 4 weeks, if desired response is achieved, continue weekly; or 1–2 mg/day for 3 months until desired response or toxicity occurs. *Intense dosage:* 3–5 mg/day for 7 days, not to exceed 0.5 mg/kg/day (irreversible bone marrow damage may occur). *Maintenance dose:* 1 mg/day for 3 out of 4 weeks. *Child:* PO: 0.3 mg/kg/wk for 4 weeks, if desired response is achieved, continue weekly.

Contraindications/Precautions

PREG
X

Contraindicated in hypersensitivity to uracil mustard, and in aplastic anemia, thrombocytopenia, and leukopenia. Do not give until 3 weeks after the effectiveness of other cytotoxic agents or radiation has been determined. *Use with caution* in renal or hepatic impairment and in malignant cell infiltration of the bone marrow (hematopoietic toxicity may be increased) and allergy to tartrazine (FD&C Yellow No. 5).

✋ **Contraindicated for pregnant or nursing mothers. Use with caution for children and the elderly.**

Side effects/Adverse reactions

Hypersensitivity: fever, hives, bronchial asthma (due to tartrazine dye), anaphylaxis. *Hem:* anemia, thrombocytopenia, leukopenia (bone marrow depression may be delayed for 2–4 weeks), hyperuricemia. *GI:* anorexia, nausea and vomiting, diarrhea, abdominal and epigastric pain, hepatotoxicity. *Skin:* dermatitis, pruritus, hyperpigmentation, alopecia. *CNS:* anxiety, irritability, depression. *GU:* amenorrhea, azoospermia.

Nursing implications/Documentation

Possible nursing diagnoses: Potential for infection; Potential for injury; Fatigue; Altered oral mucous membrane; Fluid volume deficit; Diarrhea; Altered nutrition: less than body requirements.

◆ *See important Nursing implications in Antineoplastic agents overview on page 72, which apply to all antineoplastics. The interventions that follow are additional and specific to this drug only.*

◆ Assess for ASA allergy (bronchial asthma reactions often occur to those with this allergy).

◆ Increase fluid intake to 2–3 L a day to prevent renal tubular damage from hyperuricemia secondary to cell lysis.

◆ Expect that WBC, platelet, and erythrocyte count will drop to the nadir (lowest point) at 2–3 weeks after treatment is discontinued.

◆ Be aware that therapeutic response is often accompanied by toxicity.

Patient & family teaching/Home care

Possible nursing diagnoses: Knowledge deficit; Ineffective coping (individual and family); Hopelessness; Impaired home maintenance management.

◆ *See important Patient & family teaching in Antineoplastic agents overview on page 72, which apply to all antineoplastics. The teachings that follow are additional and specific to this drug only.*

◆ Point out that drinking 2–3 L a day helps prevent kidney complications; IV fluids may be necessary.

◆ *See Antineoplastic agents overview for more information.*

urea
yoor-ee'a

Ureaphil

Class: Osmotic diuretic

PEDS	PREG	GERI
✋	C	✋

Action Increases flow of water into extracellular fluid by elevating blood plasma osmolality. Promotes diuresis by increasing osmolality of glomerular filtrates, which promotes water and electrolyte retention in the lumen of the nephron and increases rate and volume of urine flow. Reduces intraocular pressure and intracranial pressure by creating an osmotic gradient between plasma and ocular fluids, and plasma and CSF.

Use/Therapeutic goal/Outcome

Increased intracranial pressure (ICP): Reduction in intracranial pressure. *Outcome criteria:* Intracranial pressure within normal range when measured with ICP monitor.

Increased intraocular pressure (IOC): Reduction of intraocular pressure. *Outcome criteria:*

Decreased intraocular pressure when measured with tonometer.

Dose range/Administration

Adult: IV: 1–1.5 g/kg of 30% solution at a maximum infusion rate of 4 ml/min. *Maximum dose:* 120 g/day. **Child:** IV: 0.5–1.5 g/kg of 30% solution administered over 30 min. **Infants:** IV: 0.1 g/kg at a maximum rate of 4 ml/min.

Clinical alert: Do not infuse in same IV tubing as other drugs or blood transfusion. Solution may be prepared by reconstituting with 5% or 10% Dextrose in water. Use as soon as possible after preparation.

Contraindications/Precautions

PREG
C

Contraindicated in hypersensitivity, severely impaired renal function, marked dehydration, liver failure, intracranial bleeding. **Use with caution** in impaired cardiovascular, renal, or hepatic function.

✋ **Use with caution for children and the elderly. Safe use for pregnant or nursing mothers has not been established.**

Side effects/Adverse reactions

Hypersensitivity: rash. **CNS:** headache, confusion. **CV:** pulmonary edema, tachycardia, CHF, dehydration. **Hem:** electrolyte imbalances. **GI:** nausea, vomiting. **Misc:** necrotic sloughing at IV site with extravasation.

Nursing implications/Documentation

Possible nursing diagnoses: Fluid volume deficit; Altered patterns of urinary elimination; Potential for injury.

◆ Ascertain that baseline CBC, sodium, potassium, chloride, carbon dioxide, calcium, magnesium, BUN, creatinine, uric acid, and liver function studies have been obtained before giving first dose; report abnormalities and monitor closely thereafter.

◆ Monitor closely for hypokalemia and hyponatremia.

◆ Document and monitor hourly vital signs and urine output; report abnormal vital signs, urine output less than 30 cc/hr, and significant negative or positive balance in cumulative summaries.

◆ Monitor for and report signs of fluid overload (auscultate lungs for rales; check feet, ankles, and sacrum for edema).

◆ Monitor for extravasation and phlebitis, because this drug is very irritating to the tissues.

◆ Keep patients in bed with side rails up and call bell in reach until stable.

Patient & family teaching/Home care

Possible nursing diagnoses: Fear; Knowledge deficit.

◆ Before giving first dose, explain that the drug will enhance the work of the kidneys and reduce the workload of the heart by reducing fluid overload.

◆ Explain that vital signs and urine output will be monitored frequently to ensure safe dosage and fluid replacement.

◆ Stress that fluid intake limitations may be necessary, even though the patient is thirsty.

◆ Explain that changing positions slowly helps prevent dizziness.

◆ Encourage voicing of questions and concerns.

◆ *See Diuretics overviews for more information.*

urokinase

your-owe-kye'naze

Abbokinase, ♠Ukidan, Win-Kinase

Class: Thrombolytic enzyme (fibrinolytic)

Antidote: Aminocaproic acid

PEDS	PREG	GERI
✋	B	✋

Action Dissolves existing clots (thrombi) by directly converting plasminogen to plasmin (the enzyme that degrades fibrin).

Use/Therapeutic goal/Outcome

Emergency treatment of massive pulmonary emboli: Lysis of thrombi obstructing pulmonary arteries, reperfusion of ischemic tissue, prevention of tissue infarction. **Outcome criteria:** Normal blood gases; absence of infarction on lung scan.

Venous catheter occlusion: Lysis of occluding thrombus, restoration of catheter patency. **Outcome criteria:** Blood flow into syringe with catheter aspiration.

Emergency treatment of coronary artery thrombosis (not used more than 4 hr after onset of symptoms of coronary artery occlusion): Lysis of thrombi obstructing coronary arteries, reperfusion of ischemic cardiac tissue, prevention (or reduction in size) of acute myocardial infarction. **Outcome criteria:** Abrupt cessation of chest pain (often accompanied by sudden onset

▶

U

of hypotension and reperfusion arhythmias); smaller Q waves, and return of ST segment to baseline on EKG; cardiac enzyme *washout* (cardiac enzymes peak faster than they do in untreated myocardial infarction); absence of coronary occlusion upon cardiac catheterization (may be performed days later when risk of bleeding has diminished).

Dose range/Administration

Interaction alert: Do not mix any other IV drugs with urokinase solution. Risk of bleeding increases with concurrent oral anticoagulants, heparin, other thrombolytics, or drugs that affect platelet function (salicylates, dipyridamole, nonsteroidal anti-inflammatories); however, heparin is usually given during and immediately after infusion of urokinase.

Pulmonary embolism: *Adult:* IV: Using an IV pump, administer a loading dose of 4,400 IU/kg over 10 min, followed by an infusion of 4,400 IU/kg/hr for 12 hr.

Coronary artery thrombosis: *Adult:* Intracoronary artery: Following an IV heparin bolus, the physician will administer 6,000 IU per min into the occluded artery for up to 2 hr. Average total dose is 500,000 IU.

Venous catheter occlusion: *Adult:* IV: Instill 5,000 IU into occluded catheter, wait 5 min, then aspirate. If blood does not enter syringe, attempt to aspirate every 5 min for 30 min. If still occluded, cap line and let drug work for 30–60 min before aspirating again. If necessary, repeat procedure.

Clinical alert: This drug is used if the patient is allergic to streptokinase, has had a recent streptococcal infection, or has been given streptokinase in the past. It should only be administered by professionals who are well educated in all aspects of its administration. Follow package insert instructions for reconstituting urokinase carefully, because special care must be taken to prevent precipitation of medication. Check hospital policy and procedure for administration. Be sure that three IVs and other invasive lines are established **before** administration of urokinase, and have the following at the patient's bedside:

♦ Electrocardiogram machine

♦ Emergency medications

♦ Advanced cardiac life support (ACLC) cart (with defibrillator)

♦ IV pump.

Contraindications/Precautions

Contraindicated in hypersensitivity to urokinase, chest pain lasting longer than 4 hr, active internal bleeding or known potential bleeding source (e.g., ulcer disease), cerebrovascular accident (CVA), intracranial neoplasm, arteriovenous malformation, intracranial aneurysm, known bleeding diathesis, diabetic retinopathy, recent cranial or spinal surgery (or trauma), organ biopsy, or cavity aspiration within 8 weeks; surgery, trauma, or CPR (especially with rib fractures) within 10 days; traumatic endotracheal intubation, persistent hypertension (with systolic blood pressure greater than 180 mm Hg, or diastolic greater than 110 mm Hg) after treatment, subacute bacterial endocarditis. *Use with caution* for patient with recent puncture (within 10 days) of a noncompressible vessel, prothrombin time greater than 15 seconds, aspirin consumption within 72 hr, known (or suspected) left heart thrombus (risk of cerebral infarction).

♨ **Contraindicated in known or suspected pregnancy. Use with caution for those over 75 years (physician may deem to be contraindicated). Safety for children has not been established.**

Side effects/Adverse reactions

Hypersensitivity: itching, rashes, nausea, flushing, temperature elevation, respiratory difficulties, angioneurotic edema. *CNS:* Cerebral hemorrhage. *GI:* nausea, vomiting, bleeding. *CV:* bleeding of surgical or traumatic injury or puncture sites, hypotension, dysrhythmias. *Misc:* fever.

Nursing implications/Documentation

Possible nursing diagnoses: Potential for Injury; Pain.

♦ Obtain a careful history of pain, and monitor level of pain closely before, during, and after administration of urokinase.

♦ Assess carefully for contraindications to urokinase.

♦ For coronary artery thrombosis, attach patient to cardiac monitor and select the lead that shows the highest ST-segment elevation (also attach patient to a 12-lead EKG; periodic electrocardiograms will be necessary during administration).

♦ Monitor closely for hypersensitivity reactions and report to physician immediately if they occur.

- *Check hospital policy and procedure to determine variations in the following interventions.*

  - Be sure baseline and other "stat" lab studies are drawn before initiating urokinase (PT, PTT, CBC, fibrinogen level, renal lab studies, cardiac enzymes, type and crossmatch for 2 units of blood and other hospital policy routine coronary admission studies).

  - Have the necessary equipment ready for three large-bore peripheral intravenous lines (one for urokinase; another for other drugs, such as heparin and lidocaine, and the third for drawing blood samples; one of these may be needed for blood transfusion if hemorrhage occurs).

  - Before, during, and after administration of urokinase, document and report presence of abnormal pulses, abnormal neurological findings, or skin lesions (may indicate coagulation defects).

  - Document vital signs every 15 min during infusion and for 1–2 hr after infusion, then every 30 min until ordered otherwise; also document EKG strips to have a record of changes in ST segments.

  - Document neurological signs on a flow sheet every 30 min for at least 2 hr (check policy).

  - Be prepared to treat reperfusion dysrhythmias (ventricular tachycardia or fibrillation; atrial tachycardia or fibrillation) according to hospital protocol or individual physician orders; have emergency drugs and defibrillator readily available (some protocols will include starting a lidocaine drip and a heparin drip when urokinase is initiated).

  - Keep all needle punctures to an absolute minimum; apply manual pressure for 10 min to all venous puncture sites, and 30 min to arterial puncture sites; follow this with pressure dressing, and observe all intravenous and intra-arterial sites every 15 min for 1 hr, every 30 min for 2 hr, every hour for 4 hr, then every 2 hr until removed.

  - Place a sign on the door and over bed to alert staff and phlebotomist of bleeding precautions.

  - Maintain patient on complete bedrest until otherwise ordered, and monitor closely for bleeding: hemoptysis, CVA hematuria, hematemesis, melena, pain or swelling from closed space bleeding, and signs and symptoms of cardiac tamponade (distended neck veins and sig-

nificant pulsus paradoxus). Report immediately if these are observed.

  - Keep aminocaproic acid available as antidote in case of hemorrhage.

  - Check for the following lab orders post infusion: CPK, CPK Isoenzymes (q4h × 3, then qd × 2); Hgb and Hct (q4h × 24 hr, then once the next day); PTT (stat and q4h × 2, then daily throughout heparin therapy; should be maintained in the 80–120 second range).

Patient & family teaching/Home care

Possible nursing diagnoses: Anxiety; Fear; Knowledge deficit.

  - Explain the rationale for prompt initiation of treatment, and for routine procedures that ensure patient safety.

  - Encourage the person to voice questions and concerns, and to keep nurses informed of new symptoms (headache, dizziness, chest discomfort, abdominal discomfort).

  - Reinforce that symptoms associated with hypotension and dysrhythmias are likely to be transient.

  - Emphasize the need to remain in bed.

- *See Anticoagulants and Thrombolytic Enzymes overview for more information.*

valproic acid

val-proe'ic

valproic acid: *Dalpro, Depa, Depakene, Myproic Acid*

valproate sodium: *Depakene Syrup, ✦Epilim, Myproic Acid Syrup*

divalproex sodium: *Depakote, ✦Epivall, ♦Valcote*

Class: Anticonvulsant

PEDS	PREG	GERI
🖐	D	🖐

Action Precise mechanism of action is not established. Believed to limit seizure activity by increasing brain levels of GABA, a neurotransmitter in inhibitory nerves in the CNS.

Use/Therapeutic goal/Outcome

Simple and complex absence (petit mal) seizures, mixed seizures that do not respond to other anticonvulsants, and (investigational use) grand mal (tonic-clonic) seizures: Limitation of seizure activity. **Outcome criteria:** Marked decrease or absence of seizure activity.

V

Dose range/Administration

Interaction alert: Antacids and aspirin may cause valproic acid toxicity (monitor serum levels closely). Valproic acid increases serum phenobarbital levels by as much as 40 percent, and it may decrease *total* serum phenytoin levels, but increase *free* (active drug) levels. The effects of alcohol, tricylic antidepressants, anticonvulsants, and other drugs that depress the CNS may be potentiated.

🍃 **Give with meals.**

Adult and Child: PO: 15 mg/kg/day in divided doses bid or tid, with weekly increments of 5–10 mg/kg/day prn, to a maximum of 60 mg/kg/day.

Clinical alert: To avoid mouth irritation, capsules should not be chewed and syrup should not be mixed with carbonated beverages. Avoid using syrup for those on sodium restriction. Divalproex, an enteric-coated compound of valproic acid and valproate sodium, may benefit those experiencing GI symptoms. Report tremors, if noted (dose may need to be reduced).

Contraindications/Precautions
PREG D

Contraindicated in hypersensitivity to valproic acid, and in liver disease. ***Use with caution*** in kidney disease, bleeding disorders, angina pectoris, recent myocardial infarction, concomitant use with other anticonvulsants.

✋ **Use with caution for children, the elderly, and pregnancy (has shown risk to the fetus). Women taking this drug should not nurse their infants.**

Side effects/Adverse reactions

Hypersensitivity: itching, rash. ***GI:*** nausea, vomiting, indigestion, diarrhea, cramps, pancreatitis, liver failure. ***CNS:*** depression, sedation, headache, muscle weakness, incoordination, tremor, psychosis, mental deterioration. ***Hem:*** hyperammonemia, thrombocytopenia, leukopenia, anemia, increased bleeding time. ***MS:*** bone marrow depression. ***GU:*** menstrual irregularities, false positive for ketonuria. ***Misc:*** change in appetite and weight.

Nursing implications/Documentation

Possible nursing diagnoses: Potential for injury; Potential for aspiration.

◆ Document history of seizures (type, frequency, duration, usual time they occur, precipitating factors, presence of an aura); initiate seizure precautions as indicated.

◆ Monitor serum drug levels periodically to assure therapeutic range (50–100 mcg/ml).

◆ Check liver function studies, platelet counts, and prothrombin time before starting this drug; every month for at least 6 months; then every 2–3 months.

◆ Report signs of hematological side effects (persistent fatigue, sore throat, fever, infections, bleeding, easy bruising).

Patient & family teaching/Home care

Possible nursing diagnoses: Fear; Self-esteem disturbance; Knowledge deficit; Impaired home maintenance management.

◆ Advise taking this drug with meals; warn against chewing tablets or mixing syrup with carbonated beverages.

◆ Stress the need for close medical follow-up; emphasize that persistent fatigue, weakness, fever, sore throat, mouth ulcers, infections, bleeding, and easy bruising are signs of side effects that should be reported.

◆ Warn that nonspecific complaints of anorexia, malaise, fever, and lethargy may indicate serious liver toxicity and should be reported immediately.

◆ Point out that stopping anticonvulsants suddenly can cause an increase in severity and frequency of seizures.

◆ Caution against using alcohol and using OTC drugs unless approved by physician.

◆ Teach significant others—and have them demonstrate—how to protect the individual should a seizure occur.

◆ Encourage wearing a medical alert bracelet; remind the patient to inform the dentist and other physicians that he or she is taking this drug.

◆ *See Anticonvulsants overview for more information.*

vancomycin
van'koe-mye-sin

vancomycin hydrochloride: ***Vancocin***

Class: Anti-infective, Glycopeptide antibiotic, Antibacterial

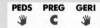

PEDS	PREG	GERI
✋	C	✋

Action Kills bacteria (bactericidal) or limits their growth (bacteriostatic) (depending upon concentration and susceptibility of the organism) by hindering cell wall synthesis, which makes the

V

bacteria more susceptible to osmotic pressure and lysis.

Use/Therapeutic goal/Outcome

Infections (severe staphylococcal infections unresponsive to other antibiotics; antibiotic-associated pseudomembranous enterocolitis caused by *Clostridium difficile*, endocarditis prophylaxis for dental procedures): Resolution or prevention of infection. *Outcome criteria:* Absence of pathogenic growth on cultures, absence of clinical manifestations of infection (fever, pain, swelling, redness, heat, odor, drainage, productive cough, dysuria, diarrhea), normal WBC count, normal X rays.

Dose range/Administration

Interaction alert: Amphotericin B, cisplatin, pentamidine, and aminoglycosides increase risk of nephrotoxicity.

Severe staphylococcus infections: Adult: IV: 500 mg q6h or 1 g q12h. *Child:* IV: 40 mg/kg/day, in divided doses q6h. *Neonate:* IV: 10 mg/kg/day, in divided doses q6h or q12h.

Endocarditis: Adult: IV: *Prophylaxis:* 1 g as single dose over 1 hr (start 1 hr before procedure). *Treatment:* continue therapy for at least 4 wks.

Antibiotic-associated pseudomembranous colitis: Adult: PO: 125–500 mg q6h for 7–10 days. *Child:* PO: 40 mg/kg/day, in divided doses q6h.

Clinical alert: To avoid side effect of hypotension, give IV doses *slowly* over 1 hour; dilute in 200 cc NS or D5W. Never give IM. Monitor closely for extravasation (may cause tissue necrosis).

Contraindications/Precautions

PREG C

Contraindicated in hypersensitivity to vancomycin, and in hearing loss. *Use with caution* in impaired kidney function.

✋ **Use with caution for children and the elderly. Safe use for pregnant or nursing mothers has not been established; use only when benefits outweigh risks.**

Side effects/Adverse reactions

Hypersensitivity: itching, rashes, facial flushing, fever, difficulty breathing, anaphylaxis. *GI:* nausea. *CV:* (with IV administration) hypotension; pain, redness, swelling, thrombophlebitis at injection site. *GU:* nephrotoxicity. *Ear:* ototoxicity (hearing loss), tinnitus. *Misc:* superinfection.

Nursing implications/Documentation

Possible nursing diagnoses: Potential for infection; Fluid volume deficit.

◆ Obtain culture specimens and baseline lab studies (CBC, BUN, creatinine, electrolytes, liver function) before administering first dose; monitor closely thereafter if therapy is prolonged.

◆ Monitor for and report hearing loss (serum levels of 60–80 mcg/ml are associated with ototoxicity).

◆ Provide preferred fluids, and record and monitor intake and output to ensure adequate hydration and urine output; report decreased urinary output.

◆ Monitor for and report symptoms of superinfection (mouth lesions, thrush, vaginal irritation, diarrhea).

◆ Hold dose and report if *red neck syndrome* (rash over face, neck, trunk, and extremities) is noted.

◆ Schedule blood drawing for peak serum levels 1 hour after completion of IV dose; schedule blood drawing for trough levels 30 minutes before IV dose.

Patient & family teaching/Home care

Possible nursing diagnoses: Knowledge deficit.

◆ Explain the importance of reporting ear symptoms (full feeling, ringing of the ears) immediately.

◆ Advise reporting new symptoms of illness (e.g., fever, mouth lesions, vaginal irritation, diarrhea); medication change may be necessary.

◆ Explain the importance of taking antibiotics for the entire time prescribed, even if symptoms abate.

◆ Stress the need to drink plenty of fluids to maintain adequate hydration.

◆ *See Anti-infectives overview for more information.*

vasopressin

vay-soe-press'in

V

vasopressin: *Pitressin*

vasopressin tannate: *Pitressin Tannate*

Class: Posterior pituitary hormone, Antidiuretic hormone, Peristaltic stimulant

PEDS	PREG	GERI
✋	B	✋

Action Decreases urine output by increasing water reabsorption in kidneys; promotes vasoconstriction by direct action on smooth muscles of vessels; stimulates gastrointestinal motility by direct action on gastrointestinal smooth muscles.

Use/Therapeutic goal/Outcome

Neurogenic diabetes insipidus: Prevention or control of dehydration. **Outcome criteria:** Reduction in volume and frequency of urination, especially during sleeping hours; increased osmolality and specific gravity of urine.

Abdominal distention: Prevention or treatment of discomfort related to atony of bowel; elimination of intestinal gas prior to diagnostic radiography of abdomen. **Outcome criteria:** Report of decreased abdominal discomfort, presence of bowel sounds and passage of gas by rectum, improved visualization of abdominal organs by radiography.

Dose range/Administration

Interaction alert: Demeclocycline, lithium, or norepinephrine may decrease antidiuretic effect; carbamazepine, chlorpropamide, or clofibrate may increase antidiuretic effect.
Antidiuretic: Adult: IM, SC: *Aqueous:* 5–10 U 2–3 times a day. *Oil suspension:* 1.5–5 U q1-3 days. **Child:** IM, SC: *Aqueous:* 2.5–10 U 2–4 times a day. *Oil suspension:* 1.25–2.5 U q1-3 days.
Abdominal distention: Adult: IM: 5–10 Uq3-4h.
Abdominal radiography: Adult: IM, SC: 10 U 2 hr before, then 30 min before study.
Clinical alert: Aqueous preparations may be administered by any parenteral route. Vasopressin tannate should be administered by intramuscular route only. For tannate in oil suspension, warm vial between hands or in warm water, and shake thoroughly to obtain a uniform suspension.

Contraindications/Precautions

PREG B

Contraindicated in hypersensitivity to vasopressin, and in chronic nephritis, and nephrogenic diabetes insipidus. **Use with caution** in hypertension, congestive failure, coronary artery or peripheral vascular disease, asthma, and history of seizures or migraines.

☞ **Contraindicated for children under 3 years. Use with caution for other young children, pregnant or nursing mothers, and the elderly.**

Side effects/Adverse reactions

Hypersensitivity: fever, rashes, hives; swelling of face, feet, hands, or mouth; wheezing, bronchoconstriction, dyspnea; anaphylaxis. **CV:** elevated blood pressure, angina, myocardial infarction. **CNS:** dizziness, lightheadedness, trembling, headaches, drowsiness, confusion, seizures, coma. **GI:** nausea, vomiting, abdominal cramps or diarrhea, increased urge for bowel movement, flatus. **Hem:** hyponatremia. **Skin:** blanching, sweating; pain, redness or swelling at injection site. **Misc:** water intoxication.

Nursing implications/Documentation

Possible nursing diagnoses: Fluid volume excess; Pain; Diarrhea; Impaired tissue integrity.

♦ Give 1–2 glasses of water with each dose to minimize transient side effects such as blanching of skin, abdominal cramps, and nausea.

♦ Record intake and output, daily weight, and specific gravity of urine; report significant discrepancies.

♦ Record blood pressure twice daily.

♦ Monitor for return of polyuria and nocturia, which may indicate need for more frequent administration.

♦ Assess for and report early signs of water intoxication and hyponatremia (drowsiness, listlessness, headache, confusion, weight gain), especially with long-acting tannate oil suspension.

♦ When ordered for abdominal distention, document bowel sounds and passage of flatus and stool; use a rectal tube to facilitate expulsion of gas.

♦ Be aware that elderly patients and children are at greater risk for water intoxication and hyponatremia.

Patient & family teaching/Home care

Possible nursing diagnoses: Impaired home maintenance management; Fluid volume excess.

♦ Stress the importance of not using more medication than the prescribed amount.

♦ With vasopressin in oil, teach to warm vial in hands and to shake vigorously to suspend the drug.

♦ Advise drinking 1 or 2 glasses of water at time of injection to minimize side effects such as blanching of skin, abdominal cramps, and

V

nausea; inform that these effects are not serious and usually last only a few minutes.

♦ Teach to measure and record fluid intake and output to identify decreased or increased response to drug; point out the need to report significant changes in response.

♦ Stress the need to report signs of water intoxication and hyponatremia (drowsiness, listlessness, headache, confusion, weight gain).

♦ Advise reporting excessive urination, angina, or dyspnea immediately.

vecuronium

vek-yoo-roe'nee-um

vecuronium bromide: *Norcuron*

Class: Nondepolarizing neuromuscular blocker, skeletal-muscle relaxant

Antidote: Neostigmine methylsulfate

PEDS	PREG	GERI
✋	C	✋

Action Relaxes or paralyzes skeletal muscles (depending on dose) by competing for cholinergic receptor sites at myoneural junction, thus blocking neuromuscular transmission and producing paralysis. This is a potent drug with shorter duration than most drugs in this classification, in addition to minimal histamine release. Does not alter consciousness, pain threshold, or thought processes.

Use/Therapeutic goal/Outcome

Endotracheal intubation and adjunct to general anesthesia: Promotion of endotracheal tube and mechanical ventilation tolerance; relaxation of skeletal muscle. *Outcome criteria:* Tolerance of endotracheal intubation and mechanical ventilation; diminished or absent voluntary and reflexive movement.

Dose range/Administration

Interaction alert: Enflurane, isoflurane, aminoglycosides, bacitracin, colistimethate, colistin B, polymyxin B, tetracyclines, magnesium salts, quinidine and succinylcholine may potentiate or prolong the action of this drug.

Adult/Child 10–17 yrs: IV: 0.04–0.1 mg/kg; then 0.01–0.15 mg/kg in 25–40 min, may repeat q12–15 min.

Clinical alert: This drug should be given only by physicians and nurses who are familiar with its use, and in the presence of a physician, nurse anesthetist, or respiratory therapist who is qualified to manage endotracheal intubation.

Contraindications/Precautions

Contraindicated in hypersensitivity to vecuronium bromide. ***Use with caution*** in severe hepatic impairment, acid/base imbalance, electrolyte imbalance, dehydration, myasthenia gravis, edema, obesity, cardiovascular impairment, and history of malignant hyperthermia.

✋ **Use with caution for infants under 1 year and the elderly. Use for children 1–10 years is controversial. Safe use for pregnant or nursing mothers has not been established.**

Side effects/Adverse reactions

Hypersensitivity: this drug is generally well tolerated. ***MS:*** skeletal muscle weakness. ***Resp:*** respiratory depression. ***CNS:*** malignant hyperthermia.

Nursing implications/Documentation

Possible nursing diagnoses: Impaired communication; Pain; Potential for aspiration; Potential for injury.

♦ Ascertain that baseline CBC, electrolytes, BUN, creatinine, liver function, chest X ray, and EKG studies are posted on chart before drug administration (report abnormalities).

♦ Protect airway, position for drainage of oropharyngeal secretions (if possible), and keep suction at bedside until the patient is fully alert; have emergency equipment and drugs available.

♦ Monitor and record vital signs every 15 min until stable; report abnormalities that might indicate potential complications.

♦ Recognize that this drug may *paralyze*, but does not relieve pain (provide analgesics if pain is suspected, anticipate human needs).

♦ Monitor for potential for injury; protect eyes if there is no blink reflex (tape shut); watch positioning of all extremities (provide range of motion exercises if therapy is prolonged).

♦ Document intake and output every 2–4 hr for 24 hr.

♦ Monitor and document response (vital signs, respiratory status, movement).

♦ Anticipate respiratory problems in the obese and those with neuromuscular disease.

Patient & family teaching/Home care

Possible nursing diagnoses: Anxiety; Fear.

- ◆ Explain all procedures, even if the person seems unconscious (the ability to hear may be present).
- ◆ Reassure that muscle weakness or stiffness will subside.
- ◆ For use with mechanical ventilation, stress that you are aware that the patient cannot move, and that this drug is being given to control breathing; reassure that breathing is being closely monitored to be sure that the lungs are being adequately oxygenated, and that ability to move will return as soon as drug is stopped. Also reassure that medication for pain and anxiety will be given to help tolerate the endotracheal tube.

verapamil
ver-ap'a-mill

verapamil hydrochloride: *Calan, Calan SR, ♠Cordilox Oral, Isoptin, Isoptin SR, ♠Veradil*

Class: ★Calcium channel blocker antianginal prototype, Antiarrhythmic, Antihypertensive

PEDS	PREG	GERI
✋	C	✋

Action Inhibits calcium ion influx across the cell membrane, which results in increased availability of oxygen to the myocardium (by dilating coronary arteries) and decreased workload and oxygen demand of the heart (by reducing heart rate and force of contraction). Vasodilation causes a drop in blood pressure and systemic vascular resistance (afterload). As an antiarrhythmic, it slows atrioventricular (AV) conduction and prolongs effective refractory period of AV node.

Use/Therapeutic goal/Outcome

Supraventricular tachyarrhythmias: Suppression of atrial ectopy. *Outcome criteria:* Regular sinus rhythm on EKG.

Angina pectoris (vasospastic and chronic stable): Promotion of myocardial oxygenation, prevention of anginal (ischemic) attacks, improved activity tolerance. *Outcome criteria:* Patient reports decreased frequency and severity of angina, and demonstrates increased activity tolerance.

Hypertension: Reduction in blood pressure. *Outcome criteria:* Blood pressure within normal limits.

Dose range/Administration

Interaction alert: Concurrent use with beta-blockers (including ophthalmic timolol), or with digitalis, may have a cardiodepressant effect (significant bradycardia or AV block can result from the additive effect of these drugs on sinus and AV nodes). Use with quinidine in hypertrophic cardiomyopathy may cause significant hypotension. Additive hypotensive effect occurs with concurrent use of antihypertensives; alpha-adrenergic blockers may cause significant bradycardia. Increased serum levels of carbamazepine and digoxin are common; dosage of these drugs may need to be lowered to prevent toxicity. Rifampin increases hepatic enzyme activity, increases verapamil metabolism, and thus decreases verapamil effect.

Angina, arrhythmias, and hypertension: **Adult:** PO: 80–120 mg tid or qid (maximum of 240–480 mg/day. *Sustained release* preparation 240 mg daily.

Supraventricular tachyarrhythmias: **Adult:** IV: Initially give 5–10 mg (0.075 to 0.15 mg/kg) over at least 2 min. May repeat in 30 min with 10 mg if necessary. **Child 1–15 yrs:** IV: 0.1–0.3 mg/kg over at least 3 min. May repeat after 30 min. Maximum dose is 5 mg. **Child < 1 yr:** IV: 0.1–0.3 mg/kg in bolus over 3 min.

Clinical alert: Check blood pressure prior to giving dose; **hold and report** if hypotension is noted. Give IV only if patient is attached to a monitor; keep resuscitative drugs and equipment nearby.

Contraindications/Precautions

PREG
C

Contraindicated in hypersensitivity to verapamil, and in Wolff-Parkinson-White syndrome, second- or third-degree heart block, or sick sinus syndrome (unless a ventricular pacemaker is in place). *Use with caution* in congestive heart failure, and dilated cardiomyopathy.

✋ Use with caution for children and the elderly; duration of action may be prolonged in the elderly. Safe use for pregnant and nursing mothers has not been established.

Side effects/Adverse reactions

Hypersensitivity: rash. *CV:* transient hypotension, congestive heart failure, bradycardia, heart block, asystole. *CNS:* headache, nervousness, dizziness, fatigue. *GI:* constipation, nausea, elevated liver enzymes. *Skin:* peripheral edema.

V

Nursing implications/Documentation

Possible nursing diagnoses: Potential for injury; Activity intolerance.

◆ Keep a record of pulse and blood pressure before and after drug administration.

◆ If patient is on a cardiac monitor, produce rhythm strip at least every 8 hours; measure PR and QRS intervals, and report any prolongation in these intervals.

◆ Be aware that episodes of angina may increase during initial therapy; treat as ordered.

◆ Observe for postural hypotension; take blood pressure in both arms, and with patient sitting and standing if possible.

◆ Keep patients receiving IV verapamil in bed with side rails up; once patient is allowed out of bed, supervise ambulation until response is determined.

◆ Coordinate care to provide frequent rest periods.

Patient & family teaching/Home care

Possible nursing diagnoses: Fear; Knowledge deficit; Impaired home maintenance management.

◆ Explain that verapamil decreases blood pressure, reduces the workload of the heart, and improves coronary blood supply.

◆ Stress the need to follow dose regimen closely (the drug should be taken at the same time each day) and the need to return for medical follow-up.

◆ Emphasize the need to pace activities, avoid stress (emotional and physical), and plan for rest periods.

◆ Explain that an extra sublingual dose of nitroglycerin may be necessary during stress, or at night if angina is nocturnal.

◆ Advise changing positions slowly to avoid dizziness.

◆ Encourage keeping a record of angina attacks to observe pattern; stress that an increase in frequency or severity should be reported.

◆ Warn that drinking alcohol may cause fainting and hypotension.

◆ *See Calcium Channel Blockers, Antihypertensives, and Antianginals overviews for more information.*

vinblastine

vin-blast'een

vinblastine sulfate (VLB): *Alkaban-AQ, Velban,* ✦⚕*Velbe, Velsar*

Class: Antineoplastic agent (plant alkaloid)

PEDS	PREG	GERI
✋	D	✋

Action Kills rapidly growing cells (cancer, hair follicles, bone marrow, GI lining, ova, and sperm) by interfering with cell division (arrests mitosis in metaphase) and inhibiting RNA synthesis. Drug is cell-cycle specific during the M-phase with limited activity in the G_2- and S-phases.

Use/Therapeutic goal/Outcome

Disseminated Hodgkin's disease and non-Hodgkin's lymphomas, testicular or breast cancer, mycosis fungoides, Kaposi's sarcoma, choriocarcinoma, and histiocytosis: Elimination or suppression of malignant cell proliferation. *Outcome criteria:* After 12 weeks, tumor and disease regression or stabilization on radiologic and physical examination.

Dose range/Administration

Interaction alert: Mitomycin may cause life-threatening bronchospasm. Do not use with radiation. May increase methotrexate levels and decrease phenytoin levels.

Adult and Child > 1 yr: IV: 3.7 mg/m² as a single dose, every 7 days; increase weekly by 1.8 mg/m², according to response. *Maximum dose:* 18.5 mg/m²/wk.

Clinical alert: This drug should be given only by nurses who are knowledgeable in the comprehensive management of the administration of antineoplastic agents. Doses may vary at physician's discretion. Repeat doses are held until it is ascertained that the patient has recovered sufficiently from toxicities of previous doses. Established protocols/policies for drug preparation, administration, and accidental skin contamination *must be followed closely* (gloves or double gloves are worn when handling drug; if the drug touches the skin, the area is washed immediately with plenty of soap and water). Vinblastine sulfate is given IV push over 1 min or diluted in 50–100 ml saline over 3–8 hr to minimize inflammation and pain along the vein. This drug is a *potent* vesicant (can cause severe damage to tissues). *Prevention* of extravasation is essential. The drug is given by administering only when it is clear that the

▶

needle is in the vein (good blood return), and the infusion site is monitored *closely* for early signs of extravasation (pain and swelling at infusion site). If extravasation is suspected, the infusion is stopped *immediately,* the physician is notified, and protocols/policies for treatment are followed.

Contraindications/Precautions

PREG D

Contraindicated in hypersensitivity to vinblastine sulfate, and in bacterial infections, or severe leukopenia. **Use with caution** in decreased bone marrow reserve, chronic debilitating illnesses, and hepatic impairment.

👋 **Contraindicated for pregnant or nursing mothers. Use with caution for children and the elderly.**

Side effects/Adverse reactions

Hypersensitivity: chills, fever, dermatitis, bronchospasm, and anaphylaxis. **Hem:** thrombosis and thrombophlebitis with insufficient drug dilution; leukopenia, thrombocytopenia, hyperuricemia. **MS:** cumulative myelosuppression, muscle pain. **GI:** nausea, vomiting, anorexia, constipation, ileus, abdominal pain, hepatotoxicity, stomatitis, pharyngitis, rectal bleeding, enterocolitis. **CNS:** neurotoxicity (numbness, paresthesia, peripheral neuropathy, mental depression, loss of deep tendon reflexes, seizures). **Skin:** dermatitis and vesiculation; alopecia; pain, inflammation, and induration at injection site; cellulitis, ulceration, and sloughing if extravasation occurs.

Nursing implications/Documentation

Possible nursing diagnoses: Potential for infection; Potential for injury; Fatigue; Altered oral mucous membrane; Fluid volume deficit; Diarrhea; Altered nutrition: less than body requirements.

♦ *See important Nursing implications in Antineoplastic agents overview on page 72, which apply to all antineoplastics. The interventions that follow are additional and specific to this drug only.*

♦ Monitor closely for and report immediately early signs of bronchospasm; keep emergency drugs and equipment readily available (bronchospasm is most common when the patient is also receiving mitomycin).

♦ Prevent constipation and ileus by monitoring bowel elimination, encouraging fluids and ambulation, and providing laxatives before problem is severe (may require prophylactic

stool softeners; constipation may be an early sign of neurotoxicity).

♦ Observe for and report early signs of CNS toxicity (numbness or tingling of extremities, muscle weakness, wristdrop or footdrop); assess for neuropathy by having the person sign his or her name before each dose.

♦ Be aware that WBC drops to the nadir (lowest point) on days 4–10 and may last another 7–14 days.

Patient & family teaching/Home care

Possible nursing diagnoses: Knowledge deficit; Ineffective coping (individual and family); Hopelessness; Impaired home maintenance management.

♦ *See important Patient & family teaching in Antineoplastic agents overview on page 72, which apply to all antineoplastics. The teachings that follow are additional and specific to this drug only.*

♦ Explain that therapeutic response takes about 12 weeks.

♦ Stress the need to monitor bowel function and prevent constipation by maintaining adequate hydration, eating enough fiber, and using stool softeners or laxatives before the problem is severe (advise reporting abdominal distention and pain, as it may indicate an ileus).

♦ Advise reporting numbness or tingling of the extremities, muscle weakness, or coordination problems, as they may indicate neurotoxicity.

♦ Counsel women to use nonhormonal contraception; stress that suspected pregnancy should be reported immediately.

♦ *See Antineoplastic agents overview for more information.*

vincristine

vin-kris'teen

vincristine sulfate: **Oncovin, Vincasar PFS**
Class: ★Antineoplastic agent (plant alkaloid) **prototype**

PEDS 👋 **PREG** D **GERI** 👋

Action Kills rapidly growing cells (cancer, hair follicles, bone marrow, GI lining, ova, and sperm) by interfering with cell division (arrests mitosis in metaphase). Is cell cycle specific in the M-phase.

Use/Therapeutic goal/Outcome

Cancer (acute leukemia, Hodgkin's disease, malignant lymphomas, neuroblastoma, rhabdomyosarcoma, Wilms' tumor, Kaposi's sarcoma, lung, and breast cancers): Elimination or suppression of malignant cell proliferation. *Outcome criteria:* Tumor/disease regression or stabilization on radiologic and physical examination; for leukemias, absence of blasts in peripheral blood specimen.

Dose range/Administration

Interaction alert: If the patient has previously received mitomycin, life-threatening bronchospasm may occur. Asparaginase decreases hepatic clearance of vincristine, whereas calcium channel blockers enhance vincristine cellular accumulation. Decreases effects of digoxin.

Adult: IV: 1–2 mg/m^2/wk *Maximum dose:* 2 mg. **Child:** IV: 1.5–2 mg/m^2/wk *Maximum dose:* 2 mg.

Clinical alert: This drug should be given only by nurses who are knowledgeable in the comprehensive management of the administration of antineoplastic agents. Doses may vary at physician's discretion. Doses are given weekly only; repeat doses are held until it is ascertained that the patient has recovered sufficiently from toxicities of previous doses. Intrathecal use can cause *death*. Established protocols/policies for drug preparation, administration, and accidental skin contamination *must be followed closely* (gloves or double gloves are worn when handling drug; if the drug touches the skin, the area is washed immediately with plenty of soap and water). Vincristine sulfate is given IV push over 1 min or injected into side-arm of running IV infusion. This drug is a potent vessicant (can cause severe damage to tissues). *Prevention* of extravasation is essential. The drug is given by administering only when it is clear that the needle is in the vein (good blood return), and the infusion site is monitored *closely* for early signs of extravasation (pain and swelling at infusion site). If extravasation is suspected, the infusion is stopped *immediately,* the physician is notified, and protocols/policies for treatment are followed.

Contraindications/Precautions

PREG
D

Contraindicated in hypersensitivity to vincristine sulfate. **Use with caution** in neuromuscular disease, those receiving neurotoxic drugs, decreased bone marrow reserve, chronic debilitating disease, or obstructive jaundice or hepatic dysfunction (dose reduction necessary). ☜ **Contraindicated for pregnant or nursing mothers. Use with caution for children and the elderly.**

Side effects/Adverse reactions

Hypersensitivity: chills, fever, urticaria, bronchospasm, anaphylaxis. **CNS:** peripheral neuropathy, asymptomatic depression of the Achilles reflex, diminished deep tendon reflexes, paresthesia, wristdrop, footdrop, cranial nerve palsies (hoarseness, vocal cord paresis, ptosis, diplopia), autonomic and CNS toxicity (constipation, adynamic ileus). **CV:** thrombosis and thrombophlebitis with insufficient drug dilution. **GI:** nausea, vomiting, ileus (mimics acute surgical abdomen), constipation, weight loss, stomatitis, dysphagia. **Hem:** thrombocytopenia, leukopenia, anemia, hyperuricemia, hyponatremia, SIADH (syndrome of inappropriate antidiuretic hormone). **GU:** urinary retention. **Skin:** pain, inflammation, and induration at injection site; cellulitis, ulceration, sloughing if extravasation occurs, alopecia.

Nursing implications/Documentation

Possible nursing diagnoses: Potential for infection; Potential for injury; Fatigue; Altered oral mucous membrane; Fluid volume deficit; Diarrhea; Altered nutrition: less than body requirements.

◆ *See important Nursing implications in Antineoplastic agents overview on page 72, which apply to all antineoplastics. The interventions that follow are additional and specific to this drug only.*

◆ Monitor closely for and report immediately early signs of bronchospasm; keep emergency drugs and equipment readily available (bronchospasm is most common when the patient is also receiving mitomycin).

◆ Prevent constipation and ileus by monitoring bowel elimination, encouraging fluids and ambulation, and providing laxatives before problem is severe (may require prophylactic stool softeners; constipation may be an early sign of neurotoxicity).

◆ Observe for and report early signs of CNS toxicity (numbness or tingling of extremities, muscle weakness, wristdrop or footdrop, coordination problems). Assess for neuropathy by

V

having the person sign his or her name before each dose.

◆ Maintain a fluid intake of 2–3 L a day to prevent renal tubular damage from hyperuricemia; monitor for and report significant positive or negative fluid balance.

◆ Be aware that WBC may stay at the nadir (lowest point) for 1 week (may occur at any point in course of therapy).

Patient & family teaching/Home care

Possible nursing diagnoses: Knowledge deficit; Ineffective coping (individual and family); Hopelessness; Impaired home maintenance management.

◆ *See important Patient & family teaching in Antineoplastic agents overview on page 72, which apply to all antineoplastics. The teachings that follow are additional and specific to this drug only.*

◆ Stress the need to monitor bowel function and prevent constipation by maintaining adequate hydration, eating enough fiber, and using stool softeners or laxatives before the problem is severe; advise reporting abdominal distention and pain, as this may indicate an ileus.

◆ Explain that numbness or tingling of the extremities, muscle weakness, or coordination problems should be reported, as they may indicate neurotoxicity.

◆ Counsel women to use nonhormonal contraception; stress that suspected pregnancy should be reported immediately.

◆ *See Antineoplastic agents overview for more information.*

vindescine

vin'deh-seen

vindescine sulfate: *DAVA,* ✿*Eldisine*

Class: Antineoplastic (plant alkaloid) agent

PEDS	PREG	GERI
🖐	D	🖐

Action Kills rapidly growing cells (cancer, hair follicles, bone marrow, GI lining, ova, and sperm) by interfering with cell division (arrests mitosis in metaphase). Is cell-cycle specific in the M-phase.

Use/Therapeutic goal/Outcome

Acute lymphoblastic leukemia, cancer of the breast, lymphosarcoma, malignant melanoma, and non-small-cell lung cancer): Elimination or suppression of malignant cell proliferation. **Outcome criteria:** Tumor and disease regression or stabilization on radiologic and physical examination; for leukemias, absence of blasts in peripheral blood specimen.

Dose range/Administration

Interaction alert: Do not mix IV with other drugs. Mitomycin may increase pulmonary toxicity. May increase cellular retention of methotrexate.

Adult: IV: *Bolus:* 3–4.5 mg/m² every 1–2 weeks; Ascertain vein patency before dose, and flush tube with NS after dose. *Infusion:* 1–2 mg/m² for 2–10 days, every 2–3 weeks (use a central line for continuous infusion).

Clinical alert: This drug should be given only by nurses who are knowledgeable in the comprehensive management of the administration of antineoplastic agents. Doses may vary at physician's discretion. Repeat doses are held until it is ascertained that the patient has recovered sufficiently from toxicities of previous doses. Established protocols/policies for drug preparation, administration, and accidental skin contamination *must be followed closely* (gloves or double gloves are worn when handling drug; if the drug touches the skin, the area is washed immediately with plenty of soap and water). Vindescine sulfate is given IV push over 1 min (followed by a saline flush) or diluted in 50–100 ml fluid and administered via a central line. This drug is a potent vessicant (can cause severe damage to tissues). *Prevention* of extravasation is essential. The drug is given by administering only when it is clear that the needle is in the vein (good blood return), and the infusion site is monitored *closely* for early signs of extravasation (pain and swelling at infusion site). If extravasation is suspected, the infusion is stopped *immediately,* the physician is notified, and protocols/policies for treatment are followed.

Contraindications/Precautions

PREG
D

Contraindicated in hypersensitivity to vindescine sulfate. **Use with caution** in hepatic dysfunction or neuromuscular disease.

✿ **Contraindicated for pregnant or nursing mothers. Use with caution for children and the elderly (greater risk of neurotoxicity).**

Side effects/Adverse reactions

Hypersensitivity: urticaria, fever, dyspnea, bronchospasm, hypotension, anaphylaxis. **Hem:**

leukopenia, anemia, thrombocytopenia. **CNS:** peripheral paresthesia, decreased deep tendon reflexes, muscle weakness, myalgia, headache, parotid and jaw pain, hoarseness. **GI:** anorexia, nausea, vomiting, stomatitis, constipation, paralytic ileus, hepatotoxicity. **Skin:** alopecia; pain, inflammation, and induration at injection site; cellulitis, ulceration, and sloughing if extravasation occurs. **Misc:** pain, syndrome of inappropriate antidiuretic hormone secretion (SIADH).

Nursing implications/Documentation

Possible nursing diagnoses: Potential for infection; Potential for injury; Fatigue; Altered oral mucous membrane; Fluid volume deficit; Diarrhea; Altered nutrition: less than body requirements.

◆ *See important Nursing implications in Antineoplastic agents overview on page 72, which apply to all antineoplastics. The interventions that follow are additional and specific to this drug only.*

• Monitor closely for and report immediately early signs of bronchospasm; keep emergency drugs and equipment readily available (bronchospasm is most common when the patient is also receiving mitomycin).

• Prevent constipation and ileus by monitoring bowel elimination, encouraging fluids and ambulation, and providing laxatives before problem is severe (may require prophylactic stool softeners; constipation may be an early sign of neurotoxicity).

• Observe for and report early signs of CNS toxicity (numbness or tingling of extremities, muscle weakness, wristdrop or footdrop, coordination problems); assess for neuropathy by having the person sign his or her name before each dose.

• Be aware that WBC drops to the nadir (lowest point) 3–5 days after a single infusion and 11–13 days after continuous therapy; hold drug for platelet count <100,000/mm³ or WBC <4000/mm³.

Patient & family teaching/Home care

Possible nursing diagnoses: Knowledge deficit; Ineffective coping (individual and family); Hopelessness; Impaired home maintenance management.

◆ *See important Patient & family teaching in Antineoplastic agents overview on page 72, which apply to all antineoplastics. The*

teachings that follow are additional and specific to this drug only.

• Stress the need to monitor bowel function and prevent constipation by maintaining adequate hydration, eating enough fiber, and using stool softeners or laxatives before the problem is severe; advise reporting abdominal distention and pain as it may indicate an ileus.

• Explain that numbness or tingling of extremities, muscle weakness, or balance problems should be reported, as they may indicate neurotoxicity.

◆ *See Antineoplastic agents overview for more information.*

Vitamin D

cholecalciferol (D₃), ergocalciferol (D₂): *Calciferol, Drisdol, ✦Radiostol, ✦Radiostol Forte*
Class: Fat-soluble vitamin

PEDS	PREG	GERI
🖐	🖐	🖐

Action Necessary for normal calcium and phosphate blood levels, bone development, parathyroid activity, and neuromuscular functioning.

Use/Therapeutic goal/Outcome

Renal osteodystrophy, rickets, and other vitamin D deficiency diseases: Promotion of normal calcium and phosphate blood levels, bone development, parathyroid activity, and neuromuscular activity. **Outcome criteria:** Calcium and phosphate blood levels within normal range; X-ray evidence of normal bone development and absence of osteomalacia; patient report of absence of bone pain.

Dose range/Administration

Interaction alert: Mineral oil and cholestyramine inhibit absorption; separate doses from Vitamin D by at least 6 hours. If given with diuretics, monitor for increased risk of Vitamin D toxicity.

Renal osteopathy/Rickets/Other Vitamin D deficiencies: **Adult:** PO, IM: 12,000 IU/day; may increase daily as needed (usual 500,000 IU/day, but 800,000 IU may be needed for vitamin D resistant rickets). **Child:** PO, IM: 1500–5000 IU/day for 2–4 wk, or a single 600,000 IU dose; may repeat after 2 wk.

Hypoparathyroidism: **Adult and Child:** PO, IM: 50,000–200,000 IU/day with 4 g calcium supplement.

V

Clinical alert: Monitor calcium blood levels closely to ensure appropriate dosage. With high doses, monitor urine calcium, potassium, and urea. Patients who cannot absorb oral Vitamin D can have IM injections of Vitamin D dispersed in oil. May be given IV, but use only water-miscible solutions used for large-volume IV administration.

Contraindications/Precautions

PREG ♇

Contraindicated in hypersensitivity to Vitamin D, and in hypercalcemia, hypervitaminosis A, and renal osteodystrophy with hyperphosphatemia. **Use with caution** in cardiovascular disease and renal calculi.

♇ Use with caution for children and the elderly. Use with caution in recommended daily allowances (RDA) for pregnant women (preg A); safe use in doses greater than RDA has not been established (preg D).

Side effects/Adverse reactions

Hypersensitivity: itching, rashes. **Hem:** hypercalcemia. **Misc:** Vitamin D toxicity (headache, dizziness, ataxia, weakness, drowsiness, psychosis, decreased libido, seizures, soft tissue calcification, dry mouth, metallic taste, runny nose, conjunctivitis, photophobia, tinnitus, anorexia, nausea, vomiting, constipation, diarrhea, polyuria, albuminuria, hypercalciuria, nocturia, renal calculi, impaired renal function).

Nursing implications/Documentation

Possible nursing diagnoses: Potential for injury; Altered nutrition: less than body requirements.

♦ Establish baseline serum calcium, phosphate, magnesium, BUN, creatinine, alkaline phosphatase and urine calcium; then monitor closely thereafter.

♦ Monitor Vitamin D levels every 2 weeks.

♦ Report symptoms of dry mouth, nausea, vomiting, metallic taste, and constipation (may indicate Vitamin D toxicity).

♦ Patients with liver dysfunction or inadequate bile production may need bile salts to absorb oral Vitamin D.

♦ Monitor diet to ensure compliance with restrictions and intake of sufficient Vitamin D.

Patient & family teaching/Home care

Possible nursing diagnoses: Knowledge deficit; Impaired home maintenance management.

♦ Explain that Vitamin D is necessary for normal calcium levels, bone growth and maintenance, and neuromuscular function.

♦ Stress the need to stick to prescribed diet; provide a list of foods high in Vitamin D that are included in prescribed diet.

♦ Warn of the dangers of increasing doses; provide a list of symptoms that may indicate Vitamin D toxicity (see Nursing implications).

♦ Advise avoidance of magnesium-containing antacids.

warfarin

(war'far-in)

warfarin sodium: **Coumadin, Panwarin, Warfilon Sodium**

Class: ★**Oral anticoagulant prototype**

Antidote: Vitamin K

PEDS	PREG	GERI
♇	**D**	♇

Action Inhibits blood coagualation by inhibiting activity of vitamin K, thus blocking synthesis of Vitamin K–dependent clotting factors in the liver (factors II, VII, IX, and X). Does **not** dissolve existing clots.

Use/Therapeutic goal/Outcome

Pulmonary emboli, deep vein thrombosis, myocardial infarction, cardiac valve problems, atrial dysrhythmias: Prevention of thrombus formation. **Outcome criteria:** Prothrombin time (PT) within therapeutic range (1.5 to 2 times the normal).

Dose range/Administration

Interaction alert: Since this drug's effects are altered by numerous other drugs, monitor PT closely whenever *any* medications are added to or deleted from the regimen.

Adult: PO: Individualized dose depends on PT and clinical status, and should be given at the same time every day. *Loading dose:* usually 10–15 mg/day for 2–5 days (may be as high as 40–60 mg). *Maintenance dose:* usually 2–10 mg/day. For elderly or debilitated patients, dose should be reduced by half.

Clinical alert: Ascertain that baseline PT has been drawn before giving first dose; monitor daily until maintenance dose is established. Be aware of the high incidence of bleeding if the PT exceeds 2.5 times the normal; risk of thrombus formation increases if PT falls below therapeutic range.

W

Contraindications/Precautions

Contraindicated in hypersensitivity to warfarin; and in active bleeding or conditions that cause a bleeding tendency (e.g., hemophilia); blood dyscrasias; thrombocytopenia purpura; leukemia with bleeding tendency; anticipated impending surgery; threatened abortion; hemorrhagic cerebrovascular accident (CVA); severe hypertension; recent surgery of the eye, brain, or spinal cord; GI ulcers; open wounds; subacute bacterial endocarditis; impaired kidney or liver function.

🖐 **Use with caution for infants, pregnant or nursing mothers, the elderly, and the debilitated.**

Side effects/Adverse reactions

Hypersensitivity: itching, rashes, fever (may indicate severe reaction). **Hem:** bleeding or hemorrhage. **Skin:** with excessive doses; petechiae, bruising. **GI:** diarrhea, vomiting, cramps, nausea.

Nursing implications/Documentation

Possible nursing diagnoses: Potential for injury; Altered oral mucous membrane.

♦ Assess for history of bleeding conditions before giving first dose.

♦ Check for baseline PT studies before giving first dose; monitor daily thereafter to ascertain therapeutic range until maintenance dose is established.

♦ Report PT below therapeutic range because of potential for thrombus formation, and PT above therapeutic range because of potential for bleeding.

♦ Chart anticoagulant therapy on the same record all medications are charted to avoid an oversight that the patient is being anticoagulated; use a flow sheet to monitor PT levels to ascertain safe dosage.

♦ Monitor for and report signs of occult or overt bleeding: check gums for bleeding, assess skin for bruising, and observe for tarry stools, GI bleeding, or hematuria (may signify onset of hemorrhage).

♦ Ensure anticoagulant therapy is discontinued prior to surgical or invasive procedures.

♦ Be aware that, because the action of warfarin is delayed, heparin is often given during the first few days of therapy.

♦ Hold drug and report immediately if the patient demonstrates fever and skin rash (may signify severe adverse reaction).

♦ Avoid IM injections, if possible.

♦ Recognize that PT levels return to normal within 2–10 days after warfarin doses are stopped.

Patient & family teaching/Home care

Possible nursing diagnoses: Knowledge deficit; Impaired home maintenance management.

♦ Emphasize the importance of taking warfarin at the same time every day, of recording the dose on the calendar, and of returning for medical follow-up. (A forgotten dose should be taken as soon as possible.)

♦ Explain that warfarin should be withheld and physician notified immediately if bleeding, bruising, petechiae, black stools, or fever accompanied by a rash occurs.

♦ Teach that aspirin, other salicylates and ibuprofen also have anticoagulant effects and should be avoided; warn against use of OTC drugs unless specifically approved by physician.

♦ Explain the importance of informing dentists and other physicians of anticoagulant therapy.

♦ Recommend using a soft toothbrush to avoid gum injury, and an *electric* razor to prevent cuts.

♦ Warn against performing activities that may result in cuts, bumps or bruises.

♦ Encourage wearing a bracelet or carrying an ID card that states that the person is taking an anticoagulant.

♦ *See Anticoagulants and Thrombolytic Enzymes overview for more information.*

zidovudine

zye-doe'vyoo-deen

(azidothymidine, AZT): *Retrovir*

Class: Anti-infective, Antiviral agent

PEDS	PREG	GERI
🖐	C	🖐

Action Prevents replication of human immunodeficiency virus (HIV), probably by inhibiting the enzyme *reverse transcriptase*; in vitro, it is incorporated into growing DNA strands (thus halting the strand's growth).

Use/Therapeutic goal/Outcome

Management of HIV infection (AIDS [acquired immune deficiency syndrome] or ARC [aids-related complex]): Alleviation of signs and symptoms. *Outcome criteria:* Decrease in signs and symptoms of AIDS; elevated T4 lymphocyte count; report of improved sense of well-being.

Zidovudine has also been used for prophylaxis in known HIV exposure (research is ongoing; check with physician and pharmacist).

Dose range/Administration

Interaction alert: Trimethoprim-sulfamethoxazole, acetaminophen, aspirin, indomethacin, and probenecid may decrease hepatic metabolism of zidovudine and increase its toxicity. Other cytotoxic drugs may increase bone marrow depression effects. *Use cautiously* with acyclovir (may cause neurotoxicity).

Adult: PO: 100–200 mg q4h (on a strict schedule, sometimes required around the clock). *Asymptomatic patients:* 100 mg 3–5 times a day. *Child:* PO: 120mg/m^2 q6h. *Adult:* IV: 1–2 mg/kg infused over 1 hour q4h around the clock until oral doses can be given. *Child:* IV: 120 mg/m^2 infused over 1 hour q6h.

Clinical alert: Keep in mind that people with AIDS or ARC are at risk for opportunistic infections, and that you are at risk of contracting HIV whenever you come in contact with the patient's bodily fluids. Follow strict body substance isolation (BSI).

Contraindications/Precautions
PREG C

Contraindicated in life-threatening hypersensitivity reactions to any of the drug's components. *Use with caution* in bone marrow depression, or kidney or liver impairment.

✋ **Contraindicated for nursing mothers. Use with caution for the elderly because elimination rate may be decreased. Safe use for children under 3 months and pregnant women has not been established.**

Side effects/Adverse reactions

Hypersensitivity: itching, rashes, stomatitis, anaphylaxis. *Hem:* anemia (secondary to severe bone marrow depression), granulocytopenia, increased platelets, thrombocytopenia. *GI:* nausea, vomiting, hepatotoxicity. *CNS:* headache, insomnia, restlessness, agitation, confusion, anxiety. *MS:* myalgia. *Misc:* bluish-brown nails.

Nursing implications/Documentation

Possible nursing diagnoses: Potential for infection; Altered oral mucous membrane.

♦ Weigh patient and obtain baseline lab studies (CBC, T4 lymphocyte count, granulocyte count, electrolytes, BUN, creatinine, liver function studies) before administering first dose; monitor at least weekly initially, then every 2–4 weeks.

♦ Encourage fluid intake, and document and monitor intake and output, to assure adequate hydration and urine output.

♦ Monitor for and report symptoms of *superinfection* (mouth lesions, thrush, vaginal irritation, diarrhea, respiratory symptoms) or CHF (dyspnea, ankle swelling).

♦ Monitor for and report oral inflammation; establish a program of gentle, rather than aggressive, mouth care.

♦ Recognize that erythropoietin or blood transfusion may be given to treat anemia.

Patient & family teaching/Home care

Possible nursing diagnoses: Knowledge deficit; Impaired home maintenance management; Altered patterns of sexuality; Social isolation.

♦ If indicated by the physician, stress the importance of taking zidovudine on a strict q4h schedule without missing doses (use an alarm clock if necessary).

♦ Explain that zidovudine provides disease management, not cure; and that the individual is still at risk for transmitting the disease.

♦ Point out that although it is not yet clear how long zidovudine must be taken, it has been demonstrated to be beneficial in the management of AIDS and ARC.

♦ Warn against taking any other drugs (including "street cures") without checking with physician (may decrease effectiveness of zidovudine).

♦ Explain that periodic blood transfusions are often necessary when taking zidovudine (side effect of bone marrow depression often results in decreased RBC production), and that periodic drug interruption may be needed.

♦ Stress the need for safe sex, explore concerns, and recommend counseling as needed.

♦ *See Anti-infectives overview for more information.*

Combination products

Acne-Aid cream: sulfur 2.5%, resorcinol 1.25%, and parachlorometaxylenol 0.375% in a microporous cellulose base.

Acnomel cream: sulfur 8%, resorcinol 2%, and alcohol 11% in a greaseless base.

Actifed: pseudoephrine hydrochloride 60 mg and triprolidine HCl 2.5 mg.

Agoral: mineral oil 28% and white phenolphthalein 1.3% in emulsion with tragacanth, agar, egg albumin, acacia, and glycerin.

Alazide: spironolactone 25 mg and hydrochlorothiazide 25 mg.

Albalon-A Liquifilm: naphazoline hydrochloride 0.05% and antazoline phosphate 0.5%.

Aldactazide: spironolactone 25 mg and hydrochlorothiazide 25 mg.

Aldactazide 50/50: spironolactone 50 mg and hydrochlorothiazide 50 mg.

Aldoclor-150: chlorothiazide 150 mg and methyldopa 250 mg.

Aldoclor-250: chlorothiazide 250 mg and methyldopa 250 mg.

Aldoril-15: hydrochlorothiazide 15 mg and methyldopa 250 mg.

Aldoril-25: hydrochlorothiazide 25 mg and methyldopa 250 mg.

Aldoril D30: hydrochlorothiazide 30 mg and methyldopa 500 mg.

Aldoril D50: hydrochlorothiazide 50 mg and methyldopa 500 mg.

Alka-Seltzer: sodium bicarbonate 1916 mg, aspirin 325 mg, and citric acid 1000 mg.

Alka-Seltzer without Aspirin: sodium bicarbonate 958 mg, citric acid 832 mg, and potassium bicarbonate 312 mg.

Allerest Tablets: phenylpropanolamine HCl 18.7 mg and chlorpheniramine maleate 2 mg.

Allergesic: phenylpropanolamine 18.7 mg and chlorpheniramine maleate 2 mg.

Altexide: spironolactone 25 mg and hydrochlorothiazide 25 mg.

Aludrox Suspension: aluminum hydroxide 307 mg and magnesium hydroxide 103 mg.

Amacodone: hydrocodone bitartrate 5 mg and acetaminophen 500 mg.

Amaphen: acetaminophen 325 mg, caffeine 40 mg, and butalbital 50 mg.

Angijen No. 1: pentaerythritol tetranitrate 20 mg and phenobarbital sodium 15 mg.

Anoquan: acetaminophen 325 mg, caffeine 40 mg, and butalbital 50 mg.

Apresazide 25/25: hydrochlorothiazide 25 mg and hydralazine HCl 25 mg.

Apresazide 50/50: hydrochlorothiazide 50 mg and hydralazine HCl 50 mg.

Apresazide 100/50: hydrochlorothiazide 50 mg and hydralazine HCl 100 mg.

Apresodex: hydrochlorothiazide 15 mg and hydralazine HCl 25 mg.

Apresoline-Esidrix: hydrochlorothiazide 15 mg and hydralazine HCl 25 mg.

Aralen Phosphate with Primaquine Phosphate: chloroquine phosphate 500 mg (300 mg base) and primaquine phosphate 79 mg (45 mg base).

Arcotrate No. 3: pentaerythritol tetranitrate 20 mg and phenobarbital sodium 8 mg.

Arthralgen: acetaminophen 250 mg and salicylamide 250 mg.

Augmentin: amoxicillin 250 mg and clavulanate potassium 125 mg per tablet; amoxicillin 500 mg and clavulanate potassium 125 mg per tablet; amoxicillin 125 mg and clavulanate 31.5 mg per 5-ml oral suspension; amoxicillin 250 mg and potassium clavulanate 31.5 mg per 5-ml oral suspension; amoxicillin 125 mg and potassium clavulanate 31.5 mg per chewable tablet; amoxicillin 250 mg and potassium clavulanate 31.5 mg per chewable tablet.

Axotal: aspirin 650 mg and butalbital 50 mg.

Azo Gantanol: sulfamethoxazole 500 mg and phenazopyridine HCl 100 mg.

Azo Gantrisin: sulfisoxazole 500 mg and phenazopyridine HCl 50 mg.

Azo Sulfamethoxazole: sulfisoxazole 500 mg and phenazopyridine HCl 50 mg.

Bancap HC: hydrocodone bitartrate 5 mg and acetaminophen 500 mg.

Barbidonna Elixir: atropine sulfate 0.034 mg/5 ml, phenobarbital 21.6 mg/5 ml, hyoscyamine hydrobromide or sulfate 0.174 mg/5 ml, hyoscine hydrobromide 0.01 mg/5 ml, and alcohol 15%.

Barbidonna Tablets: atropine sulfate 0.025 mg, hyoscine hydrobromide 0.0074 mg, hyoscyamine hydrobromide or sulfate 0.1286 mg, and phenobarbital 16 mg.

Barbidonna No. 2 Tablets: atropine sulfate 0.025 mg, hyoscine hydrobromide 0.0074 mg, hyoscyamine hydrobromide or sulfate 0.1286 mg, and phenobarbital 32 mg.

BC Powder: aspirin 650 mg, salicylamide 195 mg, and caffeine 32 mg.

BC Tablets: aspirin 325 mg, salicylamide 95 mg, and caffeine 16 mg.

Belladenal Tablets: L-alkaloids of belladonna 0.25 mg and phenobarbital 50 mg.

Bilron: bile salts and iron.

Biphetamine 12 1/2: dextroamphetamine 6.25 mg and amphetamine 6.25 mg.

Biphetamine 20: dextroamphetamine 10 mg and amphetamine 10 mg.

Bitrate: pentaerythritol tetranitrate 15 mg and phenobarbital sodium 20 mg.

Blanex: chlorzoxazone 250 mg and acetaminophen 300 mg.

Blephamide S.O.P. Sterile Ophthalmic Ointment: sodium sulfacetamide 10% and prednisolone acetate 0.2%.

Blephamide Liquifilm Suspension: phenylephrine hydrochloride 0.12% and sulfacetamide sodium 10%.

Bromfed-DM: brompheniramine maleate 2 mg, dextromethorphan hydrobromide 10 mg, and pseudoephedrine HCl 30 mg/5 ml.

Bronchial Capsules: 150 mg theophylline and 90 mg guaifenesin.

Bronchobid Duracaps: theophylline 260 mg and ephedrine HCl 35 mg.

Brondecon Tablets: 200 mg oxtriphylline and 100 mg guaifenesin.

Buff-A-Comp No. 3: codeine phosphate 30 mg, aspirin 325 mg, caffeine 40 mg, and butalbital 50 mg.

Butal: aspirin 325 mg, caffeine 40 mg, and butalbital 50 mg.

Cafergot: ergotamine tartrate 1 mg and caffeine 100 mg.

Cafergot Suppositories: ergotamine tartrate 2 mg and caffeine 100 mg.

Caladryl Lotion: diphenhydramine HCl 1%, calamine, camphor, and alcohol 2%.

Cama, Arthritis Strength: aspirin 500 mg, magnesium oxide 150 mg, and aluminum hydroxide 150 mg.

Camalox Tablets: aluminum hydroxide 225 mg, magnesium hydroxide 200 mg, and calcium carbonate 250 mg.

Cam-AP-ES: hydrochlorothiazide 15 mg, hydralazine HCl 25 mg, and reserpine 0.1 mg.

Capozide 50/25: hydrochlorothiazide 25 mg and captopril 50 mg.

Capozide 50/15: hydrochlorothiazide 15 mg and captopril 50 mg.

Capozide 25/25: hydrochlorothiazide 25 mg and captopril 25 mg.

Capozide 25/15: hydrochlorothiazide 15 mg and captopril 25 mg.

Carmol HC: urea 10% and hydrocortisone acetate 1%.

Cetacaine Liquid: benzocaine 14%, tetracaine HCl 2%, benzalkonium chloride 0.5%, butyl aminobenzoate 2%, and cetyl dimethyl ethyl ammonium bromide in a bland water-soluble base.

Cetapred Ointment: sodium sulfacetamide 10% and prednisolone acetate 0.25%.

Chardonna-2: belladonna extract 15 mg and phenobarbital 15 mg.

Cherapas: hydrochlorothiazide 15 mg, hydralazine HCl 25 mg, and reserpine 0.1 mg.

Chlor-Trimeton Decongestant: chlorpheniramine maleate 4 mg and pseudoephedrine sulfate 60 mg.

Chlor-Trimeton Decongestant Repetabs: chlorpheniramine maleate 8 mg and pseudoephedrine sulfate 120 mg.

Chlorofon-F: chlorzoxazone 250 mg and acetaminophen 300 mg.

Chloromycetin Hydrocortisone Ophthalmic: chloramphenicol 0.25% and hydrocortisone acetate 0.5% (as the prepared solution).

Chlorzone Forte: chlorzoxazone 250 mg and acetaminophen 300 mg.

Chymoral-100: 100,000 units enzymatic activity; trypsin and chymotrypsin in ratio 6:1.

Clavulin: amoxicillin 250 mg and clavulanate potassium 125 mg per tablet; amoxicillin 500 mg and clavulanate potassium 125 mg per tablet; amoxicillin 125 mg and clavulanate 31.5 mg per 5-ml oral suspension; amoxicillin 250 mg and potassium clavulanate 31.5 mg per 5-ml oral suspension; amoxicillin 125 mg and potassium clavulanate 31.5 mg per chewable tablet; amoxicillin 250 mg and potassium clavulanate 31.5 mg per chewable tablet.

Clearasil Cream: benzoyl peroxide 10% and bentonite.

Codimal-DH: hydrocodone bitartrate 1.66 mg, phenylephrine HCl 5 mg, pyrilamine maleate 8.33 mg, potassium guaiacolsulfonate 83.3 mg, sodium citrate 216 mg, and citric acid 50 mg.

Colbenemid: probenecid 500 mg and colchicine 0.5 mg.

Coly-Mycin S Otic: Each ml contains neomycin sulfate 3.3 mg, colistin sulfate 3 mg, hydrocortisone acetate 10 mg, and thronzonium bromide 0.05%.

Combipres 0.1: chlorthalidone 15 mg and clonidine HCl 0.1 mg.

Combipres 0.2: chlorthalidone 15 mg and clonidine HCl 0.2 mg.

Compound W: salicylic acid 14%, acetic acid 11%, in castor oil, alcohol, ether, and collodion.

Condrin-LA: phenylpropanolamine HCl 75 mg and chlorpheniramine maleate 12 mg.

Congespirin: phenylephrine HCl 1.25 mg and aspirin 81 mg.

Contac Capsules: phenylpropanolamine 75 mg and chlorpheniramine maleate 8 mg.

Contac 12-Hour Caplets: phenylpropanolamine 75 mg and chlorpheniramine maleate 12 mg.

Cope: aspirin 421 mg, caffeine 32 mg, magnesium hydroxide 50 mg, and aluminum hydroxide 25 mg.

Cordran-N (cream, ointment): flurandrenolide 0.05% and neomycin sulfate 0.5%.

Coricidin Tablets: chlorpheniramine maleate 2 mg and aspirin 325 mg.

Cortisporin Ophthalmic Ointment: polymyxin B sulfate 10,000 units, bacitracin zinc 400 units, neomycin sulfate 0.35%, and hydrocortisone 1%.

Cortisporin Ophthalmic Suspension: polymyxin B sulfate 10,000 units, neomycin sulfate 0.35%, and hydrocortisone 1%.

Cortisporin Otic: Each ml contains neomycin sulfate 5 mg, polymyxin B 10,000 units, and hydrocortisone 1%.

Corzide: nadolol 40 mg or 80 mg and bendroflumethiazide 5 mg.

Cyclomydril Ophthalmic: cyclopentolate HCl 0.2% and phenylephrine HCl 1%.

Cystex: methenamine 165 mg, salicylamide 65 mg, sodium salicylate 97 mg, and benzoic acid 32 mg.

Darvocet-N 50: propoxyphene napsylate 50 mg and acetaminophen 325 mg.

Darvocet-N 100: propoxyphene napsylate 100 mg and acetaminophen 650 mg.

Darvon Compound: propoxyphene HCl 32 mg, aspirin 389 mg, and caffeine 32.4 mg.

Darvon Compound-65: propoxyphene HCl 65 mg, aspirin 389 mg, and caffeine 32.4 mg.

Darvon-N with ASA: propoxyphene napsylate 100 mg and aspirin 325 mg.

Darvon with ASA: propoxyphene HCl 65 mg and aspirin 325 mg.

Decadron Phosphate with Xylocaine: dexamethasone phosphate 4 mg and lidocaine HCl 10 mg/ml.

Deconade: phenylpropanolamine HCl 75 mg and chlorpheniramine maleate 12 mg.

Deconamine: pseudoephedrine HCl 60 mg and chlorpheniramine maleate 4 mg.

Deladumone: testosterone enanthate 90 mg/ml, estradiol valerate 4 mg/ml, and chlorobutanol 0.5% in sesame oil.

Delcid Suspension: aluminum hydroxide 600 mg, magnesium hydroxide 665 mg.

Demerol APAP: meperidine HCl 50 mg and acetaminophen 300 mg.

Demi-Regroton: chlorthalidone 25 mg and reserpine 0.125 mg.

Depo-Testadiol (OIL): testosterone cypionate 50 mg, estradiol cypionate 2 mg, and chlorobutanol 0.5%.

Deprol: meprobamate 400 mg and benactyzine HCl 1 mg.

Dermoplast Spray: benzocaine 20% and menthol 0.5%.

Di-Gel Liquid: aluminum hydroxide 200 mg, magnesium hydroxide 200 mg and simethicone 20 mg.

Dialose Plus: docusate potassium 100 mg and casanthranol 30 mg.

Dilantin with Phenobarbital: phenytoin sodium 100 mg and phenobarbital 16 mg.

Dilantin with Phenobarbital: phenytoin sodium 100 mg and phenobarbital 32 mg.

Dilor-G Tablets: 200 mg dyphylline and 200 mg guaifenesin.

Dimetapp Extentabs: bromopheniramine maleate 12 mg and phenylpropanolamine hydrochloride 75 mg.

Dimycor: pentaerythritol tetranitrate 10 mg and phenobarbital sodium 15 mg.

Diolax: docusate sodium 100 mg and casanthranol 30 mg.

Disophrol Chronotabs: dexbrompheniramine maleate 12 mg and phenylpropanolamine HCl 75 mg.

Ditate-DS: estradiol valerate 8 mg and testosterone enanthate 180 mg.

Diupres-250: chlorothiazide 250 mg and reserpine 0.125 mg.

Diupres-500: chlorothiazide 500 mg and reserpine 0.125 mg.

Diurese-R: trichloromethiazide 4 mg and reserpine 0.1 mg.

Diurigen with Reserpine: chlorothiazide 250 mg and reserpine 0.125 mg.

Diutensen: methyclothiazide 2.5 mg and cryptenamine 2 mg (as tannate).

Diutensen-R: methyclothiazide 2.5 mg and reserpine 0.1 mg.

Dolacet: propoxyphene HCl 65 mg and acetaminophen 650 mg.

Dolene AP-65: propoxyphene HCl 65 mg and acetaminophen 650 mg.

Dolene Compound-65: propoxyphene HCl 65 mg, aspirin 389 mg, and caffeine 32.4 mg.

Donnagel-PG: powdered opium 24 mg, kaolin 6 g, pectin 142.8 mg, hyoscyamine sulfate 0.1037 mg, atropine sulfate 0.0194 mg, hyoscine hydrobromide 0.0065 mg, and alcohol 5% in 30-ml suspension.

Donnagel Suspension: kaolin 6 g, pectin 142.8 mg, hyoscyamine sulfate 0.1037 mg, atropine sulfate 0.0194 mg, hyoscine hydrobromide 0.0065 mg, and alcohol 3.8% in 30-ml suspension.

Donnatal Elixir: atropine sulfate 0.0194 mg/5 ml, hyoscine hydrobromide 0.0065 mg/5 ml, alcohol 23%, hyoscyamine hydrobromide or sulfate 0.1037 mg/5 ml and phenobarbital 16 mg/5 ml.

Donnatal Extentabs: atropine sulfate 0.0582 mg, Ehyoscine hydrobromide 0.0195 mg, hyoscyamine sulfate 0.3111 mg, and phenobarbital 48.6 mg.

Donnatal Tablets and Capsules: atropine sulfate 0.0194 mg, hyoscine hydrobromide 0.0065 mg, hyoscyamine hydrobromide or sulfate 0.1037 mg, and phenobarbital 16 mg.

Donnatal No. 2 Tablets: atropine sulfate 0.0194 mg, hyoscine hydrobromide 0.0065 mg, hyoscyamine hydrobromide or sulfate 0.1037 mg, and phenobarbital 32.4 mg.

Donnazyme Tablets: pancreatin 300 mg, pepsin 150 mg, bile salts 150 mg, hyoscyamine sulfate 0.0518 mg, atropine sulfate 0.0097 mg, hyoscine hydrobromide 0.0033 mg, and phenobarbital 8.1 mg.

Doxaphene Compound: propoxyphene HCl 65 mg, aspirin 389 mg, and caffeine 32.4 mg.

Doxidan: docusate calcium 60 mg and phenolphthalein 65 mg.

Dristan: phenylephrine HCl 5 mg, chlorpheniramine maleate 2 mg, aspirin 325 mg, and caffeine 16.2 mg.

Drixoral: dexbrompheniramine maleate 6 mg and pseudoephedrine sulfate 120 mg.

Drize: phenylpropanolamine HCl 75 mg and chlorpheniramine maleate 12 mg.

D-S-S Plus: docusate sodium 100 mg and casanthranol 30 mg.

Duo-Medihaler: isoproterenol HCl 0.16 mg and phenylephrine bitartrate 0.24 mg per dose.

Duradyne: acetaminophen 180 mg, aspirin 230 mg, and caffeine 15 mg.

Duradyne DHC: hydrocodone bitartrate 5 mg and acetaminophen 500 mg.

Dyazide: triamterene 50 mg and hydrochlorothiazide 25 mg.

Dyflex-G Tablets: 200 mg dyphylline and 200 mg guaifenesin.

Dyline-GG Tablets: 200 mg dyphylline and 200 mg guaifenesin.

EDTA: 1.4% polyvinyl alcohol, polysorbate 80, sodium thiosulfate, and benzalkonium chloride.

Empirin with Codeine No. 2: aspirin 325 mg and codeine phosphate 15 mg.

Empirin with Codeine No. 3: aspirin 325 mg and codeine phosphate 30 mg.

Empirin with Codeine No. 4: aspirin 325 mg and codeine phosphate 60 mg.

Empracet with Codeine No. 3: codeine phosphate 30 mg and acetaminophen 300 mg.

Empracet with Codeine No. 4: codeine phosphate 60 mg and acetaminophen 300 mg.

Enduronyl: methyclothiazide 5 mg and deserpidine 0.25 mg.

Enduronyl Forte: methyclothiazide 5 mg and deserpidine 0.5 mg.

Entozyme Tablets: pancreatin 300 mg, pepsin 250 mg, and bile salts 150 mg.

E-Pilo: epinephrine bitartrate 1% and pilocarpine HCl 1%, 2%, 3%, 4%, or 6%.

Equagesic: meprobamate 200 mg and aspirin 325 mg.

Ergocaff: ergotamine tartrate 1 mg and caffeine 100 mg.

Esgic: acetaminophen 325 mg, caffeine 40 mg, and butalbital 50 mg.

Esimil: hydrochlorothiazide 25 mg and guanethidine monosulfate 10 mg.

Estratest: esterified estrogens 1.25 mg and methyltestosterone 2.5 mg.

Estratest H.S.: esterified estrogens 0.625 mg and methyltestosterone 1.25 mg.

Etrafon 2-10: perphenazine 2 mg and amitriptyline HCl 10 mg.

Etrafon: perphenazine 2 mg and amitriptyline HCl 25 mg.

Etrafon-A: perphenazine 4 mg and amitriptyline 10 mg.

Etrafon Forte: perphenazine 4 mg and amitriptyline 25 mg.

Euthroid-1/2: levothyroxine sodium 30 mcg and liothyronine sodium 7.5 mcg.

Euthroid-1: levothyroxine sodium 120 mcg and liothyronine sodium 15 mcg.

Euthroid-2: levothyroxine sodium 120 mcg and liothyronine sodium 30 mcg.

Euthroid-3: levothyroxine sodium 180 mcg and liothyronine sodium 45 mcg.

Eutron Filmtabs: methyclothiazide 5 mg and pargyline HCl 25 mg.

Excedrin P.M.: acetaminophen 500 mg and diphenhydramine citrate 38 mg.

Excedrin Tablets: aspirin 250 mg, acetaminophen 250 mg and caffeine 65 mg.

Exna-R Tablets: benzthiazide 50 mg and reserpine 0.125 mg.

Extra Strength Maalox Tablets: aluminum hydroxide 400 mg and magnesium hydroxide 400 mg.

Fansidar: sulfadoxine 500 mg and pyrimethamine 25 mg.

Fedahist: pseudoephedrine HCl 60 mg and chlorpheniramine maleate 4 mg.

Femcaps: acetaminophen 324 mg, caffeine 32 mg, ephedrine sulfate 8 mg, and atropine sulfate 0.0325 mg.

Fermalox: ferrous sulfate 200 mg, and magnesium hydroxide, and dried aluminum hydroxide gel 200 mg.

Ferocyl: iron (as fumarate) 50 mg and docusate sodium 100 mg.

Ferro-Sequels: iron (as fumarate) 50 mg and docusate sodium 100 mg.

Fioricet: acetaminophen 325 mg, butalbital 50 mg, and caffeine 40 mg.

Fiorinal: aspirin 325 mg, caffeine 40 mg, and butalbital 50 mg.

Fiorinal with Codeine No.1: codeine phosphate 7.5 mg, aspirin 325 mg, caffeine 40 mg, and butalbital 50 mg.

Fiorinal with Codeine No. 2: codeine phosphate 15 mg, aspirin 325 mg, caffeine 40 mg, and butalbital 50 mg.

Fiorinal with Codeine No. 3: codeine phosphate 30 mg, aspirin 325 mg, caffeine 40 mg, and butalbital 50 mg.

Fluress: sodium fluorescein 0.25% and benoxinate HCl 0.4%.

4-Way Nasal Spray: phenylephrine HCl 0.5%, naphazoline HCl 0.05%, and pyrilamine maleate 0.2%.

G-1: acetaminophen 500 mg, caffeine 40 mg, and butalbital 50 mg.

Gaviscon: aluminum hydroxide 31.7 mg and magnesium carbonate 137 mg.

Gelusil: aluminum hydroxide 200 mg, magnesium hydroxide 200 mg, and simethicone 25 mg.

Gelusil-II: aluminum hydroxide 400 mg, magnesium hydroxide 400 mg, and simethicone 30 mg.

Gelusil-M: aluminum hydroxide 300 mg, magnesium hydroxide 200 mg, and simethicone 25 mg.

Gemnisyn: aspirin 325 mg and acetaminophen 325 mg.

Glyceral-T Capsules: 150 mg theophylline and 90 mg guaifenesin.

Gramcal: calcium lactate-gluconate 3080 mg, calcium carbonate 1500 mg, and potassium 390 mg; provides 1000 mg of elemental calcium.

Granulex Aerosol: trypsin 0.1 mg, balsam Peru 72.5 mg, and castor oil 650 mg/0.82 ml.

Haley's M-O: mineral oil (25%) and magnesium hydroxide.

Hexalol: methenamine 40.8 mg, phenyl salicylate 18.1 mg, atropine sulfate 0.03 mg, hyoscyamine 0.03 mg, benzoic acid 4.5 mg, and methylene blue 5.4 mg.

H.H.R: hydrochlorothiazide 15 mg, hydralazine HCl 25 mg, and reserpine 0.1 mg.

Histabid Duracaps: phenylpropanolamine 75 mg and chlorpheniramine maleate 8 mg.

Histaspan-D: chlorpheniramine maleate 8 mg, phenylephrine hydrochloride 20 mg, and methscopolamine nitrate 2.5 mg.

Histaspan-PLUS: phenylephrine hydrochloride 20 mg and chlorpheniramine maleate 8 mg.

Hycodaphen: hydrocodone bitartrate 5 mg and acetaminophen 500 mg.

Hydergine: dihydroergocornine mesylate 0.167 mg, dihydroergocristine mesylate 0.167 mg, and dihydroergocryptine mesylate 0.167 mg.

Hydromox R: quinethazone 50 mg and reserpine 0.125 mg.

Hydropine: hydroflumethiazide 25 mg and reserpine 0.125 mg.

Hydropine HP: hydroflumethiazide 50 mg and reserpine 0.125 mg.

Hydro plus: hydrochlorothiazide 50 mg and reserpine 0.125 mg.

Hydropres-25: hydrochlorothiazide 25 mg and reserpine 0.125 mg.

Hydro-Reserp: hydrochlorothiazide 50 mg and reserpine 0.125 mg.

Hydro-Serp: hydrochlorothiazide 50 mg and reserpine 0.125 mg.

Hydroserpine: hydrochlorothiazide 50 mg and reserpine 0.125 mg.

Hydrotensin-25 Tablets: hydrochlorothiazide 25 mg and reserpine 0.125 mg.

Inderide 40/25: propranolol HCl 40 mg and hydrochlorothiazide 25 mg.

Inderide 80/25: propranolol HCl 80 mg and hydrochlorothiazide 25 mg.

Inderide LA 80/50: propranolol HCl 80 mg and hydrochlorothiazide 50 mg.

Innovar Injection: fentanyl (as citrate) 0.05 mg and droperidol 2.5 mg per ml.

Isollyl: aspirin 325 mg, caffeine 40 mg, and butalbital 50 mg.

Isopto Cetapred: sulfacetamide sodium 10% and prednisolone acetate 0.25%.

Isopto P-ES: pilocarpine HCl 2% and physostigmine salicylate 0.25%.

Kaochlor-EFF: 20 mEq potassium, 20 mEq chloride (from potassium chloride, potassium

citrate, potassium bicarbonate, and betaine hydrochloride).

Kinesed Tablets: atropine sulfate 0.02 mg, hyoscine hydrobromide 0.007 mg, hyoscyamine hydrobromide or sulfate 0.1 mg, and phenobarbital 16 mg.

Klorvess: 20 mEq each potassium and chloride (from potassium chloride, potassium bicarbonate, and l-lysine monohydrochloride).

Kolyum: 20 mEq potassium and 3.4 mEq chloride (from potassium gluconate and potassium chloride).

Kondremul with Cascara: heavy mineral oil 55%, cascara sagrada 660 mg/15 ml, and Irish moss as emulsifier.

Kondremul with Phenolphthalein: heavy mineral oil 55%, white phenolphthalein 150 mg/ 15 ml, and Irish moss as emulsifier.

Lanabiotic: polymyxin B sulfate 5000 units, neomycin sulfate 5 mg, bacitracin 500 units, and lidocaine 40 mg/g.

Lanophyllin-GG Capsules: 150 mg theophylline and 90 mg guaifenesin.

Lavatar: tar distillate 33.3% in water-miscible emulsion base.

Librax Capsules: chlordiazepoxide HCl 5 mg and clidinium bromide 2.5 mg.

Limbitrol 5–12.5: chlordiazepoxide 5 mg and amitriptyline (as HCl) 12.5 mg.

Limbitrol 10–25: chlordiazepoxide 10 mg and amitriptyline (as HCl) 25 mg.

Lobac: chlorzoxazone 250 mg and acetaminophen 300 mg.

Lopressor HCT 50/25: metoprolol tartrate 50 mg and hydrochlorothiazide 25 mg.

Lopressor HCT 100/25: metoprolol tartrate 100 mg and hydrochlorothiazide 25 mg.

Lotrisone Cream: clotrimazole 1% and betamethasone dipropionate 0.05%.

Maalox No. 1: aluminum hydroxide 200 mg and magnesium hydroxide 200 mg.

Maalox Plus Tablets: aluminum hydroxide 200 mg, magnesium hydroxide 200 mg, and simethicone 25 mg.

Maalox TC Tablets: aluminum hydroxide 600 mg and magnesium hydroxide 300 mg.

Magnatril: aluminum hydroxide 260 mg, magnesium hydroxide 130 mg, and magnesium trisilicate 455 mg.

Marax: theophylline 130 mg, ephedrine sulfate 25 mg, and hydroxyzine HCl 10 mg.

Maxitrol Ointment/Ophthalmic Suspension: dexamethasone 0.1%, neomycin sulfate 0.35%, and polymixin B sulfate 10,000 units.

Maxzide: triamterene 75 mg and hydrochlorothiazide 50 mg.

Medicone Dressing Cream: benzocaine 0.5%, 8-hydroxyquinoline sulfate 0.05%, cod liver oil 12.5%, zinc oxide 12.5%, and menthol 0.18% with petrolatum, lanolin, talcum, and paraffin.

Medi-Seltzer: sodium bicarbonate 1916 mg, aspirin 325 mg, and citric acid 1000 mg.

Menrium 5–2: chlordiazepoxide 5 mg and esterified estrogens 0.2 mg.

Menrium 5–4: chlordiazepoxide 5 mg and esterified estrogens 0.4 mg.

Menrium 10–4: chlordiazepoxide 10 mg and esterified estrogens 0.4 mg.

Metatensin Tablets: trichlormethiazide 2 or 4 mg and reserpine 0.1 mg.

Metimyd Ophthalmic Ointment/Suspension: sodium sulfacetamide 10% and prednisolone acetate 0.5%.

Midol: aspirin 454 mg, caffeine 32.4 mg, and cinnemedrine HCl 14.9 mg.

Migral: ergotamine tartrate 1 mg, caffeine 50 mg, and cyclizine HCl 25 mg.

Milprem-200: meprobamate 200 mg and conjugated estrogens 0.45 mg.

Milprem-400: meprobamate 400 mg and conjugated estrogens 0.45 mg.

Minizide 1: polythiazide 0.5 mg and prazosin 1 mg.

Minizide 2: polythiazide 0.5 mg and prazosin 2 mg.

Minizide 5: polythiazide 0.5 mg and prazosin 5 mg.

Mixtard Injection: 100 mg/ml isophane purified pork insulin suspension and purified pork insulin injection.

M-YKA: quinine sulfate 64.8 mg and Vitamin E 400 units (as d,l alphatocopheryl acetate).

Modane Plus: docusate sodium 100 mg and phenolphthalein 60 mg.

Moduretic: amiloride HCl 5 mg and hydrochlorothiazide 50 mg.

Murocoll-2: scopolamine HBr 0.3% and phenylephrine HCl 10%.

Mus-Lax: chlorzoxazone 250 mg and acetaminophen 300 mg.

Mycitracin Ophthalmic Ointment: polymyxin B sulfate 5000 units, neomycin sulfate 3.5 mg, and bacitracin 500 units.

Mycitracin Ointment: polymyxin B sulfate 5000 units, bacitracin 500 units, and neomycin sulfate 3.5 mg/g.

Mycolog II Cream and Ointment: triamcinolone acetonide 0.1%, and nystatin 100,000 units/g.

Mylanta Tablets: aluminum hydroxide 200 mg, magnesium hydroxide 200 mg, and simethicone 20 mg.

Mylanta-II Tablets: aluminum hydroxide 400 mg, magnesium hydroxide 400 mg, and simethicone 40 mg.

Naldecon: phenylpropanolamine HCl 40 mg, phenylephrine HCl 10 mg, chlorpheniramine maleate 5 mg, and phenyltoloxamine citrate 15 mg.

Naquival: trichloromethiazide 4 mg and reserpine 0.1 mg.

Naturetin W/K 2.5 mg: bendroflumethiazide 2.5 mg and potassium chloride 500 mg.

Naturetin W/K 5 mg: bendroflumethiazide 5 mg and potassium chloride 500 mg.

Neo-corteff Ointment: hydrocortisone acetate 1% and neomycin sulfate 0.5%.

NeoDecadron Ophthalmic Ointment: dexamethasone phosphate 0.1% and neomycin sulfate 0.35%.

NeoDecadron Cream: dexamethasone phosphate 0.1% and neomycin sulfate 0.5%.

Neo-Polycin Ointment: polymyxin B sulfate 5000 units, neomycin sulfate 5 mg, and zinc bacitracin 400 units/g.

Neosporin G.U. Irrigant: 40 mg neomycin sulfate and 200,000 units polymixin B sulfate/ml.

Neosporin Ophthalmic: polymyxin B sulfate 10,000 units, neomycin sulfate 1.75 mg, and gramicidin 0.025 mg.

Neosporin Ophthalmic Ointment: polymyxin B sulfate 10,000 units, neomycin sulfate 3.5 mg, and bacitracin zinc 400 units/g.

Neosporin Cream: polymyxin B sulfate 5000 units, bacitracin zinc 400 units, and neomycin sulfate 5 mg/g.

Neosporin Ointment: polymyxin B sulfate 5000 units, bacitracin zinc 400 units, and neomycin sulfate 5 mg/g.

Neotal: polymyxin B sulfate 5000 units, neomycin sulfate 5 mg, and bacitracin zinc 400 units.

Neotep-Granucaps: chlorpheniramine maleate 9 mg and phenylephrine HCl 21 mg.

Neothylline-GG Tablets: 200 mg dyphylline and 200 mg guaifenesin.

Neotrizine: sulfadiazine 167 mg, sulfamerazine 167 mg, and sulfamethazine 167 mg.

Neutra-Phos: phosphorus 250 mg, sodium 164 mg, and potassium 278 mg (from dibasic and monobasic sodium and potassium phosphate).

Nitrotym-Plus: nitroglycerin 2.5 mg and butabarbital sodium 48 mg.

Nolamine: chlorpheniramine maleate 4 mg, phenindamine tartrate 24 mg, and phenylpropanolamine HCl 50 mg.

Norgesic: orphenadrine citrate 25 mg, aspirin 385 mg, and caffeine 30 mg.

Norgesic Forte: orphenadrine citrate 50 mg, aspirin 770 mg, and caffeine 60 mg.

Normozide 100/25: labetalol 100 mg and hydrochlorothiazide 25 mg.

Normozide 200/25: labetalol 200 mg and hydrochlorothiazide 25 mg.

Normozide 300/25: labetalol 300 mg and hydrochlorothiazide 25 mg.

Novafed A: pseudoephedrine HCl 120 mg and chlorpheniramine maleate 8 mg.

Novahistine Elixir: phenylephrine 5 mg, chlorpheniramine maleate 2 mg, and alcohol 5%/5 ml.

Ophtha P/S Ophthalmic Suspension: prednisolone acetate 0.5% and sodium sulfacetamide 10%.

Ophthocort: chloramphenicol 1.0%, polymixin B sulfate 10,000 units, and hydrocortisone acetate 0.5%.

Optimyd: prednisolone phosphate 0.5% and sodium sulfacetamide 10%.

Orahist: phenylpropanolamine HCl 75 mg and chlorpheniramine 12 mg.

Orenzyme Bitabs Enteric-coated Tablets: 100,000 units trypsin and 8000 units chymotrypsin.

Oreticyl 25: hydrochlorothiazide 25 mg and deserpidine 0.125 mg.

Oreticyl 50: hydrochlorothiazide 50 mg and deserpidine 0.125 mg.

Oreticyl Forte: hydrochlorothiazide 25 mg and deserpidine 0.25 mg.

Ornade Spansule Capsules: phenylpropanolamine HCl 75 mg and chlorpheniramine maleate 12 mg.

Ornex: phenylpropanolamine HCl 18 mg and acetaminophen 325 mg.

PAC New Revised Formula: aspirin 400 mg and caffeine 32 mg.

P_1E_1, P_2E_1, P_3E_1, P_4E_1, P_6E_1: epinephrine bitartrate 1% and pilocarpine HCl 1%, 2%, 3%, 4%, or 6%.

Pancrease Capsules: lipase 4000 units, protease 25,000 units, and amylase 20,000 units, in enteric-coated microspheres.

Pantopon: hydrochlorides of opium alkaloids; 20 mg is therapeutically equivalent to 15 mg of morphine.

Paracet-Forte: chlorzoxazone 250 mg and acetaminophen 300 mg.

Parepectolin: opium 15 mg (equivalent to paregoric 3.7 ml), kaolin 5.85 g, pectin 162 mg, and alcohol 0.69% in 30-ml suspension.

Pediazole: sulfisoxazole 600 mg and erythromycin ethylsuccinate 200 mg per 5 ml.

Perbuzem: pentaerythritol tetranitrate 10 mg and butabarbital sodium 15 mg.

Percocet: acetaminophen 325 mg and oxycodone hydrochloride 5 mg.

Percodan: oxycodone HCl 4.5 mg, oxycodone terephthalate 0.38 mg, and aspirin 325 mg.

Percodan-Demi: oxycodone HCl 2.25 mg, oxycodone terephthalate 0.19 mg, and aspirin 325 mg.

Peri-Colace Capsules: docusate sodium 100 mg and casanthranol 30 mg.

Peri-Colace Syrup: docusate sodium 60 mg and casanthranol 30 mg/15 ml.

Phenaphen-650 with Codeine: codeine phosphate 30 mg and acetaminophen 650 mg.

Phenaphen with Codeine No. 3: codeine phosphate 30 mg and acetaminophen 325 mg.

Phenaphen with Codeine No. 4: codeine phosphate 60 mg and acetaminophen 325 mg.

Phenergan-D: pseudoephedrine HCl 60 mg and promethazine HCl 6.25 mg.

Phenylzin: zinc sulfate 0.25% and phenylephrine HCl 0.12%.

Phrenilin: acetaminophen 325 mg and butalbital 50 mg.

Phrenilin Forte: acetaminophen 650 mg and butalbital 50 mg.

Phrenilin with Codeine No. 3: codeine phosphate 30 mg, acetaminophen 325 mg, and butalbital 50 mg.

P-I-N Forte: isoniazid 100 mg and pyridoxine HCl 5 mg.

PMB 200: meprobamate 200 mg and conjugated estrogens 0.45 mg.

PMB 400: meprobamate 400 mg and conjugated estrogens 0.45 mg.

Polycillin-PRB: ampicillin trihydrate 3.5 g and probenecid 1 g per bottle.

Polyflex: chlorzoxazone 250 mg and acetaminophen 300 mg.

Polysporin Ophthalmic Ointment: polymixin B sulfate 10,000 units and bacitracin zinc 500 units.

Polysporin Ointment: polymyxin B sulfate 10,000 units and zinc bacitracin 500 units/g.

Prefrin-A: phenylephrine HCl 0.12%, pyrilamine maleate 0.1%, and antipyrine 0.1%.

Premarin with Methyltestosterone: conjugated estrogens 0.625 mg and methyltestosterone 5 mg.

Principen with Probenecid: ampicillin trihydrate 3.5 g and probenecid 1 g per 9-capsule regimen.

Proben-C: probenecid 500 mg and colchicine 0.5 mg.

Probenemid with Colchicine: probenecid 500 mg and colchicine 0.5 mg.

Provol No. 3: codeine phosphate 30 mg and acetaminophen 325 mg.

Quadrinal: theophylline calcium salicylate 65 mg, ephedrine HCl 24 mg, potassium iodide 320 mg, and phenobarbital 24 mg.

Quibron Capsules: 150 mg theophylline and 90 mg guaifenesin.

Quibron Plus: theophylline 150 mg, ephedrine HCl 25 mg, guaifenesin 100 mg, and butabarbital 20 mg.

Q-Vel: quinine sulfate 64.8 mg and Vitamin E 400 U (as d, l alphatocopheryl acetate).

Rauzide: bendroflumethiazide 4 mg and powdered rauwolfia serpentina 50 mg.

Regroton: chlorthalidone 50 mg and reserpine 0.25 mg.

Renese-R: polythiazide 2 mg and reserpine 0.25 mg.

Rezide: hydrochlorothiazide 15 mg, hydralazine HCl 25 mg, and reserpine 0.1 mg.

R-HCTZ-H: hydrochlorothiazide 15 mg, hydralazine HCl 25 mg, and reserpine 0.1 mg.

Rhinex D-Lay: acetaminophen 300 mg, salicylamide 300 mg, phenylpropanolamine HCl 60 mg, and chlorpheniramine maleate 4 mg.

Rifamate: isoniazid 150 mg and rifampin 300 mg.

Rimactane/INH Dual Pack: Thirty 300-mg isoniazid tablets and sixty 300-mg rifampin capsules.

Riopan Plus Chew Tablets: magaldrate 540 mg and simethicone 20 mg.

Riopan Plus Suspension: magaldrate 540 mg and simethicone 20 mg/5 ml.

Robaxisal: methocarbamol 400 mg and aspirin 325 mg.

Robinul Forte Tablets: glycopyrrolate 2 mg and phenobarbital 16.2 mg.

Robinul Tablets: glycopyrrolate 1 mg and phenobarbital 16.2 mg.

Rondec: carbinoxamine maleate 4 mg and pseudoephedrine HCl 60 mg.

Salutensin: hydroflumethiazide 50 mg and reserpine 0.125 mg.

Salutensin-Demi: hydroflumethiazide 25 mg and reserpine 0.125 mg.

Senokot-S: docusate sodium 50 mg and standardized senna concentrate 187 mg.

Ser-A-Gen: hydrochlorothiazide 15 mg, hydralazine HCl 25 mg, and reserpine 0.1 mg.

Seralazide: hydrochlorothiazide 15 mg, hydralazine HCl 25 mg, and reserpine 0.1 mg.

Ser-Ap-Es: hydrochlorothiazide 15 mg, reserpine 0.1 mg, and hydralazine HCl 25 mg.

Serpasil-Apresoline No. 1: reserpine 0.1 mg and hydralazine HCl 25 mg.

Serpasil-Apresoline No. 2: reserpine 0.2 mg and hydralazine HCl 50 mg.

Serpasil-Esidrix No. 1: hydrochlorothiazide 25 mg and reserpine 0.1 mg (called Serpasil-Esidrix 25 in Canada).

Serpasil-Esidrix No. 2: hydrochlorothiazide 50 mg and reserpine 0.1 mg.

Serpazide: hydrochlorothiazide 15 mg, hydralazine HCl 25 mg, and reserpine 0.1 mg.

Silain-Gel: aluminum hydroxide 282 mg, magnesium hydroxide 285 mg, and simethicone 25 mg per 5 ml.

Simron: iron (as gluconate) 10 mg and polysorbate 20, 400 mg.

Sinutab: acetaminophen 325 mg, chlorpheniramine 2 mg, and pseudoephedrine HCl 30 mg.

Sinutab II Maxmium Strength: acetaminophen 500 mg and pseudoephedrine HCl 30 mg.

Skelex: chlorazoxazone 250 mg and acetaminophen 300 mg.

Soma Compound: carisoprodol 200 mg and aspirin 325 mg.

Soma Compound with Codeine: carisoprodol 200 mg, aspirin 325 mg, caffeine 32 mg, and codeine phosphate 16 mg.

Spironazide: spironolactone 25 mg and hydrochlorothiazide 25 mg.

Spirozide: spironolactone 25 mg and hydrochlorothiazide 25 mg.

Statrol: neomycin sulfate 3.5 mg and polymixin B sulfate 10,000 units.

Sudafed Plus: pseudoephedrine HCl 60 mg and chlorpheniramine maleate 4 mg.

Sulfapred: sodium sulfacetamide 10%, prednisolone acetate 0.25%, and phenylephrine HCl 0.125%.

Sulfoxyl Lotion Regular: benzoyl peroxide 5% and sulfur 2%.

Sulfoxyl Lotion Strong: benzoyl peroxide 10% and sulfur 5%.

Synalgos: aspirin 356.4 mg and caffeine 30 mg.

Talacen: pentazocine HCl 25 mg and acetaminophen 650 mg.

Talwin Compound: pentazocine HCl 12.5 mg and aspirin 325 mg.

Teebaconin and Vitamin B_6: isoniazid 100 mg and pyridoxine HCl 10 mg.

Tedral: theophylline 130 mg, ephedrine HCl 24 mg, and phenobarbital 8 mg.

Tedral SA: theophylline 180 mg, ephedrine HCl 48 mg, and phenobarbital 25 mg.

Tenoretic 50: atenolol 50 mg and chlorthalidone 25 mg.

Tenoretic 100: atenolol 100 mg and chlorthalidone 25 mg.

Terfonyl: sulfadiazine 167 mg, sulfamerazine 167 mg, and sulfamethazine 167 mg.

Thalfed: theophylline 120 mg, ephedrine HCl 25 mg, and phenobarbital 8 mg.

Thiosulfil-A: sulfamethizole 250 mg and phenazopyridine HCl 50 mg.

Thyrolar-1/4: levothyroxine sodium 12.5 mcg and liothyronine sodium 3.1 mcg.

Thyrolar-1/2: levothyroxine sodium 25 mcg and liothyronine sodium 6.25 mcg.

Thyrolar-1: levothyroxine sodium 50 mcg and liothyronine sodium 12.5 mcg.

Thyrolar-2: levothyroxine sodium 100 mcg and liothyronine sodium 25 mcg.

Thyrolar-3: levothyroxine sodium 150 mcg and liothyronine sodium 37.5 mcg.

Timentin for Injection: ticarcillin disodium 3 g and clavulanate potassium 100 mg per vial.

Timolide 10/25: timolol maleate 10 mg and hydrochlorothiazide 25 mg.

Titralac Liquid: calcium carbonate 1000 mg in glycine.

Titralac Tablets: calcium carbonate 420 mg and glycine 150 mg.

Triaminic: phenylpropanolamine HCl 50 mg, pyrilamine maleate 25 mg, and pheniramine maleate 25 mg.

Triaminic-12: phenylpropanolamine HCl 75 mg and chlorpheniramine maleate 12 mg.

Triaminic Tablets: phenylpropanolamine HCl 50 mg, pheniramine maleate 25 mg, and pyrilamine maleate 25 mg.

Triavil 2–10: perphenazine 2 mg and amitriptyline HCl 10 mg.

Triavil 2–25: perphenazine 2 mg and amitriptyline HCl 25 mg.

Triavil 4–10: perphenazine 4 mg and amitriptyline HCl 10 mg.

Triavil 4–25: perphenazine 4 mg and amitriptyline HCl 25 mg.

Triavil 4–50: perphenazine 4 mg and amitriptyline HCl 50 mg.

Tri-Barbs Capsule: phenobarbital 32 mg, butabarbital sodium 32 mg, and secobarbital sodium 32 mg.

Trigesic: acetaminophen 125 mg, aspirin 230 mg, and caffeine 30 mg.

Tri-Hydroserpine: hydrochlorothiazide 15 mg, hydralazine HCl 25 mg, and reserpine 0.1 mg.

Trilisate: choline salicylate 293 mg and magnesium salicylate 362 mg.

Trinalin Repetabs: azatadine maleate 1 mg and pseudoephedrine sulfate 120 mg.

Triple Sulfa: sulfadiazine 167 mg, sulfamerazine 167 mg, and sulfamethazine 167 mg.

Tuinal 50 mg Pulvules: amobarbital sodium 25 mg and secobarbital sodium 25 mg.

Tuinal 100 mg Pulvules: amobarbital sodium 50 mg and secobarbital sodium 50 mg.

Tuinal 200 mg Pulvules: amobarbital sodium 100 mg and secobarbital sodium 100 mg.

TWIN-K-CL: 15 ml supplies 15 mEq of potassium ions as a combination of potassium gluconate, potassium citrate, and ammonium chloride.

Tylenol with Codeine No. 1: acetaminophen 300 mg and codeine phosphate 7.5 mg.

Tylenol with Codeine No. 2: acetaminophen 300 mg and codeine phosphate 15 mg.

Tylenol with Codeine No. 3: acetaminophen 300 mg and codeine phosphate 30 mg.

Tylenol with Codeine No. 4: acetaminophen 300 mg and codeine phosphate 60 mg.

Tylox: acetaminophen 500 mg and oxycodone HCl 5 mg.

Unasyn Injection: ampicillin sodium 1 g and sublactam sodium 500 mg per vial; ampicillin sodium 2 g and sublactam sodium 1 g per vial.

Unipres: hydrochlorothiazide 15 mg, reserpine 0.1 mg, and hydralazine HCl 25 mg.

Univol: aluminum hydroxide and magnesium carbonate co-dried gél 300 mg and magnesium hydroxide 100 mg.

Urobiotic-250: sulfamethizole 250 mg, oxytetracycline (as the hydrochloride) 250 mg, and phenazopyridine HCl 50 mg.

Uro Gantanol: sulfamethoxazole 500 mg and phenazopyridine 50 mg.

Uro-Phosphate: methenamine 300 mg and sodium acid phosphate 500 mg. Sugar coated.

Uroquid-Acid: methenamine mandelate 350 mg and sodium acid phosphate 200 mg.

Uroquid-Acid No. 2: methenamine mandelate 500 mg and sodium acid phosphate 500 mg.

Vanoxide: benzoyl peroxide 5% and chlorhydroxyquinoline 0.25%.

Vanoxide-HC: benzoyl peroxide 5%, chlorhydroxyquinoline 0.25%, and hydrocortisone 0.5%.

Vanquish: aspirin 227 mg, acetaminophen 194 mg, caffeine 33 mg, aluminum hydroxide 25 mg, and magnesium hydroxide 50 mg.

Vaseretic: enalapril maleate 10 mg and hydrochlorothiazide 25 mg.

Vasocidin Ophthalmic Ointment: phenylephrine HCl 0.125%, sodium sulfacetamide 10%, and prednisolone sodium phosphate 0.25%.

Vasocidin Ophthalmic Solution: phenylephrine HCl 0.125%, sodium sulfacetamide 10%, and prednisolone sodium phosphate 0.25%.

Vasocon-A Ophthalmic Solution: naphazoline HCl 0.05% and antazoline phosphate 0.5%.

Vasosulf: sodium sulfacetamide 15% and phenylephrine HCl 0.125%.

Vicodin: hydrocodone bitartrate 5 mg and acetaminophen 500 mg.

Vistrax 10 Tablets: oxyphencyclimine HCl 10 mg and hydroxyzine HCl 25 mg.

Wigraine: ergotamine tartrate 1 mg, caffeine 100 mg, levorotatory belladonna alkaloids 0.1 mg, and phenacetin 130 mg.

Wigraine Suppositories: ergotamine tartrate 2 mg, caffeine 100 mg, and tartaric acid 21.5 mg.

Wingel: aluminum hydroxide 180 mg and magnesium hydroxide 160 mg.

Wygesic: propoxyphene HCl 65 mg and acetaminophen 500 mg.

Zeasorb Powder: parachlorometaxylenol 0.5%, aluminum dihydroxyallantoinate 0.2%, and microporous cellulose 45%.

Zetar Emulsion: 30% colloidal whole coal tar in polysorbates.

Zetar Shampoo: whole coal tar 1% and parachlorometaxylenol 0.5% in foam shampoo base.

Zincfrin: phenylephrine HCl 0.12% and zinc sulfate 0.25%.

Zoxaphen: chloroxazone 25 mg and acetaminophen 300 mg.

Zydone: hydrocodone bitartrate 5 mg and acetaminophen 500 mg.

Bibliography

Abrams A. *Clinical Drug Therapy*. 3rd ed. Philadelphia: J.B. Lippincott, 1991.

Abrams R. *Will It Hurt My Baby? The Safe Use of Medications During Pregnancy and Breastfeeding*. Menlo Park, California: Addison-Wesley, 1990.

Alfaro R. *Nursing Diagnosis and Nursing Process*. Philadelphia: J.B. Lippincott, 1990.

Benner P. *From Novice to Expert*. Redwood City, California: Addison-Wesley, 1984.

Benner P, Wrubel J. *The Primacy of Caring: Stress and Coping in Health and Illness*. Redwood City, California: Addison-Wesley, 1984.

Brunner L, Suddarth D. *Medical-Surgical Nursing*. 6th ed. Philadelphia: J.B. Lippincott, 1990.

Carpenito L. *Nursing Diagnosis: Application to Clinical Practice*. 4th ed. Philadelphia: J.B. Lippincott, 1991.

Carpenito L. *Nursing Care Plans and Documentation*. Philadelphia: J.B. Lippincott, 1991.

Fischbach F. *A Manual of Laboratory Diagnostic Tests*. 3rd ed. Philadelphia: J.B. Lippincott, 1991.

Kuhn M. *Pharmacotherapeutics: A Nursing Process Approach*. Philadelphia: F.A. Davis, 1991.

Kozier B, Erb G. *Fundamentals of Nursing*. 3rd ed. Redwood City, California: Addison-Wesley, 1991.

Schlafer M, Marieb E. *The Nurse, Pharmacology, and Drug Therapy*. Redwood City, California: Addison-Wesley, 1989.

Spencer R, Nichols L, et al. *Clinical Pharmacology and Nursing Management*. Philadelphia: J.B. Lippincott, 1989.

Taylor C, Lillis C, LeMone P. *Fundamentals of Nursing: The Art and Science of Nursing Care*. Philadelphia: J.B. Lippincott, 1989.

USP Dispensing Information (USP DI). 10th ed. Rockville, Maryland: The United States Pharmacopeial Convention, Inc., 1990.

Guidelines:
Overdose Management

🖐 These are general guidelines for management of drug overdose. Most standards of care mandate that regional poison control centers be consulted as soon as possible whenever there is any doubt about treatment. These centers have access to POISINDEX, the most up to date toxicology data base available. POISINDEX is designed to provide detailed treatment and management protocols for inhaled, ingested, or absorbed toxic substances (whether the substance is known or unknown). They also can help to identify the ingredient information on pharmaceutical, industrial, commercial, or botanical substances.

1 Identify life-threatening problems (e.g. respiratory distress, shock) and begin immediate treatment:

❑ Provide oxygen and respiratory support; attach to monitor or EKG; have emergency resuscitation equipment and medications ready for use.

❑ Start at least one intravenous line.

❑ Anticipate the possibility of vomiting (use suction if necessary to prevent aspiration; have nasogastric tube ready for insertion).

2 Obtain pertinent history from most reliable individual (family members, friends, paramedics, or patient, or a combination of these).

❑ Determine patient age and weight.

❑ Determine drugs taken, doses, and route of administration. *Have significant others bring in empty bottles and ask whether other medications are being taken (to rule out interactions).*

❑ Identify allergies to medications.

3 Expect that blood and urine specimens will be needed for toxicology screens and other pertinent studies (e.g. electrolytes, blood gases).

4 Anticipate that available pharmacological antagonists (e.g. narcan for narcotic overdose) or specific antidotes (e.g. protamine sulfate for heparin overdose) may be administered to neutralize drug effects.

5 Monitor closely for (and be prepared to treat) adverse effects of the drugs taken.

6 Prepare to institute measures to prevent absorption of ingested toxic substance.

❑ Expect that an emetic or gastric lavage may be ordered to empty stomach contents. *Remember that emetics are contraindicated if the patient is somnolent, comatose, or without gag reflex, if the substance is a caustic acid or base.*

❑ Have activated charcoal on hand, ready for administration via nasogastric tube after stomach contents have been emptied by emesis or lavage. *Activated charcoal absorbs the drug and prevents systemic absorption. Initial dose for adults 20–50 g, repeated every 2 to 6 hrs; for children 15–30 g in one dose.*

❑ Expect that a cathartic may be ordered to hasten transit of drug through intestine after stomach contents have been emptied and activated charcoal has been administered. *Contraindicated when caustic substances have been ingested, or if gastro-intestinal bleeding is suspected.*

7 Continue to monitor the patient closely for signs and symptoms of adverse reactions until the drug has been eliminated from the body.

❑ Presence of drug may be determined by serum or urine toxicology screens.

Guidelines:
Emergency management of anaphylactic drug reactions

1 Discontinue drug or minimize its absorption.

❑ Stop IV drug infusions.

❑ Apply a tourniquet above the level of injections. If unable to apply a tourniquet, apply ice to injection site.

❑ Wash off topical applications.

2 Support airway, administer oxygen, and get help immediately.

❑ Activate the emergency medical service system.

3 Establish an IV route.

❑ Have emergency equipment available at the bedside (endotracheal tube, suction, and cardiac monitor).

❑ Have commonly needed drugs readily available at the bedside (epinephrine, diphenhydramine, steroids, vasopressors).

4 Assess and record respirations, pulse, and blood pressure every 1–5 min.

❑ Be ready to treat hypotension with vasopressors and IV fluids.

5 Once the patient is stable, observe carefully for additional symptoms.

❑ Anticipate that additional doses of antihistamines or steroids may be necessary for 1–2 days.

Index

NOTE: Drugs are listed under their generic names. Trade names are listed in *italics*.

Benzylpenicillin benzathine, 556–557
Benzylpenicillin potassium, 556–557
Benzylpenicillin procaine, 556–557
Beriberi, thiamine for, 666
Beta-1 (selective) beta-blockers, 80, 81. *See also individual drugs*
Beta-2 (nonselective) beta-blockers, 80, 81. *See also individual drugs*
Beta-2. See Isoetharine hydrochloride, 407–408
Beta-adrenergic blockers, 44, 48, 66, 67, 80–82. *See also individual drugs*
Betalin 12. See Cyanocobalamin, 258–259
Betalin S. See Thiamine hydrochloride, 666
Betaloc. See Metoprolol, 489–490
Betamin. See Thiamine hydrochloride, 666
Betapen-VK. See Penicillin V potassium, 558
Beta-Sol. See Thiamine hydrochloride, 666
Bethanechol chloride, 86, 165–166
Bex. See Aspirin, 148–149
Biamine. See Thiamine hydrochloride, 666
Bicarbonate. *See* Sodium bicarbonate, 634–635
Bicillin L-A. See Penicillin G, benzathine, 556–557
BiCNU. See Carmustine, 194–195
Bile duct cancer, floxuridine for, 348
Biliary colic, papaverine for, 550
Biliary obstruction, pruritus from, cholestyramine for, 229
Bilron, 722
Bioglan B12 Plus. See Cyanocobalamin, 258–259
Biological response modifier/hormone, for anemia, 43
Biosone. See Hydrocortisone acetate, 384–386
Biosynthetic human insulin, 61
Biperiden, 50, 166–167
Biperiden hydrochloride, 166–167
Biperiden lactate, 166–167
Biphetamine 20, 722

Bipolar disorder (manic-depression)
  carbamazepine for, 188
  chlorpromazine for, 222
  lithium for, 433–434
  maprotiline for, 445
Birth control pills, 330–332
Bisacodyl, 91, 167–168
Bisacolax. See Bisacodyl, 167–168
Bisalax. See Bisacodyl, 167–168
Bisco-Lax. See Bisacodyl, 167–168
Bisorine. See Isoetharine, 407–408
Bitolterol mesylate, 39, 82, 168–169
Bitrate, 722
Black-Draught. See Senna, 633
Bladder
  cancer of
    cisplatin for, 236
    doxorubicin for, 310
    teniposide for, 654
    thiotepa for, 669
  neurogenic, bethanechol for, 165
  spasms of, oxybutynin for, 540
Blanex, 722
Blastomycosis, ketoconazole for, 417
Bleeding
  abnormal uterine
    estrogen for, 329
    medroxyprogesterone for, 450
  control of
    aminocaproic acid for, 129
    desmopressin for, 277
    epinephrine for, 319, 320
    menadiol for, 454
    phytonadione for, 579
  postabortion, methylergonovine for, 480
  postpartum
    methylergonovine for, 480
    oxytocin for, 547
Blenoxane. See Bleomycin sulfate, 169–170
Bleomycin sulfate, 72, 169–170
Bleph-10 Liquifilm Ophthalmic. See Sulfacetamide sodium, 647
Blephamide, 722
Blepharitis, gentamicin for, 364
Blepharoconjunctivitis, gentamicin for, 364

Blocadren. See Timolol, 674–676
Blood infections
  cefamandole for, 199
  cefazolin for, 200
  cefoperazone for, 202
  ceforanide for, 203
  cefotaxime for, 203
  cefoxitin for, 205
  ceftazidime for, 206
  ceftizoxime for, 207
  ceftriaxone for, 208
  cefuroxime for, 208
  cephalothin for, 210
  cephapirin for, 211
  moxalactam for, 506
Blood pressure, drugs for reduction of, 66–68. *See also individual drugs*
Body surface area, nomogram for calculation of, 19
Bonamine. See Meclizine hydrochloride, 448–449
Bone formation, calcitonin for promotion of, 183
Bone infections
  cefamandole for, 199
  cefazolin for, 200
  cefonicid for, 201
  ceforanide for, 203
  cefotetan for, 204
  cefoxitin for, 205
  ceftizoxime for, 207
  cephalexin for, 209
  cephalothin for, 210
  cephapirin for, 211
  ciprofloxacin for, 235–236
  imipenem-cilastatin sodium for, 391
  metronidazole for, 491
Bone marrow failure, oxymetholone for anemia caused by, 542
Bonine. See Meclizine hydrochloride, 448–449
Bordetella pertussis infections, erythromycin for, 325
Bowel prep, preoperative or preprocedure
  bisacodyl for, 167
  cascara sagrada for, 197
  kanamycin for, 414
  magnesium salts for, 442
  neomycin for, 517
  senna for, 633
Bradycardia
  anticholinergics for, 51
  atropine for, 153
  theophylline for, 664
Brain tumors
  carmustine for, 194
  floxuridine for, 348
  lomustine for, 435

with amoxicillin, 136–137

Clearasil Cream, 723

Clemastine fumarate, 64, 238

Cleocin. See Clindamycin phosphate, 239–240

Cleocin HCl. See Clindamycin hydrochloride, 239–240

Cleocin Pediatric. See Clindamycin palmitate hydrochloride, 239–240

Cleocin Phosphate. See Clindamycin phosphate, 239–240

Clindamycin, 239–240
  IV compatibility of, 33–34

Clindamycin hydrochloride, 69, 239–240

Clindamycin palmitate hydrochloride, 69, 239–240

Clindamycin phosphate, 69, 239–240

Clinoril. See Sulindac, 651–652

Clistin. See Carbinoxamine maleate, 191–192

Clofibrate, 71, 240

Clomid. See Clomiphene citrate, 240–241

Clomiphene citrate, 240–241

Clomipramine hydrochloride, 56, 241–242

Clonazepam, 54, 242–243
  seizure-type used for, 55

Clonidine, 66, 243–244

Clorazepate, 45, 244–246

Clostridium difficile pseudomembranous enterocolitis, vancomycin for, 709

Clot formation
  aminocaproic acid for promotion of, 129
  aspirin in prevention of, 148, 149

Clotrimazole, 246

Cloxacillin sodium, 68, 247

Cloxapen. See Cloxacillin sodium, 247

Clozapine, 78, 247–249

Clozaril. See Clozapine, 247–249

Cluster headaches, methysergide for, 485

CNS infections. *See* Central nervous system infections

CNS stimulants. *See* Cerebral stimulants, 84–86

Coactin. See Amdinocillin, 124–125

Coccidioidomycosis
  ketoconazole for, 417

miconazole (parenteral) for, 495

Codeine, 79, 95, 249–250
  IM compatibility of, 30
  terpin hydrate with, 658

Codeine phosphate, 249–250

Codeine sulfate, 249–250

Codesol. See Prednisolone sodium phosphate, 592–594

Codimal-A. See Brompheniramine maleate, 172–173

Codimal-DH, 723

Codoxy. See Oxycodone, with aspirin, 541–542

Codroxomin. See Hydroxocobalamin, 387–388

Cogentin. See Benztropine mesylate, 164–165

Colace. See Docusate sodium, 306

Colbenemid, 723

Colchicine, 250–251

Colchicine MR. See Colchicine, 250–251

Colds. *See* Nasal congestion

Colestid. See Colestipol hydrochloride, 251–252

Colestipol hydrochloride, 71, 251–252

Colgout. See Colchicine, 250–251

Colisceril palmitate, 252–253

Colitis
  anticholinergics for, 51
  collagenous, sulfasalazine for, 649
  ulcerative
    mesalamine for, 460
    sulfadiazine for, 648
    sulfasalazine for, 649

Collaborative problems, identification of, 8–9

Cologel. See Methylcellulose, 478

Colon cancer
  amsacrine for, 142
  carmustine for, 194
  fluorouracil for, 351
  levamisole for, 423
  methotrexate for, 473
  mitomycin for, 500

Colorectal cancer
  lomustine for, 435
  streptozocin for, 643

Colorectal surgery, and metronidazole for prophylaxis of contamination, 491

Coloxyl. See Docusate sodium, 306

Colrex. See Guaifenesin, 375

Colsalide. See Colchicine, 250–251

Coly-Mycin S Otic, 723

Coma, hepatic, neomycin in adjunctive treatment of, 517

Combantrin. See Pyrantel embonate, 613–614; Pyrantel pamoate, 613–614

Combined immunodeficiency syndrome, immune globulin for, 394

Combipres, 723

Compazine. See Prochlorperazine, 602–603

Complex partial seizures, drugs for, 55

Compound W, 723

Compoz Diahist. See Diphenhydramine, 299–300

Condrin-LA, 723

Condylomata acuminata, interferon for, 401

Congespirin, 723

Congespirin for Children. See Dextromethorphan hydrobromide, 282–283

Congestion
  ephedrine for, 318
  pseudoephedrine for, 612
  triprolidine for, 701

Congestive heart failure (CHF)
  amiloride for, 126
  amrinone lactate for, 141
  benzthiazide for, 163
  bumetanide for, 173
  captopril for, 187
  digoxin/digitoxin for, 293
  dopamine for, 307
  enalapril for, 316
  ethacrynic acid and ethacrynic sodium for, 332
  furosemide for, 360
  hydralazine for, 382
  metolazone for, 488
  nitroglycerin for, 526
  prazosin for, 591
  spironolactone for, 638

Conjec-B. See Brompheniramine maleate, 172–173

Conjugated estrogens, 328–330

Conjunctivitis. *See also* Keratoconjunctivitis
  erythromycin for, 325
  gentamicin for, 364
  sulfacetamide for, 647

Conscious sedation, midazolam for, 496
Constant-T. See Theophylline, 664–665
Constilac. See Lactulose, 421–422
Constipation, drugs for, 91–92. *See also individual drugs*
Contac, 723. *See also* Dextromethorphan hydrobromide, 282–283
Contraception, estrogen with progestin for, 330–331
Convulsions. *See* Seizures
COPD. *See* Chronic obstructive pulmonary disease
Cope, 723
Cophene-B. See Brompheniramine maleate, 172–173
Cordarone. See Amiodarone hydrochloride, 132–133
Cordilox Oral. See Verapamil hydrochloride, 712–713
Cordran-N, 723
Corgard. See Nadolol, 508–509
Coricidin Tablets, 723
Corneal ulcers
 gentamicin for, 364
 sulfacetamide for, 647
Coronary artery thrombosis
 streptokinase for, 640
 urokinase for, 705–706, 706
Coronex. See Isosorbide dinitrate, 411–412
Corophyllin. See Aminophylline, 130–131
Cortaid. See Hydrocortisone acetate, 384–386
Cortalone. See Prednisolone, 592–594; Prednisone, 594–595
Cortamed. See Hydrocortisone acetate, 384–386
Cortate. See Cortisone acetate, 254–255
Cort-Dome. See Hydrocortisone, 384–386
Cortef. See Hydrocortisone, 384–386
Cortenema. See Hydrocortisone, 384–386
Corticosteroids, 40. *See also individual drugs*
Corticotropin, 253–254
Corticreme. See Hydrocortisone acetate, 384–386
Cortifoam. See Hydrocortisone acetate, 384–386
Cortigel. See Corticotropin, 253–254
Cortinal. See Hydrocortisone, 384–386

Cortisone, 40, 254–255
 uses for, 41
Cortisone acetate, 40, 72, 254–255
Cortisporin, 723
Cortizone 5. See Hydrocortisone, 384–386
Cortone. See Cortisone acetate, 254–255
Cortril. See Hydrocortisone, 384–386
Cortrophin. See Corticotropin, 253–254
Cortropic. See Corticotropin, 253–254
Corynebacterium diphtheriae infections, erythromycin for, 325
Coryphen. See Aspirin, 148–149
Corzide, 723
Cosmegen. See Dactinomycin, 269–270
Cotazym. See Pancrelipase, 548–549
Cotrim. See Co-trimoxazole (sulfamethoxazole/trimethoprim), 255–256
Co-trimoxazole (sulfamethoxazole/trimethoprim), 68, 255–256
 IV compatibility of, 34–35
Cough, drugs for prevention/relief of, 79–80. *See also individual drugs*
Coumadin. See Warfarin sodium, 718–719
Creeping eruption, thiabendazole for, 665
Cremacoat-1. See Dextromethorphan hydrobromide, 282–283
Cremacoat-2. See Guaifenesin, 375
Cremesone. See Hydrocortisone, 384–386
Creon. See Pancrelipase, 548–549
Cretinism
 desiccated thyroid for, 672
 levothyroxine for, 426, 427
 thyroglobulin for, 671
Crohn's disease, sulfasalazine for, 649
Cromolyn sodium, 64, 257–258
Cronetal. See Disulfiram, 304–305
Cryonine. See Liothyronine sodium, 430–431
Cryptococcal meningitis, fluconazole for, 349

Cryptococcus infections (cryptococcosis)
 flucytosine for, 350
 miconazole (parenteral) for, 495
Crystalline zinc insulin, 398–400
Crystamine. See Cyanocobalamin, 258–259
Crystapen. See Penicillin G, sodium, 556
Crysticillin A.S.. See Penicillin G, procaine, 556–557
Crystodigin. See Digitoxin, 293–294
C.S.D.. See Conjugated estrogens, 328–330
Cuprimine. See Penicillamine, 555–556
Curretab. See Medroxyprogesterone acetate, 450–451
Cushing's syndrome
 aminoglutethimide for, 129
 trilostane for, 696
Cutaneous candidiasis, clotrimazole for, 246
Cutaneous larva migrans, thiabendazole for, 665
CVA (cerebrovascular accident). *See* Stroke
Cyanabin. See Cyanocobalamin, 258–259
Cyanide poisoning, amyl nitrate for, 144
Cyanocobalamin, 258–259
Cyano-Gel. See Cyanocobalamin, 258–259
Cyclacillin, 68, 259–260
Cyclan. See Cyclandelate, 260
Cyclandelate, 260
Cyclapen-W. See Cyclacillin, 259–260
Cyclidox. See Doxycycline hydrochloride, 311–313
Cyclobenzaprine hydrochloride, 99, 260–261
Cyclomen. See Danazol, 270–271
Cyclomydril Ophthalmic, 723
Cyclopar. See Tetracycline hydrochloride, 662–663
Cyclophosphamide, 72, 261–262
Cycloplegia, scopolamine for, 630
Cycloserine, 68, 263
Cyclospasmol. See Cyclandelate, 260
Cyclosporine, 90, 263–265

Depakene Syrup. See Valproate
    sodium, 707–708
Depakote. See Divalproex
    sodium, 707–708
depAndro. See Testosterone
    cypionate, 659–660
Depen. See Penicillamine, 555–
    556
Dependence. See Drug
    dependence
depMedalone. See
    Methylprednisolone
    acetate, 482–483
Depoject. See
    Methylprednisolone
    acetate, 482–483
Depo-Medrol. See
    Methylprednisolone
    acetate, 482–483
Deponit NTG Film. See
    Nitroglycerin, 525–527
Depopred. See
    Methylprednisolone
    acetate, 482–483
Depo-Predate. See
    Methylprednisolone
    acetate, 482–483
Depo-provera. See
    Medroxyprogesterone
    acetate, 450–451
Depotest. See Testosterone
    cypionate, 659–660
Depo-Testadiol (OIL), 723
Depo-Testerone. See
    Testosterone cypionate,
    659–660
Depression, drugs for, 56–58.
    See also individual drugs
Deprol, 723
Deptran. See Doxepin
    hydrochloride, 309–310
Deralin. See Propranolol
    hydrochloride, 607–608
Dermacort. See Hydrocortisone
    acetate, 384–386
Dermatophyte infections
    ketoconazole for, 417
    miconazole nitrate for, 496
DermiCort. See Hydrocortisone,
    384–386
Dermolate. See Hydrocortisone,
    384–386
Dermoplast Spray, 723
Deronil. See Dexamethasone,
    278–280
DES. See Diethylstilbestrol,
    290–292
Deseril. See Methysergide
    maleate, 484–485
Desiccated thyroid, 100, 672–
    673
Desipramine hydrochloride, 56,
    275–276

Desmopressin, 276–278
Desoxyn. See
    Methamphetamine
    hydrochloride, 467–468
Desyrel. See Trazodone
    hydrochloride, 684–685
Detensol. See Propranolol
    hydrochloride, 607–608
Dex. See Dexamethasone
    sodium phosphate, 278–
    280
Dexacen. See Dexamethasone
    sodium phosphate, 278–
    280
Dexacen LA. See
    Dexamethasone acetate,
    278–280
Dexamethasone, 40, 72, 278–
    280
  IM compatibility of, 30
  IV compatibility of, 34–35
Dexamethasone acetate, 40,
    278–280
Dexamethasone sodium
    phosphate, 40, 278–280
Dexasone. See Dexamethasone,
    278–280; Dexamethasone
    sodium phosphate, 278–
    280
Dexasone-LA. See
    Dexamethasone acetate,
    278–280
Dexchlor. See
    Dexchlorpheniramine,
    280–281
Dexchlorpheniramine, 64, 280–
    281
Dexedrine. See
    Dextroamphetamine
    sulfate, 281–282
Dexitac. See Caffeine, 181
Dexon. See Dexamethasone
    sodium phosphate, 278–
    280
Dexone. See Dexamethasone,
    278–280; Dexamethasone
    sodium phosphate, 278–
    280
Dexone LA. See
    Dexamethasone acetate,
    278–280
Dexon LA. See Dexamethasone
    acetate, 278–280
Dextroamphetamine sulfate,
    84, 281–282
Dextromethorphan
    hydrobromide, 79, 282–
    283
Dextrothyroxine sodium, 71,
    283–284
Dey-Dose Isoetharine. See
    Isoetharine
    hydrochloride, 407–408

Dey Dose Isoproterenol. See
    Isoproterenol, 409–411
Dey-Dose Metaproterenol. See
    Metaproterenol sulfate,
    462–463
Dey-Lute Isoetharine. See
    Isoetharine
    hydrochloride, 407–408
Dey-Med Metaproterenol. See
    Metaproterenol sulfate,
    462–463
D.H.E. 45. See
    Dihydroergotamine
    mesylate, 295–296
DiaBeta. See Glyburide, 367–
    369
Diabetes insipidus
    desmopressin for, 277
    vasopressin for, 710
Diabetes mellitus
    drugs for, 58–62. See also
        individual drugs
    vascular disease and,
        nylidrin for, 532
Diabinese. See Chlorpropamide,
    224–226
Diachlor. See Chlorothiazide,
    219–220
Diagnosis, nursing, medication
    administration and, 7–9
Dialose. See Docusate
    potassium, 306
Dialose Plus, 723
Dialume. See Aluminum
    hydroxide, 121–122
Diamine T.D.. See
    Brompheniramine
    maleate, 172–173
Diamox. See Acetazolamide,
    107–108; Acetazolamide
    sodium, 107–108
Diapril. See Ergoloid
    mesylates, 321
Diarrhea
    anticholinergics for, 51
    diphenoxylate for, 301
    doxycycline for, 312
    kaolin and pectin for, 415
    loperamide for, 436
    neomycin for, 517
Diazemuls. See Diazepam, 284–
    285
Diazepam, 45, 54, 284–285
  IM compatibility of, 30
  IV compatibility of, 34–35
  seizure-type used for, 55
Diazepam Intensol. See
    Diazepam, 284–285
Di-Azo. See Phenazopyridine
    hydrochloride, 567–568
Diazoxide, 66, 285–286

infection caused by
amikacin for, 125
cinoxacin for, 235
gentamicin for, 364
imipenem-cilastatin
sodium for, 391
kanamycin for, 414
nalidixic acid for, 512
neomycin for, 517
nitrofurantoin for, 524
tobramycin for, 676
trimethoprim for, 698
Eserine. See Physostigmine
salicylate, 578–579
Esgic, 725
Esidrix. See
Hydrochlorothiazide,
383–384
Esimil, 725
Eskalith. See Lithium
carbonate, 433–435
Esmolol hydrochloride, 48, 80,
327–328
Esophageal candidiasis,
fluconazole for, 349
Esophageal carcinoma,
amsacrine for, 142
Estratest, 725
Estrogen, 328–330
with progestin, 330–332
Estrogenic substances,
conjugated, 328–330
Ethacrynic acid, 87, 332–333
Ethacrynic sodium, 332–333
Ethambutol hydrochloride, 68,
333–334
Ethanolamine derivatives
(aminoacyl ethers), 64.
See also individual drugs
Ethaquin. See Ethaverine
hydrochloride, 334–335
Ethatab. See Ethaverine
hydrochloride, 334–335
Ethaverine hydrochloride, 334–
335
Ethavex. See Ethaverine
hydrochloride, 334–335
Ethinyl estradiol
and ethynodiol diacetate,
330–332
and levonorgestrel, 330–332
and norethindrone, 330–332
and norethindrone acetate,
330–332
and ferrous fumarate,
330–332
and norgestrel, 330–332
Ethosuximide, 54, 335–336
seizure-type used for, 55
Ethotoin, 54, 336
seizure-type used for, 55

Ethylenediamine derivatives,
64. *See also individual
drugs*
Ethylestrenol, 336–337
Ethynodiol diacetate, and
ethinyl estradiol, 330–
332
Etibi. See Ethambutol
hydrochloride, 333–334
Etidocaine hydrochloride, 93,
338–339
Etoposide, 72, 339–340
Etrafon, 725
Euflex. See Flutamide, 359
Euglucon. See Glyburide, 367–
369
Eulexin. See Flutamide, 359
Eustachian tube congestion,
pseudoephedrine for, 612
Euthroid, 724. *See also* Liotrix,
431–432
Eutron Filmtabs, 725
Evaluation, medication
administration and, 22
Everone. See Testosterone
enanthate, 659–660
Ewing's sarcoma, dactinomycin
for, 269
Excedrin, 725
Exdol. See Acetaminophen,
106–107
Exentabs. See Quinidine
sulfate, 618–620
Exercise-induced muscle pain,
dantrolene for, 272
Exna. See Benzthiazide, 163–
164
Exna-R Tablets, 725
Exosurf Neonatal. See
Colisceril palmitate, 252–
253
Expectorants, 79–80. *See also
individual drugs*
ammonium chloride as, 134,
135
Extended zinc suspension, 58,
398–400
pharmacokinetics of, 59
Extrapyramidal drug reactions,
drugs for treatment of,
76–77. *See also
individual drugs*
Extra Strength Maalox Tablets,
725
Extravasation, phentolamine
mesylate for, 573
Eye drops, 31
Eye infection/inflammation
atropine for, 153, 154
flurbiprofen for, 357
gentamicin for, 364
sulfacetamide for, 647
tetracycline for, 662, 663

Eye ointments, 31
Eye refraction. *See* Ophthalmic
examination
Eye surgery, miosis and,
flurbiprofen for
prevention of, 357

Factor IX complex (human),
340–341
Famotidine, 89, 341
Fansidar, 725
Fat emulsions, 342–343
Fatigue, caffeine for relief of,
181
Fatty acid deficiency, fat
emulsions for, 342
5-FC. *See* Flucytosine (5-FC),
350–351
Fedahist, 725
Fedrine. See Ephedrine
hydrochloride, 318–319
Feldene. See Piroxicam, 584–
585
Female castration
diethylstilbestrol for, 291
estrogen for, 329
Female hypogonadism
diethylstilbestrol for, 291
estrogen for, 328, 329
Female infertility, clomiphene
for, 241
Femcaps, 725
Fenicol. See Chloramphenicol,
215–217
Fenoprofen calcium, 98, 343–
344
Fentanyl citrate, 95, 344–345
with droperidol, 344
IM compatibility of, 30
Fenylhist. See
Diphenhydramine, 299–
300
Feosol. See Ferrous sulfate,
345–346
Fergon. See Ferrous gluconate,
345–346
Fer-in-Sol. See Ferrous sulfate,
345–346
Feritard. See Ferrous sulfate,
345–346
Fermalox, 725
Ferndex. See
Dextroamphetamine
sulfate, 281–282
Ferocyl, 725
Fero-Grad. See Ferrous sulfate,
345–346
Fero-Gradumet. See Ferrous
sulfate, 345–346
Ferolix. See Ferrous sulfate,
345–346
Ferospace. See Ferrous sulfate,
345–346

Gastric stasis, metoclopramide for, 486
Gastric ulcers
  misoprostol for, 499
  omeprazole for, 535
Gastrocrom. See Cromolyn sodium, 257–258
Gastroesophageal reflux
  aluminum hydroxide for, 121
  aluminum and magnesium combinations for, 120
  magaldrate for, 440
  metoclopramide for, 486
  omeprazole for, 535
  ranitidine for, 621
Gastrointestinal cancer, floxuridine for, 348
Gastrointestinal candidiasis, nystatin for, 533
Gastrointestinal colic, papaverine for, 550
Gastrointestinal infections
  cephalothin for, 210
  cephapirin for, 211
  ciprofloxacin for, 235–236
  mezlocillin for, 494
  ofloxacin for, 534
Gastrointestinal spasm, ethaverine for, 334
Gastrostomy tube, guidelines for administering medication via, 28
Gas-X. See Simethicone, 633–634
Gaviscon, 725
Gee-Gee. See Guaifenesin, 375
Gelusil, 725. *See also* Aluminum hydroxide, with magnesium hydroxide, 120–121
Gemfibrozil, 71, 363–364
Gemnisyn, 725
Genabid. See Papaverine hydrochloride, 550–551
Genalac. See Calcium carbonate, 185
Genallerate. See Chlorpheniramine maleate, 221–222
Genapap. See Acetaminophen, 106–107
Genaphed. See Pseudoephedrine hydrochloride, 612
Genasoft. See Docusate sodium, 306
Genebs. See Acetaminophen, 106–107
General anesthesia. *See* Anesthesia
Genitourinary infections (urogenital infections).

See also Urinary tract infections
  cefamandole for, 199
  cefazolin for, 200
  cefoxitin for, 205
  cephalexin for, 209
  cephalothin for, 210
  cephapirin for, 211
  erythromycin for, 325
Genitourinary spasm, ethaverine for, 334
Genoptic. See Gentamicin sulfate, 364–365
Genora. See Ethinyl estradiol, and norethindrone, 330–332; Mestranol, and norethindrone, 330–332
Gentabs. See Acetaminophen, 106–107
Gentacidin. See Gentamicin, 364–365
Gentafair. See Gentamicin sulfate, 364–365
Gentamicin, 68, 364–365
  IV compatibility of, 34–35
Gentamicin sulfate, 68, 364–365
Gen-Xene. See Clorazepate, 244–246
Geocillin. See Carbenicillin indanyl sodium, 189–190
Geopen. See Carbenicillin disodium, 189–190
Geopen Oral. See Carbenicillin indanyl sodium, 189–190
Geridium. See Phenazopyridine hydrochloride, 567–568
GFR. *See* Glomerular filtration rate
GG-CEN. See Guaifenesin, 375
Giardiasis
  metronidazole for, 491
  quinacrine for, 616
Glaucoma
  acetazolamide for, 107
  dichlorphenamide for, 287
  epinephrine for, 319, 320
  methazolamide for, 468
  physostigmine for, 578
  pilocarpine for, 580
  timolol for, 675
Glipizide, 58, 365–366
  pharmacokinetics of, 59
Glomerular filtration rate (GFR), mannitol in measurement of, 444
Glossopharyngeal neuralgia, carbamazepine for, 188
Glucagon, 367
  as acetohexamide antidote, 108
  as tolazamide antidote, 678
  as tolbutamide antidote, 680

Glucamide. See Chlorpropamide, 224–226
Glucocorticoids, 40–41. *See also individual drugs and* Adrenocorticosteroids
Glucose, blood levels of, drugs for control of, 58–62. *See also individual drugs*
Glucotrol. See Glipizide, 365–366
Glyburide, 58, 367–369
  pharmacokinetics of, 59
Glycate. See Calcium carbonate, 185
Glyceral-T Capsules, 725
Glycerol, iodinated, 79, 402
Glycopyrrolate, 50, 369–370
  IM compatibility of, 30
Glycotuss. See Guaifenesin, 375
Glytuss. See Guaifenesin, 375
Goals, determining, 10
Goiter, nontoxic
  levothyroxine for, 426
  liothyronine for, 430
Gold-50. See Aurothioglucose, 155–156
Gold sodium thiomalate, 370–371
Gonorrhea
  bacampicillin for, 160
  carbenicillin disodium for, 189
  cefuroxime for, 208
  demeclocycline for, 274
  doxycycline for, 312
  minocycline for, 497
  oxytetracycline for, 546
  penicillin G procaine for, 557
  spectinomycin for, 638
  tetracycline for, 662, 663
Gouty arthritis
  allopurinol for, 116
  colchicine for, 250
  indomethacin for, 397
  meclofenamate for, 449
  naproxen for, 516
  oxyphenbutazone for, 545
  phenylbutazone for, 574
  probenecid for, 596
Gramcal, 725
Gram-negative infections
  aztreonam for, 159
  carbenicillin disodium for, 189
  chloramphenicol for, 216
  demeclocycline for, 274
  doxycycline for, 312
  minocycline for, 497
  nalidixic acid for, 512
  oxytetracycline for, 546
  penicillin G benzathine and procaine for, 556
  tetracycline for, 662, 662–663

anesthetic, 428–429
IV compatibility of, 34–35
systemic, 429–430
Lidoject-2. See Lidocaine
hydrochloride, anesthetic,
428–429
Lido-Pen Auto-Injector. See
Lidocaine hydrochloride,
systemic, 429–430
Limbitrol, 726
Lioresal. See Baclofen, 160–161
Liothyronine sodium, 100, 430–
431
Liotrix, 100, 431–432
Lipid-lowering agents, 71–72.
See also individual drugs
and
Hypercholesterolemia;
Hyperlipidemia;
Hypertriglyceridemia
Lipo Gantrisin. See
Sulfisoxazole, 650–651
Lipoproteins, very low density,
clofibrate for reduction of
levels of, 240
Liposyn. See Fat emulsions,
342–343
Lipoxide. See Chlordiazepoxide
hydrochloride, 217–218
Liquaemin Sodium. See
Heparin sodium, 379–381
Liquid Pred. See Prednisone,
594–595
Liquids, guidelines for
administering, 28
Liquiprin. See Acetaminophen,
106–107
Lisinopril, 66, 432–433
Listeria monocytogenes
infections, erythromycin
for, 325
Lithane. See Lithium
carbonate, 433–435
Lithicarb. See Lithium
carbonate, 433–435
Lithium, 56, 433–435
Lithium carbonate, 433–435
Lithium citrate, 433–435
Lithizine. See Lithium
carbonate, 433–435
Lithobid. See Lithium
carbonate, 433–435
Lithonate. See Lithium
carbonate, 433–435
Lithotabs. See Lithium
carbonate, 433–435
Liver abscess, amoebic,
metronidazole for, 491
Liver amebiasis, metronidazole
for, 491
Liver cirrhosis. *See* Cirrhosis

Liver failure, kanamycin in
adjunctive treatment of,
414
Lixolin. See Theophylline, 664–
665
Lobac, 726
Local anesthesia, drugs for,
93–95. *See also
individual drugs*
Lodrane. See Theophylline,
664–665
Loestrin. See Ethinyl estradiol,
and norethindrone
acetate, 330–332
Loestrin Fe. See Ethinyl
estradiol, and
norethindrone acetate,
and ferrous fumarate,
330–332
Lofene. See Diphenoxylate with
atropine, 301–302
Logen. See Diphenoxylate with
atropine, 301–302
Lomanate. See Diphenoxylate
with atropine, 301–302
Lomotil. See Diphenoxylate
with atropine, 301–302
Lomustine, 72, 435–436
Lonavar. See Oxandrolone,
538–539
Long-acting insulins, 398–400
Loniten. See Minoxidil, 498–
499
Lonox. See Diphenoxylate with
atropine, 301–302
Loop (high-ceiling) diuretics,
87, 88. *See also
individual drugs*
Lo/Ovral. See Ethinyl estradiol,
and norgestrel, 330–332
Loperamide, 436–437
Lopid. See Gemfibrozil, 363–
364
Lopressor. See Metoprolol, 489–
490
Lopressor HCT, 726
Lopurin. See Allopurinol, 116–
117
Loraz. See Lorazepam, 437–438
Lorazepam, 45, 54, 437–438
Lorelco. See Probucol, 597–598
Losec. See Omeprazole, 535–
536
Lotrimin. See Clotrimazole, 246
Lotrisone Cream, 726
Lo-Trol. See Diphenoxylate
with atropine, 301–302
Lovastatin, 71, 438–439
Low back disorders,
carisoprodol for, 193
Low-density lipoproteins,
dextrothyroxine for

reduction of serum levels
of, 283
Low-Quel. See Diphenoxylate
with atropine, 301–302
Lowsium. See Magaldrate,
440–441
Loxapac. See Loxapine
hydrochloride, 439–440;
Loxapine succinate, 439–
440
Loxapine hydrochloride, 78,
439–440
Loxapine succinate, 78, 439–
440
Loxitane. See Loxapine
succinate, 439–440
Loxitane C and IM. See
Loxapine hydrochloride,
439–440
Lozide. See Indapamide, 395–
396
Lozol. See Indapamide, 395–
396
L-phenylalanine mustard, 453–
454
L-thyroxine sodium. *See*
Levothyroxine sodium,
426–427
Lucrin. See Leuprolide acetate,
422–423
Ludiomil. See Maprotiline
hydrochloride, 445–446
Luminal. See Phenobarbital,
569–571
Luminal Sodium. See
Phenobarbital sodium,
569–571
Lung cancer
amsacrine for, 142
carboplatin for, 192
carmustine for, 194
cisplatin for, 236
cyclophosphamide for, 261
doxorubicin for, 310
etoposide for, 339
ifosfamide for, 390
lomustine for, 435
methotrexate for, 473
mitomycin for, 500
procarbazine for, 600
teniposide for, 654
thiotepa for, 669
vincristine for, 715
vindescine for, 716
Lung congestion, postoperative,
acetylcysteine for, 111
Lung disease. *See also*
Respiratory infections
acetylcysteine for, 111
aminophylline for, 130
doxapram for, 308
ipratropium for, 404
theophylline for, 664

daunorubicin for, 273
mercaptopurine for, 459
teniposide for, 654
thioguanine for, 667
uracil mustard for, 703
Myeloma, multiple. *See*
Multiple myeloma
Myidyl. See Triprolidine
hydrochloride, 701–702
M-YKA, 727
Mylanta, 727. *See also*
Aluminum hydroxide,
with magnesium
hydroxide, 120–121
Myldone. See Primidone, 595–
596
Myleran. See Busulfan, 179–
180
Mylicon. See Simethicone, 633–
634
Mymethasone. See
Dexamethasone, 278–280
Myocardial infarction
alteplase for, 118
anistreplase for, 144
atenolol for, 150, 151
dopamine for, 307
heparin for, 379
metoprolol for, 489
propranolol for, 607
warfarin for, 718
Myocardial infarction
prophylaxis
aspirin for, 149
timolol for, 675
Myocardial ischemia,
papaverine for, 550
Myochrysine. See Gold sodium
thiomalate, 370–371
Myodine. See Iodinated
glycerol, 402
Myolin. See Orphenadrine
citrate, 536–537
Myproic acid. See Valproic
acid, 707–708
Myproic Acid Syrup. See
Valproate sodium, 707–
708
Myrosimide. See Furosemide,
360–361
Mysoline. See Primidone, 595–
596
Mytelase. See Ambenonium
chloride, 123–124
Myxedema
desiccated thyroid for, 672
thyroglobulin for, 671
Myxedema coma
levothyroxine for, 426, 427
liothyronine for, 430, 431

Nadolol, 44, 66, 80, 508–509

Nadopen-V. See Penicillin V
potassium, 558
Nadostine. See Nystatin, 532–
533
Nafcil. See Nafcillin sodium,
509–510
Nafcillin sodium, 68, 509–510
IV compatibility of, 34–35
Naftifine hydrochloride, 510–
511
Naftin. See Naftifine
hydrochloride, 510–511
Nalbuphine hydrochloride, 95,
511–512
Nalcrom. See Cromolyn
sodium, 257–258
Naldecon, 727
Naldecon Senior-EX. See
Guaifenesin, 375
Nalfon. See Fenoprofen
calcium, 343–344
Nalidixic acid, 68, 512–513
Nallpen. See Nafcillin sodium,
509–510
Naloxone hydrochloride, 513–
514
as alfentanil antidote, 115
as buprenorphine antidote,
176
as butorphanol tartrate
antidote, 180
as codeine antidote, 249
as diphenoxylate antidote,
301
as fentanyl antidote, 344
as hydromorphone antidote,
386
as levorphanol tartrate
antidote, 425
as meperidine antidote, 455
as methadone antidote, 466
as morphine antidote, 504
as nalbuphine antidote, 511
as oxycodone antidote, 541
as oxymorphone antidote,
543
as pentazocine antidote, 561
as propoxyphene antidote,
606
Naltrexone hydrochloride, 514–
515
Nandrobolic. See Nandrolone
phenpropionate, 515–516
Nandrobolic L.A.. See
Nandrolone decanoate,
515–516
Nandrolone decanoate, 515–516
Nandrolone phenpropionate,
515–516
Napamide. See Disopyramide
phosphate, 302–304
Naprogesic. See Naproxen
sodium, 516–517

Naprosyn. See Naproxen, 516–
517
Naproxen, 98, 516–517
Naproxen sodium, 98, 516–517
Naptrate. See Pentaerythritol
tetranitrate, 558–559
Naqua. See Trichlormethiazide,
690–691
Naquival, 727
Narcan. See Naloxone
hydrochloride, 513–514
Narcolepsy
amphetamine sulfate for, 138
dextroamphetamine for, 281
drugs for, 85. *See also*
individual drugs
methylphenidate for, 481
Narcotic abstinence syndrome,
methadone for, 466
Narcotic addiction, naltrexone
for, 514
Narcotic depression,
postoperative, naloxone
for, 513
Narcotic-induced respiratory
depression, naloxone for,
513
Narcotics, 95–98. *See also*
individual drugs
Nardil. See Phenelzine sulfate,
568–569
Narrow-spectrum anti-
infectives, 69
Nasahist B. See
Brompheniramine
maleate, 172–173
Nasal congestion
ephedrine for, 318
pseudoephedrine for, 612
triprolidine for, 701
Nasal constriction,
phenylephrine for, 575
Nasalcrom. See Cromolyn
sodium, 257–258
Nasal medications, 31
Nasal sprays, 31
Nasogastric tube, guidelines
for administering
medication via, 28
Natrilix. See Indapamide, 395–
396
Natrimax. See
Hydrochlorothiazide,
383–384
Natulan. See Procarbazine
hydrochloride, 600–602
Naturacil. See Psyllium, 612–
613
Naturetin, 727
Nausea, drugs for, 63–64. *See
also individual drugs*
Nauseatol. See
Dimenhydrinate, 297–298

Prostate cancer
   aminoglutethimide for, 129
   cisplatin for, 236
   diethylstilbestrol for, 290, 291
   estrogen for, 329
   flutamide for, 359
   leuprolide for, 423
Prostatitis (prostate infections)
   carbenicillin indanyl sodium for, 189
   ofloxacin for, 534
Prostigmin. See Neostigmine methylsulfate, 518–519
Prostigmin Bromide. See Neostigmine bromide, 518–519
Prostin E₂. See Dinoprostone, 298–299
Protamine, Zinc, and Iletin. See Protamine zinc suspension/PZI, 398–400
Protamine sulfate, 610
   as heparin antidote, 379, 610
Protamine Zinc Insulin MC. See Protamine zinc suspension/PZI, 398–400
Protamine zinc suspension/PZI, 58, 398–400
   pharmacokinetics of, 59
Protaphane. See Isophane insulin suspension, NPH, 398–400
Protenate. See Plasma protein fraction (human), 585
Proteus infections
   amikacin for, 125
   cinoxacin for, 235
   gentamicin for, 364
   imipenem-cilastatin sodium for, 391
   kanamycin for, 414
   nalidixic acid for, 512
   nitrofurantoin for, 524
   tobramycin for, 676
   trimethoprim for, 698
Prothazine. See Promethazine hydrochloride, 604–605
Protostat. See Metronidazole, 490–492
Protran. See Chlorpromazine hydrochloride, 222–224
Protrin. See Co-trimoxazole (sulfamethoxazole/trimethoprim), 255–256
Protriptyline hydrochloride, 56, 610–611
Proventil. See Albuterol sulfate, 114–115
Provera. See Medroxyprogesterone acetate, 450–451
Providencia infections

amikacin for, 125
   tobramycin for, 676
Provocholine. See Methacholine chloride, 465
Provol No. 3, 729
Prozac. See Fluoxetine, 352–353
Pruritus
   in biliary obstruction, cholestyramine for, 229
   trimeprazine tartrate for, 696
Pseudoephedrine hydrochloride, 39, 612
Pseudoephedrine sulfate, 39, 612
Pseudomembranous enterocolitis, vancomycin for, 709
Pseudomonas infections
   amikacin for, 125
   gentamicin for, 364
   imipenem-cilastatin sodium for, 391
   tobramycin for, 676
Psittacosis, chloramphenicol for, 216
Psoriasis, methotrexate for, 473
Psychiatric disorders, drugs for, 78–79. *See also individual drugs and* Depression, drugs for
Psychomotor seizures
   carbamazepine for, 188
   mephenytoin for, 456
   phenacemide for, 566
   primidone for, 595
Psychosis, drugs for, 78–79. *See also individual drugs*
Psyllium, 91, 612–613
PTU. *See* Propylthiouracil, 608–609
Pulmonary artery catheter flush, heparin for, 379
Pulmonary edema
   ethacrynic acid and ethacrynic sodium for, 332
   furosemide for, 360
Pulmonary embolism
   heparin for, 379
   streptokinase for, 640
   urokinase for, 705, 706
   warfarin for, 718
Pupillary dilatation
   atropine for, 153
   phenylephrine for, 575
Purinethol. See Mercaptopurine, 459–460
Purpura, idiopathic thrombocytopenic, immune globulin for, 394

P.V. Carpine Liquifilm. See Pilocarpine nitrate, 580–581
PVCs. *See* Premature ventricular contractions
PVF K. See Penicillin V potassium, 558
PVK. See Penicillin V potassium, 558
Pyelitis, nitrofurantoin for, 524
Pyelonephritis, nitrofurantoin for, 524
Pynbenzamine. See Tripelennamine hydrochloride, 700–701
Pyopen. See Carbenicillin disodium, 189–190
Pyranistan. See Chlorpheniramine maleate, 221–222
Pyrantel embonate, 69, 613–614
Pyrantel pamoate, 69, 613–614
Pyrazinamide, 68, 614–615
Pyridium. See Phenazopyridine hydrochloride, 567–568
Pyridostigmine bromide, 86, 615–616

Q-Pam. See Diazepam, 284–285
Quadrinal, 729
Quelicin. See Succinylcholine chloride, 644–645
Questran. See Cholestyramine, 229–230
Quibron, 729. *See also* Theophylline, 664–665
Quick Pep. See Caffeine, 181
Quinacrine hydrochloride, 69, 616–617
Quinaglute. See Quinidine gluconate, 618–620
Quinalan. See Quinidine gluconate, 618–620
Quinate. See Quinidine gluconate, 618–620
Quine. See Quinidine sulfate, 618–620
Quinethazone, 87, 617–618
Quinidex. See Quinidine sulfate, 618–620
Quinidine, 48, 618–620
Quinidine gluconate, 48, 618–620
Quinidine polygalacturonate, 48, 618–620
Quinidine sulfate, 48, 618–620
Quinora. See Quinidine sulfate, 618–620
Q-Vel, 729

Tolazamide, 58, 678–679
pharmacokinetics of, 59
Tolazoline hydrochloride, 679–680
Tolbutamide, 58, 680–681
pharmacokinetics of, 59
Tolectin. See Tolmetin sodium, 682–683
Tolinase. See Tolazamide, 678–679
Tolmetin sodium, 98, 682–683
Toloxan. See Tolazoline hydrochloride, 679–680
Tolzol. See Tolazoline hydrochloride, 679–680
Tonic-clonic seizures, drugs for, 55
Tonocard. See Tocainide hydrochloride, 677–678
Topicycline. See Tetracycline hydrochloride, 662–663
Toradol. See Ketorolac, 419
Tornalate. See Bitolterol mesylate, 168–169
Totacillin. See Ampicillin trihydrate, 140–141
Totacillin-N. See Ampicillin sodium, 140–141
Total parenteral nutrition, fat emulsions in, 342
Tourette's syndrome, haloperidol for, 378
Toxemia of pregnancy, magnesium sulfate for, 443
Toxoplasmosis, sulfadiazine for, 648
t-PA. *See* Tissue plasminogen activator (alteplase), 118–120
Trachoma
demeclocycline for, 274
doxycycline for, 312
minocycline for, 497
oxytetracycline for, 546
tetracycline for, 662, 662–663, 663
Tracrium. See Atracurium besylate, 151–152
Tramacort. See Triamcinolone acetonide, 686–688
Trandate. See Labetalol hydrochloride, 420–421
Tranquilizers. *See* Antianxiety agents, 45–48
Transderm-Nitro. See Nitroglycerin, 525–527
Transderm-Scop. See Scopolamine transdermal, 630–631
Transderm-V. See Scopolamine transdermal, 630–631
Transient ischemic attacks

aspirin for, 149
dipyridamole for, 302
Transplantation, organ
azathioprine for, 157
cyclosporine for, 264
immunosuppressants for, 90–91. *See also individual drugs*
muromonab-CD3 for, 157
Tranxene. See Clorazepate, 244–246
Tranylcypromine sulfate, 56, 683–684
Travamine. See Dimenhydrinate, 297–298
Travamulsion. See Fat emulsions, 342–343
Travasol. See Amino acid solution, 127–128
Traveler's diarrhea, doxycycline for, 312
Travs. See Dimenhydrinate, 297–298
Trazodone hydrochloride, 56, 684–685
Trazon. See Trazodone hydrochloride, 684–685
Trendar. See Ibuprofen, 389–390
Trental. See Pentoxifylline, 563–564
Tretinoin, 685–686
Trexan. See Naltrexone hydrochloride, 514–515
Triadapin. See Doxepin hydrochloride, 309–310
Trialodine. See Trazodone hydrochloride, 684–685
Triam-A. See Triamcinolone acetonide, 686–688
Triamcinolone, 40, 686–688
Triamcinolone acetonide, 40, 686–688
Triamcinolone diacetate, 40, 686–688
Triamcinolone hexacetonide, 40, 686–688
Triam-Forte. See Triamcinolone diacetate, 686–688
Triaminic, 730
Triaminicol Multi-Symptom Cold. See Dextromethorphan hydrobromide, 282–283
Triamonide. See Triamcinolone acetonide, 686–688
Triamterene, 87, 688–689
Triaphen-10. See Aspirin, 148–149
Triavil, 730
Triazolam, 45, 689–690

Trib. See Co-trimoxazole (sulfamethoxazole/ trimethoprim), 255–256
Tri-Barbs Capsule, 730
Trichinosis, thiabendazole for, 665
Trichlormethiazide, 87, 690–691
Trichomoniasis
drugs for, 69. *See also individual drugs*
metronidazole for, 491
Trichophyton infections, griseofulvin for, 371
Tricilone. See Triamcinolone, 686–688
Tricyclic antidepressants, 56, 57. *See also individual drugs*
overdose of, physostigmine for, 578
Triderm. See Triamcinolone acetonide, 686–688
Tridil. See Nitroglycerin, 525–527
Triethylenethiophosphoramide (thiotepa), 72, 669–670
Trifluoperazine hydrochloride, 78, 691–693
Triflupromazine hydrochloride, 693–694
Trigeminal neuralgia
carbamazepine for, 188
chlorphenesin for, 221
Trigesic, 730
Triglyceride-lowering agents, 71–72. *See also individual drugs and* Hyperlipidemia; Hypertriglyceridemia
Trihexane. See Trihexyphenidyl hydrochloride, 694–695
Trihexy. See Trihexyphenidyl hydrochloride, 694–695
Trihexyphenidyl hydrochloride, 50, 694–695
Tri-Hydroserpine, 730
Tri-Kort. See Triamcinolone acetonide, 686–688
Trilafon. See Perphenazine, 565–566
Tri-Levlen. See Ethinyl estradiol, and levonorgestrel, 330–332
Trilisate, 730. *See also* Choline magnesium trisalicylate, 230–231
Trilog. See Triamcinolone acetonide, 686–688
Trilone. See Triamcinolone diacetate, 686–688
Trilostane, 72, 695–696

Trimeprazine tartrate, 64, 696–697
Trimethaphan, 66, 697
Trimethobenzamide hydrochloride, 63, 697–698
Trimethoprim, 69, 698–699
 with sulfamethoxazole (co-trimoxazole), 68, 255–256
 IV compatibility of, 34–35
Trimipramine maleate, 56, 699–700
Trimox. See Amoxicillin trihydrate, 136–137
Trimpex. See Trimethoprim, 698–699
Trinalin Repetabs, 730
Trind-DM Liquid. See Dextromethorphan hydrobromide, 282–283
Tripelennamine citrate, 64, 700–701
Tripelennamine hydrochloride, 64, 700–701
Triphasil. See Ethinyl estradiol, and levonorgestrel, 330–332
Triple Sulfa, 730
Tripramine. See Imipramine hydrochloride, 392–394
Triprim. See Trimethoprim, 698–699
Triprolidine hydrochloride, 64, 701–702
Triptil. See Protriptyline hydrochloride, 610–611
Triptone Caplets. See Dimenhydrinate, 297–298
Tristoject. See Triamcinolone diacetate, 686–688
Trobicin. See Spectinomycin dihydrochloride, 638
Trophoblastic neoplasms, methotrexate for, 473
Trymegan. See Chlorpheniramine maleate, 221–222
Tubarine. See Tubocurarine chloride, 702–703
Tuberculosis, drugs for, 68. *See also individual drugs*
 streptomycin in adjunctive treatment of, 642
Tubex (Heparin Lock Flush Solution). See Heparin sodium, 379–381
Tubocurarine chloride, 702–703
Tuinal, 730, 731
Tums. See Calcium carbonate, 185
Turbinaire. See Dexamethasone sodium phosphate, 278–280

Tusal. See Sodium thiosalicylate, 637–638
Tussi-Organidin-DM Liquid. See Dextromethorphan hydrobromide, 282–283
Tusstat. See Diphenhydramine, 299–300
Twilite. See Diphenhydramine, 299–300
TWIN-K-CL, 731
Ty Caplets; Ty Caps; Ty-Tabs. See Acetaminophen, 106–107
Tylenol. See Acetaminophen, 106–107
Tylenol with Codeine, 731
Tylox, 731. *See also* Oxycodone, with acetaminophen, 541–542
Tyramine rich foods, and monoamine oxidase inhibitor therapy, 57

Ukidan. See Urokinase, 705–707
Ulcerative colitis
 mesalamine for, 460
 sulfadiazine for, 648
 sulfasalazine for, 649
Ulcers
 cimetidine for, 234
 corneal
  gentamicin for, 364
  sulfacetamide for, 647
 famotidine for, 341
 glycopyrrolate in adjunctive therapy for, 369
 misoprostol for, 499
 mouth, sucralfate for, 645
 nizatidine for, 528
 omeprazole for, 535
 propantheline for, 605
 ranitidine for, 621
 skin, gentamicin for, 364
 sucralfate for, 645
Ultracef. See Cefadroxil monohydrate, 198–199
Ultralente. See Extended zinc suspension, 398–400
Unasyn, 731. *See also* Ampicillin sodium, with sulbactam sodium, 140–141
Unicaprin-Ca. See Heparin calcium, 379–381
Unicort. See Hydrocortisone, 384–386
Uniparin. See Heparin sodium, 379–381
Unipen. See Nafcillin sodium, 509–510
Uniphyl. See Theophylline, 664–665

Unipres, 731
Uniserts (Acetaminophen). See Acetaminophen, 106–107
Unisom. See Doxylamine succinate, 45, 64
Univol, 731
Upper motor neuron disorders, dantrolene for, 272
Urabeth. See Bethanechol chloride, 165–166
Uracel-5. See Sodium salicylate, 636–637
Uracil mustard, 72, 703–704
Urea, 87, 704–705
Ureaphil. See Urea, 704–705
Urecholine. See Bethanechol chloride, 165–166
Ureteral colic, papaverine for, 550
Urethral infections
 demeclocycline for, 274
 doxycycline for, 312
 tetracycline for, 663
Urethral medications, 32
Urethral surgery, and oxybutynin for bladder spasms, 540
Urex. See Furosemide, 360–361; Methenamine hippurate, 469–470
Urgency, urinary, flavoxate for, 346
Uridon. See Chlorthalidone, 227–228
Urinary crystallization, sodium bicarbonate for, 634
Urinary frequency, flavoxate for, 346
Urinary incontinence
 baclofen for, 161
 flavoxate for, 346
Urinary retention
 bethanechol for, 165
 neostigmine for, 518
Urinary tract analgesics, 95. *See also individual drugs*
Urinary tract infections. *See also* Genitourinary infections
 drugs for, 68. *See also individual drugs*
Urinary urgency, flavoxate for, 346
Urispas. See Flavoxate hydrochloride, 346
Uritol. See Furosemide, 360–361
Urobiotic-250, 731
Urocarb. See Bethanechol chloride, 165–166
Urodine. See Phenazopyridine hydrochloride, 567–568
Uro Gantanol, 731

Doxycycline
hydrochloride, 311–313
Vibra-Tabs. See Doxycycline
hyclate, 311–313;
Doxycycline
hydrochloride, 311–313
Vinblastine sulfate, 72, 713–
714
Vincasar PFS. See Vincristine
sulfate, 714–716
Vincent's Powders. See Aspirin,
148–149
Vincristine sulfate, 72, 714–
716
Vindescine sulfate, 72, 716–
717
Viokase. See Pancrelipase,
548–549
VIPoma. *See* Vasoactive
intestinal peptide tumor
Viral infections, drugs for, 69.
See also individual drugs
Viridium. See Phenazopyridine
hydrochloride, 567–568
Virilon. See
Methyltestosterone, 483–
484
Virilon IM. See Testosterone
cypionate, 659–660
Visken. See Pindolol, 581–582
Vistrax 10 Tablets, 731
Vitamin B1, 666
Vitamin B9 (folic acid), 359–
360
Vitamin B12
cyanocobalamin, 258–259
hydroxocobalamin, 387–388
Vitamin D, 717–718
Vitamin K1, 579–580
Vitamin K4, 454
Vivactil. See Protriptyline
hydrochloride, 610–611
Vivarin. See Caffeine, 181
Vivol. See Diazepam, 284–285
VLB. *See* Vinblastine sulfate,
713–714
VLDL. *See* Very low density
lipoproteins
VM-26. *See* Teniposide, 654–
655
Voltaren. See Diclofenac
sodium, 287–288
Vomiting
drugs for, 63–64. *See also
individual drugs*
ipecac syrup to induce, 403
Von Willebrand's disease,
desmopressin for, 277
VP-16. *See* Etoposide, 339–340
Vulva, cancer of, bleomycin for,
169

Vulvovaginal candidiasis
(monilia)
clotrimazole for, 246
miconazole nitrate for, 496
nystatin for, 533
Vumon. See Teniposide, 654–
655

Warfarin sodium, 52, 718–719
Warfilone Sodium. See
Warfarin sodium, 718–
719
Warfilon Sodium. See Warfarin
sodium, 718–719
Wehamine. See
Dimenhydrinate, 297–298
Wehdryl. See
Diphenhydramine, 299–
300
Wellbutrin. See Bupropion
hydrochloride, 177–178
Wellcovorin. See Leucovorin
calcium, 422
Wernicke's encephalopathy,
thiamine for, 666
Westcort Cream. See
Hydrocortisone valerate,
385–386
Whipworms
mebendazole for, 446
thiabendazole for, 665
Wigraine, 731
Wilms' tumor
dactinomycin for, 269
doxorubicin for, 310
vincristine for, 715
Wilson's disease, penicillamine
for, 555
Wingel, 731. *See also*
Aluminum hydroxide,
with magnesium
hydroxide, 120–121
Win-Kinase. See Urokinase,
705–707
Winpred. See Prednisone, 594–
595
Winsprin Capsules. See
Aspirin, 148–149
Withdrawal. *See* Alcohol,
withdrawal from; Drug
withdrawal
Wolff-Parkinson-White
syndrome, amiodarone
for, 132
Wolfina. See Rauwolfia
serpentina, 622–623
Wounds. *See also* Skin
infections
neomycin for, 517

Wyamycin E. See
Erythromycin, 325–326
Wycillin. See Penicillin G,
procaine, 556–557
Wygesic, 731
Wymox. See Amoxicillin
trihydrate, 136–137
Wytensin. See Guanabenz, 372–
373

Xanax. See Alprazolam, 117–
118
X-Prep Liquid. See Senna, 633
Xylocaine. See Lidocaine
hydrochloride, 428–429,
429–430
Xylocard. See Lidocaine
hydrochloride, 428–429,
429–430

Yodoxin. See Iodoquinol, 403
Yutopar. See Ritodrine
hydrochloride, 626–628

Zadine. See Azatadine maleate,
156–157
Zanosar. See Streptozocin,
643–644
Zantac. See Ranitidine, 621–
622
Zapex. See Oxazepam, 539–540
Zarontin. See Ethosuximide,
335–336
Zaroxolyn. See Metolazone,
488–489
Zeasorb Powder, 731
Zendole. See Indomethacin,
396–397
Zestril. See Lisinopril, 432–433
Zetar, 731
Zetran. See Diazepam, 284–285
Zidovudine, 69, 719–720
Zinacef. See Cefuroxime
sodium, 208–209
Zinamide. See Pyrazinamide,
614–615
Zincfrin, 731
Zollinger-Ellison syndrome
cimetidine for, 234
famotidine for, 341
omeprazole for, 535
ranitidine for, 621
Zorprin. See Aspirin, 148–149
Zoster (herpes), acyclovir for,
112
Zovirax. See Acyclovir, 112–113
Zoxaphen, 731
Zydone, 731
Zyloprim. See Allopurinol,
116–117

Compatibility of drugs for IV administration

★ Compatible at Y-site
24 Number of hours compatible
☆ Compatible in syringe for 15 minutes only
○ Conflicting information
● Incompatible
Blank means no data is available

	amikacin	aminophyll.	ampicillin	calcium chl.	calcium glu.	cefamandole	cefazolin	cefoperazone	cefotaxime	cefoxitin	cephalothin	cephapirin	chloramphen.	cimetidine	clindamycin	dexameth.	diazepam	digoxin	dobutamine	dopamine	furosemide	gentamicin	heparin
amikacin		★	●	24	24		8	●	●	●		●	●	24	24	★	24	●			●		●
aminophylline	★		★		24	★	○		●		●	★	24	●	●	24	●	24	★	○	8	24	○
ampicillin	●	★		●	●	24						●	24	●		●			★			●	★
calcium chloride	24		●			●						●	24	24				●		★	24		
calcium gluconate	24	24	●									●	24	24				●		●			24
cefamandole		★							●	●			●	24	★				●				★
cefazolin	8	○	24		●							24	○	24	24				●			●	24
cefoperazone	●																	●			●		
cefotaxime	●	●													24			●			●		
cefoxitin	●													★	24			●				●	8
cephalothin	●	●											24	○	24			●			●	24	24
cephapirin	●	★		24	24								24	★				●					24
chloramphenicol	24	24	●	24	24		24				24	24				24		24		24			24
cimetidine	24	●	24			●	○			★	○	★			★	★	●	★	24		★	★	24
clindamycin	★	●	●		●	24	24		24	24	24			★				●				24	24
dexamethasone	24	24			●	★	24					24		★				●					★
diazepam	●	●	●	●	●	●	●	●	●	●	●	●	●	●	●	●		●	●	●	●	●	●
digoxin		24										24		★			●		24				★
dobutamine		★		★	●	●			●					24			●	24		★			★
dopamine		○	★	24					24			24							★			★	24
furosemide	●	8												★					●			●	●
gentamicin		24	●				●	●	●	●	●	●		★	24			●		★	●		
heparin	●	○	★		24	★	24			8	24	24	24	24	24	★	●		★	●	24	★	
hydrocortisone sodium phosphate	24	24			●						○	★	●					●				●	○
lidocaine	24			24	24	○	●			24		24		★			24	●	24	★	24		24
magnesium sulfate	★		★	○	○	○	★	★	★	★		★	★		★		●		★			★	★
mannitol	24				24				24		8	24					●			24	20		
morphine sulfate	★	●	★			★	★	★	★	★		★	★	☆	★		●		★				★
multivitamins/12		●	★	24	24	★	★	★		★				★			●					●	★
nafcillin		●											24			24	●		●			●	24
nitroglycerin		★															●		★	24			
nitroprusside	●	●	●	●	●	●	●	●	●	●	●	●	●	○	●	●	●	●	●	●	●	●	●
norepinephrine	24	●	●	24	24							●		★			●		★	★			24
oxytocin	★	24	★			★	24	★	★	★		★	24		★		●					★	★
penicillin gk+	8	★		24	24		24					24	●	★	24	24			●		6		○
phenobarbital	24	24	●	24	24		24					24			●	●	●						24
phentolamine																	●		★				
phenytoin	●	●	●	●	●	●	●		●	●	●	●	●	●	●	●	●	●	●	●	●	●	●
potassium chloride	24	24	24	24	24	24	24					24	24	24	24	★		●	★	24	24	★	24
procainamide		24			24									24			●		★				★
ranitidine	★		★			★	★			★					★	★	●		★			★	★
sodium bicarbonate	24	24	●					●		24			24	24	24	24		●		●		●	
tobramycin			★	●			●	●	●					24		24	●		24				●
trimethoprim/sulfamethoxazole																	●						
vancomycin	★	●			24								●	★			●	●					
verapamil	★	○	★	★	★	★	★	★		★	★		★	★	★	★	★	●	★	★	★	★	★